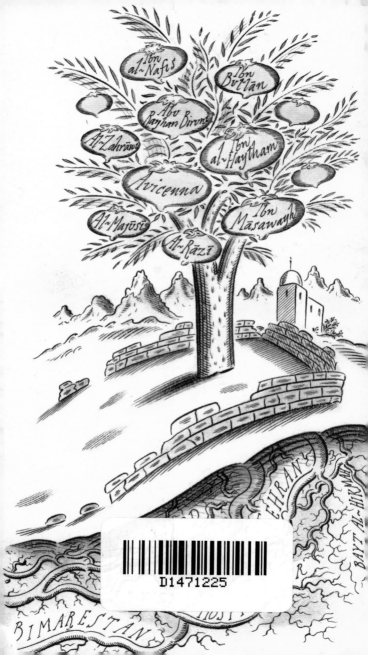

OXFORD HANDBOOK OF CLINICAL SPECIALTIES

TENTH EDITION

ANDREW BALDWIN
NINA HJELDE
CHARLOTTE GOUMALATSOU
GIL MYERS

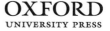

OXFORD
UNIVERSITY PRESS

Oxford University Press, Great Clarendon Street, Oxford OX2 6DP

Oxford University Press is a department of the University of Oxford. It furthers
the University's objective of excellence in research, scholarship, and education by
publishing worldwide. Oxford is a registered trade mark of Oxford University Press
in the UK and certain other countries.

Published in the United States by Oxford University Press Inc., New York

First published 1987	Sixth edition 2003	**Translations:**	Greek
Second edition 1989	Seventh edition 2006	Spanish	Romanian
Third edition 1991	Eighth edition 2008	German	Russian Polish
Fourth edition 1995	Ninth edition 2013	Hungarian	Portuguese
Fifth edition 1999	Tenth edition 2016		

British Library Cataloguing in Publication Data

Data available

Library of Congress Control Number: 2015958817

Typeset by GreenGate Publishing Services, Tonbridge, UK; printed
in China on acid-free paper through C&C Offset Printing Co. Ltd

ISBN 9780198719021

Drugs

Except where otherwise stated, recommendations are for the **non-pregnant
adult** who is **not breastfeeding**.

We have made every effort to check this text, but it is still possible that drug or
other errors have been missed. OUP makes no representation, express or implied,
that doses are correct. Readers are urged to check with the most up-to-date
product information, codes of conduct, safety regulations and latest BNF/BNFC. The
authors and the publishers do not accept responsibility or legal liability for any errors in the text, or for the misuse or misapplication of material in this work.

►For updates/corrections, see oup.co.uk/academic/medicine/handbooks/updates.

Contents

The content of each chapter is detailed on each chapter's first page.

Preface to the tenth edition

This is the first medical book to take the health of its readers seriously on the grounds that the health of one person (a patient) must not be bought at the expense of another (their doctor). It is an unsettling paradox that when we study medicine our own health may be forgotten, with long hours of hard work—often without joy or sustenance—as our health is shattered by the weight of an over-loaded curriculum (no doubt because we are over-stimulated by the too many receptors, organs, and systems, about which we know far too much).

What can a book do about this dilemma? Whilst we strive to guide you through the realms of the specialties with a concise overview of exactly what you need to know, we also place prominence on developing your skills beyond just pure facts, since these may quickly be forgotten. We want to furnish your mind with anecdotes which will remind you of the value of your hard work to inspire and motivate you to learn more. It is the quirks of medicine which we remember best; the bits that make you smile and make you realize that the work we do can be truly inspiring. The spiral symbol [۞] throughout the book, and at the start of each chapter, is your reminder to connect with and enjoy your patients; to discover what is important to them, and in so doing, make a real difference to their health and well-being. Few people receive such privileged insight into another's life. Few other professions can reflect on their day—and from the mundane, the routine, even the stressful—bring forth such engaging or thought-provoking episodes from their encounters at work.

We also hope our writings inspire you that further work can be accomplished. Do not think that a student's or junior doctor's work goes unnoticed—you are in the ideal position to make astute and objective observations uncluttered by previous baggage. Two medical students were instrumental in the journey of discovery of insulin: in 1869, German student Paul Langerhans found clusters of cells within the pancreas whose function were unknown, but were later shown to be insulin producing β-cells. Canadian student Charles Best's work with Frederick Banting led to the discovery of insulin in 1921—a miracle treatment for a previously feared and deadly disease. You may think the world of discovery is exhausted, especially for such junior members of the team, but in 2014 a medical student was the lead author for research which revealed the extent of aspergillosis in cystic fibrosis. Take heart!

So in bringing these thoughts together, try to make a habit of treasuring those unique quirks that come your way, and regularly bring them to mind as a refreshing antidote to the demands of our profession. And be aware of the possible line of enquiry that your studies or work may present, bearing in mind the dictum of Albert Szent-Gyorgyi, the physiologist who is credited with isolating vitamin c: 'Discovery is to see what everybody else has seen, and to think what nobody else has thought'.

ANDREW BALDWIN, NINA HJELDE, CHARLOTTE GOUMALATSOU, & GIL MYERS
Preface to the tenth edition—2016

Preface to the first edition

When someone says that he is 'doing obstetrics'—or whatever, this should not hide the fact that much more is being done besides, not just a little of each of medicine, psychiatry, gynaecology and paediatrics, but also a good deal of work to elicit and act upon the patient's unspoken hopes and fears. At the operating table he must concentrate minutely on the problem in hand; but later he must operate on other planes too, in social and psychological dimensions so as to understand how the patient came to need to be on the operating table, and how this might have been prevented. All the best specialists practise a holistic art, and our aim is to show how specialism and holism may be successfully interwoven, if not into a fully watertight garment, then at least into one which keeps out much of the criticism rained upon us by the proponents of alternative medicine.

We hope that by compiling this little volume we may make the arduous task of learning medicine a little less exhausting, so allowing more energy to be spent at the bedside, and on the wards. For a medical student coming fresh to a specialty the great tomes which mark the road to knowledge can numb the mind after a while, and what started out fresh is in danger of becoming exhausted by its own too much. It is not that we are against the great tomes themselves—we are simply against reading them too much and too soon. One starts off strong on 'care' and weak on knowledge, and the danger is that this state of affairs becomes reversed. It is easier to learn from books than from patients, yet what our patients teach us may be of more abiding significance: the value of sympathy, the uses of compassion and the limits of our human world. It is at the bedside that we learn how to be of practical help to people who are numbed by the mysterious disasters of womb or tomb, for which they are totally unprepared. If this small book enables those starting to explore the major specialties to learn all they can from their patients, it will have served its purpose—and can then be discarded.

Because of the page-a-subject format, the balance of topics in the following pages may at first strike the reader as being odd in places. However, it has been our intention to provide a maximally useful text rather than one which is perfectly balanced in apportioning space according to how common a particular topic is—just as the great *Terrestrial Globes* made by George Phillips in the 1960s may seem at first to provide an odd balance of place names, with Alice Springs appearing more prominently than Amsterdam. To chart a whole continent, and omit to name a single central location out of respect for 'balance' is to miss a good opportunity to be useful. George Phillips did not miss this opportunity, and neither we hope, have we. It is inevitable that some readers will be disappointed that we have left out their favoured subjects (the Phillips' Globe does not even mention Oxford!). To these readers we offer over 300 blank pages by way of apology.

JABC & JML—*Preface to the first edition*—Ferring, 1987

Conflicts of interest: none declared

No pharmaceutical company employs us in any capacity and we have not received any financial input or gifts bearing upon our research for this publication. We assert that the drugs recommended in this book have been selected on the basis of the best available evidence.

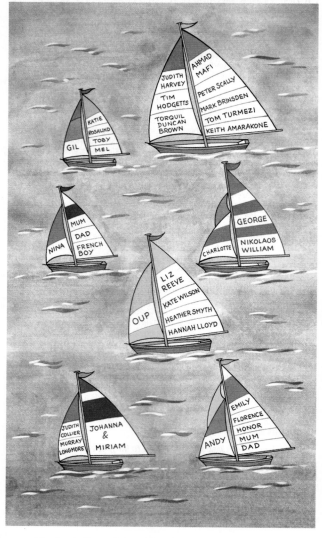

'He who studies medicine without books sails an uncharted sea, but he who studies medicine without patients does not go to sea at all.'
William Osler
Canadian physician, 1849–1919

Acknowledgements

This book was conceived and inspired by Judith Collier and Murray Longmore, who as lead authors presided over it for more than 25 years—from publication of the first edition in 1987, until publication of the ninth edition in 2013. Their knowledge, wisdom, and creativity lives on in the pages of this edition and their work has been loved and trusted by generations of doctors.

We thank all the authors who have contributed to previous editions: Judith Harvey, Tim Hodgetts, Duncan Brown, Peter Scally, Mark Brinsden, Ahmad R. Mafi, Tom Turmezei, and Keith Amarakone.

We thank those who have contributed their time and wisdom to previous editions: Dr Steven Emmet, Professor Tor Chiu, Natalie Langdown, and Professor Mark Lowenthal.

Specialist Readers We are hugely indebted to our Specialist Readers for their advice, encouragement, and constructive criticism. Each chapter in this book has benefitted from their trustworthy oversight. They are thanked individually at the beginning of each chapter.

Junior Readers It was our great pleasure to welcome a new team of Junior Readers to the tenth edition of this book. Our Junior Readers showed commitment, intelligence, and ingenuity in their contributions to the referencing and cross-referencing of this edition. We have a better book for it. They are also thanked individually at the beginning of each chapter.

Reader participation We have been very fortunate to receive so many well-considered suggestions and corrections to the book from readers all over the globe. Their contributions have enhanced the book and we are grateful.

If you would like to give us feedback, correct a mistake, or make a suggestion, you can do so at **www.oup.com/uk/academic/ohfeedback**.

How to use this book

This book has some useful features to help you get the most out of the information inside.

Quick chapter look-ups The index on the back cover refers to and aligns with the coloured tabs on the sides of the pages.

References (¹) Every reference has an individual identification indicated by a pink superscript number. The full details of every reference are held online at **www.oup.com/ohcs10refs**.

Further reading Throughout the book you will find 'Further reading' sections which are intended to guide you to sources that will further your learning, understanding, and clinical practice.

Cross references There are cross references to other topics within the book, to the *Oxford Handbook of Clinical Medicine* (*OHCM*), and to other titles in the Oxford Medical Handbooks series.

Reference intervals for common laboratory values are included inside the back cover. Conversion factors to and from SI units are given on the bookmark.

Symbols and abbreviations See page ix.

Corrections and suggestions Found a mistake? Have a suggestion for the next edition? Let us know at **www.oup.com/uk/academic/ohfeedback.** Major changes are announced online at **www.oup.co.uk/academic/series/oxhmed/updates.**

A note on the use of pronouns

For brevity, the pronoun '*he*' or '*she*' has been used in places where '*he or she*' would have been appropriate. Such circumlocutions do not aid the reader in forming a vivid visual impression, which is one of the leading aims of good authorship. Therefore, for balance and fairness, and where sense allows, we have tried alternating *he* with *she*.

Symbols and abbreviations

▶▶	don't dawdle! Prompt action saves lives
▶	this phrase is important
†† (†)	more (or less) vital topic; a rough guide for 1st-time readers
✺	an opportunity for holistic/non-reductionist thinking
●☀	conflict (controversial topic)
1,2,3	references at oup.co.uk/ohcs10refs
1,2,3	drug dose not in *BNF*, see oup.co.uk/ohcs10refs
#	fracture
Δ	diagnosis
ΔΔ	differential diagnosis
♂:♀	male to female ratio
↓	decreased
↔	normal (eg plasma level)
↑	increased
~	about
≈	approximately equal
–ve	negative
+ve	positive
∵	on account of/because of
∴	therefore
A2A	angiotensin 2 receptor (blockers)
ABC	air, breathing, circulation
A(P)LS	advanced (paediatric) life support manuals
ABR	audiological brainstem responses
AC	*ante cibum* (before food)
ACE(i)	angiotensin-converting enzyme (inhibitor)
ACTH	adrenocorticotrophic hormone
ADD	attention deficit disorder
ADH	antidiuretic hormone
AED	anti-epileptic drug
AFP	α-fetoprotein (α=alpha)
AIDS	acquired immunodeficiency syn.
AKI	acute kidney injury
Alk	alkaline (phos=phosphatase)
ALL	acute lymphoblastic leukaemia
ALS	advanced life support
ALT	alanine aminotransferase
ANA	antinuclear antibody
ANF	antinuclear factor
ANS	autonomic nervous system
AP	anteroposterior
APH	antepartum haemorrhage
APLS	advanced paediatric life support
APM	auto-premotor syndrome
ARM	artificial rupture of membranes
ASD	atrioseptal defect
ASO	antistreptolysin O (titre)
ASW	approved social worker
ATLS®	Advanced Trauma Life Support®, see www.trauma.org
ATN	acute tubular necrosis
AV	atrioventricular
AVM	arteriovenous malformation
βHCG	β-human chorionic gonadotrophin
BJGP	*British Journal of General Practice*
BMI	body mass index
BMJ	*British Medical Journal*
BNF	*British National Formulary*
BNFc	children's *BNF*
BP	blood pressure

©	courtesy of the copyright holder
C3	complement
Ca	carcinoma
CBRN	chemical, biological, radiological, nuclear
CBT	cognitive-behavioural therapy
CCDC	consultant in communicable disease control
CCF	combined (right- & left-sided) cardiac failure
ChVS	chorionic villus sampling
CI	contraindications
CIN	cervical intra-epithelial neoplasia
CMV	cytomegalovirus
CNS	central nervous system
CoC	combined oral contraceptive
COM	chronic otitis media
CPA	care programme approach
CPAP	continuous +ve airways pressure
CPR	cardiopulmonary resuscitation
CRP	C-reactive protein
CRPS	complex regional pain syndrome
CS	caesarean section
CSF	cerebrospinal fluid
CT	computed tomography
CVP	central venous pressure
CVS	cardiovascular system
CXR	chest x-ray
D	dimension (or dioptre)
D&C	dilatation (cervix) & curettage
D&V	diarrhoea and vomiting
dB	decibel
DHS	dynamic hip screw
DIC	disseminated intravascular coagulation
DIP	distal interphalangeal
DKA	diabetic ketoacidosis
dL	decilitre
DM	diabetes mellitus
DMSA	dimercaptosuccinic acid
DNA	deoxyribonucleic acid
DOH	Department of Health (NHS)
DPL	diagnostic peritoneal lavage
DRG	dorsal root ganglion
DSM-5	*Diagnostic and Statistical Manual of Mental Disorders, 5e*
DUB	dysfunctional uterine bleeding
DVT	deep venous thrombosis
EBM	evidence-based medicine
EBV	Epstein–Barr virus
ECG	electrocardiogram
ECT	electroconvulsive therapy
ED	emergency department
EDD	expected delivery date
EEG	electroencephalogram
EIA	enzyme immunoassay
ENT	ear, nose and throat
ERPC	evacuation of retained products of conception
ESR	erythrocyte sedimentation rate
ET	endotracheal
FB	foreign body
FBC	full blood count
FCR	flexor carpi radialis
FDP	flexor digitorum profundus
FDS	flexor digitorum sublimis

FH	family history
FNA	fine-needle aspiration
FNT	fetal nuchal translucency
FSH	follicle-stimulating hormone
G	gauge
g	gram
G(γ)GT	gamma(γ)glutamyl transpeptidase
G6PD	glucose-6-phosphate dehydrogenase
GA	general anaesthesia
GAS	group A Streptococcus
GBS	group B Streptococcus
GCS	Glasgow coma scale
GFR	glomerular filtration rate
GH	growth hormone
GI	gastrointestinal
GP	general practitioner
GU	genitourinary
h	hour
Hb	haemoglobin
HBsAg	hepatitis B surface antigen
HBV	hepatitis B virus
hCG	human chorionic gonadotrophin
HCV	hepatitis C virus
HDL	high-density lipoprotein
HFOV	high-frequency oscillatory ventilation
HIV	human immunodeficiency virus
HLA	human leucocyte antigen
HPA	Health Protection Agency
HPO	hypothalamic–pituitary–ovarian
HPV	human papilloma virus
HRT	hormone replacement therapy
HVS	high vaginal swab
ibid	*ibidem* (Latin, in the same place)
IBW	ideal body weight
ICP	intracranial pressure
IE	infective endocarditis
Ig	immunoglobulin
IHD	ischaemic heart disease
IM	intramuscular
INR	international normalized ratio of prothrombin time
IOP	intraocular pressure
IP	interphalangeal
IPPV	intermittent positive pressure ventilation
IPT	interpersonal therapy
IQ	intelligence quotient
ISQ	*in status quo* (Latin, no change)
ISS	injury severity score
ITP	idiopathic thrombocytopenic purpura
ITU	intensive therapy unit
IU/iu	international unit
IUCD	intrauterine contraceptive device
IUCS	intrauterine contraceptive system (eg Mirena®)
IUGR	intrauterine growth restriction
IUI	intrauterine insemination
IV	intravenous
IVF	*in vitro* fertilization
IVI	intravenous infusion
IVU	intravenous urography
JVP	jugular venous pressure
K+	potassium
kg	kilogram

kpa	kilopascal
L	litre
LA	local anaesthesia
LBC	liquid-based cytology
LCR	ligase chain reaction
LDH	lactate dehydrogenase
LFT	liver function test
LH	luteinizing hormone
LHRH	luteinizing hormone-releasing hormone
LMP	day 1 of last menstrual period
LMWH	low molecular weight heparin
LP	lumbar puncture
LSCS	lower segment caesarean section
LVH	left ventricular hypertrophy
MAOI	monoamine oxidase inhibitor
MCG	microgram
MCP	metacarpophalangeal
MCV	mean cell volume
MEA	microwave endometrial ablation
MET	meta-analysis
mg	milligrams (µg=microgram=mcg)
MHA	Mental Health Act
MI	myocardial infarction
ML	millilitre
mmHg	millimetres of mercury
MRI	magnetic resonance imaging
MRSA	meticillin-resistant *Staphylococcus aureus*
MSE	mental state examination
MSU	midstream urine culture
MTP	metatarsophalangeal
mU	milliunit(s)
MVA	motor vehicle accident
N=20*	reference to a randomized trial of 20 patients (* or whatever number follows N)
n=63*	reference to a non-randomized trial of 63 patients (* or whatever number follows n)
N2O	nitrous oxide
NaCl	sodium chloride
NAI	non-accidental injury
NBM	nil by mouth (no solids or fluids)
ND	notifiable disease
NEJM	*New England Journal of Medicine*
NEPE	non-epileptic paroxysmal events
NGT	nasogastric tube
NHS	National Health Service
NICE	National Institute for Health and Care Excellence
NICU	neonatal intensive care unit
NMJ	neuromuscular junction
NOF	neck of femur
NSAID	non-steroidal anti-inflammatory drug(s)
OAE	otoacoustic emissions
OED	*Oxford English Dictionary*, OUP
OGTT	oral glucose tolerance test
OHCM	*Oxford Handbook of Clinical Medicine* 9e, OUP
OM	otitis media
OME	otitis media with effusion
OMV	open mouth view
ON	*omni nocte* (take at night)
ORh–ve	blood group O, Rh negative
ORIF	open reduction and internal fixation

OT	occupational therapist
PA	posteroanterior
P_aCO_2	partial pressure of CO_2 in arterial blood
PAN	polyarteritis nodosa
pANCA	perinuclear antineutrophil cytoplasmic antibody
P_aO_2	partial pressure of oxygen in arterial blood
PC	*post cibum* (after food)
PCA	patient-controlled anaesthesia
PCOS	polycystic ovarian syndrome
PCR	polymerase chain reaction *or* protein:creatinine ratio
PCV	packed cell volume
PDA	patent ductus arteriosus
PE	pulmonary embolus
PET	positron emission tomography
PG	pemphigoid gestationis
PGD	preimplantation genetic diagnosis
PICU	paediatric intensive care unit
PID	pelvic inflammatory disease
PIP	proximal interphalangeal
PKU	phenylketonuria
PMB	postmenopausal bleeding
PMS	premenstrual syndrome
PO	*per os* (Latin for by mouth)
PoP	progesterone-only pill
POP	plaster of Paris
PPH	postpartum haemorrhage
PR	*per rectum*
PTR	prothrombin ratio
PUO	pyrexia of unknown origin
PUVA	psoralen-ultraviolet A
PV	*per vaginam* (via the vagina)
QOF	quality & outcomes framework
Rx	treatment (prescribing drugs)
RA	rheumatoid arthritis; regional anaesthesia
RBC	red blood cell
RCGP	Royal College of General Practitioners
RCOG	Royal College of Obstetricians and Gynaecologists
RCT	randomized controlled trial
REM	rapid eye movement
Rh	rhesus
RMO	registered medical officer
RR	relative risk
RSD	reflex sympathetic dystrophy
RSI	repetitive strain injury; rapid sequence induction
RTA	road traffic accident(s)
RTS	revised trauma score
RUQ	right upper quadrant
RVH	right ventricular hypertrophy
$S_1 S_2$	1st and 2nd heart sounds
SAD	seasonal affective disorder
SALT	speech and language therapist
S_aO_2	arterial blood O_2 saturation, ≈SpO_2 (allows for carboxyhaemoglobin)
SBE	subacute bacterial endocarditis

SC	subcutaneous
SCBU	special care baby unit
SE	side-effects
sec	second(s)
SERM	selective (o)estrogen receptor modulator
SFH	symphysis fundal height
SGA	small for gestational age
SLE	systemic lupus erythematosus
SNHL	sensorineural hearing loss
SpO_2	pulse oximetry estimated S_aO_2; no allowance for carboxyhaemoglobin
SSRI	selective serotonin reuptake inhibitor(s)
stat	*statim* (Latin for once); single dose
STD	sexually transmitted disease
STI	Sexually transmitted infection
SUFE	slipped upper femoral epiphysis
SVC	superior vena cava
SVP	saturation vapour pressure
syn	syndrome
T°	temperature, degrees Centigrade
t½	half life
T_3	triiodothyronine
T_4	thyroxine
TB	tuberculosis
TBW	tension band wiring
TCRE	transcervical resection of endometrium
TED	transverse elastic graduated
TENS	transcutaneous electrical nerve stimulation
TFT	thyroid function tests
TIA	transient ischaemic attack
ToP	termination of pregnancy
TPH	transplacental haemorrhage
TPR	temperature, pulse, and respirations
TRTS	triage revised trauma score
TSH	thyroid-stimulating hormone
TSOH	transient synovitis of the hip
TVS	transvaginal ultrasound
U	unit(s)
U&E	urea and electrolytes
UK	United Kingdom
URTI	upper respiratory tract infection
US	ultrasound
UTI	urinary tract infection
UV	ultraviolet
VF	ventricular fibrillation
VLBW	very low birthweight infant
VSD	ventriculoseptal defect
VT	ventricular tachycardia
VTE	venous thromboembolism
VUR	vesico-ureteric reflux
WCC	white blood cell count
WHO	World Health Organization
wt	weight
yrs, y	years
ZN	Ziehl–Neelsen (stain for TB)

1 Obstetrics

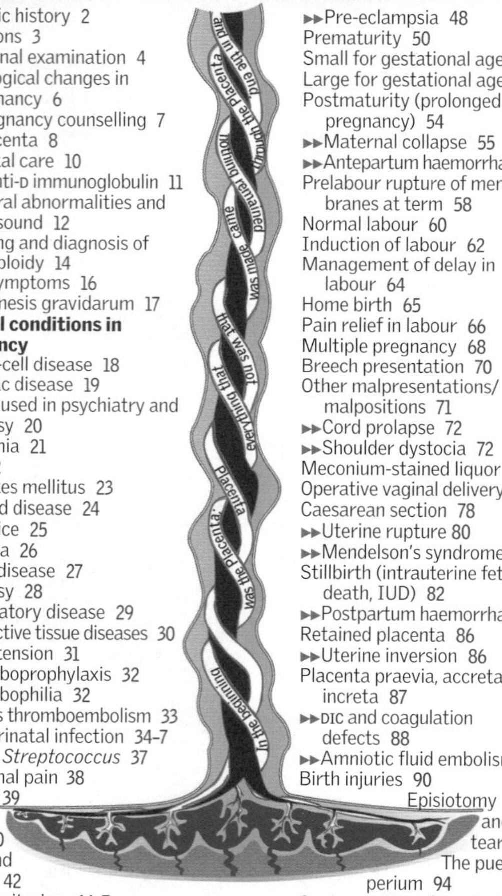

Fig 1.1 The uterine spiral arteries sustain life *in utero*, bathing the placenta with nutrients which twist and wind their way down the umbilical vein to the baby, to be returned to the placenta by the coiling umbilical arteries.

Sources RCOG Green Top guidelines; MBRACE-UK: *Saving Lives, Improving Mothers' Care* (2014).[1] **Relevant topics elsewhere** Neonatology, p107-28; breastfeeding, p124-6; rhesus disease, p116; miscarriage/termination, p258-61; preterm babies, p128, perinatal psychiatry, p386-7.

With many thanks to Miss Sarah Flint FRCOG, our specialist reader, and junior readers Mairead Kelly and Nusiba Taufik, for their contribution to this chapter.

⁘The essence of reproductive health

Pregnancy is a risky affair for babies and mothers. The direct causes of maternal mortality in the UK are sepsis (increasingly group A *Streptococcus*), pre-eclampsia, venous thromboembolism, and haemorrhage with all the other causes being rare. The most common causes of indirect deaths are cardiac disease, neurological disease, and psychiatric illnesses, including suicide. But if an obstetrician could be granted one wish, it would not be to abolish these; rather, it would be to make every pregnancy *planned* and *desired by the mother*. Worldwide, a woman dies every minute from the effects of pregnancy, and most of these women never wanted to be pregnant in the first place—but either had no means of contraception, or were without the skills, authority, and self-confidence to negotiate with their partners. So the real killers are poverty, ignorance, and the sexual desires of men, and the real solutions entail literacy, economic growth, and an equality of dialogue between the sexes. Any obstetric or governmental initiatives in reproductive health which do not recognize these facts are doomed.[2]

School-based sex education This *can* be effective, if linked to easy access to contraceptive services. Improving access to contraception reduces conception and termination of pregnancy rates in teenagers. *Adolescent pregnancy rates:* USA: 68/1000; UK: 28/1000; Canada: 25/1000. In 2012 in England & Wales, 140 pregnancies were terminated in those <14 years old (out of ~185,000 terminations and ~810,000 live births).[3]

Team work, obstetric emergencies, and debriefing

There is no finer example of interdisciplinary working than when midwife, obstetrician, and paediatrician (with porters, lab staff, and others) unite to achieve optimal outcomes in difficult obstetric practice. But outcomes are frequently not optimal, and the reason is usually poor team-work—not always because of overwork: 25% of obstetricians and 58% of midwives freely admit goals are not shared between professions.[4]

One way forward is regular meetings, agreement on spheres of leadership, auditable standards, simulations, and debriefing after emergencies, emphasizing that we cannot control the ever-present threat of disasters, and that when these occur it is processes not individuals that need interrogating.[5]

We should also debrief patients after disasters and near-misses. This can help avoid post-traumatic stress disorder and fear of future births.[6]

This can be a difficult skill to master and takes experience and practice. There are more components than for a normal medical history but each step is important. Remember to use a translator if needed, not a family member and bring out your sensitive side. Privacy and confidentiality are of utmost importance and the woman may not be willing to divulge intimate details with family members present.

Current pregnancy Include name, age, occupation, relationship status, gravidity and parity, LMP and EDD (preferably dated by 1st-trimester scan). See BOX. Irregular cycles, long cycles, and hormonal contraception make dating by LMP inaccurate. Ask about how the pregnancy is going, general health and symptoms, and fetal movements if >20 weeks. Ask about admissions or problems in this pregnancy as well as tests and scans. The woman may not know if everything is normal—this information is found in the pregnancy health record. Every woman will usually have had routine blood tests, a 1st-trimester scan, and an anomaly scan at 20 weeks.

Past obstetric history should include details of all previous pregnancies including miscarriages and terminations (plus reason for termination eg fetal abnormality). Antenatal problems eg pre-eclampsia, date and place of delivery, mode and gestation at delivery, sex, birth weight, delivery complications including shoulder dystocia, haemorrhage and stillbirth. Don't forget to ask about the postnatal period and neonatal life.

Gynaecological, medical, and surgical history Ask about contraception, pre-conception, difficulties with conception, smear history, and previous gynaecological problems or procedures. Establish any pre-existing medical disorders eg asthma, diabetes, epilepsy, or heart disease and if under the care of other medical specialists or GP. Psychiatric history is also important. Surgical history may impact on antenatal care or mode of delivery eg midline laparotomy for bowel resection for Crohn's or hip surgery limiting hip abduction.

Drug history Always check allergies and reaction. Include regular and as-required medication, as well as over-the-counter drugs. Some drugs may not be safe in pregnancy or breastfeeding.

Family history of diseases or congenital abnormalities enables adequate screening and antenatal care. Remember to ask about problems with any children the woman already has, and consanguinity.

Social history Drug and alcohol use, smoking, support at home. 'Ask the question' about domestic violence at each visit (domestic violence affects women of each social class equally). Domestic violence often escalates in pregnancy.

Definitions and obstetric shorthand

Gravidity refers to the number of pregnancies that a woman has had, to any stage, including the current one.

Parity refers to pregnancies that resulted in delivery beyond 24 weeks' gestation. An example of the shorthand way of expressing pregnancies before and after 24 weeks is para 2+1. This means that she has had 2 pregnancies beyond 24 completed weeks' gestation, and 1 which ended prior to 24 weeks. If she is not pregnant at the time of describing her she is gravida 3, but if she is pregnant now she is gravida 4. Twins present a problem as there is controversy as to whether they count as 1 for both parity and gravidity or should count as 2 for parity.

In general, aim to use proper English rather than the shorthand described above, which is open to ambiguity. For example, when presenting a patient try something like: 'Mrs Cottard is a 32-year-old lady who is 15 weeks into her 4th pregnancy; the 3rd ended in a miscarriage at 17 weeks, and the others came to term with normal deliveries of children who are now 2 & 8.' The bald statement 'Para 2+1' is ambiguous, incomprehensible to the patient, and misses the point that the patient is now approaching the time when she lost her last baby.

Dating a pregnancy Normal pregnancy is 40 weeks from the LMP. Naegele's rule: expected delivery date (EDD) ≈ 1yr and 7 days after LMP minus 3 months (not if last period was a withdrawal bleed; for cycles shorter than 28 days, subtract the difference from 28; if longer, add the difference). A revised rule suggests that the addition of 10 days rather than 7 is more accurate. In the UK, pregnancies are dated in the first trimester by US; this is accurate and based on the premise that the fetus grows at a known rate.

The labour ward runs on a combination of shorthand, acronyms, and many, many cups of tea. This list should help for your first few shifts:

APH: Antepartum haemorrhage: bleeding >24/40
ARM: Artificial rupture of membranes
CTG: Cardiotocography
FM: Fetal movements
GBS: Group B *Streptococcus*
GDM: Gestational diabetes mellitus
IUD: Intrauterine death or stillbirth
IOL: Induction of labour
Mec: Meconium-stained liquor, either thin or thick
MROP: Manual removal of placenta
NND: Neonatal death
NVD: Normal vaginal delivery
OC: Obstetric cholestasis
PET: Pre-eclampsia (used to be known as pre-eclamptic toxaemia)
PIH: Pregnancy-induced hypertension
PPH: Postpartum haemorrhage: bleeding >500mL postpartum
PPROM: Preterm prelabour rupture of membranes <37/40
PROM: Usually refers to prelabour rupture of membranes
SROM: Spontaneous rupture of membranes
SFH: Symphyso-fundal height
SPD: Symphysis pubis dysfunction
SVD: Spontaneous vaginal delivery
VBAC: Vaginal birth after caesarean section.

The uterus occupies the pelvis and cannot be felt *per abdomen* until ~12 weeks' gestation. By 16 weeks, its fundus lies half way between the symphysis pubis and the umbilicus. By 20–24 weeks it reaches the umbilicus. In a primip, the fundus is under the ribs by 36 weeks. At term the uterus lies a bit lower than at 36 weeks, as the head descends into the pelvis. From 16 weeks the SFH increases ~1cm/week.

The symphysis fundal height during pregnancy		
As a rule of thumb: at	16–26 weeks	the SFH (cm) ≈ dates (in weeks)
	26–36 weeks	the SFH (cm) ± 2cm ≈ dates
	36 weeks to term	the SFH (cm) ± 3cm ≈ dates

SFH is used as a screening tool to find babies small for gestational age (p52). Suspect this if the measurement lies >1-2cm outside these ranges given above. NB: more false positives will occur with the simpler rule of *weeks of gestation = cm from pubic symphysis to fundus.* The SFH should be plotted on a customized growth chart (p53).

Other reasons for discrepancy between fundal height and dates: •Inaccurate menstrual history •Multiple gestation •Fibroids •Polyhydramnios •Adnexal mass •Maternal size •Hydatidiform mole.

On inspecting the abdomen note size, asymmetry, and fetal movements. Signs consistent with pregnancy include a line of pigmentation, the linea nigra, extending in the midline from pubic hair to umbilicus. This darkens during the 1st trimester (the first 13 weeks). Striae gravidarum (stretch marks) can either be purple (new) or silvery-white (old). Note surgical scars, particularly from previous caesarean, laparotomy, and laparoscopy.

Palpating the abdomen *Measure the SFH* after 20 weeks (palpate <20 weeks). *Estimate number of fetuses.* Then *assess fetal lie* (longitudinal, oblique, transverse) in relation to the uterus. *Presentation* is the part of the fetus overlying the pelvic brim and is most commonly cephalic or breech. *Engagement* of the head is measured in fifths palpable eg by Pawlik's grip (examining the lower pole of the uterus between the thumb and index fingers of the right hand) Watch the patient's face during palpation and stop it if it causes pain. Obesity, polyhydramnios, and tense muscles make it difficult to feel the fetus. Midwives are skilled at palpation, and under 32 weeks of pregnancy it is often difficult, so ask them if you need help.

Auscultation The fetal heart may be heard by Doppler US (eg Sonicaid™) from ~12 weeks and with a Pinard stethoscope from ~24 weeks. Listen over the anterior shoulder of the fetus for rate and rhythm for 1 minute.

Fetal movements[7] First noted by mothers at 18-20wks, movements ↑ until 32wks then plateau at average 31/h. Fetuses sleep for 20-40-min cycles day and night (rarely >90mins). Maternal posture affects detection (lying> sitting>standing). If fetal movements are reduced, the woman should contact her midwife. If >28 weeks this should include CTG (p44) as soon as possible, and if risk factors for IUGR (p52) or stillbirth, or movements still reduced, urgent US for growth and liquor volume ± umbilical artery Dopplers (p12).

Engagement The level of the head is assessed in 2 ways: engagement, or fifths palpable abdominally. Engagement entails passage of the biggest diameter of the presenting part through the pelvic inlet. Fifths palpable abdominally states what you can feel, and makes no degree of judgement on degree of engagement of the head. In primigravida, the head usually enters the pelvis by 37 weeks, otherwise causes must be excluded (eg placenta praevia or fetal abnormality). In multips the head may not enter the pelvis until onset of labour.

Position—ie which way is the fetus facing?		
Occipitoanterior	**Occipitolateral**	**Occipitoposterior**
Back easily felt	Back can be felt	Back not felt
Limbs not easily felt	Limbs lateral	Limbs anterior
Shoulder lies 2cm from midline on opposite side from back	Midline shoulder	Shoulder 6–8cm lateral, same side as back
Back from midline=2–3cm	6–8cm	>10cm
(See figs 1.2 & 1.3.)		

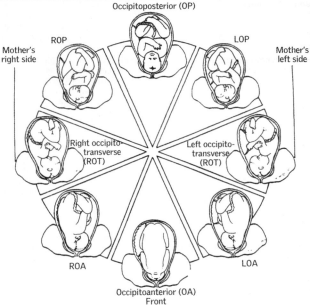

Fig 1.2 Fetal positions.

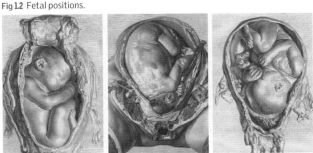

Fig 1.3 Use fig 1.2 to help determine the lie, the presentation, and the position from these dissections by William Hunter (1718–83).

William Hunter (1718-1783). *Anatomia uteri humani gravidi tabulis illustrata* (The anatomy of the human gravid uterus exhibited in figures). Courtesy of the U.S. National Library of Medicine.

Obstetrics

Hormonal changes Progesterone, synthesized by the corpus luteum until 35 post-conception days and by the placenta mainly thereafter, decreases smooth muscle excitability (uterus, gut, ureters) and raises body temperature. *Oestrogens* (90% oestriol) increase breast and nipple growth, water retention, and protein synthesis. The maternal thyroid often enlarges due to increased colloid production. Thyroxine levels, see *Thyroid disease in pregnancy*, p24. Pituitary secretion of *prolactin* rises throughout pregnancy. Maternal *cortisol* output is increased but unbound levels remain constant.

Genital changes The 100g non-pregnant uterus weighs 1100g by term. Muscle hypertrophy occurs up to 20 weeks, with stretching after that. The cervix may develop an ectropion ('erosion') (p270). Late in pregnancy, cervical collagen reduces. Vaginal discharge increases due to cervical ectopy, cell desquamation, and ↑ mucus production from a vasocongested vagina.

Haemodynamic changes *Blood:* From 10 weeks the plasma volume rises until 32 weeks when it is 3.8 litres (50% >non-pregnant). Red cell volume rises from 1.4 litres when non-pregnant to 1.64 litres at term if iron supplements are not taken (↑18%), or 1.8 litres at term (↑ 30%) if supplements are taken—hence Hb falls due to dilution (physiological 'anaemia'). WCC (mean 10.5×10^9/L), platelets, ESR (up 4-fold), cholesterol, β-globulin, and fibrinogen are raised. Albumin and gamma-globulin fall. Urea and creatinine fall.

Cardiovascular: Cardiac output rises from 5 litres/min to 6.5-7 litres/min in the first 10 weeks by increasing stroke volume (10%) and pulse rate (by ~15 beats/min). Peripheral resistance falls (due to hormonal changes). BP, particularly diastolic, falls during the 2nd trimester by 10–20mmHg, then rises to non-pregnant levels by term. With increased venous dispensability, and raised venous pressure (as occurs with any pelvic mass), varicose veins may form. Vasodilatation and hypotension stimulate renin and angiotensin release—an important feature of BP regulation in pregnancy.

Aorto-caval compression From 20 weeks the gravid uterus compresses the inferior vena cava (and to a lesser extent the aorta) in supine women, reducing venous return. This reduces cardiac output by 30–40% (so-called supine hypotension). ►Placing the woman in left lateral position or wedging her tilting 15° to the left relieves the pressure and restores cardiac output to more normal levels.

Other changes Ventilation increases 40% (tidal volume rises from 500 to 700mL), the increased depth of breath being a progesterone effect. O_2 consumption increases only 20%. Breathlessness is common as maternal $PaCO_2$ is set lower to allow the fetus to off-load CO_2. Gut motility is reduced, resulting in constipation, delayed gastric emptying, and, with a lax lower oesophageal sphincter, heartburn. Renal size increases by ~1cm in length during pregnancy.

Frequency of micturition emerges early (glomerular filtration rate ↑ by 60%), later from bladder pressure by the fetal head. The bladder muscle is lax but residual urine after micturition is not normally present. Skin pigmentation (eg in linea nigra, nipples, or as chloasma—brown patches of pigmentation seen especially on the face), palmar erythema, spider naevi, and striae are common. Hair shedding from the head is reduced in pregnancy but the extra hairs are shed in the puerperium.

Pregnancy tests Increasingly sensitive and may be positive from 9 days post-conception (or from day 23 of a 28-day cycle). The false +ve rate is low. They detect the β-subunit of human chorionic gonadotrophin in early morning urine, so are positive in trophoblastic disease (p264).

Pre-pregnancy counselling

The aim is to minimize the risks to the mother, neonate, or fetus by modifying pre-pregnancy conditions and risk factors. This may involve advising against pregnancy or delaying conception until a safer time. Babies conceived 18-23 months after a live birth have the lowest rate of perinatal problems.
Ensure rubella immune.

Stop smoking Smoking reduces ovulation and Fallopian tube function, causes abnormal sperm production (less penetrating capacity), ↑ rates of miscarriage (×2), and is associated with preterm labour and fetal growth restriction, placenta praevia, and abruption. Women should be encouraged and supported to stop smoking, and if this is not possible, to reduce the amount they smoke.

Weight loss for both partners increases conception rate and reduces risks (p39). Aim for BMI >18.5 and <30kg/m².

Exercise should be encouraged. It improves fitness and self esteem. Avoid contact sports and sports where abdominal trauma is possible.

Folic acid supplementation To prevent neural tube defects (NTDs) and cleft lip, all should have folate-rich foods + folic acid 0.4mg daily >1 month pre-conception till 13wks (5mg/day if past NTD, on antiepileptics, p28, obese (BMI >30), HIV+ve on co-trimoxazole prophylaxis, diabetic, or sickle cell disease p18). Avoid liver & vit. A (vit. A embryopathy) & limit caffeine to 200mg/day, cook meat and eggs thoroughly, avoid pâté, soft cheese, shellfish, and raw fish.

Vitamin D supplementation in at-risk ethnic groups, the obese, and those with chronic medical disease and reduced mobility.

Alcohol High levels of consumption are known to cause fetal alcohol syndrome (p138). Minimal drinking eg 1–2u/wk has not been shown to adversely affect the fetus but alcohol does cross the placenta and may affect the fetal brain. Miscarriage rates are higher among drinkers of alcohol. NICE recommends <1u/24h. Binge drinking (>5u/session) is especially harmful. To cut consumption: see *Managing alcohol consumption*, p512.

Recreational drug use is associated with miscarriage, preterm birth, poor fetal development, and intrauterine death; refer the woman for help early.

Pre-existing medical disorders may worsen during pregnancy, or be worsened by pregnancy. This may be transient or permanent. As a general rule, poorly controlled disease will remain the same or worsen with poorer outcomes, and well controlled disease remains the same or improves, with a better outcome. Refer for specialist help early: this enables optimal control of the disease and reduces risk (eg fetal malformation in diabetes mellitus, or deterioration with SLE). If the disease is severe or pregnancy involves risk to life, conception may be discouraged eg pulmonary hypertension, end-stage renal failure. If the woman is already pregnant, termination may be offered.

Medication should be changed pre-conception to reduce the risk of teratogenesis eg AEDs (anti-epileptic drugs), ACEI, immune-modulators. Seek expert help and use lowest effective dose with minimal polypharmacy. Don't forget over-the-counter preparations, including homeopathic or herbal (eg St John's wort).

Genetic counselling should be offered at a regional centre if relevant personal or family history (p154).

Spontaneous miscarriage (SM) Risk of miscarriage 15-20% all pregnancies, rising at extremes of age (>3 miscarriages = recurrent miscarriage, p261).

Obstetrics

The placenta is the organ of respiration, nutrition, and excretion for the fetus. It produces hormones for maternal well-being. It immunologically protects the fetus from rejection and allows the passage of maternal IgG antibodies.

Development The placenta develops when the blastocyst implants into the decidua and forms from trophoblastic cells. Some of these cells are invasive, penetrating endometrial blood vessels, forming sinuses (lacunae). These trophoblastic cells become primitive villi, then secondary and tertiary villi, the core being fetal blood vessels. Villi formation starts at 6 weeks, and stem villi are established by 12 weeks. The placenta continues to grow both in circumference and thickness until 16 weeks (hence the need to start aspirin in those at risk by 16 weeks to prevent pre-eclampsia), and after this, circumferentially.

Placental villi are the functional units of the placenta (fig 1.4). Each placenta has around 60, grouped into cotyledons containing 3–4 villi. On the maternal (outer or uterine) surface is the syncytiotrophoblast which is in direct contact with maternal blood, then cytotrophoblast, basement membrane, mesenchymal stroma, and then the basement membrane of fetal blood vessels. The maternal surface looks raw, rough, and spongy. The fetal surface is smooth and shiny, covered by the amnion, and the umbilical cord attached at the centre. Look for the branching of the umbilical vessels to and from the placenta. A monochorionic twin placenta is more interesting—examine closely to see if any vessels interconnect (as with twin-to-twin transfusion syndrome).

Circulation in the placenta consists of two different systems: uteroplacental and fetoplacental. *Uteroplacental* circulation is maternal blood travelling through the intervillous spaces. The uterus at term receives 500–600mL/min of blood, with the potential for torrential blood loss either as antepartum or postpartum haemorrhage. The circulation is set up so as to favour transfer of oxygen and other nutrients to the fetus. The spiral arteries become dilated and low-pressure, high-flow vessels to maximize blood flow. The first change occurs in the first trimester with structural modification, and the second wave in the second trimester with myometrial segments of these spiral arteries being invaded. If this mechanism fails for some reason, and the uteroplacental circulation becomes high resistance with low flow, the result is varying degrees of IUGR and pre-eclampsia. The *fetoplacental* circulation consists of two *umbilical arteries* which carry deoxygenated blood from the fetus to the placenta. These arteries subdivide into many branches, entering the stem of the chorionic villus, then into arterioles and capillaries. The blood is then oxygenated and picks up nutrients, flowing into its relevant venous drainage system, eventually becoming the singular *umbilical vein*. The maternal and fetal circulations coexist as a form of countercurrent, and never mix.

Functions The placenta attaches the fetus, is the organ of gaseous exchange, endocrine (hCG, growth factors, oestrogens, progestogens, and many more), barrier (infection, drugs), transfers nutrients to and from the fetus.

At term the placenta weighs 1/6th the weight of the baby. The placenta changes throughout pregnancy as calcium is deposited in the villi and fibrin on them. Excess fibrin may be deposited in diabetes and rhesus disease, so ↓ fetal nutrition.

After delivery Examine the placenta for abnormalities (clots, infarcts, vasa praevia, single umbilical artery). Blood may be taken from the cord for pH, (especially if abnormal CTG pre-delivery), Hb, Coombs' test, LFTs, and blood group (eg for rhesus disease), or for infection screens, if needed.

For placenta praevia see p87.

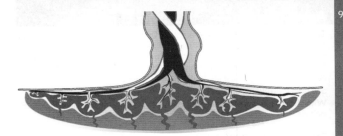

Fig 1.4 The placenta and umbilical cord. Seven spiral arteries are here seen to have been successfully invaded by trophoblast and they are now flooding the vast intervillous spaces with hot maternal blood—producing the slow whooshing crescendos heard by the US probe as the backdrop to the faster fetal heart beat. To get to the fetus proper, nutrients have a 6-part journey: maternal blood space → syncytiotrophoblast → trophoblast basement membrane → capillary basement membrane → capillary endothelium → fetal blood.

In pre-eclampsia, trophoblast invasion is too shallow: there is no progress beyond the superficial portions of the uterine spiral arterioles. So these spiral arterioles retain their endothelial linings and remain narrow-bore, high-resistance vessels, resulting in poor maternal blood flow. The mother may raise her blood pressure to compensate for this—but the price may be eclampsia (p49).

Plasma chemistry in pregnancy

	Non-pregnant		Trimester 1		Trismester 2		Trimester 3	
Centile	2.5	97.5	2.5	97.5	2.5	97.5	2.5	97.5
Na⁺ mmol/L	138	146	135	141	132	140	133	141
Ca²⁺ mmol/L	2	2.6	2.3	2.5	2.2	2.2	2.2	2.5
*corrected	2.3	2.6	2.25	2.57	2.3	2.5	2.3	2.59
Albumin g/L	44	50	39	49	36	44	33	41
AST IU/L	7	40	10	28	11	29	11	30
AST IU/L	0	40	6	32	6	32	6	32
TSH	0	4	0	1.6	1	1.8	7	7.3

*Calcium corrected for plasma albumin (*OHCM* p670)

Other plasma reference intervals (not analysed by trimester)		
	Non-pregnant	Pregnant
Alk phos IU/L	3–300	≤450 (can be ↑↑ in normal pregnancies)
Bicarbonate mmol/L	24–30	20–25
Creatine µmol/L	70–150	24–68
Urea mmol/L	2.5–6.7	2–4.2
Urate µmol/L	150–390	116–276 (24wks), 110–322 (32wks), 120–344 (36wks)

- C-reactive protein does not change much in pregnancy.
- Platelets ≥150 ×10⁹/L (beware if 120 ×10⁹/L see p48).
- *For anaemia in pregnancy, see p21.
- TSH may be low <20wks in normal pregnancy (suppressed by HCG); see above & p24.
- Protein S falls in pregnancy, so protein S deficiency is difficult to diagnose.
- Activated protein C (APC) resistance is found in 40% of pregnancies so special tests are needed when looking for this. Genotyping for factor V Leiden and prothrombin G20210A are unaffected by pregnancy.

The aims of antenatal care are to: •Detect any disease in the mother •Monitor and promote fetal well-being •Prepare mothers for birth and make a plan of care •Monitor trends to prevent or detect any early complications of pregnancy: BP is the most important variable (pre-eclampsia, p48). •Is thromboprophylaxis (p32) or aspirin (p31) needed?

See p795 for trauma in pregnancy.

Who should give antenatal care? Midwives manage care, calling in obstetricians if risks *or specific needs are identified*. Book by 12 weeks: see within 2 weeks if already ≥12 weeks pregnant.

The 1st antenatal (booking) visit is very comprehensive. ►Find a language interpreter if she needs one. Avoid using relatives (confidentiality issues). *Full obstetric history* (p2): Particularly, is there a family history of diabetes, BP↑, fetal abnormality, inheritable disease, or twins?

- •Does she have concurrent illness (p18–35)? Has she been 'cut' (FGM p247)? Risk assess for venous thromboembolism and if high risk refer to obstetrics; may need antenatal and postnatal LMWH (p32).
- •Is gestational diabetes (GDM) a risk? Screen (75g glucose tolerance test) at 28wks if BMI >30, previous baby >4.5kg, 1st-degree relative diabetic, family origin (FO) from area of high risk for diabetes. If previous GDM, screen at 16+28wks.
- •Past mental illness? If serious (schizophrenia, bipolar disorder, self-harm) or past postnatal depression, get antenatal assessment by perinatal mental health team and put management plan in notes.
- •*Women* born outside the UK are at higher risk of haemoglobinopathies, blood-borne viruses, and pre-existing cardiac disease.
- •*Unsupported women*: those with unplanned pregnancies or unemployed likely to need more support. Always *ask the question* about domestic violence (p518). Check for *substance abuse* (p374). 'Healthy Start Vitamins for Women'—folic acid + vitamins C & D (10mcg/d) are free to some during pregnancy and for 1 year after birth (Healthy Start Scheme [UK]).

Examination: Check heart, lungs, BP, weight (record BMI), and abdomen. Is a cervical smear needed? Varicose veins? Sensitively ask if genitally 'cut' (p247).

Tests: Blood: Hb, blood group, and antibody screen (p116), syphilis & rubella (±chicken-pox) serology, HBsAg (p36 & p25) HIV test; sickle test depending on family origin, Hb electrophoresis (p21) and 25-hydroxyvitamin D if relevant.[8] Take an *MSU* (protein; bacteria). If she is from an area endemic for TB or a TB contact, consider referral for Mantoux test and *CXR*.

Screening for chromosomal and structural abnormalities should be offered at booking. The 12-week scan also confirms EDD (p12).

Advise on: Smoking, alcohol, diet, correct use of seat belts (above or below the bump, not over it). Offer antenatal classes, information on maternity benefits, including free dental care. Usual exercise and travel are OK (avoid malarious areas) up to 36 weeks (singleton):[9] but check with airline; many require a 'fit to fly' letter beyond 32 weeks. Intercourse OK if no vaginal bleeding.

Later visits Discuss screening results and treat anaemia or UTI. At each visit, check urine for protein, BP, fundal height. Visits are at <12 weeks then at 16, 25, 28, 31, 34, 36, 38, 40, and 41 weeks (primip).

28wks: Do Hb and Rh antibodies at 28 weeks and give anti-D if needed (p11). Weigh only if clinically indicated.

34wks: Discuss labour and birth, pain relief.

36wks: Discuss breastfeeding, neonatal vitamin K, postnatal care, postnatal depression, and the baby blues.

40wks: Discuss post-dates pregnancy and its management (p62).

41wks: Offer membrane sweep and book IOL by 42 weeks.

Dose 250u for gestations <20 weeks, 500u if >20 weeks, (1500u if no Kleihauer). Give in deltoid (buttock absorption too slow); IV^{10}_{RCOL} or SC if bleeding disorder; as soon as possible after incident, by 72h (some protection if by 10d). From 20^{+0} weeks do Kleihauer test (FBC bottle of maternal blood; fetal RBCs less susceptible to lysis, so can be counted to measure the bleed's volume). Don't give anti-D if already sensitized ie antibodies to anti-D are present.

Postnatal use 500u is the normal dose after 20^{+0} weeks' gestation. 37% of Rh–ve women give birth to Rh–ve babies and these women do not need anti-D.

• Anti-D should be given to all Rh–ve women where the baby's group cannot be determined (eg macerated stillbirths), or if the baby's group is unknown 72h post delivery.

• Do a Kleihauer test on all eligible for anti-D. 500u anti-D can suppress immunization by up to 4mL of fetal red cells (8mL of fetal blood), but 1% of women have transplacental haemorrhage (TPH) of >4mL, especially after manual removal of placenta, and with caesarean section. A Kleihauer test is especially important in stillbirth, as massive spontaneous transplacental haemorrhage can be the cause of fetal death. Where >4mL TPH is suggested by the Kleihauer screen, a formal estimation of the TPH volume is required and 500u anti-D given for every 4mL fetal cells transfused (maximum 5000u anti-D at 2 IM sites/24h). Note: Kleihauer tests can be negative where there is ABO incompatibility as fetal cells are rapidly cleared from the maternal circulation. Liaise with the transfusion service. Check maternal blood every 48h to determine clearance of cells and need for continuing anti-D.

• Any mother receiving anti-D prenatally (see below), should also receive it postnatally unless she delivers an Rh–ve baby.

Use of anti-D in miscarriage in Rh–ve mothers

1 Anti-D should be given to all having surgical or medical terminations of pregnancy, evacuation of hydatidiform mole (p264), and ectopic pregnancies, unless they are already known to have anti-D antibodies. Give 250u if <20 weeks; 500u (and Kleihauer) if >20^{+0} weeks' gestation.

2 Anti-D should always be given where spontaneous miscarriage is followed by medical or surgical evacuation.

3 Anti-D should be given where spontaneous complete miscarriage occurs after 12^{+0} weeks' gestation.

4 Threatened miscarriage ≥12^{+0} weeks give anti-D; if bleeding continues intermittently give anti-D 6-weekly until delivery.

5 Routine anti-D is not recommended with threatened miscarriage before 12 weeks' gestation (but consider if viable fetus, heavy or repeated bleeding, and abdominal pain).

Use of anti-D in pregnancy in Rh–ve mothers

1 Give anti-D 500u at 28 and 34 weeks to Rh–ve women (primip antenatal sensitization falls from 0.95% to 0.35%). Anti-D may still be detectable in maternal blood at delivery. Still give postnatal anti-D, if indicated (as above). Take 28-week blood sample for antibodies before 28-week anti-D is given.

2 When significant TPH may occur: with chorionic villus sampling; external cephalic version; APH; uterine procedures (eg amniocentesis, fetal blood sampling); abdominal trauma; intrauterine death. Use 250u before 20 weeks' gestation, 500u (and do Kleihauer) after 20 weeks.

3 For threatened miscarriage, see above.

'The first half of pregnancy can become a time of constant "exams" to see if the baby can be allowed to graduate to the second half of pregnancy'. Congenital abnormalities, including aneuploidy, affect 2% of newborns. They are responsible for 21% of perinatal mortality and the outcome may involve physical and/or mental disability. Most congenital abnormalities are in low-risk patients with uncomplicated pregnancies. Women at higher risk are those with a previously affected fetus or child, pre-existing diabetes, epilepsy (even if not on AEDs). Everyone in the UK should be offered screening tests for structural and chromosomal abnormalities. Prenatal identification of problems allows decision-making for timing, mode, and place of delivery; meeting the neonatal team; ongoing fetal surveillance; time for the parents to come to terms with having an affected child; and in cases in which the problem would have a major impact on the child, termination of pregnancy may be offered. Remember that screening is not diagnostic, and can be declined by the woman.

Ultrasound can detect a pregnancy from approximately 5 weeks' gestation. *Early pregnancy scans* at <11 weeks are used to determine location, viability, and dating of the pregnancy. These are not routinely carried out unless there is bleeding, pain, or hyperemesis gravidarum (to exclude a molar pregnancy or twins). To *date a pregnancy,* crown–rump length between 6 and 12 weeks is most accurate—the growth is constant across the population. After 14 weeks, biparietal diameter (BPD) is the most accurate up to 20 weeks. After 34 weeks, BPD is unreliable. A woman who books for the first time in the 3rd trimester will require two growth scans, 2 weeks apart, to give the best estimate of gestation.

Nuchal translucency is carried out at 11^{+0}–13^{+6} weeks and determines viability (excludes miscarriage), dates pregnancy, and diagnoses multiple pregnancy and chorionicity (p68). 59% of those with major structural abnormalities can be detected at this stage eg anencephaly, and up to 81% with the later anomaly scan.[11] Screening for chromosomal abnormalities is carried out using the nuchal fold measurement + blood test (p14). Increased fetal nuchal translucency (NT) may reflect fetal heart failure,[12] and be seen in serious anomaly of the heart and great arteries.[13] The fetus should be in the neutral position as degree of neck flexion influences measurements. Taking the 99th percentile as a cut off for cardiac screening enables 33% of heart abnormalities to be detected antenatally.[14] Referring 99th percentile fetuses for echocardiography may show 106 cardiac abnormalities per 1000 fetuses examined.[15] There is a strong association between chromosomal abnormality and NT. In one study, 84% of karyotypically proven trisomy 21 fetuses had a NT >3mm at 10–13 weeks' gestation (as did 4.5% of chromosomally normal fetuses). The greater the extent of NT, the greater the risk of abnormality. Together with the blood screening tests, NT screening is used to calculate risk of chromosomal abnormality and if high risk (<1:150) invasive testing is offered (p15). Of all chromosomally normal fetuses (euploid) with significant nuchal thickening, 70–90% have normal outcome, 2.2–10.6% miscarry, 0.5–12.7% have neurodevelopmental problems, and 2.1–7.6% of malformations were undiagnosed before birth.[16]

The anomaly scan is a detailed US undertaken at 18–22 weeks' gestation to detect structural malformations. It takes approximately 30 minutes to complete and sensitivity varies depending on gestation, maternal BMI, operator skill, quality of the US machine, and the fetal structure involved (eg fetal heart defects are harder to detect than CNS defects).

Anomaly scan requirements

- *Skull shape and internal structures* including the cerebellum, ventricular size, and nuchal fold
- *Spine* in longitudinal and transverse views
- *Abdomen* for shape and content at the level of the stomach, kidneys, umbliicus/abdominal wall, and bladder
- *Arms and legs* for three bones and a hand or foot
- *Heart* in four-chamber view, with outflow tracts, and lungs
- *Face and lips*.

Lethal anomalies are anencephaly (absence of skull and cerebral cortex), bilateral renal agenesis, some major cardiac abnormalities, and trisomies 13 and 18. Offer a second opinion in a fetal medicine unit. Some anomalies have better survival rates than others and counselling must be supportive and informative no matter what the decision.

Fetal echocardiography is offered to those at high risk of fetal cardiac abnormality: family or personal history, NT of >3.5mm, suspected abnormality, drugs in pregnancy eg lithium, pre-existing diabetes, monochorionic twins. It is carried out in tertiary centres or by fetal medicine specialists.

Soft markers are findings on the anomaly scan that are in themselves of little significance, but are slightly more common in chromosomally abnormal fetuses. Choroid plexus cysts are seen in 1% of 20-week scans and are not significant; weak association with trisomy 18. Echogenic bowel has echogenicity similar to adjacent bone with the same US settings and is associated with increased risk of chromosomal abnormalities, congenital infection, CF and bowel obstruction. Others include 2-vessel umbilical cord, echogenic intracardiac foci and mild renal pelvic dilatation.

Fetal growth scans require accurate gestational age. Head circumference and abdominal circumference (sometimes with femur length) are used to calculate estimated fetal weight. Along with liquor volume (single deepest vertical pocket or amniotic fluid index) this is used to determine pattern of growth. Scans should be at least 2 weeks apart and used when there is increased risk of growth abnormality eg previous growth restriction, pre-eclampsia, measuring small for dates. A scan finding of a SGA fetus (p52) should prompt umbilical artery Doppler to distinguish between a fetus who is small and coping from those who are beginning to decompensate and require early delivery.

Doppler us measures blood flow in the uterus, placenta, and fetus. In an unselected population, it has not been shown to be of value but it is useful in high-risk pregnancies. *Uterine artery Doppler* measures resistance within the placenta. It is usually carried out at 23 weeks. High resistance increases risk of maternal pre-eclampsia and fetal growth restriction and requires extra maternal and fetal surveillance during pregnancy. *Umbilical artery Doppler* measures resistance in the placenta. High resistance indicates placental failure, and these fetuses are at higher risk of intrauterine death. If very preterm (<28 weeks) this can be used to time delivery. In absent or reversed end-diastolic flow, delivery by caesarean section should be considered, depending on gestation. Dopplers of fetal vessels (middle cerebral artery and ductus venosus) may be used for gestations <32 weeks to time delivery. MCA dopplers are also used to detect fetal anaemia eg with rhesus disease and parvovirus infection. Computerized CTG is helpful in monitoring of the compromised fetus (p44).

Screening in the UK NHS is offered to all women at booking. Most units use the combined test for trisomy 21 (Down's syndrome) screening, which has a detection rate of 75% with a false +ve rate of <3%. A risk of 1:150 or less is high risk and the woman is offered invasive testing eg amniocentesis. Screening tests estimate risk of trisomies 21, 13, and 18 taking into account results from NT, blood tests, and the woman's age. Results are modified further by smoking status, multiple pregnancy, IVF, maternal weight, ethnicity, and diabetes.

Trisomy 21 is the commonest cause of learning disability and the most common chromosomal abnormality. 10% die before age 5, and life expectancy is ~55 years. More fetuses at 16 weeks will have T21 than at term due to the increased rate of spontaneous miscarriage. Prevalence increases with increasing maternal age, and most occur secondary to non-disjunction of chromosome 21 at meiosis. Congenital cardiac malformations are common and 46% have VSD or ASD. Duodenal

Risk of trisomy 21 with rising maternal age	
<25 years	1:1500
30 years	1:910
35 years	1:380
40 years	1:110
45 years	1:30

atresia is also common. **Trisomy 18** (Edwards' syndrome) is the second most common trisomy after T21. Most die soon after birth and survival after 1 year is rare. Features include small chin, low-set ears, rocker-bottom feet, and VSD. **Trisomy 13** (Patau's syndrome) is rare, and babies die soon after birth. Features include microcephaly, holoprosencephaly, exomphalos and cleft lip and palate.

The combined test is the recommended screening test in the UK. It uses NT + free human chorionic gonadotrophin (HCG) + pregnancy-associated plasma protein (PAPP-A) + the woman's age. Used between 11 and 13 weeks + 6 days. It achieves detection rates of 90% of all aneuploides, 86% trisomy 21, and higher for trisomy 18 and trisomy 13. PAPP-A levels are ~19.6% lower in smokers.[17] In multiple pregnancy, risk is calculated per pregnancy if monochorionic; or per fetus when dichorionic or trichorionic.[18][NICE] Absent or hypoplastic nasal bone, and significant tricuspid regurgitation modifies the risk. The result is available in the 1st trimester, allowing for surgical termination of pregnancy.

The integrated test is a better screening test than the combined test but expensive and rarely used. It involves NT + PAPP-A in the 1st trimester + the quadruple test in the 2nd trimester. Do not use 2nd-trimester tests for triplets.[18][NICE]

The quadruple test is a blood test at 16 weeks and uses a dating scan (not a NT scan) plus maternal α-fetoprotein (AFP) + unconjugated estriol + free βhCG or total βhCG + inhibin-A + the woman's age in the 2nd trimester. Use between 15 weeks + 0 days and 20 weeks + 0 days, so useful for women presenting in the 2nd trimester.

Alpha-fetoprotein AFP is a glycoprotein synthesized by the fetal liver and GI tract. In 10% with a high AFP there is a fetal malformation, eg an open neural tube defect (but closed defects are missed), exomphalos, posterior urethral valves, nephrosis, GI obstruction, teratomas, Turner's syndrome (or normal twins). In ~30% of those with no malformation, there is an adverse outcome, eg IUGR, preterm delivery, placental abruption and 3rd-trimester deaths.

Pregnancy-associated plasma protein A (PAPP-A) is a large glycoprotein produced by the placenta that may have functions including matrix mineralization and angiogenesis. Therefore, low levels (<0.4 multiples of the median (MoM)) reflect poor early placentation. Low levels in 1st-trimester screening are associated with trisomies 18 and 21, pre-eclampsia, growth restriction, preterm delivery, and fetal demise.

Preimplantation genetic diagnosis (PGD) is an early form of prenatal diagnosis in which embryos created *in vitro* are analysed for well-defined genetic diseases eg monogenic disorders such as CF or beta-thalassaemia, or chromosome structural abnormalities. One to two cells are extracted at the 6-10-cell stage of the embryo. Fluorescence *in situ* hybridization (FISH) is used for analysis of chromosomes and polymerase chain reaction (PCR) for analysis of genes in monogenic diseases. One or two disease-free embryos are then used for implantation.

PGD selection of embryos by HLA type so that a child born after using this technology can be used as a stem cell donor to save a sibling from certain conditions (eg with Fanconi anaemia, thalassaemia, or leukaemia) is possible. Sex selection, unless to avoid sex-linked diseases, is illegal in the UK.

Pregnancy rates following PGD are 17% after testing for structural chromosome abnormality (including translocations), 16% after sexing, 21% after testing for monogenic diseases. This is lower than the expected rate of 20–25% expected for regular IVF.

Invasive testing This is offered if screening suggests an increased risk of aneuploidy (and may therefore be declined). DNA can by analysed for single-gene disorders such as CF or sickle cell disease.

Chorionic villus biopsy Carried out at 10–13 weeks. The placenta is sampled by transabdominal or occasionally transcervical approach under continuous US control. Karyotyping takes 2 days, enzyme and gene probe analysis 3 weeks, so termination for abnormality is earlier, safer, and is done before the pregnancy is apparent, compared with amniocentesis. Risks are an excess miscarriage rate of 1–2%, increased transmission of blood-borne viruses (HIV, hepatitis B & C), rarely contamination by maternal cells, and false positives or negatives from placental mosaicism (1%). It is not recommended in dichorionic multiple pregnancy. Is anti-D needed (p11)?

Amniocentesis is undertaken from 16 weeks onwards and involves the aspiration of fluid containing fetal cells shed from skin and gut. A small needle is passed transabdominally under continuous US, preferably not transplacentally. Fetal loss rate is ~1% at ~16 weeks' gestation. Anti-D is needed in all Rh–ve women (p11). Amniocentesis has the advantage of being able to diagnose fetal infections such as CMV and the excess miscarriage rate is lower than for CVS. Full cell culture for karyotyping may take as long as 3 weeks, but rapid results are possible within 2 days by FISH and PCR.

Cell-free fetal DNA (cffDNA) is a method of non-invasive prenatal testing for chromosomal abnormality. Fetal DNA is produced by the placenta from the 1st trimester, released into the maternal circulation and is cleared rapidly following delivery. Current methods cannot completely extract fetal DNA from maternal blood, and so the primary focus is on differing certain sequences eg Y chromosome of the male fetus, or Rh-D sequences in a Rh–ve woman. It can therefore be used to guide anti-D use in Rh–ve women, and the need for invasive testing in x-linked diseases—no need for invasive testing in female fetuses. There are good data to show that detection of trisomy 18 and 21 have sensitivity and specificity rates approaching 100%.

Dichorionic twins, maternal obesity, gestation <10 weeks, and placental mosaicism are known to affect results due to lower levels of cffDNA in maternal blood. The use of cffDNA is likely to be offered in the future within the NHS to high-risk women (high-risk combined screening, previous affected fetus) and has clear advantages in reducing the risks associated with invasive testing. [43] RCOL

▶Before prescribing any drug, think—is it safe? Check the BNF.

Symptoms and signs in the first 12 weeks Early symptoms are amenorrhoea, nausea, vomiting, and bladder irritability. Breasts engorge, nipples enlarge (darken at 12 weeks), Montgomery's tubercles (sebaceous glands on nipples) become prominent. Vulval vascularity increases and the cervix softens and looks bluish (4 weeks). At 6-10 weeks the uterine body is more globular. Temperature rises (<37.8°C).

Headaches, palpitations, and fainting are all commoner in pregnancy. Dilated peripheral circulation ↑sweating and feeling hot. Management: Increase fluid intake. If she feels faint from postural hypotension, stand slowly.

Urinary frequency is due to pressure of the fetal head on the bladder in later pregnancy. GFR also increases, increasing urine output. Exclude UTI.

Abdominal pain See p38.

Breathlessness is common. Are there risk factors for VTE? See p33.

Constipation tends to occur as gut motility decreases. Adequate oral fluids and a high-fibre diet help combat it. Avoid stimulant laxatives—they increase uterine activity in some women. Increased venous distensibility and pelvic congestion predispose to *haemorrhoids* and *varicose veins*. Resting with feet up and properly worn elastic stockings help.

Gastro-oesophageal reflux (heartburn) occur as progesterone-mediated pyloric sphincter relaxation allows irritant bile to reflux into the stomach. This is then worsened week-by-week from an ever-enlarging fetus pressing on the upper GI tract. Cigarettes and spices should be avoided, cold, small meals, and antacids and H$_2$- receptor antagonists may be used. Use more pillows, and a semi-recumbent position.

Musculoskeletal Symphysis pubis dysfunction (SPD), due to pelvic ligament and muscle relaxation may affect 10% (usually mild). Management: simple analgesia, physiotherapy. Not an indication for IOL or CS. Backache is common-manage as for SPD.

Carpal tunnel syndrome (p749) in pregnancy is due to fluid retention. Advise wrist splints until delivery.

Itch/itchy rashes are common (up to 25%) and may be due to the usual causes (*OHCM* p64, check LFT—see p25) or to pruritic eruption of pregnancy (PEP—an intensely itchy papular/plaque rash on the abdomen and limbs. PEP is most common in first pregnancies beyond 35 weeks' gestation. Emollients and weak topical steroids ease it. Delivery cures it. If vesicles are present, think of *pemphigoid gestationis* (PG): a rare (1:50,000) condition which may cause fatal heat loss and cardiac failure; the baby may be briefly affected; refer early (prednisolone may be needed). PG may recur in later pregnancies.

Ankle oedema This is a very common, almost normal, manifestation of pregnancy. Measure BP and check urine for protein (pre-eclampsia, p48). Check legs for DVT. It often responds to rest and leg elevation. Reassure that it is harmless (unless pre-eclampsia).

Leg cramps 33% get cramp, often in the latter half of pregnancy, which is severe in 5% and worse at night. Raising the foot of the bed by 20cm will help. More rarely is restless leg syndrome which is very difficult to treat, and poorly understood.

Chloasma This is a patch of darker pigmentation, usually on the face: p586.

Nausea affects ~80%. **Vomiting** occurs in ~50%. It may start by 4 weeks and decline over the following weeks. At 20 weeks 20% may still vomit. Most respond to frequent small meals, reassurance, and a stress-free environment. It is associated with good outcome (fewer fetal losses). Hyperemesis: p17.

This is defined as persisting vomiting in pregnancy which causes weight loss (>5% of pre-pregnancy weight) and ketosis. It is rare and affects 0.1-1% of pregnant women. Risk is increased in multiple pregnancies, molar pregnancies, and those with previous HG. May be fatal if no access to help (Charlotte Bronte died from it). It is thought to be related to high levels of hCG.

Presentation Inability to keep food or fluids down; weight ↓ ± nutritional deficiency, dehydration, hypovolaemia, tachycardia, postural hypotension, electrolyte disturbance with hypokalaemia and hyponatraemic shock, polyneuritis (B vitamins ↓), behaviour disorders, haematemesis from Mallory–Weiss tears, liver and renal failure. There may be ptyalism (inability to swallow saliva) and spitting.

Tests Urine dip for ketones and UTI (send MSU). FBC may reveal raised haematocrit; U&E to exclude hypokalaemia or hyponatraemia. Transaminases may be abnormal and albumin low. TFTs are often abnormal and should only be performed if other symptoms of hyperthyroidism. US should be carried out to diagnose multiple pregnancy and exclude a mole.

Treatment Admit to hospital if unable to keep anything down despite oral anti-emetics, for rehydration and correction of metabolic disturbance. Aggressively fluid replace with either 0.9% NaCl + K or Hartmann's. Glucose can precipitate Wernicke's encephalopathy. Remember, maintenance fluids are 2-3L/day and these women are fluid-depleted. Daily U&E to guide potassium and sodium replacement. Anti-emetics regularly eg promethazine, cyclizine, or metoclopramide PO/IV/IM. Ondansetron PO/IV is reserved if these measures fail but is not licensed in pregnancy (data so far reassuring). If vomiting still intractable, consider a course of corticosteroids eg prednisolone 40-50mg daily or hydrocortisone 100mg/12h IV. Some women are so badly affected by HG that they opt for TOP. Also remember to prescribe high-dose folic acid 5mg/day and thiamine to prevent Wernicke's encephalopathy (50mg PO TDS or IV B vitamins eg Pabrinex®). These women are high risk for VTE and while in hospital should have daily thromboprophylaxis (eg **enoxaparin** 40mg/24h sc) and anti-thromboembolic stockings.

Hyperemesis gravidarum: Amy's story

Suffering from hyperemesis was worse than anything I had experienced. It's not morning sickness that just lasts longer—other people saying that becomes frustrating! I vomited every single day from 6 weeks' gestation until 4 hours after my baby was born.

I was admitted 5 times for fluid rehydration and that was whilst taking 4 different types of anti-emetics. Some days rolling over in bed caused continuous vomiting. I couldn't work for 2 months and even after that I only managed mornings. Even working in the medical profession some people didn't understand the illness and thought I was using pregnancy as an excuse to lighten the workload.

I had a Mallory–Weiss tear at 7 weeks and developed hyperemesis-induced hyperthyroidism. I felt like nothing was ever going to help. I was scared every day and became pretty much house-bound due to always vomiting in public. I become isolated and every day was a struggle. My son is 100% worth it but my pregnancy felt like a lifetime! Even now I worry about the affects of so many medications on my baby but as Charlotte Bronte died of hyperemesis I took all medical advice, admissions, and medications to get myself and my son to term!

Sickle cell disease (SCD) is caused by a group of haemoglobin disorders (single-gene recessive) which predispose to 'sickling' of red cells in low oxygen conditions causing vaso-occlusion in small vessels, and cells prone to increased haemolytic breakdown. There are increased risks of painful crises, perinatal mortality, premature labour, and fetal growth restriction.[44] Some studies suggest ↑ spontaneous miscarriage, maternal infection, thromboembolic events, pre-eclampsia, and APH. Most prevalent in those of African descent it is also prevalent in the Caribbean, Middle East, Mediterranean, parts of India, and South and Central America. There are 100–200 pregnancies in women with SCD in the UK annually.

Preconception Women with SCD should be under annual clinic review to monitor disease. Arrange sickle specialist preconception review. Advice should cover factors affecting sickling crises (cold, hypoxia, dehydration—hence nausea and vomiting of pregnancy, over-exertion, stress). Pregnancy worsens anaemia, so ↑ risk of crises and acute chest syndrome—chest pain, cough, tachypnoea, and new infiltrates on CXR: treat as for pneumonia+blood transfusion. Screen for red cell antibodies (if present ↑risk of haemolytic disease of newborn). Pregnancy ↑ risks of infection (especially UTI). Address chance of fetus being affected (partner's blood to check carrier/haemoglobinopathy status: genetic counselling if needed). Assess current disease: echocardiography if not done in last year to exclude pulmonary hypertension (tricuspid regurgitant jet velocity >2.5m/sec high risk, p19); BP & urinalysis, U&E, LFT; retinal screening (proliferative retinopathy common); screen for iron overload if multiply transfused (if significantly overloaded, preconception chelation therapy is advised). SCD is a hyposplenic state; advise daily penicillin or erythromycin and update vaccines: hepatitis B, single-dose haemophilus influenza B & meningococcal C, 5-yearly pneumococcal, and annual H1N1 with seasonal influenza. Stop ACE/A2A drugs & hydroxycarbamide ≥3 months, preconceptually. Give 5mg folic acid daily (p7) preconceptually and throughout pregnancy .

Antenatal care Ensure preconception measures addressed. Manage by specialist multidisciplinary team if possible; if not, by 'high-risk' team using protocols. If fetus has haemoglobinopathy risk, offer prenatal testing by 8–10 weeks. From 12 weeks give 75mg aspirin daily to reduce risk of developing pre-eclampsia. Suggest TEDs in pregnancy. If hospitalized, give heparin thromboprophylaxis. Check BP at all antenatal visits and an MSU monthly. Offer viability scan at 7–9 weeks, dating scan at 11–14, anomaly scan at 20, and growth scan 4-weekly from 24 weeks. Only supplement iron if proven deficiency. Blood transfusion is not routine; if needed for sickling complication use fully compatible rhesus C,D,E and Kell typed CMV-negative blood (if so, transfusion regimen may be needed for rest of pregnancy). Top up transfusions may be needed if Hb falls to 60g/L. *Crises* affect 27–50%. Admit if fever, severe or atypical pain, chest pain, or breathless. If pain needs IV opiates use morphine/diamorphine (not pethidine, it risks fits); give nasal O₂ if oxygen sats <95% (take to ITU if O₂ sats not maintained), and adequate fluid intake 60mL/kg/h PO/IV unless pre-eclampsia (then specialist advice). Exchange transfusion is needed for acute chest syndrome or if stroke.

Intrapartum and postpartum care[44] Aim for delivery at 38–40 weeks at hospitals able to manage SCD. Keep warm and hydrated in labour/post-partum. Continuous monitoring of fetus, and maternal O₂ sats. Avoid pethidine (as for antenatal care). Give 7 days of heparin thromboprophylaxis post vaginal delivery, 6 weeks if CS. Progestogenic contraception is first choice; oestrogen-containing contraceptives are used as second-line agents.

Further reading
RCOG (2011). *Management of Sickle Cell Disease in Pregnancy* (Green-top Guideline No. 61). London: RCOG.

Cardiac disease is the leading indirect cause of maternal death in the UK, affecting <1% of pregnant women. Examine the heart in all pregnancies, but especially in those from an immigrant population.

The key is preconception counselling to identify and address risks, but much heart disease is undiagnosed, along with pregnancies being unplanned. Risk depends on presence of pulmonary hypertension, effect on haemodynamics, NYHA functional class I–IV, and presence of cyanosis. Also, history of arrhythmia, TIA, heart failure, left heart outflow tract obstruction (mitral or aortic stenosis with valve area <2cm^2 and 1.5cm^2 respectively), and ejection fraction <40% predict poorer outcome. *Never ignore* even asymptomatic cases of Marfan syndrome, pulmonary hypertension, and mitral stenosis.

Pulmonary hypertension has a mortality rate of 25–40% in pregnancy. Due to lung disease, connective tissue disease, primary, veno-occlusive, and Eisenmenger syndrome. Advise against pregnancy and offer ToP. Manage pregnancy in a tertiary centre. *Congenital heart disease:* More women survive to adulthood. Most commonly PDA, ASD, and VSD. If cyanotic and uncorrected, increased risk of IUGR. Refer for fetal echocardiography. *Marfan syndrome:* Autosomal dominant with 80% cardiac involvement with mitral valve prolapse, regurgitation, and/or aortic root dilatation. Risk of aortic dissection and rupture (esp. if root >4cm). Offer root replacement pre-pregnancy and LSCS if root >4.5cm. *Mitral stenosis* can be dangerous. Watch for dyspnoea, orthopnoea, and PND. Monitor with echo, aggressively treat AF (digoxin and β-blockers safe), treat pulmonary oedema. Valve area <1cm^2 has poor prognosis. *Arrhythmias:* If sinus tachycardia, exclude anaemia and hyperthyroidism. SVT is the commonest arrhythmia and can be treated with vagal manoeuvres and/or adenosine. *Artificial heart valves:* Warfarin risks fetal harm (p640); heparin risks valve thrombosis. Options include warfarin throughout pregnancy (INR 2.5–3.5), treatment-dose LMWH 6–12 weeks then warfarin, or LMWH throughout. *Ischaemic heart disease* is increasingly common with rising maternal age and obesity. Symptoms may be atypical and go unrecognized or be mistaken for PE. ECG, troponin, and manage as for non-pregnant women. *Peripartum cardiomyopathy* is rare and defined as heart failure without known cause and no previous history of heart disease. Onset 1 month pre- and 5 months postpartum. Diagnosis by echocardiography. Manage with elective delivery if antenatal, anticoagulants, conventional treatment for heart failure, and may require intra-aortic balloon pumps/left ventricular assist devices and/or cardiac transplantation. *Cardiac failure* is managed with diuretics, vasodilators, cardioselective β-blockers, inotropes, and once delivered, ACEI. Beware new-onset asthma in a pregnant woman—pulmonary oedema causes wheezing too.

Antenatal management Regular visits to cardiologist/obstetric combined clinic. Prevent anaemia, obesity, and smoking. Treat hypertension. Examine to exclude pulmonary oedema and arrhythmias at all visits. Refer for echocardiography. Heart failure requires admission. **Labour** Outcome is worst for mothers unable to ↑ their cardiac output (rare). Have O$_2$ and drugs to treat cardiac failure to hand. Aim for vaginal delivery at term. Shorten 2nd stage if fixed cardiac output state and offer LSCS as per cardiology advice. Epidurals are safe if hypotension is avoided. Beware IV fluids. Avoid ergometrine (use oxytocin). Most cardiac deaths are in immediate postpartum period.

Normal findings in pregnancy Ejection systolic murmur in >90% of pregnant women. CXR: slight cardiomegaly, ↑ pulmonary vascular markings. ECG: ectopics, Q-wave and inverted T in lead III, and T-wave inversion in lateral leads. The QRS shows left shift.

Further reading

Nelson-Piercy C (2015). *Handbook of Obstetric Medicine* (5th ed). Boca Raton, FL: CRC Press.

Obstetrics

Decisions about medication in pregnancy and breastfeeding should take into account the risks and benefits of treatment versus no treatment. Whilst fetal toxicity and anomalies are a concern, the primary duty is to protect and treat the mother. Have a higher threshold for drug treatment and use psychotherapy and counselling. Use the lowest effective dose and consider drugs which have previously been effective. Few drugs are regarded as contraindicated, but none can be regarded as entirely safe due to a lack of good quality data. Older drugs have traditionally been favoured as the evidence base is greater. With severe depression, bipolar affective disorder, schizophrenia, or other mental health diagnoses requiring specialist input, do not stop or change medication without their help. Remember the high risk of rapid postpartum relapse with significant associated risks to mother and infant, particularly in women with bipolar disorder (up to 50%).

Antidepressants See p346/386. Ante- and postnatal depression are common. Try to wait until the 2nd trimester before prescribing but do not delay if severe symptoms. 1st line therapy is with SSRIs (usually sertraline); available data suggest risk of fetal anomaly similar to that of obese mothers. There is a very small risk of persistent fetal pulmonary hypertension and neonatal withdrawal (breastfeeding can ease this). Avoid paroxetine (1st trimester use may be associated with cardiac malformations, and increased risk of neonatal withdrawal). Breastfeeding should be supported where it is not detrimental to maternal well-being (eg worsening sleep deprivation and stress). Fluoxetine and citalopram are present in relatively high concentrations in breast milk. Sertraline, paroxetine, imipramine, and nortriptyline have low concentrations. For all drugs, exposure through breastfeeding is lower than that *in utero*.

Mood stabilizers (AEDs) have varying malformation rates (also used as antiepileptics). Valproate and carbamazepine should not be prescribed to women of childbearing age and urgent advice sought with a view to stopping them if a woman taking them is pregnant. Valproate has the highest malformation rate (10%) with NTDs, craniofacial abnormalities, and neurodevelopmental problems (30–40%). Carbamazepine (2.2%) is also known to have increased rates of NTDs. Lamotrigine has a malformation rate of 2.1%, check blood levels regularly. All should be avoided in breastfeeding.

Lithium (p349) is linked with teratogenicity (heart defects, including Ebstein's anomaly), neonatal thyroid abnormalities, and floppy baby syndrome. Lithium should only be prescribed to women of childbearing age when alternatives have been ineffective and with appropriate counselling regarding risks. Offer specialist fetal echocardiography in those women electing to stay on lithium. Monitor drug levels 4-weekly to 36wks, then weekly, aiming for the individual's therapeutic window. Do not change brands (bioavailability varies). Signs of toxicity are tremor, drowsiness, visual disturbance. Stop lithium during labour. Check a 12h post-dose level and restart lithium based on this result. Women with bipolar disorder are at high risk of postpartum relapse which can evolve rapidly and is associated with morbidity and mortality for mother and infant. Breastfeeding is contraindicated due to the risk of neonatal toxicity.

Antipsychotics NB: rates of fetal abnormality are increased in schizophrenia, even in those taking no drugs. NICE warns of possible raised prolactin levels with amisulpride, sulpiride, and risperidone. Women taking antipsychotics associated with weight gain should have an OGTT. Women taking clozapine should not breast-feed due to risk of fetal agranulocytosis. Depot medication should be avoided where possible in women of childbearing age.

Benzodiazepines may be linked to cleft lip and palate and should be avoided. Avoid diazepam during delivery, as neonatal withdrawal may occur.

With thanks to Dr Sarah Ashurst-Williams MRCPsych.

►Even a small PPH (p84) may become life-threatening if the mother is anaemic. Anaemia predisposes to PPH, infection, makes heart failure worse, and is the main cause of perinatal problems associated with malaria. Above all, anaemia is a leading mechanism by which poverty exacts its morbid toll in pregnancy.

Definition of anaemia of pregnancy Hb <105g/L. The fall in Hb is steepest around 20 weeks' gestation, and is physiological (p6).

Who is prone to anaemia? Those who start pregnancy anaemic, eg from menorrhagia, hookworm, malaria, with haemoglobinopathies; those with frequent pregnancies, twin pregnancy, or a poor diet.

Antenatal screening includes Hb estimation at booking and at 28 weeks. In black patients do sickle-cell tests; in others at risk consider Hb electrophoresis for other haemoglobinopathies. From malarious areas consider malaria, and thick films. See p26.

Investigation should include FBC (MCV reduced, and later MCHC). serum iron, TIBC and serum ferritin are low in iron deficiency. In folate deficiency, MCV is raised, serum and red cell folate reduced.

Causes By far the most common is iron deficiency—many women enter pregnancy with low iron stores. The next most common is folate deficiency. Also consider coeliac disease, chronic kidney disease, and autoimmune disease.

Treatment Pregnancy increases iron needs by 700–1400mg (throughout pregnancy), provided for by a pregnancy-induced 9-fold increase in iron absorption. Iron and folate supplements (and prevention against hookworm and malaria) are recommended in many developing countries.

Offer *oral iron* (eg ferrous sulfate 200mg BD PO); alternate days or even twice weekly may prevent gastrointestinal side effects. In women who would refuse blood transfusion (see BOX, p85), prevention is key so prescribe iron. *Parenteral iron* may be given (to those with iron deficiency anaemia not tolerating oral iron) as iron dextran or iron sucrose. Beware anaphylaxis. Use only if cardiopulmonary resuscitation facilities to hand. Hb rises by 8g/L/week over 6 weeks, so late severe anaemia (Hb <90g/L) may need blood transfusion. One unit of blood increases the Hb by ~7g/L.

Thalassaemias (*OHCM* p336) These globin chain production disorders are found in Mediterranean, Indian, and South-east Asian populations. Although anaemic, never give parenteral iron as iron levels are usually high. Seek expert advice as to use of oral iron and folate. β-thalassaemia does not affect the fetus but in homozygotes regular transfusions sustain life only until young adulthood. There are α chains in fetal HbF, so in α-thalassaemias the fetus may be anaemic or, if severe, stillborn. Mothers carrying lethally affected hydropic fetuses risk severe pre-eclampsia, and delivery complications due to a large fetus and bulky placenta. Prenatal diagnosis is possible by chorionic villus sampling (p15) for thalassaemias anticipated by parental blood studies.

Sickle cell disease See p18. *Sickle-cell haemoglobin c disease* is a milder variant of SCD. Hb levels are usually near normal so women may be unaware they are affected. They are still susceptible to sickling crises in pregnancy and the puerperium, so antenatal diagnosis is essential. Prenatal sickle-cell diagnosis is possible by chorionic villus sampling.

►Aim for diagnosis at birth (cord blood) at the latest so that penicillin pneumococcal prophylaxis may be started (*OHCM* p334).

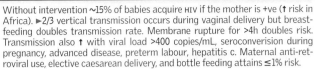

Without intervention ~15% of babies acquire HIV if the mother is +ve (↑ risk in Africa). ►2/3 vertical transmission occurs during vaginal delivery but breast-feeding doubles transmission rate. Membrane rupture for >4h doubles risk. Transmission also ↑ with viral load >400 copies/mL, seroconverision during pregnancy, advanced disease, preterm labour, hepatitis C. Maternal anti-retroviral use, elective caesarean delivery, and bottle feeding attains ≤1% risk.

Antenatal care Offer HIV tests at booking, if declined, again at 28wks. If HIV status unknown in labour rapid (20min) tests are recommended. If positive in labour; use drugs to reduce maternal–fetal transmission (below; seek expert advice). If HIV+ve arrange multidisciplinary care with HIV physician to monitor viral loads, drug regimens, and toxicity monitoring. Check for hepatitis B & C, varicella zoster, measles & toxoplasmosis antibodies. Offer hepatitis B, pneumococcal and influenza vaccines (safe in pregnancy). Screen for genital infections at booking and at 28wks. Treat infections, even if asymptomatic (to reduce risk of pre-term birth). Women needing highly active antiretroviral treatment (HAART) for their own health (symptomatic HIV/falling or low CD4 lymphocyte count <350×10⁶/L) should continue treatment throughout pregnancy and postpartum. If on HAART at booking; screen for gestational diabetes and warn of ↑risk of premature labour. If on co-trimoxazole for *Pneumocystis jirovecii* prophylaxis (CD4 <200×10⁶/L) add pre-pregnancy/1st trimester 5mg folic acid/day. Women not needing antiretrovirals for their own health should start HAART by 24wks, taking until delivered. (If good CD4 levels, viral load <10,000 copies/mL, and elective caesarean delivery planned zidovudine monotherapy orally from 20–28wks, IV in labour is an alternative.) Plan mode of delivery by 36wks.

Premature labour If membranes rupture >34wks expedite delivery, whatever the maternal viral load. If membranes rupture <34wks give steroids (p51), give erythromycin (p50), ensure mother takes usual HAART regimen, seek HIV specialist advice on how to optimize her regimen to reduce fetal transmission eg maternal nevirapine crosses placenta with long fetal plasma concentration, plus zidovudine infusion. Determine delivery balancing risks of prematurity, and infection. Manage preterm labour without membrane rupture as if HIV–ve.

Intrapartum care *Vaginal delivery:* Offer to women with viral loads <50 copies/mL, (<400 copies/mL if on HAART).⁴⁵ₙᵢcₑ Continue HAART in labour. Avoid fetal blood sampling/scalp electrodes. Avoid amniotomy unless delivery imminent. Oxytocin can be used for augmentation. Low cavity forceps are preferred over ventouse (less fetal trauma). Avoid mid-cavity or rotational forceps. *Caesarean section:* Offer elective caesarean section at 38 weeks' gestation to women if on zidovudine monotherapy (above), if on HAART with viral loads > those above, or if co-infected with hepatitis C and not on HAART. If viral load is <50 copies/mL, and elective section needed, plan for 39+ weeks.

Postpartum Avoid breastfeeding in resource-rich countries (breastfeeding doubles HIV transmission risk). Cabergoline 1mg PO within 24h of birth is recommended to suppress lactation. Newborns are treated within 4h of birth eg zidovudine twice daily for 4 weeks; HAART if high risk eg untreated mothers; mother with viral loads >50 copies/mL despite being on HAART. Co-trimoxazole (PCP) prophylaxis is given to babies at high risk of transmission. Babies are tested at day 1, 6wks, and 12wks for HIV with confirmatory test at 18 months. Affected women should have annual smears. Condoms, intrauterine systems (eg Mirena®), and depot progesterone injections are all suitable for women on HAART. Some antiretrovirals are enzyme inducers so may affect efficiency of progesterone only, and combined pills. Check if maternal MMR vaccine (if CD4 count >200/mL, contraindicated if lower), and varicella zoster vaccine (only if CD4 count >400/mL) required.

Further reading
BHIVA (2012). *Guidelines for the Management of HIV in Pregnant Women* 2012. London: BHIVA.

Classified as pre-existing (type 1 or type 2) or gestational (GDM).

Preconception Avoid unplanned pregnancy: planning reduces the risks. Adjust insulin to optimize control preconception (values as antenatally, below). Aim for HbA1c of ≤43mmol/mol (6.1%) (avoid pregnancy if HbA1c >85mmol/mol (10%)). Give 5mg folic acid daily preconception. Arrange dietitian review. Stop oral hypoglycaemics (except metformin), statins, ACE and A2A inhibitors (use other antihypertensive p31, if needed). Treat retinopathy pre-pregnancy. Retinopathy screen; ≤20% develop proliferative retinopathy. Nephropathy may worsen; if severe, avoid pregnancy. Glycosuria unrelated to DM is common (GFR ↑ and tubular glucose reabsorption ↓). Fetal glycaemia follows maternal. Compensatory fetal hyperinsulinaemia promotes fetal growth.

Complications *Maternal:* Hypoglycaemia unawareness (esp. 1st trimester) so warn about it. Increased risk of pre-eclampsia and infection, as well as higher rates of LSCS. *Fetal:* Miscarriage, malformation rates ↑ ×3 but this is reduced with good glycaemic control (fetal sacral agenesis, pathognomonic of maternal diabetes, is rare; CNS & CVS malformations much commoner). Babies may be macrosomic (risk of shoulder dystocia) or growth restricted. Polyhydramnios (?fetal polyuria), preterm labour, stillbirth.

Antenatal care Use care plan & review in joint clinic. Confirm gestation with early us. Detailed anomaly scan at 18–20 weeks. Fetal echo at 18–20 weeks. Educate about benefits of normoglycaemia. Aim for home monitored glucose 1h after every meal (postprandial) and before bed. Insulin needs increase by 50–100% as pregnancy progresses so review regularly. Aim for fasting level 3.5–5.9mmol/L; 1h post-prandial level <7.8mmol/L. Give GlucoGel® and glucagon kit (ensure partner knows how to use). Exclude ketoacidosis if unwell (poorly tolerated by fetus). Assess renal function; refer to nephrologist if creatinine >120μmol/L, protein excretion >2g/24h (use thromboprophylaxis if >5g/24h). Admit if adequate control unachievable at home and consider conversion to insulin pump (CSII) if ongoing problematic hypoglycaemia. Metformin can be used in pregnancy. Monitor fetal growth by growth scans every 4 weeks from 28 weeks.

Delivery should take place in hospital with good neonatal facilities. NICE recommends elective delivery at 38 weeks (by 40 weeks if GDM).[46][NICE] Corticosteroids to promote fetal lung maturity if preterm labour (use sliding scale for 24h after last dose of steroid). *In labour:* Continuous fetal monitoring. Avoid hyperglycaemia (causes neonatal hypoglycaemia) and use sliding scale if DM on insulin, or CBG >7mmol/L in GDM. Aim for glucose level of 4–7mmol/L. Halve rate of insulin infusion on delivery of placenta in T1DM. Insulin needs fall as labour progresses and immediately postpartum. Stop infusions at delivery in GDM and T2 if not on insulin pre-pregnancy. Return to pre-pregnancy regimen.

Postnatal • Encourage breastfeeding (insulin, metformin, and glibenclamide are compatible with breastfeeding) • Encourage pre-pregnancy counselling *before* next pregnancy • If preproliferative retinopathy review ophthalmologically for 6 months • Discuss contraception.

Gestational diabetes (OGTT glucose ≥7.8mmol/L, *OHCM* p198) *Incidence:* 3–6% depending on population studied. Screen if 1st degree relative, previous baby >4.5kg, BMI >30, ethnicity (South Asian, Caribbean, Middle Eastern), previous GDM. Monitor glucose and fetal growth if diagnosed. If levels not controlled by diet and exercise over 1–2 weeks consider oral hypoglycaemics (metformin, glibenclamide—note NICE and product characteristic sheets give conflicting advice) or insulin. 50% develop T2DM, so give lifelong dietary advice and follow-up.[47] Check fasting glucose 6 weeks postpartum and screen annually.

Further reading

(2015). *Diabetes in Pregnancy: Management from Preconception to the Postnatal Period* (NG3). London: NICE.

▶Whenever a mother isn't quite right postpartum, check her TSH & free T₄—but note that any apparent hypothyroidism may be transitory.

Biochemical changes in normal pregnancy NB: normal pregnancy mimics hyperthyroidism (pulse ↑, warm moist skin, slight goitre, anxiety).

• Thyroid binding globulin & T₄ output rise to maintain free T₄ levels.
• High levels of hCG mimic TSH.
• There is reduced availability of iodine (in iodine-limited localities).
• TSH may fall below normal in the 1st trimester (suppressed by hCG).
• The best thyroid tests in pregnancy are free T₄, free T₃, and TSH.

Pre-pregnancy hyperthyroidism Treatment options include antithyroid drugs (but 60% relapse on stopping treatment), radioactive iodine (contra-indicated in pregnancy or breastfeeding: avoid pregnancy for 4 months after use), or surgery. Fertility is reduced by hyperthyroidism.

Hyperthyroidism in pregnancy (Usually Graves' disease.) If severe, it is associated with infertility. There is ↑ risk of prematurity, fetal loss, and, maybe, malformations. Severity of hyperthyroidism often falls in pregnancy. Transient exacerbations may occur (1st trimester & postpartum). Carbimazole and propylthiouracil (PTU) are commonly used. PTU crosses the placenta less and is used in newly diagnosed thyrotoxicosis in pregnancy. Monitor ≥monthly. PTU is preferred postpartum (less concentrated in breast milk). Partial thyroidectomy can be done in the 2nd trimester—most commonly for dysphagia, stridor, large goitre, suspected carcinoma, or antithyroid drug allergy.

TRAb (TSH-receptor stimulating antibodies): ↑ levels can cause *fetal thyrotoxicosis* (1%) after 24wks causing premature delivery; goitre so polyhydramnios; extended neck in labour and fetal tachycardia. If mother has been on antithyroid drugs signs may not be manifest until the baby has metabolized the drug (7–10 days postpartum). Test thyroid function in affected babies frequently. Antithyroid drugs may be needed. It resolves spontaneously at 2–3 months, but perceptual motor difficulties, and hyperactivity can occur later in childhood.

Note labour, delivery, surgery, and anaesthesia can precipitate *thyroid storm* (fever, tachycardia, altered mental state—agitation, psychosis, coma) requiring urgent treatment.

Hypothyroidism Untreated hypothyroidism is associated with infertility, oligomenorrhoea or menorrhagia, ↑ rates of miscarriage, stillbirth, anaemia, pre-eclampsia, and IUGR. Also, reduced IQ and neurodevelopmental delay in offspring. Optimize T₄ preconception. Monitor replacement by T₄ and TSH measurement in each trimester or 6 weeks post dose adjustment. Use pre-pregnancy levothyroxine doses postpartum.

Postpartum thyroiditis Prevalence: 5%. Hyperthyroidism is followed by hypothyroidism (~4 months postpartum). The hyperthyroid phase does not usually need treatment as it is self-limiting. If treatment is required, β-blockers are usually sufficient. Antithyroid drugs are ineffective as thyrotoxicosis is from thyroid destruction releasing thyroxine, rather than increased synthesis. Monitor the hypothyroid phase for >6 months, and treat if symptomatic. Withdraw treatment after 6–12 months for 4 weeks to see if long-term therapy is required. 90% have thyroid antiperoxidase antibodies; 5% of antibody-positive women become permanently hypothyroid each year so monitor annually. Hypothyroidism may be associated with postpartum depression, so check thyroid status of women with postpartum depression.

Further reading
Nelson-Piercy C (2015). *Handbook of Obstetric Medicine* (5th ed). Boca Raton, FL: CRC Press.

Obstetrics

▶Get expert help *promptly*. Jaundice in pregnancy may be lethal. Know exactly what drugs were taken and when (*prescribed* or *over-the-counter*). Where has she travelled to? Jaundice occurs in 1 in 1500 pregnancies. Viral hepatitis and gallstones may cause jaundice in pregnancy and investigation is similar to the non-pregnant. Those with Gilbert's and Dubin–Johnson syndrome (*OHCM* p712) do well in pregnancy (jaundice may be exacerbated with the latter).

Tests Do all the usual tests (*OHCM* p250), eg urine tests for bile, serology, LFTs, and US. Bile acids are a test usually only requested in pregnancy and if raised, diagnose obstetric cholestasis.

Obstetric cholestasis[48][NICE]. Incidence: 0.7% pregnancies in UK. There is pruritus, especially of palms and soles in the second half of pregnancy, without a rash and worse at night. Diagnosis of exclusion—test for viral hepatitis, autoimmune screen, and US of liver. Liver transaminases are mildly ↑ (<300U/L) in 60%, ↑ bilirubin in 25%, and ↑ bile acids. There is risk of preterm labour, fetal distress, meconium, and stillbirth (but recent research suggests risk of stillbirth lower than previously thought)—offer IOL from 37-38 weeks. Give **vitamin K** 10mg PO/24h to the mother if abnormal clotting screen, and 1mg IM to the baby at birth. **Ursodeoxycholic** acid reduces pruritus and abnormal LFTs. Symptoms resolve within days of delivery. It can recur with oestrogen-containing contraceptive pills and in 40-70% of subsequent pregnancies.

Acute fatty liver of pregnancy Incidence: 1:6600-13,000 deliveries—so it is rare but extremely serious. The mother develops abdominal pain, jaundice, headache, vomiting, ± thrombocytopenia and pancreatitis. There is associated pre-eclampsia in 30-60% (±postpartum). It usually occurs after 30 weeks. There is hepatic steatosis with micro-droplets of fat in liver cells. Deep jaundice, uraemia, severe hypoglycaemia, and clotting disorder may develop causing coma and death. Manage in HDU or ITU (may need tertiary centre support). Monitor BP. Give supportive treatment for liver and renal failure and treat hypoglycaemia vigorously (CVP line). Correct clotting disorders. Enlist haematologist's help. Expedite delivery. Epidural and regional anaesthesia are CI. Monitor postpartum. Beware PPH and neonatal hypoglycaemia. ▶Maternal mortality is 18% (higher with delayed diagnosis) and 23% for the fetus.

Some other causes of jaundice in pregnancy

- Viral hepatitis; ALT ↑, eg >200u/L; maternal mortality ↑ (~20%) in E virus.[45][NICE] treatment is supportive. Hepatitis C is thought to affect <1% of women in the UK at present. Vertical transmission affects about 5% of babies. Elective caesarean delivery is only recommended for those with coexistent HIV not on HAART[45][NICE] Passive antibodies transferred from the mother wane by 18 months. Check babies for HCV RNA at 2-3 months (& 12 months, and anti HCV antibody at 12-18 months), refer baby to paediatric hepatologist if HCV RNA positive.[49] Refer infected women for specialist treatment to clear the viral infection after birth (*OHCM* p470).
- Jaundice of severe pre-eclampsia (hepatic rupture and infarction can occur); ALT <500u/L; bilirubin <86μmol/L.
- Hepatitis may occur if halothane is used for anaesthesia (so avoid it).
- HELLP syndrome (p49) (haemolysis, elevated liver enzymes, and low platelet count). Incidence in pregnancy: 0.1-0.6%; in pre-eclampsia: 4-12%. It causes upper abdo pain, malaise, vomiting, headache, jaundice, microangiopathic haemolytic anaemia, DIC, LDH ↑, ALT ↑ <500u/L, bilirubin <86μmol/L. It recurs in 20%. *Treatment*: get expert help. Admit; deliver if severe.

Hepatitis B Check HBsAG in all women with jaundice and look for IgM anti-HBc to detect acute infection. Babies need immunoglobulin and vaccination at birth (p151). Offer vaccination to all the family. Avoid FSE/FBS.

In any woman who presents with odd behaviour, fever, jaundice, sweating, DIC, fetal distress, premature labour, seizures, or loss of consciousness, always ask yourself: ▶ *Could this be malaria?* If so, do thick and thin films. Confirm (or exclude) pregnancy. Seek expert help, eg from Liverpool, below.

Plasmodium falciparum malaria is dangerous (and complicated) in pregnancy, particularly in those with no malaria immunity. Cerebral malaria has a 50% mortality in pregnancy. 3rd-stage placental autotransfusion may lead to fatal pulmonary oedema. Hypoglycaemia may be a feature (both of malaria itself and secondary to quinine). There is ↑ susceptibility to sepsis. Women with coexistent HIV have less good pregnancy outcomes (fetal and maternal).

Other associations between *falciparum* malaria and pregnancy are anaemia, miscarriage, stillbirth, low birth weight, and prematurity. PPH is also more common. Hyperreactive malaria splenomegaly (occurs typically where malaria is holoendemic) may contribute to anaemia via ↑ haemolysis.

Vivax malaria is less dangerous, but can cause anaemia and ↓ birth weight.

Treating malaria ▶OHCM p396; ▶▶cerebral malaria, *OHCM* p397. In severe *falciparum* artesunate 2.4mg/kg IV at 0, 12, & 24h then daily until can take oral **artesunate+clindamycin** is 1st line, if available (tel 08451 555000 tropical medical registrar for advice/supply), or load with **quinine** 20mg/kg IVI over 4h in 5% glucose (max 1.4g) (do not load if on quinine/mefloquine). Then 10mg/kg IVI over 4h in 5% glucose every 8h with 450mg **clindamycin**/8h IV. Beware hypoglycaemia with quinine. Switch to artesunate regimen as soon as it is available.ᴮᶜᴼᴸ When severe treat on ITU. If haematocrit <20% give slow transfusion of packed cells, with 20mg furosemide. Include the volume of packed cells in fluid balance calculations. Consider exchange transfusion. Beware hyperpyrexia (fan, give paracetamol); renal failure; pulmonary oedema; and sepsis (if shock do blood cultures give IV **ceftriaxone**). Get expert help. Uncomplicated *falciparum* and resistant *vivax* are treated for 7 days with **quinine** 600mg with **clindamycin** 450mg/8h PO. Non-resistant *vivax*, *ovale*, and *malariae* are treated with **chloroquine** orally over 3 days with weekly dose to prevent relapse during pregnancy. 3 months after delivery (and G6PD testing) **primaquine** is then given for *ovale* and *vivax* prevention of relapse.

If infection peripartum, anticipate fetal distress, fluid-balance problems, and hypoglycaemia in labour. Monitor appropriately. After any infection send placenta for histology and placental, cord, and baby blood (weekly×4) for blood films to check if baby infected (0.3–4% are), and treat baby if infected.

Prevention in UK women Advise against visiting malarious areas. If it is unavoidable, give prophylaxis (*OHCM* p396). Emphasize importance of preventive measures such as mosquito nets and insect repellents. Normal dose chloroquine and proguanil if *P. falciparum* strains are sensitive. With proguanil, give concurrent folic acid 5mg/day. If chloroquine resistance, mefloquine is best.

Mefloquine is recommended for 2nd and 3rd trimester use.[51] Heed strict contraindications (eg epilepsy, neuropsychiatric disorder). If unsuitable atovaquone-proguanil, with folic acid (eg Malarone®) is an alternative in 2nd and 3rd trimesters for chloroquine- or mefloquine-resistant areas. 1st-trimester prophylaxis is a problem. Seek expert advice (eg tel National Travel Health Network and Centre 0845 602 6712).

Mothers living in endemic areas Chemoprophylaxis improves birthweight (by ~250g, with fewer very low birthweight babies). Red cell mass also rises. WHO advises intermittent preventive treatment (IPT) eg with 2 or 3 doses of **sulfadoxine-pyrimethamine** (SP) during pregnancy, but monthly doses are better if HIV +ve.[52] But SP causes Stevens–Johnson syndrome in 1 in 7000, and resistance to SP has spread fast, so new IPT regimens need urgent evaluation in pregnancy.[53] Dihydroartemisinin-piperaquine (eg Artekin®) is a good candidate.[54]

▶If in doubt, phone an expert, eg, in the UK, at Liverpool (tel. 0151 705 3100).

Note Values considered normal when not pregnant may reflect decreased renal function in pregnancy. Creatinine >75μmol/L and urea >4.5mmol/L merit further investigation. See TABLE on p9. Glycosuria in pregnancy usually reflects altered renal physiology rather than hyperglycaemia.

Asymptomatic bacteriuria Found in 2% of sexually active women, it is commoner (up to 7%) during pregnancy—especially in diabetics and in those with renal transplants. With the dilatation of the calyces and ureters that occurs in pregnancy, 30% will go on to develop pyelonephritis, which can cause fetal growth restriction, fetal death, and premature labour. This is the argument for screening all women for bacteriuria at booking. If present on MSU, treatment is given (eg cefalexin 500mg TDS PO). Trimethoprim and nitrofurantoin are safe alternatives but avoid trimethoprim in the 1st trimester (antifolate action) and nitrofurantoin in the 3rd (neonatal haemolytic anaemia). Check MSU on a regular basis eg at each visit to ensure eradication. 15% develop recurrent asymptomatic bacteriuria. Acute cystitis affects 1%, characterized by urinary frequency, urgency, dysuria, haematuria, and lower abdominal pain. Most infections are due to *E. coli* and urine dip positive for nitrites and leucocytes suggests UTI. Send MSU and treat as per asymptomatic bacteriuria.

Pyelonephritis Affects 1-2% of pregnant women and is more common due to dilatation of upper renal tract in pregnancy. Also more common in congenital renal abnormalities, neuropathic bladder, and stones. This may present as malaise with urinary frequency or as a more florid picture with raised temperature, tachycardia, vomiting, and loin pain. Urinary infections should always be excluded in those with hyperemesis gravidarum and those admitted with premature labour. After blood and urine culture give IV antibiotics (eg **cefuroxime** 1.5g/8h IV, awaiting sensitivities, and if septic consider stat dose of gentamicin). Continue IV antibiotics for at least 24h and orals for 2-3 weeks. MSUs should be checked for eradication of infection. Check renal function regularly and carry out US of renal tract to exclude stones and abnormalities. In those who suffer repeated infection, **low-dose oral amoxicillin or cefalexin** may prevent recurrences. If two or more confirmed UTIs in pregnancy, perform renal US and consider antibiotic prophylaxis for the rest of pregnancy.

Chronic renal disease With mild renal impairment (pre-pregnancy creatinine <125mmol/L) without hypertension there is little evidence that pregnancy accelerates renal disorders. Patients with marked anaemia, hypertension, retinopathy, or heavy proteinuria should avoid pregnancy as further deterioration in renal function may be expected. Risks include miscarriage, pre-eclampsia, fetal growth restriction, preterm delivery, and fetal death.

Pregnancy for those on dialysis is fraught with problems (fluid overload, hypertension, pre-eclampsia, polyhydramnios). A 50% increase in dialysis is needed. Live birth outcome is 50%. Outcome is better for those with renal transplants, but up to 10% of mothers die within 7 years of giving birth.

Obstetric causes of acute kidney injury Most commonly occurs postnatally and is rare. Anuria is uncommon—check for retention, blocked catheters, and ureteric damage.
• Sepsis (septic miscarriage, puerperal sepsis, urinary)
• Haemolysis (eg HELLP syndrome, acute fatty liver, sickle cell crisis, malaria)
• Hypovolaemia (blood loss from PPH or abruption)
• Volume contraction (pre-eclampsia, hyperemesis gravidarum)
• Don't forget drugs—especially NSAIDs

Whenever these situations occur, monitor urine output and fluid balance carefully (catheterize the bladder). Aim for >30mL/h output. Monitor renal function (U&E, creatinine). Management depends on the cause. Avoid using diuretics unless under specialist advice. Dialysis may be needed (*OHCM* p304).

Epilepsy affects ~0.5% of women of childbearing age and is the commonest neurological condition in this age group. It is categorized according to seizure type: primary generalized epilepsy (tonic–clonic seizures, absences, myoclonic jerks), and partial or focal seizures which may progress to secondary generalization (complex partial seizures) of which temporal lobe epilepsy is a part. *Other causes of seizures in pregnancy:* Eclampsia is the most important (p49); cerebral vein thrombosis, intracranial mass, stroke, hypoglycaemia, hyponatraemia, drugs and withdrawal, infection, postdural puncture, pseudoseizures (may overlap with genuine epilepsy).

Most women have no change in seizure frequency in pregnancy. Those with poorly controlled epilepsy are most likely to experience a deterioration (check drug compliance). Status epilepticus is a medical emergency and dangerous for both mother and fetus, and complicates 1.8% of pregnancies. Overall, the risk of seizure is highest peripartum (1–2% fit intrapartum).

Preconception

- Neurologist involvement to confirm diagnosis
- Optimize treatment: aim for seizure control on lowest dose with avoidance of polypharmacy to minimize risk of congenital malformation (CM: note CM rate depends on AED used but is increased even if on no treatment). Can consider stopping if no seizures for 2 years. See p20 for risks of AEDs
- Folic acid 5mg daily for >3 months prior to conception, until delivery
- Increased risk of epilepsy in offspring (4–5% but higher risk with maternal, and 15–20% if both parents have it).

Antenatal care

- Attendance at consultant-led obstetric clinic with aim for vaginal delivery
- Attendance at NT and anomaly scans (may need fetal echocardiography)
- If epilepsy well controlled, stay on AED. If the woman has stopped medication and has regular seizures, advise her to restart. If on valproate she may wish to change (highest risk of CM)
- Check she is taking 5mg folic acid
- Use bath only if others home and door unlocked
- Drug levels if increased seizures, especially with lamotrigine due to alteration in free drug concentration in pregnancy (salivary or serum)
- Vitamin K (10mg daily PO) in last 4 weeks of pregnancy if on hepatic enzyme-inducing AEDs: carbamazepine, ethosuximide, phenytoin, primidone, phenobarbital. In the baby, vitamin K-dependent clotting factors may be reduced, leading to haemorrhagic disease of the newborn.

Intrapartum care

- Aim for vaginal delivery unless obstetric indications occur for LSCS. A fit in labour is not an indication for LSCS unless in status
- Delivery should take place in a hospital
- Continue AEDs in labour
- Epidural anaesthesia is safe in women with epilepsy
- Benzodiazepines if seizure not self-terminating (lorazepam 4mg IV, diazepam 10–20mg rectally or IV)
- Seizures are more common intrapartum and postpartum due to sleep deprivation, reduced drug absorption, and hyperventilation.

Postnatal care

- Give baby vitamin K 1mg IM to reduce haemorrhagic disease of the newborn
- Avoid early discharge: stay in hospital for 24 hours when seizure risk highest
- Strategies for avoiding dropping the baby during a seizure ie changing the baby on the floor
- Encourage breastfeeding
- Gradually reduce AED dose back to pre-pregnancy levels
- Discuss contraception (high-dose oral contraceptives if on enzyme inducers).

Obstetrics

Oxygen demand increases significantly in pregnancy, due to raised metabolic rate and consumption. Tidal volume increases more than respiratory rate. Arterial pO_2 increases, and pCO_2 falls, along with bicarbonate, giving a compensated respiratory alkalosis. This is normal. PEFR is unchanged in pregnancy, along with FEV_1. Breathlessness is a common symptom affecting 75% of women and is usually worse in the 3rd trimester.

Asthma is common, affecting up to 7% of women in pregnancy and is due to reversible bronchoconstriction of airways from smooth muscle spasm, along with inflammation and increased mucous production. *Symptoms* include cough, breathlessness, wheeze, and chest tightness, often with a diurnal variation (worse at night and early morning). Coexistent atopy (hay fever, eczema) is common. *Diagnosis* is based on history, >20% diurnal variation in PEFR for 3+ days/week during 2-week period, or >15% improvement in FEV_1 after inhaled bronchodilators. For most women asthma remains unchanged or improved, but it may worsen (especially if poorly controlled to start with). Severe and/ or poorly controlled asthma may result in fetal growth restriction and preterm labour. *Management* should focus on preventing acute attacks. Follow British Thoracic Society guidelines and use a stepwise approach. Most medication is safe in pregnancy (but do not start leukotriene receptor antagonists). Remember to check inhaler technique and give smoking cessation advice. Asthma attacks in pregnancy are rare due to endogenous steroid production; continue usual medication and treat as for non-pregnant patient. In PPH use prostaglandin F2a with caution unless life-threatening haemorrhage.

Pneumonia is no more common than in non-pregnant women, but has a higher mortality rate, especially with varicella zoster pneumonia. Smokers, those with chronic lung disease and the immunosuppressed are more at risk. *Symptoms* often start with a dry cough, progressing to productive, fever, rigors, breathlessness and pleuritic chest pain. Listen for coarse crackles on auscultation and look for signs of consolidation. Take FBC, U&E, CRP, sputum culture, ABG, and CXR (very small dose of radiation—a fraction of the maximum dose allowed in pregnancy). *Management:* Maintain O_2 sats >96%, ensure hydrated, arrange chest physiotherapy and give antibiotics (amoxicillin 500mg TDS or clarithromycin 500mg BD). Severe pneumonia requires IV treatment with cefuroxime 1.5g TDS ± clarithromycin 500mg BD. Treat for 7 days. Call for help if adverse features: RR >30/min, sats <92% or pO_2 <8kPa, systolic BP <90mmHg, acidosis; bilateral or multiple lobe involvement on CXR.

Tuberculosis (TB) is on the increase in the UK, Europe, and America partly due to HIV+ve patients having higher susceptibility. In the UK, ethnic minority women in pregnancy are most commonly affected. *Onset* is insidious, with cough, haemoptysis, weight loss, and night sweats, and may cause coarse crackles in the upper lobes and lymphadenopathy. *Diagnosis* is confirmed on sputum for acid-fast bacilli, but culture takes 6 weeks. The Mantoux test is not affected by pregnancy. Congenital infection via placenta is rare. Refer to a respiratory physician. *Treat* with rifampicin, isoniazid (plus pyridoxine), and pyrazinamide and/ or ethambutol. Infectious until 2 weeks of treatment. The baby should be given the BCG ± isoniazid in high-risk cases. Encourage breastfeeding.

Cystic fibrosis (CF) has improving life expectancy (41 years at present), so pregnancy is more common. Prenatal genetic counselling is important and paternal screening should be carried out. Obstetric care jointly with CF physicians, dietician, and physiotherapist. Optimize status pre-pregnancy. Cardiac echo, admit for O_2 if sats <90%, and treat infections aggressively. Increased risk of IUGR due to hypoxia therefore growth scans every 4 weeks from 28 weeks. Maintain high-calorie diet and screen for GDM. Aim for vaginal delivery but limit second stage (increased risk of pneumothorax).

Rheumatoid arthritis is usually alleviated by pregnancy (but exacerbations may occur in the puerperium). Methotrexate use is contraindicated (terato-genic); sulfasalazine may be used (give extra folate). Azathioprine use may cause IUGR and penicillamine may weaken fetal collagen. Non-steroidal anti-inflammatories can be used in the first and second trimesters but are not recommended in the third as they can cause premature closure of the ductus arteriosus and late in pregnancy have been associated with renal impairment in the newborn. Anti-tumour necrosis factor TNF-alpha therapies have not shown problems; but experience is limited.[55] Congenital heart block is a rare fetal feature. Deliver babies with heart block as below for SLE.

Systemic lupus erythematosus SLE exacerbations are commoner in pregnancy and the puerperium. Most are mild to moderate involving skin, but those with renal involvement and hypertension may deteriorate and are prone to pre-eclampsia. Of those with SLE glomerulonephritis and a creatinine >130μmol prior to conception only 50% achieve a live birth. Pre-eclampsia, oligohydramnios, and IUGR may occur. Both hydralazine and methyldopa can be used in pre-eclampsia.

Planned pregnancy should be embarked on after 6 months' stable disease without requiring cytotoxic suppression. Disease suppression may be maintained with azathioprine and hydroxychloroquine. Aspirin 75mg daily should be started prior to conception and continued throughout pregnancy, and the fetus should be carefully monitored.

Rarely, the fetus is affected by maternal antibodies that cause a self-limiting, sunlight-sensitive rash (usually face and scalp) for which no treatment is required; or anti-Ro or anti-La antibodies irreversibly damage the fetal heart conduction system causing congenital heart block (~65% require a pacemaker). Deliver by caesarean or monitor fetal blood gases in labour.

Mothers requiring ≥7.5mg daily prednisolone in the 2 weeks before delivery should receive **hydrocortisone 100mg/6h IV** in labour.

Antiphospholipid syndrome Those affected have antiphospholipid antibodies (lupus anticoagulant and/or anticardiolipin antibodies on 2 tests taken >8 weeks apart) ± past arterial thrombosis, venous thrombosis, or recurrent pregnancy loss. It may be primary, or follow other connective tissue disorder (usually SLE in which it occurs in 10%). *Outcome:* Untreated, <20% of pregnancies proceed to a live birth due to 1st trimester loss or placental thrombosis (causes placental insufficiency, leading to IUGR and fetal death).

Regular fetal assessment (Doppler flow studies and US for growth) is required from 20 weeks as appropriate obstetric intervention can substantially increase the number of live-born babies.

Management: Affected women are treated from conception with aspirin 75mg daily and heparin eg enoxaparin 40mg sc/24h from when fetal heart identified (~6 weeks). Those who have suffered prior thromboses receive heparin throughout pregnancy. See p32.

Postpartum, use either heparin or warfarin (breastfeeding contraindicated with neither) as risk of thrombosis is high.

Pregnancies in those with SLE (especially with renal disease) and antiphospholipid syndrome require specialist management.

BP falls in early pregnancy until 24 weeks due to a fall in vascular resistance. Stroke volume then increases after this time, leading to a rise in BP. It tends to fall again after delivery (often leading to an improvement and tricking doctors into stopping antihypertensives too early) peaking again at day 3–4 postpartum. Remember to use the correct cuff size—using a small cuff on a large arm leads to a falsely elevated reading. Automated BP monitors tend to under-record BP; best practice is to use a sphygmomanometer. Hypertensive disorders in pregnancy account for a significant proportion of maternal morbidity and mortality due to stroke, as well as neonatal problems from iatrogenic prematurity. ►A BP of >160/110 in pregnancy is a medical emergency (p48-9). If proteinuria develops, this is super-imposed pre-eclampsia (p48).

Chronic hypertension affects 3–5% pregnancies and pre-dates the pregnancy. Women who develop hypertension before 20 weeks' gestation or have a high booking BP (130–140/80–90mmHg) are more likely to have chronic hypertension. These women have a higher risk of developing pre-eclampsia (double if on treatment), fetal growth restriction, and placental abruption. If it is a new finding, exclude other causes of hypertension (coarctation, renal artery stenosis, other renal disease, rarely Cushing's syndrome, Conn's, and phaeochromocytoma). *Preconception:* ACE inhibitors, A2A blockers, and thiazide risk congenital abnormality so change these pre-conception to labetalol or methyldopa. *Antenatal:* Ensure suitable antihypertensive is being used (above). Aim for BP <150/90 (140/90 if end-organ damage), but with diastolic ≥80. If hypertension is secondary to another disorder involve a specialist in hypertensive disorders. Give aspirin 75mg/24h/PO from conception until the baby is born. Admit if BP >160/110. Fetal US every 4 weeks from 28 weeks to assess fetal growth, amniotic fluid volume, and umbilical artery Dopplers. If fetal activity is abnormal, arrange cardiotocography (CTG). Aim for induction of labour around the EDD. *Intrapartum:* During labour, monitor BP hourly if BP <159/109, continuously if ≥160/100. If severe hypertension does not respond to treatment, advise operative delivery. Give oxytocin alone at 3rd stage of labour (ergometrine causes severe hypertension, risking stroke). *Postnatally* check BP on days 1, 2, and once on days 3–5 and at 2 weeks. Change methyldopa to another antihypertensive post delivery as risk of postnatal depression. Avoid diuretics if breastfeeding (labetalol, atenolol, metoprolol, captopril, and enalapril are safe).

Pregnancy-induced hypertension (PIH) affects 6–7% of pregnancies. It is defined as hypertension in the second half of pregnancy (BP >140/90) in the absence of proteinuria or other features of pre-eclampsia. There is an increased risk of developing pre-eclampsia (15–26%) especially with earlier onset of hypertension. *Management:* Assessment in secondary care, with urine testing for proteinuria with automated reagent strip readings or urine protein/creatinine ratio testing to rule out pre-eclampsia. Check urine and BP weekly if mild (BP 140/90–149/99) but start treatment eg with labetalol PO if >150/100 and check BP and urine twice weekly. If BP ≥ 160/110 admit to hospital, measure BP 4 times daily and check urine daily and check FBC, U&E, AST/ALT and bilirubin at presentation and weekly. If hypertension is mild do 4-weekly fetal growth scans; if severe and cannot stabilize on oral treatment make plans for delivery. Aim for delivery after 37 weeks unless pre-eclampsia (p48) supervenes. During labour continue antihypertensives, monitor BP hourly (continuously if >160/110). If BP is outside target range despite antihypertensives (>160/110) advise operative delivery. Continue antenatal antihypertensives postnatally (as above), reducing treatment if BP <130/80. Review at 2 and 6 weeks. If treatment is still needed at 6 weeks arrange review with specialist in hypertensive disorders.

Venous thromboembolism (vte) is a leading cause of morbidity and mortality in pregnancy in developed countries and is preventable. It includes deep vein thrombosis (dvt) of the legs, pelvis, and pulmonary embolism (pe). Every woman should have vte risk assessed at booking, each antenatal admission, in labour, and postnatally. Basic steps should also be taken to reduce vte: avoid immobility and dehydration (don't forget hyperemesis). Pregnancy alone is a risk factor due to a combination of venous stasis, trauma to pelvic veins at delivery, procoagulant changes to the clotting cascade (higher levels of factors x, viii, and fibrinogen, reduced endogenous anticoagulation activity, and reduction in protein s activity). These changes occur from early in the first trimester until 6 weeks postpartum. lmwhs are drugs of choice in pregnancy and safer than unfractionated. If in doubt as to whether a woman needs it, seek senior advice or refer to haematology.

Risk factors for vte: *High risk (give antenatal lmwh prophylaxis):* History of > 1 vte, unprovoked or oestrogen-related vte, single provoked vte + thrombophilia or family history, antithrombin iii deficiency (30% risk of vte in pregnancy). *Intermediate risk (consider antenatal lmwh prophylaxis):* Thrombophilia but no vte, single provoked vte, medical comorbidities eg cancer, inflammatory conditions, significant cardiac or respiratory conditions, sle, sickle cell disease, nephrotic syndrome, iv drug user, any antenatal surgery. *Other risk factors:* if 3 or more consider antenatal prophylaxis: age >35, obesity, parity 3 or more, smoker, large varicose veins, current infection, pre-eclampsia, immobility, dehydration, multiple pregnancy, assisted reproduction techniques.

Indications for lmwh thromboprophylaxis: See list for vte risk factors. For any woman requiring antenatal lmwh it must be given 6 weeks postpartum. Any woman undergoing emergency lscs need 7 days' postpartum lmwh. If other risk factors are also present it may need to be given for longer. Other postpartum risk factors include mid-cavity or rotational instrumental delivery, postpartum haemorrhage and blood transfusion. Check local trust guidelines. Often the postnatal drug chart or notes will have a colour-coded vte risk assessment which will help you assess need for thromboprophylaxis.

Dosing of lmwh depends on body weight. Enoxaparin 40mg sc/24h 50–90kg, 60mg sc/24h if 91–130kg, 80mg/24h if 131–170kg. Postnatally, enoxaparin can be given as soon as possible as long as no ongoing postpartum haemorrhage, and >4h since epidural sited or removed.

Thrombophilia in pregnancy

Thrombophilia is the tendency to increased clotting and there are many underlying causes. Whether or not women need antenatal lmwh depends on presence of other risk factors and expert advice. *Factor v Leiden* (4% population) increases risk 5–8 times if heterozygote and 10–34 times if homozygous. *Protein c deficiency* (0.3% population) risk increased by 2–4.8 times. *Protein s deficiency* (2% population) increases risk 3.2 times. *Antithrombin iii deficiency* (0.02%) increases risk 4.7–10 times. *G20210A prothrombin gene mutation* (1% population) increases risk 3–10 times in heterozygotes and 26 times in homozygotes. *Acquired thrombophilia* is lupus anticoagulant ± cardiolipin antibody and increases risk of both arterial and venous thrombosis.

Screening of women should occur if there is a past history of vte and should be carried out when the woman is not pregnant. Those with a family history or those with second trimester pregnancy loss and early onset pre-eclampsia.

Further reading

rcog (2015). *Reducing the Risk of Venous Thromboembolism during Pregnancy and the Puerperium* (Green-top Guideline No. 37a). London: rcog.

rcog (2015). *Thromboembolic Disease in Pregnancy and the Puerperium: Acute Management.* (Green-top Guideline No. 37b). London: rcog.

▶ *This is a medical emergency and is one of the leading causes of maternal morbidity and mortality in the UK.* VTE can happen in any trimester and occurs in 1–2:1000 pregnancies. Symptoms may be atypical; DVT is 3 times more common than PE and a DVT will lead to PE in 16% of untreated patients. Overall, VTE is most common in the postnatal period.

Symptoms and signs of VTE *Deep vein thrombosis:* Leg swelling (left more often than right), pain, redness. Look for swelling (2cm greater diameter than other leg), tenderness, pyrexia, erythema, oedema, and in pelvic DVT lower abdominal pain. WBC count may be raised. *Pulmonary embolism:* Shortness of breath, chest pain, haemoptysis. Think of PE in any collapsed pregnant or postpartum woman. She may feel faint, have a raised JVP, and also have symptoms or signs of DVT. On auscultation there may be a pleural rub or fine crepitations, but more likely no chest signs at all. She may be hypoxic with a raised respiratory rate. In massive PE there is hypoxia, low blood pressure, tachycardia, and collapse leading to cardiac arrest.

Investigations should include FBC, U&E, LFTs, and a clotting screen. Thrombophilia screens may be falsely positive in pregnancy. If PE is suspected carry out ABG (may be normal in 20% of those with PE), ECG (look for signs of right heart strain), and CXR.

Imaging for DVT is compression or duplex US of the deep veins. If there is high clinical suspicion of DVT or PE and investigations are negative, continue treatment dose LWMH and repeat imaging in 1 week. Seek expert advice from haematology in these cases. In PE, if the CXR is normal, first arrange compression or duplex US of deep veins (if positive for DVT, PE can be presumed if chest symptoms, and further radiation of chest avoided). If negative, go on to perform ventilation/perfusion lung scanning (V/Q). If the CXR is abnormal, seek advice from radiology about imaging. Spiral CT or MRI may be the recommended next option.

D-dimers are tricky in pregnancy. Generally speaking, they are not helpful as they are commonly raised due to changes in the coagulation system. However, if they have been taken and are negative, a low level is likely to suggest no VTE. A raised level means nothing.

Treatment should start as soon as there is clinical suspicion of VTE and only stopped once it is ruled out. *Massive PE* necessitates immediate expert help. The woman may need thrombolysis or percutaneous catheter thrombus fragmentation. Embolectomy can only be carried out in centres with cardiothoracics. Consider unfractionated heparin (loading dose 5000IU then 1000–2000IU/h. Take blood for APTT 6h post loading dose, aiming for 1.5–2.5× laboratory control value. *LMWH* is more effective and safer than unfractionated heparin. Treat twice daily eg enoxaparin or dalteparin—see BNF and local guidelines. Refer to haematologist for follow up—they will want anti-Xa activity measuring 3h post injection to ensure correct dosage. Continue anticoagulation for 6 months and 6 weeks postpartum. Consider switching to warfarin post-delivery (safe in breastfeeding). Remember that in the next pregnancy, the woman needs thromboprophylaxis throughout, and for 6 weeks postpartum. *During labour* LMWH should be stopped. Keep well hydrated. Avoid regional anaesthesia (spinal/epidural) until at least 12h after last dose of prophylactic, and 24h after therapeutic LMWH. Wait >4h until epidural catheter removed until next dose, and do not remove catheter until >12h after last dose. Those at high risk on stopping anticoagulation: consider unfractionated heparin; can also consider IVC filter.

Investigating rash in pregnancy[56] Rashes can be either infectious or non-infectious. Investigate maculopapular rashes for rubella and parvovirus B19 (p142) (both can infect the fetus) and measles. Also consider causes of rash such as *Streptococcus*, meningococcus, Epstein–Barr virus, and syphilis.

Measles is unfortunately on the increase due to reduced numbers of people having the MMR vaccine. Measles in pregnancy can be dangerous, leading to mortality and severe morbidity from encephalitis and pneumonia. It is an RNA paramyxovirus, spread by respiratory droplets and is highly infectious. Incubation is 9–12 days, with the infectious period 2–5 days before and after the rash develops. Symptoms include fever, generalized maculopapular erythematous rash, Koplik's spots (pathognomonic, see p142). Look for cough, coryza, and conjunctivitis as well as corneal scarring. Diagnosis is on serology with paired samples in the acute and convalescent phase (10–14 days later). IgM in serum is positive >4 days but <1 month after the rash, and viral RNA in saliva. Measles in pregnancy is associated with fetal loss and preterm delivery, but not congenital infection or abnormality. If maternal rash appears 6 days pre- or post-delivery, give human normal immune globulin immediately after birth or exposure, to prevent neonatal subacute sclerosing panencephalitis.

Rubella Childhood vaccination prevents rubella susceptibility and routine antenatal screening finds those needing postpartum vaccination (avoid pregnancy for 1 month: vaccine is live). Spread is by respiratory droplets, with an incubation period of 14–21 days. Symptoms (p142) are absent in 50%. The fetus is most at risk in the 1st 16 weeks' gestation. 80% of fetuses are affected if maternal primary infection is in the 1st 12 weeks of gestation: <5% are affected if infection is after 16 weeks. Risk of fetal damage is much lower (<5%) with reinfection. Cataract is associated with infection at 8–9 weeks, deafness at 5–7 weeks (can occur with 2nd-trimester infection), cardiac lesions at 5–10 weeks. *Other features*: purpura, jaundice, hepatosplenomegaly, thrombocytopenia, cerebral palsy, microcephaly, IQ↓, cerebral calcification, microphthalmia, retinitis, growth disorder. Miscarriage or stillbirth may occur. If suspected in the mother seek expert help. Take antibody levels 10 days apart and look for IgM antibody 4–5 weeks from incubation period or date of contact. If infection is confirmed in the 1st trimester, TOP is offered without invasive prenatal diagnosis.

Cytomegalovirus (CMV) In the UK, CMV causes more motor and cognitive impairment than rubella. Maternal infection is mild (or ↑T°, lymphadenopathy, rash & sore throat). Up to 5:1000 live births are infected; with primary maternal infection, 40% fetuses are infected irrespective of gestation. Of these, 90% are normal at birth of which 20% develop late and usually minor problems. Of the 10% symptomatic babies, 33% will die and 67% have long-term problems. CMV-associated congenital defects include IUGR, microcephaly, hepatosplenomegaly and thrombocytopaenia, jaundice, chorioretinitis. Later-onset problems include motor and cognitive impairment and sensorineural deafness. Δ: (Tricky; ask lab). Paired sera. Are IgM and IgG antibodies found? Amniocentesis at >20wks + shell viral culture can detect fetal transmission. Also do throat swab, urine culture, and baby's serum after birth. Reducing exposure to toddlers' urine (the source of much infection) in pregnancy limits spread. NB: reactivation of old CMV may occur in pregnancy; it rarely affects the baby. One way to know that +ve serology does not reflect old infection is to do serology (or freeze a sample) pre-pregnancy.

Toxoplasmosis 40% of fetuses are affected if the mother has the illness (2–7:1000 pregnancies); the earlier in pregnancy the more the damage but the lower the transmission rate. Symptoms are similar to glandular fever. Fever, rash, and eosinophilia also occur. If symptomatic, the CNS prognosis is poor.

Diagnose by reference laboratory IgG and IgM tests. *Maternal, ℞ (Royal College regimen):* Start **spiramycin** promptly in infected mothers, eg 1.5g/12h PO. In symptomatic non-immune women test every 10 weeks through pregnancy. If infected, consider amniocentesis to see if the fetus is infected. If the fetus is infected, give the mother **pyrimethamine** 50mg/12h as loading doses on day 1, then 1mg/kg/day + **sulfadiazine** 50mg/kg/12h + **calcium folinate** 15mg twice weekly all until delivery. *Affected babies:* (diagnose by serology—>90% asymptomatic). Intracranial calcification, hydrocephalus, choroidoretinitis if severely affected. Encephalitis, epilepsy, mental and physical developmental delay, jaundice, hepatosplenomegaly, thrombocytopenia, and skin rashes occur. Treat with 4-weekly courses of pyrimethamine, sulfadiazine, and calcium folinate × 6, separated by 4 weeks of **spiramycin**. **Prednisolone** is given until signs of CNS inflammation or choroidoretinitis abate. *Prevention:* Avoid eating raw meat, wash hands if raw meat touched, wear gloves if gardening or dealing with cat litter, and avoid sheep during lambing time.

Parvovirus B19 is a DNA virus, spread by respiratory droplets with a 4-20-day incubation period. 50% of women in the UK are immune. In pregnancy often no symptoms occur, but may include 'slapped cheek' rash, a maculopapular rash, fever, and arthralgia. Diagnosis is again on paired samples in the acute and convalescent phases (>10 days apart). IgM antibodies appear and IgG titres increase. Consequences in the woman herself are minimal unless she is immunocompromised, in which case watch for sudden haemolysis requiring blood transfusion. 30% fetuses are infected, causing fetal suppression of erythropoiesis and cardiac toxicity. This leads to cardiac failure and fetal hydrops. 10% of fetuses infected at <20 weeks' gestation will die. Parvovirus is not teratogenic. Manage with serial US looking for signs of fetal anaemia (fetal hydrops and abnormal middle cerebral artery dopplers). If the fetus does develop anaemia, manage in a tertiary fetal medicine unit and consider *in utero* red cell transfusion.

Intrauterine syphilis Maternal screening occurs (UK screen 55,700 to prevent 1 case. In some parts of London 2:1000 women are infected); if infection found, treat the mother with **benzylpenicillin** 600mg/24h IM daily for 10 days. ~⅓ are stillborn. Neonatal signs: rhinitis, snuffles, rash, hepatosplenomegaly, lymphadenopathy, anaemia, jaundice, ascites, hydrops, nephrosis, meningitis, ±keratitis, and nerve deafness. Nasal discharge exam: spirochetes; x-rays: perichondritis; *CSF:* ↑ Monocytes and protein with +ve serology. *Treatment:* Give benzylpenicillin 37mg/kg/24h IM for 3 weeks.

Listeria Affects 6-15:100,000 pregnancies. Maternal symptoms: fever, shivering, myalgia, headache, sore throat, cough, vomiting, diarrhoea, vaginitis. Miscarriage (can be recurrent), premature labour, and stillbirth may occur. Infection is usually via infected food (eg milk, soft cheeses, pâté). ►Do blood cultures in any pregnant patient with unexplained fever for ≥48h. Serology, vaginal and rectal swabs do not help (can be commensal). See *OHCM* p409.

Perinatal infection usually occurs in 2nd or 3rd trimester. 20% of affected fetuses are stillborn. Fetal distress in labour is common. An early postnatal feature is respiratory distress from pneumonia. There may be convulsions, hepato-splenomegaly, pustular or petechial rashes, conjunctivitis, fever, leucopenia. Meningitis is commoner after perinatal infection. Diagnose by culture of blood, CSF, meconium, and placenta. Infant mortality: 30%. Isolate baby (nosocomial spread can occur). Treat with **ampicillin** 50mg/kg/6h IV and **gentamicin** 3mg/kg/12h IV until 1 week after fever subsides. Monitor levels.

Further reading

Health Protection Agency (2011). *Guidance on Viral Rash in Pregnancy.* London: HPA.

Hepatitis B virus (HBV) All mothers should be screened for HBsAg. Carriers have persistent HBsAg for >6 months. High infectivity is associated with HBeAg so anti-HBe antibodies are negative. Without immunization 95% of babies born to these mothers might develop hepatitis B, and 93% of the babies would be chronic carriers at 6 months. If the mother develops acute infection in the mid- or 3rd trimester there is high risk of perinatal infection. Her risk of death is 0.5-3%. Most neonatal infections occur at birth but some (especially in the East) are transplacental; hence the seeming failure of vaccination in up to 15% of neonates adequately vaccinated. Most infected neonates will develop chronic infection and in infected males lifetime risk of developing hepatocellular cancer is 50%; 20% for ♀. Most will develop cirrhosis, so immunization is really important. ►Give immunoglobulin (200u IM) and vaccinate babies of carriers and infected mothers at birth. See p151. In uncomplicated hepatitis, HBV DNA is cleared, anti-core antibodies develop, followed by anti-HBe antibodies with the decline and disappearance of HBeAg and HBsAg at 3 months. Do serology of vaccinated baby at 12-15 months old. If HBsAg−ve and anti-HBs is present, the child is protected.

Hepatitis C See p25.

Hepatitis E Risk of maternal mortality is ↑ (25% if in 3rd trimester); death is usually postpartum, preceded by fulminant hepatic failure, coma, and massive PPH. 33-50% of babies become infected. A vaccine is being developed.

Herpes simplex (HSV) Neonatal infection can cause blindness, IQ↓, epilepsy, jaundice, respiratory distress, DIC, and death (in 30%, even if treated).

Prevalence of past (2°) HSV infection is ~25% and recurrence in pregnancy is not usually a problem thanks to maternal antibodies. If a mother develops primary (first-ever) genital herpes in pregnancy, refer to a genitourinary clinic to screen her (and her partners) for other infections and confirm it is 1°. If in last trimester, give her oral aciclovir or valaciclovir ± elective caesarean if 1° infection within 6 weeks of her due date. Type-specific HSV diagnosis: PCR.

If active 1° infection lesions at time of delivery, recommend LSCS, even if membranes have ruptured up to 4h previously. If a mother with 1° lesions does deliver vaginally, risk of infection to the baby is 41%, so give mother (by IVI in labour) and newborn high-dose aciclovir (p200; do PCR at birth). Try to avoid fetal blood sampling, scalp electrodes, and instrumental delivery. Neonatal infection usually appears at 5-21 days with grouped vesicles/pustules on a red base, eg at the presenting part or sites of trauma (eg scalp electrode) ± periocular and conjunctival lesions. Non-vesicular rashes also occur.

Varicella zoster If mothers develop chickenpox near delivery, aim for delivery after 7 days, give babies varicella immune immunoglobulin (VZIG) at birth and monitor for 28 days; and treat with aciclovir if neonate develops chickenpox. Babies of non-immune mothers also need VZIG if contacts in 1st 7 days of life. Earlier in pregnancy, if women with no personal history of chickenpox have had significant (eg 15min) chickenpox contact; check blood for varicella antibodies; if none, give VZIG, and manage as still potentially infectious 8-28 days later and notify doctor if develops rash. Women developing chickenpox in pregnancy should avoid contact with pregnant women, and have oral aciclovir 800mg 5×daily PO for 7 days if >20wks pregnant if presenting within 24h of rash. Hospitalize if chest, CNS symptoms, dense/haemorrhagic rash, or immunocompromised. Fetal varicella syndrome (FVS) complicates ~1% fetuses of mothers infected at 3-28 weeks of pregnancy by reactivation *in utero*. FVS features: skin scarring, eye defects (microphthalmia, chorioretinitis, cataracts), neurological abnormalities (microcephaly, cortical atrophy, IQ↓, bowel and bladder sphincter disturbances). Refer to fetal medicine specialist for detailed US at 16-20wks, or 5wks post-infection.

Chlamydia trachomatis Associations: low birthweight, premature membrane rupture, fetal death. ~30% of infected mothers have affected babies. Conjunctivitis develops 5–14 days after birth and may show minimal inflammation or purulent discharge. The cornea is not usually involved. *Complications:* Chlamydia pneumonia, pharyngitis, or otitis media. *Tests: Special swabs are available but may be unreliable.* See p285. *Treatment:* Local cleansing of eye + **erythromycin** 12.5mg/kg/6h PO for ~3 weeks eliminates lung organisms. Give parents/partners **erythromycin**[58] or **azithromycin** 1g PO single dose.

Gonococcal conjunctivitis Occurs within ~4 days of birth, with purulent discharge and lid swelling, ± corneal hazing, corneal rupture, and panophthalmitis. Note, 50% will also have concurrent chlamydial infection. *Treatment:* Infants born to those with known gonorrhoea should have **cefotaxime** 100mg/kg IM stat, and **chloramphenicol** 0.5% eye-drops within 1h of birth. For active gonococcal infection give **benzylpenicillin** 50mg/kg/12h IM and 3-hourly 0.5% **chloramphenicol** drops for 7 days. Isolate the baby.

Ophthalmia neonatorum This is purulent discharge from the eye of a neonate <21 days old. There are many causes: chlamydiae, herpes virus, staphylococci, streptococci, pneumococci, *E. coli*. *Tests:* Swab for bacterial and viral culture, microscopy (look for intracellular gonococci), and chlamydia (eg immunofluorescence). Treat gonococcus and chlamydia as above; other infections with neomycin drops or ointment (allows chlamydia detection—not so with chloramphenicol).

Clostridium perfringens Suspect this in any complication of illegal termination of pregnancy and when intracellular encapsulated Gram +ve rods are seen on genital swabs. It may infect *in utero* deaths or any other anaerobic site (eg haematomas). *Signs:* Endometritis→septicaemia/gangrene→myoglobinuria→renal failure→death. *Treatment:* • Surgically debride all devitalized tissue • Hyperbaric O_2 • High-dose IV **benzylpenicillin** (**erythromycin** if serious penicillin allergy). The use of gas gangrene antitoxin is controversial. Seek expert help.

TB All babies born into households with TB, to immigrant mothers from areas with a high TB prevalence, or who will travel to such areas should have BCG (Bacillus Calmette–Guérin) vaccination after birth, 0.05mL intradermally at deltoid's insertion: 0.03mL if using a multiple puncture gun. Babies not vaccinated in hospital are unlikely to be vaccinated in the community.[59] Give other vaccinations as usual, avoiding the BCG vaccinated arm for 3 months. Separate babies from mothers with active or open TB until she has had 2 weeks of R_x and is sputum –ve. BCG vaccinate the baby and treat with isoniazid until he or she has a +ve skin reaction (Mantoux). Consider CXR in pregnant women with cough, fever, or weight loss. Encourage breastfeeding.

Group B *Streptococcus* (GBS)

GBS is a common bowel commensal carried by up to 20% of women vaginally. There is no screening for it in the UK but it may be found on routine high vaginal swabs or on urine culture. Neonatal risks include severe, early-onset infection which has 20% mortality, presenting as pneumonia, meningitis, and/or septicaemia.

In labour give all women IV antibiotics if: •+ve GBS high vaginal swab at any time in pregnancy • Any baby previously infected with GBS • Any documented GBS bacteriuria in this pregnancy • Gestation <37wks • Any intrapartum fever • If a woman is GBS+ve (swab or bacteriuria), with prelabour rupture of membranes at term, treat with GBS antibiotic prophylaxis and induce labour • If culture result unknown and membranes are ruptured at term for >18h: GBS prophylaxis (eg **penicillin**).[60] Give benzylpenicillin 3g IV as loading dose then 1.5g 4-hourly throughout labour. If penicillin allergic, give clindamycin 900mg IV 8-hourly.

▶With any pain in pregnancy think, is this labour? If pain is in the second half of pregnancy, is this pre-eclampsia (p48)? ▶Women with chest, back, or epigastric pain severe enough for opiates need full investigation: cardiac causes (ECG, CXR, troponin, echocardiography, CT angiography + CT/MRI chest scan).

Abdominal pain may be from ligament stretching or from symphysis pubis strain. In early pregnancy remember miscarriage (p260) and ectopics (p262).

Abruption The triad of abdominal pain, uterine rigidity, and vaginal bleeding suggests this. It occurs in between 1 in 80 and 1 in 200 pregnancies. Fetal loss is high if >50% of placenta affected. A tender uterus is highly suggestive. US is poor at diagnosis—rely on clinical signs. A live viable fetus merits rapid delivery as demise can be sudden. Prepare for DIC, which complicates 33–50% of severe cases, and beware PPH, which is also common. See p84.

Uterine rupture See p80.

Uterine fibroids For torsion and red degeneration, see p277.

Uterine torsion The uterus rotates axially 30–40° to the right in 80% of normal pregnancies. Rarely, it rotates >90° causing acute uterine torsion in mid or late pregnancy with abdominal pain, shock, a tense uterus, and urinary retention (catheterization may reveal a displaced urethra in twisted vagina). Fibroids, adnexal masses, or congenital asymmetrical uterine anomalies are present in 90%. Diagnosis is usually at laparotomy. Deliver by LSCS.

Ovarian tumours Torsion, rupture, see p280. **Pyelonephritis** See p27.

Appendicitis Incidence: ~1:1000 pregnancies. It is not commoner in pregnancy but mortality is higher (esp. from 20wks). Perforation is commoner (15–20%). Fetal mortality is ~1.5% for simple appendicitis; ~30% if perforation. The appendix migrates upwards, outwards, and posteriorly as pregnancy progresses, so pain is less well localized (often para-umbilical or subcostal—but right lower quadrant still commonest) and tenderness, rebound, and guarding less obvious. Peritonitis can make the uterus tense and woody-hard. ▶Don't delay surgery!—laparotomy over site of maximal tenderness with patient tilted 30° to the left by an experienced general surgeon (laparoscopy also appears to be safe).

Cholecystitis Incidence 1–6 per 10,000 pregnancies. Pregnancy encourages gallstone formation due to biliary stasis and increased cholesterol in bile. Symptoms are similar to the non-pregnant with subcostal pain, nausea, and vomiting. Jaundice is uncommon (5%). US confirms the presence of stones. The main differential diagnosis is appendicitis, and laparotomy or laparoscopy is mandatory if this cannot be excluded. Surgery should be reserved for complicated non-resolving biliary tract disease during pregnancy as in >90% the acute process resolves with conservative management. For patients requiring surgery, laparoscopic cholecystectomy can be a safe and effective method of treatment, but miscarriage/preterm labour is a risk.

Rectus sheath haematoma Very rarely, bleeding into the rectus sheath and haematoma formation can occur with coughing (or spontaneously) in late pregnancy causing swelling and tenderness. US is helpful. ΔΔ: Abruption. *Management:* Laparotomy (or perhaps laparoscopy—but not in late pregnancy) is indicated if the diagnosis is in doubt or if there is shock.

Pancreatitis in pregnancy is rare, but mortality is high (37% maternal; 5.6% fetal). Diagnose by serum amylase.

Urinary tract infection See p27.

Gastroenteritis is common and symptoms may be severe. If otherwise well, try and manage at home. Most settle with rehydration salts and rest. Always think—could diarrhoea and vomiting be a symptom of severe sepsis (p40)?

✪Pregnancy and obesity (BMI >30 at booking)

Maternal obesity is continually increasing in the developed world, such that 1 in 5 pregnant women are now obese in the UK. A normal body mass index (BMI) is 18.5–24.9, overweight 25–29.9, and obesity is defined as a BMI over 30. Obesity is known to carry a higher risk of maternal death (p514).

►Ideally, women should lose weight to a healthy BMI pre-pregnancy. The woman should not diet as such once pregnant, but should be discouraged to gain further weight and encouraged to eat a balanced diet, as well as take regular exercise. Remember that 'eating for two' is a myth and calorie intake only needs to increase a small amount from the 2nd trimester.

Maternal and fetal risks

Pregnancy-induced hypertension and pre-eclampsia is twice as likely, especially if there is excessive weight gain. *Gestational diabetes* is three times more common. *Venous thromboembolism* is doubled. *Other risks* include (subfertility), miscarriage, stillbirth, maternal cardiac disease, induction of labour, failed induction, caesarean section, instrumental delivery, macrosomia, shoulder dystocia, 3rd- and 4th-degree perineal tears, difficulty siting regional anaesthesia, higher risks during general anaesthetic, higher failure rate of VBAC, wound infection, endometritis, chest infection, postpartum haemorrhage, and higher rates of postnatal depression.

Management of a pregnant woman with obesity

2010 CMACE/RCOG guidelines recommend:
- Referral for consultant-led care
- 5mg folic acid from 1 month before conception and for the first trimester to prevent increased risk of NTDs
- Obese women are more prone to vitamin D deficiency so ensure they are taking 10mcg vitamin D supplementation while pregnant and breastfeeding
- Screen for diabetes, eg oral glucose tolerance test (OGTT) at 24–28 weeks and consider LMWH thromboprophylaxis for 7 days postnatally if one additional thrombotic risk factor (p32)
- Mobilize all obese women early
- If women with BMI ≥30 require caesarean section and if subcutaneous fat is >2cm thick, suture that separately, to prevent infection
- Consider serial growth scans (SFH measurement may not be accurate)
- *Women with BMI >40* should always receive 7-day postnatal heparin prophylaxis and TED stockings whatever the mode of delivery. They should have an antenatal consultation with an obstetric anaesthetist with an anaesthetic plan made for labour and delivery, and need 3rd-trimester assessment to plan manual handling requirements and provision of appropriate TED stockings. When in labour, inform anaesthetist. They should have continuous midwifery care and should have an IV sited early in labour. If operative delivery is required, the attending anaesthetist should be a consultant (or signed off obese-competent) obstetric anaesthetist.

Obstetrics

Sepsis in pregnancy is one of the leading direct causes of maternal death in the UK, with many caused by group A *Streptococcus* caught in the community. The mortality rate of severe sepsis with organ dysfunction is 20–40%, reaching 60% with septic shock. In the non-pregnant population, surviving sepsis is clearly linked to its early recognition and treatment.

Definitions *Sepsis:* Infection plus systemic manifestations of infection. *Severe sepsis:* Sepsis with sepsis-induced organ dysfunction or evidence of tissue hypoperfusion. *Septic shock:* Persistent tissue hypoperfusion despite adequate fluid replacement. *Risk factors:* Obesity, impaired glucose tolerance/diabetes, impaired immunity, immunosuppressants, anaemia, vaginal discharge, pelvic infection, history of group B *Streptococcus*, invasive procedures such as amniocentesis, cervical cerclage, prolonged rupture of membranes (more than 24 hours), group A *Streptococcus* infection in close contacts, black or other ethnic minority group origin. *Organisms:* Lancefield group A beta-haemolytic *Streptococcus* and *E. coli* are most common. Mixed Gram-negative and Gram-positive organisms occur in chorioamnionitis. Coliforms are associated with UTI, preterm prolonged rupture of membranes, and cervical cerclage. Anaerobes such as *Clostridium perfringens* are less common, with *Peptrostreptococcus* and *Bacterioides* predominating.

Clinical features Fever, rigors, diarrhoea or vomiting (may indicate endotoxin production), rash (generalized maculopapular streptococcal rash or purpura fulminans indicates toxic shock syndrome), abdominal or pelvic pain, offensive vaginal discharge (smelly suggests anaerobes; serosanguinous *Streptococcus*), productive cough and urinary symptoms.

Diagnostic criteria for sepsis •Fever (>38°C) or hypothermia (<36°C) •Tachycardia •Tachypnoea •Systolic hypotension (<90mmHg) or mean arterial pressure <70mmHg •Impaired mental state •Significant oedema or positive fluid balance •Hyperglycaemia (plasma glucose >7.7mmol/L). *Inflammatory markers:* •Raised WCC (>12×10⁹/L) but be aware that leucocytosis is common in labour •Leucopaenia (<4×10⁹/L) •CRP >7mg/L. *Tissue perfusion:* •Raised lactate (>4mmol/L) •Decreased capillary refill or mottling. *Organ dysfunction:* •Arterial hypoxaemia •Oliguria (<0.5mL/kg/h for 2h despite adequate fluid resuscitation) •Creatinine rise of >44μmol/L (severe sepsis if creatinine >176μmol/L) •INR >1.5; APTT >60s •Thrombocytopaenia (platelets <100×10⁹/L) •Hyperbilirubinaemia (>70umol/L) •Ileus. ►These signs are often unreliable in the pregnant woman and develop late and far more rapidly than in the non-pregnant state.

Investigations Blood cultures are key—take before giving antibiotics. Other cultures (eg throat, high vaginal swab, mid-stream urine) should also be taken but should not delay therapy. Take FBC, U&E, CRP, LFTs and clotting as well as serum lactate to guide management. An ABG will determine if there is hypoxia. Do not delay imaging on the grounds of pregnancy.

Treatment Give IV broad-spectrum antibiotics (eg piperacillin-tazobactam 4.5g/8h) within 1h of recognition (fig 1.5: the 'Golden Hour of Sepsis')—see BOX for alternatives. If lactate >4mmol/L and/or hypotensive, give an initial fluid bolus of 20mL/kg of crystalloid. Give vasopressors if BP does not respond to initial fluid bolus; aim for mean arterial pressure (MAP) of >65mmHg. Oxygen should be given. The woman may require central venous access. Immunoglobulin may be helpful in severe streptococcal or staphylococcal infection if other therapies have failed. It neutralizes exotoxin and inhibits production of tumour necrosis factor and interleukins. It has no effect on endotoxins. Use the multidisciplinary team and involve critical care outreach. Early consultant obstetrician, anaesthetic, and microbiologist review is recommended. Sepsis is associated with preterm labour so warn the neonatal unit. If chorioamnionitis is suspected, expedite delivery.

Transfer to intensive care if •Persistent hypotension or raised lactate suggesting need for inotropes •Pulmonary oedema •The woman requires mechanical ventilation or airway adjuncts •Decreased conscious level •Renal dialysis •Hypothermia •Uncorrected acidosis •Multi-organ failure. Some units can manage high-dependency patients within the labour ward setting.

Fetal monitoring Continuous fetal monitoring in labour is recommended (neonatal encephalopathy and cerebral palsy is increased with intrauterine infection). If the mother is pyrexial, the fetus will be about a degree hotter leading to uncomplicated fetal tachycardia. Fetal blood sampling may be less reliable and results valid for a significantly shorter time period than usual due to increased fetal metabolic rate. Spinal and epidural anaesthesia should be avoided and general anaesthesia used for caesarean section. If preterm delivery is anticipated, consider giving maternal corticosteroids. Unless the source of sepsis is intrauterine, stabilize the woman first. At delivery of the baby, take arterial and venous cord blood gases.

Choice and limitations of antibiotic therapy

- *Cefuroxime:* Associated with *c. difficile*; no cover for MRSA, *Pseudomonas*, or ESBL
- *Metronidazole:* Anaerobic cover only
- *Co-amoxiclav:* No MRSA or *Pseudomonas* cover, concern about increased risk of necrotizing enterocolitis in neonates exposed *in utero*
- *Clindamycin:* Covers most streptococci and staphylococci. Switches off ex- otoxin production. Not renally excreted or nephrotoxic. Useful in penicillin- allergic patients.
- *Piperacillin-tazobactam and carbapenems:* Covers all except MRSA; renal sparing
- *Gentamicin:* Nephrotoxic with abnormal renal function; requires regular monitoring of levels after 3 doses.

Sepsis in the puerperium The source is most commonly the genital tract and uterus, resulting in endometritis. Don't forget mastitis and breast abscess. Check caesarean and episiotomy wounds. If the degree of pain appears beyond clinical signs, consider necrotizing fasciitis. Organisms include group A *Streptococcus*, E. *coli*, *Staphylococcus aureus*, *Streptococcus pneumoniae* and MRSA. Signs to look for are fever, rigors, diarrhoea, breast engorgement, abdominal pain, offensive vaginal discharge, cough, urinary symptoms, delay in uterine involution, heavy or offensive lochia (postpartum vaginal blood loss), lethargy, and reduced appetite. Investigate and treat as previously. The neonate may require treatment with IV antibiotics, especially if the mother is infected with group A *Streptococcus*.

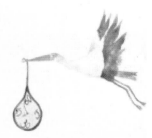

Fig 1.5 The Golden Hour of Sepsis.
© Charlotte Goumalatsou.

Further reading
RCOG (2012). *Bacterial Sepsis in Pregnancy* (Green-top Guideline No. 64a). London: RCOG.
RCOG (2012). *Bacterial Sepsis following Pregnancy* (Green-top Guideline No. 64b). London: RCOG.

The ideal pelvis This has a rounded brim, a shallow cavity, non-prominent ischial spines, a curved sacrum with large sciatic notches, and sacrospinous ligaments >3.5cm long. The angle of the brim is 55° to the horizontal, the AP diameter at least 12cm, and transverse diameter at least 13.5cm. The subpubic arch should be rounded and the intertuberous distance at least 10cm. A *clinically favourable* pelvis is one where the sacral promontory cannot be felt, the ischial spines are not prominent, the subpubic arch and base of supraspinous ligaments both accept 2 fingers, and the intertuberous diameter accepts 4 knuckles when the woman is examined.

The true pelvis Anteriorly there is the symphysis pubis (3.5cm long) and posteriorly the sacrum (12cm long). See fig 1.6.

Zone of inlet: Boundaries: Anteriorly lies the upper border of the pubis, posteriorly the sacral promontory, laterally the ileopectineal line. Transverse diameter 13.5cm; AP diameter 11.5cm.

Zone of cavity: This is the most roomy zone. It is almost round. Transverse diameter 13.5cm; AP diameter 12.5cm.

Zone of mid-pelvis: Boundaries: Anteriorly, the apex of the pubic arch; posteriorly the tip of the sacrum, laterally the ischial spines (the desirable distance between the spines is >10.5cm). Ovoid in shape, it is the narrowest part.

Zone of outlet: The pubic arch is the anterior border (desirable angle >85°). Laterally lie the sacrotuberous ligaments and ischial tuberosities, posteriorly the coccyx.

Head terms The *bregma* is the anterior fontanelle. The *brow* lies between the bregma and the root of the nose. The *face* lies below the root of the nose and supraorbital ridges. The *occiput* lies behind the posterior fontanelle. The *vertex* is the area between the fontanelles and the parietal eminences.

Moulding The frontal bones can slip under the parietal bones which can slip under the occipital bone so reducing biparietal diameter. The degree of overlap may be assessed vaginally.

Presentation	Relevant diameter presenting	
Flexed vertex	Suboccipitobregmatic	9.5cm
Partially deflexed vertex	Suboccipitofrontal	10.5cm
Deflexed vertex	Occipitofrontal	11.5cm
Brow	Mentovertical	13cm
Face	Submentobregmatic	9.5cm

Movement of the head in labour (normal vertex presentation)

1 Descent with increased flexion as the head enters the cavity. The sagittal suture lies in the transverse diameter of the brim.
2 Internal rotation occurs at the ischial spine level due to the grooved gutter of the levator muscles. Head flexion increases. (The head rotates 90° if occipitolateral position, 45° if occipitoanterior, 135° if occipitoposterior.)
3 Disengagement by extension as the head comes out of the vulva.
4 Restitution: as the shoulders are rotated by the levators until the bisacromial diameter is anteroposterior, the head externally rotates the same amount as before but in opposite direction.
5 Delivery of anterior shoulder by lateral flexion of trunk posteriorly.
6 Delivery of posterior shoulder by lateral flexion of trunk anteriorly.
7 Delivery of buttocks and legs.

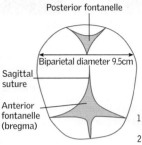

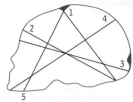

1 Suboccipitobregmatic 9.5cm
  flexed vertex presentation
2 Suboccipitofrontal 10.5cm
  partially deflexed vertex
3 Occipitofrontal 11.5cm deflexted vertex
4 Mentovertical 13cm brow
5 Submentobregmatic 9.5cm face

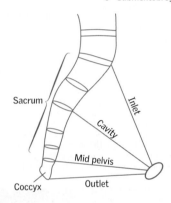

Fig 1.6 Pelvic diameters vs fetal head.

'*Life forced her through this gate of suffering.*' DH Lawrence, *Sons and Lovers.*

Fetal monitoring in labour aims to detect signs of fetal compromise and is carried out either by intermittent auscultation (IA) or by continuous cardiotocograph (CTG), also known as electronic fetal monitoring (EFM). Approximately 10% of cerebral palsy is due to intrapartum hypoxia. Uterine contractions restrict the blood supply to the fetus, especially those in the second stage. A healthy, well-grown fetus with a good reserve should withstand labour, but one that has started to decompensate pre-labour (for example, in absent or reversed end diastolic flow in umbilical artery Dopplers, p13) is unlikely to manage the stress of regular contractions and reduction in blood supply.

Intermittent auscultation (IA) with Doppler US (Sonicaid™) for a full minute after a contraction in low-risk women:
• Every 15min in 1st stage,
• Every 5min throughout 2nd stage.
If abnormality noted or intrapartum problems occur, start CTG monitoring.

Electronic fetal monitoring/continuous cardiotocograph is carried out for certain maternal and fetal risk factors which, if present, increase the risk of fetal compromise in labour (see BOX). It results in higher rates of intervention and operative delivery (instrumental and LSCS) without a convincing reduction in rates of cerebral palsy. CTG is sensitive but not specific in detecting fetal hypoxia: a fetus with an abnormal CTG will be hypoxic (acidotic) on fetal blood sampling (FBS) 50% of the time. The interpretation of CTG is probably another factor, and doctors and midwives working on the labour ward should undergo yearly CTG training with regular group teaching to maintain skills. The monitoring itself is carried out either through an abdominal probe (US) or via a fetal scalp electrode (FSE, producing a fetal ECG). FSE is a metal clip or tiny screw in direct contact with the fetus and is useful if there is doubt about the source of the heartbeat, poor contact of the abdominal probe, obesity, and very mobile women but requires ruptured membranes. When FSE is used, some centres have the facility to measure the fetal ECG ST waveform (STAN) which can reduce the need for FBS and instrumental delivery, but not caesarean section. Like FBS, STAN should be approached with caution in any woman with fever.

Indications for electronic fetal monitoring

• Induction of labour
• Post-maturity (>42 weeks)
• Previous LSCS
• Maternal cardiac problems
• Pre-eclampsia or hypertension
• Prolonged rupture of membranes >24h
• Prematurity <37 weeks
• Diabetes of any type
• Antepartum or intrapartum haemorrhage
• Small for gestational age
• Oligohydramnios
• Abnormal umbilical artery Dopplers
• Multiple pregnancy
• Meconium-stained liquor
• Abnormal lie (eg breech)
• Oxytocin augmentation
• Epidural anaesthesia
• Pyrexia
• Abnormality heard on intermittent auscultation

The language used should be standardized and you may be asked to describe a trace using 'DR C BRAVADO'. This useful mnemonic is broken down as follows: *DR,* determine risk; why is the woman having EFM? *C* for contractions; how many in 10 minutes? *BRA* meaning baseline rate; *V* for variability, *A* for accelerations, *D*ecelerations, and *O* verall (normal, non-reassuring, abnormal).

Baseline rate is the average level of the fetal heart rate when any accelerations or decelerations have been excluded. It appears as a straight-ish line between other features on the trace. Normal is 100–160bpm. Bradycardia is a baseline of <100bpm; tachycardia >160bpm can be associated with maternal fever. BR >180bpm is abnormal.

Variability is thought of best as the 'bandwidth' of the baseline. Take a small square on the CTG; each one should contain a variation in FHR of >5bpm. Reduced variability is <5bpm (but this can be normal if <30min and can happen when the baby is sleeping). Other causes of reduced variability include fetal hypoxia, malformation, magnesium, and prematurity <28 weeks.

Accelerations are an upward spike of >15bpm for >15 seconds. They are a reassuring feature and commonly occur when the fetus is moving.

Decelerations appear as downward spikes of >15bpm for >15 seconds. These may be a normal feature of labour, and how concerning they are depends on the shape of them, and when they appear relative to a contraction. *Early* decelerations mimic the shape and timing of the contraction and are caused by head compression. They are therefore seen in breech presentation in labour and the second stage. *Late* decelerations reach their nadir after the peak of the contraction has passed and are a sign of acidosis especially with other abnormal features. *Shallow* decelerations together with reduced variability represent an abnormal trace that warrants intervention. *Typical variable* decelerations are v-shaped with shoulders on either side, and are associated with cord compression and are not usually associated with hypoxia. *Atypical* variables have loss of shouldering, last >60s, >60 beats from the baseline, may be slow to recover, be a 'w' shape, and lose variability within the deceleration. They may be a sign of fetal hypoxia. See figs 1.7–1.11 on p46–7.

Classification of CTG

	Baseline (bpm)	Variability (bpm)	Decelerations	Accelerations
Reassuring	100–160	>5	None or early	Present
Non-reassuring	161–180	<5 for 30–90min	Variable decelerations for >50% contractions for >90min, taking <60s to recover, or drop from BR of >60 beats, or taking >60s to recover, for <30min	
Abnormal	<100 >180	<5 for >90min	Late decelerations >50% contractions for >30min Single prolonged deleration >3min	
NICE 2014. Intrapartum care: CG190				

Normal: All four features are in the reassuring category.

Non-reassuring: One non-reassuring feature, but the rest reassuring.

Abnormal: Two or more non-reassuring or one abnormal feature.

Improving a CTG Correct any possible insults: left lateral position to shift weight off maternal vessels and correct cord compression; IV fluids if hypotensive after epidural or dehydrated; reduce or stop oxytocin infusion if contracting >5:10 (5 contractions in 10min) or bradycardia.

Fetal blood sampling is used to improve the specificity of CTG in detecting fetal hypoxia. It should be taken when the trace is abnormal, unless immediate delivery is required (eg bradycardia >3min, suspected LSCS scar rupture). FBS involves taking a small sample of blood from the fetal scalp. The woman is placed in the left lateral position and a speculum with a light attached placed against the fetal scalp. A small scratch is made on the fetal scalp and fetal blood collected in a capillary tube and analysed in a blood gas machine. The woman ideally should be at least 4cm dilated with ruptured membranes. If FBS fails, the baby should be delivered as soon as possible—by LSCS if not fully dilated. Do not attempt FBS/FSE if the woman has suspected ITP, any blood-borne viruses and use with caution in pyrexia. In units where STAN is used (p44) a normal FBS result is required prior to this method of EFM commencing when the CTG is abnormal.

- Normal pH: >7.25 (repeat in 1h if CTG remains abnormal)
- Borderline pH: 7.21–7.24 (repeat in 30min if CTG remains abnormal)
- Abnormal pH: <7.20 (immediate delivery).

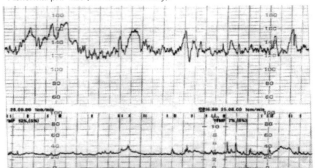

Fig 1.7 Normal CTG. All characterisitics (see p45) are within normal limits.

Reproduced from Sarris et al, *Training in Obstetrics and Gynaecology* (2009) with permission from OUP.

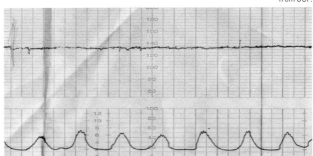

Fig 1.8 Significantly reduced variability (almost a pencil line). This can be normal in sleep-cycling but if >90min is ominous; can also occur with narcotic agents.

Reproduced from Sarris et al, *Training in Obstetrics and Gynaecology* (2009) with permission from OUP.

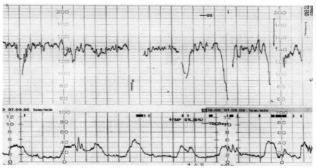

Fig 1.9 Typical variable decelerations. Note the presence of shouldering on either side of the deceleration, and the clear 'v' shape. These are usually a sign of cord compression, head or eyeball compression during labour and are due to a fetal reflex and are not ominous.

Reproduced from Sarris et al, *Training in Obstetrics and Gynaecology* (2009) with permission from Oxford University Press.

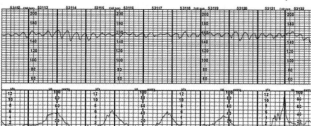

Fig 1.10 Sinusoidal pattern which if >10min can indicdate fetal anaemia but if <10min could be due to thumb-sucking.

Reproduced with permission from periFACTS OB/GYN Academy.

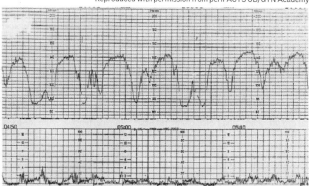

Fig 1.11 Abnormal CTG with reduced variability and atypical variable decelerations. There is loss of shouldering, reduced variablity within the decel and some have a 'w' shape.

Reproduced from Sarris et al, *Training in Obstetrics and Gynaecology* (2009) with permission from Oxford University Press.

Pre-eclampsia is characterized by hypertension and proteinuria in pregnancy and affects up to 5% of pregnancies. It is a multisystem disorder originating in the placenta; the primary defect is failure of trophoblastic invasion of spiral arteries leaving them vasoactive—properly invaded they cannot clamp down in response to vasoconstrictors and this protects placental flow. Increasing BP partially compensates for this. Pre-eclampsia also affects hepatic, renal, and coagulation systems. It develops after 20 weeks and resolves within 6 weeks of delivery. Pre-eclampsia is a major cause of maternal morbidity (from cerebral haemorrhage, multi-organ failure, and adult respiratory distress syndrome) and mortality, as well as iatrogenic prematurity (the only cure is delivery of the baby). **Risk factors** *High risk:* •Previous severe or early-onset pre-eclampsia (<20 weeks) •Chronic hypertension (p31) or hypertension in previous pregnancy •Chronic kidney disease •Diabetes mellitus •Autoimmune disease (SLE, antiphospholipid, thrombophilia). *Moderate risk:* •1st pregnancy •≥40y •Pregnancy interval >10y • BMI ≥30kg/m² •FH pre-eclampsia •Multiple pregnancy •Low PAPP-A (p25) •Uterine artery notching on Doppler US at 22–24 weeks. If 1 high-risk or 2 moderate-risk factors take aspirin 75mg/24h PO from 12th week of pregnancy until delivery to prevent pre-eclampsia. *Fetal:* Hydatidiform mole; multiple pregnancy; fetal hydrops (eg rhesus disease). **Effects of pre-eclampsia** Plasma volume ↓; peripheral resistance ↑; placental ischaemia. If the BP is >180/140mmHg microaneurysms develop in arteries. DIC may develop. Oedema may develop suddenly. The liver may be involved (contributing to DIC)—and HELLP syndrome may be present with placental infarcts. *Severe complications* are eclampsia, HELLP syndrome (p49), cerebral haemorrhage, IUGR, renal failure, and placental abruption.

Symptoms may be absent, especially with mild pre-eclampsia. Ask about headache, flashing lights, epigastric or right upper quadrant pain, nausea and vomiting, and swelling of face, fingers, and lower limbs. **Signs** may include pregnancy-induced hypertension, proteinuria, epigastric or right upper quadrant tenderness, brisk reflexes, >2 beats of clonus, confusion, fits, placental abruption, IUGR and stillbirth. **Investigations** Protein-creatinine ratio (PCR) >30mg/ mmol; raised serum uric acid, thrombocytopaenia, prolonged PT&APTT, raised creatinine, anaemia if haemolysis (LDH raised), abnormal LFTS (particularly transaminases), fetal growth restriction, oligohydramnios, notching of uterine arteries on Doppler, abnormal umbilical artery Dopplers.

Management depends on disease severity. All women with pre-eclampsia should deliver on a labour ward. NICE recommends admission of all women with pre-eclampsia, but units are increasingly managing mild disease as outpatients. *Mild pre-eclampsia:* BP 140–149/90–99mmHg. Urine PCR >30mg/ mmol is diagnostic in the presence of hypertension and does not need to be repeated—it is not reflective of severity of pre-eclampsia. 4-hourly BP; twice-weekly bloods to monitor renal function, LFTS, FBC. Fetal growth scans every 2 weeks. Do not start antihypertensives unless BP >150/100mmHg. IOL after 37/40. *Moderate pre-eclampsia:* BP 150–159/100–109mmHg. Admit to hospital until delivery. Measure BP 4-hourly; check bloods 3 times per week; fortnightly fetal growth scans, and twice-daily CTG. Start antihypertensives. Aim for IOL at 37/40. *Severe pre-eclampsia:* BP >160/110, or symptoms/signs (eg clonus), or end-organ damage. Call for senior help from obstetrics, anaesthetic and midwifery staff. Stabilize BP with antihypertensives eg nifedipine 10mg PO twice 30 min apart. If BP still remains high, start IV antihypertensives (labetalol or hydralazine). Prophylactic magnesium sulphate 4g IV loading dose then 1g IV/hour. Bloods every 12–24h. Maintain strict fluid balance, catheterize, give steroids for fetal lung maturity and if >34 weeks deliver. For women <34 weeks, time delivery according to senior advice but will generally need to be once woman is stable, but ideally within 24–48h.

Eclampsia

▸▸ *This is an obstetric emergency.* It is a tonic–clonic seizure + pre-eclampsia. It occurs in 1% of pregnancies diagnosed with pre-eclampsia.

▸▸ 38% fit antenatally, 18% intrapartum, and 44% postnatally. It may be the first presentation of pre-eclampsia. If death occurs it is usually due to cerebral haemorrhage, HELLP, or organ failure.

▸▸ Call for help: senior obstetrics staff, senior midwives, anaesthetic registrar and consultant, a scribe, and neonatal team should delivery be required.

▸▸ Don't forget to manage airway, breathing, circulation, and IV access. Continuously monitor maternal oxygen saturation, and BP.

▸▸ Magnesium sulfate is used to prevent and treat seizures. Give 4g IV over 5–10min then 1g/h for 24h. Treat further fits with 2g bolus.

▸▸ Repeated seizures should be treated with diazepam and intracranial haemorrhage needs to be ruled out.

▸▸ Catheterize for hourly urine output (with urometer). HR, BP, respiratory rate and oxygen saturations every 15min. FBC, U&E, LFTs, creatinine, and clotting studies every 12–24h.

▸▸ Stop magnesium sulfate IVI if respiratory rate <12/min or tendon reflex loss, or urine output <20mL/h. Have IV calcium gluconate ready in case of MgSO4 toxicity: 1g (10mL) over 10min if respiratory depression.

▸▸ Restrict fluids to 80mL/h. Hourly urine output. Renal failure is rare. Maintain fluid restriction until postpartum diuresis. Fluid restriction is inappropriate if there is haemorrhage—may need CVP line for accurate assessment.

▸▸ Monitor fetal heart rate with CTG.

▸▸ Deliver once the mother is stable; vaginal delivery is not contraindicated but LSCS is the quickest route as IOL is likely to take a long time eg if preterm.

▸▸ *Manage the third stage with oxytocin. Syntometrine® and ergometrine are contraindicated due to risk of severe hypertension leading to stroke.*

Treatment of hypertension Beware: automated BP devices underestimate BP.

▸▸ If BP >160/110mmHg or mean arterial pressure >125mmHg, use labetalol 20mg IV increasing after 10min intervals to 40mg then 80mg until 200mg total is given. Aim for BP 150/80–100mmHg. Alternative is hydralazine 5mg slowly/20min til 20mg given (unless pulse >120bpm) after 500mL colloid IV.

HELLP syndrome

This is a severe variant of pre-eclampsia and consists of *H*aemolysis, *E*levated *L*iver enzymes, and *L*ow *P*latelets. Pregnancies affected by pre-eclampsia can develop HELLP in varying degrees, and liver enzymes usually rise first, followed by a drop in platelets (may be severe) and then haemolysis. As with pre-eclampsia, cure is with delivery of the fetus.

Symptoms are epigastric or right upper quadrant pain, nausea and vomiting, and dark urine due to haemolysis. The woman may have right upper quadrant tenderness and raised BP. It may be discovered after eclampsia.

Treatment is as for eclampsia and is an indication for delivery. Involve the anaesthetist and senior help. Regional anaesthesia is contraindicated if platelets <80, and if platelets are <50 and surgery is required, cover with platelet transfusion.

Further reading

NICE (2010). *The Management of Hypertensive Disorders during Pregnancy* (CG107). London: NICE.

▶This is a leading cause of perinatal mortality and morbidity—5–10% births but 50% of perinatal deaths.

Premature infants are those born before 37 weeks' gestation. Prevalence: ~6% of singletons, 46% of twin, 79% of triplet or higher-order deliveries. About 1.4% are before 32^{+0} weeks—when neonatal problems are greatest. In 25%, delivery is elective (p62). 10% are due to multiple pregnancy; 25% are due to APH, cervical incompetence, chorioamnionitis, uterine abnormalities, diabetes, polyhydramnios, pyelonephritis, or other infections. In 40% the cause is unknown, but abnormal genital tract colonization (bacterial vaginosis) with ureaplasma and *Mycoplasma hominis* is implicated, as either a risk factor or risk marker.

Risk factors are previous preterm birth, multiple pregnancy, cervical surgery (eg LLETZ or cone biopsy), uterine anomalies, pre-existing medical conditions, pre-eclampsia, and IUGR.

Managing preterm rupture of membranes (PROM)

Admit for 48h (highest risk of preterm labour); rule out any evidence of chorioamnionitis and sepsis. If there is evidence of chorioamnionitis, expedite delivery irrespective of gestation. Take T°, MSU, and HVS—using a sterile bivalve speculum. Signs such as raised CRP develop late and should not be relied upon. Give corticosteroids for fetal lung maturity (see p51) and erythromycin 500mg PO QDS for 10 days (reduces neonatal morbidity). In 80%, membrane rupture initiates labour. The problem with the 20% who do not go into labour is balancing advantages of remaining *in utero* (maturity and surfactant ↑) against the threat of infection (causes 20% of neonatal deaths after PROM). Intrauterine infection supervenes after membranes have ruptured in 10% by 48h, 26% by 72h, 40% by >72h. If infection develops, take blood cultures and give IV antibiotics (include cover for group B *Streptococcus*) and expedite labour (p62). The risks to the fetus from PROM are those of prematurity, infection, pulmonary hypoplasia, and limb contractures. If labour does not occur spontaneously, discharge after 48h and manage as an out-patient avoiding intercourse, tampons and swimming, with weekly follow-up in the day unit for FBC and CRP. Aim for IOL after 34 weeks if cephalic.

Management of preterm labour In 50% contractions cease spontaneously. Treating the cause (eg pyelonephritis) may help it cease. Give corticosteroids (p51). Trials of tocolytic drugs have shown them to be of almost no clinical benefit, and only nifedipine is associated with improvement of fetal outcome. It is quite reasonable not to use tocolytic drugs; though they may be considered desirable in certain circumstances eg to give time for corticosteroids to work, or for *in utero* transfer. Consider transfer to hospital with NICU facilities. Check presentation (breech more common with increasing prematurity). Check FBC, CRP, HVS, MSU. Speculum to rule out PROM, take fetal fibronectin (see p51) and if no PROM gentle vaginal exam to assess dilatation. If in labour, give IV antibiotics to prevent GBS (eg benzylpenicillin 3g loading dose followed by 1.5g 4-hourly). Call paediatrician to attend to the baby at birth. See cord-cutting recommendations on p51.

Tocolytics Absolute CI: chorioamnionitis, fetal death or lethal abnormality, condition (fetal or maternal) needing immediate delivery. Relative CI: fetal growth restriction or distress, pre-eclampsia, placenta praevia, abruption, cervix >4cm. Atosiban (licensed in Europe) has fewer maternal effects, but has not been shown to benefit the fetus. Nifedipine is as effective, and associated with less newborn respiratory distress and admission to intensive care. Regimen: **nifedipine** 20mg PO then 10–20mg/6–8h according to uterine activity (unlicensed use). Use up to 48h. SE: ↓ BP; headache; flushing; pulse ↑ (transient); myocardial infarction (very rare); CI: heart disease (use with caution in diabetes, and multiple pregnancy as pulmonary oedema risk).

Fetal fibronectin is a protein not usually detected in vaginal secretions between 22 and 36 weeks. It is used to rule out preterm labour and is a bedside test. Those with positive fFN have a 10% chance of preterm delivery and should be admitted and given corticosteroids. Falsely positive if intercourse, significant bleeding, speculum, or vaginal exam within 48 hours.

Glucocorticoids *Dose:* Betamethasone 12mg IM with a 2nd dose 12-24h later (or dexamethasone 6mg/12/h ×4 doses).

These help fetal surfactant production, lowering mortality (by 31%) and complications of RDS (p118) by 44%. They also help close patent ductuses and protect against periventricular malacia, a cause of cerebral palsy.
• Use in all women at risk of iatrogenic or spontaneous preterm birth between ~24^{+0} and ~34^{+6} weeks.
• If growth restriction too, use up to 35^{+6} weeks.
• If risk at 23^{+0}-23^{+6} weeks use only on senior advice.
• Use before all elective cs up to 38^{+6} weeks.
• Consider use at 35–36 weeks if delivery expedited for pre-eclampsia (NICE).[120]
• If diabetic, monitor glucose (may need admission and insulin infusion).

Benefit occurs within 24h. Repeat doses are not beneficial. A further 'rescue' dose is only recommended if the first course was given before 26 weeks and a new obstetric indication arises.

Magnesium sulfate Studies show a neuroprotective effect if given antenatally for babies <34 weeks' gestation. It is estimated that 63 women will need treatment to prevent one case of cerebral palsy. Australian draft national clinical guidelines recommend a maternal loading dose of 4g IV over 20-30 minutes followed by 1g/h maintenance infusion for up to 24h (or birth, if earlier), and use if fetus <30 weeks' gestation.[62]

Delivery Babies delivered at <28 weeks' gestation should be delivered in a room with temperature of 26°c, wrapped in food-grade plastic wrap or bag without drying after birth and be placed under heat whilst stabilizing (keep wrapped until temperature checked in NICU).[63] Older babies are wrapped in dry towels. A 3min delay in cutting the cord, (if premature babies are vigorous and not needing active resuscitation), and holding the baby 20cm below the introitus, results in higher haematocrit levels, and reduces transfusion and oxygen supplement requirements in premature babies, and reduces rates of intraventricular haemorrhage, but increases the need for phototherapy.[63]

Prematurity, survival, and disability—the figures
• Cerebral palsy is present in 20% of surviving babies born at 24–26 weeks' gestation (compared with 4% at 32 weeks) in a large French study.[64]

Viability thresholds for very premature babies have reduced by 1 week per decade for the last 40 years. Survival before 22 weeks is very rare. In 1995, 1% of babies born at 22–23 weeks survived to leave hospital, 11% at 23–24; 26% at 24–25; 44% at 25–26. Of surviving babies born between 23–24 weeks two-thirds had moderate or severe disability; by 25 to 26 weeks two-thirds had no or only mild disability. These figures have lead to guidelines for consideration of treatment at different gestations, eg not resuscitating babies of less than 22 weeks' completed gestation unless specifically requested by parents after discussion with senior paediatrician; but normally admitting babies of >23 weeks' completed gestation to neonatal intensive care.[65] The figures for England, Wales, and Northern Ireland were that 58% of babies born at 24 weeks' gestation survived the neonatal period, increasing to 77% at 25 weeks; (85% at 26 weeks; 92% at 27 and 28 weeks; 96% at 29 weeks; 97% at 33 weeks).[66]

Further reading
RCOG (2010). *Antenatal Corticosteroids to Reduce Neonatal Morbidity and Mortality* (Green-top guideline No. 7). London: RCOG.

Obstetrics

▶All women should be assessed at booking for risk factors for the SGA fetus in order to identify those at increased risk who require increased monitoring. At booking, every woman should have a customized growth chart for SFH which takes into account maternal age, parity, BMI, ethnicity and birthweights of previous children. A single SFH measurement <10th centile or static growth should prompt referral for fetal US (fig 1.12). Those women at high risk (see below) should be referred for consultant-led care and have serial US measurement of fetal size including umbilical artery Doppler from 26–28 weeks. Women with 3 or more minor risks factors should have uterine artery Doppler at 20–24 weeks, and if abnormal, serial growth scans. Identifying the SGA fetus is important because they have a higher mortality (both intrauterine and neonatal), higher incidence of cerebral palsy, and are more likely to have intrapartum fetal distress, meconium aspiration, and emergency LSCS.

Definition Estimated fetal weight <10th centile for their gestational age or abdominal circumference <10th centile. *Placental factors:* Abnormal trophoblast invasion eg pre-eclampsia, infarction, abruption. Tends to cause asymmetrical growth restriction with head sparing and reduced abdominal circumference. *Fetal factors:* Genetic abnormalities especially trisomies 13, 18, and 21, and Turner syndrome; congenital anomalies and infection such as CMV, rubella; multiple pregnancy.

Major risk factors • Maternal age >40 • Smoker • Cocaine use • Previous SGA baby • Previous stillbirth • Maternal/paternal SGA • Chronic hypertension • Diabetes • Renal impairment • Antiphospholipid syndrome • Heavy antepartum bleeding • Echogenic bowel • Pre-eclampsia • Low PAPP-A. **Minor risk factors** • Maternal age >35 • Nulliparity • BMI <20 • IVF •Pregnancy-induced hypertension.

Management Once a fetus is identified as SGA, if the umbilical artery Dopplers are normal, growth scans should be carried out every 2–3 weeks. If Dopplers remain normal, aim for IOL at 37 weeks. If abnormal Dopplers and preterm, delivery depends on other indices such as ductus venosus Doppler (<32 weeks). If absent or reversed end-diastolic flow in umbilical artery Doppler, consider delivery by LSCS. Offer corticosteroids for fetal lung maturity up to 35⁺⁶ weeks. Growth restricted fetuses are more susceptible to hypoxia and even if Dopplers are normal, intervention rate in labour is higher. After birth, temperature regulation may be a problem, so ensure a warm welcome and encourage skin-to-skin contact with the mother. Neonates have little stored glycogen so are prone to hypoglycaemia. Feed within 2h of birth *Effects of IUGR in adult life:* As adults, higher risk of hypertension, coronary artery disease, type 2 diabetes, and autoimmune thyroid disease.

Large for gestational age

These are babies above the 95th centile in weight for gestation.

Causes Constitutionally large (usually familial—the largest 10% of the population); maternal diabetes (p23); obesity is a major cause.

Labour and aftercare Large babies risk birth injury (see *Shoulder dystocia*, p72) but IOL does not reduce it. They are prone to hypoglycaemia and hypocalcaemia. Polycythaemia may result in jaundice. They are also prone to left colon syndrome: a self-limiting condition clinically mimicking Hirschsprung's disease (p130) whereby temporary bowel obstruction (possibly also with meconium plug) occurs.

Further reading

RCOG (2013). *The Investigation and Management of the Small-for-Gestational-Age Fetus* (Green-top Guideline No. 31). London: RCOG.

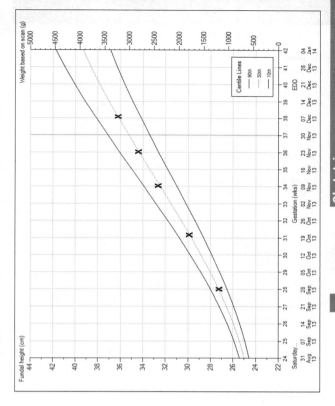

Obstetrics

Fig 1.12 Customized antenatal growth chart. The sfh should follow the same centile throughout pregnancy. Deviation from this should prompt referral for a fetal growth scan.

With permission from the Perinatal Institute, www.perinatal.org.uk.

Obstetrics

Definition Prolonged pregnancy is defined as that exceeding 42 completed weeks of pregnancy.

Incidence 5–10% of pregnancies (30% if previous prolonged pregnancy).

Problems
• Intrapartum deaths 4 times more common
• Early neonatal deaths 3 times more common
• Increased rates of induction of labour and operative delivery
• Possible placental insufficiency
• Macrosomia (25% >4000g), shoulder dystocia, and fetal injury
• Fetal skull more ossified so less mouldable
• Increased meconium passage in labour (25–40%) (p73)
• Increased fetal distress in labour
• Increased caesarean rates for labours after 41 completed weeks.

Management Confirm EDD. At 38-week visit discuss what is recommended if spontaneous labour does not occur by 41 completed weeks, including membrane sweep and induction. Arrange for visit at 41 weeks if not delivered.

1 Membrane sweep. On vaginal examination as much membrane is swept from the lower segment as possible by a finger inserted through the cervix. It is thought to induce natural prostaglandins. This may cause discomfort and a little bleeding but may induce labour 'naturally'. 8 women are membrane swept for 1 formal induction avoided. Offer at 40- and 41-week visit in nullips, at 41 weeks in multips.

2 A policy of induction after 41 completed weeks' pregnancy does reduce fetal death rate. NICE says to offer induction between 41^{+0} and 42^{+0} weeks.$_{NICE}^{87}$ Induction is with vaginal prostaglandin followed by oxytocin (p62). After induction, monitor the fetus in labour (p44). It is estimated that 500 inductions are needed to prevent 1 perinatal death.

3 If the woman declines induction then arrange twice-weekly CTG (p44), and US estimation of amniotic fluid depth to try to detect fetuses who may be becoming hypoxic. Doppler studies of cord blood flow may be used to look for absent end-diastolic flow as a predictor of fetal compromise.

Signs of postmaturity in the baby : Dry, cracked, peeling, loose skin; decreased subcutaneous tissue; scaphoid (hollow) abdomen; meconium staining of nails and cord.

Immediate resuscitation is key. Broadly speaking, follow the Advanced Life Support algorithm. Call for help, and put out a maternal collapse call via switchboard (2222 in the UK). Senior staff including obstetric and anaesthetic consultants and registrars, senior midwives, medical registrar, and neonatal teams as well as a porter should come quickly.

Airway Open the airway with head tilt and chin lift.

Breathing Look for chest movement and listen for breath sounds.

Circulation Check carotids for pulse; if pulse present check BP. If no pulse and/or no breathing, put out cardiac arrest call and start CPR. CPR after 20 weeks should be carried out in left lateral position (place a wedge under the woman or tilt the table). After 20 weeks, if no return of spontaneous circulation after 5 minutes, perform LSCS. This is not to save the fetus—it is essential for maternal resuscitation. In obstetrics, haemorrhage is a common cause of collapse so check vaginally for bleeding.

Drugs Think of overdose, drugs to maintain circulation or to dissolve massive thromboembolism. Remember to check blood glucose to exclude hypoglycaemia.

Environment Avoid injury of the patient and staff, especially if defibrillating.

The history may help ascertain the cause. Check observations every 15 minutes and catheterize for urine output. Take blood for FBC, U&E, LFTs, coagulation screen, uric acid (pre-eclampsia or eclampsia, p48-9), group and save, and cross-match if suspicion or confirmed bleeding. Other investigations depend on the suspected cause but may include ABG, CXR, V/Q scan or CTPA, ECG, CT/MRI brain. Anaesthetic and general medical colleagues are invaluable in these situations especially if she has a cardiac arrest or is sick enough to require ITU.

Causes of maternal collapse

Obstetric causes
- Massive obstetric haemorrhage: may be ante- or postpartum (p56&84)
- Eclampsia (p49)
- Intracranial haemorrhage (especially if preceding severe pre-eclampsia)
- Amniotic fluid embolism (p89)
- Uterine inversion causing neurogenic shock (p86)
- Post-surgical haemorrhage eg intra-abdominal following LSCS
- Severe sepsis (p40)
- Peripartum cardiomyopathy.

Non-obstetric causes
- Massive pulmonary embolism (p33)
- Pre-existing cardiac disease; never dismiss myocardial infarction as a possibility, or aortic dissection
- Anaphylaxis (check the drug chart; could it be latex allergy?)
- Stroke
- Meningitis
- Overdose
- Diabetic ketoacidosis; hypoglycaemia
- Has the woman been abroad? Think about malaria (p26).

Genital tract bleeding from 24^{+0} wks' gestation complicates 3–5% of pregnancies. Any bleeding in pregnancy is associated with increased perinatal mortality. Severe bleeds can cause maternal death. Ask about domestic violence.

▶Speculum examination is safe in placenta praevia.

Dangerous causes Abruption, placenta praevia, vasa praevia (here the baby may bleed to death).

Other uterine sources: Circumvallate placenta, placental sinuses.

Lower genital tract sources: Cervical polyps, erosions and carcinoma, cervicitis, vaginitis, vulval varicosities.

Placental abruption Part of the placenta becomes detached from the uterus. The outcome depends on the amount of blood loss and degree of separation. It may recur in subsequent pregnancies (4%: 19–24% if twice). *Associations* pre-eclampsia, smoking, IUGR (p52), PROM (p58), multiple pregnancy, polyhydramnios, ↑ maternal age, thrombophilia, abdo trauma, assisted reproduction, cocaine/amphetamine use, infection, non-vertex presentation. Bleeding may be well localized to one placental area and there may be delay before bleeding is revealed.

Consequences: Placental insufficiency may cause fetal anoxia or death. Compression of uterine muscles by blood causes tenderness, and may prevent good contraction at all stages of labour, so beware a PPH (which occurs in ~25%). Posterior abruptions may present with backache. There may be uterine hypercontractility (>5 contractions per 10min). Thromboplastin release may cause DIC (10%). Concealed bleeding may cause maternal shock after which beware renal failure and Sheehan's syndrome.

Placenta praevia (For terminology and complications, see p87.) The placenta lies in the lower uterine segment. Bleeding is always revealed (fig 1.13).

Distinguishing *abruption*	From *placenta praevia*
Shock out of keeping with visible loss	Shock in proportion to visible loss
Pain constant	No pain
Tender, tense uterus	Uterus not tender
Normal lie and presentation	Both may be abnormal
Fetal heart: absent/distressed	Fetal heart usually normal
Coagulation problems	Coagulation problems rare
Beware pre-eclampsia, DIC, anuria	Small bleeds before large

Note: the risk of PPH is increased in both conditions. The lower segment may not contract well after a placenta praevia.

Management of APH *Admit* (unless spotting which has stopped, and the placenta is not low-lying). ▶▶If bleeding is severe, put up IVI, take bloods, and raise legs. Give O$_2$ at 15L/min via mask with reservoir. On admission, if shocked give fresh ABO Rh compatible or O Rh–ve blood (eg 6U, 2 IVIs) stat until systolic BP >100mmHg. Send blood for clotting screen. Catheterize bladder; keep urine output >30mL/h. Call anaesthetist to monitor fluids (CVP lines help). *Summon expert help urgently.* If bleeding is severe, *deliver*—caesarean section for placenta praevia (sometimes for abruption, or induction). Beware PPH (manage 3rd stage with Syntometrine®).

For milder bleeding, set up IVI, do Hb, crossmatch, coagulation studies, and U&E. Check pulse, BP, and blood loss regularly. Establish diagnosis (US of placenta, speculum examination). If placenta praevia is the diagnosis, keep in hospital until delivery (usually by caesarean section at 37–38 weeks). If pain and bleeding from a small abruption settles and the fetus is not compromised the woman may go home (after anti-D, if indicated; 6-weekly if recurrent bleeds), but then treat as 'high-risk' pregnancy (serial scans). IOL if APH at term.

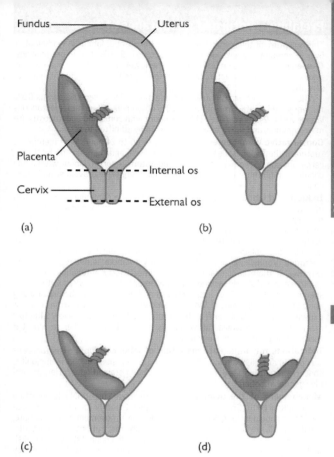

Fig 1.13 (a) Grade I placenta praevia, encroaches the lower segment but does not reach the os. (b) Grade II placenta praevia reaches the os but does not cover it. (c) Grade III placenta praevia partially covers the os and (d) Grade IV completely covers the os. Placenta praevia may also be classified minor (a and b) or major (c and d).

With permission from Angel RK Shere.

This is rupture of the membranes prior to the onset of labour in women at or over 37 completed weeks' gestation. It occurs in 8–10% of term pregnancies.

Causes Mostly unknown; infection of the lower genital tract or amnion is a known aetiological factor; polyhydramnios; multiple pregnancy; malpresentation.

When there is PROM risk of serious infection is increased (1% versus 0.5% for women with intact membranes). 60% of women will go into spontaneous labour within 24 hours. After 24 hours chorioamnionitis and endometritis are more common, and the baby is more likely to be admitted to SCBU.

Conservative management is appropriate up to 24 hours post membrane rupture if the liquor is clear, the mother is well, and there are no fetal concerns. She should regularly take her temperature, report to labour ward if any change in fetal movements, colour or smell of liquor, and avoid sexual intercourse.

Induction of labour If spontaneous labour has not commenced by 24h then NICE recommends induction of labour. Vaginal prostaglandin is the preferred method of trying to induce labour eg prostaglandin E_2 gel 1–2mg for 6 hours followed by an oxytocin infusion if contractions have not started. Those giving birth after 24h of ruptured membranes should deliver where there are neonatal care facilities, and advised to stay in hospital for 12h after birth.

Routine prophylactic use of IV antibiotics in labour is not recommended. However, if there is clinical evidence of infection, IV antibiotics should be commenced and should include cover for group B *Streptococcus* with broad-spectrum antibiotics. Take HVS, send MSU and blood cultures before starting antibiotics. *If induction of labour is declined:* Offer advice from a senior midwife or doctor. Monitor fetal heart rate at 1st contact and every 24h after membrane rupture whilst the woman is not in labour. Ask her to report if there are reduced fetal movements.

Indications for immediate induction of labour Group B *Streptococcus* carriers; HIV carriers aiming for a vaginal delivery; signs of chorioamnionitis; concerns regarding fetal movements; meconium-stained liquor; Herpes simplex genital infection.

Management of the neonate Babies are most susceptible to infection within 12h of birth. Observe at 1h, 2h, and then 2-hourly for further 10h. Observations should include general well-being, chest movement and nasal flare, capillary refill, feeding, muscle tone, temperature, respirations, and heart rate. If there is any suggestion of sepsis in the baby, call a neonatal care specialist. Mothers should also be advised to report any health concerns about the baby in the 1st 5 days of life.

Further reading

NICE (2008). *Induction of Labour* (CG70). London: NICE

'Labour is one of the shortest yet most hazardous journeys humans make in their lifetime.' From the 1st trimester, the uterus has Braxton Hicks contractions (ie non-painful 'practice' contractions, eg to ≤15mmHg pressure; in labour pressure is ~60mmHg). They are commonest after 36 weeks.

Normal labour (fig 1.14) ~60% of births are normal and need no intervention. Normal labour occurs after 37wks' gestation and results in spontaneous vaginal delivery of the baby within 24h of the onset of regular spontaneous contractions. It is often heralded by a 'show', ie a plug of cervical mucus and a little blood as the membranes strip from the os (membranes may then rupture).

The first stage of labour *Latent phase:* There are painful, often irregular contractions, the cervix initially *effaces* (becomes shorter and softer) then dilates to 4cm. *Established phase:* regular contractions with dilatation from 4cm. A satisfactory rate of dilatation from 4cm is 0.5cm/h. The 1st stage generally takes 8–18h in a primip, and 5–12h in a multip. During the first stage check maternal BP, and T° 4-hourly, pulse hourly; assess the contractions every 30min, their strength (you should not be able to indent the uterus with the fingers during a contraction) and their frequency (ideally 3–4 per 10min, lasting up to 1min). Note frequency of bladder emptying. Offer vaginal examination eg every 4h to assess the degree of cervical dilatation, the position, and the station of the head (measured in cm above or below the ischial spines) and note the degree of moulding and caput (p42). Note the state of the liquor (p73). Auscultate fetal heart rate (if not continuously monitored), by Pinard or Doppler every 15 min, listening for 1 min after a contraction. For fetal monitoring, see p44.

The second stage *Passive stage* is complete cervical dilatation but no pushing. This is seen particularly in women with epidural anaesthesia where 1–2 hours of passive stage is recommended to reduce the instrumental delivery rate. In *active stage,* maternal pushing uses abdominal muscles and the Valsalva manoeuvre until the baby is born (see *Movement of head in labour,* p42). Discourage supine maternal position in 2nd stage. Encourage mother to adopt a comfortable position. Check BP and pulse hourly, T° 4-hourly , assess contractions half-hourly, auscultate for 1min after a contraction every 5 min, offer vaginal examination hourly, and record urination during 2nd stage. If contractions wane, oxytocin augmentation may be needed.

As the head descends, the perineum stretches and the anus gapes. Expect birth within 3h from active 2nd stage in primips (refer to obstetrician if not imminent at 2h); expect birth within 2h in a multip (refer if birth not imminent at 1h). Prevent a precipitate delivery (and so intracranial bleeding) by pressure over the perineum. 1-min delay in clamping the cord is recommended in vigorous term babies. 3-min delay benefits premature babies (↓ anaemia).[68]

The third stage is delivery of the placenta. As the uterus contracts to a <24-week size after the baby is born, the placenta separates from the uterus through the spongy layer of the decidua basalis. It then buckles and a small amount of retroplacental haemorrhage aids its removal.

Signs of separation: Cord lengthening → rush of blood (retroplacental haemorrhage) *per vaginam* → uterus rises → uterus contracts in the abdomen (felt with hand as a globular mass). Physiological (natural) 3rd stage takes ≤1h.

Use of Syntometrine® (**ergometrine maleate** 500mcg IM + **oxytocin** 5U IM) as the anterior shoulder is born decreases third stage time (to ~5min), and decreases the incidence of PPH. It can precipitate myocardial infarction and is contraindicated in those with pre-eclampsia, severe hypertension, severe liver or renal impairment, and severe heart disease. If BP not measured in labour give just **oxytocin**. Examine the placenta to check it is complete.

▶Is thromboprophylaxis needed? (p32)

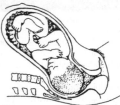

(1)
First stage of labour. The cervix
dilates. After full dilatation
the head flexes further and
descends further into the pelvis.

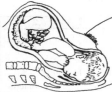

(2)
During the early second
stage the head rotates at
the levels of the ischial spine
so the occiput lies in the
anterior part of pelvis.
In late second stage the
head broaches the vulval ring
(crowning) and the perineum
stretches over the head.

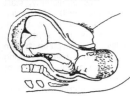

(3)
The head is born. The shoulders still lie
transversely in the midpelvis.

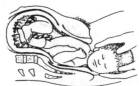

(4)
Birth of the anterior shoulder.
The shoulders rotate to lie in the
anteroposterior diameter of the
pelvic outlet. The head rotates
externally, 'restitutes', to its
direction at onset of labour.
Downward and backward traction
of the head by the birth attendant
aids delivery of the anterior shoulder.

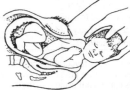

(5)
Birth of the posterior
shoulder is aided by lifting
the head upwards whilst
maintaining traction.

Fig 1.14 Normal labour.

~20% of UK labours are induced artificially, usually because it has been decided that to remain *in utero* is relatively more risky for the fetus than to be born, but in some it is because of risk to the mother. 75% of inductions are for hypertension, pre-eclampsia, prolonged pregnancy, or rhesus disease. Other indications are diabetes, previous stillbirth, abruption, fetal death *in utero*, and placental insufficiency.

▶Inducing mothers at 41+ weeks aims to reduce stillbirth rates.

Contraindications Malpresentations (including breech), fetal distress, placenta praevia, cord presentation, vasa praevia, pelvic tumour eg cervical fibroid.

Cervical assessment When an induction is being planned the state of the cervix will be assessed. If primips are induced with an unripe cervix (Bishop's score ≤3, see TABLE) the rates of prolonged labour, fetal distress, and caesarean section are increased. This is less marked in multips.

Modified Bishop score	0	1	2
Cervical dilation (cm)	0	1-2	3-4
Length of cervix (cm)	>2	1-2	<1
Station of head (cm above ischial spines)	-3	-2	-1
Cervical consistency	Firm	Medium	Soft
Position of cervix	Posterior	Middle	Anterior

A score of >5 is favourable and if >7, induction with artificial rupture of membranes should be possible, thereby avoiding prostaglandins. Induction of labour is carried out using prostaglandin PGE2 in the form of a 10mg/24h pessary or vaginal gel 1-3mg 6-hourly. The fetus should be monitored on CTG prior to prostaglandin use, and for 30min post-insertion. PGE2 may stimulate uterine contractions or precipitate labour. Failed induction prompts reassessment of the cervix by someone senior. If rupture of membranes is not possible, induction can be reconsidered 48 hours later or LSCS offered.

After artificial or spontaneous rupture of membranes (amniotomy), start intrapartum fetal heart rate monitoring using CTG (p44). If the liquor is clear, allow the woman to mobilize for 2-4 hours to allow spontaneous contractions to start. If she is not contracting after this time, start oxytocin IV in 0.9% saline using a pump system (eg Ivac®). Infusions start at 1-4 milliunits (MU) per min, increasing every 30min until 4 contractions occur every 10min (usually at a rate of 4-10MU/min: occasionally 20MU/min may be needed).

Monitor the fetal heart and stop if fetal distress or uterine hyperstimulation (>5 contractions in 10min with fetal compromise). Beware using large volumes of IV fluid (if >4 litres, there is risk of water intoxication—ie confusion, seizures, and coma). Use standard strength solutions as per *BNF*. Induction of labour in a woman with a previous caesarean section is controversial and senior advice should be sought due to the increased risk of scar rupture with prostaglandins and oxytocin infusions. Misoprostol (a prostaglandin E1 analogue) PO or PV is as effective at cervical ripening and inducing labour as PGE2 and oxytocin. Oral route (eg 50mcg 4-hourly) has fewer problems with uterine hyperstimulation.[69] NICE says only use this for labour induction after intrauterine death.

Problems with induction • Failed induction (15%) • Uterine hyperstimulation (1-5%) • Iatrogenic prematurity • Infection • Bleeding (vasa praevia) • Cord prolapse (eg with a high head at amniotomy) • Caesarean section (22%) and instrumental delivery rates (15%) are higher • Uterine rupture (rare).

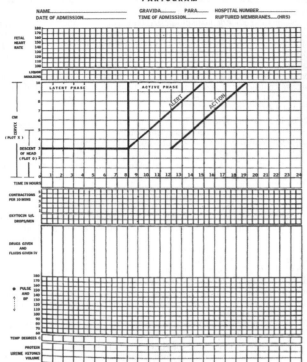

PARTOGRAM

NAME_____ GRAVIDA_____ PARA_____ HOSPITAL NUMBER_____
DATE OF ADMISSION_____ TIME OF ADMISSION_____ RUPTURED MEMBRANES____(HRS)

Fig 1.15 Example of a partogram. It has a steep x/y gradient of ratio 1:1. Less steep ratios (eg 2:1) may predispose to premature intervention, as does inclusion of the 'latent' phase on the partogram.

Reproduced from Collins et al, *Oxford Handbook of Obstetrics and Gynaecology* (2013) with permission from Oxford University Press.

The first stage of labour is divided into two stages: the latent phase and the active phase (p60). Adequate progress is that of 2cm dilatation per 4 hours of active labour (also see partogram (fig 1.15) on p63). However, other markers of progress are descent of the head and effacement of the cervix and these should also be taken into consideration. There is no absolute time limit for labour and progress is assessed dynamically throughout. The causes of poor progress are described according to *power, passenger, and passage*; poor uterine contractions (power) are the commonest cause; malpresentation or malposition or a large fetus (passenger); inadequate pelvis (passage) or a combination thereof.

Delay in 1st stage of labour This is <2cm/h dilatation in 4h in any woman; or slowing in progress in 2nd or subsequent labours.
• *Assess the woman*: Review her notes and obstetric / past obstetric history
• Palpate her abdomen for lie, head palpable, and contractions
• Check fetal heart rate and colour of amniotic fluid (meconium, blood stained)
• Vaginal assessment of dilatation, effacement, caput, moulding, station of the head, and position
• Does she need analgesia and rehydration?
• *Management:* Offer amniotomy and reassessment in 2 hours.
• If membranes are already ruptured, oxytocin infusion (to correct malposition and/or inefficient uterine activity) and reassessment in 4 hours. 8 hours of oxytocin may be needed before seeing a significant change. Start continuous fetal heart rate monitoring with oxytocin infusion.
• If the woman is multiparous or has had a previous LSCS, get senior advice; this is because oxytocin use in a multiparous uterus with no previous LSCS is associated with increased rates of rupture. Oxytocin use in a woman attempting vaginal birth after caesarean section also increases uterine rupture (from 50:10,000 with spontaneous labour to 8:1000 with oxytocin and 24:1000 with prostaglandin).
• If there are fetal heart rate concerns, perform FBS prior to commencing oxytocin augmentation.
• If there is slow progress after the above, consider LSCS.
• Offer epidural before starting oxytocin; also change maternal position to upright or left lateral if she is lying flat on her back!

Delay in 2nd stage of labour The active 2nd stage starts when the woman starts pushing. There is delay in a primip if delivery is not imminent after 1 hour of active pushing. She should be reviewed and if progress is being made and there are no fetal heart rate concerns she can push for up to 2 hours. If delivery not imminent at this point, she requires obstetric review for consideration of instrumental delivery or LSCS. A multiparous woman requires review after 1 hour of active pushing for consideration of instrumental delivery or LSCS.

Causes of delay are as for delay in the first stage, but also maternal exhaustion. For instrumental delivery, see p74.

Further reading

NICE (2014). *Intrapartum Care for Healthy Women and Babies* (CG190). London: NICE.

Pregnant women in the uk have a choice of giving birth at home, in midwifery-led units (MLU), or in a hospital. For those women wanting a home or MLU birth, they must have a low-risk pregnancy. Those women with risk factors are safer having a hospital delivery. Overall, home birth now accounts for ~2% of births in the uk, compared with 80% in the 1930s, but this varies significantly by area. GPs in practice rarely provide care for home births, although this is more likely in a very rural area.

Reasons to choose a home birth
• Own home where the woman is more likely to feel relaxed
• Fear of hospitals
• Continue care with a named midwife (labour wards are not staffed with community midwives as a rule, whereas her community midwife would be on call for her)
• Support from family members (hospitals limit the number of people allowed to be in the labour room and/or present for delivery)
• Previous home birth
• Previous bad experience in a hospital setting or with a hospital delivery
• To avoid intervention.

If a woman is booked for a home birth
• 29% change to consultant-led care (eg she develops a risk factor such as hypertension, or the baby is SGA)
• 30% of nulliparous woman and 15% of multiparous women transfer to hospital in labour, mostly for slow progress or pain relief
• Should there be an acute complication such as fetal hypoxia or maternal haemorrhage, the delay caused by transfer to hospital could lead to a worse outcome
• Neonatal resuscitation facilities are more limited at home
• Overall, perinatal mortality is slightly increased
• Maternal mortality is the same
• Obstetric intervention is lower, even in women transferred to hospital (but remember they are low risk and so at lower risk of intervention to start with)
• Apgar scores are higher with fewer neonatal respiratory problems.

Other things to consider include that the home environment is clean and that there is easy access for an ambulance. Midwives at a home delivery usually work as a pair, especially during the second stage.

Obstetrics

►Pain relief in labour is our greatest gift to womankind; labour is painful, especially if it has been induced or is being augmented with oxytocin. In the antenatal period, educating women on what to expect in labour, and the options for pain relief, help to reduce fear. The ideal analgesia must be harmless to mother and baby, must allow good maternal cooperation, and must not affect uterine contractility or maternal mobility.

Non-pharmacological methods

Education about labour reduces fear; breathing exercises and relaxation techniques teach the mother ways to cope with pain herself. The presence of a supportive *birth partner* reduces the need for pain relief as well as intervention. *Acupuncture, homeopathy, and hypnosis* may be helpful, but are not offered by the NHS. *Transcutaneous electrical nerve stimulation (TENS)* is safe and useful especially in shorter labours, and postpones use of stronger analgesia. NICE does not recommend its use in established labour. A TENS machine is a small, battery-operated device that connects to electrodes, which attach to the skin via self-adhesive pads. *Water birth:* Labouring in water has been shown to reduce need for regional anaesthesia. It is recommended by NICE with the advice that water temperature be checked hourly and kept <37.5°C to prevent maternal pyrexia. However, it is usually not possible for a high-risk woman on continuous monitoring to labour in water due to technical difficulties with CTG equipment underwater. Newer machines have waterproof attachments or remote monitoring facilities; not every room on a labour ward has a birthing pool.

Pharmacological methods

Nitrous oxide (50% in O_2 = Entonox®) can be inhaled throughout labour and is self-administered using a demand valve. CI: pneumothorax. It has a short onset of action and half-life, but SE include nausea, vomiting and feeling faint.

Narcotic agents such as pethidine and diamorphine should be available in all birth settings. They can provide limited pain relief during labour but may have significant SE for both mother (drowsiness, nausea, vomiting) and baby (short-term respiratory depression, and drowsiness which may last several days). They may also interfere with breastfeeding, and if given intramuscularly or intravenously should be given with an anti-emetic. Narcotic analgesia is a contraindication to entering the birthing pool within 2 hours of administration. Pethidine 50–150mg IM given with cyclizine 50mg IM is most commonly used. If regional anaesthesia is contraindicated (sepsis, low platelets, recent LMWH), consider setting up a PCA eg remifentanil, which is rapidly metabolized and unable to cross the placenta—get anaesthetic advice.

Pudendal nerve block (sacral nerve roots 2, 3, and 4) uses 8–10mL of 1% lidocaine (lignocaine) injected 1cm beyond a point just below and medial to the ischial spine on each side. It is used with perineal infiltration for instrumental delivery, but analgesia is insufficient for rotational forceps.

Local anaesthetic (lidocaine) infiltrated into the perineum is used before episiotomy at the time of delivery, and before suturing vaginal tears.

Regional anaesthesia

Epidural analgesia (fig 1.16) Pain relief is by anaesthetizing pain fibres carried by T10–S5. The woman should be fully consented before regional anaesthesia is given due to the small complication rate. Epidurals are safe and offer effective analgesia. There is reduced maternal catecholamine secretion. Epidurals can be regularly topped up (a catheter is left in the epidural space) and can help lower BP in pre-eclampsia. *Complications* include failure to site, patchy block, hypotension, dural puncture (<1:100) and post-dural puncture headache, transient or permanent nerve damage (extremely rare), and increased risk of operative vaginal delivery. Before siting an epidural, check platelet count is >75×10⁹, insert wide-bore IV access and gain consent. It can be inserted with the woman sitting or lying on her side. Full aseptic technique must be followed and L3/4 space is usually used. Once the epidural has been inserted, monitor BP every 5min for 20min, and record block height and density. Continuous electronic fetal monitoring is required. It is not uncommon to see a fetal bradycardia following epidural insertion due to maternal hypotension. Give IV fluids—it almost always recovers. Top-ups are required ~2-hourly. Recall anaesthetist if inadequate pain relief within 30min. If the epidural is used for LSCS, remember that the block will take longer to establish compared with spinal. *Epidurals, spinals, and LMWH:* Wait 12h after heparin dose before inserting block or removing catheter (24h if on therapeutic rather than prophylactic dose of heparin).₇ₒ Wait at least 4h after block siting before next dose of LMWH.

Combined spinal epidural (CSE) anaesthesia gives quicker pain relief, with the option of prolonging the anaesthesia with the epidural. CSE is sometimes used to cover a caesarean section with the potential to take more time than usual eg placenta praevia, or previous difficult surgery.

Spinal anaesthesia (fig 1.16) is used for most LSCS performed in the UK. They are relatively easier to insert than epidurals, produce a reliably dense block but because they are a single injection, may wear off if the procedure is prolonged (>2h) and can cause more profound hypotension compared with epidural.

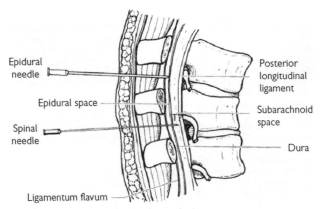

Fig 1.16 Epidural versus spinal regional anaesthesia.
Reproduced from Allman et al, *Oxford Handbook of Anaesthesia* (2011) with permission from Oxford University Press.

Further reading
NICE (2007) *Intrapartum Care: Management and Delivery of Care to Women in Labour.* (NICE Guideline CG55). London: NICE.

Incidence[uk] Twins: 3:200 pregnancies; triplets: 1:5000.

Predisposing factors Previous twins; FH of twins (dizygotic only); ↑ maternal age (<20yrs 6.4:1000, >25yrs 16.8:1000); induced ovulation and IVF (1% of all UK pregnancies of which 25% are ≥twins); race origin (1:150 pregnancies for Japanese, 1:23 in Nigerian Yoruba women). The worldwide rate for monozygotic (of which 75% monochorionic ie shared placenta) twins is constant at ~4:1000.

Features Early pregnancy: uterus large for dates; hyperemesis. Later there may be polyhydramnios. The signs are: >2 poles felt; a multiplicity of fetal parts felt; 2 fetal heart rates heard (reliable if rates differ by >10 beats/min). US confirms diagnosis (at 11^{+0}-13^{+6} weeks distinguishes monochorionic from dichorionic twins by placental masses, lambda sign in dichorionic).

Complications during pregnancy • Polyhydramnios • Pre-eclampsia (10% in singleton pregnancies; 30% in twins) • Anaemia commoner (iron and folate requirements increased) • APH incidence rises (6% for twins vs 4.7% for singletons) from both abruption and placenta praevia (large placenta) • Gestational diabetes • Operative delivery.

Fetal complications Perinatal mortality ↑ (8:1000 singletons; 36.7:1000 for twins; 73:1000 for triplets; 204:1000 for higher multiples). The main problem is prematurity. Mean gestation for twins is 37 weeks, for triplets 33 weeks. Growth restriction (p52) is commoner (growth rate=singletons until 24 weeks, may slow thereafter). Malformation rates ↑ ×2-4, especially if monozygotic. Selective feticide (eg with intracardiac potassium chloride)[1] is best used before 20 weeks in the rare instances where it is indicated. With monochorionic pregnancies, placental vascular anastomoses may result in disparate twin size and one twin acting as the 'donor' and the other the 'recipient' ie twin-twin transfusion syndrome (TTTS)[1]. Placental anastomoses can be ablated by laser coagulation *in utero*. Rarely, a fetus dying *in utero* shrinks and mummifies (fetus papyraceous) which may be delivered prematurely.

Complications of labour PPH (4-6% in singletons, 10% in twins). Malpresentation is common (cephalic (Ce)/Ce 40%, Ce/breech (Br) 40%, Br/Br 10%, Ce/transverse (Tr) 5%, Br/Tr 4%, Tr/Tr 1%). Vasa praevia rupture; cord prolapse (0.6% singleton, 2.3% twins); placental abruption and cord entanglement (especially monoamniotic).

Management
- US at 11^{+0}-13^{+6} weeks for viability, chorionicity, nuchal translucency, malformation: monthly from 20wks (2-weekly if monochorionic: membrane folding suggests TTTS). Name twins eg left, right. Discordant growth of ≥25% (suggests TTTS) indicates tertiary centre referral. Check FBC at 20-24 weeks. Give aspirin >12wks if other risks for pre-eclampsia.
- High-risk pregnancy for consultant-led care.
- More antenatal visits, eg weekly from 30 weeks (risk of eclampsia ↑).
- Tell the mother how to identify preterm labour, and what to do.
- Offer elective birth at 37^{+0}wks for uncomplicated dichorionic twins; at 36^{+0}wks (+steroids p51), for uncomplicated monochorionic twins; at 35^{+0} weeks (+steroids) for uncomplicated triplets.[18][NICE] Use IV access in labour and anaesthetist availability at delivery. Have paediatricians (one per baby) present at delivery in case resuscitation needed (2nd twins have a higher risk of asphyxia). Most newborns spontaneously deliver before these dates.
- Postnatal support groups for multiple pregnancy eg for breastfeeding.

Terminology *Monochorionic* twins or triplets share the placenta. If *monoamniotic* they share one amniotic sac; if di-amniotic there are 2 sacs, triamniotic, there are 3. One placenta risks fetofetal transfusion, 1 sac risks entanglements.

---

1 In monochorionic twins, total cord coagulation is required to avoid haemorrhage from the co-twin into the dying fetus. Potassium is CI (could pass to other twin).[71] Ethical and legal considerations are complex.

With >4 million IVF babies born worldwide since 1978 it is apparent that there are increased problems for pregnancy and offspring, not merely those of multiple pregnancy.[72] These are:

- Multiple birth: affects 1 in 4 IVF pregnancies. Monozygotic twins are also commoner. The rate of triplets was 5× pre-IVF rates by 1998 but are now only twice, as only 2 embryos are implanted into women <40 years old. Meta-analysis shows that 1 fresh embryo transfer with a frozen embryo months later if unsuccessful gives as good results as 2 embryos transfer.[73]
- Older mother effects: so more pre-eclampsia, pregnancy-induced hypertension, caesarean section delivery, and diabetes in the mothers (all of which have implications for offspring).
- Donor egg problems: pregnancy-induced hypertension is 7.1 times more common if nulliparous women receive donated eggs than for standard IVF.
- Genetic defects: Beckwith–Wiedemann syndrome is 6 times commoner in IVF babies and there is concern that intracytoplasmic sperm injection (ICSI) techniques could encourage chromosomal abnormalities or CF in offspring of men with azoospermia or oligospermia. Men with low sperm counts are now screened for CF carrier status and chromosomal abnormalities before referral for ICSI.
- Low birthweight is 1.75 times commoner for singleton IVF babies compared to naturally conceived babies (and very low birthweight 2.7-3 times commoner). Part of this is due to prematurity, part to growth restriction. Interestingly low birthweight is particularly correlated to the number of gestation sacs at earliest scan, even if a baby ends up as a singleton. IVF twins are less commonly low birthweight compared to naturally conceived twins. There is also some evidence to suggest a slightly higher rate of stillbirth.
- Vasa praevia (p8) rates increased, possibly up to 1:300.[74]
- Prematurity is twice as common in IVF singleton babies compared to those naturally conceived, 3 times more common for prematurity <32 weeks. Again it is commoner if there was originally >1 gestation sac. There is less difference between IVF and naturally conceived twins.
- Perinatal mortality is ↑ 60% in IVF conceived singletons (but natural conception after delay ↑ mortality ×3 compared to quick conception).
- Abnormality rates are slightly increased (in singletons too).

Bringing up one child is difficult: twins are often very very difficult—but triplets is more than very very very difficult—and are frequently a source of significant psychopathology. Even 4 years after their birth, all mothers in one triplets study[75] suffered from exhaustion and emotional distress. The relationship with the children was often difficult (aggression and conflicts). One-third of mothers had sufficient depression to require psychotropic medication, and one-third spontaneously expressed regrets about having triplets. If triplets are reduced to twins *in utero*, subsequently one-third of mothers will suffer emotional problems (persistent sadness and guilt) up to 1 year. However, adjustment had occurred in ~90% by 2 years after birth.[76]

Legislation in most developed countries is trying to limit the numbers of embryos that may be implanted at IVF in order to reduce higher-order pregnancies (already there has been a reduction by 25% since 1998). The UK current practice is moving to single embryo transfer in mothers <35yrs.

Breech presentation The commonest malpresentation: 40% of babies are breech at 20 weeks, 20% at 28 weeks, but only 3% at term. In pregnancy, it is normal for the buttocks to come to lie in the fundus. *Causes and associations:* • Idiopathic • Uterine abnormalities eg bicornuate uterus, fibroids • Prematurity • Placenta praevia • Oligohydramnios • Fetal abnormalities eg hydrocephalus. US may show the cause and influence the management.

Extended breech presentation is commonest (70%)—ie flexed at the hips but extended at the knees. *Flexed breeches* (15%) sit with hips and knees both flexed so that the presenting part is a mixture of buttocks, external genitalia, and feet. *Footling breeches* (15%) have the greatest risk of cord prolapse (5-20%).

Diagnosis of breech presentation Try to diagnose antenatally, but 30% present undiagnosed in labour. The mother may complain of pain under the ribs. On palpation the lie is longitudinal, no head is felt in the pelvis, and in the fundus there is a smooth round mass (the head) which can be ballotted, a sensation akin to quickly sinking an apple in water. Ultimately the diagnosis is made by US, or if the woman is labouring, feeling the breech vaginally.

External cephalic version (ECV)[77][RCOG]—turning the breech by manoeuvring it through a (usually forward), somersault. Turn the baby only if vaginal delivery planned, after 36-37 weeks. Success rate 40% primips, 60% multips. *ECV contraindications:* • Placenta praevia • Multiple pregnancy (except delivery of 2nd twin) • APH in last 7 days • Ruptured membranes • Growth restricted babies • Abnormal CTG • Mothers with uterine scars, uterine abnormality • Fetal abnormality • Pre-eclampsia, or hypertension (risk of abruption is increased). Monitor CTG (p44). Give anti-D (500U) to Rh–ve patients. Emergency caesarean rate after ECV is 1:200.

Mode of delivery The risk of fetal hypoxia and birth trauma is increased with vaginal delivery. Neonatal morbidity and mortality are increased irrespective of mode of delivery, possibly due to higher risk of congenital abnormalities and preterm babies being breech. Planned caesarean section may provide better outcome for the fetus and evidence suggests that the neonate is less likely to go to SCBU. Most breeches are delivered by LSCS and as a result, there is less experience with vaginal delivery. Evidence is less clear for preterm singletons and twins. (RCOG recommends caesarean if 1st twin breech; vaginal delivery if 2nd twin breech.) If vaginal delivery occurs, attendants experienced at breech delivery should be present. Contraindications to vaginal breech include inexperienced clinician, footling or kneeling breech, estimated fetal weight >3800 OR <2000g, previous LSCS and hyperextended fetal neck .

Vaginal breech delivery Approach with a 'hands-off' technique: the baby is not touched by the birth attendant until the scapulae are visible. Encourage the baby to remain so that the spine is anterior (may need to be gently rotated). Once the scapulae are visible, hook the arms at the elbow; if arms not visible, rotate the body in each direction to allow delivery of the arms. Allow the body to hang and once the nape of the neck is visible, place two fingers of the right hand over the maxilla, and two fingers from the left hand over the occiput to flex the head (Mauriceau–Smellie–Veit manoeuvre). If this fails, forceps are used to deliver the head. A neonatal doctor should be present for a vaginal breech delivery because the most difficult and risky part is delivery of the head.

▶Check baby for hip dislocation at birth and by US at 6 weeks (↑incidence): also, if vaginal delivery, for Klumpke's paralysis (p750) and signs of CNS injury.

Obstetrics

Obstetrics

Occipitoposterior position (OP) In 50% of patients the mothers have a long 'anthropoid' pelvis. Diagnosis may be made antenatally by palpation (p4). On vaginal examination the posterior fontanelle will be found to lie in the posterior quadrant of the pelvis. Labour tends to be prolonged because of the degree of rotation needed, so adequate hydration and analgesia (consider epidural) are important. During labour 65% rotate 130° so that the head is occipitoanterior at the time of birth, 20% rotate to the transverse and then arrest ('deep transverse arrest'), 15% rotate so that the occiput lies truly posterior and birth is by flexion of the head from the perineum. Although in 73% delivery will be a normal vaginal delivery, 22% will require forceps and 5% a caesarean section.

Face presentation (fig 1.17) Incidence 1:600–1:1500. 15% are due to congenital abnormality such as anencephaly, tumour of or shortened fetal neck muscles. Most occur by chance as the head extends rather than flexes as it engages. On early vaginal examination, the nose and eyes may be felt but later this will not be possible because of oedema. Most engage in the transverse (mentobregmatic diameter ≈9.5cm). 90% rotate so that the chin lies behind the symphysis (mentoanterior) and the head can be born by flexion. If the chin rotates to the sacrum (mentoposterior), caesarean section is indicated. Ventouse is contraindicated but forceps delivery is possible if the head is well below the spines.

Brow presentation (fig 1.17) This occurs in 1:1000–1:3500 deliveries. The head is between full flexion and full extension, and may revert to either. If it persists, vaginal delivery is not possible. Most of the time, it is diagnosed in advanced labour. On vaginal examination the anterior fontanelle and supraorbital ridges may be felt. Management is expectant; if progress is slow or brow presentation persists, delivery by LSCS is indicated.

Transverse lie (compound shoulder presentation) Antenatal diagnosis: ovoid uterus wider at the sides, the lower pole is empty, the head lies in one flank, the fetal heart is heard in variable positions. On vaginal examination with membranes intact no distinguishing features may be felt, but if ruptured and the cervix dilated, ribs, shoulder, or a prolapsed hand or cord may be felt. The risk of cord prolapse is high. If malpresentation persists or ECV at 37 weeks fails, caesarean section will be necessary. Those with persistent instability of lie need hospital admission from 37 weeks (to prevent cord prolapse at home when the membranes rupture) and decision as to elective caesarean section.

Typical causes
• Multiparity
• Multiple pregnancy
• Polyhydramnios
• Placenta praevia
• Arcuate/septate uterus
• Contracted pelvis.

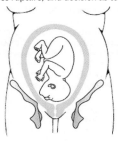

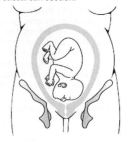

(a) Brow presentation   (b) Face presentation

Fig 1.17 (a) Brow presentation; (b) face presentation.

This is descent of the cord through the cervix, below the presenting part, after rupture of membranes. It is an emergency because cord compression and vasospasm from exposure of the cord causes fetal asphyxia.

Incidence 0.1–0.6%; ↑ if: 2nd twin, footling breech, prematurity, polyhydramnios, unengaged head, transverse or unstable lie, male. If cord presentation is noted prior to membrane rupture, carry out caesarean section. Whenever you rupture membranes, remember that cord prolapse is possible, eg if the presenting part is poorly applied.

Presentation The problem is obvious if the cord is at the introitus. But the only sign may be fetal bradycardia or variable fetal heart decelerations: always do a vaginal exam in this context to exclude prolapsed cord.

Action Get senior help. Activate alarms. Tell labour ward. Keep cord in vagina (minimal handling prevents spasm). Stop the presenting part from occluding the cord: The aim is to deliver the fetus as quickly as possible, either by LSCS or instrumental if the woman is fully dilated. The steps below are to minimize cord compression and vasospasm:

▶▶ Displace the presenting part by putting a hand in the vagina; push it back up (towards mother's head) during contractions. NB: there is little evidence that replacing the cord above the presenting part helps (*not* recommended).[78 RCOG]

▶▶ Knee-to-chest position so that her bottom is higher than her head.

▶▶ Infuse 500mL saline into bladder via an IVI giving set taped to a catheter(16G). Remember to empty the bladder before any attempt at delivery/extraction.

▶▶ Tocolysis (**terbutaline** 0.25mg sc) reduces contractions and helps bradycardia.

If cervix fully dilated and the presenting part is low in pelvis, delivery by ventouse/forceps (if cephalic) or by breech extraction (by an experienced obstetrician) is best if it leads to birth in <15min. The neonatal team should be present at delivery and paired cord blood samples taken for pH and base excess (if normal, intrapartum hypoxic brain injury is 'excluded').

▶▶Shoulder dystocia

RCOG definition A delivery requiring additional obstetric manoeuvres to release the shoulders after gentle downward traction has failed. The incidence is 1:200 deliveries (UK and USA). There can be high rate of fetal mortality and morbidity. Postpartum haemorrhage occurs in 11% of mothers and 3.8% get 4th degree perineal tears whether or not manoeuvres are used. Brachial plexus injuries occur in 4–16% (1:2300 live births UK) of which 10% are left with permanent disability. A common cause of litigation: note which shoulder is anterior as posterior shoulder injuries are not considered due to the birth attendant (maternal propulsive forces may contribute to injuries).

Associations •Large/postmature fetus (but most babies >4800g do not develop it and 48% that do weigh <4000g), maternal BMI >30kg/m² •Induced or oxytocin augmented labours •Prolonged 1st or 2nd stage or secondary arrest •Assisted vaginal delivery •Previous shoulder dystocia (1–16%). Most occur in women with no risk factors. •Diabetes mellitus. ▶Suggest caesarean delivery to diabetic mothers with fetuses >4500g; discuss antenatally if previous shoulder dystocia.

Management The danger is death from asphyxia. ▶▶Speed is vital as the cord is usually squashed at the pelvic inlet; prompt and rehearsed shoulder dystocia drills (part of every labour ward mandatory training) improves outcome.

•*Help*: extra midwives, labour ward coordinator, senior obstetrician, neonatologist, anaesthetist and a scribe for timing of manoeuvres.

•*Episiotomy*: to give space for internal manoeuvres. The episiotomy itself won't relieve the shoulder dystocia.

•*Legs:* place in McRoberts (hyperflexed lithotomy) position. It is successful in 90%. Abduct, rotate outwards, and flex maternal femora so each thigh touches the abdomen (1 assistant to hold each leg). This straightens the sacrum relative to the lumbar spine and rotates the symphysis superiorly helping the impacted shoulder to enter the pelvis without manipulating the fetus.

- *Suprapubic pressure* with flat of hand laterally in the direction baby is facing, and towards mother's sacrum, continuously or with a rocking motion. Apply steady traction to the fetal head. This aims to displace the anterior shoulder allowing it to enter the pelvis.
- *Enter the pelvis* for internal manoeuvres; these aim to rotate the fetal shoulders to the oblique diameter. If this fails, rotation by 180° so posterior shoulder now lies anteriorly may work, as may *delivery of the posterior arm*.
- *Roll* the mother on to all fours if these fail.
- In practice, if McRoberts and suprapubic pressure fails, attempt whichever internal manoeuvre you are most confident with.
- *Other manoeuvres* include maternal symphysiotomy; or replacement of the fetal head by firm pressure of the hand to reverse the movements of labour and return the head to the flexed occipito-anterior position and caesarean delivery (Zavanelli). The baby is likely to be severely acidotic at this stage.
- If the baby dies prior to delivery, cutting through both clavicles (cleidotomy) with strong scissors assists delivery.
- Check the baby for damage, eg Erb's palsy (fig 1.18, p76) or fractured clavicle.
- Beware PPH or 3rd/4th degree vaginal tears in the mother.

In the notes, record time of delivery of head; direction head faced after restitution; manoeuvres (timing & sequence); time of delivery of body; who and when present; Apgar of baby at birth; umbilical cord blood acid–base measurement. Debrief both the team and the mother.

Obstetrics

Meconium-stained liquor

In late pregnancy, it is normal for some babies to pass meconium (bowel contents), which stains the amniotic fluid a dull green. This is not significant. During labour, fresh meconium, which is dark green, sticky, and lumpy, may be passed. This may be a response to the stress of a normal labour, or a sign of distress, so transfer to a consultant-led unit and commence continuous fetal heart rate monitoring (p44). Prelabour rupture of membranes with meconium-stained liquor requires immediate induction of labour in an obstetric-led unit with advanced neonatal life support available.

Aspiration of fresh meconium can cause severe pneumonitis (meconium aspiration syndrome) and occurs in 1:1000 deliveries. Routine suction of nasopharynx and oropharynx prior to birth is not recommended. Only suction airway if there is thick meconium in oropharynx and the baby requires resuscitation. Have a healthcare professional trained in advanced neonatal support in attendance (p107) to suck out pharynx and trachea under direct vision using a laryngoscope if the baby has depressed vital signs. Observe babies for 12 hours.

Further reading

NICE (2007) *Intrapartum Care: Management and Delivery of Care to Women in Labour* (NICE Guideline CG55). London: NICE.

RCOG (2012): *Shoulder Dystocia* (Green-top Guideline No.42). London: RCOG.

Operative vaginal delivery (the use of an instrument to aid delivery) occurs in 10–15% of births in the UK. A companion in labour, an upright or lateral position for delivery, and delay in pushing with epidural, reduce the need for operative deliveries. If an instrumental delivery is not possible or fails, LSCS in the second stage of labour becomes the only method to deliver the baby, and this is associated with increased morbidity to the mother. Forceps and ventouse have different characteristics and uses, and the woman should be fully informed and verbally consented before undertaking this type of delivery. Only an experienced operator may undertake an instrumental delivery. The term 'trial' may be used and refers to a situation where the operator is uncertain if instrumental vaginal delivery will be successful. A trial therefore takes place in theatre where immediate LSCS can be carried out. This requires written consent, and failure is more likely if BMI >30, suspected large baby, OP position, and with a mid-cavity delivery (head at or 1cm below spines). 2nd-stage LSCS requires senior support.

Criteria for use
• Consent for and explain the procedure
• 1/5th or less head palpable per abdomen
• Ruptured membranes
• Adequate analgesia: epidural or pudendal block
• Adequate contractions
• Bladder empty and catheter balloon deflated
• Fully dilated cervix with head at ischial spines or below
• Check presentation (must be cephalic) and position of head
• Check instrument ie forceps lock
• Once instrument applied, recheck position and that no maternal tissues are caught
• Neonatal doctor in attendance.

Indications for operative vaginal delivery

Maternal
• Prolonged second stage for any reason; this may be due to fetal malposition such as OP or OT positions, or due to dense epidural block and diminished urge to push
• Maternal exhaustion
• Medical avoidance of pushing eg severe cardiac disease
• Pushing not possible eg tetraplegia or paraplegia.

Fetal
• Suspected fetal distress
• For the after-coming head in a breech delivery.

Specific indications for forceps
• Assisted breech delivery, forceps to deliver head
• Assisted delivery of preterm infant <34 weeks' gestation
• Controlled delivery of head at caesarean section
• Assisted delivery with face presentation
• Assisted delivery with suspected coagulopathy or thrombocytopenia in fetus (but note coagulopathy is a relative CI to forceps)
• Instrumental delivery where maternal condition precludes pushing (eg cardiac disease, respiratory disease)
• Cord prolapse in second stage of labour
• Instrumental delivery under GA
• Presence of significant caput (fetal head swelling secondary to labour)

▶Abandon operative vaginal delivery if no progression with each pull and delivery not imminent with 3 pulls by experienced operator.

Forceps

These consist of curved blades designed to fit around the fetal head, allowing traction to be applied via handles. They require much less maternal effort for successful delivery than ventouse and are therefore less likely to fail. There are several different type of forceps (see fig 1.19). Forceps may be safer for the baby, but can cause significant maternal genital tract trauma (and they add 1cm to the diameter of the head).

Low cavity forceps (eg Wrigley's) are used for 'lift out' deliveries, when the head is on the perineum. They have a short shank and are lighter in weight. They are sometimes used at LSCS to help control delivery of the head.

Mid-cavity non-rotational forceps (Neville-Barnes; Simpson's) have a long shank, cephalic and pelvic curves, and must only be used when the sagittal suture lies in the AP diameter. The blades are placed one by one in-between contractions.

Mid-cavity rotational forceps (Kielland's) have a reduced pelvic curve, making them suitable for rotation (only in experienced hands).

Ventouse (vacuum extraction)

This technique uses a suction device to suck fetal scalp tissues into a ventouse cup. The artificial caput (swelling) created is called a chignon, and takes 24–48 hours to resolve (and is something the mother should be warned of). The baby must be >34 weeks' gestation with no maternal coagulopathy. Ventouse is associated with less genital tract trauma than forceps but is more likely to cause fetal trauma (cephalohaematoma and retinal haemorrhage) and more likely to fail. Like with forceps, there are different types of ventouse available (fig 1.20) including the metal cup, soft cup, and most commonly, the Kiwi OmniCup (a single use cup with hand pump).

See fig 1.19 and fig 1.20 on p77 for images.

Complications of operative vaginal delivery
- Maternal genital tract trauma, especially with forceps; includes obstetric anal sphincter injury
- Spiral vaginal tears with rotational forceps deliveries
- Fetal injuries with forceps (rare):
  - Facial nerve palsy
  - Skull fractures
  - Orbital injury
  - Intracranial haemorrhage
- Fetal injuries with ventouse:
  - Cephalhaematoma (most common)
  - Retinal haemorrhage
  - Scalp lacerations and scalp avulsions (more common if >3 pulls used).

▶ The use of sequential instruments should be avoided where possible because the rate of complications is increased, hence the need for choosing the initial instrument wisely. Women in labour and in their birth plans frequently ask for forceps to be avoided—but a well-planned and straightforward forceps delivery is much better for both mother and baby than a failed ventouse followed by a forceps.

When to abandon an operative vaginal delivery
- No descent with each subsequent pull
- Delivery not imminent after 3 pulls when the instrument is correctly applied and the operator is experienced
- Proceeding to emergency LSCS: the head may be impacted in the pelvis and difficult to deliver.

After delivery Give vitamin K (p120). Give regular analgesia. Document time and volume of 1st void urine (catheterize for 12h if epidural or spinal). Pass catheter if residual suspected. Is thromboprophylaxis needed (p32)? Discuss future delivery; >80% will be vaginal but individual plan if 3rd- or 4th-degree tear with this delivery.

Obstetric brachial plexus injury (OBPI)

OBPI complicates <0.5% of live births.

Risk factors Large birthweight; shoulder dystocia with prolonged 2nd stage of labour; forceps delivery; vacuum extraction; diabetes mellitus; breech presentation. Formerly, the cause of OBPI was excessive lateral traction applied to the fetal head at delivery, in association with anterior shoulder dystocia.

Instrumental-associated OBPI may arise because of nerve stretch injuries after rotations of >90° or from direct compression of the forceps blade in the fetal neck.[79] Not all cases of brachial plexus palsy are attributable to traction. Intrauterine factors may play some role.[80]

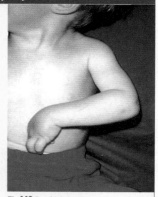

Fig 1.18 Brachial plexus injury.

Management 10–20% need surgical intervention for optimal results.[81]

Some injuries will be permanent.[82] See p750 for orthopaedic insights.

Obstetrics

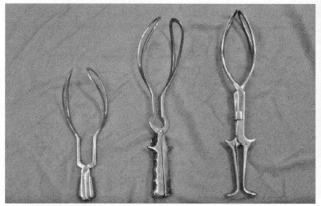

Fig 1.19 Forceps, from left to right: outlet forceps (also known as Wrigleys) for use during an outlet vaginal delivery or at cs; non-rotational forceps (Neville-Barnes or Simpson's) for direct oa or op vaginal delivery and have a pelvic curve; and rotational forceps (Kjellands)which have no pelvic curve, to enable rotation without damaging maternal tissues. Rotational forceps also have a sliding lock mechanism.

Reproduced from Collins et al, *Oxford Handbook of Obstetrics and Gynaecology* (2013) with permission from Oxford University Press.

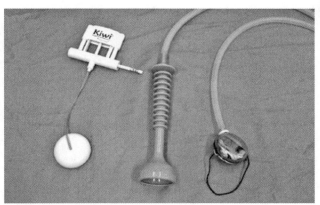

Fig 1.20 Ventouse, from left to right: the Kiwi, a plastic hand-held deivce with a hand pump, commonly used in units around the uk. The silicone cup, which is attached to a separate suction pump and foot pedal, and the metal cup, which is again attached to a separate pump and foot pedal.

With permission of Clinical Innovations Europe Ltd, 2008, and Menox AB, Goteborg, Sweden, 2008.

This is the delivery of a fetus through an incision in the abdominal wall and uterus. In the UK, 24% of nulliparous women deliver by cs (<5% in a multip with no previous cs). Having a previous caesarean is the biggest predictor of having another (67% in the next pregnancy, mostly elective).

Maternal mortality: ~1 per 100,000. Morbidity is higher with emergency operations—eg infection, ileus, and thromboembolism. For 1st operations 25% are due to failure to progress, 28% for fetal distress, 14% for breech. Use of support in labour, induction at 41 weeks, consultant involvement in decision to section, fetal blood sampling when fetal monitoring is used, and use of a 4h partogram with action line all help reduce incidence of caesarean sections. 9:1000 will require ITU care.

Types of caesarean section

Lower uterine segment incision Joel Cohen skin incision (straight incision 3cm above symphysis pubis) with blunt dissection thereafter is recommended (reduces blood loss). Transverse incision in the lower segment is associated with reduced adhesion formation, lower blood loss, and lower risk of scar dehiscence in subsequent pregnancies. Fetal laceration rate is 1-2%.

Classical cs (vertical incision on uterus, with either transverse or vertical skin incision): Rarely used. Indications: • Very premature fetus, lower segment poorly formed • Fetus lies transverse, with ruptured membranes • Structural abnormality makes lower segment use impossible • Fibroids positioned such that lower segment incision is not possible • Some anterior placenta praevias when lower segment abnormally vascular • Maternal cardiac arrest and rapid birth desired (but LSCS may be quicker if operator more experienced with this method). A classical cs is associated with more adhesion formation and infection, and is a contraindication to attempting vaginal delivery subsequently.

Indications are varied and many; here are some examples:
• Repeat cs
• Fetal compromise such as fetal bradycardia, scalp pH <7.20, cord prolapse
• Failure to progress in labour, or failed induction of labour
• Malpresentation eg breech, transverse lie
• Severe pre-eclampsia and induction of labour unlikely to be successful
• IUGR with absent or reversed end-diastolic flow
• Twin pregnancy with non-cephalic presenting twin
• Placenta praevia.

Category of cs determines the timing and is dependent on the indication.

Category 1 (crash) is for immediate threat to life of woman or fetus and the baby should be delivered within 30min of the decision being made; eg placental abruption, fetal bradycardia. *Category 2* is for maternal or fetal compromise, not immediately life-threatening (30–60min) eg failure to progress. *Category 3* is also thought of as semi-elective eg pre-eclampsia, or failed induction of labour, and *Category 4* is elective eg term singleton breech. Elective cs should be carried out after 39 weeks, unless maternal or fetal indications arise, to reduce the incidence of transient tachypnoea of the newborn. If elective delivery is planned for <39 weeks, corticosteroids should be given for fetal lung maturity.

Complications are most common with emergency cs (which itself may be considered by some to be a complication of failed vaginal delivery). *Intraoperative* complications include blood loss >1L (7–9%), uterine lacerations/extensions beyond the uterine incision, blood transfusion (2–3%), bladder laceration (0.5%), bowel injury (0.05%), ureteral injury (0.03–0.09%) and hysterectomy (0.2%). Haemorrhage is more likely with placenta praevia or abruption, extremes of birth weight and maternal obesity. *Postoperative* complications most commonly involve wound infections, endometritis, and UTI. Venous thromboembolism is more common and every woman with emergency CS should have 7 days of prophylactic LMWH. High BMI is independently associated with infection, along with chorioamnionitis, pre-eclampsia, and increased surgical blood loss. *Before undertaking any CS* check placental site to exclude praevia, and if previous LSCS, accreta, or percreta.

Before an emergency section ►Explain to the mother what is to happen and take written consent.

• Activate the anaesthetist, theatre staff, porters, and paediatrician.
• Get senior help—in the daytime, senior obstetric staff should be present.
• Neutralize gastric contents with 20mL of 0.3 molar sodium citrate, and promote gastric emptying with metoclopramide 10mg IV. (NB: there is no time for H_2 agonists to work; ranitidine is kept for elective sections, eg 150mg PO 2h before surgery). The stomach should be routinely emptied prior to extubation to minimize risk of post-operative aspiration. See Mendelson's syndrome, p80.
• Take blood for group and save and/or crossmatch, eg 2u; if for abruption; if placenta praevia insert 2nd IV line and cross-match 6u.
• Take to theatre (awake); set up IVI.
• Catheterize the bladder. Tilt 15° to her left side on operating table.
• Ensure neonatologist is present before starting.
• Offer prophylactic antibiotics and give before skin incision.[45][NICE]

►In reducing maternal mortality, the importance of having an experienced anaesthetist is vital. When appropriate, offer regional anaesthesia. Document indication for and urgency of operation. Note: in 2002-3 only 8% of caesarean sections were under GA.

Management of women already on thromboprophylaxis[70][RCOL] If on high dose or 75% of weight-adjusted therapeutic dose prophylaxis (see p32) halve to same dose/24h as was previously being given/12h, on the day before planned caesarean. For all on prophylaxis omit dose on morning of caesarean and give 3h post-op unless epidural used: see p66. 2% of women will get a wound haematoma.

After CS[NICE] Give one-to-one support in recovery unit. Aim for baby/mother skin to skin contact (beware chilling baby). Check pulse, respiratory rate (RR), BP, and sedation levels at least half hourly for 1st 2h, then hourly for 24h and until 2h after epidural or patient-controlled opiate analgesia discontinued. Use MEOWS (Modified Early obstetric warning score chart). After epidural, remove urinary catheters when mobile or 12h after last top-up dose (whichever is later). After GA, give extra midwife support to help establish breastfeeding. Mobilize early. Remove wound dressing at 24h. Give analgesia (ibuprofen + paracetamol with morphine for break-through pain). Average hospital stay is 2-3 days but mothers can be discharged after 24h if they wish and are well. Discuss reason for CS, birth options in future, and contraception.

Long-term effects of CS In subsequent pregnancies, there is a higher incidence of placenta praevia and accreta. The risk of uterine rupture is also increased to 1:200 with spontaneous labour (almost unheard of in nulliparous UK women). Risk of antepartum stillbirth in the next pregnancy doubles, and the cause is unclear. In those undergoing multiple CS, surgical risks increase with each subsequent CS.

Obstetrics

Ruptured uterus is rare in the UK (0.5–2:10 000 deliveries in an unscarred uterus but 1:100 deliveries in parts of Africa). Associated maternal mortality is 5%, and the fetal mortality 30%. ~70% of UK ruptures are due to dehiscence of CS scars. Lower-segment scars are far less likely to rupture (<0.74%) than the classical scars (2–9%)—see p78. Other risk factors: •Obstructed labour in the multiparous, especially if oxytocin is used •Previous cervical or uterine surgery •High forceps delivery (high station of head eg above the spines is a contraindication to instrumental delivery) •Internal version •Breech extraction. Rupture is usually during the 3rd trimester or in labour.

Vaginal birth after caesarean (trial of scar) Vaginal birth will be successful in 72–76%. Endometritis, need for blood transfusion, uterine rupture, and perinatal death (↑ by 2–3:10,000 births—mainly due to increased stillbirth at around 39 weeks: this increases mortality to that of a firstborn) are commoner than with elective repeat caesarean. Neonatal respiratory problems are, however, reduced. 24–28% undergo repeat emergency section. Of 9 ruptures in 4021 women undergoing VBAC there were no maternal or fetal deaths.[85] Use continuous electronic fetal monitoring in labour.

Signs and symptoms Rupture is usually in labour. In a few (usually a caesarean scar dehiscence) rupture precedes labour. Pain is variable, some only having slight pain and tenderness over the uterus. In others pain is severe. Vaginal bleeding is variable and may be slight (bleeding is intraperitoneal). Unexplained maternal tachycardia, sudden maternal shock, cessation of contractions, disappearance of the presenting part from the pelvis, and fetal distress are other presentations. *Postpartum indicators of rupture*: continuous PPH with a well-contracted uterus; if bleeding continues postpartum after vaginal repair; and whenever shock is present.

Management If suspected in labour, perform category 1 CS (p78), and explore the uterus. ▶▶ •Give O₂ at 15L/min via a tight-fitting mask with reservoir •Set up IVI •Crossmatch 6U of blood and correct shock by fast transfusion. The type of operation performed should be decided by a senior obstetrician; if the rupture is small, repair may be carried out; if the cervix or vagina are involved in the tear, hysterectomy may be necessary. Care is needed to identify the ureters and exclude them from sutures. Give post-operative antibiotic cover, eg cefuroxime 1.5g/8h IV and metronidazole 500mg/8h.

▶▶Mendelson's syndrome

This is the name given to the cyanosis, bronchospasm, pulmonary oedema, and tachycardia that develop due to inhalation of gastric acid during general anaesthesia. Clinically it may be difficult to distinguish from cardiac failure or amniotic fluid embolism. Pre-operative H₂ antagonists, sodium citrate, gastric emptying, cricoid pressure (see fig 9.9, p629), the use of cuffed endotracheal tubes during anaesthesia, and pre-extubation emptying of stomach aim to prevent it (p79).

Management ▶▶Tilt the patient head down. Turn her to one side and aspirate the pharynx. Give 100% O₂. Give aminophylline 5mg/kg by slow IVI and hydrocortisone 200mg IV stat.[86] The bronchial tree should be sucked out using a bronchoscope under general anaesthesia. Antibiotics should be given to prevent secondary pneumonia. Ventilation conducted on intensive care may be needed. Physiotherapy should be given during recovery.

Obstetrics

Stillbirths are those babies born dead after (but that were alive at—see BOX) 24 weeks' completed gestation. Rate: 1:200 total births. Death *in utero* can occur at any stage of pregnancy or labour. Delivery is an emotional strain for mother and attendant staff: labour may seem futile, mothers may feel guilty—or punished.

Some hours after a fetus has died *in utero* the skin begins to peel. At delivery such fetuses are described as *macerated*, as opposed to *fresh* stillbirths. If left, spontaneous labour usually occurs (80% within 2 weeks, 90% within 3 weeks). Coagulopathy (p88) occurs in 10% within 4 weeks of late IUD: 30% thereafter.

Causes of stillbirth (CMACE 2009) No cause found (28%), placental cause (12%), ante- or intrapartum haemorrhage (11%), major congenital anomaly (9%), infection (5%), hypertension in pregnancy (6%), maternal disease (renal, diabetes 5%), IUGR (7%), mechanical eg cord prolapse, knot in cord (8%). Multiple pregnancy ↑ risk (16.6:1000). Social deprivation, increasing maternal age, smoking, previous CS, IVF, and obesity increase incidence.

Diagnosis The mother usually reports absent fetal movements. No fetal heart sounds (unreliable). Diagnose by absent fetal heart beat on US. It may help the mother to see lack of heart beat. Mothers sometimes feel passive movements after death. Repeat US, if mother requests. If mother alone at diagnosis; offer to call a companion.

Management ▶If mother Rh−ve give anti-D (see BOX, p11). Do Kleihauer on *all* women to diagnose fetomaternal haemorrhage (FMH)—a cause of stillbirth; and to determine anti-D dose. If large FMH diagnosed; repeat Kleihauer at 48h to check fetal cells cleared. Check maternal T°, BP, urine for protein, and blood clotting screen if fetus not thought recently demised. Advise delivery if preeclampsia, abruption, sepsis, coagulopathy, or membrane rupture. If safe, the mother may want to go home after diagnosis to reflect, collect things, and make arrangements. If not induced in 48h check for coagulopathy twice weekly. Labour is induced using mifepristone orally, adding prostaglandin vaginally. Oxytocin augmentation may be needed later. If uterine scar, seek consultant advice re induction/augmentation. Deliver away from sounds of babies, if possible.

Ensure good pain relief in labour (if epidural, check clotting tests all normal and no sepsis). Do not leave the mother unattended. When the baby is born wrap it (as with any other baby) and offer to the mother to see and to hold—if she wishes. Photographs should be taken for her to take home, a lock of the baby's hair and palm-print given (keep in notes for later if not wanted). Unseen babies can be difficult to grieve for. Naming the baby and holding a funeral service may help with grief. Remember thromboprophylaxis if needed (p32). Discuss lactation suppression and contraception.

Tests to establish cause *Maternal tests:* Kleihauer (above); FBC, CRP, LFT, TFT, HbA1c, glucose, blood culture, viral screen (TORCH (Toxoplasmosis, Other, Rubella, CMV, Herpes) etc. screen p35), thrombophilia screen, antibodies (anti-red cell, anti-Ro, anti-La, alloimmune antiplatelet, if indicated[87], MSU, urine for cocaine (if indicated and permission given), cervical swabs.[87]

Fetal tests: Fetal and placental swabs. Cord blood in lithium heparin tube for infection. Thorough examination of the baby. Take time to talk to parents about how helpful a post-mortem may be to them, in understanding what happened, and planning further pregnancies. If post-mortem is refused, MRI (may miss significant pathology and is not routinely available), cytogenetics (use fetal skin, cartilage, and placenta, this can also be used for sexing babies which may be difficult in macerated and very premature stillbirths) ± small volumes of tissue for metabolic studies, and placental histology may be acceptable but are less informative and still need written parental consent.

Further reading
RCOG (2010). *Late Intrauterine Fetal Death and Stillbirth* (Green-top Guideline No. 55). London: RCOG.

- Give parents a follow-up appointment to discuss causes found by the tests described on p82. Consider a home visit if parents prefer. Refer for genetic counselling if appropriate.

- In England, a *Certificate of Stillbirth* is required (issued by obstetrician or midwife attending birth), that the mother or father is required to take to the Registrar of Births and Deaths within 42 days (21 days in Scotland, 5 days in Northern Ireland) of birth for fetuses born after 24 weeks' completed gestation. If there is developmental or us evidence that the fetus was not alive at 24 completed weeks' gestation (eg in cases of fetus papyraceous, or after selective fetal reduction before 24 weeks), then such a certificate is not issued,[88][RCOG] but evidence for the fact why the fetus is not believed to have been alive at 24 completed weeks should be written in the woman's notes. The father's name only appears in the register if the parents are married, or if both parents make the registration, or the father signs a Form of Declaration (available from Registrar). Registration can be delegated to a health care professional or hospital bereavement officer.

- The Registrar then issues a Certificate of Burial or Cremation which the parents then give to the undertaker (if they have chosen a private funeral—in which case they bear the cost of the funeral), or to the hospital administrators if they have chosen a hospital funeral—for which the hospital bears the cost. Parents are issued with a Certificate of Registration to keep which has the name of the stillborn baby (if named), the name of the informant who made the registration, and the date of stillbirth.

- UK hospitals are directed by the Department for Work and Pensions to offer 'hospital' funerals for stillborn babies (arranged through an undertaker). If the parents offer to pay for this, the hospital may accept. The hospital should notify the parents of the time of the funeral so that they may attend, if they wish. With hospital funerals a coffin is provided and burial is often in a multiple-occupancy grave in a part of the graveyard set aside for babies. The hospital should inform parents of the site of the grave. Graves are unmarked, so should the parents not attend the funeral and wish to visit later it is recommended that they contact the graveyard attendants for the grave to be temporarily marked. Parents may buy a single occupancy grave, if they wish, on which they can later erect a headstone. Hospitals can arrange cremations, but the parents pay for this. Tell parents that there may not be any ashes after cremation.

- Arrange a follow-up appointment with the obstetrician to discuss implications for future pregnancy, and the cause (if known) of the stillbirth. Give parents the address of a local branch of an organization for bereavement counselling, eg SANDS.[89] Grief may take a long time to resolve (p498) and parents may find it difficult to contact ordinary medical staff.

Each maternity unit should have a bereavement counsellor to support the parents, and help guide them through the formalities, as well as ensuring they are aware of the resources and support available.

In the UK, statutory maternity pay and the maternity allowance and social fund maternity payments are payable after stillbirth.

After stillbirth Be vigilant to possible depression. In next pregnancy after stillbirth recommend obstetrician antenatal care and delivery, and screen for diabetes. If there was evidence of growth restriction, assess growth by serial us biometry in subsequent pregnancies.[87][RCOG]

Primary PPH is the loss of >500mL in the first 24h after delivery. This occurs after ~6% of deliveries; major PPH (>1 litre) in 1.3%. *Causes (4 Ts): Tone:* uterine atony (90%); *Tissue:* retained products of conception; *Trauma:* genital tract trauma (7%); *Thrombin:* clotting disorders—p88 (3%). Death rate: 2/yr in the UK; 125,000/yr worldwide. Massive obstetric haemorrhage is the loss of >1500mLs and should prompt a hospital alert (2222 call, see BOX).

Secondary PPH This is excessive blood loss from the genital tract after 24h from delivery. It usually occurs between 5 and 12 days and is usually due to retained placental tissue or clot, often with infection. Uterine involution may be incomplete. Treat with antibiotics, US to look for retained products (difficult to interpret postpartum).

Risk factors for PPH *Antenatal:* • Previous PPH or retained placenta • BMI >35kg/m² • Maternal Hb <85g/L at onset of labour • Antepartum haemorrhage • Multiparity >4 • Maternal age >35 • Uterine malformation or fibroids • A large placental site (twins, severe rhesus disease, large baby) • Low placenta, • Overdistended uterus (polyhydramnios, twins) • Extravasated blood in the myometrium (abruption). *In labour:* • Prolonged labour (1st, 2nd or 3rd stage) • Induction or oxytocin use • Precipitate labour • Operative birth or caesarean section. ▶Book mothers with risk factors for obstetric unit delivery.

Management of postpartum haemorrhage

- Call for help—this is a life-threatening emergency. Ask for senior midwife, obstetrics registrar and SHO, anaesthetic registrar, a scribe, and if massive haemorrhage put out 2222 call to alert haematologist, blood bank, porters, and theatres.
- High-flow oxygen.
- Assess airway and intubate if decreased conscious level.
- Insert two large-bore cannulae (14G/grey or above) and take blood for FBC, U&E, LFTs, clotting screen, and cross-match 4–6 units. If blood loss torrential and mother unstable use group O Rh–ve blood until cross-matched available. Transfuse 1 unit packed red cells to 1 unit fresh frozen plasma.
- Start IV fluids eg 1 litre Hartmann's stat.
- Catheterize and use urometer for hourly urine output.
- Deliver placenta, empty the uterus of clots or retained tissue.
- Massage uterus to generate contraction/perform bimanual compression.
- Give drugs to contract uterus:
    - Syntometrine® IM 1 ampoule
    - Oxytocin infusion 40 units at 10 units/hour
    - Ergometrine 500mcg IV/IM
    - Misoprostol 1000mcg PR
    - Carboprost 250mcg every 15min up to 8 doses.
- Repair vaginal or cervical tears.
- If ongoing bleeding after 2nd dose of carboprost, or suspicion of uterine rupture or retained tissue, take to theatre for examination under anaesthesia, including laparotomy if necessary.
- In theatre, insert Rusch balloon (fig 1.21 —large balloon which sits inside the uterus, exerting pressure on placental bed).
- If uterus still atonic despite empty bladder and drugs, and bleeding responds to compression, insert B-lynch suture (fig 1.22). This is a compression suture inserted through lower segment, over the top of the uterus including the posterior surface and looks like a belt and braces.
- If bleeding is still ongoing, consider internal iliac or uterine artery ligation.
- Uterine artery embolization helpful but not available in all units at all times.
- Subtotal or total hysterectomy: the decision should not be delayed because maternal death may result.

Managing those refusing blood transfusion in pregnancy

- Document maternal attitude to transfusion at booking.
- Give oral iron and folate to mother to maximize haemoglobin stores (parenteral iron if does not respond—p21 (not if thalassaemia)).
- Book for delivery where there are good facilities to deal with haemorrhage promptly (including facilities for hysterectomy, and interventional radiology techniques such as uterine artery embolization), and with critical care facilities and cell salvage if the mother is high risk, eg if placenta praevia.
- Ensure consultant obstetrician and anaesthetist assess antenatally to make plans for labour.
- The woman should make an Advanced Directive, making clear her views on which blood products she will and won't accept.
- Arrange us to know placental site.
- Inform consultant when admitted in labour. Ensure experienced staff conduct labour. Give oxytocin as soon as the baby is delivered. Do not leave the mother alone for first hour post-delivery.
- Consultant obstetrician and anaesthetist should perform caesarean section if required.
- Cell savers which wash the woman's own blood so that it may be returned may be acceptable to some women (suitable for intra-abdominal blood not contaminated by amniotic fluid).[89]
- Haemorrhage should be dealt with promptly, and clotting disorders excluded early. Involve a consultant obstetrician early (to decide if intervention may be needed eg embolization of uterine arteries, B-Lynch suture, internal iliac ligation or hysterectomy), and a consultant anaesthetist (for help with fluid replacement and for use of intensive care facilities). Liaise with a consultant haematologist. Avoid dextran (adversely affects haemostasis), but Gelofusine® is useful. Erythropoietin is not an effective alternative to transfusion as it takes 10–14 days to work.
- Ensure the woman does not want to change her mind and receive a transfusion.
- Should the woman die of exsanguination, both bereaved relatives and distressed staff should be offered support.

Obstetrics

Fig 1.21 Bakri and Rusch balloons.
Reproduced from Georgiou, C. (2009), Balloon tamponade in the management of postpartum haemorrhage: a review. *BJOG: An International Journal of Obstetrics & Gynaecology*, 116: 748–757.

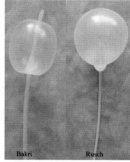

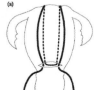

Fig 1.22 B-lynch suture.
Reproduced from Clyburn et al, *Obstetric Anaesthesia for Developing Countries* (2010) with permission from Oxford University Press.

The third stage of labour (p60) is considered delayed if not complete by 30 minutes with active management, by 60min with physiological 3rd stage. A placenta not delivered by then will probably not be expelled spontaneously. The danger with retained placenta is haemorrhage. Associations: •Previous RP or uterine surgery •Preterm delivery •Maternal age >35y •Placental weight <600g •Parity >5 •Induced labour •Pethidine used in labour.

Management If the placenta does not separate readily, avoid excessive cord traction—the cord may snap or the uterus invert. Check that the placenta is not in the vagina. Palpate the abdomen. Rub up a contraction, put the baby to the breast (stimulates oxytocin production). Give 20IU oxytocin in 20mL saline into umbilical vein and proximally clamp cord. Empty the bladder (a full bladder causes atony). If the placenta still does not deliver within further 30min, offer examination to see if manual removal is needed (delay may precipitate a PPH). Stop if examination is painful. Insert IV access and take FBC and group&save. Take written consent. Transfer to theatre for regional anaesthesia (or epidural top-up) and manual removal of the placenta.

Manual removal With the mother in lithotomy position, using aseptic technique, place one hand on the abdomen to stabilize the uterus. Insert the other hand through the cervix into the uterus. Following the cord assists finding the placenta. Gently work round the placenta, separating it from the uterus using the ulnar border of the hand. When separated it should be possible to remove it by cord traction. Check that it is complete. Give oxytocic drugs and one dose of antibiotic eg cefuroxime 1.5g and metronidazole 500mg IV.

Rarely, the placenta will not separate (placenta accreta)—call for senior help.

►►Uterine inversion

Inversion of the uterus is rare. It may be due to mismanagement of the third stage, eg with cord traction in an atonic uterus (between contractions) and a fundal insertion of the placenta. It may be completely revealed, or partial when the uterus remains within the vagina. Even without haemorrhage the mother may become profoundly shocked, due to increased vagal tone.

Management The ease with which the uterus is replaced depends on the amount of time elapsed since inversion, as a tight ring forms at the neck of the inversion.
• Call for help: senior midwife, obstetrician and anaesthetist, and theatre staff
• Immediate replacement: push the fundus through the cervix with the palm of the hand
• If this fails, insert 2 large-bore IV cannulae and take blood for FBC, U&E, clotting and crossmatch 4–6 units (94% have postpartum haemorrhage)
• IV fluid
• Transfer to theatre for anaesthesia
• If the placenta is still attached, leave it there as removing it will increase the bleeding
• Tocolytic drugs eg terbutaline to relax the uterus and make replacement easier. Agents used for general anaesthesia are also helpful
• Try manual replacement but if this fails, replace using hydrostatic pressure: infuse warm saline into the vagina, sealing the labia with the other hand
• If this fails, laparotomy to try and pull the uterus up.

Obstetrics

Placental types

- *Velamentous* insertion (1%): umbilical vessels go within the membranes before placental insertion.
- *Placenta succenturia* (5%): There is a separate (succenturiate) lobe away from the main placenta which may fail to separate normally and cause a PPH or puerperal sepsis.
- *Vasa praevia:* Fetal vessels from velamentous insertion or between lobes (succenturia, or bilobe placenta) risk damage at membrane rupture causing fetal haemorrhage. Caesarean delivery is needed (urgent if fetal compromise at membrane rupture, elective if detected antenatally by US).
- *Placenta membranacea* (1:3000): A thin placenta surrounds the baby. Some is in the lower segment so predisposes to APH. It may fail to separate in the 3rd stage.
- *Placenta accreta:* There is abnormal (morbid) adherence of all or part of the placenta to the uterus, termed *placenta increta* if myometrium infiltrated, *placenta percreta* if penetration reaches the serosa. These 3 types predispose to PPH and there is an increased need for caesarean hysterectomy. Incidence ↑ with the number of previous caesarean sections. Diagnose prenatally (colour Doppler US/MRI p78).

Placenta praevia (see also p56–7) The placenta lies in the lower uterine segment. It is found in ~0.5% of pregnancies. Risks are of significant haemorrhage by mother and fetus. Avoid digital PV examinations (speculum examination is safe), and advise against penetrative intercourse.

Associations: Caesarean section; sharp curette TOP; multiparity; multiple pregnancy; mother >40 years; assisted conception; deficient endometrium-manual removal of placenta, D&C, fibroids, endometritis. US at <24 weeks' gestation shows a low-lying placenta in 28% but with lower segment development only 3% lie low at term. Transvaginal US is superior to transabdominal for localizing placentas accurately, especially when the placenta is posterior, and, if combined with 3D power Doppler/MRI, diagnoses vasa praevia and placenta accreta. It has not been shown to increase bleeding. Repeat US at 32wks if major praevia, 36wks if minor.

Major placenta praevia (placenta covering the internal os) requires caesarean section for delivery. Minor placenta praevia (placenta in lower segment but does not cross the internal os): aim for normal delivery unless the placenta encroaches within 2cm of the internal os (especially if posterior or thick). Presentation may be as APH (separation of the placenta as the lower segment stretches causes bleeding) or as abnormal fetal lie. Problems are with bleeding and with mode of delivery as the placenta obstructs the os and may shear off during labour, or may be accreta (5%), especially after a previous CS (>24%). Poor lower segment contractility predisposes to postpartum haemorrhage. Caesarean section should be consultant-performed or supervised with consultant anaesthetic attendance at 38wks, (36–7wks with steroid cover, crossmatched blood + haematologist available,[NICE] if accreta suspected), at a hospital with blood bank and level 2 critical care beds.[RCOG] Admitting those with major placenta praevia at ≤35wks' gestation so that immediate help is available, is controversial, and not practised by many UK units but consider admission at 34wks if there has been significant bleeding.

Obstetrics

DIC in pregnancy is always secondary to stimulation of coagulation by pro-coagulant substance release in the maternal circulation. Known triggers are: retention of a dead fetus (of >20 weeks' gestation which has been dead for >3 weeks); pre-eclampsia; placental abruption; endotoxic shock; amniotic fluid embolism; placenta accreta; hydatidiform mole; prolonged shock from any cause; acute fatty liver of pregnancy (p25). *Pathogenesis:* Thromboplastins are released into the circulation, fibrin and platelets are consumed as intra-vascular clotting occurs. *Tests:* Kaolin–cephalin clotting time ↑ (↓ factors II, V, VII), fibrinogen ↓, fibrin degradation products ↑. In situations where DIC is a possibility send blood for crossmatch, platelets, partial thromboplastin time or accelerated whole blood clotting time, prothrombin time, fibrinogen estimation, and fibrin degradation products. Preliminary results should be available in 30min. *Management:* Presentation may be as heavy bleeding and shock, and the first measures must be the correction of shock. ▶▶Give O₂ at 15L/min via a tight fitting mask with reservoir. Set up 2 wide-gauge IVIs, take bloods as above, and give blood fast (group-compatible blood—available in 5–10min or O Rh−ve blood if desperate). Stored blood is deficient in clotting factors. Give fresh frozen plasma to normalize the kaolin–cephalin clotting time and the prothrombin time. Platelets are indicated with prolonged bleeding and low platelet count. Calcium is sometimes needed to counteract citrate in stored blood (eg 10mL of 10% **calcium gluconate** IVI, eg after 6u of blood). Seek expert help from a haematologist. The condition is usually self-limiting if the stimulus can be removed. In the case of intrauterine death and abruption (p56) removal of the uterine contents is the way to correct the stimulus, and this should be done as promptly as possible. *Mortality:* <1% if placental abruption; 50–80% if infection/shock.

Autoimmune idiopathic thrombocytopenic purpura (AiTP) Incidence 1–2:1000 pregnancies. IgG antibodies cause thrombocytopenia (associated with increased bone marrow megakaryocytes) in the mother and, being able to cross the placenta, they cause thrombocytopenia in ~10% of fetuses. Exclude systemic lupus erythematosus in the mother (thrombocytopenia may be an early presentation; do DNA binding, *OHCM* p540). Consider maternal HIV. If maternal platelets fall below 50 × 10⁹/L near delivery, give steroids. Splenectomy is rarely necessary during pregnancy. IgG 0.4g/kg IV for 5 days is sometimes used near expected date of delivery, inducing maternal and fetal remission for up to 3 weeks, but it is extremely expensive. Aim for non-traumatic delivery for both mother and baby: avoid FBS, FSE, ventouse and rotational forceps delivery. Neonatal platelet count may fall further in the first days of life, then gradually rise to normal over 4–16 weeks. Treatment is not needed unless surgery is contemplated. Maternal mortality due to AiTP is now negligible, but fetal mortality remains (due to intracranial bleeding). Take cord blood at delivery. If platelets <20 × 10⁹/L give baby IgG 1g/kg IVI at birth.

Causes of thrombocytopenia in pregnancy
1 Spurious (send repeat sample in citrated bottle)
2 Gestational thrombocytopenia—usually mild and self-limiting
3 Idiopathic thrombocytopaenic purpura
4 Pre-eclampsia (platelets may fall early, preceding clotting abnormality)
5 DIC (above) and haemolytic uraemic syndrome (p176)/thrombotic thrombocytopenic purpura (2 ends of a microangiopathic spectrum, *OHCM* p332)
6 Folate deficiency
7 Congenital (May–Heggin anomaly, hereditary macrothrombocytopenia)
8 Bone marrow disease; hypersplenism
9 HELLP syndrome (p49).

Amniotic fluid embolism

This condition is thankfully rare but carries a high mortality of up to 61% (20% in 2006-8 UK). 8% of direct maternal deaths were caused by AFE in the UK and of those who survive, 85% have permanent neurological damage. The incidence is 1:8000-1:30,000 births and it tends to occur with rupture of membranes (70%), at CS (19%), during delivery, and rarely during termination of pregnancy, manual removal of placenta, and amniocentesis.

Risk factors include multiple pregnancy, maternal age >35y, CS, instrumental delivery, eclampsia, polyhydramnios, placental abruption, uterine rupture, and induction of labour.

Clinical features Symptoms and signs evolve rapidly and the first sign may be maternal collapse.

• Dyspnoea, chest pain, hypoxia and/or respiratory arrest leading to acute respiratory distress syndrome (ARDS) (*OHCM* p178)
• Hypotension
• Fetal distress
• Seizures (20%)
• Reduced conscious level
• Cardiac arrest
• Almost all women go on to develop DIC within 48h.

An anaphylactic type of response occurs to amniotic fluid in the maternal circulation.

Management

▸▸ The first priority is to prevent death from respiratory failure. Give mask oxygen and call an anaesthetist urgently. Endotracheal intubation and ventilation may be necessary. Set up IVI in case DIC should supervene. Cardiovascular collapse is due to left ventricular failure. DIC and haemorrhage then usually follow. Treatment is essentially supportive—important steps are detailed below. Diagnosis may be difficult: exclude other causes of maternal collapse (BOX, p55).

▸▸ Cardiopulmonary resuscitation if indicated.

▸▸ Give highest available O_2 concentration. If unconscious, ventilate and use 100% inspired O_2. This is to prevent neurological sequelae from hypoxia.

▸▸ Monitor for fetal distress.

▸▸ If hypotensive, give fluids rapidly IVI to increase preload. If still hypotensive consider inotropes: **dobutamine** (a better inotrope than dopamine), eg in a dose range of 2.5-10mcg/kg/min IVI may help.

▸▸ Pulmonary artery catheterization (Swan-Ganz catheter if available) helps guide haemodynamic management.

▸▸ After initial hypotension is corrected, give only maintenance requirements of fluid to avoid pulmonary oedema from ARDS. Transfer to intensive care unit as soon as possible.

▸▸ Treat DIC with fresh whole blood or packed cells and fresh frozen plasma. Use of heparin is controversial; there are insufficient data to warrant routine heparinization.

▸▸ If the mother has a cardiac arrest, it is recommended to deliver the baby via CS. Peri-mortem caesarean within 5 minutes can aid resuscitation of the mother.

Most mortality occurs in the first hour. Mortality rates reported: 26.4-61%. (In 2006-8 there were 13 deaths in England and Wales.) Report suspected cases to National Amniotic Fluid Embolism Register (at UKOSS).[2] Should the woman die, perform autopsy as soon as possible. Specifically request that the lungs be examined for amniotic squames or lanugo hair to confirm the diagnosis.

2 UKOSS The National Perinatal Unit, Old Road Campus, Old Road, Headington, Oxford, OX3 7LF, www.npeu.ox.ac.uk

Obstetrics

▶Give all babies with signs of trauma **vitamin k** 1mg IM at birth (unless already given as part of routine measures).

Birth injuries to the baby *Moulding:* This is a natural phenomenon, not an injury. The skull bones can override each other (p42) to reduce the diameter of the head. Moulding is assessed by degree of overlap of the overriding at the sutures. If moulding is absent, skull bones are felt separately. With slight moulding, the bones just touch, then they override but can be reduced; finally they override so much that they cannot be reduced.

Cephalhaematoma: This is a subperiostial swelling on the fetal head, and its boundaries are therefore limited by the individual bone margins (commonest over parietal bones). It is fluctuant. Spontaneous absorption occurs but may take weeks and may cause or contribute to jaundice.

Caput succedaneum: This is an oedematous swelling of the scalp, superficial to the cranial periosteum (which does not, therefore, limit its extent) and is the result of venous congestion and exuded serum caused by pressure against the cervix and lower segment during labour. The presenting part of the head therefore has the swelling over it. It gradually disappears in the first days after birth. When ventouse extraction is used in labour a particularly large caput (called a chignon) is formed under the ventouse cup.

Erb's palsy: See fig 1.18, p76. This can result from shoulder dystocia (p72) (so ↑ ×10 in UK diabetic pregnancies).$_{\text{Ncol}}^{92}$ The baby's arm is flaccid and the hand is in the 'porter's tip' posture (p750). Exclude a fractured clavicle and arrange physiotherapy. Most resolve, but if it has not resolved by 6 months, it is unlikely to improve further.

Subaponeurotic haematoma: Blood lies between the aponeurosis and the periosteum. As haematoma is not confined to the boundaries of one bone, collections of blood may be large enough to result in anaemia or jaundice. They are associated with vacuum extractions.

Skull fractures: These are associated with difficult forceps delivery and may also occur after a difficult second-stage CS delivery where the head is impacted. They are commonest over parietal or frontal bones. If depressed fractures are associated with CNS signs, ask a neurosurgeon if the bone should be elevated.

Intracranial injuries: Intracranial haemorrhage is especially associated with difficult or fast labour, instrumental delivery, and breech delivery. Premature babies are especially vulnerable. Normally a degree of motility of intracranial contents is buffered by cerebrospinal fluid. Excessive moulding and sudden changes in pressure reduce this effect and are associated with trauma. In all cases of intracranial haemorrhage check babies' platelets. If low, check mother's blood for platelet alloantibodies (PLA1 system). Subsequent babies are at equal risk. IV maternal immunoglobulin treatment is being evaluated.

Anoxia may cause intraventricular haemorrhage (p108). Asphyxia causes intracerebral haemorrhage (often petechial) and may result in cerebral palsy. Extradural, subdural, and subarachnoid haemorrhages can all occur. Babies affected may have convulsions, apnoea, cyanosis, abnormal pallor, low heart rate, alterations in muscle tone, restlessness, somnolence, or abnormal movements. Treatment is supportive and expectant. See p108 & p110.

Fetal laceration occurs in 1–2% of CS deliveries. It is more common with breech CS delivery and with CS after membrane rupture (the baby's skin may lie flush against the uterus). Most are superficial and heal without scarring but the parents should be warned of this risk when consent is taken for CS.

Anal sphincter injury

Approximately 85% of vaginal deliveries are complicated by perineal trauma, and of these 60–70% will require suturing. The vast majority are 1st- and 2nd-degree tears (affecting perineal skin and/or muscles) but 3–4% will be 3rd- or 4th-degree injuries. A 3rd-degree tear is one affecting part or all of the anal sphincter muscle, and a 4th the anal mucosa. Primary repair of obstetric anal sphincter injuries (OASI) significantly reduces the risk of ongoing flatus and stool incontinence but doesn't alleviate it completely. Faecal incontinence is a source of misery, and requires expert attention.

Risk of mechanical injury is greatest after the first vaginal delivery (4% primip vs 1% multip). Traumatic stretching of the pudendal nerves occurs in >30% of primips, but is mostly asymptomatic, or mildly/transiently so. These patients are at ↑ risk in subsequent deliveries (cumulative pudendal nerve injury is well recognized). Other risk factors: • Baby >4kg • Persistent occipito-posterior position • Induced labour • Epidural • 2nd stage >1h • Midline episiotomy • Instrumental delivery (6–7% OASI in primip, 2.5% multip).

After repair, prescribe laxatives (eg lactulose 15mL OD or BD depending on stool softness) and antibiotics (cefuroxime 500mg PO/8h and metronidazole 400mg PO/8h for 7–10 days). Arrange follow-up at 6–12 weeks post delivery to check healing and continence. If flatus or faecal incontinence occurs, get expert help. Referral for specialist physiotherapy is essential, along with endoanal US. Whether symptomatic or not, there is an argument for elective CS delivery next time but the mother will need counselling. If asymptomatic, there is still an increased risk of repeat OASI. If symptomatic despite specialist help, the woman requires a secondary sphincter repair post-delivery of any subsequent children—this fact will not be altered by offering elective CS. Elective caesarean may not protect against symptoms caused by pudendal nerve neuropathy.[93]

Vesicovaginal fistula

This abnormal opening between bladder and vagina leading to urinary incontinence, a common sequel to obstructed labour is thought to affect 3 million women worldwide,[94] now almost exclusively in developing countries.

Obstructed labour is particularly a problem for malnourished girls who become pregnant before full pelvic maturation. In obstructed labour, the pelvic head progressively compresses the soft tissues of vagina, bladder, and rectum against the pelvis causing ischaemic damage to these tissues and fetal asphyxiation. 2 days after the fetus dies it becomes macerated, softens, and can be vaginally expelled. A few days later, the mother passes sloughed ischaemic tissue leaving a fistula between bladder, urethra, and vagina or rectum and vagina (or both). Damaged tissues adjacent to the sloughed tissue heal poorly, often with fibrosis. Vagina and rectum may later stenose; chronic pyelonephritis and renal failure can ensue. Incontinent women are often shunned by family, divorced by their husbands, and stigmatized (especially in cultures where the affliction is believed to be punishment by a god).

Treatment is with continuous urinary drainage for 3 months if presenting with vesicovaginal fistula early (<3 months postpartum) or surgery if later. Operation is most successful for 1st operation and small defects (<2cm) with successful closure rates of up to 85% (but 16–32% of these women remain incontinent).

Good obstetric management of obstructed labour prevents fistulas. Early treatment can allow healing without recourse to surgery. Sadly it is those parts of the world where there is poor access to obstetric facilities where women develop fistulas and where the chance of having subsequent repair is also limited.

Further reading

Aliyu F et al. (2011). A patient's journey: Living with obstetric fistula. *BMJ* 342:1360.

▶Examine gently. Unless marked bleeding, allow the mother some bonding time with baby before examination and repair (but it should be completed within an hour of delivery; endorphins from delivery also help reduce pain)._{NICE}

Perineal tears These are classified by the degree of damage caused. Risk factors for development are discussed in the BOX on p91.

Labial tears Common; these heal quickly; suturing is required if both labia are torn to prevent them fusing together. These tears are particularly painful.

First-degree tears These tears are superficial and do not damage muscle. Suture unless skin edges well apposed to aid healing._{NICE}

Second-degree tears These lacerations involve perineal muscle. Repair is similar to that of episiotomy (see below).

Third-degree tears Damage involves the anal sphincter muscle. Classification:
3a External anal sphincter (circular fibres) thickness <50% torn
3b External anal sphincter thickness >50% torn
3c Both external and internal anal sphincters (longitudinal fibres) torn.

If anal/rectal mucosa also involved it is a **fourth-degree tear**. See p91. 3rd/4th-degree tears need repair by an experienced surgeon, under epidural or GA in theatre with intra-operative antibiotic cover. Rectal mucosa is repaired first using absorbable suture from above the tear's apex to the mucocutaneous junction. Muscle is interposed. Vaginal mucosa is then sutured. Internal anal sphincter is repaired with interrupted sutures. Overlap and repair severed ends of the external anal sphincter. Finally repair skin. Give antibiotic prophylaxis with 3rd- and 4th-degree tears. Give high-fibre diet and lactulose for 10 days to avoid constipation. Arrange pelvic floor exercise physiotherapy for 6-12 weeks. Arrange consultant obstetrician follow-up at 6-12 weeks; if pain or incontinence refer to specialist gynaecologist or colorectal surgeon for endoanal US or manometry._{RCOL}

Episiotomy This is performed to enlarge the outlet, eg to hasten birth of a distressed baby, for instrumental or breech delivery, and to try to prevent 3° tears (but anal tears are not reduced by more episiotomies in normal deliveries). Rates: 8% Holland, 12% England, 50% USA.✷

The tissues which are incised are vaginal epithelium, perineal skin, bulbocavernous muscle, superficial, and deep transverse perineal muscles. With large episiotomies, the external anal sphincter or levator ani may be partially cut, and ischiorectal fat exposed.

Technique: Hold the perineal skin away from the presenting part of the fetus (2 fingers in vagina). Infiltrate area to be cut with local anaesthetic, eg 1% lidocaine (=lignocaine). Still keeping the fingers in the introitus, cut mediolaterally towards the ischial tuberosity, starting midline (6 o'clock), so avoiding the Bartholin's glands.

Repair: (See fig 1.23) NB: use resorbable suture—eg polyglactin 910. In lithotomy, and using good illumination, repair the vaginal mucosa first. Start above the apex using continuous non-locked stitches 1cm apart, 1cm from wound edges. Then repair muscles with continuous non-locked technique_{NICE}to obliterate any dead spaces. Finally close the skin with subcuticular stitch. Perform rectal examination afterwards to check sutures have not penetrated the rectal mucosa.

Problems with episiotomy: Bleeding; infection, and breakdown; haematoma formation. For comfort some suggest ice packs, salt baths, hair dryer to dry perineum. 60% of women suffer perineal damage (episiotomy or tear) with spontaneous vaginal delivery; rectal diclofenac can provide effective analgesia. Superficial dyspareunia: see p310. If labia minora are involved in the skin bridge, the introitus is left too small.

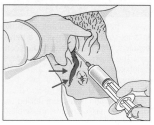

(1) Swab the vulva towards the perineum. Infiltrate with 1% lidocaine (→arrows).

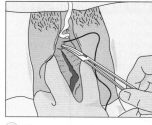

(2) Place tampon with attached tape in upper vagina. Insert 1st suture above apex of vaginal cut (not too deep as underlying rectal mucosa nearby).

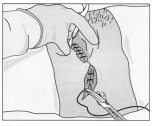

(3) Bring together vaginal edges with continuous stitches placed 1cm apart. Knot at introitus under the skin. Appose divided levator ani muscles.

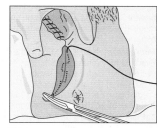

(4) Close perineal skin (subcuticular continuous stitch is shown here).

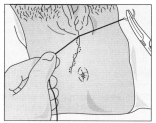

(5) When stitching is finished, remove tampon and examine vagina (to check for retained swabs). Do a PR to check that apical sutures have not penetrated rectum.

Fig 1.23 Repairing an episiotomy.

The puerperium is the 6 weeks after delivery. The uterus involutes, from 1kg weight at delivery to 100g. Felt at the umbilicus after delivery, it is a pelvic organ at 10 days. Afterpains are felt (especially while breastfeeding) as it contracts. The cervix becomes firm over 3 days. The internal os closes by 3 days, the external os by 3 weeks. Lochia (endometrial slough, red cells, and white cells) is passed *per vaginam*. It is red (*lochia rubra*) for the 1st 3 days, then becomes yellow (*lochia serosa*) then white over the next 10 days (*lochia alba*), until 6 weeks. The breasts produce milky discharge and colostrum during the last trimester. Milk replaces colostrum 3 days after birth. Breasts are swollen, red, and tender with physiological engorgement at 3 to 4 days.

The first days Is thromboprophylaxis needed? (p32) If Rh−ve, give anti-D, within 72h (see BOX, p11). Check T°, BP, breasts, legs, lochia, fundal height if heavy PV loss. Teach pelvic floor exercises. Persistent *red lochia*, failure of *uterine involution*, or *PPH* (p84) suggest endometritis or retained products. *Sustained hypertension* may need drugs (*OHCM* p134). ▶Check rubella immunity. Vaccinate if non-immune (simultaneously but different limb from anti-D, or wait 3 months).⁹⁶ *Check Hb* on postnatal day 1 or ≥day 7: postpartum physiological haemodilution occurs from days 2–6. Discuss contraception (see BOX, p95).

Puerperal pyrexia is T° >38°C in the first 14 days after delivery or miscarriage. Examine fully (chest, breasts, legs, lochia, and bimanual vaginal examination). Culture MSU, high vaginal swabs, blood, and sputum. 90% of infections will be urinary or of the genital tract. Superficial perineal infections occur around the second day. *Endometritis* gives lower abdominal pain, offensive lochia, and a tender uterus (on bimanual vaginal exam). Endometritis needs urgent IV antibiotics (below). For breast infection give **flucloxacillin 500mg/6h PO** early for ≥10 days, to prevent abscesses. Breastfeeding or breast expression should continue to prevent milk stagnation. Even if the cause of pyrexia is unknown, it is wise to treat with **cefalexin 500mg/8h + metronidazole 400mg/8h**.

Superficial thrombophlebitis This presents as a painful tender (usually varicose) vein. Give NSAID, eg **ibuprofen 400mg/8h PO**. Use anti-thromboembolic stockings. Recovery is usual within 4 days. *Deep vein thrombosis:* see p33.

Puerperal psychosis (1:500 births) ▶See p386. This is distinguished from the mild depression that often follows birth by a high suicidal drive, severe depression (p342), mania, and more rarely schizophrenic symptoms (p336) with delusions. Exclude puerperal infection causing delirium. Presentation is by day 7 postpartum in 50%, by 3 months in 90%. Onset is usually sudden and deterioration rapid. Refer to heath trust's community psychiatric team for pregnancy. Admission to specialist mother and baby unit may be needed. See p386 for a fuller discussion of postnatal depression. 10% of mothers develop postnatal depression; in ⅓–½ of these depression is severe.

The 6-week postnatal examination gives a chance to: •See how mother and baby are •Do BP & weight •Do FBC if anaemic postnatally •Arrange a cervical smear if due •Check contraceptive plans are enacted (see BOX, p95) •Ask about depression, backache, incontinence. Ask: 'Have you resumed intercourse?' (CEMACE recommends abstinence or 'gentle intercourse' for first 6 weeks postpartum to prevent fatal air embolism).⁹⁷ Sexual problems are common, and prolonged: ~50% report that intercourse is less satisfactory than pre-pregnancy, with major loss of libido, and dyspareunia the chief complaints. At 1 year post-delivery, there is no difference between those who have had a vaginal versus CS delivery. Vaginal examination to check healing is *not* usually needed unless the woman has concerns or she reports incontinence.

Obstetrics

Contraception after a baby

Lactational amenorrhoea (LAM)[98] This is Nature's contraception. Breast-feeding delays return of ovulation (breastfeeding disrupts frequency and amplitude of gonadotrophin surges so that although there is gonadotrophin rise in response to falling placental sex steroids after delivery, ovulation does not occur). Women who are fully breastfeeding day and night (ie breast milk is baby's sole nutrient), and are less than 6 months postpartum, and amenorrhoeic can expect this method to be 98% effective. Average 1st menstruation in a breastfeeding mother is at 28.4 weeks (range 15–48). Contraceptive efficacy of LAM is decreased after 6 months, if periods return, if breastfeeding frequency reduces, night feeding stops, there is separation from the baby (eg return to work), if the baby receives supplements, or if mother or baby become ill or stressed. In the UK although 69% of mothers initiate breastfeeding only 21% still feed at 6 months. Aim for additional contraception once decreased efficacy is anticipated.

Progesterone-only pill (PoP, p304) These may be started any time postpartum but if started after day 21 additional precautions are needed for 2 days. They do not affect breast milk production. Low doses (<1%) of hormone are secreted in the milk but have not been shown to affect babies.

Combined pills Start at 3 weeks if not breastfeeding. They affect early milk production and are not recommended if breastfeeding until 6 months (but can be used from 6 weeks if other methods unacceptable). Levels of hormone in breast milk are similar to that of ovulatory cycles.

Emergency contraception Use of progesterone method (p299) is suitable for all. It is not needed before 21 days postpartum.

Depot injections These are not recommended until 6 weeks in those breastfeeding (theoretical risk of sex steroid to baby's immature nervous system and liver). Medroxyprogesterone acetate 150mg given deep IM 12-weekly can start 5 days postpartum if bottle feeding, or norethisterone enantate 200mg into gluteus maximus 8-weekly (licensed for short-term use only, but can be given immediately postpartum when medroxyprogesterone use can cause heavy bleeding).

Progesterone implants Insertion is not recommended until 6 weeks in those who are breastfeeding. 0.2% of daily dose of etonogestrel is excreted in breast milk. Implant at 21–28 days in those bottle feeding.

Intrauterine contraceptive devices (IUCD) These should be inserted within the first 48h postpartum or delayed until 4 weeks. This is to minimize risk of uterine perforation at insertion. Levonorgestrel-releasing intrauterine devices are also inserted at 4 weeks.

Diaphragms and cervical caps The woman needs to be fitted at 6 weeks as different sizes may be required from previously. Alternative contraception is needed from day 21 until the new ones are confidently handled.

Sterilization Unless sterilization highly advisable at caesarean section (eg repeated sections, family complete), it is best to wait an appropriate interval as immediate postpartum tubal ligation has possible increased failure rate and is more likely to be regretted.

Obstetrics

Worldwide perspective In North Europe, a woman's lifetime risk of dying in pregnancy or childbirth is 1:30,000; in the world's poorest parts it is 1:6.[99]

Definition The death of a mother while pregnant or within 42 days of the pregnancy ending, from any cause related to or aggravated by the pregnancy or its management, but not from accidental or incidental causes. *Direct deaths* result from obstetric complications of the pregnant state (including pregnancy, labour, and the puerperium) from interventions, omissions, incorrect treatment, or a chain of events resulting from any of the above eg eclampsia, haemorrhage, or amniotic fluid embolism. *Indirect death:* A death which has arisen from pre-existing disease or disease that developed during pregnancy which was not due to direct obstetric causes, but which was aggravated by pregnancy, eg diabetes, heart disease, epilepsy, or hormone-dependent malignancies. *Coincidental death:* Accidental or incidental death which would have happened even if the woman was not pregnant, eg domestic violence or road traffic accidents. *Late deaths* are those occurring between 42 days and 1 year after termination, miscarriage, or delivery that are due to direct or indirect maternal causes.

History Since 1952 there have been 3-yearly confidential enquiries into maternal deaths. Maternal deaths are reported by the obstetric unit involved, and then investigated by a team of experts. Reports allow analysis, reflection, and recommended actions so each death should improve future care. Maternal mortality has reduced since reports started, (deaths per 100,000 *maternities* (live birth, or stillbirth ≥24wks' gestation) were 67.1 in 1955-7, 33.3 in 1964-6 & 10.12 in 2009-12 of which direct deaths were 3.25/100,000).

Currently In 2009-12 (MBRACE-UK report from 2014[1]), 357 women died during, or within 6 weeks of the end of their pregnancy, 321 of which were from direct (26%) or indirect causes (74%). The decrease seen since the previous Confidential Enquiry is primarily due to a fall in direct maternal deaths. However, deaths from indirect (medical and psychiatric) causes are not being effectively addressed and have remained static for the past 10 years.

In 2009-12, thrombosis was the chief cause of direct death in the UK, followed by genital tract sepsis and haemorrhage. Deaths from complications of pre-eclampsia are at their lowest level since monitoring began and those from sepsis have halved since the last report. 'Other indirect causes' were the leading cause of indirect deaths and this was chiefly due to non-genital tract sepsis and influenza. Over half of deaths due to influenza occurred after a vaccine became available and were therefore preventable. Cardiac disease remains the leading single cause of indirect death, which is unchanged from the previous report. Neurological disease is the third-highest and also remains static. Deaths from psychiatric disease are relatively uncommon but they make up a significant proportion of late maternal deaths (95 of 419).

30% of mothers were still pregnant at the time of their deaths, a third of these under 20 weeks' gestation. 74% of infants survived. Of the babies delivered by perimortem cs, 30% survived. Maternal mortality rates remain highest in older women, those from the most deprived areas, and from some ethnic minorities. A third of women were born outside the UK. 74% had pre-existing medical conditions and 17% mental health problems. 27% were obese and almost a quarter smoked during pregnancy. Only 29% received the level of antenatal care recommended by NICE and 25% did not receive the minimum level of care. *Key messages* from the report: • Pre-pregnancy advice for women with pre-existing medical or mental health problems • Early joint specialist antenatal care • Prompt treatment of sepsis • Early involvement of senior clinicians • Encouraging women to take up the influenza vaccination.

This is the number of stillbirths and deaths in the 1st week of life (early neonatal deaths)/1000 births. Stillbirths only include those fetuses of >24 weeks' gestation; if a fetus of <24 weeks' gestation is born showing signs of life, and then dies, this is counted as a perinatal death in the UK (if dying within the 1st 7 days). Neonatal deaths are those infants dying up to and including the 28th day after birth. Other countries use different criteria—including stillbirths from 20 weeks and neonatal deaths up to 28 days after birth, so it is not always easy to compare statistics.

Perinatal mortality is affected by many factors. Rates are high for *small* (61% of deaths are in babies <2500g) and *preterm* babies (70% of deaths occur in the 5% who are preterm). See p50 & p128. *Regional variation* in the UK is quite marked. There is a *social class variation* with rates being less for social classes 1 and 2 than for classes 4 and 5. *Teenage mothers* have higher rates than mothers aged 20–29. From 35yrs rates rise until they are 1.5-fold higher than the low-risk group (25–35yrs) by age >40. *Second babies* have the lowest mortality rates. Mortality rates are doubled for 4th and 5th children, trebled by 6th and 7th (this effect is not independent of social class as more lower social class women have many children). Rates are lower for *singleton births* than for multiple (↑×10 for triplets vs singletons).[100] Time to conception also has an influence with mortality rates being 3 times more if it has taken a long time to conceive compared with a short time (in Denmark).[101] Perinatal mortality in UK* (*figures exclude Scotland) is twice as high in offspring of mothers of black ethnicity; 1.5 times commoner if of Asian ethnicity.[102]

Perinatal mortality rates in the UK have fallen over the years from 62.5:1000 in 1930–5 to 7.6:1000 in 2009 for UK*. Declining mortality reflects improvement in standards of living, improved maternal health, and declining parity, as well as improvements in medical care. The main causes of stillbirth were congenital abnormalities (9%), antepartum/intrapartum haemorrhage (11%), placental conditions (12%) in 2009. The cause in 28% of stillbirths was unexplained. The main causes of neonatal death were prematurity (48%) and malformation (22%).

Examples of how changed medical care may reduce mortality

- Worldwide, treatment of syphilis, antitetanus vaccination (of mother during pregnancy), and clean delivery (especially cord techniques) have the greatest influence in reducing perinatal mortality.
- Antenatal detection and termination of malformed fetuses.
- Reduction of mid-cavity procedures and vaginal breech delivery.
- Detection of placenta praevia antenatally.
- Prevention of rhesus incompatibility.
- Preventing progression of preterm labour.
- Better control of diabetes mellitus in affected mothers.
- Antenatal monitoring of 'at-risk' pregnancies.

While we must try to reduce morbidity and mortality still further, this must not blind us to other problems that remain, such as the 'over-medicalization' of birth; the problem of reconciling maternal wishes to be in charge of her own delivery with the immediate needs of the baby; and the problem of explaining risks and benefits in terms that both parents understand, so that they can join in the decision-making process.

Other relevant pages Orthopaedics (Chapter 11); Infectious disease (*OHCM* p372–447);
perinatal infection p34–7; child psychiatry p368–73; pain p718.

*With many thanks to our Specialist Reader, Dr Stuart Crisp FRCPCH FRACP, and Kushalinii
Ragubathy and MF Niroshan, our Junior Readers, for their contribution to this chapter.*

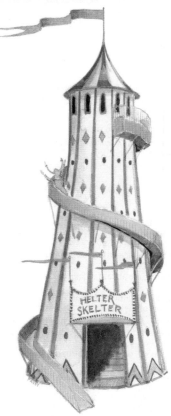

Fig 2.1 Helter Skelter (© Carolyn Pavey; watercolour, pen and ink). Helter skelters should be fun—as should our childhood. Pushing off at the top requires bravery and boldness, and so do many new adventures and experiences in childhood. The spiral shape of the slide is an illustration of the journey of discovery and learning that we travel through childhood towards adolescence. These years are about finding our way in life—from being completely dependent for all our care needs, to gaining the skills required to live independently and with success. In order to do this we need the boundaries, love, and protection that allow us to flourish in a positive and safe way (helter skelters would not be fun without the protective side wall). Good health allows us to grow and develop, yet there should be access to healthcare and treatment when required. Not all children have good health, access to healthcare, or a safe and loving home. It is our job to try and ensure we identify those in need—whether lacking in vitamins, minerals, or a parent's love, and put in place what is needed to help them climb back up to the top of the slide and continue on their journey.

There are 3 aims when taking a history:

1 Establish rapport with the child and their (extended) family. This builds trust and is critical to subsequent communication.

2 Formulate a differential diagnosis and ask questions to refute/support this.

3 Consider the above in the context of the child and family.

To facilitate this, remember to:

• Introduce yourself and explain what is to happen
• Talk first to the child, then to the carers, then to any relevant others
• Smile!
• Get down to the child's level
• Use non-medical language with no jargon.

Always record the date and time when you undertook the consultation, who was present, and who gave the history.

Presenting complaints Record the child's, parents', and GP's own words.

The present illness
• When and how did it start?
• Was he/she well before?
• How did it develop?
• What aggravates or alleviates it?
• Has there been contact with infections?
• Has the child been overseas recently?
• Have the carers sought medical attention before now?
• Which treatments have been tried?
• Especially in infants, enquire about feeding, wet and dirty nappies, alertness, and weight gain.
• After ascertaining the presenting complaint, use further questioning to test the various hypotheses of the differential diagnosis.

Past medical history *In utero:* Any problems (eg abnormal bleeding, infections, Rh disease); medication, alcohol, or recreational drug exposure? Were US normal?

At birth: Gestation, mode of delivery, birthweight, resuscitation required, birth injury, malformations.

As a neonate: Jaundice, fits, fevers, bleeding, feeding problems. Did the baby receive vitamin K? How long did the baby spend on the special care baby unit? Ask about later illnesses, operations, accidents, newborn screening tests, drugs, allergies, immunization and travel. Check the Red Book (UK only).[1]

Development (p219) Ask about the age the child learned to sit, crawl, walk, and talk.

Drugs Prescribed, recreational, *in utero*, and over-the-counter. Drug intolerances, adverse drug reactions, and true allergies (ie rashes, anaphylaxis).

Family history Are there any medical problems that run in the family? Is there anyone in the wider family with medical, psychiatric, or learning difficulties? Has anyone had a child die? Consanguinity is common in some cultures and may be relevant to disease.

Social history Who is at home? Note ages of siblings. Do they all have the same father? Ask about play, eating, sleeping, schooling, and pets. Who looks after the child if the parents work? What work do they do? Ask about their hopes, fears, and expectations about the child's illness and hospital stay.

Ensure privacy whenever discussing sensitive issues.

►If the family does not speak your language, find an interpreter.

1 The Red Book (and e-book) is a personal child health record given to parents in the UK at birth.

Systems review			
	Neonate	**Toddler**	**Older child**
General condition	Weight gain, appetite, sleep	Weight gain, appetite, sleep, milestones, is the child its normal self?	Do they feel unwell, tired, or fatigued? How is school?
Cardiorespiratory	Tachypnoea, grunting, wheeze, cyanosis, cold sweats (heart failure), exposure to TB, smokers in the family? Is there a family history of heart murmur?	Cough, exertional dyspnoea, sputum, haemoptysis, exposure to TB, smokers in the family. Family history of heart murmur or rheumatic fever?	Exercise limitation? Cough, wheeze, sputum, haemoptysis, chest pain, exposure to TB, smokers in the family? Family history of heart murmur or rheumatic fever?
Gut	Appetite, D&V, feeding problems, jaundice, bleeding, appropriate weight gain?	Appetite, D&V, stool frequency, rectal bleeding, weight gain?	Appetite, D&V, abdominal pain, stool frequency, rectal bleeding, weight loss.
Genitourinary	Wet nappies (how often?)	Wet nappies (how often?) Is there a history of infection? Any haematuria?	Haematuria, dysuria, discharge, sexual development. History of infection? Any history of bedwetting? Menarche? polydipsia/polyuria?
Neuromuscular	Seizures; attacks; jitters	Seizures, drowsy hyperactive hearing↓ vision↓ gait	Headaches, fits, odd sensations, drowsy, schooling, vision hearing, co-ordination
ENT; teeth	Noisy breathing. Did the baby have a newborn hearing test?	Are there problems with hearing or balance? Problems with ear infections or discharge? Any difficulty breathing? Nasal discharge, snoring or bleeding? Any lumps or glands?	Earache, discharge, recurrent infections? Problems with hearing or balance? Difficulty breathing? Nasal discharge, snoring, or bleeding? Lumps or glands? Sore throat, dental problems, or mouth ulcers?
Skin	Is there a rash? Birthmarks or other marks on the skin?	Is there a rash? Is it itchy? Birthmarks or other marks on the skin?	Is there a rash? Is it itchy? Birthmarks or other marks on the skin?

Paediatrics

Physical examination

A single routine will not work for all children. Gaining the confidence of the child and family during history taking will help. Convincing the child to let you examine them may be best done by the family. If the child is very ill, examination still needs to be thorough (p103). There is no correct order: *be opportunistic*, eg with younger children on a lap listen to heart when there are gaps in crying. You may not need to examine each system each time. Talk to the child and explain what you are doing. Sometimes it helps to examine their toy.

1 Wash and warm your hands. Encourage both parents to be present.

2 *General health:* Is the child ill or well? Alert, lethargic, or uncomfortable/ in pain? Playing is a good sign. If crying, is it high pitched or normal? Behaving normally and interacting with the parents? Any jaundice, cyanosis, rashes, anaemia, or dehydration (p234)? Neck stiffness is a rare sign in infants.

3 *Vital signs*: Temperature, heart rate, respiratory rate, BP, capillary refill time (press on the sternum for 5sec; capillary refill should be <2sec).

4 *Respiratory system:* Is the shape of the chest normal? Any intercostal, subcostal, or sternal recession, or nasal flaring? Use of accessory muscles? Is there grunting or any other audible noise breathing in (stridor) or out (wheeze)? Percuss the chest for dullness. Auscultate the chest, listening for breath sounds, fine crackles, rhonchi, wheeze, and pleural rub.

5 *Cardiovascular system:* Check for peripheral and central cyanosis; look for clubbing and peripheral oedema. Compare strength of femoral and right brachial pulse. Is the apex beat displaced? Auscultate the heart with the child sitting and in supine positions. Listen over the apex, the 2nd intercostal space to the left of the sternum (pulmonary valve), and the right of the sternum (aortic valve), and the 4th intercostal space over the sternum (tricuspid valve). Fixed splitting of the second heart sound occurs with an atrial septal defect. A gallop rhythm suggests congestive cardiac failure.

6 *Gastrointestinal system:* The child should be supine and relaxed, with the knees bent. Look for distension, visible peristalsis, and hernias. Listen for bowel sounds, and percuss for hepatosplenomegaly and ascites. Palpate looking for tenderness and masses (during inspiration and deep expiration). Never perform a PR—this should be done once only and by a senior. If relevant check for anal patency, fissures, and prolapse.

7 *Genitourinary system:* If relevant, examine external genitalia for evidence of ambiguity, congenital abnormality, and size. Examine once only using a chaperone and maintain the child's dignity and privacy. Note Tanner stage.

8 *Musculoskeletal system:* Watch the child walk and play. Examine all limbs and digits for congenital anomaly. Are there symmetrical skin creases on both thighs? If <6 months check for congenital hip dislocation. Inspect the spine looking for dimples, hair tufts, masses, or cysts at the base. Is there any abnormal curvature or posture?

9 *Ears, nose, and throat:* Always best to leave until the end with young children. Ask the mother to hold the child on their lap with one of her arms around the upper body and the other holding their head firmly against her. Is there evidence of otitis externa? Post-auricular rash is a sign of measles, rubella, and eczema. Look at the tympanic membrane using an otoscope noting colour and lucency. Is it perforated? Use a spatula to check the tonsils, as well as inspect the teeth and oral mucosa (plaques, white patches, spots, ulcers). Can the child breathe through both nostrils? Is there a runny nose? Check for neck lumps and lymphadenopathy.

10 Is there anything else the parents would like you to see or check?

11 *Height, weight, and head circumference;* plot on centile charts.

Is this child seriously ill?

Recognizing the need for prompt help is a central skill of paediatrics. Watch and learn from an experienced paediatrician in action. (See also APLS, p239.)

Airway, breathing, circulation: then inverse 'traffic light' assessment.

   Taking most feeds OK; normal colour (lips, tongue, skin); responds to social cues, alert or wakens quickly, lusty cry, or playing. Breathing calmly.

Taking ≤50% of feeds; pale; not responding to social cues; hard to wake; ↓activity; no smiling; tachypnoea; SaO₂ <95%; crepitations; nasal flaring if <1yr; capillary refill time >3sec. Don't rely on BP.³

Pale; mottled; ashen; blue. Doesn't stay awake when roused.² Consciousness↓ (not engaging; apathy; coma); skin turgor↓. Any GRUNTING signs?

➤➤ Grunting; weak or continuous high-pitched cry; tachypnoea.

➤➤ Rib recession; retraction of sternomastoid, nasal flaring; wheeze; stridor.

➤➤ Unequal or unresponsive pupils; focal CNS signs, fits, marked hypotonia.⁴

➤➤ Not using limbs/lying still; odd or rigid posture decorticate (flexed arms, extended legs); or decerebrate (arms + legs extended).

➤➤ T° ≥38°c if <6 months or ≥39° especially if cold or shutdown peripheries.

➤➤ I have a bad feeling about this baby. ►Learn to trust your judgement.

➤➤ Neck rigidity, non-blanching rash, meningism, bulging fontanelle, etc.

➤➤ Green bile in vomit⁵(≈GI obstruction,⁶ eg atresia, volvulus, intussusception).⁷

When assessing response level, use AVPU. A=alert; V=responds to voice; P=responds to pain; U=unresponsive.

Causes
• Sepsis, meningitis
• Seizures
• D&V/gastroenteritis
• Viraemia
• Obstruction, eg volvulus
• FPIES (food protein-induced enterocolitis syndrome)
• DKA (p188)
• Hypoglycaemia
• U&E imbalance
• Myocarditis
• Congenital heart dis.
• Cardiomyopathies
• Intussusception (p172)
• Arrhythmias
• DIC (p120 & ОНСМ p346)
• Haemolytic uraemic syn.
• Reye's syndrome (p652)
• Metabolic errors

Age—reference interval for:	Breathing rate	Pulse	Systolic BP
<1yr	30–40/min	110–160/min	70–90mmHg
2–5yr	20–30/min	95–140/min	80–100mmHg
5–12yr	15–20/min	80–120/min	90–110mmHg
>12yr	2–16/min	60–100/min	100–120mmHg

Beware an inappropriately normal heart rate or respiratory rate in a tiring and peri-arrest child.

Action ➤➤ Manage A, then B, before moving on to C.

• Call for help.
• Basic life support.
• Establish an airway; use 100% O₂. Use jaw lift if necessary; suction nasopharynx and mouth as needed. Provide oral or nasopharyngeal airway. Do not force a distressed patient to lie down.
• Identify level of respiratory severity and if resuscitation is needed eg bronchodilators for acute severe asthma. Work of breathing can be assisted by non-invasive ventilatory suport.
• Start pulse oximetry and cardiac monitoring. Establish IV access. Have a low threshold for intraosseus access if IV access is difficult (p236). Take relevant bloods. Provide IV fluids (20mL/kg normal saline) if volume depleted. Review and repeat until clinical improvement occurs. Early involvement of seniors is imperative. If no response to initial fluid bolus get specialist help—inotropes may be required.
• Treat the cause.

Paediatrics

Crying Up to 20% report problems with crying in the 1st 3 months of life; usually no cause is found. Crying peaks at 6–8 weeks old (~3h/day, worse in the evenings) and subsides by 4 months.[8] Cries of hunger and thirst are indistinguishable. The demand feeding vs routine feeding debate rages amongst parents, with each group convinced that they have the happier babies. Crying worsens 'postnatal blues' and may be the last straw for a parent with few reserves. Aim to offer help before this stage (www.purplecrying.info, www.cry-sis.org.uk). Don't make parents feel inadequate; encourage parents to take it in turns to sleep. Explain normal crying and sleeping.

- Baby-centred approach to help parents help the baby deal with discomfort.
- Take parents' concerns seriously.
- Help parents recognize when their baby is tired and hungry ('read-your-baby' lessons may be needed), and to apply a consistent approach to care.
- Involve the health visitor.
- Vocal (singing), vestibular (rocking, going for a drive) or tactile stimulation (hugs) may help. Encourage help from friends/family. Simplify daily living.
- If not coping, admit to a parenting centre or hospital;[9] don't over-medicalize!

Colic (Paroxysmal crying with pulling up of the legs, for >3h on ≥3days/wk.) There is an association with feeding difficulties.[10] *R:* *Movement* (carry-cot on wheels) is often tried and may help.[11] Let the baby *finish the first breast first* (hindmilk is easier to digest).[12] If breastfeeding, a low-allergen diet may help, as may probiotics. *Reassure strongly; reduce stress;*[13] encourage *grandparent* involvement. Remember: a crying baby may be a sign of major relationship problems.

Fisher's rule

Cows' milk protein allergy is a separate entity to colic, and is either IgE or non-IgE-mediated. It causes colic symptoms, but also gastro-oesophageal reflux disease, blood/mucus in stools, and may result in faltering growth. In exclusively breastfed babies, ask the mother to completely exclude cows' milk protein from her diet. In formula-fed babies, change to a hypoallergenic extensively hydrolysed or amino acid formula.

Nappy rash/diaper dermatitis 4 types (may co-exist):[14]

1 The common 'ammonia dermatitis'—red desquamating rash, sparing skin folds (as opposed to seborrhoeic dermatitis, which doesn't), is due to moisture retention, not ammonia.[15] It responds to frequent nappy changes (cloth nappies retain more moisture than disposables), or nappy-free periods, careful drying, and emollient creams. Best treatment: leave nappy off. Use barrier cream: eg **Sudocrem**® (zinc oxide cream).

2 Candida/thrush is isolatable from ~½ of all nappy rashes. Its hallmark is satellite spots beyond the main rash. Mycology: see p598. Treatment: as above, + **clotrimazole** (± **1% hydrocortisone** cream, no stronger, eg as Canesten HC®). Avoid oral antifungals (hepatotoxic) and gentian violet (staining is disliked).

3 Seborrhoeic dermatitis: a diffuse, red, shiny rash extends into skin folds, often occurs with other seborrhoeic areas, eg occiput (cradle cap). *R:* as for 1.[16]

4 Isolated, psoriasis-like scaly plaques (p594), which can be hard to treat.

Sleep problems See p392.

Further reading

NICE (2015). *Clinical Knowledge Summaries: Cows' Milk Protein Allergy in Children.*
http://cks.nice.org.uk/cows-milk-protein-allergy-in-children#!scenariorecommendation:1

Vomiting

- Effortless regurgitation of milk is common during feeds ('posseting')
- Vomiting between feeds is also common. Ask about carpets: significant vomiting in a baby will have caused lots of damage to the parents' carpets. No damage: unlikely to be pathological
- Gastro-oesophageal reflux, gastritis
- Over-feeding (150mL/kg/day is normal)
- Pyloric stenosis (projectile, at ~8 weeks old). Observing feeding is helpful in deciding if vomiting is projectile (eg over the end of the cot)
- Any infection, eg UTI
- Adverse food reaction
- Infective gastroenteritis.

Rarer causes
- Pharyngeal pouch
- Poisoning
- Raised intracranial pressure
- Metabolic conditions eg diabetic ketoacidosis, acute intermittent porphyria
- Almost any other illness
- *Bilious (green) vomiting:* Get urgent help, p130; consider duodenal obstruction or volvulus.

Paediatrics

Chronic childhood illness, and family support

Diseases such as asthma, CNS disease, and neoplasia may cause disintegration of even the most apparently secure families: ►*Consequent strife and marital breakdown may be more severe and have far-reaching consequences.*

Remember that illness makes families poor, and movement down the social scale leads to unpredictable consequences in housing and (un)employment. Families experiencing housing instability and food insecurity (without homelessness or hunger) are known to miss out on healthcare.[17][n=12,746]

Marital disharmony may seem to be beyond the scope of paediatrics, but any holistic view of child health *must* put the family at the centre of *all* attempts to foster child health and well-being.

We see many families coping well with severe, prolonged illness in a child. But don't presume that because things are OK in clinic today, you can afford to neglect the fostering of family life. Given a certain amount of stress almost *all* families will show psychopathology, in time. Your job is to prevent this if possible. Counselling skills are frequently needed. Ensure the GP is fully informed so that they are able to look after the parents' mental health.

Fever (meningitis, p202; pneumonia, p160; UTI, p174.) Most children with a fever have a self-limiting viral infection which resolves without any long-term consequences. However, it is important to exclude the possibility of underlying serious infection—bacteraemia occurs in 4% of febrile children. A thorough history and examination are required to determine the source.

Be concerned when:
• Less than half the usual amount of feed has been taken in the last day.
• There is breathing difficulty, or high-pitched continuous moans or cries.
• There is a history of being pale, mottled, cyanosed, and hot.
• Dull expression; apathetic; disinterested in you; drowsy; dehydrated.
• A significant reduction in the number of wet nappies in the last 24h.
• Blood in stool, or seizures, or tachycardia not explained by pain or fever.
The 3rd question is: *Is neutropenia possible* (eg on chemotherapy)?

Assess the *'traffic light' way*, p103, paying especial attention to red signs (pale, mottled, ashen blue, not staying awake when roused). Beware inappropriately normal vital signs. Always listen to your sixth sense: discuss with a senior doctor if you are uneasy about a patient. Then observe the limbs: pain causes *pseudoparalysis*, eg with legs in a frog position (hips & knees semi-flexed, feet rotated outward), eg in osteomyelitis, or septic arthritis. The above signs carry extra weight if immunocompromised.

Management of a child with fever is according to the traffic light system (p103) but use clinical judgement too. Discussion with seniors is essential. Once a diagnosis is reached treat accordingly.

Green features
• Manage at home (but consider social and family circumstances, parental instinct or concerns, contact with serious illness and recent travel)
• Parents should be instructed to check on their child during the night, offer regular drinks (seek medical advice if the child stops drinking), to look for signs of dehydration (dry mouth, no tears), look for a non-blanching rash by rolling a glass over the rash (seek immediate medical advice if present). If the child is well, but the fever continues for >4 days parents should be reviewed in the emergency department (GPs cannot diagnose Kawasaki's disease). Parents should not tepid-sponge their child and should keep their child off school or nursery.

Red or amber features
• These children need admission
• Red features: life-threatening illness—child needs urgent treatment
• If there is no apparent source of infection, carry out the following:
  • Blood—culture, FBC, CRP, electrolytes
  • Urine—test for UTI
  • Lumbar puncture—if clinical assessment dictates it and no contraindications
  • CXR—if respiratory symptoms/signs and no other focus
• Antibiotics: maximum dose third-generation cephalosporins (not ceftriaxone due to risk of calcium chelation) should be given to children with fever and signs of shock or coma, and/or signs of meningococcal disease, or suspected *N. meningitidis, Streptococcus pneumoniae, E. coli, Staphylococcus aureus,* or *Haemophilus influenzae* type B
• If herpes simplex encephalitis is suspected, give IV aciclovir
• If bacterial meningitis confirmed, some give IV corticosteroid if >3 months.

Further reading

NICE (2013). *Fever in Under 5s: Assessment and Initial Management* (CG150). London: NICE. http://www.nice.org.uk/guidance/cg160

Paediatrics

Most neonates are perfectly healthy: the best plan is to return these babies to the mother to help bonding. Mother-and-baby skin-to-skin contact is ideal, rather than swaddling or nursery cots, and is the best way to maintain temperature. A paediatrician or nurse trained in advanced neonatal resuscitation should attend the following births, and whenever there is concern about the fetus: emergency caesareans, breeches, twins, instrumental deliveries, prematurity, eclampsia, and thick meconium-stained liquor. Hypoxia is the cause of most neonatal cardiac arrests.

Before birth Check and heat the resuscitaire, and have at least 2 towels available.

At birth
- Baby pink and crying: give back to mother
- If not, rub vigorously and get a brief antenatal history, and check gestation
- If no spontaneous breathing, start bag and mask ventilation using air (eg Neopuff at 6mmHg)
- Ensure the chest is expanding; if not, readjust the head position and consider airway adjuncts or a second person to ensure an adequate seal. Once 5 inflation breaths have caused chest movement, if the baby is still not making any respiratory effort, aim for 40-60 breaths/min. If not pinking up, add oxygen step-wise
- Check heart rate and if <60/min start chest compressions (1/3 depth of AP diameter and rate of 100/min)
- Adequate ventilation usually ensures that the heart rate improves
- If not, give IV or IO adrenaline 0.3mL 1:1000; if no response repeat with 1mL followed by 20mL/kg 0.9% saline. If maternal APH use O negative blood
- Check glucose and treat hypoglycaemia with 10% glucose; repeat sugar level
- If meconium and baby unresponsive, suck out oropharynx under direct vision, and suction/wash out under vocal cords. If baby vigorous, do nothing
- Naloxone is rarely helpful and is dangerous if the mother is on methadone.

Endotracheal intubation is a key skill: use 3.5mm uncuffed, unshouldered tubes on term infants; 3mm if 32-36 weeks, 2.5mm if smaller. Learn from experts.

Dry and stimulate baby (unless <28wks); place under radiant heat

↓

Start clock; assess *colour, tone, breathing,* & *heart rate*. Place head in neutral position

↓

If not breathing
Give 5 inflation breaths and reassess

↓

If no increase in HR look for chest wall movement

Call for help

↓

If no chest wall movement, re-check *head position* and try airway manoevres and/or 2-person airway control. Repeat 5 inflation breaths. Confirm response: visible chest movements or ↑ HR

↓

Any sucking out of the pharynx should be under direct vision.[18]
- Repeat 5 inflation breaths
- Insert oropharyngeal airway
- Repeat inflation breaths
Consider intubation. Confirm response: visible chest movements or ↑ HR

↓

When chest is moving, continue with ventilation breaths if no spontaneous breathing

↓

Check heart rate; if absent or <60 *start chest compressions*. Do 3 chest compressions to 1 breath, for 30sec

↓

Reassess HR: if HR still absent or <60 consider venous access (IV, umbilical venous catheter or intra-osseous) and drugs (adrenaline). Continue ventilation & chest compressions

↓

At all stages ask: *Do I need help?*

Paediatrics

Apgar[3]	Pulse	Respirations	Muscle tone	Colour	On suction
2	>100	Strong cry	Active	Pink	Coughs well
1	<100	Slow, irregular	Limb flexion	Blue limbs	Depressed cough
0	0	Nil	Absent	All blue or white	No response

3 Apgar score: A score is given for each vital sign at 1, 5, and 10 minutes of age using the above scoring system

Neonatal intensive care is a technological development of the basic creed of first aid— ABC; airway, breathing, and circulation. There is also an E. Epithelial cells determine whether low birthweight babies survive outside the uterus. They manage all interactions with the *ex utero* world: • Lung mechanics/gas exchange • Renal tubular balance of fluid and electrolytes • Barrier functions of the gut and skin for keeping bacteria out and water in, plus enabling digestion • Intact neuroepithelium lining of the ventricles of the brain and retina.[19]

Monitor T°, pulse, BP (intra-arterial if critical), respirations, blood gases ($SaO_2 \pm$ intra-arterial electrode), U&E, bilirubin, FBC, weight, weekly head circumference.

Problems facing babies on NICU

- Hypothermia: incubators allow temperature to be controlled
- Hypoxia (ventilatory support, p110)
- Hypoglycaemia (p112)
- Respiratory distress syndrome (p118)
- Infection (p112)
- *Intraventricular haemorrhage* occurs in 25% if birthweight ≤1500g.[20] Preterm infants are at risk of IVH due to unsupported blood vessels in the subependymal germinal matrix and the instability of blood pressure associated with birth trauma and respiratory distress. Delayed cord clamping in prems may ↓risk.[21] *Signs:* Seizures, bulging fontanelle and cerebral irritability but many will have no clinical symptoms.[22] *Tests:* US; MRI. *Complications:* IQ↓, cerebral palsy, hydrocephalus Many survive without any sequelae.
- *Apnoea:* prevalence is 25% of neonates <2.5kg, higher with lower birthweights. Common causes are prematurity, infection, hypothermia, aspiration, congenital heart disease. Caffeine is used in babies <28 weeks. *Prevention:* Maternal corticosteroids for fetal lung maturation to increase surfactant production in those at risk of preterm delivery (23-34⁺⁶ weeks' gestation) (p51).
- Necrotizing enterocolitis (p120).
- *You* may become the problem: overzealous investigation/handling is damaging,[23] as is under-intervention.[24]
- *Retinopathy of prematurity* is a disorder of the developing retina. Abnormal fibrovascular proliferation or retinal vessels may lead to retinal detachment and visual loss. Major risk factors are low birth weight and prematurity. Exposure to supplemental oxygen is a cause, in particular large fluctuations in PaO_2, so careful titration of O_2 levels has led to a decrease in the incidence of ROP. *Prevalence (lower limits):* <750g: 62%, >1000g: 10%[25] *Classification:* There are 5 stages, depending on site involved, the degree of retinal detachment, and extent. *Treatment:* Diode laser therapy causes less myopia than cryotherapy. Screening: see BOX below:

Screening for retinopathy of prematurity[26]

Screening is performed by indirect opthalmoscopy (a light attached to a headband with a small handheld lens, giving a better view of the fundus than direct fundoscopy), or wide field digital retinal screening.

Screening criteria

If ≤27 weeks, screen at 30-31 weeks postmenstrual age.

If born at 27-32 weeks, screen at day 28-35 of life.

Screening is repeated 2-weekly depending on severity of disease.

With our first breath, pulmonary vascular resistance falls, and there is a rush of blood to our lungs. This is partly mediated by endogenous nitric oxide (NO). This breath initiates changes from fetal to adult circulation—a process which may be interrupted in various conditions, eg meconium aspiration, pneumonia, respiratory distress syndrome, diaphragmatic hernia, group B strep infection, and pulmonary hypoplasia.

Pulmonary hypertension arises as a consequence of these adverse events. It may also be due to hypertrophy of the muscular layer in the pulmonary arteries (primary pulmonary hypertension).

The chief diagnostic features are an underlying cause (eg meconium aspiration) and persisting desaturation despite intensive O_2 use. When it is suspected, arrange echocardiography, and get help. Echo will show right-to-left shunting at the ductus arteriosus in the absence of structural heart disease.

Ventilate (p110) gently, and correct reversible contributory factors (hypothermia, polycythaemia, hypocalcaemia, hypoglycaemia). Give surfactant as indicated (p118). Inhaled nitric oxide has a role in promoting adult circulation and may improve outcomes from premature babies.

Extracorporeal membrane oxygenation (ECMO) ECMO is a complex procedure available in tertiary units providing life support for respiratory failure, which obviates the need for lung gas exchange.

Paediatrics

This is a skill to be learned at the cot side. Nurses and specialist respiratory therapists will help you. Needs of apparently similar babies vary, so what follows is only a guide to prepare your mind before teaching. Continuous refinement in the light of transcutaneous and blood gas analysis is needed. The aims are to improve gas exchange, decrease work of breathing, and enable ventilation for those with respiratory depression or apnoea.

Non-invasive ventilation

CPAP (continuous positive airways pressure) Pressure is delivered throughout the respiratory cycle, assisting spontaneous ventilation. It prevents airway collapse and loss of lung volume. Complications include pneumothorax, nasal trauma, feed intolerance, and reflux. It is used in RDS and respiratory support, particularly in preterm infants, post-extubation, and in upper airway obstruction. CPAP is delivered by nasal mask or binasal prongs, or rarely via face mask.

NIPPV (nasal intermittent positive pressure ventilation) This combines nasal CPAP with superimposed ventilator breathing at a set pressure—it can be used as a bridge between invasive ventilation and nasal CPAP.

HFNC (high-flow nasal cannula) A high flow nasal cannula delivers a distending positive pressure to the airways similar to CPAP. Humidifying the gas delivered reduces side effects of mucosal dryness. Use of HFNC may reduce the number of ventilated days compared to CPAP, but it is not yet considered as standard practice.[29]

Invasive ventilation

Invasive ventilation is broadly composed of *conventional mechanical ventilation* (CMV) (AKA intermittent mandatory ventilation (IMV)) and *high-frequency ventilation* (HFV).

TCPL (time-cycled pressure limited ventilation) Continuous flows of heated and humidified gas pass via an endotracheal tube. The breath delivered is set by peak inspiratory pressure (PIP) and either the absolute inspiratory time (T_I), or the inspiratory:expiratory ratio (I:E ratio). The delivered tidal volume is dependent on lung compliance and resistance. Nasotracheal siting is best (fewer tube displacements).[30] TCPL allows the infant to make respiratory efforts between ventilator breaths which can lead to dysynchrony between the ventilator and the baby. *Initial settings:* Choose to give good chest inflation and air entry on auscultation and adequate oximetry readings. Typical settings might be T_I 0.32sec, 40 cycles/min, inspiratory pressure 14–18cmH$_2$O, and PEEP 5cmH$_2$O. Adjust in the light of blood gas analysis.

PTV (patient-triggered ventilation), including SIMV and SIPPV. PTV combines TCPL ventilation with a sensor which detects spontaneous breaths. The ventilator then delivers a breath which is synchronized with the infant's own inspiratory effort. In PTV, inspiratory and end-expiratory pressure is set by the operator, but the rate (within limits) set by the baby. PTV is associated with a shorter duration of ventilation.[31,32] Hiccups cause problems if abdominal movement is used to detect inspiration.

HFV (high-frequency ventilation) delivers small volumes of gas at very rapid rates. Its aim is to reduce ventilator-associated lung injuries. There are several different types—high-frequency positive pressure ventilation (HFPPV), jet ventilation, flow interrupted and oscillatory ventilation (HFOV). HFPPV may reduce incidence of air leak compared to CMV (see 'Other factors' BOX).[33]

Sedation is given prior to elective intubation with an opiate such as morphine or fentanyl, with a muscle relaxant (suxamethonium). For ventilated preterm infants, evidence does not support routine use of morphine infusion. Most babies do not need long-term paralysis.

Factors associated with a good outcome from ventilation

Factors associated with a better outcome: antenatal corticosteroids, singleton pregnancy, ♀ sex, and higher birthweight.[34] In this study of infants born at 22 to 25 weeks' gestation, 49% died, 61% died or had profound impairment (eg neurosensory disability, IQ↓, or cerebral palsy), and 73% died or had some impairment.

Complications of mechanical ventilation of neonates

Lung Pneumothorax; pulmonary haemorrhage; bronchopulmonary dysplasia (p119); interstitial pulmonary emphysema; pneumonia. Multidrug-resistant organisms may be the cause of late-onset ventilator-associated pneumonia (cefepime has a role here).[35] Post extubation atelectasis may be more frequent after nasal intubation (esp. in very-low-birthweight infants).[36]

Airways Upper airway obstruction (worse in inspiration and may cause stridor). Consider bronchoscopy (may show supraglottic lesions). Laryngomalacia and gastro-oesophageal reflux also occur, but more rarely.[37]

Others Patent ductus arteriosus; ↑intracranial pressure ± intraventricular haemorrhage (p108); retinopathy of prematurity (p108); subcutaneous emphysema; pneumomediastinum; pneumopericardium; pneumoperitoneum; air embolus (very rare and not clinically significant).

Weaning from the ventilator

As the baby's condition improves, ventilatory support is weaned. Reduce oxygen to lowest level needed to maintain PaO_2. This reduces retinopathy risk. Decrease the rate of IMV and lower P_I by 2cmH2O at a time; try extubating if blood gas OK with ~4cmH2O PEEP and a PIP of 12-14 with spontaneous breaths over a backup rate of 5. Preterm infants benefit from starting nasal CPAP following extubation. If ventilation has been short-term, extubation without CPAP is appropriate.

Other factors

Pain relief/sedation Consider 5% glucose IVI with morphine 25-50mcg/kg over ≥5min, then 5-40mcg/kg/h. This is thought safe, and lowers catecholamine concentrations.

Air leak Air ruptures alveoli tracking along vessels and bronchioles (pulmonary interstitial emphysema), and may extend intrapleurally (pneumothorax + lung collapse), or into the mediastinum or peritoneum. Associated with high PIP, it is less common with HFOV. *Signs:* Tachypnoea, cyanosis, chest asymmetry. The lateral decubitus CXR is often diagnostic if you have time. ▶▶Prompt 'blind' needle aspiration of a pneumothorax may be needed in an acute deterioration. Aspirate through the second intercostal space in the midclavicular line with a 25G 'butterfly' needle and a 50mL syringe on a 3-way tap. Following this, insert a chest drain.

Sepsis More common in premature than term babies. Acquired transplacentally, via ascent from vagina, during birth, or from the environment. Mortality up to 15% (30% if low birthweight). Categorized as early onset (within 48h birth) or late onset. *Presentation:* Signs may be non-specific and subtle. Labile temperature, lethargy, poor feeding, respiratory distress, collapse, DIC.

Management
- ABC (p108)
- Supportive (may require ventilation, volume expansion, inotropes)
- Take blood for FBC, CRP (may be normal; helpful if raised; bacterial sepsis unlikely if CRP normal 12h later), glucose
- Blood cultures (results take 48h)
- CXR
- Lumbar puncture for culture, glucose, protein count, WCC and Gram stain
- If there is a failure to respond within 24h, investigate further with stool sample for virology, throat swab, serology for herpes virus, urine CMV culture, VDRL.

Antibiotics in early-onset neonatal infection
- Give broad-spectrum antibiotics eg benzylpenicillin + gentamicin until blood culture results are available. Stop if well and cultures negative; continue treatment for 7 days if cultures positive
- If meningitis is suspected, give cefotaxime. If confirmed, treat for 14-21 days
- If *Listeria* suspected (purulent conjunctivitis, maternal infection), give ampicillin/amoxicillin.

Antibiotics in late-onset neonatal infection
- Broad-spectrum antibiotics eg flucloxacillin + gentamicin
- Give cefotaxime if meningitis likely
- Coagulase –ve Staph sepsis is more likely in preterm infant with CVP line— treat with vancomycin and discuss removal and use of the line with senior
- Consider fungal sepsis if failure to respond to standard treatment.

Risk factors for neonatal sepsis

Risk factors for early-onset neonatal sepsis
- Prolonged rupture of membranes >18h
- Maternal infection; maternal pyrexia, chorioamnionitis, UTI
- Mother known carrier of group B *Streptococcus* (GBS) from vagina or urine, or previous infant affected by it (prevention: p37, obstetrics)
- Preterm labour
- Fetal distress
- Breaks in neonatal skin or mucosa.

Infection is caused by organisms acquired from the mother—usually GBS, *E. coli* or *Listeria*. Other agents include herpes simplex (highest risk to neonate-from primary vulval herpes infection within 6 weeks of delivery), *Chlamydia trachomatis*, anaerobes and *H. influenza*.

Risk factors for late-onset neonatal sepsis
- Central lines and catheters
- Congenital malformations eg spina bifida
- Severe illness
- Malnutrition
- Immunodeficiency.

Infection tends to be caused by environmental organisms, eg coagulase-negative staphylococci, *Staph. aureus*, *E. coli* and GBS. Fungal sepsis (from *Candida* sp.) should be considered in any infant who fails to respond to standard therapy.

Neonatal seizures (~4/1000 births) Most occur 12–48h after birth, and may be generalized or focal, and tonic, clonic, or myoclonic.

Causes
• Hypoxic-ischaemic encephalopathy (due to antenatal or intrapartum hypoxia/respiratory distress etc.)
• Infection (meningitis/encephalitis)
• Intracranial haemorrhage/infarction
• Structural CNS lesions (focal cortical dysplasia/tuberous sclerosis)
• Metabolic disturbance (hypoglycaemia; ↓Ca^{2+}; ↑↓Na^+; ↓Mg^{2+})
• Metabolic disorders (urea cycle disorders/amino acid metabolism)
• Neonatal withdrawal from maternal drugs or substance abuse
• Kernicterus
• Idiopathic seizures eg benign 5th day fits.

Diagnosis: Can be difficult as there may only be subtle clinical signs of seizures, eg lip-smacking, limb-cycling, eye deviation, apnoeas. EEG can confirm seizure activity.

Treatment: ABC. Turn on the side. Ask an experienced nurse to help.
• Rule out or treat reversible causes such as hypoglycaemia
• Start on empirical antibiotics
• Insert IV access and take blood for FBC, U&E, LFTS, calcium, magnesium, glucose and blood gas
• If available, commence cerebral function analysis monitoring (CFAM)
• Radiological investigation may include cranial US, and MRI
• Specialist tests include toxicology screening, serum ammonia, urine organic acids, serum amino acids, karyotype and TORCH screen
• Treat the cause. A single short seizure does not need to be treated with anticonvulsants. If prolonged (>3–5min) or repeated seizures consider anticonvulsants. *First line:* Phenobarbital Loading dose: 20mg/kg IV as slow injection. *Second line:* Phenytoin 18mg/kg IVI. Other agents: clonazepam; midazolam; paraldehyde. If intractable seizures consider pyridoxine 50mg IV + 50–100mg/day PO in case of pyridoxine deficiency.[Autosomal 38 recessive] *Hypocalcaemia:* Calcium gluconate 10%, 4.4mL/kg/day PO (IV: 0.5mL/kg diluted in 4.8mL/kg of saline over 5–10min). Monitor ECG. *Hypomagnesaemia:* Give 100mg/kg of $MgSO_4$ 10% (=100mg/mL),[1] IV over >10min.[39]

Hypoxic-ischaemic encephalopathy (HIE) is a clinical syndrome of brain injury secondary to a hypoxic-ischaemic insult. In developed countries, the incidence is 2–5/1000 live births, of which 1–2/1000 are moderate to severe. The cause may be antenatal, intrapartum, or postpartum, eg cord prolapse, placental abruption, any cause of maternal hypoxia, or inadequate postnatal cardiopulmonary circulation. Presentation varies depending on the severity of cerebral hypoxia. The baby will have respiratory depression at birth, and a need for resuscitation, including IPPV. pH soon after birth is <7.0 and base excess worse than −12. Encephalopathy develops within 24h of birth. Management is with resuscitation, avoidance of hyperthermia, exclusion of other causes of encephalopathy, and monitoring and treatment of seizures (eg using CFAM, cerebral function analysis monitoring). Therapeutic hypothermia is standard for term babies with moderate to severe HIE, because it reduces death and disability.

Shock *Causes:* Blood loss (placental haemorrhage, twin–twin transfusion; intraventricular haemorrhage; lung haemorrhage); capillary plasma leaks (sepsis, hypoxia, acidosis, necrotizing enterocolitis); fluid loss (D&V; inappropriate diuresis); cardiac causes (hypoxia, L-to-R shunts, valve disease, coarctation). *Signs:* Pulse ↑; BP ↓; urine output ↓; coma. *Management:* ABC. Ventilate as needed. Give colloid 10–20mL/kg IV as needed. Inotropes may be used, eg dopamine 3–20mcg/kg per min[2] ± dobutamine 5–20mcg/kg/min as needed[40] (*may* act synergistically; detailed dosing: p203). Treat causes.

Paediatrics

The aim is to screen for abnormality, and to see if the mother has any questions or difficulties.[4] The following is a recommended routine before the baby leaves hospital—or during the 1st week of life for home deliveries. Before the examination find out if the birthweight was normal. Was the birth and pregnancy normal? Is mother Rh-ve? Find a quiet, warm, well-lit room. Enlist the mother's help. Explain your aims. Listen if she talks. Examine systematically, eg head-to-toe. Wash your hands meticulously. Note observations (eg τ°).[41,42]

Head Circumference (50th centile=35cm, p224), shape (odd shapes from a difficult labour soon resolve), fontanelles (tense if crying or intracranial pressure↑; sunken if dehydrated). *Eyes:* Red reflex (absent in cataract & retinoblastoma); corneal opacities; conjunctivitis. *Ears:* Shape; position. Are they low set (ie below eyes)? The tip of the nose, when pressed, shows jaundice in white babies. Breathing out of the nose (shut the mouth) tests for choanal atresia. Ensure oto-acoustic screening is done (p548). Are follow-up brainstem-evoked responses needed?[43] *Complexion:* Cyanosed, pale, jaundiced, or ruddy (polycythaemia)? *Mouth:* Look inside; insert a finger: is the palate intact? Is suck good? Does the baby's face look normal? Dysmorphism can be difficult to detect soon after birth as the baby may have some puffiness in the face.

Arms & hands Single palmar creases (normal or trisomy 21). Does the baby look like the parents? Waiter's tip sign of Erb's palsy of C5 & 6 trunks (p76; p766). Number of fingers. Clinodactyly (5th finger is curved towards the ring finger, eg in normal or trisomy 21).

Thorax Watch respirations; note grunting and intercostal recession. Palpate the precordium and apex beat. Listen to the heart and lungs. Inspect the vertebral column for neural tube defects.

Abdomen Expect to feel the liver. Any other masses? Inspect the umbilicus. Is it healthy? Next, lift the skin to assess skin turgor. Inspect genitalia and anus. Are the orifices patent? Ensure in the 1st 24 hours the baby passes urine (consider posterior urethral valves in boys if not) and stool (consider Hirschprung's, cystic fibrosis, hypothyroidism). Is the urinary meatus misplaced (hypospadias), and are both testes descended? The neonatal clitoris often looks rather large, but if very large, consider CAH, p134. Bleeding PV may be a normal variant following maternal oestrogen withdrawal.

Legs Test for developmental dysplasia of the hip (p684). Avoid repeated tests as it hurts, and may induce dislocation. Can you feel femoral pulses (to 'exclude' coarctation)? Note talipes (p684). Toes: too many, too few, or too blue?

Buttocks/sacrum Is there an anus? Are there 'mongolian spots'? (blue—and harmless). Tufts of hair ± dimples suggest bifida occulta. If you can't see the bottom of a dimple, arrange US. Any pilonidal sinus?

CNS Assess posture and handle the baby. Intuition can be most helpful in deciding if the baby is ill or well. Is he jittery (hypoxia/ischaemia, encephalopathy, hypoglycaemia, infection, hypocalcaemia)? There should be some control of the head. Do limbs move normally? Is the tone floppy[5] or spastic? Are responses absent on one side (hemiplegia)? The Moro reflex is done by sitting the baby at 45°, supporting the head. On momentarily removing the support the arms will abduct, the hands open and then the arms adduct. Stroke the palm to elicit a grasp reflex. Is the baby post-mature, small for dates, or premature (p128)?

▶Discuss any abnormality with the parents *after liaising with a senior doctor.*

4 The neonatal period is the 1st 28 days of life; if prem, 44 completed weeks of the infant's conceptional age (=the chronological age plus gestational age at birth).[44]
5 Causes of floppiness: Sepsis; hypoglycaemia; dehydration; hypothermia; trauma/abuse; myopathy; poor nutrition; botulism (may look like near sudden infant death syndrome)[45]; maternal drugs (lorazepam; clozapine); alcohol withdrawal; rickets; trisomy 21, Ehlers–Danlos, or Prader–Willi syndromes; cerebral palsy; CNS syndromes—eg muscular dystrophy, myasthenia, Zellweger leukodystrophy, Guillain–Barré—or myotonic dystrophy (shake hands with the mother: she may have delayed release of grip).[46]

Neonatal jaundice is common, occurring in 60% of neonates.[47] Most do not need any treatment. Jaundice is caused by raised bilirubin levels. When severe, or not properly managed, kernicterus, a permanent form of brain damage, may occur. Transcutaneous bilirubin levels measured by midwives in homes may prevent kernicterus in babies discharged early by allowing early detection of jaundice. In non-Caucasians, the device needs recalibration.[48] Management of severe neonatal jaundice typically involves phototherapy, and exchange transfusion if very severe. The threshold levels for these treatments varies with gestational age, and post-natal age. (see NICE guidelines at www.nice.org.uk/cg98)

Hyperbilirubinaemia (<200µmol/L) after 24h is usually 'physiological':
1 Increased bilirubin production in neonates due to shorter RBC lifespan.
2 Decreased bilirubin conjugation due to hepatic immaturity.
3 Absence of gut flora impedes elimination of bile pigment.
4 Exclusive breastfeeding (esp. if there are feeding difficulties→↓intake→ dehydration→↓bilirubin elimination + ↑enterohepatic circulation of bilirubin—not a reason to stop[49]).

Visible jaundice within 24h of birth is always abnormal. *Causes:* ►Sepsis or:
• *Rhesus haemolytic disease:* +ve direct Coombs test (DCT, p117).
• *ABO incompatibility:* (mother O; baby A or B, or mother A and baby B, or vice versa) DCT +ve in 4%; indirect Coombs +ve in 8%. Maternal IgG anti-A or anti-B haemolysin is 'always' present.[50]
• *Red cell anomalies:* congenital spherocytosis (fragility tests/EMA binding, p196); glucose-6-phosphate dehydrogenase deficiency (do enzyme test).[51]

Tests: FBC; film; blood groups (eg rare group incompatibility); Coombs test.[52]

Prolonged jaundice (not fading after 14 days in term babies, or 21 days in prems) *Causes:* breastfeeding; sepsis (UTI & TORCH, p34); hypothyroidism; cystic fibrosis; biliary atresia if conjugated and pale stools. *Galactosaemia:* urine tests for reducing agents (eg Clinitest®) are +ve, but specific tests (Clinistix®) for glycosuria are –ve (an insensitive test; galactose-1-phosphate uradyl transferase levels diagnostic).

Phototherapy uses light energy to convert bilirubin to soluble products (lumirubin and other isomers) that can be excreted without conjugation. Efficacy depends on irradiance (measured in µW/cm²)—so exposing baby will lead to more rapid reduction in serum bilirubin, as will using light from above and below. Breast feeds should be brief to maximize time under the lights. SE: T°↑↓; eye damage (baby will need eye protection); diarrhoea; separation from mother; fluid loss. *Intense phototherapy* is an adjunct to exchange transfusion.[53,54] To decide when to start phototherapy/exchange transfusion use NICE guidelines (www.nice.org.uk/cg98), or your unit's protocol.

Exchange transfusion Uses warmed blood (37°c), 160mL/kg (double volume), given ideally via umbilical vein IVI, with removal via umbilical artery. The aim is to remove bilirubin in those with severe or rapidly rising hyperbilirubinaemia.

Kernicterus refers to the clinical features of acute bilirubin encephalopathy (ABE): lethargy/poor feeding/hypertonicity/opisthotonus/shrill cry—and chronic bilirubin encephalopathy, as well as the yellow staining in the brain associated with ABE. Risk is increased with extremely high bilirubin levels (360µmol/L; lower in prems). Long-term sequelae include athetoid movements, deafness, and ↓IQ. It is prevented by phototherapy (below) ± exchange transfusion.[55]

Further reading
NICE (2010). *Neonatal Jaundice* (CG98). London: NICE. https://www.nice.org.uk/guidance/cg98

Physiology When a RhD–ve mother delivers a RhD+ve baby a leak of fetal red cells into her circulation may stimulate her to produce anti-D IgG antibodies (isoimmunization). In subsequent pregnancies these can cross the placenta, causing worsening rhesus haemolytic disease (*erythroblastosis fetalis*) with each successive Rh+ve pregnancy. First pregnancies may be affected due to leaks, eg: •Threatened miscarriage •APH •Mild trauma •Amniocentesis •Chorionic villous sampling •External cephalic version.

There is a wide clinical spectrum. A severely affected oedematous fetus (with stiff, oedematous lungs) is called a *hydrops fetalis*. Anaemia-associated CCF causes oedema, as does hypoalbuminaemia (the liver is preoccupied by producing new RBCs). *ΔΔ:* Thalassaemia; infection (eg toxoplasmosis, CMV, p34); maternal diabetes.

Clinical Rh disease ►*Test for D antibodies in all Rh–ve mothers, at booking, 28 & 34 weeks' gestation.* Anti-D titres <4u/mL (<1:16) are very unlikely to cause serious disease; it is wise to check maternal blood every 2 weeks. If >10u/mL, get the advice of a referral centre: fetal blood sampling ± intra-peritoneal (or, with fetoscopy, intravascular via the cord) transfusion may be needed.

Signs
• Jaundice—eg on day 1
• Yellow vernix
• CCF (oedema, ascites)
• Hepatosplenomegaly
• Progressive anaemia
• Bleeding
• CNS signs
• Kernicterus (p115)

Expect fetal Hb to be <7g/dL in 10% of those with titres of 10–100u/mL (75% if titres >100u/mL).

Do regular US (+amniocentesis if anti-D titre >4u/mL). Timing is vital. Do it 10 weeks before a Rh-related event in the last pregnancy (eg if last baby needed delivery at 36 weeks, expect to do amniocentesis at 26 weeks). Fetuses tolerating high bilirubins may be saved risky transfusions (fatality 2–30%) if monitored by serial measurements of fetal Hb (by fetoscopy or non-invasive middle cerebral artery peak velocity) and daily US to detect oedema, cardiomegaly, pericardial effusion, hepatosplenomegaly, or ascites.[56]

Anti-D is the chief antibody. Others: Rh C, E, c, e, Kell, Kidd, Duffy (all are IgG). Low concentrations sometimes produce severe disease.

Prognosis is improving. Mortality is <20% even for hydropic babies. Note that maternal antibodies persist for some months, and continue to cause haemolysis during early life.[57]

Exchange transfusion *Indications/technique:* If Hb <7g/dL, give 1st volume of the exchange transfusion (80mL/kg) as packed cells, and subsequent precise exchanges according to response. ►*Keep the baby warm.*

Phototherapy (ultraviolet somerization of bilirubin to its soluble form) may be all that is needed in less than severe disease. Give extra water (30mL/kg/24h PO). Avoid heat loss. Protect the eyes. Keep the baby naked. Keep breastfeeds short to maximize time under the phototherapy lights.

Giving Rh–ve mothers anti-D immunoglobulin (see BOX, p11) This strategy has markedly reduced need for exchange transfusion (cost per QALY ≈£11,000–52,000, see *OHCM* p12).[58,59]

ABO incompatibility 1 in 45 of group A or B babies born to group O mothers will have haemolysis from maternal antibodies. Exchange transfusion may be needed, even in first-borns.

- Get expert help.
- At birth, take cord blood for Hb, PCV, bilirubin (conjugated and unconjugated), blood group, Coombs test,[6] serum protein, LFT, and infection screen (p112) to find the cause—eg isoimmunization; thalassaemia; infection (eg toxoplasmosis, syphilis, parvoviruses, CMV p34); maternal diabetes; twin-twin transfusion; hypoproteinaemia.
- Expect to need to ventilate with high inspiratory peak pressure and positive end pressure. HFOV may have a role, p110.▶※
- Monitor plasma glucose 2–4-hourly, treating any hypoglycaemia.
- Drain ascites and pleural effusions if affecting ventilation.
- Correct anaemia.
- Vitamin K 1mg IM, to reduce risk of haemorrhage.
- If CCF is present, **furosemide** may be needed, eg 1–2mg/kg/12h IV.
- Limit IV fluids to 60mL/kg/24h (crystalloid); if exchange transfusing, aim for a deficit of 10–20mL/kg. Monitor urine output.
- Prognosis: 90% of those with non-immune hydrops die *in utero*; 50% die postnatally. Babies with non-immune hydrops not secondary to infection have a good neurological outcome.[60]

Biliary atresia

Incidence 1:17,000. This is rare but serious. Apparently healthy term babies have jaundice, yellow urine, and pale stools due to biliary tree occlusion by angiopathy at around week 3 of life. The spleen becomes palpable after the 3rd or 4th week—the liver may become hard and enlarged. Early surgery (Kasai procedure = hepatoportoenterostomy—the extrahepatic biliary tree is identified, a cholangiogram performed to check diagnosis, and an intestinal limb (Roux-en-Y) is attached to drain bile from the porta hepatis) has a good chance of restoring flow of bile to bowel (60% success if done <60 days of age) but if presenting for operation late (eg at 100 days) Kasai procedure is unlikely to be successful due to advanced liver damage and cirrhosis; and the baby will likely need liver transplant in 1st year of life. It can occur in premature babies. 20% have associated cardiac malformations: polysplenia and situs inversus. Refer all term babies jaundiced beyond 2 weeks (preterm at 3) for conjugated/unconjugated bilirubia. Breast milk jaundice has ↑ unconjugated bilirubin. Conjugated bilirubin >25 (or >5% of total bilirubin) may reflect serious liver disease (<20μmol is normal). US may help with diagnosis. Percutaneous liver biopsy may show bile duct proliferation and bile plugs. Babies suspected of biliary atresia should be urgently assessed in a liver unit.

---

6 The direct Coombs test (DCT) identifies red cells coated with antibody or complement and a positive result usually indicates an immune cause of haemolysis (*OHCM* p330).

RDS is due to a deficiency of alveolar surfactant, which is commonest in premature babies. Insufficient surfactant leads to atelectasis; re-inflation with each breath exhausts the baby, and respiratory failure follows. Hypoxia leads to ↓cardiac output, hypotension, acidosis, and renal failure. It is the major cause of death from prematurity. *Infants at risk:* 91% if 23–25 weeks; 52% if 30–31 weeks.[61] Also commoner in maternal diabetes, males, 2nd twin, caesareans.

Signs Increased work of breathing shortly after birth (1st 4h)—tachypnoea (>60/min), grunting, nasal flaring, intercostal recession, and cyanosis. CXR: diffuse granular patterns (ground glass appearance) ± air bronchograms.

Differential diagnosis Sepsis (p112).*Transient tachypnoea of the newborn (TTN)* is due to excess lung fluid. It usually resolves after 24h. *Meconium aspiration* (p120); congenital pneumonia (GBS); tracheo-oesophageal fistula (rare; suspect if respiratory problems after feeds); congenital lung abnormality.

Prevention Betamethasone or dexamethasone should be offered to all women at risk of preterm delivery from 23–35 weeks (p51); mothers at high risk should be transferred to perinatal centres with experience in managing RDS.

Treatment[61] Delay clamping of cord (p51) to promote placento–fetal transfusion. Give oxygen via an oxygen–air blender, starting with 21%, and increasing if no improvement in heart rate, despite good chest movement. Attach oxymeter and follow local guidelines for required saturations. Sats of 85% are normal in first 5–10min of life if baby active. If not, increase O_2 by 10% every minute until improving. If spontaneously breathing stabilize with CPAP (5–6cm H_2O). If gestation ≤26wks, intubate and give prophylactic surfactant via ET tube ± 2 further doses if ongoing O_2 demand/ventilation requirement. Monitor O_2, as needs may suddenly↓.[62] Aim for sats between 85–93% to reduce risk of retinopathy of prematurity and bronchopulmonary dysplasia.[61] Some centres give a dose of surfactant then extubate to non-invasive CPAP; others keep the baby intubated and wean as tolerated.

• Wrap up warmly and take to NICU/SCBU incubator.
• If blood gases worsen, intubate and support ventilation (p110). ↑$PaCO_2$ suggests that the minute volume is too low, so increase rate.
• *Traditional ventilator settings:* (p110) On connecting the endotracheal tube, check chest movement is adequate and symmetrical. Listen for breath sounds. PaO_2 is increased by ↑mean pressure (not too high). $PaCO_2$ is decreased by ↑minute volume (↑ breath frequency) by lessening expiratory time. Always check with a CO_2 monitor. Ask a senior colleague for advice.[63,64]
•▶ If any deterioration, check *DOPE:* Displaced ET tube, Obstructed (secretions, blood), Pneumothorax, Equipment failure (ventilator, tubing).
• *Fluids:* Give 10% glucose IVI (p123). *Nutrition:* Get help. Inositol is an essential nutrient promoting surfactant maturation and plays a vital role in neonatal life. Supplementing nutrition of prems with inositol reduces complications (IVH, p108; bronchopulmonary dysplasia, p119).[65] Full parenteral nutrition can be started on day 1. *Minimal* enteral feeding with expressed breast milk can also be started on day 1.[61]

Signs of a poor prognosis ☼ If, despite everything, the baby is still deteriorating, enlist senior help. It may be appropriate to not escalate treatment any further, or even to withdraw treatment; this is a consultant decision. Explain what is happening to the parents, and that the baby will feel no pain. Encourage christening, or what is congruent with parents' beliefs. Relieve pain (p172); keep the baby comfortable. In the light of dialogue with parents and nurses it may be appropriate to disconnect the tubes, so allowing the parents to hold the baby, and, in so doing, to aid their grief. NB: contact your Trust's head and defence organization if legal issues beckon.[66]

Communicating with parents

Take time to explain to parents exactly what is happening to their baby—not just for the RDS, but for *any* serious diseases. Structured, tested interviews yield these guidelines:[67]
• Ask both parents to be present (plus a nurse whom they trust).
• Elicit what the parents now know. Clarify or repeat as needed.
• Hand your bleep to a colleague. Allow time. Call the parents by name.
• Look at the parents (mutual gaze promotes trust).
• Name the illness concerned with its complications. Write it down.
• Give support group details: www.cafamily.org.uk tel: 020 7240 0671 for a list.
• Answer any questions. Arrange follow-up (<50% may be remembered).

Doctors' decisions are increasingly being questioned by parents. If you and your team are sure your actions are in the child's best interests, and the parents take a different view, take any steps you can to resolve the issue in a non-confrontational way. Violent fights between doctors and parents endanger other children (some UK units have had to be evacuated while police are called). You should know emergency procedures for contacting the High Court to settle the issue (go through the on-call manager: your Trust can make applications day or night). Failure to get Court approval will leave you open to criticism from the European Court of Human Rights, which is likely to take the view that 'do not resuscitate' notices fail to guarantee respect for the child's 'physical and moral integrity'—guaranteed by Article 8 of the Convention on Human rights—see Glass *vs* United Kingdom, 2004 (61827/00).[68]

Bronchopulmonary dysplasia (BPD)

This complicates ventilation for RDS in 40% of babies of <1kg birthweight.[69] There is persistent hypoxia ± difficult ventilator weaning—eg still requiring ventilation at 36 weeks' postmenstrual age (eg SaO_2 ≤88% in air). BPD is mainly from barotrauma and oxygen toxicity, whereas surfactant-related BPD is multifactorial with airway infections triggering inflammatory cascades. (Without surfactant, many would not survive to get BPD.)[70] Oxidative processes may also play a key role, but antioxidants are unproven.[71]
Tests *CXR:* Hyperinflation, rounded, radiolucent areas, alternating with thin denser lines. *Histology:* Necrotizing bronchiolitis with alveolar fibrosis.
Mortality Variable, ∴ complex interaction with surfactant use.[72]
Early sequelae Feeding problems. O_2 desaturation during feeds is not uncommon; severe RSV bronchiolitis; gastro-oesophageal reflux.
Late sequelae ↓IQ; cerebral palsy; by adolescence/early adulthood the main changes remaining are asthma and exercise limitation.
Prevention Steroids (antenatal & postnatal); surfactant and 'suitably high' calorie feeding.[73]

Pulmonary hypoplasia

This is very rare. Suspect this in all infants with persisting neonatal tachypnoea ± feeding difficulties, particularly if prenatal oligohydramnios. Hypoplasia may be a consequence of oligohydramnios, eg in Potter's syndrome or premature rupture of the membranes. In diaphragmatic hernia it is a consequence of the 'space-occupying lesion'. Cystic adenomatoid malformations are another cause. They are often detected on the fetal anomaly US. CXR may be misleadingly reported as normal. The condition need not be fatal: postnatal catch-up growth occurs.

Differential RDS, meconium aspiration, sepsis, or primary pulmonary hypertension.[74] Some degree of pulmonary hypoplasia is the price of adopting an early elective delivery for early spontaneous rupture of the membranes, but despite this, expectant management leads to fewer deaths.[75]

Necrotizing enterocolitis (NEC) is an inflammatory bowel necrosis. Prematurity is the chief risk factor: if weight <1500g, 5–10% develop NEC. Other risk factors: enteral feeds, bacterial colonization, mucosal injury.[76] *Signs:* If mild, just some abdominal distension. A little blood/mucus may be passed PR. If severe, there is sudden abdominal distension, tenderness (± perforation), shock, DIC & mucosal sloughing. Pneumatosis intestinalis (gas in the gut wall seen on x-ray) is pathognomonic for NEC. *R:* Stop oral feeding (except oral probiotics, eg *Bifidobacteria infantis*, which may help);[77] barrier nurse; culture faeces; cross-match (may get anaemic); give antibiotics: eg **cefotaxime + vancomycin**.[78] Liaise early with surgeon; repeated AXR and girth measurement. Platelets mirror disease activity; <100×10⁹/L is 'severe'.[79] *Laparotomy indications:* Progressive distension, perforation (up to 50% die). *Prophylaxis:* Expressed breast milk; probiotics.

Meconium aspiration syndrome (MAS) occurs in the term/near term infant when meconium, the faecal material that accumulates in the fetal colon during pregnancy, is passed *in utero,* leading to meconium-stained amniotic fluid (MSAF). MSAF occurs in ~8–25% of births, due to fetal maturity or fetal distress. MAS occurs in only 5% of these infants;[80] it is defined as respiratory distress in the infant born through MSAF which cannot otherwise be explained. Aspiration of meconium mostly occurs *in utero*.[81] It may lead to airway obstruction, surfactant dysfunction, pulmonary vasoconstriction, infection, and chemical pneumonitis. Intrapartum suctioning of the oro/naso pharynx wastes time and makes no difference.[82] Endotracheal suctioning is only needed for those infants who aren't vigorous at birth.[82] Cricoid and/or chest compression at birth to prevent aspiration have not been shown to be useful.[83] Surfactant, ventilation, inhaled nitric oxide, and antibiotics may be required.[42]

Vitamin K deficiency bleeding (VKDB=haemorrhagic disease of the newborn) occurs from days 2-7 postpartum. *Cause:* No enteric bacteria to make vit K. The baby is usually well, apart from bruising/bleeding. Prothrombin & partial thromboplastin times (PT & PTT)↑; platelets ↔. *Prevention:* (Many regimens) vit K 1mg (0.4mg/kg if prem) IM (if at ↑risk[7])—or 2 doses of oral colloidal (mixed micelle) **phytomenadione** 2mg at birth, repeated in ≤7d; if breastfed, give a 3rd dose at 1 month old; not needed if bottle-fed (already fortified). NB: a weak correlation[84] with cancers caused a scare, but there is no hard evidence. *R:* Plasma, 10mL/kg IV & vit K (≤1mg slow IV) for active bleeding (monitor coagulation).[85]

Disseminated intravascular coagulation (DIC) *Signs:* Septic signs (ill); petechiae; venepuncture oozings; GI bleeding. *Tests:* Platelets↓; schistocytes (fragmented RBCs); INR↑; fibrinogen↓; partial thromboplastin time↑; D-dimer↑ (hard to interpret if birthweight low).[86,87] *Treatment:* Get help; treat cause (eg NEC, sepsis, etc); give **vit. K** ≤1mg slow IV± **platelet transfusion** (aim for >30×10⁹/L).
• Fresh **plasma±cryoprecipitate**,[3] 10mL/kg IV± **heparin** IV ± **protein** C.[88,89]
• If bleeding still continues, consider **exchange transfusion**.

Autoimmune thrombocytopenia (ITP) <10% of babies of women with ITP are thrombocytopenic (p88). *Alloimmune thrombocytopenia* (1:2000 births; via fetomaternal incompatibility of platelet antigens). It develops *in utero.* 50% are 1st born (it recurs in ~80% of later pregnancies with same or ↑severity). If affected *in utero* 25% have CNS problems. Platelets fall for 48h post-delivery. Treat severe thrombocytopenia with *compatible platelets* or *irradiated maternal platelets.* IVIg 400mg/kg/day[4] for 48h and steroids may help. *Platelet transfusion via cordocentesis* from 24wks may be needed in later pregnancies. Diagnose by detecting *maternal platelet allo-antibody* against father's platelets.

***

7 Asphyxia, bleeding problems, cholestasis—or mother with liver disease or on carbamazepine, phenobarbital, phenytoin, rifampicin, or warfarin.

Minor neonatal problems

Most neonates have a few minor lesions; the more you examine neonates the better you will become at reassuring mothers.

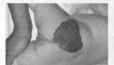

Fig 2.2 Strawberry naevus.

Strawberry naevus (fig 2.2) May not be present at birth, and increase in size over first few months, then fade again. Some may ulcerate or bleed. If large or in critical area (over eye or joint), consider early **propranolol** to shrink the lesion.

Milia 1–2mm pearly white/cream papules caused by retention of keratin in dermis. Found on forehead, nose, cheeks. Will resolve spontaneously.

Erythema toxicum (neonatal urticaria) These are harmless red blotches, often with a central white pustule which come and go in crops. Described as 'flea bitten' in appearance. They last ~24h, in contrast to septic spots which are smaller and not mobile. *Miliaria crystallina* (a prickly-heat-like-rash) develops due to transient sweat-pore disruption[90] or immaturity[91]—hence its characteristic 1–2mm retention vesicle.[92] Prevalence: ≤ 8%.[93] In *miliaria rubra* there is a surrounding flush.

Stork mark These are areas of capillary dilatation on the eyelids, central forehead, and back of the neck—where the baby is deemed to have been held in the stork's beak. They blanch on pressure and fade with time.

Peeling skin/desquamation Common in postmature babies, it does not denote future skin problems. Olive oil prevents skin folds from cracking.

Petechial haemorrhages, facial cyanosis, subconjunctival haemorrhages These temporary features generally reflect suffusion of the face during delivery (sometimes inaccurately referred to as 'traumatic asphyxia').

Swollen breasts These occur in both sexes and occasionally lactate (witch's milk). They are due to maternal hormones and gradually subside if left alone, but if infected need antibiotics. Milk may persist until 2 months old.

The umbilicus It dries and separates through a moist base at about day 7. Signs of infection: odour, pus, periumbilical red flare, malaise. Take swabs and blood cultures, give antibiotics. Granuloma: exclude a patent urachus and cauterize with a silver nitrate stick.

Sticky eye (Commonly from a blocked tear duct, p418.) Swab to exclude *ophthalmia neonatorum* (p36)/chlamydia (special swab). When vertically transmitted sexual infections occur, liaise with your microbiologist and local genitourinary medicine (GUM) clinic.

Feeding anxieties Healthy term babies require little milk for the first few days and early poor feeding is not an indication for investigation or bottle top-ups. The exceptions are babies of diabetic mothers who develop hypoglycaemia. New babies may have difficulty co-ordinating feeding and breathing, and briefly choke, gag, or turn blue. Exclude disease, check feeding technique (too much? too fast?) and reassure. Regurgitation is often due to overfilling a tiny stomach with milk and air. Check feeding technique; if bottle fed, is the teat too big for the mouth or the hole too small or the amount too great? Winding during feeds may help but is not essential to health.

Red-stained nappy This is usually due to urinary urates but may be blood from the cord or baby's vagina (oestrogen withdrawal bleed).

Neonatal sneezing clears nasal amniotic fluid. If jittery ± τ°t/ muscle hypertonia, suspect fluoxetine or opiate withdrawal.[94,95]

Harlequin colour change Transient, episodic, demarcated erythema on left or right, with simultaneous contralateral blanching—occasionally related to use of systemic alprostadil (no need to stop: the condition is self-limiting).

Breastfeeding (± expressed breast milk, p124–6) is the ideal way to feed term babies. Small babies may remain small and this is not helped by over-feeding. Adequate incremental weight gain is more important than overall size—a good rule of thumb is 'an ounce (25g) a day with a day off on Sundays.'

Nasogastric tube feeding *Indications:* Any sick infant who is too ill or too young to feed normally (eg respiratory distress syndrome). Expressed breast milk or formula milk is fed via a naso- or orogastric tube either as a bolus or as a continuous infusion. ☞ If gastro-oesophageal reflux or aspiration is a problem, then a silastic naso-jejunal tube can be used. After entering the stomach, the tube enters the jejunum by peristalsis: confirm its position on x-ray. When the baby improves, start giving some feeds by mouth (PO), eg by increasing the ratio of oral to nasogastric feeds, either in whole feeds, or by fractions of each feed. If during oral feeds, cyanosis, bradycardia, or vomiting supervene, you may be trying too soon.

Trophic feeding *Synonyms:* Minimal enteral or hypocaloric feeding; gut priming.

Rationale: If prems go for weeks with no oral nutrition, normal GI structure and function are lost despite an anabolic body state. Villi shorten, mucosal DNA is lost, and enzyme activity is less. Early initiation of subnutritional enteral feeding may help by promoting gut motility and bile secretion, inducing lactase activity, and by reducing sepsis and cholestatic jaundice.[96] See fig **2.3**.

Technique: Typically, milk volumes of ~1mL/kg/h are given by tube starting on day 2–3. Use expressed breast milk (or a preterm formula, eg Nutriprem®).

Effects: Studies show that weight gain and head growth is better, and that there are fewer episodes of neonatal sepsis, fewer days of parenteral nutrition are needed, and time to full oral feeding is less. If too much is given, NEC (p120) may ensue.[97]

Eligibility: Experience shows that almost all prems with non-surgical illness tolerate at least some milk as trophic feeds.[98]

Parenteral nutrition (PN, via a central vein). Indications: post-op; trauma; burns; if oral nutrition is poor (eg in ill, low-birthweight babies) and necrotizing enterocolitis (when the gut must be 'rested'). ▸*Sterility is vital*; prepare using laminar flow units. Monitoring of electrolytes must be meticulous.[8]

Daily checks: Weight; fluid balance; U&E; blood glucose; Ca^{2+}. Test for glycosuria. Change IVI sets/filters; culture filters, Vamin®, and Intralipid® samples.

Weekly: Length; head circumference; skinfold thickness. LFT; Mg^{2+}; PO_4^{3-}; alk phos; ammonia; triglycerides; FBC; ESR/CRP (helps determine if there is sepsis).

Complications: Infection; acidosis; metabolic imbalances; thrombophlebitis; hepatobiliary stenosis; cholelithiasis; osteopenia.[99]

Stopping IV nutrition Do in stages to prevent hypoglycaemia.

Fig 2.3 'Gavage' (from an old French word meaning 'to gorge') denotes a controversial farming and gastronomic method entailing insertion of a long funnel into a goose's throat. Down this funnel is pumped a slurry of ground corn and water, to produce obesity—and, to some palates, a delicious (if unnaturally fatty) pâté—*pâté de foie gras*). On the neonatal unit, gavage feeding should not be quite so enthusiastic. But French farmers were right about one thing: *bolus* gavage feeding is better than *continuous* tube feeds, at least with regard to trophic feeding.[100]

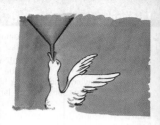

It is better to talk to a breastfeeding mother whilst pregnant than to rely on simple encouragement and leaflets.[101]

Reflexes Rooting (searching, with wide-open mouth)→suckling (jaw goes up and down while the tongue compresses the areola against the palate)→swallowing reflex (as milk hits the oropharynx, the soft palate rises and shuts off the nasopharynx; the larynx rises, and the epiglottis falls, closing the trachea).

Skill Don't assume this comes naturally; it can be difficult for both mother and baby to get the hang of, and can be anxiety-provoking. The best way to learn is from an experienced person in comfortable surroundings—eg sitting in an upright chair, rather than inadequately propped up in bed. Reassure that a few problematic feeds do not mean that the baby will starve, and that bottle feeding is needed. *Most term babies have plenty of fuel reserves*—and perseverance will almost always be rewarded. Furthermore, 'top-up' bottle feeds may undermine confidence, and, by altering the GI milieu, diminish the benefits of breastfeeding.

A good time to start breastfeeding is just after birth (good bonding; PPH risk↓), but labour procedures may make this hard, eg intrapartum opiate analgesia ± operative delivery, T° and BP measurements, washing, weighing, going to a postnatal ward. ▶*It is never too late to put to the breast.*

From the baby's viewpoint, breastfeeding entails taking a large mouthful of breast-with-nipple, which he or she gets to work on with tongue and jaw. Ensure the baby is close to the mother with the shoulders as well as the head facing the breast—which, if large, may need supporting (mother's fingers placed flat on the chest wall at the base of the breast: avoid the 'scissors' grip which stops the baby from drawing the lactiferous sinuses into his mouth).

• Avoid forcing the nipple into the mouth; so do not place a hand over his occiput and press forwards. Cradle the head in the crook of the arm.

• Explain the signs of correct attachment:
  • Mouth wide open, and chin touching the breast (nose hardly touching).
  • The baby should be seen to be drawing in breast, not just nipple.
  • Lower lip curled back, maximally gobbling the areola (so angle between lips >100°). (Don't worry about how much areola can be seen above the top lip: this gives little indication of where the tongue and lower jaw are.)
  • Slow, rhythmic, and deep jaw movements, as well as sucking movements. The 1st few sucks may be fast, shallow, and non-nutritive: here the baby is inducing the 'let-down' reflex, which promotes flow.

• When helping with placing, it is quite appropriate to 'tease' the baby by brushing his lip over the nipple, and then away. This may induce a nice big gape. With one movement bring to the breast, aiming his tongue and lower jaw as far as possible from the base of the nipple—so his tongue can scoop in the nipple and a good mouthful of breast.

• Keeping on the postnatal ward for a few days, and having the mother learn with an experienced, friendly midwife is very helpful, but this is rare in the UK, as cost and other pressures make admissions shorter. Most hospitals have a breastfeeding expert (usually a senior midwife) who can help troubleshoot if problems persist.

Paediatrics

It is good for every breastfeeding mother to learn this skill (access to teaching is *required* before the accolade of 'baby-friendly' can be granted to UK hospitals). There are at least 4 times when expressing is valuable:
• To relieve (sometimes very) painful breast engorgement between feeds.
• To keep milk production going when it is necessary to give nipples a rest owing to soreness—which is quite a common problem.
• To aid nutrition if sucking is reduced for any reason (eg prematurity or cleft lip).
• If the mother is going to be separated from her baby for a few feeds, eg going out to work.

The best way to learn is from a midwife, and by watching a mother who is already successfully expressing milk. Pumps are available from any chemist. If not, wash hands, and dry on a clean towel. Then, try to start flow by:
• Briefly rolling the nipple: this may induce a let-down reflex, especially if the baby is nearby.
• Stroke the breast gently towards the nipple.
• With circular movements, massage the breast gently with the 3 middle fingers.

Applying warm flannels, or expressing in the bath may aid flow, eg while the mother is learning, and only a few drops are being expressed.

Teach the mother to find the 15 or so ampullae beneath the areola: they feel knotty once the milk comes in. Now with the thumb above the areola and the index finger below, and whole hand pressing the breast back on the chest wall, exert gentle pressure on the ampullae. With rhythmic pressure and release, milk should flow. Use a sterile container.

Take care that the fingers do not slip down on to the nipple, and damage the narrowing ducts. Fingers tire easily: practice is the key. Concentration is also needed to be sure to catch oddly angled jets.

If kept in a fridge, the milk lasts 5 days. Frozen milk should be used within 6 months. It is thawed by standing it in a jug of warm water. Any unused milk should be discarded after 24 hours, not refrozen. NB: it is known that the antioxidant level of stored breast milk falls, but it is not known if this matters. Refrigeration is better than freezing and thawing.[102]

Mastitis

This is a common reason to give up breastfeeding and is easily treatable.
Symptoms
• Tender, hot, reddened area of breast
• Fever may be present or absent.
Treatment
• Flucloxacillin 500mg QDS PO for 7-10 days
• Ibuprofen 400mg TDS PO
• Continue breastfeeding
• If breastfeeding too painful, express the milk
• Consider checking breastfeeding technique with a breastfeeding expert.

Factors which make starting breastfeeding harder • Family pressures, including partner's hostility (10% breastfeed vs ~70% if he approves).
• If mother and baby are separated at night in hospital.
• Unfriendly working environments.
• Cultural reframing of breasts as sex objects; no non-sexual role models.
• The commitment a breastfeeding mother makes is huge and sustained—24/7 for many months (WHO advises exclusive breastfeeding for 6 months).[9] ☛

Breastfeeding advantages ► Mutual gaze ↑emotional input from mother.
• Sucking promotes uterine contractions, so avoiding some PPHs.
• Breastfeeding-induced oxytocin surges promote trust and diminish fear.[103,104]
• Less insulin resistance, BP↑, & obesity (growth is less rapid, p181)[105] due to ↑breast milk long-chain polyunsaturated fatty acids.[106] ►LCPUFAs *may* also ↑IQ.[107]
• Breast milk is free and clean, and gives babies an attractive smell.
• Colostrum has endorphins: good for birth-associated stress?[108]
• IgA, macrophages, lymphocytes (with interferon), and lysozyme protect from infection. Acids in breast milk promote growth of friendly lactobacilli in the baby's bowel. Gastroenteritis may be less severe if the mother makes and transfers antibodies (an 'immune dialogue').
• Infant mortality, otitis media, pneumonia, & diarrhoea are less if breastfed.[109]
• Breast milk contains less Na^+, K^+, and Cl^- than other milk, so aiding homeostasis. If dehydration occurs, risk of fatal hypernatraemia is low.
• Exclusive breastfeeding ↓risk of: type 1 DM, rheumatoid arthritis, inflammatory bowel disease, food allergy/atopy (if family history +ve).[110–112]
• Breastfeeding helps mothers lose weight, and is contraceptive (unreliable!).
• Some protection in premenopausal years against maternal breast cancer.

Why is feeding on demand to be encouraged?
• It keeps the baby happy, and enhances milk production.
• Fewer breast problems (engorgement, abscesses).

NB: feeding by routine is possible with a structured plan (see *The New Contented Little Baby Book*),[113] which may help to promote a diurnal sleep cycle.

NB: although co-sleeping (a baby sleeping in the parental bed) can aid parental sleep, there is a risk of inadvertent smothering (p148).

Contraindications to breastfeeding • An HIV +ve mother in developed countries • Amiodarone • Antimetabolites • Antithyroid drugs • Opiates. See *BNF*.

Problems Treat *breast engorgement* by better breast technique and better latching-on; aim to keep breasts empty, eg by hourly feeds or milk expression. If a *breast abscess* forms, discard the milk if it is pus-like. Give the mother flucloxacillin 500mg/6h PO (it is safe for her baby). Surgery may be needed. Treat *sore nipples* by ensuring optimal attachment (p124), and moist wound healing (paraffin gauze dressing or glycerin gel)[114] *not* by resting, except in emergency.

Prematurity Preterm breast milk is the best food for prems. Give unheated, via a tube (p122). Add vitamins D 1000U/day and K (p122). Phosphate supplements may be needed. Even term babies may (rarely) develop rickets ± hypocalcaemia (eg fits, recurrent 'colds', lethargy, or stridor) if exclusively breastfed, unless vitamin supplements are used (p150).

9 However, evidence is insufficient to say confidently 'Breastfeed exclusively for 6 months' in developed countries, as breast milk may not meet full energy needs of some infants at 4-6 months old—and there may be risk of specific nutritional deficiencies. Further evidence is awaited.[115]

There are few contraindications to breastfeeding but many pressures not to (p126). In many communities >50% mothers are breastfeeding at 2 weeks but this reduces to ≤40% at 6 weeks. Most change to bottle because of lack of knowledge or no encouragement. Advertising also has a role. The WHO/UNICEF *International Code of Marketing of Breastmilk Substitutes* bans promotion of bottle feeding and sets out requirements for labelling and information on feeding.[116] The advantage of bottle feeding is that fathers and others can help; Knowing how much milk the baby is taking can be reassuring to mothers.

Teats Babies fed with a cross-cut teat 'lets the baby determine rate' cry less and spend more time awake and content than babies fed with standard teats.

Standard infant formulas (Cows' milk 'humanized' by reducing the solute load and modifying fat, protein, and vitamin content.) As with breast milk, the protein component is whey-based. Brands are similar so shopping around for a brand which 'suits better' is unlikely to be an answer to feeding problems.

Follow-on formula milks are like standard formulas, but the protein component is casein-based (∴ delays stomach emptying and allows less frequent feeds). These are marketed to satisfy hungrier babies before they start weaning. Typical age of use: 6–24 months.

Soya milks These are no longer recommended. They contain high levels of phyto-oestrogens which have oestrogen-like properties. This could affect immunity and thyroid function, as well as the more obvious hormonal disruption, especially in boys. Soya milks are still on sale in the supermarket: try to discourage parents from their use. Soya milk is *not* indicated in re-establishing feeding (regrading) after gastroenteritis.

Hydrolized formula is a cows' milk formula where protein is hydrolized into short peptides (eg Nutramigen®). Indications: *cows' milk allergy* (seen in 1% of babies, eg with bloody diarrhoea ± perioral rash) or *soya allergy*. Cows' milk can be reintroduced eg at 1 year.

Specialist milks Many types exist (eg for gastro-oesophageal reflux, malabsorption, metabolic diseases, etc). Get help from a paediatric dietician.

Preparing feeds Hands must be clean, equipment sterilized, and boiled water used—infective gastroenteritis causes many deaths in poor countries and considerable morbidity in the UK. Powder must be accurately measured. Understrength feeds lead to poor growth and overstrength feeds have caused dangerous hypernatraemia, constipation, and obesity.

Feeding After the first few days, babies need ~150mL/kg/24h (30mL=1oz) over 4–6 feeds depending on age and temperament. If small-for-dates up to 200mL/kg/day is needed; if large-for-dates, <100mL/kg. Feeds are often warmed; there is no evidence that cold milk is bad. Flow should almost form a stream; check before each feed as teats silt up. The hole can be enlarged with a hot needle. Bottles are best angled so that air is not sucked in with milk.

Weaning Introduce solids at 6 months by offering a selection of finger foods with or without puree. Avoid adding salt or sugar. Encourage home cooking and eating together as a family. Normal supermarket cows' milk *may* be used from when the baby is ~1 year old, but it may still be too rich in protein, Na⁺, K⁺, phosphorus—and is poor in iron, trace elements, linoleic and alpha-linolenic acids[10] and vitamins C & B complex. Infants must be able to cope with its higher solute load.[117]

---

10 Docosahaenoic acid (DHA) is the main lipid in our brain-derived endogenously via α-linolenic acid (ALA). Several studies have tried to improve blood DHA concentrations of formula-fed infants by ↑ ALA in feeds and measuring changes in growth & development. Results are far from clear.[118]

Some definitions *Preterm:* A neonate whose calculated gestational age from the last menstrual period is <37 completed weeks—ie premature.

Low birth weight (LBW): Birth weight of <2500g regardless of gestational age. Thus a LBW baby may not be small for gestational age (see below) if they are born preterm. 6% of UK infants are <2500g at birth, and 50% of these are preterm. 10% of pregnancies end in spontaneous preterm delivery, and 70% of all perinatal deaths occur in preterm infants.

Very low birth weight (VLBW): Birth weight of <1500g regardless of age.

Extremely low birth weight (ELBW): Birth weight <1000g regardless of age.

Small for gestational age (SGA): Typically SGA refers to a birth weight below the 10th percentile for gestational age (SGA). In *intrauterine growth restriction (IUGR)* there is a failure of growth in utero, which may or may not result in the baby being SGA. *Symmetric (proportional)* SGA: all growth parameters are symmetrically small, suggesting that the fetus was affected from early pregnancy. This is seen in babies with chromosomal abnormalities and in the constitutionally small. *Asymmetric (disproportional)* SGA: the weight centile is < length and head circumference. It is usually due to IUGR and an insult later in pregnancy eg pre-eclampsia. These babies have a higher risk of complications. *Chief causes:* ▶Poverty/poor social support may account for 30% of variance in birthweights.[119] *Other causes:* Constitutional factors; malformation; twins; congenital infection; placental insufficiency (maternal heart disease, BP↑, smoking, diabetes, sickle-cell disease, pre-eclampsia).[120] Gestational age (based on US) is more important for predicting survival than the birthweight alone. *Are SGA effects permanent?* 90% of SGA catch up growth in the first 2 yrs, however as adults they are on average 1 standard deviation shorter than the mean adult height.[121] There may be an association between SGA and adult risk of coronary heart disease and obesity.[121]

Complications: Increased risk of fetal death; risks from congenital infection or malformations if present, hypoglycaemia, hypothermia, polycythaemia (secondary to chronic intrauterine hypoxia), NEC, meconium aspiration.

Causes of prematurity are mostly unknown (40%); smoking tobacco, poverty, and malnutrition play a part. Others: past history of prematurity; genitourinary infection/chorioamnionitis; pre-eclampsia; diabetes mellitus; polyhydramnios; closely spaced pregnancies; multiple pregnancy; uterine malformation; placenta praevia; abruption; premature rupture of the membranes. Labour may be induced early on purpose or accidentally (p62).

Estimating the gestational age Check EDD on 12 week scan (later scans less accurate). If no scans in pregnancy or LMP, use the Dubowitz score (p228).

Management Delivery should take place in a centre capable of caring for preterm babies; arrange *in utero* transfer if necessary (better outcomes than *ex utero*). Once born, ensure adequate resuscitation (p107). Take to NICU/SCBU. Plan supplemental breast milk or low-birth-weight formula if <2kg. Monitor and maintain blood glucose. Encourage mother to express from day 1. Tube feed if oral feeds are not tolerated. If oral feeding is contraindicated (eg respiratory distress) IV feeding is needed (p122). Support parents.

Survival if very premature 40% of infants born before 23 weeks die on labour ward. Of those surviving labour ward, 75% died on the neonatal unit. 47% survive at 24 weeks and 67% at 25 weeks. [EPICure2] Mortality is associated with intracranial abnormalities seen ultrasonically.

Disability *As a percentage of live births:* if 23 weeks' gestation: 5% had no or minor subsequent disability (24 weeks ≈ 12%; 25 weeks ≈ 23%). Morbidity relates to cerebral palsy, squint, and retinopathy (p108).[123,149,150] Disability may be subtle but specific: one pattern is ↓numeracy if gestation is <30/40, associated with ↓grey matter in the left parietal lobe.[123] ADD risk↑ (p212).

Is this baby small for gestational age?

Use centile charts which take into account that first-borns are lighter than subsequent births: the TABLE gives sample data.

Weeks of gestation	Tenth centile weight (grams)				
	First born: Boy	Girl	Subsequent births:	Boy	Girl
32	1220	1260		1470	1340
33	1540	1540		1750	1620
34	1830	1790		2000	1880
35	2080	2020		2230	2100
36	2310	2210		2430	2310
37	2500	2380		2600	2480
38	2660	2530		2740	2620
39	2780	2640		2860	2730
40	2870	2730		2950	2810

Very low birthweight: 1–1.5kg; *extremely low birthweight:* 500–999g.

Preventing neonatal deaths—worldwide[124]

Each year, of the 130 million babies who are born, ~4 million die in the 1st 4 weeks of life (the neonatal period)—most from preventable causes. Two-thirds occur in India, China, Pakistan, Nigeria, Bangladesh, Ethiopia, DRC, Indonesia, Afghanistan, and Tanzania. Most of the deaths are caused by pre-term births, infections, respiratory problems, and tetanus. (Malaria and some diarrhoeal diseases are less important in the neonatal period except in those areas of the highest neonatal mortality.) Prevention depends on:
- Tetanus vaccination, access to antibiotics and breastfeeding advice.
- Sanitary delivery rooms with basic emergency services (caesarean sections and blood transfusion; obstructed labour is a major problem).
- Preventing and managing low birthweight. Low birthweight affects 14% of births worldwide, but accounts for ~70% of neonatal deaths. Managing low birthweight babies need not require expensive technology. Much could be achieved by application of known primary care principles of warmth, feeding, and the prevention and early treatment of infection.
- Preventing maternal mortality (0.5 million maternal deaths/yr) is a prerequisite for preventing many neonatal deaths. In one small but harrowing study from Gambia *all* the children born to mothers who died from pregnancy-related causes were themselves dead at 1 year.[125]

MDG-4 *Millennium Development Goals* are internationally 'agreed' commitments to reduce poverty and ill-health. The 4th goal aimed to reduce mortality in under-5s by ⅔ by 2015. 17,000 fewer children die every day in 2015 compared with 1990, but 6 million children still die before reaching their 5th birthday. The developing world spends $2 billion annually on this. It is estimated that another $4 billion is needed to do the job.

Non-pharmacological methods to reduce pain in neonates

Pain relief through non-nutritive sucking (NNS), rocking, massage, 20% sucrose (12mg may be enough),[126] distilled water, and expressed breast milk (EBM) have been studied in a randomized way—in the context of a heel-prick. Duration of cry and pain score were used as objective measures of pain. Pain scores and duration of crying were lowest in the NNS and rocking groups compared with sucrose, distilled water, expressed breast milk and massage.[127] Other trials show that for venepuncture, breastfeeding or glucose plus use of a pacifier provides good analgesia.[128,129] Other alternatives: kangaroo care (skin-to-skin with mum); morphine; fentanyl. Whenever you hear *siren cry* (sequence of almost identical cries with a period of 1sec) think: 'How can I help this baby? What is going wrong?'[130]

►Bilious (green) vomiting in neonates always needs urgent help (paediatric surgeon + neonatology team) for prompt investigation and management.

Hirschsprung's disease Occurs in 1 in 5000 births.[131] Congenital absence of ganglia in a segment of colon (or in the rare 'long-segment' disease, can be all the way up to the stomach) leading to functional GI obstruction, constipation and megacolon. Faeces may be felt *per abdomen*, and PR exam may reveal tight anal sphincter and explosive discharge of stool and gas. ♂:♀ ≈ 3:1. *Complications:* GI perforation, bleeding, ulcers, enterocolitis (may be life-threatening). Short-gut syndrome after surgery. *Tests:* Diagnosis through rectal suction biopsy of the aganglionic section, staining for acetylcholinesterase-positive nerve excess, is most accurate.[132] Excision of the aganglionic segment is needed ± colostomy.

Oesophageal atresia (OA) + tracheo-oesophageal fistula (TOF) A spectrum of abnormalities with OA plus a distal TOF being the most common (86%). Isolated OA (7%) and TOF without OA (4%) can also occur.[133] *Prenatal signs:* Polyhydramnios; small stomach. *Postnatal:* Cough, airway obstruction, ↑secretions, blowing bubbles, distended abdomen, cyanosis, aspiration. *Δ:* Inability to pass a catheter into the stomach; x-rays show it coiled in the oesophagus. Avoid contrast imaging. *R:* Stop feeding, suck out oesophageal pouch. Primary surgical repair is possible in the majority of cases.[134] 50% have other anomalies.

Congenital diaphragmatic hernia (CDH) A developmental defect in the diaphragm allowing herniation of abdominal contents into the chest. Leads to impaired lung development (pulmonary hypoplasia and pulmonary hypertension). *Incidence:* 1:2400. *Diagnosis:* Prenatal: US; postnatal: CXR. *Signs:* Difficult resuscitation at birth; respiratory distress; bowel sounds in one hemithorax (usually left so heart is best heard on the right). pH <7.3 and cyanosis augur badly (∵ lung hypoplasia).[135] *Associations:* other malformations (neural tube); trisomy 18; chromosome deletions eg at 15q2, Pierre Robin (p138).[136] *Treatment:* • *Prenatal:* Referral to tertiary fetal medicine centre for consideration of fetal surgery (tracheal obstruction by balloon: it encourages lung growth, pushing out other viscera)—but premature birth may be caused.[137] • *Postnatal:* Insert a large-bore nasogastric tube when diagnosis suspected: at birth if prenatal diagnosis. The aim is to keep all air out of the gut. Facemask ventilation is contraindicated (so immediately intubate, ventilate, and paralyse, with minimal pressures). Surgery in an appropriate centre.

Inguinal hernias These are due to a patent processus vaginalis (the passage which ushers the descending testicle into the scrotum). They present as a bulge lateral to the pubic tubercle, eg during crying. In one series (n=6361), ♂:♀×5:1; there were 59% right, 29% left, and 12% bilateral hernias (almost all indirect), with a hydrocele in 19%.[138] Incarceration occurred in 12%. Most surgeons aim to repair these promptly (laparoscopic repair is possible)[139] to avoid incarceration. Six/two rule: baby <6 weeks, operate within 2 days; <6 months, operate within 2 weeks; <6 years, within 2 months. Hydroceles are hard to distinguish from incarceration.

Hydroceles in infancy A processus vaginalis patent at birth, and allowing *only fluid* from the peritoneal cavity to pass down it, generally closes during the first year of life—so no action is usually needed. If it persists until the age of 2 it may need surgical correction.[140] If the fluid-filled sac is adjacent to the spermatic cord, it is called an encysted hydrocele or a spermatic cord cyst. If the proximal opening of the processus vaginalis is wide, a true inguinal hernia is formed, and action is always required.[141]

Imperforate anus Covers a variety of anorectal abnormalities. Babies may have an associated fistula starting in the rectum. Most girls have a posterior fourchette fistula; boys have a posterior urethral fistula (may pass meconium in urine). Absence of perineal fistula in boys indicates communication with the urethra (so colostomy may be required). Do GU imaging to show commonly associated GU abnormalities. Posterior sagittal anorectoplasty is possible.[142] Babies with trisomy 21 commonly have imperforate anus without fistula.

Mid-gut malrotations ▶Bilious neonatal vomiting merits immediate surgical referral (pass NGT).[143] Absent attachment of the small intestine mesentery can cause mid-gut volvulus or obstruction of the third part of the duodenum by fibrotic bands. Presentation may be late; passage of blood per rectum heralds mid-gut necrosis—and is an indication for emergency surgical decompression.

Acute gastric volvulus causes non-bilious vomiting, epigastric distention, and signs of pain, and is often associated with abnormalities of adjacent organs. There may also be feeding difficulty. Anterior fixation of the stomach to the anterior abdominal wall may be needed after upper GI imaging.

Anterior abdominal wall defects

Gastroschisis: (figs 2.4 & 2.5) A paraumbilical defect with evisceration (extrusion of viscera) of abdominal contents. Most are diagnosed antenatally on US. *Incidence:* ~1:3000; rising (especially in babies of young parents—or, in multips, if there has been a new father for this pregnancy

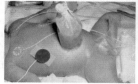

Fig 2.4 Gastroschisis.

(hence the idea that maternal immune factors play a role).[144] Corrective surgery has a good outcome in 90% (so deliver where there are good paediatric surgical facilities). At delivery, cover exposed bowel in clingfilm, keep the baby warm and hydrated and aim to close the defect surgically as soon as possible. This may involve a staged procedure using a silo, because the abdomen at birth is too small to accommodate the gut. Intestinal function is slow to resume and the baby may require TPN for several weeks.

Exomphalos (omphalocele): (fig 2.5) Ventral defects of the umbilical ring with herniation of abdominal viscera (which are covered in peritoneum) are common and often associated with malformations such as chromosomal, cardiac, or genitourinary abnormalities. A small exomphalos may contain only a Meckel's diverticulum while a large defect may contain the stomach, liver and bladder. The growth of viscera outside the abdominal cavity may lead it to be proportionately small making reduction of visera more difficult. *Antenatal:* Most are identified by routine fetal anomaly scans (AFP↑ too).[145] *Postnatal management:* •Protect herniated viscera •Maintain fluids and electrolytes. •Prevent hypothermia, gastric decompression, prevention of sepsis, and maintenance of cardiorespiratory stability. •Primary or staged closure may be used to repair the defect. With big defects, closure can cause respiratory insufficiency, haemodynamic compromise, dehiscence, and inability to close the abdomen and subsequent death.[145] After pulmonary and other comorbidities have stabilized, the omphalocele may gradually be reduced with a loose elastic bandage, with *delayed closure* at 6 to 12 months old.[145,146]

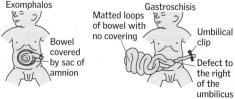

Exomphalos — Bowel covered by sac of amnion

Gastroschisis — Matted loops of bowel with no covering — Umbilical clip — Defect to the right of the umbilicus

Fig 2.5 Exomphalos and gastroschisis.

Pre-auricular tags are markers of GU problems; consider GU US.[147]

Undescended testis—cryptorchidism (2–3% of neonates, 15–30% of prems; bilateral in 25% of these). On cold days, retractile testes may hide in the inguinal pouch, eluding all but the most careful examination (eg while squatting, or with legs crossed, or in a warm bath they may be 'milked' down into position). These retractile testes need no surgery. If truly undescended it will lie along the path of descent from the abdominal cavity. Early (eg at 1 year) fixing within the scrotum (orchidopexy) may prevent infertility and reduces later neoplasia (untreated, risk is ↑ >5-fold).

Posterior urethral valves affect male fetuses and occurs from folds of bladder mucosa blocking the bladder neck, causing outflow obstruction. Usually diagnosed antenatally with oligohydramnios and renal tract dilatation or postnatally with absent or feeble voiding (± uraemia and a palpable bladder). *Micturating cystogram:* posterior urethral dilatation.

Hypospadias affects 1:350 male births. Characterized by abnormal position of external urethral meatus on the ventral penis. Most commonly causes difficulty urinating while standing and cosmetic appearance that is different to other boys. Occasionally, ventral curvature of the penis occurs (chordee). Avoid circumcision: use foreskin for preschool repair in one or more procedures.

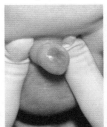

Epispadias (fig 2.6) (meatus on dorsum of penis) May occur with bladder exstrophy (see below).

Fig 2.6 Epispadias.

Some congenital/genetic disorders

Horseshoe kidney (crossed-fused kidney): Symptoms: Silent or obstructive uropathy ± renal infections. US diagnosis: kidneys 'too medial'; lower pole 'too long'; anterior-rotated pelvis; poorly defined inferior border; isthmus often invisible.[148] Absence of one kidney or horseshoe kidney is associated with Mullerian anomalies in girls (such as unicornuate uterus).

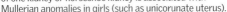

Autosomal recessive polycystic kidney disease and congenital hepatic fibrosis (ARPKD-CHF) is characterized by cystic dilations of the collecting ducts associated with biliary dysgenesis and periportal fibrosis. PKHD1 is the responsible gene (on short arm of chromosome 6). Typically diagnosed by prenatal US (hyperechogenic, large kidneys ± oligohydramnios). Affects 1 in 40,000. Severe cases lead to pulmonary hypoplasia. 80% of those infants that survive the 1st month of live will live to 15. Affected children tend to develop hyponatraemia, hypertension and renal failure. The histology of the liver is always abnormal. Survivors risk UTIs and portal hypertension with haematemesis.[149]

Ectopic kidney: May be seen on US (eg pelvic mass) or renal scintigraphy. Associations: anorectal abnormalities, UTIs; calculi.[150]

Renal agenesis causes oligohydramnios, Potter's facies + death if bilateral. VACTERL association (vertebral, anal, cardiac, tracheoesophageal, renal and limb anomalies). *Diagnosis:* prenatal US.[151]

Patent urachus: Urine leaks from the umbilicus. *Image:* excretory urogram.

Bladder exstrophy: Congenital anomaly which involves extrusion of the bladder through a defect in the abdominal wall. It is a spectrum of disease and can also involve the pelvic bones, ureters, bladder neck and sphincters, and can be associated with other problems, such as inguinal and umbilical herniae, and undescended testes.[152]

Double ureter: Associations: ureterocele, UTI, pyelonephritis; may be symptomless.

Renal tubular defects: (eg renal glycosuria, cystinuria, or diabetes insipidus). In *renal tubular acidosis* conservation of fixed base is impaired, causing metabolic acidosis + alkaline urine. *Symptoms:* Failure to thrive; polyuria; polydipsia. [153]

Wilms' nephroblastoma This is the commonest renal tumour of childhood (6–7% of all malignancies). [154] It is an undifferentiated mesodermal tumour of the intermediate cell mass. It may be sporadic, familial (2%), or associated with Beckwith–wiedemann syndrome (BWS, p638), aniridia, GU malformations (eg cryptorchidism), and retardation (WAGR). One of the Wilms' tumour genes (WT1 on chromosome 11) encodes a protein which is a transcriptional repressor downregulating IGF-II, an insulin-like growth factor. [155]

Median age at presentation: 3.5yrs. 95% are unilateral. *Staging:*
  I Tumour confined to the kidney
  II Extrarenal spread, but resectable
  III Extensive abdominal disease
  IV Distant metastases
  V Bilateral disease

The patient: 75% present <4yrs of age, mostly with a painless, palpable abdominal mass. Other features include fever, flank pain, and more rarely haematuria and hypertension. Metastases occur in 10%, most commonly in the lungs. US: renal pelvis distortion; hydronephrosis. CT/MRI provide the detailed anatomical information needed for surgical planning. [156]

Management: Avoid biopsy; nephrectomy + **vincristine** and **actinomycin** for 4 weeks pre-op can cure. Chemotherapy is used in all tumours. A 2-drug regimen is recommended for early Wilms' (without radiotherapy); more advanced stages need a 3-drug regimen + radiotherapy. [157] Genetic and biological factors guide risk categorization and help individualize care. [158,159] N=382

Prognosis: ~90% long-term survival. [160]

This is rare, but devastating for the parents. It can be an endocrinological emergency: *refer promptly.* ►Think about genetic, gonadal, phenotypic (affected by sex hormone secretion etc), psychological, and social-role sexualities. Male sex differentiation depends on SRY genes (on Y chromosomes) transforming an indifferent gonad into a testis; its products (testosterone & anti-Mullerian hormone) control fetal sex differentiation.[11][161]

Ask about exposure to progesterone, testosterone, phenytoin, aminogluteth-amide? Past neonatal deaths? Note penis size and urethral position (fig 2.7) . Are the labia fused? Is there a vaginal opening? Have the gonads descended? Preterm girls have relatively prominent labia and clitoris; preterm boys have undescended testicles until 34wks' gestation.

Tests Parents and relatives will be anxious to know the sex of their baby. However, any decision regarding the infant's sex must be delayed until a multidisciplinary team assessment has been carried out (including birth registration). Investigations include genetic sex determination (FISH for X and Y chromosomes plus karyotype (3–5 days). Test blood for serum electrolytes, glucose, adrenal androgens (urine for steroid profile), LH/FSH.

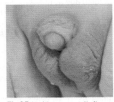

Fig 2.7 Ambiguous genitalia.

Don't rely on appearances whenever there is: bilateral cryptorchidism (at term), even if a penis is present; unilateral cryptorchidism with hypospadias; penoscrotal or perineo-scrotal hypospadias. Genetic tests are also vital: eg terminal deletion of 10q deletes genes essential for normal male genital development.[162]

Congenital adrenal hyperplasia (From deficiency of 21-hydroxylase, 11-hy-droxylase, 17-α-hydroxylase or 3-β-hydroxysteroid dehydrogenase from a defect on the gene *CYP21*). Cortisol is inadequately produced, leading to a rise in adrenocorticotrophic hormone, adrenal hyperplasia and overproduction of androgenic cortisol precursors (particularly 17OH-progesterone, leading to ↑testosterone production). Most affected infants are also salt losers, as 21-hy-droxylase is needed for aldosterone biosynthesis. In boys this is usually the sole early manifestation (excess virilization may be early or in adulthood). Biochemical screening is carried out in some centres in boys, to diagnose before life-threatening adrenal hyperplasia. Girls are detected by finding virilization at neonatal examination; prenatal diagnosis is possible and treatable by giving the mother dexamethasone from early in pregnancy. The variation in time of onset and clinical presentation despite identical CYP21 mutations, makes adrenal hyperplasia a continuum of disorders. Treatment is medical (glucocorticoid replacement in all; mineralocorticoid replacement if salt-wasting form) and surgical (clitoral reduction and vaginoplasty). Growth and fertility are also impaired.[163] *Incidence:* 1:14,000.[164] *Signs:* Vomiting, dehydration, and ambiguous genitalia. Girls may be masculinized. Boys may be normal at birth, but have precocious puberty, or ambiguous genitalia (↓androgens in 17-hydroxylase deficiency), or incomplete masculinization (hypospadias with cryptorchidism from ↓3β-hydroxysteroid dehydrogenase). *Hyponatraemia* (with paradoxically ↑urine Na⁺) and *hyperkalaemia* are common. ↑Plasma 17-hydroxyproges-terone in 90%; urinary 17-ketosteroids↑ (not in 17-hydroxylase deficit).

Aromatase deficiency Rare. CYP19 genes are needed for normal oestrogeni-zation: recessive mutations cause ambiguous genitalia in 46,XX individuals; at puberty there is hypergonadotropic hypogonadism, with no secondary sexual characteristics, except for progressive virilization. Boys have normal male sexual differentiation but are tall with brittle bones. Oestrogen receptor gene mutations are similar.[165]

►►Emergency treatment of adrenocortical crisis

Babies may present with an adrenocortical crisis (circulatory collapse) in early life. This is an acute exacerbation of an underlying adrenal insufficiency brought on by stressors (typically infection, trauma, or surgery) and is a life-threatening emergency. The adrenal gland is unable to respond to the stressor by increasing production/secretion of cortisol. Other presentations include hyponatraemic seizures in infancy (often misdiagnosed as a febrile convulsion).

Symptoms/signs
• Nausea/vomiting
• Abdominal pain
• Lethargy
• Hypotension.

►►Urgent treatment is needed with:
• Hydrocortisone—neonate: 10mg slow IV stat, then 100mg/m² daily by IVI; child 1 month–12yrs: 2–4mg/kg/6h; if >12yrs: 100mg/6–8h slow IV
• 0.9% saline IVI
• Glucose
• Fludrocortisone 0.1mg/day PO.

Assigning sex and gender

►There are two pieces of information every new parent is asked: the weight and the sex. It is traumatic for them not to be able to tell. However, don't shy away from telling patients that you do not know whether their baby is a boy or girl, and that tests must be done. This is unsatisfactory, but much better than having to re-assign gender. This is why a neonate with ambiguous genitalia is an emergency for the parents and the well-being of the wider family. Choice of gender must take into account chromosomal and gonadal sex, the hormonal milieu during fetal life, surgical aspects, internal anatomy, fertility issues, psychosexual development, and adult sexual function. NB: ♀ karyotype does not guarantee absence of intra-abdominal testes—so future risks of malignancy have to be assessed too.[166]

The MDT: paediatric endocrinologist with psychological expertise, a neonatologist, paediatric urologist, gynaecologist, geneticist, radiologist, psychologist, and clinical biochemist.

Prenatal preparation entails comparing prenatal karyotype with US genital scans to formulate a differential diagnosis—but US is unreliable in >50% of ♀ pseudohermaphroditism.[167,168] NB: it is common to assign ♀ gender when in doubt,[169] but while some favour a gender compatible with the chromosomal sex, if possible, others point out that this is a simplification as we don't fully understand determinants of gender role (social sex).[170,171] It is important not to think simply in terms of what promotes the greatest efficiency in the act of sexual intercourse.[172]

Advise against registering the birth until a definite treatment plan is in place. Once registered, legal sex cannot be changed in most countries.

---

11 Androgens cause maleness in 46, XY individuals, provided no mutations in the X-linked androgen receptor occur. Mutations cause more or less complete androgen insensitivity and female phenotype, with normal levels of testosterone and dihydrotestosterone (DHT). If there is partial insensitivity, topical (periscrotal) DHT (Andractim®) has been used to augment maleness, but if *in vitro* functional assays show this is impossible, babies are usually brought up as girls.[173]

Incidence 8:1000 births (the most common type of birth defect).[174] 1 in 10 stillbirths have evidence of severe congenital heart disease. Many defects are identified prenatally during anomaly scan or fetal echocardiography due to family history (other indications: pre-existing diabetes and monochorionic twins). Intrauterine cardiac intervention is possible for some conditions.[175]

Symptoms can present from hours to days postnatally (hypoplastic left heart, transposition of the great arteries (TGA), shunt dependent circulations) to during adulthood (atrial septal defect (ASD), ventricular septal defect (VSD), coarctation, COA). Any defect can cause decompensation and heart failure, but only right-to-left shunts cause cyanosis. ↑ pulmonary vascular resistance or failing left ventricular function can result in reversal of left-to-right flow across a shunt: Eisenmenger's syndrome (p642). In assessing suspected congenital heart disease, ask yourself is there *acute decompensation or heart failure?* Poor feeding, dyspnoea, tachycardia (bradycardia or inappropriately normal rate suggests imminent arrest), hepatomegaly, cool peripheries, acidosis on ABG, pulmonary venous congestion on CXR. Is there cyanosis?: (TGA, tetralogy of Fallot, tricuspid or pulmonary atresia, total anomalous pulmonary venous return (TAPVR), hypoplastic left heart, truncus arteriosus).

Investigations FBC, CXR, PaO_2 (air and 100% FiO_2), ECG, echo, ± cardiac catheter/advanced imaging techniques. **Management of heart failure** Sit upright, oxygen, calories via NG feed, diuretics (furosemide 1mg/kg/24hr infusion ± spironolactone). Duct dependent cyanotic conditions will need alprostadil (PGE_1) to maintain patency. Transfer to neonatal cardiac centre.

VSD (30%) *Symptoms:* Usually mild. *Signs:* Harsh loud pansystolic blowing murmur ± thrill. ECG: Ventricular hypertrophy and strain. CXR: pulmonary engorgement, cardiomegaly. *Course:* small or muscular defects close spontaneously, 20% by 9 months. Larger defects often need surgery. **ASD** (7%) *Symptoms:* Usually none. *Signs:* Widely split fixed s_2, systolic (pulmonary flow) murmur upper left sternal edge (ULSE).[176] ECG: RVH ± partial RBBB, absence of sinus arrythmia. CXR: cardiomegaly, globular heart. *Course:* Variable depending on site (secundum vs primum vs AVSD; common in trisomy 21). **Pulmonary stenosis** (7%) Usually asymptomatic. *Signs:* ESM ULSE, thrill, soft s_2. See *OHCM* p142. **Patent ductus arteriosus (PDA)** (12%) *Persistent:* Term babies at >1 month. Patent in premature babies. *Symptoms:* Rare unless large defect causing CCF and pulmonary hypertension. *Signs:* Continuous machine murmur below left clavicle, thrill, collapsing pulse, failure to thrive, pneumonias, loud s_2. CXR & ECG: usually normal. Ensure no duct dependent circulation by echo. Closure avoids spontaneous bacterial endocarditis and circulatory overload. 'Patent' treated with oral or IV ibuprofen (10mg/kg then 5mg/kg at 24 and 48hrs).[177] 'Persistent' with ibuprofen early and endovascular surgery at 1yr. **Coarctation** (5%) Usually no *symptoms* unless severe or interrupted arch type and so duct dependent and symptomatic (shock) day 3–10. *Signs:* HTN, radio-femoral delay (femoral pulses ↓volume, feet pulseless), ejection systolic murmur at ULSE. CXR: rib notching (late), '3' sign. ECG: LVH & strain. *Course:* Stent or surgery by 5yrs to avoid pulmonary HTN and end organ damage. **TGA** (5%) *Symptoms:* Cyanosis (mixing of systemic and pulmonary venous return) day 1–2. *Course:* Maintain PDA (prostaglandin) of utmost importance; balloon catheter atrial septal perforation, surgery with arterial switch in first few days of life. **Tetralogy of Fallot** (5%) Cyanotic (decreased pulmonary blood flow with R-to-L shunt). Large VSD, overriding aorta, subpulmonary stenosis, RVH. Mainly diagnosed antenatally or on hearing a harsh ESM LLSE. Cyanosis gradually worsens or with sudden short severe exacerbations causing distress and pallor due to hypoxia with risk of MI and stroke. Corrective surgery at 6 months old with shunt formation as interim measure.

With many thanks to Dr Carol Postlethwaite MRCP DRCOG.

We hear innocent murmurs (eg parasternal low-frequency 'twangs' in early systole) in ~80% of children, at some time (eg with fever, anxiety, exercise). *Still's murmur* is an example, and may be abolished by hyperextension of the back, and neck. Lack of other features distinguishes these from malformations: *no* clubbing; *no* cyanosis; *no* thrills; *no* rib recession; *no* clicks; *no* arrhythmias; normal pulses & apex; *no* failure to thrive. When in doubt, get a skilled echocardiogram. CXR & ECG often mislead.[178] Another (validated) option is to use an electronic stethoscope and e-mail the sounds to a cardiologist.[179]

Questions to ask yourself while listening to the 2nd heart sound (s_2)
• Is it a double sound in inspiration, and single in expiration? (Normal)
• Is s_2 split all the time? (atrial septal defects, ASD)
• Is s_2 never split, ie single? Fallot's; pulmonary atresia; severe pulmonary stenosis; common arterial trunk; transposition of the great arteries (the anterior aorta masks sounds from the posterior pulmonary trunk).
• Is the pulmonary component (2nd part) too loud? (Pulmonary hypertension)
NB: the 2nd heart sound is more useful diagnostically than the first. See fig 2.8.

Points to note on hearing murmurs If you have an ear for detail! *Timing:*
• *Ejection systolic* (innocent, or peripheral arterial stenosis).
• *Pansystolic* with no crescendo–decrescendo (VSD, PDA, COA, mitral incompetence).
• *Late systolic*, no crescendo–decrescendo (mitral prolapse, *OHCM* p138).
• *Early diastolic* decrescendo (aortic or pulmonary incompetence).
• *Mid-diastolic* crescendo–decrescendo (↑atrio-ventricular valve flow, eg VSD, ASD; or tricuspid or mitral valve stenosis). An opening snap (*OHCM* p138) and presystolic accentuation suggest the latter.
• *Continuous murmurs* (PDA, venous shunt, or arterio-venous fistula).

Loudness: The 6 grades for systolic murmurs (thrills mean pathology):
1 Just audible with a quiet child in a quiet room. *2* Quiet, but easily audible.
3 Loud, but no thrill. *4* Loud with thrill.
5 Audible even if the stethoscope only makes partial contact with skin.
6 Audible without a stethoscope.

Accentuating/diminishing manoeuvres *Inspiration:* Augments systemic venous return ('negative' pressure draws blood from abdomen into the thorax), and therefore the murmurs of pulmonary stenosis and tricuspid regurgitation. *Expiration:* Augments pulmonary venous return and decreases systemic return, and therefore VSD, mitral incompetence, and aortic stenosis too. In (mild) pulmonary stenosis, the ejection click is augmented by expiration. *Valsalva manoeuvre:* ↓Systemic venous return and benign flow murmurs, but ↑ murmurs from mitral incompetence and sub-aortic obstruction. *Sitting or standing (vs lying):* ↓Innocent flow murmurs, but ↑ murmurs from subaortic obstruction or from a venous hum (places to listen: right base; below left clavicle; neck—it is abolished by gently pressing the ipsilateral jugular; PDA murmurs are similar, but no change with posture).

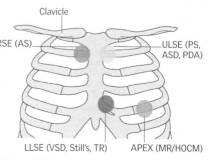

Clavicle

URSE (AS)

ULSE (PS, ASD, PDA)

LLSE (VSD, Still's, TR)   APEX (MR/HOCM)

Fig 2.8 Auscultation of heart murmurs.

Paediatrics

This is the most common facial malformation. It results from failure of fusion of maxillary and premaxillary processes (during week 5). The defect runs from lip to nostril. It may be bilateral, when there is often a cleft in the palate as well, with the premaxillary process displaced anteriorly. Palate clefts may be large or small (eg of uvula alone). **Incidence** ~1:1000. ♂·♀ > 1:1 **Causes** Genes, benzodiazepines, antiepileptics, rubella. Other malformations are common, eg trisomy 18, 13–15, or Pierre Robin short mandible (causing intermittent upper airway obstruction). **Prevention** Quit smoking pre-pregnancy.[180] Folic acid 5mg/day periconception ± multivitamins may help if the woman already has an affected child.[181,182] Avoidance of anti-epileptics. **Interdisciplinary treatment** Orthodontist, plastic surgeon, oral surgeon, GP, paediatrician, speech therapist. Feeding with special teats may be needed before plastic surgery (usually, lip repair at 3 months, and palate at 6 months). Repair of unilateral complete or incomplete lesions often gives good cosmesis. Refer to expert centres. If bilateral, there is always some residual deformity. Surgery may involve iliac bone grafts + insertion of Gore-Tex® membranes.[183] **Complications** Otitis media, aspiration, post-op palatal fistulae, poor speech (speech therapy helps). Social adjustment↓.[184] Avoid taking to NICU—may ↓bonding—a big problem (also the dopaminergic 'high' a normal baby's smile induces in the mother's putamen may be subverted by the defect)[185]

Other head & neck malformations

Eyes Anophthalmos: there are no eyes; rare; part of trisomy 13–15.
Ectopia lentis: Presents as glaucoma with poor vision. The lens margin is visible; seen in Marfan's (OHCM p720), Ehlers–Danlos (p642), homocystinuria; incidence: <1:5000; autosomal-dominant (a-Dom) or recessive (a-R). *Cataract:* Rubella, Down's. *Coloboma:* Notched iris with a displaced pupil; incidence: 2:10,000; (a-R). *Microphthalmos:* Small eyes; 1:1000; due to rubella—or genetic (autosomal dominant).
Ears Accessory auricles: seen in front of the ear; incidence: 15:1000.
Deformed ears: Treacher Collins syndrome (p655).
Low-set ears: associations—Down's syndrome; congenital heart disease.
Nose/throat Choanal atresia: *Signs:* postnatal cyanotic attacks; nasal catheter doesn't go into the pharynx because of nasal malformation. *Incidence:* ≤1:5000. *Surgery:* consider a micro-endoscopic nasal approach.[186] *Branchial fistula:* These open at the front of sternomastoid (a remnant of the 2nd or 3rd branchial pouch). *Incidence:* <1:5000. Branchial and thyroglossal cysts: p576.
Skull & spine *Brachycephaly:* Short, broad skull from early closure (craniostenosis) of the coronal suture; incidence: <1:1000; Down's-associated or a-Dom. *Cleidocranial dysostosis:* No clavicles (so shoulders meet). Slow skull ossification, no sinuses, high-arched palate; incidence <1:5000; a-Dom. *Craniofacial dysostosis:* Tower skull, beaked nose, exophthalmos. *Δ:* spiral CT. Klippel–Feil syndrome (p648): fused cervical vertebra (so the neck is short).
CNS Hydrocephalus: incidence 0.3–2:1000. Ante- or neo-neonatal injury, infection, or genes (sex-linked) may cause aqueduct stenosis. Dandy–Walker syndrome (p640); Arnold–Chiari malformation (OHCM p708). *Microcephaly: Causes:* genetic,[187] intrauterine viruses (eg rubella), hypoxia, x-rays, maternal alcohol. *Incidence:* 1:1000. Recurrence risk: 1:50.

Fetal alcohol spectrum disorder Severity depends on how much alcohol the mother has had in pregnancy. *Features:* microcephaly, short palpebral fissures, hypoplastic upper lip, absent philtrum, small eyes, IQ↓, cardiac malformations.

For spina bifida, see p140.

To outsiders, it seems as if paediatricians are obsessed with measuring head circumference and head shape, and translating the latter into Latin—as if defining the *outside* could explain what is going on *inside*. To insiders, though, ▶*it is to diagnose and treat craniostenosis that we measure heads*. So... always know where your patient is on his or her centile charts.

Plagiocephaly If fully expressed, synostosis affects coronal (rarely lambdoidal) sutures (±palpable bony ridge) with a flat forehead and elevation of the orbit on one side. Minor (unfused) plagiocephalic asymmetry is common in infants sleeping on their backs, improves with time, and is of no significance. Associations: scoliosis and pelvic obliquity (fig 2.9).

Craniostenosis=craniosynostosis=premature closure of one or more of the skull's fibrous sutures by ossification. It affects ~1:2000 of whom 2–11% have a family history. 15–40% have one of 180 recognized syndromes (with a family history it's 50%). Normal time for sutures to close is 3–9 months for the metopic (frontal) suture, 22–39 months for other sutures (sagittal, coronal, lamboid). The skull compensates for closure by growing in the direction parallel to the closed suture. If the compensatory growth allows insufficient space for the growing brain there will be ↑ICP ± visual loss, sleep impairment (obstructive sleep apnoea), eating problems and ↓IQ. Babies with insufficient head growth (centile charts p222-4) or skull deformity need assessment by a craniofacial surgeon. 4-20% of children with single suture closure have raised intracranial pressure, up to 60% if more than one suture involved. Look for papilloedema. Skull x-ray: single closed suture. CT: structural brain abnormalities and suture fusion and will diagnose deformational plagiocephaly (due to absent suture) and pansynostosis secondary to microcephaly. Subarachnoid spaces are larger in microcephaly. Surgery at 6-12 months aims to normalize the cranial vault and to allow for brain growth.

Dolicephalic The head is elongated, eg as in Marfan's, or El Greco portraits.

Dystopia canthorum Intercanthal distance is increased, but not the interpupillary or (bony) interorbital distances.

Holoprosencephaly (a whole, ie single-sphered, brain) Hypotelorism with cleft palate ± premaxillary agenesis ± cyclopia ± cebocephaly (see above)—follows failure of the lateral ventricles to separate (defective cleavage of the prosencephalon), eg with fusion of the basal ganglia.

Lissencephaly Smooth cortex with no convolutions (agyria).

Metopic suture This is the same as the frontal suture.

Micrognathia The mandible is too small.

Neurocranium That part of the skull holding the brain.

Oxycephalic (=turricephaly=acro-cephaly) The top of the head is pointed.

Rachischisis Spinal column fissure.

Sinciput Anterior, upper part of head.

Viscerocranium Facial skeleton.

Wormian bones Supernumerary bones in the sutures of the skull.

Cyclopia Extremely rare. A single eye in the area normally occupied by the root of the nose, which is missing, or present in the form of a proboscis (a tubular appendage) located above the eye. It may be part of trisomy 13 (Patau's syndrome).

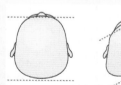

Fig 2.9 Plagiocephaly from positional flattening.
©The Royal Children's Hospital, Melbourne, Australia; Kids Health Info, www.rch.org.au/kidsinfo/fact_sheets/Plagiocephaly_misshapen_head/

NTDs result from failure of the neural tube to close between the 3rd and 4th week of *in utero* development.

Myelodysplasia Any neuroectoderm defect, eg of the cord, either multiple anterior horns, several central canals, failure of cord fusion so that there is a flat neural plaque, not a fused tube (*myelocele*), or a double neural tube (*diplomyelia*), or herniation through a bony defect as a *meningocele* (contains dura & arachnoid) or meningomyelocele (the cord is involved too, fig **2.10**). *Spina bifida* implies an incomplete vertebral arch (*spina bifida occulta* if covered by skin). *Anencephaly* is absent skull vault and cerebral cortex. It is fatal. *Encephalocele* means that part of the brain protrudes through the skull.

Incidence in Europe ~4000 preventable NTDs/yr.[188] *Risk* increases with young primips, lower social class, and homozygosity for a point mutation (c677→T; prevalence ≈10%, interfering with folate metabolism). *Recurrence risk* rises 10-fold if one pregnancy is affected, 20-fold if 2, 40-fold if 3 pregnancies affected; and 30-fold if a parent is affected. See 'Prevention' for risk reduction.

Neurological deficit is variable, depending on level of the lesion and the degree to which the lower cord functions independently from the upper cord. The defect may progress after birth; hydrocephalus gradually worsens mental performance. A child who learns to walk during his 2nd year may subsequently outgrow his ability to support (weight increases as the cube of surface area, power only as its square). Those with lumbosacral myelomeningoceles usually learn to walk with callipers by the age of 3, but ≤20% with higher lesions ever walk. When there is paralysis below L3, as unopposed hip flexors and adductors are likely to dislocate the hips; only 5–13% retain their ability to walk.[189] [n=173]

Postnatal surgery Firm guidelines on whom to treat often prove simplistic in individual infants. The final outcome of early closure of the defect depends on the state of the kidneys after multiple UTIs, and the extent of delayed hydrocephalus (requiring ventriculoperitoneal CSF shunts). Early postoperative mortality may account for ~25% of deaths. Many operations may be needed for spinal deformity (often severe and very hard to treat).

Antenatal diagnosis on US Fetuses with anencephaly have an absent cranium and bulging eyes ('frog-like' appearance); 99% will be detected by 20 weeks. Findings on US of spina bifida vary according to the severity of the lesion. A defect may be seen in the vertebral bodies or tissue overlying the spine; other signs include frontal bone scalloping (lemon sign) and a banana-shaped cerebellum. 95% of major lesions are detected. Termination of pregnancy is offered at any stage of pregnancy if an NTD is discovered.

Intrauterine surgery (*eg at 23 weeks' gestation*) This is very controversial.

Hurdles for the developing child
- Urinary and faecal incontinence. Penile appliances, urinary diversions, or intermittent self-catheterization save bed sores. Regular evaluation of bladder function is essential (surgery may or may not help).[12]
- Immobility. Mobility allowances can be of great help.
- Social and sexual isolation, if a special school is needed.[190]

Prevention Folic acid 0.4mg daily for 3 months pre-conception until 13 weeks' gestation reduces the risk. In mothers who have already had an affected baby, there is good evidence that folic acid (eg 5mg/day—or if diabetic, obese, on anti-epileptics, p7) given from before conception (as the neural tube is formed by 28 days, before pregnancy may even be recognized) reduces the risk of recurrence of neural tube defects by 72%.

Paediatrics (side margin)

---

12 Untethering the spinal cord may be indicated: seek expert advice. See *J Urol* 2007: 331.[191]

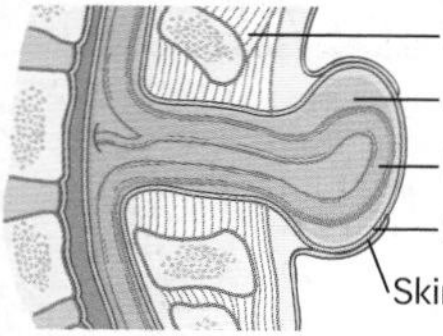

- Intraspinous ligaments
- csf in subarachnoid space
- Displaced spinal cord
- Dura mater with overlaying membranous sac
- Skin stops here

Fig 2.10 Meningomyelocele.

Should we fortify staple foods with folic acid?

This is done in many places but not in Europe. Research showing that the hoped-for decline in NTDs is not occurring—as most people are ignorant of (or do not act on) advice to take folic acid before conception.[192] Inertia is reasonable, perhaps, as some unforeseen harm may occur from fortification. If fortification is favoured, fortification of flour is one attractive option.[193] 40 countries have tried this; success in preventing NTDs ranges from 19% to 78%.[194]

So what harm could there be from folic acid? It can correct anaemia due to a low vitamin B_{12}—and hence might mask the underlying disease, and allow development or progression of B_{12}-related neuropathy and subacute combined degeneration of the spinal cord, if diagnosis depended on the presence of anaemic symptoms. This possibility may be partly overcome by educating ourselves, so that we do not believe that macrocytic anaemia is a necessary sign of B_{12}-related neurological disorders.[195] Another argument in favour of universal fortification is that significant neuropsychiatric morbidity is also preventable by folic acid supplementation.[196] the FACIT trial 2007

Measles ND (ND=notifiable disease) (RNA paramyxovirus) *Spread:* Droplets. *Incubation:* 7–12 days; infective from prodrome (the 4cs: cough, coryza, conjunctivitis, cranky), T°↑, until 5d after rash starts. *Koplik spots* on palate (fig 2.11) are pathognomonic. They are often fading as the rash appears (eg behind ears, on day 3–5, spreading down the body, becoming confluent). Δ: IgM & IgG +ve;[197] PCR for typing. *Complications:* More common if <5yrs or >20yrs. Otitis media is most common complication. Croup and tracheitis occur in infants. Pneumonia is the most common cause of death in

Fig 2.11 Koplik spots. Courtesy of the U.S. Centers for Disease Control.

measles. Older patients may develop encephalitis—of these 15% die; 25% develop fits, deafness, or ↓cognition. *Subacute sclerosing parencephalitis* is a chronic complication of measles which develops 7–13yrs after primary infection with progressive changes in behaviour, myoclonus, choreoatheotosis, dystonia, dementia, coma and death. *R̟:* Isolate—in hospital, if the patient is ill or immunocompromised or malnourished, or has pneumonitis, CNS signs, or dehydration, then:

- Ensure adequate nutrition (catabolism is very high). Continue breastfeeding, even during diarrhoea. Pass a nasogastric feeding tube if intake is poor.
- In the developing world, need for vitamin A arises; consider 2 doses, + 1 more at 6 weeks later (p460). CI: pregnancy; known not to be deficient.
- Treat secondary bacterial infection; antibiotics such as amoxicillin for otitis media and pneumonia. Prophylactic antibiotics have no role.[198]

Immunization: BOX p151. 80% effective.[199] *Prognosis:* Good in rich countries; in poor areas death rate is ~10%.[200] (0.9 million/yr, mostly in Africa).[201]

RubellaND (RNA virus) *Incubation:* 2–3wks. *Infectivity:* 5 days before to 5 days after start of rash. *Signs:* Macular rash; suboccipital lymphadenopathy. *Immunization:* Live virus, BOX p151.[202] *Complications:* Small joint arthritis. Malformations *in utero* (p34). Infection during the 1st 4 weeks of fetal development: eye anomaly (70%); wks 4–8: cardiac abnormalities (40%); wks 8–12: deafness (30%).

MumpsND (RNA paramyxovirus) *Spread:* Droplets/saliva. *Incubation:* 14–21d. *Immunity:* Lifelong, once infected. *Infectivity:* 7 days before and 9 days after parotid swelling starts. *Signs:* Prodromal malaise; T°↑; painful parotid swelling, becoming bilateral in 70% (ΔΔ: Sjögren's; leukaemia; dengue; herpes-virus; EBV; HIV; sarcoid; pneumococci; *Haemophilus*; staphs; anaphylaxis; blowing glass or trumpets; drugs; fig 2.12). *Complications:* Usually none; orchitis (± infertility), arthritis, meningitis, pancreatitis, myocarditis, deafness, myelitis. *R̟:* Rest. *Vaccine:* BOX p151, for *any* non-immune adult or child (SE: rare parotitis/pancreatitis).

Erythrovirus ('fifth disease', erythema infectiosum; parvovirus B19; fig 2.13). *Signs:* Usually a mild, acute infection, with malar erythema ('slapped cheek') and a rash mainly on the limbs (*gloves and socks syndrome*, in adults).[203] By the time this appears, infectivity has waned. Constitutional upset is mild. Arthralgia is commoner in adults—who may present as 'glandular fever' (false +ve Paul–Bunnell).[204] Spread by droplet[202] is rapid in closed communities. It can also cause the marrow to stop making RBCs (*aplastic crisis*)—serious if RBC lifespan is already short (eg sickle-cell disease, thalassaemia, spherocytosis, HIV). Δ: IgM (PCR if immunocompromised). *R̟:* Transfusions and immunoglobulins are rarely needed.[203] *Pregnancy:* Risk of fetal death is ~10% (esp. midtrimester)[205]—eg from hydrops fetalis ∵ inhibition of multiplication and lysis of erythroid progenitor cells. If pregnant woman exposed, check serum IgM/IgG for previous immunity. *Fetal/neonatal problems:* hydrops (in ~3%; treat by intrauterine transfusion if severe), growth restriction, meconium peritonitis, myocarditis, glomerulonephritis, placentomegaly, hepatomegaly, oedema, pancytopenia. Respiratory insufficiency/death is rare. 10% of those affected before 20 weeks miscarry; in the rest, risk of congenital abnormality is ~1%.[206]

Paediatrics

Hand, foot, & mouth disease The child is mildly unwell; develops vesicles on palms, soles, and mouth. They may cause discomfort until they heal, without crusting. *Incubation:* 5–7 days. *Treatment* is symptomatic. *Cause:* Coxsackie-virus A16 or enterovirus 71 (suspect in outbreaks with herpangina, meningitis, flaccid paralysis ± pulmonary oedema). Herpangina entails fever + sore throat + vesicles or macerated ulcers (on palate or uvula, which heal over 2 days) ± abdominal pain and nausea. This has nothing to do with the bovine form.

Herpes infections See *OHCM* p400–1. Varicella zoster/chickenpox: p144.

Roseola infantum This is a common, mild, self-limiting illness in infants, caus-ing T°↑, then a maculopapular rash on subsidence of fever at the end of the 4th febrile day. Uvulo-palatoglossal junctional ulcers may be a useful early sign.[207] *Cause:* Herpes virus 6 (HHV6; double-stranded DNA). It is related to other herpes viruses (HSV 1 & 2, varicella zoster, EBV & CMV). *Synonyms:* exanthem subitum, fourth disease, 3-day fever. It is neurotropic (a rare cause of encephalitis/focal gliosis on MRI, maybe accounting for why the not uncommon roseola 'febrile fits' tend to occur *after* the fever).[208]

Other causes of rashes in children See also skin diseases section (p582).
• A transient maculopapular rash is a feature of many trivial viral illnesses (but a few macules may be a sign of early meningococcaemia).
• Purpuric rashes: meningococcaemia (p202); Henoch–Schönlein purpura (p197); idiopathic thrombocytopenic purpura (check FBC and film).
• Drug rashes (maculopapular) from eg amoxicillin in glandular fever common.
• Scabies (p608); insect bites.
• Eczema (p596); urticaria (p584); psoriasis—guttate psoriasis may follow a respiratory tract infection in children (p594); pityriasis rosea (p602).
• Still's disease: transient maculopapular rash, fever, and polyarthritis.

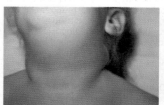 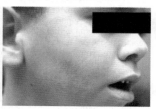

Fig 2.12 Mumps: generalized salivary swelling.
Courtesy of the US Centers for Disease Control and Prevention.

Fig 2.13 Slapped cheeks (parvovirus B19).
Courtesy of the US Centers for Disease Control and Prevention.

Managing distressing fever in viral illnesses

►Unwrap ►Rehydrate ►Antipyretics. Antipyretics aren't always needed[209] (↑mortality if used in severe sepsis).[210] Keep records of quantity used.

Ibuprofen at 10mg/kg/8h (~100mg/8h if 1–4yrs old; twice this if 7–10yrs) is better than **paracetamol** at 15mg/kg/6h, so try it first.

Oral paracetamol doses *1–3 months old:* 30–60mg/8h. Children over 3 months use maximum of 4 doses/24h then doses are: *3–6 months* 60mg/4–6h; *6 months–2yrs* 120mg/4–6h; *2–4 years* 180mg/4–6h; *4–6 years* 240mg/4–6h; *6–8 years* 240–250mg/4–6h; *8–10 years* 360–375mg/4–6h; *10–12 years* 480–500mg/4–6h; *12–16 years* 480–750mg/4–6h; *16+ years* 500mg–1g/4–6h. Maximum of 4 doses in 24h.

Paracetamol suppositories are available (60, 120, 125, 240, 250, 500mg or 1g).

Chickenpox is a primary infection with varicella-zoster virus. Shingles (*OHCM* p400) is a reactivation of dormant virus in posterior root ganglia.

Chickenpox *Signs:* Crops of skin vesicles of different ages, often starting on face, scalp, or trunk. The rash is more concentrated on the torso than the extremities. *Incubation:* 11–21 days. *Infectivity:* 4 days before the rash, until all lesions have scabbed (5 days). *Spread:* Droplets. It can be caught from someone with shingles. It is one of the most infectious diseases known. 95% of adults have been infected; immunity is lifelong. *Tests:* Fluorescent antibody tests and Tzanck smears are rarely needed. ΔΔ: Hand, foot, and mouth disease; insect bites; scabies; rickettsia. *Course:* T°↑; rash starts 2 days later, often starting on the back: macule→papule→vesicle with a red-surround→ulcers (eg oral, vaginal)→crusting. 2-4 crops of lesions occur during the illness. Lesions cluster around areas of pressure or hyperaemia. *Complications:* If spots are blackish (*purpura fulminans*) or coalescing and bluish (necrotizing fasciitis), get urgent help on ITU; avoid ibuprofen. Be alert to pneumonia, meningitis, myelitis, CNS thrombi, DIC, LFT↑, Guillain–Barré, Henoch–Schönlein, nephritis, pancreatitis, myositis, myocarditis, orchitis, cerebellar ataxia. If susceptible, *live attenuated vaccine* pre-cytotoxics/steroids may be wise. *Immunization:* occurs in the US/Japan/Australia and other countries, but is not routine in the UK. Reasons not to vaccinate include paradoxically increasing shingles/chickenpox in adults[211] and lack of cost-effectiveness.[212] *Dangerous contexts:* Immunosuppression; cystic fibrosis; severe eczema; neonates. *R*: Keeping cool may reduce lesion numbers. **Calamine lotion** soothes. Trim nails to lessen damage from scratching. Consider daily antiseptic for spots (chlorhexidine). **Flucloxacillin** 125-250mg/6h PO if bacterial superinfection—treat for septicaemia if worsening. **Antivaricella-zoster immunoglobulin** (if ≤10 days post-exposure) + **aciclovir** if immuno-suppressed or on steroids (it's licensed as a 7-day course in chickenpox); begin within 24h of the rash. In renal failure, ↓ dose. There is *no* clear evidence on aciclovir ↓complications if immunocompetent, but it may help severe symptoms, eg in adolescents, or as 2nd or 3rd family contacts. If used, use at the 1st sign of infection, or as a 7-day *attenuating dose* of 10mg/kg/6h starting 1wk post-exposure. **Famciclovir** is less well-studied.[213]

Shingles *Treatment:* Oral analgesia. Ophthalmic shingles: p420. Aciclovir may reduce pain, but also progression of zoster in the immunocompromised (may be rampant, with pneumonitis, hepatitis, and meningoencephalitis). **Aciclovir** IVI dose: 10mg/kg/8h (over 1h), with concentration <5mg/mL, over >1h.

Varicella in pregnancy Pneumonitis and encephalitis are no commoner in pregnancy, despite pregnancy being an immunocompromised state (1 in 400 and 1 in 1000, respectively). Infection in the 1st 20 weeks (esp. 13–20 weeks) may cause fetal varicella syndrome (FVS) in 2%.[214] Signs of FVS are variable, eg cerebral cortical atrophy and cerebellar hypoplasia, manifested by microcephaly, convulsions, and IQ↓; limb hypoplasia; rudimentary digits ± pigmented scars. Maternal shingles is *not* a cause. If the mother is affected from 1 week before to 4 weeks after birth, babies may suffer severe chickenpox. Give the baby zoster immunglobulin 250mg IM at birth; if affected, isolate from other babies, and give aciclovir.

Infection is preventable by pre-pregnancy vaccination with live varicella vaccine,[215] but testing for antibodies pre-conceptually is expensive, and cost-effectiveness depends on local rates of seronegativity. ~80% of those who cannot recall any previous chickenpox are, in fact, immune.[216]

Varicella zoster globulin prevents infection in 50% of susceptible contacts, eg 1000mg IM (adults). Infection in pregnancy merits **aciclovir** (it's probably OK for the fetus). Chickenpox at birth is a problem. Barrier nursing mothers causes distress and is of unproven value. Infant mortality: up to 20%.[217]

In many sub-Saharan countries, ~40% of all under-5 mortality is a result of AIDS. If an HIV +ve mother breastfeeds, this ↑risk of vertical transmission by ~50%. Mothers with HIV should bottle feed in the UK, but in countries without reliable clean water, breastfeeding is less risky than bottle feeding.[218,219] Infection can occur from the 1st trimester; ~50% of infections occur at the time of delivery, and are more likely if mothers have symptomatic HIV infection or a high viral load. Transmission rates with full intervention (ie antiretrovirals around birth, caesarean section, no breastfeeding) are <5%. For caesarean section and zidovudine in preventing vertical transmission, see p34. CMV may be fatal in infants whose mother's HIV status wasn't recognized in pregnancy.[220] HIV infection—prenatal/labour: p34/p22; adult HIV: OHCM, p408.

Diagnosing vertically acquired HIV Test at birth, 3 and 6 months of age for
- HIV viral PCR
- P24 antigen
- specific IgA.

▶*Aim to diagnose 95% of infected infants before the age of 1 month.* Monitoring CD4 counts (*OHCM* p413) helps in staging HIV. The all clear can only be given if all tests are negative at 18 months but infection unlikely if tests negative and the baby is well at 6 months.

Consider HIV in children with: PUO; lymphadenopathy; hepatosplenomegaly; persistent diarrhoea; parotid enlargement; shingles; extensive molluscum; platelets↓; recurrent slow-to-clear infections; failure to thrive; clubbing, unexplained organ disease;[221] TB; pneumocystosis; toxoplasmosis; cryptococcosis; histoplasmosis; CMV; LIP (below). *Suspect non-vertical HIV seroconversion illness if:* Tº↑, fatigue, rash, pharyngitis, lymphadenopathy, oral ulcers, D&V, headache, myalgia, arthralgia, meningism, peripheral neuropathy, thrush, weight↓, night sweats, genital ulcers, WCC↓; platelets↓; transaminases↑.[222]

HIV & the lung: TB; lymphocytic interstitial pneumonia (LIP), immune reconstitution inflammatory syndrome, malignancy, bronchiectasis.[223] *LIP:* tachypnoea; hypoxia; clubbing; diffuse reticulonodular infiltrates on CXR; bilateral hilar lymphadenopathy. It is not AIDS-defining. It is less serious than pneumocystosis.

Prognosis By 3yrs old, up to half with early-onset opportunistic infection have died vs 3% of those with no such infection. Children with slow progression of HIV have persistent neutralizing antibodies. Transplacental passage of maternal neutralizing antibody may also have a role.

Ensure full course of vaccines (+*Pneumococcus*; avoid live vaccines if very immunocompromised, and BCG if symptomatic and TB prevalence is low).[224,225]

Highly active antiretroviral therapy (HAART) Use PENTA regimen. Pediatric European Network for the Treatment of AIDS[226] (*OHCM* p413). Those with AIDS-defining conditions or CD4 <15% (esp. if falling) should start HAART at once. If few symptoms and CD4 stable at >20% get advice.[227] *Obstacles:* Poor adherence (unpleasant tasting medicine); SE (lipids↑, glucose↑, bone metabolism↓); lack of family routines.[228] Diarrhoea-related morbidity:[229] micronutrient (eg Zn) zinc supplementation helps.[230]

▶Teach HIV+ve children about safe sex and other HIV issues before puberty.

Further reading

Pediatric European Network for the Treatment of AIDS: http://penta-id.org

Paediatrics

▶Involve social services *today* when issues of abuse arise. Read what follows with local child protection and NICE guidelines,[231] and relevant legislation in your country, eg in England, the *Children's Act* (states that *the child's welfare is always paramount*). *Child abuse* is defined as deliberate infliction of harm to a child or failure to prevent harm, and may be physical, sexual, emotional, bullying and online abuse, or neglect. *Neglect* is a persistent failure to meet a child's basic physical or psychological needs that is likely to result in serious impairment of the child's health and development. In *Munchausen's by proxy*, a parent fabricates alarming symptoms in their child to gain attention via unnecessary interventions.

Risk factors for NAI Birthweight <2500g; mother <30yrs; unwanted pregnancy; stress; poverty.[232] **Prevalence:** 1% of ED work.[233]

Suspect abuse if: Disclosure by child, or:
• Odd story, incongruent with injuries; odd mode of injury; odd set of signs.
• Delayed presentation to doctor, or taken by someone who is not a parent.
• History inconsistent with the child's development. Can the baby really walk?
• Efforts to avoid full examination, eg after an immersion burn.
• Psychological sequelae (stress; depression) from sexual or emotional abuse.[13]
• Unexplained fractures, eg forearm or rib (esp. posterior, from squeezing).[234]
• It is rare for a non-ambulant baby to sustain an accidental fracture.
• Buttock, perineum or face injury; intracranial bleeds;[235] torn lingual frenulum; vitreous/retinal bleeds, hyphaema (fig 5.4, p413), lens dislocation, bulging fontanelle, head circumference↑ ± xanthochromia; ▶if in doubt, do CT.
• *Also:* Cigarette burns; whip marks (outline of belt/buckle, or double electric flex); bruised non-mobile baby; signs of suffocation; fingermark bruising; perforated pharynx; bite marks.[236]
• In suspected physical abuse, skeletal survey with x-ray can help (infants cannot localize pain). CT/MRI if suspected head injury. If there is extensive or unusual bruising, perform a clotting screen. Retinal haemorrhages are a sign of non-accidental head injury (use an experienced ophthalmologist).

▶NB: site or type of fracture can never be *relied on* to distinguish abuse from an accident (extraordinary things, even spiral fractures, can happen in play).

ΔΔ: Osteogenesis imperfecta; osteoporosis, eg from propionic acidaemia.[237,238]

The first aim is to prevent organ damage, murder, and other significant harm. ▶If this is a real concern, admit the child and *contact the duty social worker today*—eg for an emergency protection order. Offer help to the parents. Learn to listen, leaving blame and punishment to judges. Find out about local policies and referral routes. Remember that often our duty is not to diagnose child abuse, but to recognize *possible* abuse, and then to get help.

Sexual abuse Know your local guidelines. Follow them. Inform Social Services. If you do not, ask yourself with whom you are colluding. Forensic specimens (eg pubic hair, vaginal swabs) are to be taken by an expert who knows how to be gentle, and to avoid a 'second rape'. Prepubertal STI means abuse until proven otherwise. Young girls can get discharge from streptococcal infection and foreign bodies which aren't from sexual abuse. Does abuse cause psychological harm? Yes, almost always. See p323.

Repertoire of actions in primary care ▶After informing Social Services, liaise with health visitor (may be a very helpful source of information) or NSPCC (National Society for the Prevention of Cruelty to Children).
• Admission to a place of safety (eg hospital or foster home).
• Continuing support for parents and protection for siblings.
• Prevention: encourage impulses to be shared, and not acted on.
• Attend a case conference (social worker, health visitor, paediatrician; police).[14]

A possible sequence of events might be:

Unexplained signs (or disclosure, or allegations), eg odd bruising
↓
'Testing of professional hypotheses' ≈ weighing it up in your own mind
↓
'Clarification by discussion with an experienced colleague' ≈ tell your boss
↓
'Reach a critical threshold of professional concern' ≈ you're both worried
↓
'Weigh the pros and cons of breaking confidentiality' ≈ you must breach confidentiality if doing so prevents harm to a child
↓
'Sharing concerns with statutory agencies' ≈ phone Social Services/police
↓
'Act within a timeframe not detrimental to the child' ≈ aim to do it now
↓
'Contemporaneous records detailing all your sources'≈ write it down now
↓
'Preliminary consultation with all concerned': don't promise to keep secrets
↓
'Strategic multidisciplinary discussion' ≈ is an abuse investigation needed?
↓
If so, 'Instigation of child abuse investigation' ≈ plan case conference
↓
'Must parents/child be present?'
↓
Tell parents & child (if appropriate) what your report to conference will be
↓
Case conference timed to let doctors fulfil their major role ≈ ? get a locum
↓
Register your dissent (if any) to the conference conclusions in its minutes
↓
Child is placed on a Register indicating that questions of abuse are unresolved and that the child remains at risk
↓
'Establish networks for information exchange, discussion & advice' ≈ follow up by Social Services, or a national society protecting children from cruelty (NSPCC).

Not all our efforts to protect children end thus. Successes are frequent. And of course this sequence oversimplifies...the sign ≈ is not meant flippantly: it is intended as shorthand, denoting the exercise of reflection, good judgement, action, and the following of agreed procedures.

13 Hulme K (1984). *Bone People*. Auckland: Spiral/Hodder & Stoughton. This novel tests Samuel Johnson's aphorism that `it is better that a man should be abused than be forgotten'. Read it before making quick judgements about families
14 The UK Families at Risk Review (2008) specifies joined-up agencies that 'ensure' that there is 'no wrong door' that families knock on—all doors lead to getting the correct help. Also: •Confirm social services referrals in writing •Question other's opinions if you disagree. •Document all phone-calls •Record discussions if there is disagreement over risk of deliberate harm.

Definition Sudden unexplained infant death (SUID) is any infant death that is unexpected and initially unexplained. Often, a cause of death is determined after a thorough investigation and autopsy. The deaths that remain unexplained are defined as SIDS: sudden infant death syndrome is the sudden death of an infant under 1 year of age, which remains unexplained after a thorough investigation including an autopsy, examination of the death scene, and review of the clinical history.

Putative causes
Obstructive apnoea:
• Inhalation of milk
• Airways oedema
• Passive smoking
Central apnoea:
• Faulty CO_2 drive
• Prematurity
• Brainstem gliosis
Others:
• Long Q–T interval[15]
• Staph infection[16]
• Overheating
• ↑Vagal tone or Mg^{2+}↑
• Immature diaphragm
• Genetic & viral causes

Epidemiology Peak incidence: 1–4 months; risk↑ if: poor, parents are smokers, baby is male or premature, winter, previous sibling affected by SIDS; coexisting minor upper respiratory infection is common, co-sleeping. There are many causal theories (see MINIBOX).

Sleeping supine ('back to sleep', even for short naps),[239] preventing overheating, and cigarette smoke exposure are the chief preventive interventions: risk from passive smoking is dose-dependent, and often at least doubles risk.[240]

The face is an important platform for heat loss—and it is known that the incidence of SIDS is ~5–10-fold higher among infants usually sleeping prone (17-fold higher if sleeping in a room separated from parents): ►so always recommend sleeping supine. Advise as follows:

• Do not overheat the baby's bedroom. Aim for a temperature of 16–20°c.
• Do not use too much bedding, and avoid duvets if less than 1 year of age.
• If ill or feverish, consult a GP—do not increase the amount of bedding.
• Use a grow-bag; this is a modified sleeping bag for a baby, containing arm holes and prevents the baby migrating under the blanket.
• While sleeping, avoid heaters, hot water bottles, electric blankets, and hats. Do wrap up for trips out in winter, but unwrap once indoors, even if this means disturbing the baby. Never tuck in blankets higher than the armpit.[241]
• Babies >1 month do not need to be kept as warm as in hospital nurseries.
• Avoid co-sleeping and never, even if very tired (new parents!), if parents are deep sleepers, or if they have had any alcohol or drugs.[242,243]

Autopsy is unrevealing; minor changes are common; petechial haemorrhages over pleura, pericardium, or thymus, and vomit in the trachea may be agonal events. *Causes to exclude:* sepsis, metabolic defects (eg MCAD deficiency) and heart defects.

Action after failed resuscitation in the Emergency Department
• Document all interventions, venepuncture sites, and any marks on the baby. You don't have to keep all tubes *in situ*, but ensure that someone who did not intubate confirms endotracheal placement of the tube before extubation.
• Keep all clothing and the nappy.
• Explain clearly to parents that despite your best efforts, the baby has died.
• Unless the cause is obvious, be non-committal about cause of death. Explain the baby *must* have a post-mortem (this is a coroner's case).
• Contact the consultant on call, the police, child protection team, and the coroner at once; also GP, health visitor, and any other involved professions.

Paediatrics

---

15 Risk↑ if Q–T corrected for rate (QT^c) ≳440msec. QT^c=(Q–T)/($\sqrt{R-R}$).[244,245] LQTS genes are important.[246]
16 Staphs in mattress foam are implicated (∴ do not reuse).[247,248]

How the GP can help the family on the first day
• A prompt visit to express sympathy emphasizing that no one is to blame.
• Explain about the legal requirement for an autopsy and coroner's inquest. The parents may be called upon to identify the body.
• Bedding may be needed to help find the cause of death.

Subsequent help
Don't *automatically* suppress lactation, but if this becomes necessary caber-goline (250mcg/12h PO for 48h) is preferred to bromocriptine. NB: continued lactation may be an important way of grieving for some mothers.

Many parents will not want anxiolytics eg diazepam, but may want hypnotics (such as a short course of zopiclone).

Advise the parents of likely grief reactions (guilt, anger, loss of appetite, hearing the baby cry). Make sure that the coroner informs you of the autopsy result; a consultant paediatrician or GP should explain the findings to the parents.. They should already have a routine appointment with a consultant paediatrician. This can provide an opportunity for the parents to ask questions. The parents may find an electronic apnoea alarm reassuring in caring for later infants. Programmes exist to prevent a future SID—eg the CONI programme (care of next infant) and parents can contact them in future pregnancies.

Paediatrics

Further reading
Care of Next Infant: www.lullabytrust.org.uk/coni

The main aims: • Encouraging breastfeeding (p124) • Monitoring development • Immunization • Overseeing growth (p180) • Parental support • Education and reassurance about normal childhood events. • Talking to the child, and building up a good relationship.

Monitoring The most cost-effective times to screen are unknown.

Birth & 6 weeks:	Neonatal check (p114), and with GP at 6 weeks. Arrange vaccinations and vitamin drops (A, D & C) unless adequate sunlight/diet.[17]
1–9 months:	Hips, testes descent, CVS examination.
18–24 months:	*Educate* on diet, dental care, accidents; walking (look for waddling), social and linguistic milestones; Hb if *iron deficiency* likely—it may well be. *Any parental depression?*
4 years:	Testes descent, CVS examination. Nutrition, dental care.

At each visit: • Encourage questions • Ask about, and test for, squint, vision, and deafness • Chart centiles. *Beware reading too much into a single reading.* Remember to correct age for prematurity. Note the milestones in the TABLE. There is much individual variation.

6 weeks:	Smiles.
4 months:	Uses arm support when prone; holds head steady when supported while sitting; reaches out; spontaneous smiling.
6 months:	Bears some weight on legs; on pulling to sitting, there is no head lag; reaching out; transfers things from hand to hand.
8 months:	Sits unaided.
≥1 year:	Just stands; walks using a table's support; clashes cubes; pincer grip; can say 'Mummy' ± 'Daddy'. Plays 'pat a cake'.
18 months:	Can walk; scribbles; 2-cube tower. 2–4 words. NB: drooling ± throwing items on the floor is abnormal by now.
2 years:	Kicks a ball; overarm 'bowling'; gets undressed.
3 years:	Jumps; can stand on one foot; copies; can build an 8-cube tower; knows his first and last name; dressing needs help.
4 years:	Stands on 1 foot for >4sec; picks the longer of 2 lines.

Health promotion in refugee children/asylum-seekers Unaccompanied children may request asylum explicitly or implicitly. Our job is to look after them, not to interpret laws. ☜Tell immigration officers/police that children cannot be detained even if there is doubt about a child's age. UK immigration officers must abide by the UN convention on the Rights of the Child (1989). This stipulates that each State must ensure the rights of each child within its jurisdiction *without discrimination of any kind*. Any child who has been abused has the right to physical and psychological recovery and social integration. (Prison is not a form of social integration.) Take any opportunity to promote children's health. If from areas of chronic conflict, don't assume the child has been vaccinated. Start from scratch. Test for TB (skin test) and give BCG, or refer to a chest clinic if needed. See Home Office[249] & Royal College Guidelines.[250] Paediatricians and GPs can promote refugee health by:

• Documenting development, ensuring nutrition, and treating physical illness.
• Easing access to antenatal and all other preventive care activities.
• Identifying depression/anxiety, and picking up clues that torture may have taken place: nightmares; hallucinations; panic attacks; sexual problems; phobias; difficulties with relationships. These may also be signs that the child has been recruited to fight other people's wars. Treating childhood depression is controversial (SSRI, p368) *but not treating it may be worse.*[251]
• Recognizing and treating TB and HIV (look for persistent oral candida, caries, UTIs, widespread lymphadenopathy, hepatosplenomegaly; failure to thrive; developmental delay). See p145.
• Liaising with social services to ensure housing and schooling.

Paediatrics

Immunization schedule (DoH^UK 2014)[252]

2 months:	**Pediacel®**, ie 5-in-1 diphtheria + tetanus + acellular pertussis + inactivated polio + haemophilus B (HIB); if prem, still give at 2 months; can give if ≤10 yrs if missed vacs + **Prevenar13®** (13-valent pneumococcal) + **Rotarix®** (Rotavirus) + **Bexsero®** (Meningitis B)
3 months:	**Pediacel®** + **Neisvac C®** or **Meningitec®** (Meningitis C vaccine)+ **Rotarix®**
4 months:	**Pediacel®** + **Prevenar13®** + **Neisvav C®** or **Meningitec®** + **Bexsero®**
12 months:	**Menitorix®** (*H. influenzae* with meningitis C) + **Bexsero®**
13 months:	**MMR^L** or **Priorix®L** (Measles, Mumps & Rubella) + **Prevenar13®**
3¼-5yrs:	**Repevax®** or **Infanrix-IPV®** (Diphtheria, tetanus, pertussis & polio) + **Priorix®L** or **MMR^L**
13-18⁺yrs:	**Revaxis®** (low-dose diphtheria, tetanus, inactivated polio; can also be used for primary vaccination if >10yrs). **Gardasil®** (against human papilloma virus) protects against cervical cancer: see p272.
Any age:	**BCG^L** (not universal in UK) If at ↑risk of TB, eg for all from high-prevalence country, ie >40:100,000/yr, or a visitor to such a country for >1 month. May start at 3 days old. **Hepatitis B**: p263; universal (WHO advice) or if at ↑risk. **MMR^L** may be given at any age if presents late. One-off **pneumococcal vaccine** with 23-valent Pneumovax II®, as above, if <2yrs); yearly **'flu vaccine** if risk↑: see *OHCM* p390. Consider 2nd pneumococcal vaccine if at ↑risk after >5yrs.[253]
Pregnant:	Pertussis (as **Repevax®**) and flu, as indicated.

►An acute febrile illness is a contraindication to any vaccine. Note:

►Give live vaccines either together, or separated by ≥3 weeks.

►Don't give live vaccines if primary immunodeficiency, or if on steroids (≥2mg/kg/day of prednisolone); but if HIV+ve, give all immunizations (including live) except for BCG, in areas where TB prevalence is low.

Hepatitis B (Engerix B®) See *OHCM* p262. Give at birth, 1 & 2 months, if mother is HBsAg +ve—0.5mL IM in anterolateral thigh. If birthweight ≤1500g give Hep B immunoglobulin as well as vaccine, regardless of mother's e-antigen status. If at term, give Hep B Ig unless mother is anti-HBe +ve.

HPV vaccination to prevent cervical cancer: see p272.

Chickenpox vaccination In the USA this is routine and has greatly reduced incidence and hospitalizations/mortality.[254] Eradication is impossible.

Immunization in immunodeficiencies See Royal College Guidelines.

Can the pain of the injection be reduced? Topical lidocaine–prilocaine 5% cream (EMLA®) and oral glucose at the time of vaccination does decrease the latency to 1st cry, and other objective markers of pain.[255]

MMR is not just for children In the UK, in 2005, mumps rates rose 10-fold (to 5000/month), eg among students who were too old to have had full vaccination. Any non-immune adult is eligible for MMR (exclude pregnancy). If >18 months, the 2 doses of MMR should be separated by 3 months. MMR vaccine may also be offered to unimmunized, or measles-only immunized or seronegative post-partum women (avoid pregnancy for 1 month following immunization).

Does MMR vaccine cause autism? No. Large-scale studies find no link.

What sort of needle? For IM vaccination, WHO advises that needles are 25mm long (blue in the UK).[256] Stretch the skin flat between thumb and forefinger to aid a deep injection—and make the angle (needle to skin) 90°. The subcutaneous route is OK for MMR; bunch the skin up, and inject at 45° into fat.

17 Adequate sunlight to prevent rickets is a big issue, especially north of Oxford (51°45') as UV-B is too scarce to make active vitamin D in winter.[257-258] Risk of rickets↑ if: skin pigmented; sunscreens or concealing clothing used; staying indoors to play video-games●[risk too]; obesity; malabsorption; renal and liver disease; using anticonvulsants. Good vit. D status in pregnancy (p10) helps neonatal bones, immune function, and lungs (asthma risk↓ by 40%●[risk]).[260]

Gene probes use recombinant DNA technology to identify specific mutations causing genetic diseases (eg Huntington's chorea; muscular dystrophy; polycystic kidneys; cystic fibrosis; thalassaemias) to DNA markers scattered throughout our genome. Using fetal DNA from amniotic fluid cells (amniocentesis) in the 2nd trimester, or from chorionic villus sampling in the 1st.

Enzyme defects Many of the inborn errors of metabolism can be diagnosed by incubation of fetal tissue with a specific substrate.

Chromosomal studies can be undertaken on cultured cells or on direct villus preparations. The most important abnormalities are aneuploidies (abnormalities in chromosome number)—eg trisomy 21, 18, and 13.

Screening for chromosomal abnormalities (eg the fragile X syndrome, p648) may be performed on at-risk mothers who may be carriers.

Non-disjunction After meiosis one gamete contains two chromosomes 21 (say)[18] and the other gamete has no chromosome 21. After union of the 1st gamete with a normal gamete, the conceptus has trisomy 21 (50% spontaneously miscarry). This is the cause in ≥88% of babies with trisomy 21, and increases significantly in mothers over 40 (p12).

Robertsonian translocations (fig 2.14) entail a fusion between the centromeres of 2 chromosomes with loss of the short arms forming a chromosome with two long arms, one derived from each chromosome. They involve any 2 of chromosomes 13, 14, 15, 21, & 22 (all acrocentric, ie the centromere is close to one end; the short arms contain few genes). This translocation trisomy 21 is the cause in 4% of Down's syndrome (unrelated to maternal age). If the father carries the translocation, risk of trisomy 21 is 10%; if it is the mother, the risk is 50%. 0.3% of mothers have this translocation.

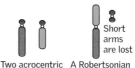

Two acrocentric chromosomes   A Robertsonian translocation

Short arms are lost

Fig 2.14 A chromosome with 2 long arms.

Balanced translocations entail no net gain or loss of chromosomal material, two chromosomes have been broken and rejoined in the wrong combination.

Mosaicism A trisomy may develop during early divisions of a normal conceptus (∴ somatic, not germline). If the proportion of trisomy 21 cells is low (eg 4%) CNS development may be 'normal'. It accounts for ≤8% of Down's babies.[261]

Other chromosomal abnormalities Edward's (p642), Klinefelter's (p646), Patau's (p650), and Turner's (p655) syndromes. In the *cri-du-chat* syndrome there is deletion of the short arm of chromosome 5, causing a high-pitched cry, CVS abnormalities, microcephaly, widely spaced eyes, and a 'moon' face.

Trisomy 21 *Causes:* See earlier in topic. *Recognition at birth:* Flat facial profile, abundant neck skin, dysplastic ears, muscle hypotonia, and x-ray evidence of a dysplastic pelvis are the most constant features. Other features: see BOX, p153. Widely spaced 1st & 2nd toes and a high-arched palate are more visible later. If uncertain, it is best to ask an expert's help, rather than baffle the mother by taking karyotype tests 'just in case it's Down's'.[19] *Associated problems:* Duodenal atresia; VSD; patent ductus; AVSD (foramen primum defects, p136); and, later, a low IQ and a short stature. Helping the mother accept her child may be aided by introducing her to a friendly mother of a baby with trisomy 21. *Prenatal diagnosis:* p12–15.

---

18 Chromosome 21 contains only 225 genes: most of its DNA is apparently meaningless.
19 Even in good hands, accuracy of suspicion is only 64%, so at some stage karyotyping is needed.[262]

Clinical features
• Single palmar crease
• Hypotonia
• Flat face/round head
• Protruding tongue
• Broad hands
• Upward slanted palpebral fissures and epicanthic folds
• Speckled irises (Brushfield spots)
• Intellectual impairment
• Short stature
• Pelvic dysplasia
• Cardiac malformations
• Hypoplasia of middle phalanx of (incurving) 5th finger
• Intestinal atresia
• High-arched palate.

Associations[263][NICE]
• Lung problems (lung capacity is reduced in almost 100%)
• Congenital heart disease (40%)
• Digestive problems (6%)
• Hypothyroidism
• Hearing loss (60%)
• Leukaemia
• Early-onset Alzheimer's disease (50%)
• 44% survive to age 60 years.

The health needs approach to someone with trisomy 21 This approach starts by asking: How can I help? Health maintenance for children with trisomy 21 is more important, not less, compared with the needs of other children—because their families are vulnerable, and many conditions are more likely in those with this condition. Examples are otitis media, thyroid disease, congenital cataracts, leukaemoid reactions, dental problems, and feeding difficulties.[264]

The patient-centred approach Different approaches are needed at different times: a key skill in becoming a good doctor is to be able to move seamlessly from one approach to another—and knowing when to adopt which approach.

Goal To provide accurate, up-to-date information on genetic conditions to enable families and patients to make informed decisions.

▶Genetic counselling is best done in regional centres to which you should refer families (nearest centre: UK tel.: 020 7794 0500). *Consider the consequences of doing any test on a child—but especially a genetic one. Discuss with a geneticist or senior doctor first—will the child be glad of the information when they are old enough to understand?*

In order to receive most benefit from referral:
- The affected person (proband) ideally comes with family (spouse, parents, children, siblings); individuals can of course be seen alone as well.
- The family should be informed that a detailed pedigree (family tree) will be constructed, and medical details of distant relatives may be asked for.
- Irrational emotions (guilt, blame, anger) are common. Deal with these sensitively, and do not ignore. *Remember:* you do not choose your ancestors, and you cannot control what you pass on to your descendants.
- Warn patients that most tests give no absolute 'yes' or 'no' but merely 'likely' or 'unlikely'. In gene tracking, where a molecular fragment near the gene is followed through successive family members, the degree of certainty of the answer will depend on the distance between the marker and the gene (as crossing-over in meiosis may separate them).
- Accept that some people will not want testing, eg the offspring of a Huntington's chorea sufferer—or a mother of a boy who might have fragile x syndrome, but who understandably does not want her offspring labelled (employment, insurance, and social reasons). Offer a genetic referral to ensure that her decision is fully informed (but remember: 'being fully informed' may itself be deleterious to health and well-being).

Naming chromosomes Autosomes are numbered 1 to 22 roughly in order of size, 1 being the largest. The arms on each side of the centromere are named 'p' (petite) for the short arm, and 'q' for the long arm (remember, there's always a long Q for a short P). Thus 'the long arm of chromosome 6' is written '6q'.

Chromosomal disorders include trisomy 21, p152, Turner's (45X0, p655) and Klinefelter's (47,XXY, p646) syndromes. Many genes are involved when the defect is large enough to be seen microscopically.

Autosomal-dominants Adult polycystic kidney (16p), Huntington's chorea, (4p). A single copy of a defective gene causes damage. Some people inheriting the defective gene are phenotypically normal (=*reduced penetrance*).

Autosomal recessives Infantile polycystic kidney; cystic fibrosis (7q), β-thalassaemia, sickle cell (11p), most metabolic conditions, and almost all which are fatal in childhood. In general, both genes must be defective before damage is seen, so carriers are common. Both parents must be carriers for offspring to be affected, so consanguinity (marrying relatives) increases risk.

X-linked Duchenne muscular dystrophy, p642; haemophilia A & B; fragile x (p648). In female (xx) carriers a normal gene on the 2nd x chromosome prevents bad effects manifesting. Males (XY) have no such protection.

NB: being pregnant and unwilling to consider termination does *not* exclude one from undergoing useful genetic counselling.

'Couple screening' A big problem with counselling is the unnecessary alarm caused by false +ve tests. In cystic fibrosis screening (analysis of cells in mouthwash samples) this is reducible by 97% (0.08% vs 3.2%) by screening mother and father together—who need only get alarmed if *both* turn out to be screen-positive. The trouble with this is false reassurance. Many forget that they will need future tests if they have a different partner, and those who do not are left with some lingering anxieties.

Three contrasting principles:
1 The parents must decide: counselling must be non-directive.
2 Every newborn child has the right to be born healthy, if possible.
3 Every child has a right to be born.

Non-directive counselling is something of a mantra among counsellors, partly because of an unwillingness to promulgate a single view of what is right in what can be a very complex area. Public health doctors are questioning this obedience to the non-directive ethic because, from their point of view, it makes attainment of their chief goal more difficult—namely to improve the health and well-being of all residents, including newborns. For example, we should tell pregnant women not to drink much alcohol, public health doctors assert, because this is necessary to prevent fetal alcohol spectrum disorder. The same goes for other syndromes. When we know what to do we should state clearly and unequivocally what the mother should do. This is our duty to her and her unborn child.

Let us examine the public health doctor's standpoint more closely. He wants to improve health. To do this, it is necessary to define health. We have done this elsewhere (p470) and have argued that health entails more than just soundness of body and mind. It is not clear that an autocratic society in which patients were told what to do would be more healthy than a society of autonomous individuals each addressing the great questions of health and existence from his or her own viewpoint.

Another problem for the public health doctors is that, in the case above, it is not clear whether the directive 'don't drink if you are pregnant' would lead to fewer children with fetal alcohol spectrum disorder. It might lead to more orphans (a mother knows she is doing wrong, feels guilty, avoids health professionals, and dies of some unforeseen consequence of pregnancy, or from guilt-borne suicide).[265]

As ever, the way forward is not by abstract thought but by getting to know our patients better. There may be rare occasions when we know our patients well enough to risk 'You are mad not to follow this advice...'. But mostly we cannot be sure that this injunction will work, and it is wiser to explore the patient's world view and their expectations, and then use this knowledge to reframe the benefits of our proposed action in a way that makes sense to the individual concerned, taking into account his or her culture and system of beliefs.

In the UK, the Children's Act states that the welfare of the child is paramount. What this means in the context of a family is open to interpretation.

Obesity in childhood has risen fast in the West, and appears now to be slowing. However, it remains a huge public health problem, not only in childhood, but also in the medium and long term: obese and overweight children are far more likely to become obese adults with the resultant effects on health.

Prevalence In the UK, the Millennium Cohort Study is a long-term study of children born in 2000–1. Aged 7, 7% had been obese, rising to 20% by age 11, with a further 15% being overweight.

Causes Essentially an imbalance between energy intake and expenditure.
• *Dietary:* Fast and processed foods, especially those high in carbohydrates.
• *Exercise:* There has been an overall decline in physical activity of children in the UK, with reduced time playing sports at school, and an increase in sedentary activities at home (TV, computer games, social networking).
• *Sleep deprivation* leads to low leptin levels (a hormone which communicates adequate fat levels) and high ghrelin levels (released by the stomach to signal hunger); this increases appetite.
• *Socioeconomic background:* The more deprived areas have almost double the prevalence of childhood obesity than the least deprived. Higher levels of parental education appear to be protective against childhood obesity.
• *Genetics:* Obese parents are more likely to have obese children; however, it is difficult to establish how much of this effect is due to genetics versus growing up in an obesogenic environment.
• *Medication* can increase weight gain; sodium valproate, carbamazepine, mirtazapine, steroids. *Others:* High or low birth weight; intrauterine exposure to maternal gestational diabetes or maternal obesity.

Medical causes include hypothyroidism, Cushing's syndrome, growth hormone deficiency, and Prader–Willi syndrome.

Diagnosis Use UK-WHO charts for children under 4; once over 4 years old use UK 1990 BMI charts. A BMI over the 91st centile is overweight; over the 98th centile obese, and above the 99.6th centile severely obese.

This needs sensitive discussion with the child and their parents. Parents do not always have the correct perception of their child's weight. Emphasize the long-term problems associated with being overweight or obese and this being a good opportunity to improve their child's health in the future. Is the child having any physical or emotional problems resulting from being overweight? Talk about factors which may be contributing—diet, exercise, lifestyle, family circumstances, disability, other medical or family problems. *Screen* for co-morbidities eg hypertension, diabetes, and lipids.

Management
• What has been tried before? It is important to involve the whole family
• The primary treatment is dietary modification and exercise
• Diet alone is not recommended
• Referral to a dietician can be very helpful; aim to eat a healthy diet
• Aim for moderate exercise of at least 60 minutes per day. Exercise not only increases energy expenditure but also increases self-esteem and helps sleep
• The MEND programme (Mind, Exercise, Nutrition...Do it)
• Refer: BMI >98th centile; weight-related morbidity; suspicion of medical cause.

Medium-term consequences: Insulin resistance, type 2 diabetes, sleep apnoea, orthopaedic problems, non-alcoholic fatty liver disease, psychosocial morbidity, polycystic ovarian syndrome, vitamin D deficiency. *Long-term problems:* Atherosclerosis, early-onset cardiovascular disease, some cancers (particularly breast and bowel), subfertility, hypertension.

Further reading
NICE (2013). *Managing Overweight and Obesity among Children and Young People: Lifestyle Weight Management Services* (PH47). London: NICE. https://www.nice.org.uk/guidance/ph47

There is no accepted UK definition of hypertension in children, but research in the USA has suggested using a cut-off of the 95th centile of average systolic/diastolic BP adjusted for gender, height, and age. Use the correct cuff size and a manual sphygmomanometer. Take ≥3 BPs (snugly fitted cuff of bladder-width >70% of upper arm length) >1 week apart (in general) before diagnosing hypertension. Use the 1st and 5th Korotkoff sounds. Ambulatory BPs can show that white coat hypertension is about as common in children as in adults.[266,267]

Prevalence in the USA is 3–4% of 3–18-year-olds.

Risk factors
- High salt intake; fast and processed foods are particularly to blame
- Obesity
- Low birth weight in those who go on to develop obesity.

Causes of raised blood pressure in children

Child <6yrs Renal parenchymal disease, renal vascular disease, coarctation of the aorta, endocrine causes, essential hypertension.

6–12yrs Renal parenchymal disease, essential hypertension, renal vascular disease, endocrine causes, coarctation, iatrogenic cause.

Adolescence Essential hypertension, iatrogenic illness, renal diseases, coarctation of the aorta, endocrine causes.

As a general rule, the younger the child, the higher the probability of identifying the cause. In 80% the cause is renal parenchymal disease.

History and examination
- Symptoms/signs are non-specific in a neonate
- In older children: headaches, fatigue, blurred vision, epistaxis, Bell's palsy, sleep-disordered breathing
- Ask about prematurity, bronchopulmonary dysplasia, head or abdominal trauma, family history of hypertension, neurofibromatosis, and multiple endocrine neoplasia; urinary tract infection, medication (especially steroids and drugs used to treat ADHD) and diet
- Examine the child from head to toe; check height and weight against centile charts. Points of interest: signs of left ventricular hypertrophy, poor amplitude of peripheral pulses (aortic coarctation); abdominal mass (Wilms' tumour); virilization (congenital adrenal hyperplasia).

Investigations
- Urine to check for albumin and blood
- U&E; creatinine; FBC (check extent of disease, evidence of anaemia from renal disease; raised potassium if aldosterone elevated)
- Renal US to exclude renal abnormalities
- Identify co-morbidities: fasting lipids and glucose; consider sleep study
- Screen for end-organ damage: ECG (LVH/strain), echocardiogram (hypertrophy); retinal screening.

Treatment
- Lifestyle modification: weight loss if necessary; a healthy, low-salt diet, regular exercise; avoidance of smoking and alcohol
- Treatment is required if the child is symptomatic, has secondary hypertension, diabetes, end-organ damage, or persistent hypertension despite lifestyle modification. This is with ACE-inhibitors, beta-blockers, thiazide diuretics and calcium channel blockers.

►**Hypertensive crisis** (p177) presents with cerebral oedema, heart failure, seizures, pulmonary oedema, or renal failure. Anti-convulsants are not effective in treating hypertensive seizures. Treat hypertension with nifedipine, labetalol, or sodium nitroprusside. Aim to gradually reduce BP over several hours.

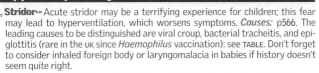

Paediatrics

Stridor Acute stridor may be a terrifying experience for children; this fear may lead to hyperventilation, which worsens symptoms. *Causes:* p566. The leading causes to be distinguished are viral croup, bacterial tracheitis, and epiglottitis (rare in the UK since *Haemophilus* vaccination): see TABLE. Don't forget to consider inhaled foreign body or laryngomalacia in babies if history doesn't seem quite right.

Investigations: This is a clinical diagnosis. Lateral neck x-ray (fig 2.15) may show an enlarged epiglottis, but should be avoided—it wastes valuable time.

Croup (acute laryngotracheobronchitis) *Signs:* Stridor, barking cough, hoarseness from obstruction in the region of the larynx. *Age:* <6yrs (but can be recurrent in older, atopic children). *Epidemics:* Autumn. *Causes:* Parainfluenza virus (1, 2, 3), respiratory syncytial virus, measles (rare). *Pathology:* Subglottic oedema, inflammation, and exudate. Croup is classified into mild/moderate and severe disease. ℞: Mild illness (minimal recession/stridor, no cyanosis, alert child, good air entry) may be sent home if settles—eg with **dexamethasone**, 0.15mg/kg PO stat (some give more[268]) *or* prednisolone 1–2mg/kg stat. *In hospital:* Aim for minimal interference and careful watching (TPR; SaO_2) by experienced nurses. *Watch for severe signs:* Restlessness; cyanosis (give O_2); recession; stridor at rest; rising pulse/respiratory rate; tiredness, altered conscious level. Use nebulized **adrenaline**[269] 1:1000 (400mcg/kg up to 5mL); if poor response, repeat, and take to ITU. Remember: volume of stridor is a factor of flow; in severe disease, stridor will be very soft. Failure to improve with steroids/nebulized adrenaline should prompt the consideration of **bacterial tracheitis**. This is defined by the presence of thick mucopurulent exudate and tracheal mucosal sloughing that is not cleared by coughing, and risks occluding the airway. There is often a history of a viral infection (such as croup) with an acute deterioration. Pronounced tracheal tenderness may be present.

Managing epiglottitis (for signs, see BOX on p159) *Avoid approaching the child and do not examine the throat.* This may precipitate obstruction. Do not cannulate the patient or upset him. Ask for senior help from an anaesthetist and ENT surgeon. Take the child to theatre for inhalation induction of anaesthesia and EUA if necessary. A tracheostomy may be required if complete obstruction occurs (A smaller diameter endotracheal tube than normal for that age may be needed). The cause is usually *Haemophilus influenzae* type B, treat with **cefotaxime**, 25–50mg/kg/8h IV). Severe bacterial tracheitis also benefits from early intubation, allowing suctioning of respiratory secretions and improved ventilation. Treat with cefotaxime + flucloxacillin. **Hydrocortisone** may be given in both, but isn't of proven value.

Diphtheria is caused by the toxin of *Corynebacterium diphtheriae*. It usually starts with tonsillitis ± a false membrane over the fauces. The toxin may cause polyneuritis, often starting with cranial nerves. Shock may occur from myocarditis, toxaemia, or cardiac conducting system involvement. *Other signs:* dysphagia; muffled voice; bronchopneumonia; airway obstruction preceded by a brassy cough (laryngotracheal diphtheria); nasal discharge with an excoriated upper lip (nasal diphtheria). If there is tachycardia out of proportion to fever, suspect toxin-induced myocarditis (do frequent ECGs). Motor palatal paralysis also occurs causing fluids to escape from the nose on swallowing.

Diagnosis: Swab culture of material below pseudomembrane; PCR.[270]

Treatment: Diphtheria antitoxin: 10,000–30,000U IM[51] (any age; more if severe, see BNF) and **erythromycin**; give contacts 7 days' erythromycin syrup: <2yrs old 125mg/6h PO (500mg per 6h if >8yrs) *before swab results are known.*

Risk ↑ if: Homeless/refugee; aged 3–6yrs old; in 'asocial' families. *Prevention:* Isolate until 3 –ve cultures separated by 48h. Vaccination: BOX, p151.

For URTI, see OHCM p390; for sore throat, see p564.

Mild croup	Bacterial tracheitis	Epiglottitis
Common	Uncommon	Rare
6 months–6 years	6 months–14 years	2–7 years
Onset over a few days	Viral prodrome for 2-5 days, then rapid deterioration	▸▸Sudden onset
Stridor only when upset	Continuous stridor	▸▸Continuous stridor
Stridor sounds harsh	Stridor may be biphasic	▸▸Stridor softer, snoring
Swallows oral secretions	Swallows oral secretions	▸▸Drooling of secretions
Voice hoarse	Very hoarse	▸▸Voice muffled
Likely to be apyrexial	Moderate–high fever, appear toxic	▸▸Toxic and feverish (eg T° >39°c)
Barking cough	Barking cough	Cough not prominent

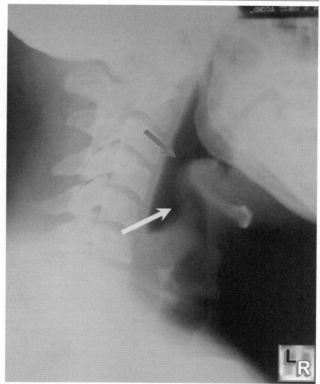

Fig 2.15 Lateral x-ray of the neck showing an enlarged epiglottis (red arrow) and thickening of the aryepiglottic folds (yellow arrow). ▸▸Do not take an x-ray in suspected epiglottitis—this is included for interest only. There is reversal of the normal lordotic curve in the cervical spine and slight dilatation of the hypopharynx. learningradiology. com NB: the aryepiglottic folds are mucous membranes extending on each side between the lateral border of the epiglottis and the summit of the arytenoid cartilage. They form the lateral border to the top of the larynx.

Courtesy of Dr William Herring.

▶If severely ill, think of staphs, streps, TB, and *Pneumocystis* (HIV) (*OHCM* p154). *In chronic cough think of:* • Pertussis • TB • Foreign body • Asthma.

Acute bronchiolitis is *the* commonest lung infection in infants; coryza precedes cough, fever (sometimes), tachypnoea, wheeze, inspiratory crackles, apnoea, intercostal recession ± cyanosis, ± fever. *Typical cause:* Respiratory syncytial virus (RSV). *Others:* Mycoplasma, parainfluenza, adenoviruses. Those <6 months old or with underlying medical conditions are most at risk. *Signs prompting admission:* Inadequate feeding, respiratory distress, hypoxia. *Tests:* PCR/fluorescent antibody tests rarely contribute. If severe: CXR to exclude pneumothorax or lobar collapse; blood gases/SpO₂; FBC.[271] *R̵:* O₂ (stop when SpO₂ ≥92%);[272] nasogastric feeds. 5% of those need respiratory support (mostly CPAP) (mortality ≈1%; 33% if symptomatic congenital heart disease). Steroids and nebulized adrenaline may reduce admission rates and/or length of stay but are not used routinely. Reserve the use of ribavirin prophylaxis for the immunocompromised and those with underlying heart or lung disease (benefit uncertain).

Pneumonia[273,274] *Signs:* T°↑, malaise, poor feeding. Respiratory distress: tachypnoea, cyanosis, grunting, intercostal recession, use of accessory muscles. Older children may have typical lobar signs (pleural pain, crackles, bronchial breathing). *Admit:* if SpO₂ <92%; signs of respiratory distress. *Tests:* Consider CXR/FBC/blood and sputum cultures if severe pneumonia. Investigations are not required in community acquired pneumonia in a child going home. Viral LRTI is more common than bacterial infection in children <2, so those with mild symptoms can typically be discharged without antibiotics (ensure follow-up if symptoms persist). *Oral R̵:* Amoxicillin is 1st-line; alternatives: co-amoxiclav, azithromycin, clarithromycin.[273] *Causes:* Pneumococcus, Mycoplasma, Haemophilus, Staphylococcus, TB, viral. *Monitor:* TPR; SpO₂.[275]

TB Suspect if: overseas contacts, HIV+ve; odd CXR *Signs:* Anorexia, low fever, failure to thrive, malaise. Cough is common (may be absent). *Diagnosis:* Tuberculin test (*OHCM* p398); interferon-gamma release assays (blood test); culture + Ziehl–Neelsen stain of sputa (×3). CXR: consolidation, cavities. Miliary spread (fine white dots on CXR) is rare but grave. *R̵:* Get expert help. 6-month supervised plan:[276] isoniazid 15mg/kg PO 3 × a week + rifampicin 15mg/kg/PO 3 times a week + pyrazinamide (1st 2 months only) 50mg/kg PO 3 times a week. Monitor U&E & LFT before and during treatment. Stop rifampicin if bilirubin↑ (hepatitis). Isoniazid may cause neuropathy (give concurrent pyridoxine). ▶Explain the need for prolonged treatment. Multiple drug resistance: *OHCM* p409. *Prophylaxis:* If TB-with-HIV, co-trimoxazole prophylaxis is likely to be needed (pneumocystosis, p145).[276]

Whooping cough (*Bordetella pertussis*) *Signs:* Apnoea; bouts of coughing ending with vomiting (± cyanosis) worse at night or after feeds. Whoops (not always heard) are caused by inspiration against a closed glottis. Co-infection with RSV (above) is common. *Peak age:* Infants, with a 2nd peak in those >14.[277] In the UK, the illness is often mild, with 1% needing admission (eg with secondary pneumonia); but severe in the very young (may be fatal).[278] *Δ:* PCR is via nasal swab; culture is unsatisfactory. Absolute lymphocytosis is common (may be very high). *Incubation:* 10–14 days. *Complications:* Prolonged illness (the '100-day cough'). Coughing bouts may cause petechiae (eg on cheek), conjunctival, retinal & CNS bleeds (rare), apnoea, inguinal hernias ± lingual frenulum tears. Deaths may occur (esp. in infants), as may late bronchiectasis. *R̵:* A macrolide such as clarithromycin is often used in those likely to expose infants to the disease (benefit unproven). Admit if <6 months old (risk of apnoea). May need ventilating and even ECMO (p109). *Vaccine:* p151, not always effective. 30% of severe infections are via a fully vaccinated sibling. Vaccinating the mother during pregnancy reduces risk in babies. Immunity wanes steadily throughout childhood.

Many children with cough and wheeze do not fit into the categories on p160, and are too young for a diagnosis of asthma to be made with confidence. These infants often end up being treated with escalating bronchodilator therapy with frequent courses of antibiotics against uncultured organisms. While it is true that asthma can begin in infancy, most of these chesty infants do not have asthma—but we tend to prescribe 'just in case'. As the natural history of symptoms is to vary from hour to hour, sometimes we *appear* to be successful. NB: *viral wheeze/virally induced respiratory distress* or *virus induced lower airways disease (VILAD)* may be the appropriate label here: it is a non-atopic disorder; *respiratory syncytial virus* is more often the culprit rather than *Haemophilus*. An alternative diagnosis is *altered awareness of minor symptoms*, or *multi-trigger wheezing* to exercise, smoke, cold air, viruses, and allergens.[279] When viruses are looked for (found in 80%), it turns out that together rhinoviruses, coronaviruses, human metapneumovirus, and human bocovirus account for 60% of viruses.[280] Although symptom scores and need for GP consultations are highest in infants with RSV, they are similar in infants infected with other viruses.[280]

Passive smoking does not trigger illness but does prolong symptoms. If the mother smoked during pregnancy, it significantly increases the risk of viral-induced wheeze in the child. 'Happy wheezers' (ie undistressed) probably need no treatment, but if chest symptoms start very early in life, a sweat test should be considered to rule out cystic fibrosis, especially if there is failure to thrive and loose stools. Between these ends of the spectrum of 'chestiness' lie those who clearly need some help. These may benefit from inhaled β_2-agonists (via a spacer) ± inhaled steroids, given for ~8 weeks in the lowest effective dose (not if this would mean almost continuous exposure). Assess benefit by ↓ in sleep disturbance. If ill enough to consider admission, 3 days' oral prednisolone 2mg/kg/day can ↓ duration of symptoms in children 6–35 months old with VILAD.[281] Other randomized trials disagree, so steroids may be best reserved for the atopic.[282]

Aim to engage in a constructive dialogue with parents so that they understand that treatment is often unsuccessful, but that their child is unlikely to come to harm, while he or she is 'growing out of it'.

If cough is a chronic problem, exclude serious causes (eg TB; foreign body; asthma) and reassure. There is no good evidence that brand name cough medicines are better than placebo—but they may help the parents.

This is one of the commonest autosomal recessive diseases (~1:2000; ~1:22 of Caucasians are carriers); it reflects mutations in the cystic fibrosis transmembrane conductance regulator gene (CFTR) on chromosome 7, which codes for a cyclic AMP-regulated sodium/chloride channel. There is a broad range of severity of exocrine gland function, leading to meconium ileus in neonates (and its equivalent in children), lung disease akin to bronchiectasis, pancreatic exocrine insufficiency, and a raised Na^+ sweat level—depending in part on the type of mutation (85% from 5 mutations, the commonest of which is ΔF_{508}) but other mutations, eg in intron 19 of CFTR, cause lung disease but no increased sweat Na^+.

Antenatal (p152) carrier-status testing is possible, as is preimplantation genetic diagnosis after *in vitro* fertilization.

Diagnosis ►In the UK, all newborns are screened looking for an abnormally raised immunoreactive trypsinogen, and 29 CFTR mutations on the Guthrie card[283] (85% coverage).[284]

• 10% present with meconium ileus as neonates.
• Later presentation is with:
  • Recurrent pneumonia (±clubbing)
  • Failure to thrive
  • Slow growth
• Fatty, oily, pale stools are reflective of steatorrhoea.

Sweat test: Sweat Cl^- <40mmol/L is normal (CF probability is low); >60mmol/L supports the diagnosis. Intermediate results are suggestive but not diagnostic of cystic fibrosis.[285] The test is technically challenging, so find an experienced worker (there are false positives and false negatives).

Pitfalls of the sweat test:[286] *False-positive sweat test:* May be seen in atopic eczema, adrenal insufficiency, ectodermal dysplasia, some types of glycogen storage diseases, hypothyroidism, dehydration, malnutrition. On the first day of life, up to 25% of normal newborns show a sweat sodium concentration >65mmol/L, but this rapidly declines on the second day after birth.
False-negative sweat test: Oedema is the most important cause. Poor technique can also give false negative results.

Other tests: IRT/DNA;[20] CXR: hyperinflation, increased antero-posterior diameter, bronchial dilatation, cysts, linear shadows, and infiltrates; malabsorption screen; random glucose; spirometry (obstructive pattern with decreased FVC and increased lung volumes); sputum culture. Mycobacterial colonization affects up to 20%; consider if rapid deterioration.

►*Genetic counselling* (p154). Long-term survival depends on care from specialist centres, antibiotics and good nutrition.

Respiratory problems (neutrophilic airway inflammation): Start physiotherapy (×3/day) at diagnosis. Teach parents percussion + postural drainage. Older children learn forced expiration techniques. Organisms are usually *Staph. aureus*, *H. influenzae* (rarer), and *Strep. pneumoniae* in younger children. Eventually >90% are chronically infected with *Pseudomonas aeruginosa*. In adolescence, aspergillosis can occur. *Burkholderia cepacia* (*Ps. cepacia*) is associated with rapid progression of lung disease (prompt diagnosis using PCR may be available: isolate the patient). Treat acute infection after sputum culture using higher than or double standard doses, and for weeks if necessary. If very ill, respiratory support becomes of utmost importance. Treat with **ticarcillin**, 80mg/kg (max 3.2g)/6-8h IV (if aged >1 month) + **gentamicin**, p175, or **ceftazidime** (50mg/kg/8h IV) alone may be needed 'blind'. Nebulizing ticarcillin and tobramycin at home *does* prevent admissions.

20 Having 2 mutations is associated with severe disease ($\Delta f508$, w1282x, g542x, n1303k, 1717-1g→a). Carrying one mutation may not be so bad (3849 + 10 kb → A T).[287]

Gastrointestinal problems & nutrition: Energy needs rise by ~130% (∵ malabsorption and chronic lung inflammation). Most have steatorrhoea from pancreatic malabsorption and need enzymes: **Pancrex v®** powder mixed with tepid food for infants—and **Pancrex v Forte®** for older children, ≤10 tabs/meal—to give regular, formed, non-greasy bowel actions. Most older children use enzymes in microspheres (eg **Creon®**) so fewer tablets are needed. **Omeprazole** (or **cimetidine, or ranitidine**) helps absorption by ↑duodenal pH.[288] If all this controls steatorrhoea, a low-fat diet is not needed, but vitamins are still needed (A & D, eg as **Abidec®** 0.6mL/24h PO for infants or as multivitamin capsules 2/24h PO for older children). Diet should be high calorie/high protein.

Complications of CF
• Haemoptysis
• Pneumonia
• Pneumothorax
• Pulmonary osteo-arthropathy
• Diabetes mellitus
• Cirrhosis
• Cholesterol gallstones
• Fibrosing colonopathy
• Male infertility

Fine-bore nasogastric feeding is needed only if weight cannot otherwise be maintained.

GI obstruction if **Creon®** is omitted/inadequate or child dehydrated (causes meconium ileus equivalent): admit urgently to a specialist centre for medical treatment (eg with **Gastrografin®**); seek advice from the CF team (avoid laparotomy unless perforation has occurred).

Impaired glucose tolerance: Risk rises with age and is higher if homozygous for ΔF508 mutations. Screen yearly with OGTT from 12yrs. Insulin may be needed; optimize diet, then optimize dose, not vice versa. Only try oral hypoglycaemics if nutrition is satisfactory.[289]

Psychological help: Parents and children need expert counselling—and transitional clinics with multidisciplinary teams when transferring from paediatric to adult services. The Cystic Fibrosis Research Trust can help here. Online resources can provide contact between other CF patients without the risk of cross-infection.

Meconium ileus Presents with failure to pass stool or vomiting in the 1st 2 days of life. Distended loops of bowel are seen through the abdominal wall. A plug of meconium may show as a firm mass in one such loop. Tiny bubbles may be seen in the meconium ('inspissated'). *Options:* • Nasogastric tube drainage • Washout enemas • Excision of the gut containing most meconium.

Prognosis Death may be from pneumonia or cor pulmonale. Most survive to adulthood (median survival is >31yrs, and possibly >50yrs for those born after 2000).[290,291] 5-year survivorship models take account of forced expiratory volume in 1sec (% of expected), gender, weight-for-age z score, pancreatic function, plasma glucose, *Staph. aureus* and *Burkholderia cepacia* infection, and number of acute lung exacerbations/yr.[292]

Newer options

Recombinant human deoxyribonuclease (rhDNase) has been shown to improve lung function and reduce the number of pulmonary exacerbations. *Ivacaftor* (CFTR potentiator) improves lung function in those with G551D mutation.

Lung transplantation (heart + lung, or double lung) is getting safer; consider in those who are deteriorating (FEV₁ <30% of expected) despite maximum therapy, provided nutrition is good, and there is no TB or aspergillus. Good results are limited by donor availability (avoid raising hopes).

Gene therapy aims to deliver normal copies of the cystic fibrosis gene into patients, so allowing them to make CFTR protein. This is still at the research stage.

Paediatrics

(See BTS guidelines.[293]) In the developed world, asthma is *the* leading chronic illness in children.[294] It implies reversible airway obstruction (peak flows vary by >20%) ± wheeze, dyspnoea, or cough. 10% of the population is affected. **Prevalence ↑ if:** Birthweight↓; family history; bottle fed; atopy; ♂; pollution;[295] past lung disease.[296] **Genetics** Asthma susceptibility genes are described (eg ADAM33).**Triggers** Pollen; house dust mite; feathers; fur; exercise; viruses; chemicals; smoke; traffic. ΔΔ Foreign body; pertussis; croup; pneumonia/TB (do CXR!);[297] hyperventilation; aspiration; cystic fibrosis (wet cough, starting at birth, failure to thrive).

Treatment Aims to minimize symptoms and their impact on life, as well as use of reliever medication and to prevent severe attacks. Use step-wise approach, achieve control, and then step down.

Exacerbations: Treat early (rescue **prednisolone** 30–40mg/day if >5yrs or 20mg/day if 2–5yrs for 5 days).

General management: Annual review of symptoms, exacerbations, oral steroid use, and time off school or nursery; check inhaler technique and medication adherence; make a personalized self-management action plan; advice regarding tobacco smoke exposure; record height and weight on centile charts.

Drug therapy
1 Occasional **β-agonists** via pMDI[21] eg **salbutamol** 100mcg. Use spacer. If needed >3× per week, add step 2 (also if >5 yrs and many exacerbations, or asthma wakes from sleep >once/wk).
2 Add inhaled steroid,[22] eg **beclometasone**: specify brand[298] as potencies vary: **Clenil Modulite®** 50mcg is a lower-potency CFC-free inhaler. Use up to 200mcg of **Clenil®**/12h.[299]
3 Review diagnosis; check inhaler use/concordance; eliminate triggers; monitor height. *If <5yrs:* Add 1 evening dose of **montelukast** 4mg as a mouth-dissolving capsule (can cause behavioural problems). *If >5yrs:* Consider respiratory review. Can try inhaled **salmeterol** 50mcg/12h (long-acting β-agonist); monitor closely; concern over reduced effectiveness of short-acting β₂-agonist in adults. If symptomatic ↑ inhaled steroid and try **montelukast** 5mg or **theophylline**, eg **Slo-Phyllin®** 125–250mg/12h PO if 6–12yrs. Check compliance.
4 Refer to specialist (± CXR).[300] ↑Inhaled steroid (**Clenil®** 400mcg/12h).
5 Add **prednisolone** (if >5yrs) at lowest dose that works; check: growth.

▶**Treating severe asthma** This is an emergency. Calmness helps. Give these treatments if life-threatening signs are present (TABLE, p165), or if not improving 15–30min after R starts.

1 Sit up; high-flow 100% O_2	6 Nebulizers continuously until improving, then eg 30min intervals, reducing frequency once improving. Give ipratropium 8-hrly if needed
2 **Salbutamol:** 5mg O_2-nebulized in 4mL saline (2.5mg if <5yr) with **ipratropium bromide** 0.25mg	
3 **Hydrocortisone** 100mg IV; or prednisolone soluble tabs, 1–2mg/kg to max 40mg (60mg if already on steroids & <12yr), 50mg >12yr	7 Consider starting CPAP in the ED. Take to ITU if exhausted, confused, coma, or refractory to R and needing IVI salbutamol (2mcg/kg/min)
4 Consider one IV dose of **magnesium sulfate**, 40mg/kg over 20min (≤2g);	
5 **Aminophylline** 5mg/kg IV over 20min (not if already on a xanthine); then IVI aminophylline infusion. Give with ondansetron (causes vomiting).	

Before discharge ensure: • Peak flow >75% of predicted • Good inhaler technique • Is stable on discharge regimen • Taking **inhaled steroids+oral prednisolone** • Written management plan • Follow-up: GP in 1 week; in clinic in ~4 weeks.

Prevention ↓Triggers.[301] A Mediterranean diet rich in fruit (esp. if eaten by the mother in pregnancy) may help.[302] Homeopathy[303] and flu vaccination don't help.

Inhaler and nebulizer questions

- If <8yrs old, pressurized metered dose inhalers (pMDI)[21] with a spacer[22] are best for routine use in stable asthma for both steroids and bronchodilators.
- Nebulizers are not more efficacious than a well-used inhaler.
- *Is there a better alternative to nebulizers* (bulky and need servicing)? Evidence supports valved holding chambers (eg AeroChamber Plus®).[22][304]
- Do combined inhalers offer added value? The SMART study Symbicort® maintenance & relief therapy shows real benefit from a fixed dose of long-acting β-agonist (formoterol) with budesonide (4.5/80mcg/day + additional puffs for symptom relief). Doctor dependency was less, and there were fewer exacerbations but the risk of asthma death was higher, therefore it should only be used under paediatric specialist advice.[305]

Pitfalls in managing asthma

- Faulty inhaler technique. Watch the patient operate the device.
- Inadequate perception of, and planning for, the severe attack.
- Unnoticed, marked diurnal variation in airways obstruction. Always ask about nocturnal waking; it is a sign of dangerous asthma.
- Being satisfied with less than total symptom control.
- Too much inhaled steroid (>400mcg beclometasone or >800mcg of budesonide)/day if ≤12yrs old;[306][23] *Consider adrenal insufficiency if ↓consciousness*; do blood glucose; IM hydrocortisone may be needed. Monitoring growth is *not* a good way to screen for adrenal suppression (cortisol ≤500nmol/L).[307]

Severity of acute asthma exacerbation	
Near-fatal / life-threatening	Respiratory acidosis and/or requiring mechanical ventilation with increased ventilation pressures
	Any one of the following: PEFR <33% predicted; Sats <92%; silent chest; cyanosis; feeble respiratory effort; bradycardia; dysrhythmia; hypotension; exhaustion; confusion; coma
Acute severe	Any one of: PEFR 33–50% predicted; RR 2–5yrs >40/min, 5–12yrs >30/min, >12yrs >25/min; pulse 2–5yrs >140bpm, 5–12yrs >125bpm, >12yrs >110bpm; inability to complete sentences; use of accessory muscles
Moderate exacerbation	Increasing symptoms; PEFR 50–70% best or predicted; no features of severe asthma
Brittle asthma	Type 1: wide variability in PEFR despite intensive therapy; Type 2: sudden severe attacks despite apparently well-controlled asthma

Paediatrics

Further reading

Asthma UK (patient information and support): www.asthma.org.uk

BTS/SIGN (2014). *British Guideline on the Management of Asthma*. Edinburgh: BTS/SIGN.

NICE (2013). *Asthma*. http://cks.nice.org.uk/asthma

21 pMDI=press-and-breathe pressurized meter dose inhaler—as recommended by NICE.
22 *Spacers:* (eg **AeroChamber®**—a responsive inspiratory valve allows opening on minimal effort to aid inhalation; it closes before exhalation disturbs retained aerosol) Static charge is a problem. Clean monthly. Wash in detergent. Dry in air. Wipe mouthpiece clean of detergent before use. Replace yearly.
23 Anti-IgE agents may ↓ need for steroids. **Omalizumab** is a recombinant humanized monoclonal antibody directed against IgE and can inhibit the immune system's response to allergen exposure. It prevents IgE from attaching to mast cells, reducing IgE mediated inflammation.[308]

Signs Fever, splenomegaly, clubbing, splinter haemorrhages, anaemia, rash, heart failure, microscopic haematuria, new murmur (eg with known congenital heart lesion or IV line *in situ*). *Typical cause:* Streps; staphs.[309] See also OHCM p144.

Tests Blood cultures (different times and different sites), echocardiogram.

Blind treatment After 3 blood cultures: benzylpenicillin 25mg/kg/4h IV + gentamicin (BOX, p175); get microbiological help.

Preventing endocarditis Prophylactic antibiotics are now generally not recommended. Advise on oral hygiene.[310]

Rheumatic fever

This is a systemic febrile illness caused by a cross-sensitivity reaction to group A β-haemolytic streps, which, in the 2% of the population that is susceptible, may result in permanent damage to heart valves. It is common in developing countries, but is rare in the West, but pockets of resurgence sometimes occur in the USA in overcrowded areas (favours streptococcal spread). *Incidence:* 500,000/yr (worldwide).[311]

Jones diagnostic criteria Elicit 2 major criteria or 1 major and 2 minor *plus* evidence of preceding strep infection: scarlet fever, a throat swab with β-haemolytic streptococci or a serum ASO titre >333U/L (reference intervals vary).[312]

Major criteria: (revised 2001)
- Carditis (1 of: changed murmur; CCF; cardiomegaly; friction rub; +ve echo)
- Polyarthritis (often migratory)
- Erythema marginatum, OHCM p564
- Subcutaneous nodules
- Sydenham's chorea (p654)

Minor criteria:
- Fever
- ESR >20mm or C-reactive protein↑
- Arthralgia, ie pain but no swelling
- ECG: PR interval >0.2sec
- Previous rheumatic fever or rheumatic heart disease.

Don't count arthralgia if polyarthritis is used as a major criterion; likewise for long P-R if carditis is used. *Joints:* Knees, ankles, elbows, & wrists may be *very* tender, but no permanent sequelae. *Echo criteria:* Mitral regurgitant jet is: >1cm; holosystolic (throughout systole); visible in 2 planes; mosaic pattern (ie chaotic flow).

The *MacCallum plaque*[24] is at the base of the posterior mitral leaflet. Aortic, pulmonary and tricuspid valves are affected in descending order of frequency.

Treatment of rheumatic fever Rest/immobilization helps joints and heart. Aspirin (high-dose, p646; but get advice *re* Reye's, p652). If severe, get help. Prednisolone (below) *may* help.[313] Phenoxymethylpenicillin for pharyngitis (~125mg/6h PO) preceded by one dose of benzylpenicillin (25mg/kg IM or IV). *Sydenham's chorea:* unless mild, consider prednisolone (2mg/kg/day[6] for 4wks, then taper; halves time to remission to ≤8 weeks; emotional and learning difficulties can take far longer to resolve).[314] Consider haloperidol; valproic acid; carbamazepine.[315]

Prevention *Primary:* Where incidence is high, this might be worthwhile, but might entail giving IM penicillin for sore throats.[316] *Secondary:* Symptoms are often worse on recurrence of rheumatic fever—eg seen in 2.6%.[317] Prevent with phenoxymethylpenicillin 125mg/12h <6y; 250mg/12y >6y.[318]

PANDAS *(paediatric autoimmune neuropsychiatric disorders associated with strep infections).* Suspect this in those with tics (or Tourette's syndrome, OHCM p692) and obsessive–compulsive disorder. Anorexia nervosa *may* also be a feature. Antibiotics and risperidone have been tried.[319–321] See p654.

---

24 MacCallum's plaque is due to subendocardial Aschoff bodies: these are a classic histological feature of rheumatic fever. They are perivascular with a necrotic core set in a layer of lymphocytes. Nodules are found in joints, tendons, heart, and blood vessels. They heal with extensive myocardial fibrosis.

Paediatrics

Diarrhoea may be an early sign of *any* septic illness. Faeces are sometimes so liquid they are mistaken for urine. NB: it is *normal* for breastfed babies to have liquid stools. Deaths/yr=1.5×10⁶ children worldwide.[322]

Gastroenteritis Rotavirus is the most common cause of gastroenteritis in infants and children. It causes ~600,000 childhood deaths/yr (a rotavirus vaccine is part of the UK immunization schedule, p151).[323] *Other enteric viruses:* Norovirus (most common cause in adults), astrovirus; adenovirus. *Treatment:*[324] ▶If dehydrated, see p234. Weigh, to monitor progress and quantify dehydration, if a recent previous weight is known. Start oral **rehydration therapy** (ORT), eg **Dioralyte®**, at 50mL/kg over 4h (≈1mL/kg every 5min). Continue breastfeeding. If child refuses ORT, offer other fluids (eg bottle milk/water—not fruit juice) or consider ORT via a nasogastric tube. IV therapy is reserved for those who deteriorate or are in shock. Reintroduce milk after 4h of rehydration with ORT (even if <6 months), or sooner if he recovers and is hungry (starving harms).[325] Use of antiemetics (**ondansetron 0.1–0.15mg/kg**) has been shown to decrease vomiting[326] and reduce need for IV fluids, hospital admission,[327] and overall costs,[328] but isn't officially recommended. *Complications:* Dehydration; malnutrition; temporary sugar intolerance after D&V with explosive watery acid stools. (Rare; manage with a temporary lactose-free diet.) Post-enteritis enteropathy resolves spontaneously after ~7wks. *Tests:* Stool: look for bacteria, ova, cysts, parasites. *Prevention:* Hygiene, good water & food, education, fly control.

Classification diarrhoea by mechanism *Secretory* (↓absorption or ↑secretion) Stool is watery even if fasting, eg: cholera, *c. difficile*, *E. coli*, carcinoid. *Osmotic:* (↑osmotic load in gut lumen) Stool is watery, acidic, and +ve for reducing substances. *Motility disorders: Increased:* Thyrotoxicosis, irritable bowel syndrome dumping syndrome. Decreased: Pseudo-obstruction, intussusception (eg <4yrs old). *Inflammatory:* (eg bloody diarrhoea), salmonella, shigella, campylobacter, rotavirus, amoebiasis, NEC (p120), Crohn's/UC (look for weight↓; anaemia; WBC↑; platelets↑; ESR↑), coeliac disease, haemolytic uraemic syndrome (p176).

Malnutrition

☁ Rising food prices + global warming + political corruption × malnutrition + war

▶Being a major cause of death and misery, this is a global issue for us all. **Kwashiorkor** is due to ↓intake of protein & essential amino acids. *Signs:* Poor growth; diarrhoea; apathy; anorexia; oedema; skin/hair depigmentation; distended abdomen; glucose↓; K⁺↓; Mg²⁺↓; Hb↓; cholesterol↓; albumin↓. ℞: Re-educate child, family, and politicians. Offer a gradually increasing, high-protein diet + vitamins. **Marasmus** is lack of calories + discrepancy between height and weight. It is HIV-associated.[329] *Signs:* Distended abdomen, diarrhoea, constipation, infection; albumin↓. Mid-arm circumference <9.9cm (any age) predicts severe malnutrition better than being <60% of median weight for age, or 85% of median height for age and 70% of median weight for height. Most can be treated at home with fortified ready-to-use foods if >6 months.[330] Parenteral feeding may be needed to restore hydration and renal function. Next offer a balanced diet with vitamins. Despite this, stature and head circumference may remain poor. Kwashiorkor and marasmus may coexist (*protein-energy malnutrition*).[331] *Prevention:* ▶Stop man-made activity contributing to climate instability. ▶Stop biofuels supplanting food crops. ▶Give to charity www.ox-fam.org (to pay for fertilizers, high-yield seeds, and simple irrigation schemes). Medically, we often target the malnourished (z-score -2, p227) at aged ½–5yrs, found by screening, but better results are achieved by giving *universal* help at ½–2yrs in at-risk places.[332]

Worldwide, poor mothers are at ↑ risk of death: there is no worse start to life than the death of one's mother (100% fatal to her babies in some places).

Poverty-associated short stature, BMI <18.5 (p514) and iron deficiency in mothers accounts for 20% of maternal mortality.

Malnutrition causing stunting causes ~2.2 million deaths/yr and 21% of disability-adjusted life years (DALYs) in children <5yrs old.[333]

Deficiencies in vitamin A and zinc cause 1 million deaths/yr. Zinc supplementation[24] cannot always be relied on to ↓morbidity in children recovering from diarrhoea and respiratory illness in developing countries.[334] Prevention of the poverty which caused the diarrhoea is more important.

Not breastfeeding for the 1st 6 months of life (especially non-exclusive breastfeeding) causes 1.4 million deaths/yr in children <5yrs old.[335] NB: the position is further complicated by the fact that proteins, fat concentrations, and caloric value in breast milk from undernourished mothers are lower than in breast milk from well-nourished mothers.

The points above account for 35% of child deaths and total global disease burden. In many other conditions (eg diarrhoeal diseases, HIV, asthma, obesity) poverty plays a leading role. But the main health issue is that it's harder to educate yourself if you live in a slum. ►No power≈no light≈no homework≈no learning≈an early death.

Southern diarrhoea is only an excuse for northern amnesia

As you read this page two events unfold: in the northern hemisphere a child is born with a silver spoon in his mouth, his future assured thanks to incubators, ventilators, wealth, and family planning. Diametrically opposed to this birth another occurs in the southern hemisphere where the silver was mined for that lovely spoon. This child, according to our stereotype, must 'Wait for his future like a horse that's gone lame *To lie in the gutter and die with no name*'.[336] We assume that this death is from diarrhoeal diseases that we are all working, more or less efficiently, towards controlling—and we are pleased to blame non-human agencies for these deaths.

This model of our imperfect world does not stand up to scrutiny—the diarrhoea was the cause of death, and the diarrhoea was caused by poverty.

The point of all this is to illustrate that if we want to do something for children it is no good just doing something about the big killers, such as diarrhoea, and it's no good simply attacking poverty, for there is something dark in our human heart which needs addressing before merely statistical or biological interventions have any chance of success. There is only one way of influencing human nature for the better, and that is through dialogue. So, in this sense, the treatment of diarrhoea is dialogue. Without such dialogue the rich wring their hands while poverty wrings necks.

25 Strategies for supplementing vit A (in neonates & late infancy), Zn, & Fe for children and universal promotion of iodized salt can improve nutrition and prevent related diseases, and may reduce stunting at 36 months by 36% and mortality between birth and 36 months by about 25%.[337]

Acute abdominal pain Children ≤8yrs old often have difficulty in localizing pain, and other factors in the history may be more important.[338] Pointers:
- Hard faeces suggest that constipation is the cause (p210).
- In those of African or Mediterranean origin, suspect sickle-cell disease.
- Do tuberculin test (*OHCM* p398) if travel or other factors suggest TB risk.
- In children with pica (p210), do a blood lead level (and ferritin).
- Abdominal migraine is suggested by periodic abdominal pain with vomiting especially if there is a positive family history.
- If any past UTI, suspect GU disease (eg renal colic, but this is rare).

Common physical causes Gastroenteritis, UTI, viral illnesses (eg tonsillitis associated with mesenteric adenitis), and appendicitis.

Rarer causes Mumps pancreatitis; diabetes; volvulus; intussusception; Meckel's diverticulum; peptic ulcer; Crohn's/ulcerative colitis, Hirschsprung's disease; Henoch–Schönlein purpura and hydronephrosis. Consider menstruation or pelvic inflammatory disease in older girls. ▶In boys always check for a torted testis.

Tests ▶Always dip the urine. *Others:* Consider plain abdominal x-ray; US; FBC; CRP; renal imaging, barium studies.

Appendicitis (*OHCM* p610) is rare if <5yrs, but perforation rates are high in this group (nearing 90%). Think: how can I tell this from other causes of abdominal pain? • Clues in the history: increasing pain in right lower quadrant, no previous episodes, anorexia, slight vomiting, absence of cough and polyuria. • Examination hint: fever and pulse↑ are likely; if the child appears well and can sit forward unsupported, and hop, appendicitis is unlikely. • Tests have very low positive and negative predictive value.

Gastro-oesophageal reflux/oesophagitis Presents with regurgitation, distress after feeds, apnoea, pneumonia, failure to thrive, and anaemia. *Tests:* Clinical diagnosis. Endoscopy if concerned about eosinophilic oesophagitis; evaluation with an oesophageal pH probe rarely carried out. US is not much help. *Treatment:* Reassurance; avoid over-feeding (a common cause). Drugs may be needed, eg an **antacid + sodium/magnesium alginate**, eg for term infants, Infant Gaviscon® dual dose sachets, 1 dose mixed with 15mL boiled (cooled) water. This paste is given by spoon after each breast feed. If bottle fed, give each half of a dual sachet dose dissolved in 4oz of feeds. **Carobel®** thickens the feeds. If this fails, some experts use **domperidone ± omeprazole** (or similar). Most resolve by 6–9 months; if not, consider fundoplication, eg if there is failure to thrive, severe oesophagitis, apnoea, or bleeding.

Abdominal distension

Causes Always remember acute GI obstruction as a cause; also consider:

Air:	Ascites:	Solid masses:	Cysts:
Faecal impaction	Nephrosis	Wilms' tumour	Polycystic kidney
Air swallowing	Hypoproteinaemia	Neuroblastoma	Hepatic; dermoid
Malabsorption	Cirrhosis; CCF	Adrenal tumour	Pancreatic

Hepatomegaly Infections: many, eg infectious mononucleosis, CMV.
Malignancy: leukaemia, lymphoma, neuroblastoma (see below).
Metabolic: Gaucher's and Hurler's diseases, cystinosis; galactosaemia.
Others: sickle-cell disease and other haemolytic anaemias, porphyria.

Splenomegaly All the above causes of hepatomegaly (not neuroblastoma).

Neuroblastoma This may be thought of as an embryonal neoplasm, derived from sympathetic neuroblasts. Presenting with decreasing frequency from birth to 5yrs of age. Some forms regress, while others present after 18 months old (eg with metastases ± DVT) are highly malignant (outlook depends on

(Paediatrics — side margin)

stage; has not improved over the last 25yrs). *Prevalence:* 1:6000–1:10,000— the most common solid tumour in the under-5s. *Signs:* Abdominal swelling. *Metastatic sites:* Lymph nodes, scalp, bone (causing pancytopenia ± osteo-lytic lesions). In 92%, urinary excretion of catecholamines (vanillylmandelic & homovanillic acids) are raised. *Treatment:* Refer to special centre. Excision (if possible) and chemotherapy (eg cyclophosphamide + doxorubicin). *Prognosis:* Worse if certain genotypes (pseudodiploid karyotypes, chromosome 1p dele-tions, N-*myc* gene amplifications), less mature catecholamine synthesis, and if >12 months old. Those <1yr do best. *Surveillance:* Pre-morbid screening by looking for excretion of catecholamines in the urine detects disease early, but may not save lives.[339] Uncertainty is added by a 2008 study which appeared to record lower mortality in a screened group, (although it was a very large study, it is dubious, being retrospective).[340]

Recurrent abdominal pain ≥10% of children >5yrs suffer recurrent abdominal pains interfering with normal activity. Is there organic disease? No cause is found in most, but don't let this encourage complacency (you may delay diag-nosis of *Crohn's* or *peptic ulcer*) or lead to underlying psychological problems (do consider it: who is present when the pain starts; what, or who, makes the pain better?). NB: long-term follow-up indicates a 4-fold ↑risk of psychological problems manifesting in adult life. Consider: gastro-oesophageal reflux, small bowel dysmotility, gastritis, duodenitis, carbohydrate malabsorption (eg lac-tose, sorbitol), abdominal migraine. *Who to investigate:* There are no rules. Do an MSU. Be suspicious if pain is unusual in terms of site, character, frequen-cy, or severity. Whenever symptoms are present for more than a few months recheck for associated features, eg in inflammatory bowel disease (Crohn's) there may be no diarrhoea in 50%, according to one careful study,[341] but poor growth is often the clue that prompts further tests.

Coeliac disease: an example of malabsorption

Malabsorption typically presents with diarrhoea, failure to thrive ± anaemia (folate↓; ferritin↓), possibly with abdominal protrusion, everted umbilicus and wasted buttocks (if late-presenting). As subclinical/latent forms exist, investigate any unexplained anaemia, fatigue, 'ir-ritable bowel' symptoms, diarrhoea, weight↓, arthralgia, eczema, and short stature. Patients may present at *any* age. Coeliac disease may cause short stature without overt gastrointestinal signs or symptoms. There may be a deceleration on the growth chart after introduction to gluten at weaning (4–6 months). See fig 2.16.

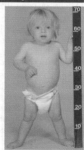

Fig 2.16 Coeliac disease.

Cause Enteropathy induced by gluten (in wheat, barley, and rye). Δ Serological tests show raised IgA anti-tissue transglutaminase (IgA-tTG), and endomysial antibodies (EMA). Also measure total IgA—if deficient measure IgG anti-gliadin antibodies.[342] Serology is less reliable if <18mths—IgA-AGA may be most useful in this age group.[343] Confirm by finding villous atrophy on small bowel biopsy via endoscopy. Villi return to normal on the special diet; avoid a gluten challenge test unless diagnosis is in doubt.[344] ℞ *Gluten-free diet*: no wheat, barley, rye (no bread, cake, pasta, pizza, pies). Rice, maize, soya, po-tato are OK (also ≤25g/day of *pure* oats).[345] Canadian Celiac Assoc. 2007 Gluten-free biscuits, flour, bread, and pasta are prescribable. Minor dietary lapses may matter.
Other causes of malabsorption Cystic fibrosis; post-enteritis enteropathy; giardia; rotaviruses; bacterial overgrowth; worms; short bowel syndrome.
Coeliac associations Type 1 diabetes, hypothyroidism.

Infantile hypertrophic pyloric stenosis Presents at 3–8 weeks (♂:♀≈4:1) with vomiting which occurs after feeds, and becomes projectile (eg vomiting over far end of cot). Pyloric stenosis is distinguished from other causes of vomiting by the following:

• The vomit does not contain bile, as the obstruction is so high.
• No diarrhoea: constipation is likely (occasionally 'starvation stools').
• Even though the patient is ill, he is rarely obtunded: he is alert, anxious, and always hungry—and possibly malnourished, dehydrated.
• The vomiting is large volume and within minutes of a feed.

Observe left-to-right LUQ (left upper quadrant) peristalsis during a feed (seen in late-presenting babies). Try to palpate the olive-sized pyloric mass: stand on the baby's left side, palpating with the *left* hand at the lateral border of the right rectus in the RUQ, during a feed from a bottle or the left breast. There may be *severe* water & NaCl deficit, making urine output & plasma Cl⁻ (also K⁺ & pH) vital tests to guide resuscitation and determine when surgery is safe (Cl⁻ should be >90mmol/L). The picture is of hypochloraemic, hypokalaemic metabolic alkalosis. NB: don't rush to theatre.[346][n=84]

Imaging: US detects early, hard-to-feel pyloric tumours, but is only needed if examination is -ve.[347] Barium studies are 'never' needed.

Management: Correct electrolyte disturbances. Before surgery (Ramstedt's pyloromyotomy/ endoscopic surgery) pass a wide-bore nasogastric tube.

Intussusception The most common cause of intestinal obstruction in children. The small bowel telescopes, as if it were swallowing itself by invagination. Patients may be any age (typically 5–12 months; ♂:♀≈3:1) presenting with *episodic* intermittent inconsolable crying, with drawing the legs up (colic) ± vomiting ± blood PR (like red-currant jam or merely flecks—a late sign). A sausage-shaped abdominal mass may be felt. He may be shocked and moribund. In between pains there may be no signs.

Tests/management: The least invasive approach is US with reduction by air enema (preferred to barium). CT may be problematic, and is less available. There may be a right lower quadrant opacity ± perforation on plain abdominal film. If reduction by enema fails, reduction at laparoscopy or laparotomy is needed. Any necrotic bowel should be resected.

Pre-op care: ➡Resuscitate, crossmatch blood, pass nasogastric tube. NB: children over 4 years old present differently: rectal bleeding is less common, and they have a long history (eg >3 weeks) ± contributing pathology (cystic fibrosis, Henoch–Schönlein or Peutz–Jeghers syndromes; ascariasis, nephrotic syndrome or tumours such as lymphomas—in the latter obstructive symptoms caused by intussusception are the most frequent mode of presentation). Recurrence rate: ~5–15% in infants.[348]

Phimosis The foreskin is too tight, eg due to circumferential scarring; retraction over the glans is impossible, eg with foreskin ballooning on voiding ± balanitis. *It is normal to have a simple non-retractile foreskin up to the age of 4yrs.* By 11yrs or older, prevalence is <8%.[349] Time or a wait-and-see policy will usually obviate the need for circumcision. *Forced* retraction may be causative, not therapeutic. Topical corticosteroids cream also helps (esp. before 8yrs). Use twice-daily with stretching exercises for 15 days, then daily for 15 days.[350]

Other surgical problems: *appendicitis, hernias, volvulus, torsion of the testis, acute abdomen:* p170, p130, *OHCM* p654; *OHCM* p608.

Presentation ▶Often the child may be *non-specifically* ill. Infants may present with collapse and septicaemia, and toddlers as vomiting, 'gastroenteritis', failure to thrive, colic, or PUO. Many with dysuria and frequency have *no* identifiable UTI, and often have vulvitis. The urinary tract is normal in most with UTI, but ~35% have vesico-ureteric reflux (VUR), ~14% have renal scars (most have reflux too), ~5% have stones, ~3% develop hypertension. Each year in the UK, 10–20 children enter end-stage renal failure programmes because of renal scarring presumed secondary to UTI ± VUR and chronic pyelonephritis complications. UTI is a common source of morbidity.[25]

Definitions *Bacteriuria:* Bacteria in urine uncontaminated by urethral flora. It may be *covert* ('no' symptoms), and can lead to renal scarring, BP↑, and, rarely, chronic renal failure. *UTI* denotes symptomatic bacteriuria that may involve different GU sites (∴ loin/suprapubic tenderness; fever; dysuria). *Chronic pyelonephritis* is a histological/radiological diagnosis. Juxtaposition of a cortex scar and a dilated calyx is the key feature. It is a cause of hypertension and can result in renal failure, eg if the kidneys are congenitally dysplastic. During micturition, urine may *reflux* up ureters, seen on a micturating cystogram (requires catheterization) or MAG3 scan (catheterization not needed)—grades: *I* Incomplete filling of upper urinary tract, without dilatation. *II* Complete filling ± slight dilatation. *III* Ballooned calyces. *IV* Megaureter. *V* Megaureter + hydronephrosis.

UTI incidence Boys: ≤0.23%/yr; girls: 0.31–1%; ratios are reversed in neonates. *Recurrence:* 35% if >2yrs old. *Prevalence of covert bacteriuria* in schoolgirls: ~3%. *Prevalence of associated GU anomalies:* 40% (½ have reflux; others: malpositions, duplications, megaureter, hydronephrosis). *Renal scars and age:* We used to concentrate on treating babies early, thinking new scars were rare after 4yrs old, but prospective ^{99m}Tc dimercaptosuccinate (DMSA) scintigraphy (the best test) shows new scars appearing on repeat scans in 43% of those <1yr old, 84% of those aged 1–5yrs, and 80% of those >5yrs old.

Tests Dipstick all urines. If nitrites or WCC +ve, UTI is very likely. Get a clean catch sample; bag urines have many false negatives and positives from vulvitis or balanitis. Wash the genitals gently with water, and tap repeatedly in cycles of 1min with 2 fingers just above the pubis, 1h after a feed, and wait for a *clean voided urine (CVU) sample*, avoiding the stream's 1st part. Do prompt microscopy[26] & culture. >10^8 organisms/L of a pure growth signifies UTI. *US:* US is cheap, non-invasive, getting more accurate, and is worthwhile in 1st UTIs (a good prenatal scan may suffice);[351] *sensitivity, specificity, positive predictive value, and negative predictive value* for detecting reflux are 18%, 88%, 23%, and 83%, respectively.[352] A right kidney longer than the left by ~10mm is a good predictor of an abnormal DMSA scan but as most scarring is visible on US, DMSA scans are rarely needed.[353] Reserve renography for: infants, *recurrent UTI* and +ve family history of GU abnormality. If these are present and US is normal, proceed to ^{99}*Technetium renography*—static for scarring (^{99m}Tc DMSA scan, dynamic for obstructive uropathy) ± *isotope cystography. Micturating cystourethrography (MCU)* is still the best way of excluding reflux—but it is said that if DMSA is negative, MCU 'never' shows significant reflux.[354] In general, it is *not* needed in over 1yr-olds if initial tests are normal, pyelonephritis is unlikely, there is no family history of reflux, and there are no *recurrent* UTIs; it is invasive and unpleasant, but careful preparation with play therapy (p402) mitigates this. NB: operating on reflux is unlikely to improve renal function.[355]

---

25 Prevalence unknown as under-reported. See Bauer R et al. (2008). New developments in the diagnosis and management of pediatric UTIs. *Urol Clin North Am* 35(1):47–58.

26 Microscopy is more reliable than stix tests for nitrites & leucocytes: *Effective Health Care* 2004 8.6.

Antibiotic treatment *Age <3 months:* IV amoxicillin + gentamicin (below) or IV cephalosporin and ampicillin (to cover *Listeria*) (p106). *Child >3 months with uncomplicated lower UTI:* 3-day course of **trimethoprim**[27] 50mg/5mL, 4mg/kg/12h (max 200mg) PO ± prophylaxis (see below), **nitrofurantoin**, or **amoxicillin/co-amoxiclav** •Avoid constipation •↑Oral fluids •Encourage full voiding •Repeat MSU. ▶Resistance to trimethoprim and ampicillin renders monotherapy insufficient in some places.[356]

If the child or infant is ill (pyelonephritis + septicaemia) and blind parenteral therapy is needed, ▸▸gentamicin (5–7mg/kg/day) may be given in a once-a-day regimen (IM if IV access fails). In one study, children and infants were randomly assigned to once-daily gentamicin 5mg/kg/day[28] or 2.5mg/kg/8h slowly IV, where kg = lean body weight if obese.[28] There was no difference in efficacy, nephrotoxicity, ototoxicity, or renal scarring.[357] If neonate >35 weeks postmenstrual age, 2.5mg/kg/12h IV, slowly: consider a longer course if premature (gestation <34 weeks).[358] Do levels.[29] IV cefotaxime and co-amoxiclav are alternatives.

Treating ureteric reflux If prophylactic antibiotics fail, ureteric reimplantation can reduce reflux, but scarring remains. Keep on antibiotic prophylaxis.

Prevention Just one episode of reflux of infected urine may initiate renal scarring, so *screening* for bacteriuria is useless: damage is too quick. But once a UTI is suggested (eg by stix) treat it *at once*, before you know culture sensitivities, as renal damage may be about to happen. Consider prophylaxis if recurrent UTI, significant GU anomaly/renal damage. *Example:* **trimethoprim prophylaxis** (2mg/kg at night, max 100mg), eg while awaiting imaging—and sometimes indefinitely (optimum duration is unknown, but may be after 2 negative cystograms, if the indication is reflux). Consider screening siblings for reflux. Prophylaxis can be stopped after reflux has been ruled out if there is no scarring.

Avoid predisposing factors:
• Treat and prevent constipation
• Clean the perineum from front to back
• Avoid nylon underwear and bubble baths
• Encourage fluid intake and double micturition.

Surgical correction of moderate reflux is 'unlikely to be beneficial', and in minor reflux is 'likely to be harmful' (carefully made EBM phrases!)

Further reading

NICE (2007). *Urinary Tract Infection in Under 16s: Diagnosis and Management* (CG54). London: NICE. https://www.nice.org.uk/guidance/cg54

27 Trimethoprim every 12h, eg if aged 6 weeks–6 months 25mg; 6 months–6yrs 50mg, 6–12yrs 100mg.
28 Assumes normal renal function; give lower dose if the patient is obese, based on *lean body weight* estimated by the 50th centile on weight-for-age charts. See *OHCM* p738.
29 Levels may not be needed if **gentamicin** is given for <72h (usually the case). One-hour post-dose (peak) serum gentamicin concentration should be 5–10mg/L (3–5mg/L for streptococcal or enterococcal endocarditis); pre-dose ('trough') concentration should be <2mg/L in neonates and <1mg/L in others on a once-daily regimen (<1mg/L for streptococcal or enterococcal endocarditis—*BNF* advice). In neonates phlebotomy is difficult and causes anaemia—so an example of monitoring advice from one NICU is: No levels before 48h of therapy unless proven infection requiring gentamicin and one of: •Perinatal asphyxia •Congenital renal defects •Renal insufficiency (creatinine >133μmol/L, ie >1.5mg/dL). www.cop.ufl.edu/wppd/research/sample7.pdf

Paediatrics

Acute kidney injury (AKI) Characterized by a rapid rise in creatinine or development of oliguria/anuria.[359] *Causes* in developed nations AKI occurs secondary to cardiac surgery, bone marrow transplantation, toxicity (NSAIDs, aminoglycosides, vancomycin, aciclovir, and contrast nephropathy) and sepsis,[360] in the tropics causes include: diarrhoea/dehydration (50%);[361] glomerulonephritis (34%); drug-induced haemolysis in G6PD deficiency (5%); snake bite (4%); haemolytic uraemic syndrome (2%); myoglobinuria (*OHCM* p307). *Severity:* The paediatric RIFLE criteria stratifies grade of AKI based on magnitude of changes in eGFR or urine output (*Risk, Injury, and Failure*), and two outcome measures (*Loss of kidney function* and *End-stage renal failure*).[362]

Acute tubular necrosis (ATN) causes: • Crush injury • Burns • Dehydration • Shock • Sepsis • Malaria.

Plasma chemistry: K$^+$↑; creatinine↑; urea↑; PO$_4^{3-}$↑ or ↔; Ca^{2+}↓; Na$^+$↓; Cl$^-$↓. *MSU:* Are there red cell casts (=GN, p178)? If no RBCs seen but Labstix +ve for RBCs, consider haemo/myoglobinuria (*OHCM* p307). *Other tests:* ECG, serum and urine osmolality, creatinine, acid–base state, PCV, platelets, clotting studies (DIC), C$_3$, ASO titre, ANA (antinuclear antibody). *Radiology:* ▶Arrange prompt abdominal US. Are the ureters dilated (eg stones: 90% radio-opaque)? If so, urgent surgery may be required. *Treatment:* Remove or reduce the cause promptly. Involve paediatric nephrology team early.

• Treat shock and dehydration (p234)—then:
• If urine/plasma (U/P) osmolality ratio is >5 the kidneys concentrate well; the oliguria should respond to rehydration. If the U/P ratio is low, try for a diuresis: **furosemide** 2–5mg/kg/6h IV slowly, (get help if more needed).
• Monitor BP. If BP↑↑: **nitroprusside** ('Hypertensive emergencies', BOX, p177).
• 24h fluid requirement: Avoid overhydration. Replace losses + insensible loss (12–15mL/kg). Aim for weight loss (0.5%/day).
• Give no K$^+$. Monitor ECG. Tall T-waves and QRS slurring prompt urgent lowering of K$^+$, with IV **salbutamol** 4mcg/kg or 5mg nebulized (2.5mg if <25kg). A less easy to use alternative (if >1month old) is glucose with soluble insulin. Also consider **polystyrene sulfonate resins** 0.5–1g/kg max 60g PO and **calcium gluconate** (10%, 0.5mL/kg IV over 10min; monitor ECG: stop IVI if heart rate↓) to counteract electrophysiological effect of hyperkalaemia.
• High-energy, low-volume infant renal formulas may prevent fluid excess.
• Consider renal replacement therapy as soon as fluid overload occurs. Many centres now prefer continuous haemofiltration to peritoneal dialysis.[360]
• ▶Improvement is ushered in with a diuretic phase.

Haemolytic uraemic syndrome (HUS) is rare. *Essence:* Acute microangiopathic haemolytic anaemia (schistocytes, burr cells, *OHCM* fig 2 p327 & fig 3 p323), thrombocytopenia, renal failure + endothelial damage to glomerular capillaries. Typical HUS (95%) is associated with diarrhoea, atypical HUS (5%) is not.[363] *Typical HUS* is more frequent in the summer months, and in children <3yrs. It is associated with Shiga toxin producing *E. coli* type 0157:H7.[364] *Signs:* Colitis→haemoglobinuria→oliguria ± CNS signs→encephalopathy→coma. LDH↑. WCC↑. Coombs -ve. PCV↓. *Mortality:* 5–30% (<5% UK). ADAMTS13 helps with risk statification. *Treatment:* Liaise early with paediatric nephrology unit as early dialysis may be required. Supportive. Get help. Antibiotics, fibrinolytics, and anticoagulation are not used.[365] Treat renal failure (see earlier in topic). Relapses in TTP may be preventable by steroids, splenectomy, or vincristine.

Chronic renal failure *Causes:* Congenital dysplastic kidneys, pyelonephritis, glomerulonephritis, recurrent infection, reflux nephropathy; AKI leading to cortical necrosis. ▶Monitor growth, BP, U&E, Ca^{2+} (often ↓), PO$_4^{3-}$ (often ↑).
The Child: Weakness, tiredness, vomiting, headache, restlessness, twitches, BP↑, hypertensive retinopathy, anaemia, failure to thrive, seizures, and coma. *Treatment:* (See BOX.) Talk with experts about haemodialysis.

Get a dietician's help. Calorie needs may not be met if vomiting is a problem. Eggs & milk may be appropriate (high biological protein value). Provide protein at a level of 2.5g/kg/24h. Vitamin drops may be needed. Nasogastric or gastrostomy tube feeding has a role. Growth hormone therapy combined with optimal dialysis improves growth: see *BNF*.

Acidosis is common, needing no treatment if serum bicarb is ≥20mmol/L.[30]

Renal osteodystrophy A bone disease resulting from poor mineralization due to renal failure, causing poor growth, muscle weakness, slipped epiphyses, bone pain, and bone deformity (±cranial nerve lesions).[366] It is like rickets and low bone turnover osteomalacia (osteoblast and osteoclast activity ↓) osteomalacia. If glomerular filtration falls to ≤25% of normal, compensatory mechanisms to enhance phosphate excretion fail; resulting hyperphosphataemia promotes hypocalcaemia, so PTH rises, which enhances bone resorption to release Ca^{2+} in an attempt to correct hypocalcaemia. PTH↑ leads to marrow fibrosis (osteitis fibrosis cystica). Also, the failing kidneys cannot convert enough 25-hydroxycholecalciferol to active 1,25-dihydroxycholecalciferol, so GI calcium absorption falls, so worsening hypocalcaemia. ℞: Aim to normalize calcium and ↓associated hyperphosphataemia. Keep PTH within normal limits in predialysis children and 2–3 times over upper normal limit in those on dialysis. Avoid aggressive use of calcium-based phosphate binders and vit D derivates to prevent PTH oversuppression and development of adynamic bone disease. NB: there is little paediatric experience with calcimimetics, eg **cinacalcet**, that directly stimulate Ca^{2+}-sensing receptors and potently suppress PTH secretion without increasing Ca^{2+}.[367]

Hyperphosphataemia is treated with phosphate binders, eg **calcium carbonate** taken just before food. Dose: see *BNF*^c section 9.5.2.2. This combines with dietary phosphate to form calcium phosphate, which is expelled in faeces. If there are episodes of Ca^{2+}↑, **sevelamer** may have a role (a synthetic calcium- and aluminium-free phosphate binder).[368]

If Ca^{2+} is low despite correcting serum phosphate, give 1,25-dihydroxycholecalciferol (**calcitriol**), eg 15 nanograms/kg/24h PO max 250 nanograms (increased in increments of 5ng/kg until Ca^{2+} and alk phos are normal, PTH level is reduced to 200–400pg/mL). x-ray evidence of healing rickets may also exist. Then reduce dose. SE: ↓renal function, hypercalcaemia, and hyperphosphataemia. Because normal bone requires adequate levels of PTH to promote bone modelling, oversuppression of PTH must be avoided to avoid adynamic osteodystrophy.

Anaemia is common, and is the result of ↓erythropoietin (± poor iron and folic acid intake). A typical Hb is 60–90g/L. Do not transfuse, as this suppresses erythropoietin production. Erythropoietin is indicated (sc in pre-dialysis and peritoneal dialysis patients, and IV if on haemodialysis).

▶▶Hypertensive emergencies

Get expert help. While awaiting this, use sodium nitroprusside 0.5mcg/kg/min IVI, increased in 200-nanogram increments as needed, up to 8mcg/kg/min IVI by pump (allows precise control). Protect from light. Monitor BP continuously; ↑dose slowly to the required level. CI: severe hepatic impairment. Withdraw over ≥20min to prevent rebound hypertension. If used for >1 day, cut dose to 4mcg/kg/min IVI. Labetalol is an easy-to-use alternative, eg 0.25mg/kg/dose IV, doubled every 15min (as needed) up to 3mg/kg/h IV; CI: phaeochromocytoma.[369,370]

---

30 If pH ≤7.2, bicarbonate may be needed (by IVI if arrhythmias): get help as response is unpredictable, and dosing is difficult.

Acute glomerulonephritis *Essence:* Haematuria & oliguria (±BP↑, ± uraemia) produced by an immune glomerulonephritis (GN) in the kidney. *Peak age:* 7yrs. *Uncomplicated presentation:* Haematuria; oliguria; BP↑ (50%); periorbital oedema; fever; GI disturbance; loin pain. *Complicated presentations:*

Causes of nephritis
• β-haemolytic strep via a preceding sore throat
• Henoch-Schönlein purpura
• Toxins or heavy metals
• Berger's dis. (OHCM p708)
• Malignancies
• Viruses
• Bacteria (IE/SBE; syphilis)
• Renal vein thrombosis

• *Hypertensive encephalopathy:* Restless; drowsy; severe headache; fits; vision↓; vomiting; coma.
• *Uraemia:* Acidosis, twitching, stupor, coma.
• *Cardiac:* Gallop rhythm, cardiac failure ± enlargement, pulmonary oedema.

Blood tests: FBC, U&E (creatinine, K, bicarbonate, calcium, phosphate and albumin), complement (low c3, normal c4), ASOT/antiDNAaseB. Antinuclear factor (ANA), anti-DNA antibodies (if SLE suspected), anti-neutrophil cytoplasmic (ANCA) antibodies (if vasculitis suspected), syphilis serology, blood cultures, virology. *MSU:* Count RBCs, WBCs, hyaline, granular casts; red cell casts mean glomerular bleeding. Check urine culture, and specific gravity (normal range: infants ~1.002-1.006; child/adult ~1.001-1.035). *Other tests:* Throat swabs, urgent renal US; CXR if fluid overload suspected. Requires supportive treatment with careful attention to fluid balance, treatment of hypertension and infection.

Poststreptococcal glomerulonephritis (PSGN) presents 7-21 days after a streptococcal infection (pharyngitis, impetigo) with gross haematuria (cola-coloured urine) and oedema + hypertension ± malaise, anorexia, fever, and abdominal pain. *Urine:* Proteinuria, RBC casts ± oliguria. *Blood:* ↑urea, ↑creatinine, ↓c3. Recent streptococcal infection should be confirmed (serum ASO titre). Typically, renal biopsy is not needed. ℞: Na+ restriction, diuretics, antihypertensives. Restrict protein in oliguric phase. Give **penicillin** orally for 10 days. Check BP often. If encephalopathy, give **nitroprusside** (p177). Oedema resolves in 5-10 days; however, hypertension, haematuria and proteinuria may last for several weeks. Prognosis is very good (95% full recovery).

Nephrotic syndrome Oedema, proteinuria (urinary protein-creatinine ratio (PCR) >200mg/mmol), albumin <25g/L ± hypercholesterolaemia. In 90% the cause is unknown, but any of the causes of nephritis (see MINIBOX) can cause nephrotic syndrome too. *Histology:* Usually minimal change GN (often associated with allergy and IgE production). *Classified* as steroid sensitive (SS), steroid-dependent (SD) or steroid-resistant (SR). *Symptoms:* Insidious onset oedema, usually periorbital, then generalized. Anorexia, GI disturbance, infections, irritability; ascites, oliguria. *Urine:* Frothy; albuminous ± casts; Na+↓ (secondary hyperaldosteronism). *Blood:* Albumin↓ (so total Ca²⁺↓); urea and creatinine usually normal. *Renal biopsy:* Reserve this for older children with any of: haematuria, BP↑, urea↑, if protein loss is unselective (ie large molecular weights as well as small), and treatment 'failures'. *Complications:* Pneumococcal peritonitis or other spontaneous infections; increased susceptibility to infection due to renal loss of immunoglobulins. Consider **pneumococcal vaccination** if >2yrs. Also ↑ risk of VTE. *Treatment:* Get help. Eat healthily with no added salt and no high protein content. Fluid restrict to 800-1000mL/day. Give diuretics if very oedematous and no evidence of hypovolaemia. Albumin infusion is only recommended in symptomatic hypovolaemia or severe diuretic-resistant oedema—discuss with senior. **Prednisolone** 60mg/m²/day (max 80mg) for 4 weeks, then 40mg/m²/48h for 4 weeks then wean over 4 months. 90% respond in 8 weeks. If steroid toxicity and relapsing NS, consider **cyclophosphamide**. Steroid-dependent NS may be treated with ciclosporin.[371] Ciclosporin is nephrotoxic.[372] ▶Monitor BP. Control minimizes later renal failure.

Steroids in nephrotic syndrome

In nephrotic syndrome, protein leaks from blood to urine through glomeruli, causing hypoproteinaemia, including loss of immunoglobulins, and oedema. Before steroids (and antibiotics), many died from infections. Most children with nephrotic syndrome respond to corticosteroids, but many experience a relapsing course with recurrent oedema and proteinuria. Corticosteroids reduce mortality to ~3%, with infection remaining the most important cause of death. NB: steroids cause obesity, poor growth, BP↑, diabetes, osteoporosis, avascular necrosis (hip), and adrenal suppression.[373]

Steroid-resistant proteinuria and ACE-i

Enalapril is used in courses of >2yrs: dose example: 1 month–12yrs: initially 100mcg/kg/day (monitor BP carefully for 1–2h; increase as needed to 0.5mg/kg/12h (maximum). In one study, urine protein electrophoresis showed a reduction of 80% and 70% in the total protein and albumin, respectively, after enalapril. Some patients become free of proteinuria. ACE-i are discontinued if renal failure occurs, eg during infections.[374,375]

Is growth normal? is a key question in determining the health of a child. Take any opportunity to weigh and measure a child. A series of plots on centile charts (p222-4) shows if growth is slow (growth curve crosses the centiles). NB: the growth rate in mid-childhood is 5-6cm/yr; this accelerates at puberty (peak height velocity) before epiphyses start to fuse.

Failure to thrive means poor weight gain in infancy (falling across centile lines). Head circumference is preserved relative to height, which is preserved relative to weight. In 95% this is due to not enough food being offered, or taken. Worldwide, poverty is *the* big cause; in the UK it is difficulty at home, neglect, unskilled feeding, or not enough breast milk (top-up bottles *may* be needed). *Idiosyncratic growth pattern* is one cause, or normal kind of short stature (↓birthweight, short siblings or parents)—likely if he is a contented child.

Features to note
• Signs of abuse (p146)
• Feeding patterns
• Behaviour
• Activity level
• Family finances
• Health and happiness
• Chart family heights
• Any parental illnesses
• Dysmorphic face

Be sceptical about reliability of data. Is the birthweight accurate? Was the child clothed during weighings? Length measurements are particularly error-prone: growth velocity is more useful than measurements done at a one time. *Issues to address:* Feeding and maternal interaction are most important. Is the child anorectic or ravenous—'hyperphagic short stature'?[376] Also:

• If breastfeeding, does he latch well and swallow repeatedly, suggesting adequate milk supply? (p124)
• If bottle feeding, does the teat's hole allow milk to flow through?
• Does weight gain return if the child is removed from the family?
• Is there evidence relevant to child protection proceedings?

Tests: Check feeding technique. It is a great skill to know *when* to investigate. It's better from the child's point of view to ask a trusted colleague's advice *before* painful tests. In one study only 39 of 4880 tests were helpful.[377]

Options are: MSU (clean catch urine); coeliac serology; U&E/glucose, LFT, Ca^{2+}, proteins, immunoglobulins, CRP, TSH; FBC; sweat test; urinary amino ± organic acid chromatography; stools (MC&S ± sugar detection); CXR, renal or CNS US; skeletal survey for dwarfism and abuse; ECG/echo. In *non-organic failure to thrive*, studies favour weekly visits from trained lay visitors.[378]

Short stature is a height <3rd centile (p224). Use the method shown on the charts to correct for mid-parental height (short stature may represent 'regression towards the mean' of their heights). ►*Any chronic disease can cause short stature.* Hypopituitarism (an important cause of short stature) usually manifests after age 2yrs: look for relative obesity, without any other explanation for low growth velocity (ie <25th centile; measure for ≥1yr, see p226). Deficiency of growth hormone (GH) is shown by an impaired rise (peak GH <15MU/L) after a stimulus (eg sleep or hypoglycaemia, induced by IV insulin (OHCM p224), or an arginine stimulation test. Preschool screening for short stature is the aim. To be effective, start synthetic GH early.

Typical causes
• Constitutional (~80%)— if both parents short
• Psychological neglect
• Poverty; physical abuse
• Drugs: eg steroids
• Genetic: eg Turner's or cystic fibrosis
• Ineffective diet (coeliac)
• Inflammatory bowel dis.
• Hypothyroidism
• Infection (eg UTI; TB)
• GH↓ (as above)
• Rarities, eg Noonan, p650

Somatotropin example: 23–39mcg/kg/day SC; expect growth velocity to ↑ by ≥50% from baseline in year 1 of treatment. Other pituitary hormones may also be deficient (OHCM p224). *Causes of height↑:* Thyrotoxic; precocious puberty; Marfan's; homocystinuria. *Causes of weight↑:* (p156) Snacks[etc]; not enough exercise; hypothyroidism; Cushings'; Prader–Willi, p652; Bardet–Biedl, p638; Cohen syndrome (hypotonia, obesity, prominent front teeth; seizures); polycystic ovary syndrome, p252.[379]

It is clear that some populations are inherently shorter than others, and this poses problems when using UK90 growth charts (i.e charts for children >4); which are based on cohorts of UK children in the 1980s (see also p224).[380] Consider these facts:

- The Dutch are the tallest *nation* on earth (mean ♂ height 1.84m): the tallest *population group* is the Masai people (eg in Tanzania and Kenya).
- African and Afro-Caribbean 5–11-yr-olds' height is ∼0.6 standard deviations scores (SDs) greater than white children living in England.
- Gujarati children and those from the Indian subcontinent (except those from Urdu- or Punjabi-speaking homes) have heights ∼0.5 SDs less than white children living in England.
- Gujarati children's weight-for-height is ∼0.9 SDs less than expected for Afro-Caribbeans, or white children in England—so Gujarati children's weight is ∼1.5 SDs less than for white children living in England.
- Urdu and Punjabi weight is ∼0.5 SDs < expected for white UK children.
- Published charts have centile lines 0.67 SDs apart; for height and weight shift the centile lines up by 1 centile line division for African-Caribbeans.
- Re-label Gujarati children's weight charts, so the 0.4th centile becomes the ∼15th centile, and the 2nd weight centile becomes the ∼30th centile.
- For most other Indian subcontinent groups, height & weight need shifting down, eg relabel the 0.4th & 2nd centile lines 1.5th & 6th respectively. NB: Sikh children are taller and heavier than Caucasians.[381]
- Body mass index centiles are said to be appropriate for African-Caribbeans, but recalculate as above for Indian subcontinent children, except for Gujarati-speaking children (0.4th & 2nd centiles→4th & 14th).

Trends towards tallness with each generation occur at varying rates in all groups, so 3rd-generation immigrants are taller than expected using 2nd-generation data. Intermarriage adds further uncertainty. NB: to print the *new CDC charts*, see www.cdc.gov/nchs/about/major/nhanes/growthcharts/clinical_charts.htm

Hypothyroidism Thyroid hormone is necessary for growth and neurologic development. Dysfunction may occur in the neonate, infant, or during childhood. *Congenital:* Thyroid scans divide these into 3 groups: athyreosis; thyroid dysgenesis; dyshormonogenesis. Also remember maternal antithyroid drugs (p24, eg propylthiouracil). *Acquired:* Prematurity; Hashimoto's thyroiditis; hypopituitarism; trisomy 21. *Signs:* May be none at birth—or prolonged neonatal jaundice, widely opened posterior fontanelle, poor feeding, hypotonia, and dry skin are common. Inactivity, sleepiness, slow feeding, little crying, and constipation may occur. Look for coarse dry hair, a flat nasal bridge, a protruding tongue, hypotonia, umbilical hernia, slowly relaxing reflexes, pulse↓, and poor growth and mental development if it has not been picked up. Other later signs: IQ↓, delayed puberty (occasionally precocious), short stature, delayed dentition.[382] *Universal neonatal screening:* Cord blood or filter paper spots (at ~7 days, from heel prick) allow early diagnosis (the 'Guthrie card'). They *do* prevent serious sequelae. Act on high *and* low TSHs (may indicate pituitary failure).[383] *Tests:* T₄↓, TSH↑ (but undetectable in secondary hypothyroidism), ^{131}I uptake↓, Hb↓. Bone age is less than chronological age. As it is unwise to x-ray the *whole* skeleton, the left wrist and hand are most commonly used. There are a large number of ossification centres. Each passes through a number of morphological stages, and using comparisons with key diagrams from 'normal' populations, a rough bone age can be determined. There is no hard-and-fast answer to the question of how much discrepancy (eg 2yrs) between skeletal and chronological years is significant.

Levothyroxine (LT4): Start neonates with ~15mcg/kg/day; adjust by 5mcg/kg every 2 weeks to a typical dose of 20–50mcg/day. <2yrs start with 5mcg/kg/day (max 50mcg) adjust by 10–25mcg every 2–4 weeks; >2yrs start with 50mcg and adjust by 25mcg every 2–4 weeks (eg to 25–75mcg/day; adult doses are reached by 12yrs).[384,385] Adjust according to growth and clinical state. *Avoid high TSH levels.* Those with athyreosis need the highest doses of T₄ and the closest monitoring early on. Those with dysgenesis and dyshormonogenesis need more attention later.

Hyperthyroidism *Typical child:* Pubertal girl with palpitations, tremor, anxiety, tachycardia. *Tests* show low TSH and high T₄. Fine-needle cytology of goitres may show *juvenile autoimmune thyroiditis.*
Carbimazole starting dose: ~250mcg/kg/8h. Adjust according to response.[386]
Propylthiouracil: 2.5mg/kg/8h (/12h in neonates) PO until euthyroid—then adjust dose; expect remission in ~67%.[387] Higher doses may be needed. Typical maintenance dose: ⅓–⅔ of remission-inducing dose.

Thyroid disease in pregnancy and neonates See p24.

The glycogen storage disorders (GSD) result from defects in enzymes required for the synthesis and degradation of glycogen. Abnormal stores are deposited in liver, muscle, heart, or kidney. In some types there are CNS effects. Most types (there are >12) are autosomal recessives. There is considerable variability in severity and prognosis. Early diagnosis and treatment are important for minimizing organ damage. Types include: von Gierke disease (type I, p655), Pompe's disease (type II, p652), Cori disease (type III—hypoglycaemia, hepatomegaly, with failure to thrive), Anderson disease (type IV), McArdle disease (type V), Hers disease (type VI) and Tauri disease (type VII) In McArdle's, (most common GSD in adolescents) the cause is myophosphorylase deficiency. Stiffness and myalgia follow exercise. Venous blood from exercised muscle shows ↓levels of lactate & pyruvate. ↓phosphorylase staining in muscle biopsy confirms diagnosis. There may be myoglobinuria. *Treatment:* No extreme exercise. Oral glucose and fructose may help.

Paediatrics

Inborn errors of metabolism and phenylketonuria (PKU)

These are often diagnosed by a urine metabolic screen (eg amino acids, organic acids, carbohydrates, mucopolysaccharides—in deciding which tests to do, get help; interest the lab in your problem). Typical signs: diarrhoea, lethargy, respiratory distress, metabolic acidosis (± odd body smells), jaundice, hypoglycaemia, U&E imbalance, fits, and coma. Features may be intermittent, and provoked by crises (eg infection; dehydration). In addition, look for:

Urine amino acids ↑ in:
• Alkaptonuria
• Canavan leucodystrophy
• Cystinosis
• Cystathioninuria
• Fructose intolerance
• Galactosaemia
• Hartnup disease
• Homocystinuria
• Hyperammonaemia

Physical sign	Possible significance
Hepatosplenomegaly	Eg amino acid and organic acid disorders, lysosomal storage diseases (Anderson–Fabry disease[31])
Coarse facies	Mucopolysaccharidoses, eg Hurler's syndrome, p646, gangliosidoses, mannosidoses
WCC↓, platelets↓	Organic acidurias
Hypoglycaemia	Many diseases, eg von Gierke's syndrome; MCADD[32]
Mental retardation	See p216
Failure to thrive	Aminoacidurias, organic aciduria, cystinuria, lactic acidosis, storage diseases

PKU **(phenylalanine ketonuria)** *Cause:* Mutation of phenylalanine hydroxylase (PAH) gene (chromosome 1—autosomal recessive) leading to absent or reduced activity of phenylalanine hydroxylase. Classic PKU leads to gradual mental impairment. The defect leads to ↓CNS dopamine, reduced protein synthesis, and demyelination.[388] Milder forms of hyperphenylalanaemia can occur with different mutations to the same gene, or mutations to cofactor tetrahydrobiopetrin (BH₄). *Clinical features:* Fair hair, fits, eczema, musty urine. The chief manifestations are ↓IQ (eg dyscalculia ± poor spelling ± ↓cognition).[389] *Tests:* Detected in UK on Newborn Screening. Hyperphenylalaninaemia (reference interval: 50–120μmol/L). Treatment instigated in infants with levels >360μmol/L—to avoid ↓IQ which may start with levels of >394μmol/L.[390] *Treatment:* Get expert help. *Diet:* protein substitute that lacks phenylalanine but is enriched in tyrosine. Aim to keep phenylalanine levels to <360μmol/L[391] by prescribing artificial food substitutes (amino acid drinks) to give <300mg–8g of natural protein/day (depending on age and severity of phenylalanine hydroxylase deficiency).[392] Hypomyelination may be proportional to degree of phenylketonaemia, but some studies fail to show stricter diets are associated with higher IQs. Despite treatment, children are more prone to depression, anxiety, phobic tendencies, isolation, and a less 'masculine' self-image.[393] Adherence to the diet may be poor (it's unpalatable).[394] Also, the diet may cause changes of questionable significance in levels of selenium, zinc, iron, retinol, and polyunsaturated fatty acids.[395]

Prevention of manifestations: Screen blood at 1 week (using a heel-prick and filter paper impregnation—the Guthrie test). *Maternal phenylketonuria* ▶Preconception counselling is vital. Effects on the baby: facial dysmorphism, microcephaly, growth retardation, IQ↓.

---

31 Anderson–Fabry disease may present with torturing, lancinating pains in the extremities (± abdomen) made worse by cold, heat, or exercise. It is a neuritis (vasculitis of the vasa nervorum). By adolescence, angiokeratomata appear (clusters of dark, non-blanching, petechiae) in the 'bathing trunk' area (esp. umbilicus & scrotum). Also: paraesthesiae, corneal opacities, hypohidrosis, proteinuria and renal failure. It may respond to enzyme R̸ (α-galactosidase A ↓). Carbamazepine may help the pain.

32 MCAD deficiency is screened for in neonates on the same sample as for PKU & hypothyroidism. It's an autosomal recessive (mutation of the **m**edium-**c**hain **a**cyl-CoA **d**ehydrogenase gene; ACADM; 1p31). Signs: hypoketotic hypoglycaemic coma; metabolic acidosis; LFT↑; medium chain dicarboxylic aciduria; 'SIDS'. ♀:♂≈1:1. R̸: avoid fasting; diet to give more calories from carbohydrates & proteins, while minimizing lipids. It is the chief inherited disorder of mitochondrial fatty acid oxidation in N. Europe. Carrier rate: 1:65.

Paediatrics

Puberty may start as early as ~8yrs in girls and ~9yrs in boys. Refer to a paediatric endocrinologist if onset before this. ♀:♂ ≈10:1.[396] Causes may be central (gonadotrophin dependent, eg craniopharyngioma or pituitary tumour) or peripheral (eg testis or adrenal problem, or HCG↑ from rare tumours 'anywhere'). For delayed puberty in girls, see p250–1.

Biology Think of each physical sign of puberty as a bioassay for a separate endocrine event. Enlargement of the testes is the 1st sign of puberty in boys, and is due to pulses of pituitary gonadotrophin. Breast enlargement in girls and penis enlargement in boys is due to gonadal sex steroid secretion. Pubic hair is a manifestation of adrenal androgen production. Growth in boys accelerates when testis volume reaches 10–12mL. Girls start to grow more quickly once their breasts have started to develop. Stage 4 breast development is a prerequisite for menarche (in most girls). The best sign that precosity is pathological is when this consonance of puberty goes awry: in Cushing's syndrome, pubic hair is 'too much' for the testicular volume; in hypothyroidism, the testes are large (FSH as TSH↑↑) while growth velocity is low.[397]

Sexual signs may be obvious or subtle.[33] Gynaecomastia may worry boys.[34] One consequence is short stature caused by early epiphyseal fusion. Premature adrenal maturity (adrenarche) may presage insulin resistance. Ask about general hypothalamic dysfunction—polyuria, polydipsia, obesity, sleep, and temperature regulation. There may be signs of ICP↑, visual disturbance. If onset before 2yrs, suspect hypothalamic hamartoma. LH receptor gene mutations cause sporadic or familial male gonadotrophin-independent precocious puberty.

Rare causes
• Stress (eg adoption)
• CNS tumours/empty sella
• Craniopharyngioma
• Thyroid disorders
• Choriocarcinoma
• Meningoencephalitis
• McCune–Albright syn.
• 21-hydroxylase deficiency
• Rare genetic defects

Tests Growth charts; puberty staging (Tanner charts, figs 2.17–2.19); CNS CT/MRI; bone age (skeletal x-ray); urinary 17-ketosteroids; karyotype; adrenal, testis & pelvic ♀ US, T4; TSH; LH; FSH; HCG; AFP; GH; pituitary tests (*OHCM* p224); oestrogen/testosterone (if no adrenal source of ↑testosterone is found, left vs right spermatic vein sampling may suggest one testis has a tiny Leydig cell tumour or hyperplasia).[398] Virilizing 21-hydroxylase deficiency is confirmed by ↑17-hydroxyprogesterone on ACTH stimulation.[399]

Management: a physiological approach Initiation of puberty depends on release from inhibition of neurons in the medial basal hypothalamus that secrete gonadotrophin-releasing hormone (GnRH), and on decreasing hypothalamic-pituitary sensitivity to –ve feedback from gonadal steroids. These changes are accompanied by ↑frequency and magnitude of 'pulses' of LH. GnRH pulses are needed for normal gonadal function. Continuous high levels of GnRH paradoxically suppress secretion of pituitary gonadotrophins; this forms the basis for treating precocious puberty with synthetic GnRH **analogues** (nasal or SC). There is a reversal of gonadal maturation and all the clinical correlates of puberty (not for pubic hair, as there is no change in the secretion of androgens by the adrenal cortex). There is deceleration in skeletal maturation. Treatment is continued eg up to 11yrs. Families need reassurance that the child will develop normally. Endogenous oestrogen accelerates growth (♂ & ♀), as well as mediating ♀ sexual characteristics: testolactone can help by ↓its biosynthesis. Anti-androgens (eg **flutamide**) and **spironolactone** also have a role.[400]

---

33 Eg in boys: rapid growth of penis and testes; ↑frequency of erections; masturbation; appearance of pubic hair; body odour; acne, ↑energy expenditure ± tantrums/impulsive anger; early occurrence of capacity for frank sexual imagery in dreams and daydreams; early capacity for erotic and sexual arousal in relation to visual imagery, visual perception, and tactile sensation.
34 There is often transient oestrogen/testosterone imbalance early in ♂ puberty. Try to avoid tests (testosterone; oestradiol; gonadotropins; karyotype if testes <6mL). Reassure.

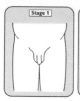

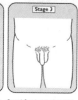

Fig 2.17 Tanner stages of puberty in males.

Reproduced from Butler & Kirk, *OSH Paediatric Endocrinology and Diabetes* (2011) with permission from Oxford University Press.

Stage 1: Prepubertal with no pubic hair.
Stage 2: Scrotum and testes have enlarged and have more textured scrotal skin. Growth of slightly pigmented downy hair sparse.
Stage 3: The penis has grown, especially in length. Hair is darker and curlier.
Stage 4: Further penile growth, in length and breadth, has occured. Glans is larger and broader, and hair is adult in type.
Stage 5: The testes and scrotum are adult in size. Pubic hair is adult in quantity and pattern, and presents along the inner borders of the thighs.

Paediatrics

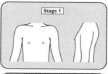
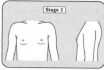

Fig 2.18 Tanner stages of breast development in females.

Reproduced from Butler & Kirk, *OSH Paediatric Endocrinology and Diabetes* (2011) with permission from Oxford University Press.

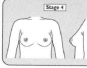
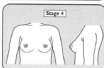
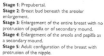

Stage 1: Prepubertal.
Stage 2: Breast bud beneath the areolar enlargement.
Stage 3: Enlargement of the entire breast with no protrusion of papilla or of secondary mound.
Stage 4: Enlargement of the areola and papillas as a secondary mound.
Stage 5: Adult configuration of the breast with protrusion of the nipple.

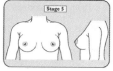

Fig 2.19 Tanner stages of pubic hair development in females.

Reproduced from Butler & Kirk, *OSH Paediatric Endocrinology and Diabetes* (2011) with permission from Oxford University Press.

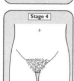

Stage 1: No pubic hair.
Stage 2: Straight hair is extending along labia.
Stage 3: Pubic hair has increased in quantity, is darker, and is present in typical female triangle, but in smaller quantity than in later stages.
Stage 4: Pubic hair is more dense, curled, and adult in distribution, but less abundant than in adults.
Stage 5: Abundant adult-type pattern; hair may extend onto the medial aspect of the thighs.

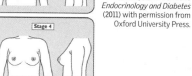

Paediatrics

Type 1 DM is the third most common chronic disease in UK children (after asthma and cerebral palsy). It is an autoimmune disorder caused by T-cell-mediated destruction of pancreatic beta-cells, leading to insulin deficiency and hyperglycaemia. Genetic and environmental factors are implicated in its development, particularly the insulin-dependent diabetes mellitus (IDDM1) gene locus, part of the HLA DR/DQ locus on the major histocompatability complex. Peak age of onset is 5-7yrs (but increasing in toddlers) and just before or at the onset of puberty, especially during winter. Good care of the child with diabetes requires involving the family unit *and* carers at school.

Typical presentation: Several weeks of polyuria, lethargy, polydipsia, and weight loss ±infection, poor growth; ketosis. *Diagnosis:* Based on *WHO* criteria:[401] signs of hyperglycaemia with ↑venous blood glucose, ie ≥11.1mmol/L (random) or ≥7mmol/L (fasting) , or raised venous blood glucose on 2 occasions without symptoms. Oral glucose tolerance tests are rarely required in children. Check autoantibodies: islet cell autoantibody, anti-insulin antibody, antiGluAD antibody and anti-IA2. Also screen for other autoimmune diseases (TFT/thyroid antibodies, coeliac disease). R̠: Should be delivered by a multidisciplinary paediatric diabetes care team—which provides 24h access to advice.[402] For diabetic ketoacidosis see p188. If non-ketotic, IV fluids are rarely needed. Inform children and parents that they may experience a partial remission phase ('honeymoon period') with the start of insulin. *Starting insulin:* Discuss with paediatric endocrinologist. One regimen would be to estimate total daily requirement of insulin (0.5-1 units/kg/24h for prepubertal children; 1.5 units/kg/24h if pubertal)—this daily dose should be ⅓ rapid acting (eg aspart or Novorapid®) and ⅔ long-acting (eg detemir). ⅔ of the daily dose should be given pre-breakfast, and ⅓ should be given pre dinner.[403] Tailor insulin regimen to your patient and their family. They may benefit from a continuous subcutaneous insulin infusion. *Diet:* Ask a paediatric dietician. Energy needs ≈1500kcal/m² or 1000kcal +100 to 200kcal for each year of age. Aiming for 30% of this with each major meal, and 10% as a bedtime snack suits some children. Giving ~20% of calories as protein, ~50% as unrefined carbohydrate, and ≤30% as fat is a rule of thumb. If the child is mildly to moderately symptomatic and clinically well, subcutaneous insulin and oral diet and fluids may be begun at diagnosis, avoiding hospital admission.[404]

Type 2 DM is rare (but increasing) in children (0.2:100,000;[405] ↑×13 if of Asian ethnicity); insulin resistance/syndrome x is burgeoning. ►See p156 for obesity in children.

Have a detailed written care plan What other things should a newly diagnosed child and his or her family know?
• Insulin: doses (eg during illness); practise self-injecting skills on oranges.
• Diet: What? When? Why important? What do you do if the child is hungry?
• Can blood glucose be monitored accurately? Watch the carer's technique.
• What does the carer do if the blood sugar is not well controlled?
• Does the parent or carer know what 'well controlled' means?
• Too much insulin? *Signs:* weakness→hunger→bolshy→faintness→sweating →abdo pain→vomiting→fits→coma. Explain symptoms as they happen, and reversal with drinks (or Glucogel® oral gel).
• What should happen if the child misses a meal, or is sick afterwards?
• What happens to insulin requirements during 'flu and other illnesses?
• Who does mother or father contact in emergency? Give written advice.
• Is the GP told of discharge/follow-up plans? His role is vital in encouraging optimism, and in keeping in touch with those who skip appointments.[406]
• Encourage membership of Diabetes UK (www.diabetes.org.uk).

MODY: maturity-onset diabetes of the young

MODY is a autosomal dominant kind of non-ketotic diabetes, in childhood or young adults.[407] The defect is one of pancreatic beta cell dysfunction—leading to impaired insulin secretion.[408] ≥6 causal genes exist. MODY is caused by single gene defects, as opposed to type 1 & type 2 diabetes which have polygenic and environmental causes. Classic MODY accounts for <5% of all childhood diabetes in white children.[409]

MODY2 (GCK subtype) is caused by mutations in the glucokinase gene on chromosome 7. Glucokinase converts glucose to glucose-6-phosphate, which is needed to stimulate insulin secretion by the beta-cells. There is mild, asymptomatic, stable hyperglycaemia from birth. Microvascular disease is rare. Drugs are rarely needed.

MODY3 (HNF1A subtype) is the most common type. It is caused by a defect on chromosome 12 leading to a progressive decrease in insulin production. It features severe hyperglycaemia after puberty, which often leads to a diagnosis of type 1 DM. Despite progressive hyperglycaemia, sensitivity to sulfonylureas is retained for years. Some children may be able to stop insulin (previously assumed to be lifelong treatment). Diabetic retinopathy and nephropathy often occur in MODY3. Frequency of cardiovascular disease is not increased. Owing to the pleiotropic character of transcription factors, most MODY subtypes are diseases with multi-organ involvement in addition to diabetes.

MODY5 (HNF-1B)is more frequent than originally thought. It is associated with pancreatic atrophy, renal abnormalities, and genital tract malformations.

MODY 1, 4, & 6 These subtypes of MODY are all rare.

Molecular diagnosis matters because it has important consequences for prognosis, family screening, and management. Although MODY is dominantly inherited, expression varies, so a family history of DM is not always present.

Hypoglycaemia

▸▸Mild or moderate episodes: give oral glucose (tablets or sugary drink). If uncooperative or unable to eat give oral glucose gel.
▸▸Severe hypoglycaemia: Get help. Get IV access. Intra-oral GlucoGel® has a role if IV access fails.
▸▸Give glucose 5mL/kg of 10% IVI, or by rectal tube if no IV access, with glucagon 0.5–1mg IM or slowly IV (0.5mg if <25kg). *Expect quick return to consciousness*. If not, recheck glucose; if low, give IV dexamethasone (p200); if normal, ask yourself *is this a post-ictal state after a hypoglycaemic fit?* Here, giving more glucose worsens cerebral oedema.
▸▸Sublingual 'kitchen' sugar may be used as an immediate 'first aid' measure in managing hypoglycaemia. Place one level teaspoon of sugar moistened with water under the tongue every 10–12 minutes until stable.

'What are the aims of routine follow-up in the diabetes clinic?'

• To approach normoglycaemia via motivational education. Group learning is better than didactic doctor-sermons.
• To prevent complications (esp. renal & retinal). Check growth & fundi (dilate pupils; retinopathy takes ~10yrs to develop). Blood: glucose, HbA₁c, microalbuminuria—present in 25% after 10yrs (50% after 20yrs): ▸reducible to 15% if glucose well-controlled; microalbuminuria may spontaneously reverse.
• If normoglycaemia is unachievable, choose the best compromise with the child's way of life and strict glucose control.
• Carbohydrate-counting and insulin dose adjustment (eg DAFNE) matches insulin dose to the amount of carbohydrate eaten. Increases dietary freedom and can help to reduce HbA₁c without increasing hypoglycaemia.
• Introduce to a friendly diabetic nurse-teacher; ask 'Is real-time *continuous* glucose monitoring indicated?'. Feedback helps motivation and safety.

Just 100 years ago, DKA was universally fatal. The first patient to receive insulin (on January 11th 1922), was Leonard Thompson—a 14-yr-old boy, who went on to live a further 13 years. DKA results from a deficiency of insulin, often in combination with increased levels of counter-regulatory hormones (catecholamines, glucagon, cortisol and growth hormone—eg due to sepsis). The big concern with childhood DKA, (as opposed to adult DKA), is the increased frequency of cerebral oedema (see BOX), which occurs in ~1% of childhood DKA and has a mortality of 25%. Other fatal events in DKA include hypokalaemia and aspiration pneumonia (use NGT if semi-conscious and protect airway).

The patient Listlessness; confusion; vomiting; polyuria; polydipsia; weight loss; abdominal pain. *Look for:* Dehydration; deep and rapid (Kussmaul) respirations; ketotic (fruity-smelling) breath; shock; drowsiness; coma.

Diagnosis Requires the combination of *hyperglycaemia* (≥11mmol/L), *acidosis* (venous pH <7.3 and bicarbonate <15mmol/L), and *ketones* in urine and blood. *Severity* is categorized by degree of acidosis: mild—pH <7.3; moderate—pH <7.2; or severe—pH <7.1

Management[35] Follow local protocols and ask for senior help. Do GCS (p778; p201 if <4yrs). True coma is rare (<10%) in DKA: exclude other causes of coma; DKA may be precipitated by sepsis. Take the following action if shocked, consciousness↓, coma, or vomiting.[35]

• *Resuscitate: ABC:* Give 0.9% saline to correct dehydration; aim to restore deficit over 48h; over-enthusiastic fluid resuscitation may cause cerebral oedema. Consider ITU if BP↓, or <2yrs or ward staff busy (all children with DKA initially require high level of nursing care—usually 1:1).

• *Rapidly confirm diagnosis* with history, finger-prick glucose + ketones; venous blood gas; urine dip for ketones/glucose.

• *Formal investigations:* Weigh; FBC; U&E; glucose; Ca^{2+}; PO_4^{3-}; blood gas; ECG monitoring (look for peaked T-waves of hyperkalaemia), lab urine.

• *Use clinical signs to assess dehydration* (BOX) Now calculate the volume of fluid to be replaced (fluid requirement): ie maintenance fluid *plus* the dehydration deficit *minus* any fluid already given as resuscitation fluid. It should be given at a constant steady rate over the 1st 48h. (see worked example).

• *Start IV fluids:* Start with 0.9% saline + 20mmol KCl/500mL. When blood glucose falls to 14mmol/L use 0.9% saline + 5% glucose + 20mmol KCl /500mL. After 12h, if plasma sodium is stable, change to 0.45% saline + 5% glucose + 20mmol KCl/500mL.

• *Start IV insulin only after 1h of IV fluids:* Cerebral oedema may be more likely if insulin is started early. There is no need for an initial bolus of insulin. Use a 1 unit/mL solution of fast acting **insulin** (eg Actrapid®). Run at 0.1 units/kg/h. Ensure there is glucose in the IV fluids when venous glucose is <14mmol/L. Do NOT stop insulin at this stage it is still required to switch off ketogenesis. Once pH >7.3 and glucose is <14mmol/L consider reducing insulin to 0.05units/kg/h.

• *Stop IV insulin:* When blood ketone levels are <1.0mmol/L, and patient is able to tolerate food, give a dose of subcutaneous insulin; feed the patient. Stop infusion 10–60min after subcutaneous insulin injection.

Avoid bicarbonate in DKA: it increases the risk of cerebral oedema. If acidosis persists, consider ↑dose of insulin .

Ongoing monitoring • Hourly blood glucose • CNS status ≥half-hourly. • Nurses must tell you of headache or behaviour change promptly as these may indicate cerebral oedema (BOX) • Hourly fluid balance • U&E + blood gases 2h after starting IVI, then 4-hourly. Have a dedicated line for drawing blood. • If a central venous catheter (CVC) is used to aid monitoring, consider DVT prophylaxis.[36,410]
• Weigh twice daily • Monitor ECG for T-wave changes • Infection screen.

Cerebral oedema (MINIBOX) is a big threat, and is almost exclusively a condition of childhood. Pathophysiology is poorly understood but more common with rapid fall in glucose or sodium: usually occurs 4–12h from start of treatment, but it may be present at onset of DKA or up to 24h afterwards, presenting as a sudden CNS deterioration after initial improvement. Major cause of death in diabetic children, not the much-feared hypoglycaemia *Leukocytosis* may occur without any infection. *Infection*: (there may be no fever). Do MSU, blood cultures, and CXR. Start broad-spectrum antibiotics (p202) if infection suspected. *Creatinine:* some assays for creatinine crossreact with ketone bodies, so plasma creatinine may not reflect true renal function. *Hyponatraemia* (from osmotic effects of glucose): if <120mmol/L, search for other causes, eg triglycerides↑↑. Hypernatraemia >150mmol/L may be treated with 0.45% saline to start with (0.9% saline thereafter). *Ketonuria* does not equate with ketoacidosis. Normal individuals may have ketonuria after an overnight fast. Not all ketones are due to diabetes—consider alcohol, if glucose normal. Test plasma with Ketostix® or Acetest® to demonstrate ketonaemia. *Acidosis* without gross elevation of glucose may occur, but consider poisoning, eg with aspirin.

Serum amylase is often raised (up to 10-fold), and non-specific abdominal pain is common even in the absence of pancreatitis.

CNS deterioration
If warning signs: headache, ↓pulse, ↑BP, restlessness, irritability, focal neuorology (CN palsies), posturing, ↑ICP, or falling consciousness: ➡ Call your senior ➡ Exclude hypoglycaemia ➡ **Mannitol** 1g/kg IVI ➡ Restrict IV maintenance fluids by ½ and replace deficit over 72h ➡ Move to PICU and do CT ➡ Treat sepsis vigorously

Degree of dehydration[35]

• *Mild*—is hard to detect; it approximates to ~**3%** weight loss
• *Moderate*—dry mucous membranes and ↓skin turgor: ~**5%**
• *Severe*—sunken eyes and ↓capillary refill time: ~**8%**.
Overestimation of dehydration is dangerous—➡ don't use an estimation of greater than 8%. NB: 8% dehydrated = water deficit of 80mL/kg.

Calculating fluid requirement in DKA

Hourly rate = (48h maintenance + deficit (never use more than 10% deficit) – fluid already given) ÷ 48

The BPSED[35] suggests the following maintenance requirements based on weight (different from standard APLS rates):

<12.9kg	80mL/kg/24h	35–59.9kg	45mL/kg/24h
13–19.9kg	65mL/kg/24h	>60kg	35mL/kg/24h
20–34.9kg	55mL/kg/24h		

A 20kg 6-year-old boy who is 8% dehydrated, and who has already had 20mL/kg of saline will require:

$$(48h\ maintenance + deficit - fluid\ already\ given) \div 48$$
$$\approx 55mL \times 20kg \times 2\ (as\ 48h) + (80mL/kg \times 20kg) - (20mL \times 20kg) \div 48$$
$$\approx (2200mL + 1600mL - 400mL) \div 48$$
$$\approx 3400mL \div 48 = 71mL/h$$

35 Guidelines for the management of DKA in children, British Society for Paediatric Endocrinology and Diabetes (BSPED) 2009—available at: www.bsped.org.uk/clinical/docs/DKAGuideline.pdf. These have been endorsed by NICE.

36 Because thrombotic complications are rare, heparin isn't usually needed and is not recommended as part of standard therapy, but see brighton-healthcare.nhs.uk/diabetes/newpage17.htm[411] SE: thrombotic thrombocytopoenia.[412]

37 Note that pooling of KCl and insulin may cause uneven delivery in some IVI containers, so repeated mixing may be needed.[413]

Paediatrics

Most commonly seen between age 2–3yrs (accidental). Consider if this could be a suicide attempt in older children. Determine *what*, *how much* and *when* poison was ingested; the number of tablets dispensed is often given on the pack—count how many are left and consider the maximum dose that could have been taken. Ask if *other medicines/chemicals* are kept in the same place and could the child have taken more than one poison? Was this child playing with any *others*? If so, they too may have shared some of the poison. If the tablets are from an unlabelled box, the dispenser may have records and be able to name the tablets; to help identify medication from loose tablets brought in by parents use sites such as www.drugs.com/pill_identification.html—this is USA based—your hospital may subscribe to a equivalent local system. Once the poison has been identified consult TOXBASE (www.toxbase.org) or local equivalent.

▶Contact a National Poisons Information Service (NPIS, eg 0844 892 0111 in UK).
Examination Look for signs of toxidromes (see BOX). Ensure complete set of vital signs are obtained. Note GCS and pupils.

Principles of management

• As always: ABC is your priority. Also check blood glucose.
• Consider intubation if GCS <8, or respiratory failure; if GCS 8–14 consider oral/nasopharyngeal airway (caution if vomiting) and put in recovery position.
• Maintain BP; correct hypoglycaemia; monitor urine output.
• Baseline studies may include: FBC, U&E; glucose; ECG.
• Do a blood gas: a metabolic acidosis with an increased anion gap can be due to drugs such as metformin; alcohol; ethylene; toluene; cyanide; isoniazid; iron; aspirin; paraldehyde or other causes (DKA; lactic acidosis).
• Certain drugs can be measured in serum—so test for paracetamol; ethanol; methanol; ethylene glycol; salicylates; iron; anti-convulsants; lithium; digoxin; theophylline; carboxyhaemaglobin if these are suspected.
• The mainstay of care is *supportive management*.
• Consider *gastric decontamination*—discuss with a toxicologist.
• *Ipecac syrup*, or any form of forced vomiting, is no longer recommended.[414] *Activated charcoal* is controversial as there is no evidence it improves clinical outcome.[415] It is most effective if given within 1h of ingestion. Concerns exist about the risk of aspiration of charcoal if the patient vomits (increased in hydrocarbon poisonings) or becomes drowsy. Avoid with lithium, alcohol, cyanide, iron ingestions or rapid acting ingestions.[415] *Cathartics* and *gastric lavage* are virtually never indicated.[416–418] *Whole-bowel irrigation* should not be routinely used, but it may be of benefit in sustained released ingestions. Only use after consulting NPIS or if specifically recommended in TOXBASE.[418]
• Determine if a *specific antidote* is available (see 'Specific antidotes' and p192–3).

Specific antidotes

• *Beta-blockers:* Cause hypotension, bradycardia, heart block and heart failure. Monitor ECG; atropine 40mcg/kg IV for bradycardia, then glucagon (50–150mcg/kg IV + infusion of 50mcg/kg/h in 5% glucose). Consider adrenaline or dopamine infusions.
• *Carbon monoxide:* High-flow oxygen and mannitol for cerebral oedema. Severe cases may benefit from hyperbaric oxygen therapy.
• *Digoxin:* Atropine is used if bradycardic. Digoxin specific antibody (Digibind®) is used in those with severe dysrhythmias/hyperkalaemia.
• *Opioids:* Use IV naloxone 10mcg/kg; if no response try 100mcg/kg (max 2mg). An infusion may be required.
• *Methanol/ethylene glycol:* Fomepizole.[419] Contact poisons unit promptly.
• *Sulfonylureas:* ?Try octreotide.[420] Other antidotes: OHCM p852.

Paediatrics

Toxidromes

- *Opioid*—eg morphine, codeine, methadone, oxycodone, heroin—bradycardia, hypotension, decreased respiratory rate, and pin-point pupils.
- *Cholinergic*—eg organophosphates; pilocarpine—*(DUMBELLS):* Diarrhoea; Urination; Miosis; Bradycardia; Emesis; Lacrimation; Lethary; Salivation.
- *Anticholinergic*—eg antihistamines, tricyclic antidepressants, deadly nightshade, atropine—these patients are *Hot as a hare, Red as a beet, Dry as a bone, Blind as a bat*, and, *Mad as a hatter*—with hyperthermia, facial flushing, dry skin, dilated pupils, and delirium. They also have tachycardia and urinary retention.
- *Sympathomimetic*—eg cocaine, amphetamines, pseudoephedrine—patient is tachycardic, hypertensive, hyperthermic and has dilated pupils. Risk of seizures.

Iron poisoning

Iron is a common childhood poison. It is absorbed as Fe^{2+}, oxidized to Fe^{3+} and bound to transferrin. Toxicity occurs when transferrin binding capacity is reached.

Identify the exact preparation, as formulations contain different amounts of elemental iron. A 200mg $FeSO_4$ tablet contains ~65mg elemental iron. 125mg/mL $FeSO_4$ drops contain 25mg iron/mL. A 300mg ferrous fumarate tablet may contain 100mg of iron (depends on brand), whereas a 300mg ferrous gluconate tablet may only contain 35mg iron. Expect mild toxicity at doses of >20mg/kg of elemental iron. Mod-severe toxicity occurs with doses of >60mg/kg.[421,422]

Presentation Patients may have ingested tablets, liquid, or multi-vitamins containing iron. He may present with nausea, vomiting, haematemesis, diarrhoea, altered mental status, or hypotension. Between 6–12 hours there may be a phase of apparent improvement. Between 12–24 hours cardiovascular collapse and massive GI bleeding can occur. Severe metabolic acidosis may develop as each Fe^{3+} ion combines with water to produce $3H^+$ and $FeOH^3$. Renal and hepatic failure may ensue. Hepatotoxicity is a marker of severity and is a common cause of death. Survivors may develop pyloric strictures after 4–6 weeks secondary to scarring. *Tests:* Baseline blood gas, serum iron concentration, U&E, FBC, glucose. Iron levels at 4–6h help determine level of severity. Levels of <350mcg/dL (~60µmol/L) are associated with minimal symptoms. Levels >500mcg/dL (~90µmol/L) are associated with serious toxicity. An abdominal x-ray may show tablets within the gut and reveal a bezoar (a mass within the gastrointestinal system). ▸In severe toxicity do not wait for tests: start desferrioxamine.

Management

- Obtain expert help as this is one of the few instances when gastric lavage/endoscopy to remove tablets in the stomach may be recommended.
- Activated charcoal is not given as it has no effect on iron absorption.
- Whole-bowel irrigation may help (esp. in slow-release preparations).[423]
- Supportive care—IV fluids and sodium bicarbonate to correct acidosis.
- Chelation with IV desferrioxamine (5–15mg/kg/h—start at higher dose then reduce after 4–6h—max 80mg/kg/24h). Therapy should be stopped when the acidosis improves. It is rarely required for >24h. Use of desferrioxamine leads to orangey-red urine which demonstrates that free iron has been bound to the desferrioxamine. It is associated with hypotension, rashes, pulmonary oedema, and acute respiratory distress syndrome.
- Haemofiltration has been used in children, in combination with desferrioxamine to rapidly reduce iron levels.[424]

The most common salicylate is acetylsalicylic acid, ie aspirin, which is not recommended in children <16y due to its association with Reye's syndrome (p652). Choline salicylate is found in Bonjela® for adults. Since 2009, Bonjela teething gel® in the UK has used lidocaine as its active ingredient, however Bonjela teething gel® in other countries (eg Australasia) continues to contain choline salicylate (8.7%) and there are reports of toxicity in children.[425] Methyl salicylate is found in oil of wintergreen (98%). As little as 3mL can be fatal in children.[426] Methyl salicylate is also found in muscle rubs such as Bengay®, Deep Heat®, and Tiger Balm® (~15–40%). **Presentation** Toxicity occurs at ~100mg/kg aspirin. Early signs include tinnitus and hearing loss. Stimulation of respiratory centres leads to tachypnoea and a respiratory alkalosis. Interference with aerobic metabolism leads to the metabolic (lactic) acidosis which is characteristic of salicylate poisoning. GI irritation (nausea, vomiting, abdominal pain is common). Central effects lead to agitation, delirium and seizures. Rhabdomyolysis, pulmonary oedema and electrolyte disturbances may also occur. **Tests** Blood gas; FBC; U&E, glucose. Salicylate levels are best obtained at 6 hours (reflects a peak level) however, do an initial level to confirm diagnosis, and then levels every 2h to confirm levels are decreasing—enteric coated (EC) preparations can lead to delayed absorption. Large bezoars of EC aspirin may be seen on x-ray. **Management** Resuscitate with boluses of 10–20mL/kg of 0.9% saline. Correct hypoglycaemia. Potassium may be needed as hypokalaemia is common. Serious poisoning is indicated by levels >2.5–3.6mmol/L—consider urinary alkalinization with IV sodium bicarbonate to enhance elimination (under expert guidance in ITU). Activated charcoal is effective in adsorbing aspirin, but as patients are liable to vomit or experience ↓GCS consider intubating first and using a NGT. Repeat doses can be given. Haemodialysis is the definitive treatment: use when evidence of end-organ injury[427] (seizures, severe acidosis, rhabdomyolysis, renal failure, pulmonary oedema). *Seek expert help.*

Paracetamol (acetaminophen) poisoning

Refer to Toxbase (www.toxbase.org). The therapeutic dose is 15mg/kg. Hepatotoxicity can occur if ≥75mg/kg ingested. The initial features are nausea and pallor. Hepatic enzymes rise after ~24h. Jaundice and an enlarged, tender liver occur after 48h. Hypoglycaemia, hypotension, encephalopathy, coagulopathy, coma may also occur.

Management of single oral paracetamol overdoses
- If you are certain the ingested paracetamol is <75mg/kg in a child, then management may be safely done at home after addressing risk of self harm.[428]
- Admit those ingesting >75mg/kg (or an unknown amount) and do a serum paracetamol concentration at ≥4h post ingestion, with venous gas, U&E, FBC, LFTs and clotting. If presenting <1h, and >150mg/kg of tablets ingested, and no contra-indication (eg vomiting; ↓GCS), give activated charcoal.[429]
- Consult the nomogram on p193 (fig **2.20**). If plasma paracetamol level is above the line, or the patient has an abnormal INR, ALT or creatinine, treat with acetylcysteine (NAC).
- The initial dose is 150mg/kg in up to 200mL (depending weight; see BNF) of 5% glucose infused over 1h, followed by 50mg/kg IVI over the next 4h, and 100mg/kg IVI over next 16h. It is very effective in preventing liver damage if given <8h after overdose.
- Patients with a delayed presentation (>15h) or in whom a staggered ingestion ≥24h, or uncertain timing, should have acetylcysteine started immediately if ingested dose is >75mg/kg, or dose is unknown.
- Consider the cause. All deliberate overdoses need psychiatric evaluation, preferably by Child and Adolescent Mental Health specialists. Causes may

be extremely complex and deep-seated: although the patient may claim a seemingly superficial cause, this may be hiding deep social or psychiatric pathology.

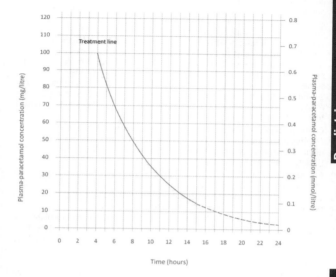

Fig 2.20 Paracetamol overdose treatment nomogram.
With permission from The Royal College of Emergency Medicine: www.rcem.ac.uk/Shop-Floor/Clinical%20Guidelines/College%20Guidelines/Paracetamol%20Overdose.

Further reading

The Royal College of Emergency Medicine (2012). *Paracetamol Overdose in Adults and Children*. www.rcem.ac.uk/Shop-Floor/Clinical%20Guidelines/College%20Guidelines/Paracetamol%20Overdose

Information relating to all poisonings: www.toxbase.org (will require an institutional login)

Paediatrics

ALL is the commonest (80%) childhood leukaemia (~500 cases/yr[uk]); it is a malignant disorder of lymphoid progenitor cells. Other forms: *OHCM* p346–53. Peak age is 2–6years, with a second peak >50y. Incidence is greater in white children than in black children. **Causes** Precise cause is unknown. There are genetic associations: ALL is concordant in ~25% of monozygotic twins; individuals with trisomy 21 have a 4-fold increased risk (also increased risk in Bloom's syndrome, ataxia-telangiectasia). Chromosomal translocations such as t(12;21) resulting in the TEL-AML fusion gene are associated with 30% of cases (only present in 1% of the general population). t(9;22)—the Philadelphia chromosom—occurs in 15–30% (mostly adults) and is associated with a poor prognosis. Environmental risk factors which have been implicated include prenatal exposure to x-rays; *in utero* exposure to infection, delayed postnatal exposure to infection, and environmental radiation.[430–432]

Classification WHO classifies ALL into either *B lymphoblastic leukaemia* or *T lymphoblastic leukaemia*.[433] Prior to 2008 the term pre-B-cell ALL was used to distinguish *B lymphoblastic leukaemia* from mature B-cell ALL which is termed Burkitt lymphoma/leukaemia.

Presentation Pancytopenia (pallor, infection, bleeding), fatigue, anorexia, fever, bone pain. Painless lumps in neck, axilla, groin. The period before diagnosis is often brief (2–4 weeks). Cranial infiltration may lead to CNS effects, eg cranial palsies. Testicular infiltration can lead to orchidomegaly.

Tests *Bloods:* WCC↑, ↓ or ↔. Normochromic, normocytic anaemia ± platelets↓, urate↑, LDH↑. *Marrow:* 50–98% of nucleated cells are blasts. *CSF:* Pleocytosis (with blast forms), protein ↑, glucose ↓. *Cytogenetic analysis:* 80% will have genetic abnormalities at diagnosis. *CXR:* May show mediastinal mass.

Prognosis depends on clinical signs, biologic features of lymphoblasts and response to induction chemotherapy. Based on these features patients can be stratified into 4 risk categories. *Standard risk:* Patients are aged 1–9.9yrs, have WCC of <50×10⁹/L; lack unfavourable cytogenetic features, show a good response to initial chemotherapy and have <5% bone marrow blasts by 14 days and <0.01% blasts by 28 days. *Low risk:* These patients meet the standard risk criteria and have favourable genetics, such as trisomy 4, 10 or 17. *High risk:* Patients do not meet standard criteria or have extra-medullary involvement (eg brain/testis). *Very high risk:* Have unfavourable genetics, such as the Philedelphia chromosome, hypodiploidy—or poor response to initial chemotherapy. *Event-free survival* at 5yr is 95% in the low risk group; 30% in the very high risk. Infant leukaemia has the worst outcome: 20%. Overall survival is 80%.

Treatment of ALL typically has 3 phases: *Induction therapy:* 3-drug induction over 4 weeks (eg **vincristine, dexamethasone,**[434] **L-asparaginase**) + intrathecal (IT) therapy (**methotrexate ± cytarabine + hydrocortisone**) results in remission of >95%. High-risk patients may get a further agent as **daunorubicin.**[433] ~2% die of infection. *Consolidation phase:* Cranial irradiation if known CNS disease. Further chemotherapy (eg **cyclophosphamide; cytarabine; mercaptopurine**). *Maintenance phase:* For ~2½yrs (daily **mercaptopurine** + weekly **methotrexate ± vincristine/steroid pulses**). 3-monthly intrathecal drugs.

Complications ▶▶*Neutropenic sepsis:* See box. **Co-trimoxazole** prevents pneumocystosis. Revaccinate (1 dose of each type, p151) 6 months after chemotherapy (as vaccine-specific antibody↓).[435] *Hyperuricaemia:* From massive cell death at induction: pre-treat with ↑ fluid intake + **allopurinol.** *Poor growth:* Monitor carefully.[436] *Cancer elsewhere:* Risk of CNS tumours or a 2nd leukaemia is 3%.

Relapses: Consider FLAG,[38] clofarabine,[437] or marrow transplant; consider if risk ↑↑, eg WCC >200×10⁹/L, MLL gene rearrangement, B-cell ALL with t(8;14). ● ● [438] [439] Tyrosine kinase inhibitors (eg **imatinib**) are used in children with t(9;22).

Pitfalls ►Ignoring quality of life; eg most cytotoxics may be given at home. • Omitting to examine the testes (►a common site for recurrence). • Thiopurine methyltransferase deficiency may cause fatal myelosuppression (?do pre-treatment pharmacogenomic analysis).[440] • Inappropriate transfusion (leukostasis, *OHCM* p346, if WCC >100×10⁹/L).[441] • SE of chemotherapy. NB: ondansetron is better than other anti-emetics.

►►Febrile neutropenic patients who may be septicaemic (eg from an infected venous catheter)

Suspect infection when untoward events happen in a neutropenic patient (WCC <2×10⁹/L, or neutrophils <1×10⁹/L). Do T° often; brief rises to ≤38°C *may* be ignored if the child is well but most would send cultures and treat early because the risk of overwhelming sepsis is so great. Emphasize to the parents and child the importance of swift routes to hospital. Take blood cultures and MSU; swab all orifices. Do FBC, CRP & serology. Get help from your senior and a microbiologist; follow local protocols.

Likely organisms In one UK study, blood cultures were +ve in 30%. Grampositive organisms predominated (80%) and most were coagulase-negative staphs. 6% were Gram-negative isolates and <1% fungal.[442]

Blind treatment Use local protocols piptazobactam (eg Tazocin®)[443] ± gentamicin[444] OR imipenem (±teicoplanin)—the broadest-spectrum β-lactam[39] antibiotic, which may have advantages over cephalosporins if an anaerobe such as *Bacteroides* is suspected (NB: imipenem is not indicated in CNS infections).[445]

Tazocin® (for example) = piptazobactam = piperacillin + tazobactam IV over 3–5min or IVI: 1 month–18yrs: 90mg/kg/6h, max 4.5g/6h. (The neonatal dose is 90mg/kg/8h.)

Gentamicin Child 1 month–12yrs: 2.5mg/kg/8h. 12–18yrs 2mg/kg/8h.

Imipenem *Dose in children <40kg:* 15mg/kg/6h max 2g/24h. Heavier children have the adult dose: 250–500mg/6h (less sensitive organisms: up to 25mg/kg/6h IVI; max, eg 1g/6h). Check U&E. If creatinine clearance <70mL/min, ↓dose frequency (see *Data sheet*). NB: do not use IM formulations IV (IM formulations are not for use in children). If blood culture *does* prove +ve, either change imipenem after microbiological advice, or continue it for 5 days, if he has been afebrile for >24h. If blood cultures are –ve, give for a few days and send home when well and afebrile for >24h. SE: (It is usually well-tolerated.) Thrombophlebitis, anuria, polyuria, seizures (eg in ~2%), confusion, psychic disturbance, encephalopathy, vertigo, tinnitus, transient hearing loss, BP↓, pruritus, taste perversion, pseudomembranous colitis; arthralgia; eosinophilia; WCC↓; Hb↓; LFT↑. There are few clinically important drug interactions, eg seizures if co-therapy with ganciclovir.[446]

Meropenem is preferred in some units (unlicensed; more active against most Gram –ves than imipenem but is less active against most Gram +ves).[447] Dose: 1 month to 12yrs: 10–20mg/kg/8h IVI over 5min. Over 50kg weight: adult dose (eg 1g/8h IVI). SE: D&V (eg antibiotic-associated colitis); abdominal pain; LFT↑; platelets↓; partial thromboplastin time↓; +ve Coombs' test; eosinophilia; WCC↓; headache; paraesthesiae; rash; pruritus; fits (rare).[448]

Teicoplanin For blind treatment of the worst infections, consider adding this to imipenem. Dose: 10mg/kg/12h IV for 3 doses, max 400mg, then 6mg/kg/24h (max 400mg); neonates: 16mg/kg on day 1, then 8mg/kg/day). SE: (few): headache; WCC↓; platelets ↓/↑; LFT↑; allergy (rare). No major interactions.[449]

If fever persists and blood cultures remain –ve ask: Is aciclovir indicated? Is a fungus possible? For amphotericin see SPC/*data sheet* & *OHCM* p168.

---

38 FLAG = Fludarabine, cytarabine (Ara-C), and G-CSF (recombinant human granulocyte-colony stimulating factor); clofarabine; it is non-standard.[450,451] A novel alternative is myeloablative chemotherapy and radiation followed by infusion of umbilical cord blood saved after delivery for this kind of eventuality.[452]
39 Named for the β-lactam ring in their structure. Examples: penicillins, cephalosporins, etc.

The clinical problem You have the results of a full blood count, showing anaemia (Hb <110g/L, p220, the WHO criterion). *How should you proceed?*

1 Take a history (including travel, diet, ethnic origin); examine the child.

2 MCV <70fL: ?IDA/iron deficiency anaemia (poor diet, poverty, bleeding, stomatitis, koilonychia) or *thalassaemia* (Mediterranean/SE Asia areas, short stature, muddy complexion, icteric sclerae, distended abdomen ∴ hepatosplenomegaly, bossed skull, prominent maxillae, from marrow hyperplasia).

3 MCV >100fL: suspect ↓folate (malabsorption; phenytoin), ↓B12 (breast milk from a vegetarian, ↓intrinsic factor, malabsorption), or haemolysis. Signs of B12↓: poor feeding, late milestones; odd movements; microcephaly, failure to thrive.

4 MCV 81–97fL (normocytic): suspect haemolysis, or marrow failure (transient, after infections, or thyroid, kidney, or liver failure, or malignancy). Causes of aplasia: chloramphenicol; Diamond–Blackfan (p640); Fanconi's anaemia (p644).

5 WCC/differential abnormal? Eosinophilia + anaemia + tropics ≈ hookworms.

6 Severe tropical anaemias (eg Hb <50g/L): malaria; bacteraemia (eg nontyphoid salmonella[453]); worms; HIV; B12↓; G6PD↓; iron deficiency; sickle cell anaemia.

7 Next look at the ESR and CRP. This may indicate some chronic disease.

8 Film + reticulocyte count ± thick film for malaria. Hypochromic microcytic RBCs ≈ IDA; target cells ≈ liver disease or thalassaemia; ferritin for IDA; sickling tests + Hb electrophoresis for thalassaemia & sickle-cell anaemia; B12; red cell folate.

9 Prevention: no cows' milk if <1yr; if formula-fed, use iron-fortified; wean at 4–6 months. Adequate vitamin C intake; iron supplements if premature.

Iron deficiency anaemia (~26% of infants, worldwide;[454] peak age ~18 months) this is despite fortification, of, formula, breakfast cereals and noodles etc.[455] Iron-deficient babies are less happy than others, with ↓psychomotor development and poor cognition.[456] In the UK, dietary causes are common, eg poverty, lack of education, or coeliac disease. In recurrent IDA, suspect bleeding (eg Meckel's diverticulum, p651, or oesophagitis). ℞: **Ferrous fumarate** syrup (140mg/5mL), 0.25mL/kg/12h PO (if <12yrs old (max. 20mL), or Sytron®. If poor compliance, try Iron Spangles which can be poured into yoghurt or ice cream. Warn of the dangers of overdosage, p191. Aim for Hb rise of >10g/L/month. In many places, the 1st step is de-worming.

Haemolysis Is malaria or sickle-cell disease possible? Get help, and try to provide the expert with sufficient information to answer these 4 questions:

1 Any evidence of ↑RBC production? (Polychromasia, reticulocytosis.)

2 Is there decreased RBC survival? (Bilirubin ↑, haptoglobins ↓.)

3 Is there intravascular haemolysis? (Haemoglobinuria.)

4 Is there an inborn error of metabolism (eg G6PD deficiency), spherocytosis, or is the defect acquired (usually with +ve Coombs' test)?

Hereditary spherocytosis is the main cause of haemolysis in north European children (mainly autosomal dominant; spontaneous mutations in 25%). It is often mild; parvovirus B19 infection can trigger transient severe anaemia. Flow cytometric analysis of eosin-5-maleimide (EMA) binding to red cells, and cryohaemolysis test have replaced osmotic fragility tests.[457] Splenectomy leads to ↑RBC survival and is sometimes indicated; gallstones may occur in the 1st decade, and if symptomatic cholecystectomy ± splenectomy may be needed.[458]

Sickle-cell disease: OHCM p334. Hydrate and give O2. *Pain relief:* Warmth, hydration, ibuprofen 10mg/kg/8h PO,[8] ± morphine sulfate solution, load with 0.4mg/kg PO,[459] then 0.3mg/kg/4h + MST® 1–1.5mg/kg/12h[9] for background analgesia; this *may* be preferred to IVI morphine, eg 0.1mg/kg (+lactulose 2.5–10mL/12h PO ± senna). *Patient-controlled analgesia:* Morphine 1mg/kg[10] in 50mL 5% glucose at 1mL/h with self-delivered extra boluses of 1mL as needed; do respiration & sedation score every ¼h + SaO2 if chest or abdominal pain.[460,461] Deferasirox (eg Exjade®) is a good but expensive oral iron chelator; needed if many transfusions are used.

▶Don't think that if a child is not anaemic he is not iron deficient. CNS iron levels fall *before* RBC mass. If in doubt, check ferritin. Treating low ferritins may improve:—• Memory • Lassitude • Developmental delay • Sleep • Mood • Cognition—in toddlers and adolescent girls, facing demands of puberty and menstruation. NB: pica (eating dirt, p210) is a sign of iron deficiency.

Purpura: 2 questions: ▶Is the child ill? ▶What is the platelet count?

• *If ill & platelets* ↓: Meningococcal septicaemia (►ceftriaxone, p202), *leukaemia*, or *disseminated intravascular coagulation* (check a visual non-automated blood film & WCC, discuss with lab). *Haemolytic uraemic syndrome* (p176).

• *If ill & platelet count* ↔ *or* ↑: Viruses eg measles; enteroviruses (95% petechial rashes will be viral);[462] vasculitis (Kawasaki, p646; platelets↑);[463] SBE. *Meningococcal septicaemia* less likely.

• *If well(ish) & platelet count* ↔ and no history of trauma: HSP (below).

• *If well & platelet count↓* consider *idiopathic thrombocytopenic purpura* (rarely, *Wiskott–Aldrich syndrome*, p655, or *aplastic anaemia*). NB: vomiting or coughing can cause petechiae in superior vena cava distribution.

Henoch–Schönlein purpura (HSP) is an acute immune complex-mediated vasculitis. Most patients have an antecedent upper respiratory tract infection. Purpura (purple spots/nodules not disappearing on palpation), arthritis/arthralgias (74%)—often knees/ankles—and abdominal pain (51%) are the classic triad. ♂:♀×1.3:1.[464] *Other signs:* Renal involvement (54%; severe nephropathy in 7%, acute renal insufficiency in 2%), scrotal oedema (13%), and intussusception (0.6%). *Tests:* ESR↑ (57%), IgA↑ (37%), proteinuria (42%) ASO titres↑ (36%). Check U&E & BP. Steroids may help resolve abdo pain,[465] but role in prevention of chronic kidney disease is less clear.[466] Most recover in ≤2 months. Recurrences, verified in 35%, correlate with ↑ESR.

Complications (worse in adults): massive GI bleeds, ileus, haemoptysis (rare), and acute renal failure (rare). One option in HSP nephritis (not usually needed) is high-dose steroids + cyclophosphamide; this decreases proteinuria (a risk factor for renal insufficiency in HSP).[467] Chronic renal failure occurs in 5%.

Idiopathic (immune) thrombocytopenic purpura (ITP) is most common acquired bleeding disorder in childhood. ITP has acute and chronic forms. *Presentation:* Acute bruising, purpura, and petechiae. Usually a history of recent URTI or gastroenteritis. May follow CMV, EBV, parvovirus, varicella zoster, or live virus vaccine (eg MMR/rubella). If there is significant mucosal bleeding, or lymphadenopathy, hepatosplenomegaly, or pancytopenia, another diagnosis is likely. *Tests:* Isolated thrombocytopenia (<20×10⁹ in 80%); do a film to ensure no other abnormalities. Marrow is unnecessary, unless:[468]

• Unusual signs are present, eg abnormal cells on a film, lymphadenopathy.
• Platelet count is not rising after ~2 weeks.
• Treatment is contemplated with steroids or immunoglobulin—may decrease period of profound thrombocytopenia.

Intracranial haemorrhage occurs in <1% (mortality is 50%)[469]—do CT if there is headache or CNS signs. *Natural history:* Most can be managed at home. Gradual resolution over ~3 months for 80% with or without therapy. 20% become chronic (>6 months); the chronic form is compatible with normal longevity, and normal activities, provided contact sports are avoided. ℞: Admit eg if: • Unusual features, eg excessive bleeding. • Life-threatening bleeding requires platelet transfusion. Splenectomy is considered for chronic ITP and failure of treatment. **Rituximab⁴⁰** and **anti-D⁴¹** (p11) reduce the need for splenectomy.

---

40 Rituximab can induce remission in ~30%.[470] SE: T°↑, pruritus, throat tightness, serum sickness.
41 Anti-D: a single dose of 50mcg/kg IV ↑ platelet count to ≥20×10⁹/L in 70% of children within 3 days.[471]

Synonym: *primary hypogammaglobulinaemia* (not secondary to protein-losing enteropathy, chronic lymphatic leukaemia, or myeloma). Bruton's agammaglobulinaemia was the first immunodeficiency syndrome to be described.[472]

Essence Antibodies (that are produced by B lymphocytes) can kill pathogens by binding to target antigens and activating complement system or facilitating their uptake by phagocyte cells. They can also neutralize the toxins secreted by the pathogens. Disorders of B cells increase susceptibility to infections by encapsulated bacteria, but not (usually) viral or fungal infections. Most are recessive, eg caused by mutations in genes on autosomal or x chromosomes.[472]

Typical signs
• Frequent infections
• Bronchiectasis
• Chronic sinusitis
• Failure to thrive
• Nodular lymphoid hyperplasia (gut)
• Absent tonsils
• Enteropathy
• Hepatosplenomegaly
• Anaemia
• Arthropathy
• Lymphopenia
• Serum total protein↓ (albumin; immunoglobulins are missing)[473]

The patient When the signs in the MINIBOX are unexplained, refer to an immunologist, to assess antibody responses to protein and carbohydrate antigens, measure IgG subclasses, specific antibodies to the immunized illnesses, and count lymphocytes involved in antibody production (CD4, CD8, CD19, CD23 +ve lymphocytes). Immunoglobulin levels are interpreted by age. There is a role for watching responses to test vaccinations. Primary immunodeficiency is more likely if there is a positive family history/parental consanguinity.[474]

Types of primary immunodeficiency See BOX, p199.

Management Aim to include the patient and the family in the process. Treat intercurrent infections promptly. This may include postural physiotherapy, and bronchodilators as well as antibiotics. Immunoglobulin replacement obviates most complications and is best delivered by an immunologist, after detailed assessment. Many patients can join a self-infusion programme. Before infusions, exclude active infection (to minimize risk of adverse reactions), and a baseline check of transaminase enzymes, creatinine, and anti-IgA antibody titres should be done. The dose of IV immunoglobulin is determined by the severity and frequency of infections, and the plasma level of IgG. Most receive ~400mg/kg/month (see *data sheet*/SPC, usually as 2 doses, 2 weeks apart).[11][475] Have hydrocortisone and an antihistamine at the ready. SE: headaches, abdominal pain, anaphylaxis, transmission of hepatitis.[476] IM immunoglobulins are not favoured, but the subcutaneous route is being investigated and appears satisfactory.[477][N=40]

Complications *Chest:* Bronchiectasis, granulomas, lymphoma. *Gut:* Malabsorption, giardia, cholangitis, atrophic gastritis, colitis. *Liver:* Acquired hepatitis, chronic active hepatitis, biliary cirrhosis. *Blood:* Autoimmune haemolysis, ITP (p197), anaemia of chronic disease, aplasia. *Eyes/CNS:* Keratoconjunctivitis, uveitis, granulomas, encephalitis. *Others:* Septic arthropathy, arthralgia, splenomegaly.

Gene therapy Autologous haematopoietic stem cells transduced with the γc gene can restore immune system in boys with severe combined immunodeficiency. A harmless retrovirus carries the replacement gene, and infects the stem cells *in vitro*. When these are replaced in the marrow an immune system develops within a few months[42]—obviating the need for intrusive anti-infection isolation measures and IV immunoglobulin. It is an alternative to marrow transplants (eg if no HLA match can be found). There is likely to be a limitation to initiation of normal thymopoiesis, so do it promptly.

---

42 T cells & repertoires of T-cell receptors were ~normal up to 2yrs post-op; thymopoiesis is shown by naive T cells. Antibody production is adequate.

IgA deficiency (IgA↓ + normal or ↑ levels of other immunoglobulins). It is the most common primary antibody deficiency. Many are asymptomatic. It may accompany cvid (below). Patients tend to develop respiratory infections which may lead to bronchiectasis. Gastrointestinal infection (eg giardiasis) and disorders such as malabsorption, coeliac disease, ulcerative colitis are associated with IgA deficiency. Although rare, all blood products/iv immuno-globulin infusion can lead to severe, even fatal, anaphylaxis due to the presence of IgA. Ideally blood products if needed should be obtained from an IgA-deficient individual—or washed red cells given. Patients are recommended to wear a medical alert bracelet because of this.[478] *Prevalence:* Varies with ethnicity: 1 in 143 in Middle East; 1 in 875 in uk; 1 in 18,500 in Japan.[478]

Transient hypogammaglobulinaemia of infancy Temporary delay in antibody production. *Onset:* 3–6 months. It is more severe than normal antibody deficiency that happens at this age. Immunoglobulin levels become normal by 2–4 yrs. *Prevalence:* ~1 in 10,000.[479]

Common variable immunodeficiency (cvid) (IgG↓, IgA↓, IgM variable). *Onset:* 2nd to 3rd decade of life. Enlarged tonsils, splenomegaly, gastrointestinal disease, liver dysfunction and cancer (esp lymphoma) may be present. *Prevalence:* ~1 in 10,000–50,000.[480]

Bruton x-linked agammaglobulinaemia Tyrosine kinase gene mutation (xq21) causes ↓ immunoglobulins and ↓mature b cells,[481] hence ↑ susceptibility to bacterial (but not viral) infections. Lymphocytes are unable to synthesize immunoglobulin. *Onset:* 3months–3years.[482] Also: arthropathy + absent Peyer's patches, tonsils and appendix. *Prevalence:* ~1 in 250,000 (the commonest inherited antibody deficiency).[481] *R:* Beware septicaemia and cns infections (may require interferon alfa and high-dose iv immunoglobulin).[483] After marrow transplantation serum immunoglobin rises to normal levels over ~3 months.[484]

IgG subclass deficiency There are ↓ levels of one or more of 4 subclasses of IgG. Total IgG levels may be normal. IgG₂↓ is the most common and often is associated with IgA↓, and ataxia-telangiectasia.

Severe combined immunodeficiency (scid) t-cell dysfunction usually causes combined immunodeficiency as t cells are necessary for b-cell differentiation. *Onset:* 1-3 months. Patients are susceptible to all types of bacterial, viral, fungal, and protozoal infections. *Treatment:* Stem cell transplant. *Prevalence:* ~1 in 50,000-75,000.[485]

Causes Meningoencephalitis; head injury; subdural/extradural bleeds (*abused?*); hypoxia (eg near-drowning); ketoacidosis; tumours; thrombosis;[43] Reye's (p652).

Signs Listless; irritable; drowsy; headache; diplopia; vomiting; tense fontanelle; ↓level of responsiveness (Children's Coma Scale if <4yrs, see p201, or use the Glasgow Coma Scale if >4yrs (p722); If unconscious look for: pupil changes (ipsilateral dilatation); abnormal posturing (decorticate/decerebrate); Cushing's triad (slow pulse, raised BP and breathing pattern abnormalities) warns of imminent coning. Chronic: papilloedema and hydrocephalus.

Management ABC is the initial priority. Aim to prevent ischaemia. Help venous drainage by keeping head in the midline, elevated at ~25°. Give O₂ if T° >40°C. Treat hypoglycaemia. Control seizures (p208). ▶*Don't do LP* until CT obtained and child is intubated. If severe, take to ITU to monitor ICP & cerebral perfusion pressure (CPP=mean arterial pressure minus ICP; if CPP <40mmHg cerebral ischaemia is likely).
▶▶Intubate. Hyperventilation is no longer recommended.
▶▶Give mannitol 20% eg 2.5mL/kg IVI over 30min[486] or 3% hypertonic saline (5mL/kg bolus) which may have fewer side effects.[487]
▶▶Dexamethasone: if <35kg, 16.7mg IV (20.8mg if >35kg) then as per BNF[c] §6.3.2.
▶▶Fluid restriction & diuresis, avoiding hypovolaemia (keep Na⁺ 145–150mmol/L, osmolarity to 300–310, and CVP to 2–5cmH₂O). ▶▶Pulse & BP continuously.
▶▶Send to neurosurgical centre.

Herpes simplex encephalitis (HSE) is the most treatable encephalitis. ▶Think of it in any febrile child with focal or general seizures and CNS (esp. temporal lobe) signs ± ↓consciousness. Signs are often non-specific.[488] Nasolabial herpes is often absent. CNS deficits may be mild or gross (eg hemiparesis). *Tests:* CT, EEG and CSF often non-specific (do PCR). MRI is better than CT. *R̠:* ▶▶Start aciclovir. If >12yrs old: 10mg/kg[IBW]/8h by IVI over 1h eg for 3wks (20mg/kg/8h in neonates).[489] Monitor U&E & urine output; *Mortality:* ~7%. 60% survive intact. *CNS sequelae:* Kluver–Bucy syndrome (hypersexuality, rage, visual agnosia); aphasia;[490] amnesia; auditory agnosia; autism.[491]

Brain tumours ▶Arrange urgent referral if unexplained headache and/or focal symptoms, eg progressive weakness or numbness, unsteadiness, difficulty speaking, or vision changes/VI nerve palsy. ⅔ are in the posterior fossa. Consider brain tumours in children with lethargy, behavioural change, visual disturbances, diabetes insipidus (polyuria/polydipsia), growth disturbances (eg growth failure , delayed/arrested/precocious puberty), nausea ± vomiting.[492]

Medulloblastoma: Midline cerebellar embryonal tumour (inferior vermis) causing ICP↑, speech difficulty, truncal ataxia ± falls. ♂:♀≈4:1. Peak age: 4yrs. Seeding is along CSF pathways. *Rx:* surgical resection + radio/chemotherapy.

Brainstem astrocytoma: Most common brain tumour in children. Associated with neurofibromatosis 1 and prior radiation. Cranial nerve palsies; pyramidal tract signs (eg hemiparesis); cerebellar ataxia; signs of ICP↑ are rare.

Midbrain and third ventricle tumours may be astrocytomas, pinealomas or colloid cysts (cause posture-dependent drowsiness). *Signs:* behaviour change (early); pyramidal tract and cerebellar signs; upward gaze defect.

Suprasellar gliomas: Visual field defects; optic atrophy; pituitary disorders (growth arrest, hypothyroidism, delayed puberty); diabetes insipidus (DI). Cranial DI is caused by ADH↓, so that there is polyuria and low urine osmolality (always <800mosmol/L) despite dehydration.

Cerebral hemispheres: Usually gliomas. Meningiomas are rare. Fits are common. Signs depend on the lobe involved (OHCM p503). *Tests:* MRI/CT ± EEG. *Options:* Excision if possible; CSF shunting; radiotherapy; chemotherapy alone.[493]

43 Venous sinus thrombosis risk↑ if: infection; perinatal problems; blood dyscrasias. Signs: ↓consciousness (50%), papilloedema (18%), cranial nerve palsy (33%), hemiparesis, hypotonia. Thrombolysis may be needed.[494]

Paediatrics

Other space-occupying lesions Aneurysms; haematomas; granulomas; tuberculomas; cysts (cysticercosis); ►abscess: suspect if ICP↑; T°↑; WCC↑. Get help.

Children's coma scale (An objective record of coma level to help quantify prognosis and monitor progress.) Use if <4yrs; if >4, use Glasgow scale, p778.

• *Best motor response* (6 grades, quantified in the following *blue numbers*):
  6 *Carrying out a request ('obeying command'):* Moves to your request.
  5 *Localizing response to pain:* Put pressure on the patient's finger nail bed with a pencil or sternal pressure: purposeful movements towards changing painful stimuli is a 'localizing' response.
  4 *Withdraws to pain:* Pulls limb away from painful stimulus.
  3 *Flexor response to pain:* Pressure on the nail bed causes abnormal flexion of limbs—decorticate posture (indicative of damage to cerebral hemispheres, thalamus, internal capsule or midbrain) .
  2 *Extensor posturing to pain:* The stimulus causes limb extension (adduction, internal rotation of shoulder, forearm pronation; decerebrate posture from brainstem damage).
  1 *No response to pain:* Score best response of any limb.

• *Best verbal response* (5 grades) If intubated *can the patient grimace?*
  5 Orientated: smiles, is orientated to sounds, fixes and follows objects.
  4 Crying but consolable (or interaction odd/inappropriate)
  3 Inconsistently consolable (or moaning)
  2 Inconsolable crying (or irritable)
  1 No response.

• *Eye opening* (4 grades)
  4 *Spontaneous eye opening.*
  3 *Eye opening in response to speech:* Any, not just a request to open eyes.
  2 *Eye opening to response to pain:* Pain to limbs as above.
  1 *No eye opening.*

Add the score in the 3 areas. Eg: no response to pain + no verbalization + no eye opening = 3. As a rule of thumb, <8≈intubation needed; 4–8≈ intermediate prognosis; 3 ≈ bad prognosis. An alternative (and easier) scale is *AVPU:* Alert; responds to voice; responds to PAIN; Unresponsive.

Paediatrics

Migraine

In children we modify migraine criteria to include moderate to severe *bilateral* or *frontal* headache lasting 1–48h with nausea/vomiting + any 2 of: photophobia, phonophobia (vertigo and abdo pain also occur), sometimes heralded by visual or sensory aura. The headache is aggravated by routine physical activity. If the headache occurs daily, use the term chronic daily headache and manage accordingly. (See *OHCM* p462.) **Prevalence** 5% (10% in adolescence). **Triggers** Diet, dehydration, overtiredness and stress. **Drugs** (as early as possible in an attack); paracetamol (p143); ibuprofen 10mg/kg PO (see p143).[495] Domperidone treats the nausea. If this fails and over 12yrs, try sumatriptan,[496] eg if weight >30kg.[495] **Prophylaxis** If migraine is disrupting social activity or schooling on a regular basis, consider starting prophylaxis. Avoid triggers and get enough sleep. Evidence for what works is poor.[497] Start with a 3 month trial of pizotifen, and if this fails, propranolol. Amitriptylline may also help. **Non-drug treatments** Relaxation training, biofeedback, self-hypnosis, and guided imagery have a role.[498] Signs for prompt referral:
• Headaches of increasing frequency or severity, or if aged <6yrs.
• Headache unrelieved by paracetamol or ibuprofen.
• Irritable; loss of interest/skills; slowing of physical or cognitive development.
• Head circumference above the 97th centile, or greatly out of line.

Other causes of headache Viruses; meningitis; sinusitis (frontal sinus not developed until >10yrs); hypertension (always do BP), stress, behavioural.

Signs Flu-like prodrome, consciousness↓; odd behaviour; vomiting; fits; T°↑; meningism. *Infective causes:* include HSV (↦aciclovir, p200); mumps (ask about parotiditis/testicular pain); varicella zoster (recent chicken pox?); rabies (dog-bite abroad); parvovirus (slapped cheek syndrome); immunocompromise (CMV, EBV, HHV-6); influenza; toxoplasmosis; TB; mycoplasma; malaria (if a possibility do a thick blood film and enlist specialist help, *OHCM* p394); dengue; Rickettsia; Lyme disease.[499] Do CSF PCR; test stool, urine, and blood. *Non-infective differential*: hypoglycaemia; DKA; kernicterus (p115), hepatic failure (eg Reye's syndrome), lead or other poisoning, subarachnoid haemorrhage, malignancy, lupus.[500] **Investigations:** CSF MC&S and PCR; bloods, stool (enteroviruses), urine

▶*Prolonged fevers*—consider: endocarditis; Still's (p654); malignancy.

▶▶Meningitis

Suspect this in any ill baby or child (APLS and NICE guidelines). Symptoms may be subtle, especially in infants—irritability, abnormal cry, lethargy and difficulty feeding. Signs include fever, seizures, apnoea, bulging fontanelle. ▶*Get expert help from your senior*. If there is any hint of meningococcal disease, ▶▶GIVE IV CEFOTAXIME (200mg/kg/24h IV/IM 6hrly). See BNF[c] §5.1.2. Sending blood/CSF cultures must not delay this.

Septic signs Commonly present before meningeal signs—include T°↑; cold hands/feet, limb/joint pain, abnormal skin colour, odd behaviour; rash (fig **2.21**, p205; don't *expect* petechiae with meningococcus); DIC; pulse↑; BP↓; RR↑.

Meningeal signs Comparatively late, and less common in young children, they are neither sensitive nor specific[501]—include stiff neck ('unable to kiss knee'; often absent if <18 months); Kernig's sign (resistance to extending knee with hip flexed); Brudzinski's sign (hips flex on bending head forward); photophobia; opisthotonus.

Other causes of stiff neck Tonsillitis, lymphadenitis, subarachnoid bleed.

Lumbar puncture May be contraindicated in initial management (see p200); if: focal signs; DIC; purpura or *brain herniation* is near (odd posture or breathing; coma scale <13, p201; dilated pupils, doll's eye reflexes, BP↑, pulse↓, papilloedema). Preliminary CT cannot show LP will be safe. If in doubt give antibiotics. *Technique:* (*OHCM* p782) Learn from an expert. •Explain everything to mother. •Get IV access first (if you are doing a procedure bigger than a cannula, you need a cannula first): acute deterioration is possible. Ask an experienced nurse to position child fully flexed (knees to chin) on the side of a bed, with his back exactly at right angles with it. •Mark a point just above (cranial to) a line joining the spinous processes between the iliac crests. •Drape & sterilize the area; put on gloves. •Infiltrate 1mL of 1% lidocaine superficially in the older child. •Insert LP needle aiming towards umbilicus. Keep the needle perpendicular to the back at all times. •Catch 4 CSF drops in each of 3 bottles for: *urgent Gram stain, culture, virology, glucose, protein* (do blood glucose too). •Do CNS observations often. *After LP:* FBC, U&E, culture blood, urine, nose swabs, stool virology. CRP: is it >20mg/L? CXR. Fluid balance, TPR & BP hourly.

Treating pyogenic meningitis before the organism is known

▶▶ Protect airway; give high-flow O₂; set up IVI: if in shock give 0.9% saline in two, 20mL/kg boluses. If persists beyond 2 boluses—give blood as 3rd bolus, consider intubation. Early inotropes improve outcome in sepsis. Call a paediatric intensivist early.

▶▶ Ceftriaxone 50–80mg/kg/day (max2–4g) IV infusion if >3months–18yrs.

▶▶ Cefotaxime 50mg/kg—/12h if <7d; /8h if 7-21d; /6h if <21 days-3months) PLUS amoxicillin/ampicillin p204.

▶▶ Dexamethasone (0.15mg/kg/6h IV eg for 4 days) with 1st antibiotic dose if child >3months and not meningococcal septicaemia (↓ hearing loss in pneumococcal meningitis but otherwise not clearly beneficial).

►►If pre-hernia signs, treat for ICP↑ (p200), eg mannitol 20%, 2.5-5mL/kg IVI.
Treat for cryptococcus if HIV+ve. After culture, check the minimum inhibitory concentration (MIC) of the antibiotics used to the organism *in vitro*.

Complications Secondary abscesses, subdural effusion, hydrocephalus, ataxia, paralysis, deafness (steroids prevent this), IQ↓, epilepsy, brain abscess.

CSF in meningitis	Pyogenic	Tubercular	Aseptic	Normal range if >1 month old
Appearance[502,503]	Often turbid	May be fibrin web	Usually clear	Clear
Predominant cell	Polymorphs eg 1000/mm³	Mononuclear 10-350/mm³	Mononuclear 50-1500/mm³	≤5 lymphocytes; ~0 neutrophils
Glucose level	<⅔ of blood	<⅔ of blood	>⅔ of blood	>⅔ of blood
Protein (mg/dL)	↑ (mean ≈300)	↑ >40 (mean ≈200)	≥40 and <1500	<40

Bacterial antigen detection for N. meningitidis, H. influenzae & streps helps in partially treated meningitis. CSF lactate typically rises before the CSF glucose falls in pyogenic meningitis.

Preventing deaths from meningococcal disease *Most children survive with prompt treatment.*
- Rapid skilled assessment of all febrile children.
- Don't expect meningeal signs; septicaemic signs are more fatal.
- Any rash (or none) will do for the meningococcus. If you wait for purpura, you may be waiting until the disease is untreatable.
- For any acutely unwell child *leave your consulting room door ajar.* Explain that a doctor can be contacted *at any time* if:
  - He seems to be worsening
  - A rash develops
  - Poor response to antipyretics
  - Cold hands or feet; odd skin colour
  - Unrousable or crying in an odd way
  - Odd features eg limb/joint pain.
- Beware fever + lethargy + vomiting, even if no headache or photophobia.
- Give parenteral penicillin *early* (p205), before admission to hospital.
- Monitor pulse, BP, respiratory rate, pupil size/reactivity, level of consciousness (AVPU, p103); WCC and platelets (both may be ↓).
- Urgent activation and transfer to paediatric intensive care unit (PICU). Do blood gases to assess degree of acidosis. Alert haematology that blood and blood products may be required. Intubation, ventilation, and vigorous IV fluid resuscitation must be prompt. Monitor catheter urine output. Crossmatch blood. Continuously monitor ECG.
- Inotropes may be needed: dopamine or **dobutamine** (same dose) eg at 10mcg/kg/min (put 15mg/kg in 50mL of 5% glucose and infuse at 2mL/h).[504] This is OK by peripheral vein, but if adrenaline is needed, use a central line (0.1mcg/kg/min, ie 300mcg/kg in 50mL of 0.9% saline at 1mL/h).[504]
- If plasma glucose <3, give 10% glucose 5mL/kg as a bolus, then as needed.

Heroic, non-standard ideas: Extracorporeal membrane oxygenation; terminal fragment of human bactericidal/permeability-increasing protein (rBPI21) to ↓cytokines; heparin with protein C concentrate to reverse coagulopathy; plasmapheresis to remove cytokines, and thrombolysis (rTPA) for limb reperfusion.[505]

Other issues Ensure immunization (protein–polysaccharide conjugate vaccine prevents type C; from April 2015 in the UK a meningitis B vaccine has been introduced). Inform your local CDC (consultant in communicable diseases). ►Stop parents smoking! 37% of cases are put down to aerosolized spread via smokers coughs.[506]

Meningococcal prophylaxis for contacts with aerosolized meningococci.[507] Rifampicin—12hrly for 4 doses PO: if <1yr, 5mg/kg; 1-12yrs: 10mg/kg (max 600mg); >12yrs: 600mg. It interacts with the contraceptive Pill, can stain contact lenses, and turns urine red. **Ceftriaxone** single IM dose: 125mg if <12yr; 250mg if >12yr. **Ciprofloxacin** 500mg PO is an option if ≥12yrs old (250mg if 5–12yrs).

Paediatrics

The meningococcus, the pneumococcus, and, in the unvaccinated, *Haemophilus influenzae* are the great killers. In the former, the interval between seeming well and coma may be counted in hours. If you suspect meningococcal disease, give **benzylpenicillin** (see BOX) before hospital admission᷄ᷓᷜᷔ (do not worry about ruining the chance of a positive blood or CSF culture later).

Neisseria meningitidis Abrupt onset ± rash (figs 2.21 & 2.23) (purpuric or not, eg starting as pink macules on legs in 20%); septicaemia may occur with no meningitis (Waterhouse–Friderichsen, *OHCM* p707), so early LPS may be normal, giving false reassurance. Arthritis, conjunctivitis, myocarditis & DIC may coexist. *Typical age:* Any. *Film:* Gram -ve cocci in pairs (long axes parallel), often within polymorphs. Drug of choice: **cefotaxime/ceftriaxone** (p202) or **benzylpenicillin** 50mg/kg/4h IV. If penicillin and cephalosporin-allergic, give **chloramphenicol** (below). Treat shock with colloid (± inotropes, p203). *Prevention:* p202.

Haemophilus influenzae (Rare if immunized). *Typical age:* <4yrs. *Drugs:* **Ceftriaxone** (p202) or, where there is no resistance, **chloramphenicol** 12–25mg/kg/6h IVI (neonates: see *BNF*) + IV **ampicillin**—if ≤1wk old, 30–60mg/kg/12h (/8h if 1wk–3wks old; /6h if 3–4wks old). If >4wks old 25mg/kg/6h (max 1g), doubled in severe infections. **Rifampicin** (below) may also be needed. With **chloramphenicol**, monitor peak levels; aim for 20–25mcg/mL; usual doses may be far exceeded to achieve this. (Trough level: <15mcg/mL.) As soon as you can, switch to PO (more effective). **Steroids** (p202) prevent hearing loss.

Strep pneumoniae Typical age: Any. *Risk factors:* Respiratory infections, skull fracture (▶is this 'minor runny nose' CSF rhinorrhoea?), meningocele, HIV.[509] *Film:* Gram +ve cocci. ℞: **Ceftriaxone**, p202 or **benzylpenicillin** 50mg/kg/4h slow IV—or, if resistance likely (eg parts of Europe and USA) ± **rifampicin**. As an add-in or an alternative, consider **vancomycin**, if >1 month old: 15mg/kg/8h (max 2g/24h) IVI over 1h, but CSF penetration is unreliable.[510] Monitor U&E.

Escherichia coli This is a major cause of meningitis in neonates (in whom signs may consist of feeding difficulties, apnoea, seizures, and shock). Drug of choice: **cefotaxime** (p202) or **gentamicin** (p175).

Group B haemolytic streptococci eg *via* mother's vagina (so swab mothers whose infants suddenly fall ill at ~24h-old). Infection may be delayed a month. Drug of choice: **benzylpenicillin** 25–50mg/kg/8–12h slow IV.

Listeria monocytogenes presents soon after birth with meningitis or septicaemia (± pneumonia). It is rare unless immunocompromised. Microabscesses form in many organs (granulomatosis infantiseptica). *Δ:* Culture blood, CSF, placenta, amniotic fluid. ℞: IV **ampicillin** (above) + **gentamicin** (p175).[511]

TB (fig 2.22) can cause CNS infarcts, demyelination with cranial nerve lesions, and tuberculomas ± meningitis (long prodrome with lethargy, malaise, and anorexia). Photophobia and neck stiffness are likely to be absent. The 1st few CSFs may be normal, or show visible fibrin webs and widely varying cell counts. *Dose examples:* **Isoniazid** 10mg/kg/24h PO max 500mg (? with vit B₆) + **rifampicin** 10mg/kg/24h (≤600mg/day) for 1yr + (for 2 months) **pyrazinamide** 35mg/kg/day with eg **streptomycin** if >4wks old, eg 20–30mg/kg once daily (max 1g) IM adjusted to give a peak plasma level <40mcg/mL and a trough of <3mcg/mL; alternative: **ethambutol** 15mg/kg/day PO if old enough to report visual problems.[512,513] Adding **dexamethasone** improves survival (at least in those >14yrs old) but probably does not prevent disability.[514] Children <14 should be given **prednisolone** 4mg/kg/24h for 4 weeks then follow a reducing course.[513]

Other bacteria Leptospiral species (canicola); *Brucella*; *Salmonella*.

Causes of 'aseptic' meningitis Viruses (eg mumps, echo, herpes, polio), partially treated bacterial infections, cryptococcus (use ink stains).

Giving IM benzylpenicillin before hospital admission

- 300mg IM up to 1 year old.
- 600mg if 1–9yrs.
- 1.2g if >10yrs.
- When in doubt, give it: it may be negligent not to do so.
- If penicillin-allergic, **cefotaxime** may be used (50mg/kg IM stat; if >12yrs 1g).[515]

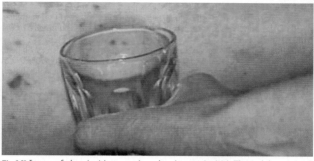

Fig 2.21 Image of glass test in purpuric rashes (eg meningitis). The rash has stained, and does not blanch. © Dr Petter Brandtzaeg, and the Meningitis Trust.

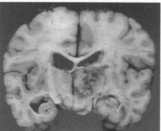

Fig 2.22 Tuberculoma. Caseous (cheese-like) necrotic material is surrounded by epithelioid cell granulomas. Rupture releases mycobacteria into the subarachnoid space, hence causing TB meningitis. © Prof. Dimitri Agamanolis.

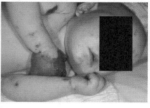

Fig 2.23 4-month-old girl with gangrene of hands due to meningococcaemia. Courtesy of the U.S. Centers for Disease Control and Prevention.

Epilepsy is a tendency to intermittent abnormal electrical brain activity. 1% of children will have had a seizure (not associated with fever) by the age of 14 years. Classification depends on whether signs are referable to one part of a hemisphere (partial epilepsy) or not (generalized), and on whether consciousness is affected (complex) or not (simple). Seizures in *generalized epilepsy* may be:

• *Tonic/clonic (grand mal):* Limbs stiffen (the tonic phase) and then jerk forcefully (clonic phase), with loss of consciousness.

• *Absences (petit mal):* Brief (eg 10sec) pauses ('he stops in mid-sentence, and carries on where he left off'); eyes may roll up; he/she is *unaware of the attack*.

• *Infantile spasms/West syndrome:* Peak age: 5 months. Clusters of head nodding ('Salaam attack') and arm jerks, every 3–30sec. IQ↓ in ~70%.[516] EEG is characteristic (hypsarrhythmia). ℞: prednisolone 1st line; 2nd line vigabatrin (SE: visual field defects);[517] some specialists prefer ACTH.[518]

• *Myoclonic seizures:* 1–4yrs; eg 'thrown' suddenly to the ground. ℞: valproate.

Partial epilepsy: Signs are referable to part of one hemisphere. Complex phenomena: (temporal lobe fits) consciousness↓; automatisms (lip smacking, rubbing face, running); fits of pure pleasure.[519,520]

Causes: Often none is found. Infection (eg meningitis); hyponatraemia, glucose↓, Ca^{2+}↓, Mg^{2+}↓; Na^+↑↓; toxins; trauma; metabolic defects; tuberous sclerosis; CNS tumour (<2%) or malformation; flickering lights, eg TV; exercise.[521]

ΔΔ: Arrhythmias eg prolonged QT, migraine, narcolepsy, night terrors, faints (reflex anoxic seizures, p207), tics, Münchausen's (eg by proxy, OHCM p720).

Tests: Expert EEG; MRI is the preferred choice—it is more sensitive and has no exposure to radiation. CT may be more available and not require an anaesthetic—use in emergent situations to look for acute haemorrhage/lesions.[522]

A simple febrile convulsion is a *single* tonic–clonic, symmetrical generalized seizure lasting <15min, occurring as T°↑ rises rapidly in a febrile illness—typically in a normally developing child (½–6yrs old). Think of meningo-encephalitis, CNS lesion, epilepsy, trauma, glucose↓, Ca^{2+}↓, or Mg^{2+}↓ if: • Focal CNS signs or CNS abnormality • Previous history of epilepsy • The seizure lasts >15min (but, a complex febrile seizure may last >15min) • There is >1 attack in 24h. *Lifetime prevalence:* ~3% of children have at least one febrile convulsion. *Examination:* Find any infection; if any neck stiffness consider meningitis. ℞: Put in recovery position; if fit is lasting >5min: lorazepam IV, buccal midazolam (p208), or diazepam PR.[523] paracetamol syrup (p143). Consider FBC, U&E, Ca^{2+}, glucose, MSU, CXR, ENT swabs.[524] *To LP or not LP?* Risk of pyogenic meningitis is as low (<1.3%) as the risk in a febrile child with no seizures[525] if *all* the above criteria are fulfilled. Avoid LP in the post ictal period as a CNS assessment will be impossible. If you suspect meningitis, then treat *now*. *Parental education:* Allay fear (a child is *not* dying during a fit). Febrile convulsions don't usually (≤3%) mean risk of epilepsy. For the 50% having recurrences, teach carers to give standard antipyretics early in any febrile illness. If the seizure lasts >10min treat as status epilepticus. *Further prevention:* There is poor evidence to support measures to prevent febrile seizures. Explain that all fevers (eg vaccination-associated) should prompt oral antipyretics (p142), but that this does not necessarily avoid another seizure, with buccal midazolam to hand if needed. *Prognosis:* In typical febrile convulsions (defined above) there is no progress to epilepsy in 97%.[526] Risk is much higher if pre-existing CNS abnormality (50%), epilepsy in a 1st-degree relative, or complex febrile seizures.

This is often a true dilemma, and it matters as epilepsy treatment can be toxic. Also, if it is harmful to label any child, it is doubly so to mislabel a child. So always get help with the diagnosis. Watching and waiting, repeat EEGs, and videos of attacks (eg on mobile phone) may be needed.[527] About a third of children diagnosed with epilepsy have non-epileptic events, and half of adolescents presenting to the emergency department in 'status epilepticus' actually have non-epileptic psychologically-induced episodes. Neonates and infants commonly get benign neonatal sleep myoclonus, where single or repetitive jerking movements of the arms and legs occur while falling asleep; they may also get shuddering attacks. Toddlers may have breath-holding attacks and reflex-anoxic seizures (see below), night terrors, febrile myoclonus, benign paroxysmal vertigo of childhood and benign paroxysmal torticollis. In childhood, daydreaming can appear similar to an absence seizure. Fainting can be followed by myoclonic jerks. **Psychologically determined paroxysmal events (PDPE)** Used to describe episodes of psychological origin; they may be triggered by specific situations, movements cannot be explained anatomically, and there is rapid return to normal. Injury and passing urine may occur. PDPE should be acknowledged by parents and the child that these attacks are non-epileptic and any gain from this behaviour should be removed. Psychological support is essential.

Some specific types of seizure

Reflex anoxic attacks Paroxysmal, self-limited brief (eg 15sec) asystole triggered by pain, fear (eg at venepuncture) or anxiety. During this time the child is deathly pale—± hypotonia, rigidity, upward eye deviation, clonic movements, and urinary incontinence. Typical age: 6 months to 2 years (but may be much older). *Prevalence:* 0.8% of preschool children. ΔΔ: Epilepsy is often misdiagnosed, as the trigger aspect to the history is ignored or unwitnessed. When in difficulty, refer to a specialist for vagal excitation tests under continuous EEG & ECG monitoring NB: tongue-biting is not described in reflex anoxic seizures. *Management:* Check ferritin >50ng/mL. Drugs are rarely needed. Atropine has been tried, to reduce sensitivity to vagal influences. Anticonvulsants are not needed. Pacemakers might be an option. *What to tell parents:* Avoid the term 'seizure', as this is all that is likely to be remembered. *White breath-holding attacks* is a useful synonym. Emphasize its benign nature, and that the child usually grows out of it (but it may occur later in life, and in older siblings).[528]

Panayiotopoulos syndrome (6% of all epilepsies) A benign focal seizure disorder occurring in early and mid-childhood (peak age: 5yrs). Autonomic symptoms may predominate. EEG: shifting and/or multiple foci, often with occipital predominance. It occurs mainly at night, with vomiting and eye deviation with impaired consciousness before the convulsion starts. Many seizures last for 30 minutes (some may last hours)—but there is no permanent brain damage. *Treatment:* As remission often occurs within 2 years, antiepileptic medication is often not needed. Reassure.[529]

Age-dependent epileptic encephalopathy Ohtahara syndrome: tonic spasms ± clustering. EEG: suppression-burst.[530] Chloral hydrate may help.[530] This transforms over time into West syndrome, and thence to Lennox-Gastaut syndrome. Think of these as age-specific epileptic reactions to non-specific exogenous CNS insults, acting at specific developmental stages.[531]

Rolandic epilepsy (benign epilepsy with centrotemporal spikes, BECTS) 15% of all childhood epilepsy. Infrequent, brief partial fits with unilateral facial or oropharyngeal sensory-motor symptoms, speech arrest ± hypersalivation. Treatment is rarely needed. Sulthiame may be used in some units.[532,533]

Stepwise ℞ of status epilepticus Call for help. ABC. Supportive therapy: •Secure airway; give O₂. •Secure IV access. Do BP, pulse, glucose, Ca²⁺ (±Mg²⁺). Set a clock in motion •Check T°; if ↑, give rectal paracetamol (it may be a febrile convulsion) ►If hypoglycaemic baby, give glucose 2mL/kg IV of 10% solution, then repeat blood glucose (rare in older children). Neonates: p112; see also APLS, p236–9.)

►►Seizure control: proceed to the next step only if fits continue	
0min	►►ABC. High-flow O₂. Estimate weight. Check blood glucose. IV access.
5min	►►Lorazepam 0.1mg/kg IV; slow bolus via a large vein *OR* buccal midazolam 0.3–0.5mg/kg; squirt half between lower gum and the cheek on each side.
15min	Repeat lorazepam. **Call for senior help. Prepare phenytoin.**
20min	►►Phenytoin 18mg/kg IVI; over 20min. Monitor ECG OR (if on regular phenytoin) ►►Phenobarbital 18mg/kg over 5min *Call PICU & your anaesthetist—prepare for intubation* locate ET tube,ᵉᵗᶜ p626.
40min	►►Rapid sequence induction. Transfer to PICU.

►These times refer to elapsed time on the clock from the 1st drug, not gaps between each drug. Some authorities recommend starting ventilation earlier, and always be ready to do this to protect the airway.

Tests SaO₂, glucose, U&E, Ca²⁺, Mg²⁺, arterial gases, FBC, ECG. Consider anticonvulsant levels, toxicology screen, blood ammonia (requires special blood bottle), lumbar puncture (after resolution), culture blood and urine, virology, EEG, MRI, CT, carbon monoxide level, lead level, amino acid levels, metabolic screen.

Once the crisis is over Refer to a specialist: is MRI or prophylaxis, eg with sodium valproate or carbamazepine (p209) needed? Aim to use one drug only. Increase dose until fits stop, or toxic levels reached. Out of the context of status, prophylaxis is typically started after the 2nd seizure. Choice of anti-epileptic drug (AED) should be based on epilepsy syndrome/presenting seizure type.

Carbamazepine SE: Rash (± exfoliation); platelets↓, agranulocytosis, aplasia (all rare). It induces its own enzymes, so increasing doses may be needed.

Sodium valproate (200mg/5mL). SE: vomiting, appetite↑, drowsiness, platelets↓ (do FBC pre-℞). Rare hepatotoxicity can be fatal (eg if coexisting unsuspected metabolic disorder). Monitor LFT, eg in 1st 6 months. When prescribing to girls of childbearing potential, warn of teratogenic risk (carbamazepine also).

Ethosuximide The syrup is 250mg/5mL. SE: D&V, rashes, erythema multiforme, lupus syndromes, agitation, headache. Indication: absence seizures.

Lamotrigine Uses: absences and intractable epilepsy as an add-on. Dose when given with valproate if 2–12yrs: 0.15mg/kg/day PO for 2wks, then 0.3mg/kg daily for 2wks, then ↑ by up to 0.3mg/kg every 1–2 weeks. Usual maintenance: 1–5mg/kg/day (higher if with non-valproate anticonvulsants: ~2.5–7mg/kg/12h).

Vigabatrin (May be 1st choice in infantile spasms and tuberous sclerosis fits.) This blocks GABA transaminase. Consider adding it to regimens if partial seizures are uncontrolled. Starting dose: 15–20mg/kg/12h increased after 2wks to a typical dose of 30–40mg/kg/12h (max 150mg/kg/day). Blood levels do not help (but monitor concurrent phenytoin: it may fall by ~20%). SE: Drowsiness, depression, psychosis, amnesia, diplopia, and field defects (test every year).

Levetiracetam licensed for used as monotherapy for focal seizures—but thought not cost-effective (NICE). Increasingly used in preference to phenytoin for status epilepticus SE: depression; lethargy; weakness.

Diet Consider a high-fat ketogenic diet under speciliast supervision if 2 drugs fail to work (it can ↓ fits by ⅔).⁵³⁴ SE: constipation, vomiting, ↓energy, hunger.

Education Showers are safer than baths. Emphasize compliance/concordance (one seizure may ↓the threshold for the next, referred to as kindling).⁵³⁵

Newer anticonvulsants NICE reserves gabapentin, lamotrigine, oxcarbazepine, tiagabine, topiramate, and vigabatrin (as an adjunct for partial seizures) for children not benefiting from (or able to tolerate) older drugs (p208) or older drugs have contraindications/interactions (the Pill)—or the child is of childbearing potential or is likely to need drugs into her childbearing years.[514]

Drug	Starting dose mg/kg/24h	Target dose for initial assessment of effect mg/kg/24h	Dose increment		Interval in days	Usually effective dose mg/kg/24h	Doses per day	Target trough drug level in plasma	
			Size mg/kg/24h					mg/L	µmol/L
Carbamazepine	5	12.5	2.5		7	10-25	2-3	4-12	
Valproate	10	20	10.0		10	15-40	1-2	Not helpful	
Phenytoin	5	7	1.0		10	5-15	2	10-20	40-80
Phenobarbital	3	6	0.5		1	4-8	1-2	15-40	60-180
Ethosuximide	10	15	5.0		5	10-20	1-2	40-99	280-700
Clonazepam	0.025	0.05	0.025		7	0.025-0.1	2-3	Not helpful	

Which drug?

Tonic–clonic fits: First try **sodium valproate**. If unsuitable try lamotrigine (may exacerbate myoclonic seizures) or carbamazepine (may exacerbate myoclonic and absence seizures). Adjunctive treatment includes clobazam, levetiracetam, or topiramate.

Absences: First choice, **ethosuximide**; second, **sodium valproate**. If neither work, try lamotrigine, then try combinations. Carbamazepine, gabapentin, oxcarbazepine, phenytoin, tiagabine, and vigabatrin are not recommended for absence seizures.

Myoclonic or akinetic fits: **Sodium valproate** is first line. Levetiracetam or topiramate are second line.

Infantile spasms: Vigabatrin (or corticosteroids).

Partial fits: First try carbamazepine or lamotrigine; then sodium valproate or oxcarbazepine.

If drugs fail Do not use ever more toxic combinations: ►refer for neurosurgical advice and MRI.[536] In drug-resistant epilepsy, surgery or a ketogenic diet may help. See p208 and *Pediatr Neurol*: 2008;38(1):38–43. ❀

Stopping anticonvulsants See *OHCM* p497. The risk of seizure recurrence during the tapering down process is no greater if the tapering period is 6 weeks compared with 9 months.

Data from Brodie MJ et al. (1996). Antiepileptic drugs. NEJM 334:168–75; and Engel J et al. (2007). *Epilepsy: A Comprehensive Textbook*. Philadelphia, PA: Lippincott Williams & Wilkins.[538]

► *Only enter battles you can win*. If the child can win, be more subtle, eg consistent rewards, not inconsistent punishments. Get a health visitor's advice; ensure everyone is encouraging the same response from the child.

Entrances *Food refusal* and *food fads* are common. Reducing pressure on the child, discouraging parental over-reaction, and gradual enlarging of tiny portions of attractive food are usually all that is needed. Check ferritin and FBC. Keep a watchful eye on growth and weight gain. *Overeating:* Eating comforts, and if the child is short on comfort, or if mother feels inadequate, the scene is set for overeating and lifelong patterns are begun. Diets may fail until the child is hospitalized (p382). If obese (p156, p226, p514), remember hypothalamic syndromes (eg the very rare Prader–Willi, p652), but the treatment remains the same.

Pica is eating things which are not food, eg plastic, or faeces (coprophagia); if persistent, look for other disturbed behaviours, autism, or ↓IQ. *Causes:* Iron or other mineral deficiency; obsessive-compulsive disorder. *Complications:* Lead poisoning; worm infestations.[539] Treating iron deficiency helps; otherwise behaviour modification.[540]

Exits *Constipation* is difficulty in defecation; it may comprise of <3 stools per week; large hard stool; 'rabbit dropping' stool; distress/straining/bleeding with passage of stool. It may lead to abdominal pain, abdominal masses, overflow soiling ± 'lavatory-blocking' enormous stools (megarectum), and anorexia. Causes: diet, poor fluid, or fibre intake—or fear, eg as a result of a fissure. Rarely Hirschprung's disease (p130). Failure to pass meconium in first 48h? Ask about onset of constipation and precipitants (fissure/change in diet/timing of potty training/fears and phobias/moving house/acute infections/family upheavals).

Red flags include:
- Constipation from birth or first few weeks.
- Failure to pass meconium within 48h.
- Faltering growth (an amber flag really; consider coeliac disease/hypothyroid).
- New weakness/abnormal reflexes in legs, delayed locomotion.
- Abnormal appearance of anus / skin in sacral/gluteal region (look for sacral dimples/hairy patches/flattening of gluteal muscles/multiple fissures).
- Gross abdominal distension with vomiting.

Action: • Find out about potty/toilet refusal • Does defecation hurt? • Is there parental coercion? Break the vicious cycle of: large faeces → pain/fissure → fear of the pot → rectum overstretched → call-to-stool sensation dulled → soiling → parental exasperation → coercion. ► Exonerate the child to boost confidence for the main task of obeying calls-to-stool to keep the rectum empty. *Treat* faecal impaction with escalating dose regimen of polyethylene glycol 3350 + electrolytes eg 'Movicol® Paediatric Plain' as 1st-line intervention (NICE suggests doses, which exceed those in the BNF^c, as follows: if <1y then ½–1 sachet daily; if aged 2–5y then 2 sachets on day 1; increase by 2 sachets every 2 days to max. of 8 sachets daily; if 5–12y start on 4 sachets and increase in steps of 2 to a maximum of 12 per day. If >12y use Movicol® or equivalent (lacks electrolytes and contains a higher dose of polyethylene glycol 3350) at 4 sachets on day 1, escalating by 2 sachets/day to a maximum of 8. Follow this with maintenance 'Movicol® Paediatric Plain' (<12y)/Movicol® (>12y) ± lactulose ± prolonged alternate-day senna, adjusting dose to produce regular soft stools.

NB: behaviour therapy in combination with laxatives is effective,[542] but biofeedback methods are not.[543] Clinics run by nurse specialists can be more effective than those run by consultants.[544] Dietary modifications to ensure a balanced diet, with sufficient fluids and fibre are necessary but not sufficient by themselves. Encourage daily physical activity. Treat perianal cellulitis with amoxicillin.

Paediatrics

Digital rectal examination and abdominal x-rays are rarely required. Do not use enemas until all attempts at oral medication have failed.

Soiling is the escape of stool into the underclothing.

Faecal incontinence is faecal soiling in the context of a physical/anatomical lesion (Hirschsprung's disease, anal malformation, anal trauma, meningomyelocele, muscle diseases).[545]

Encopresis is the repeated passage of solid faeces in the wrong place in those >4yrs old. ♂:♀≈5:1. It may be voluntary or non-voluntary. It is usually due to overflow in constipation, but may occasionally be a behavioural response to sexual abuse. Treat retentive encopresis (80% of cases) with enemas, extra dietary fibre, stool softeners, and 'mandatory' daily toilet sittings ~15–30min after eating. Try behaviour therapy and referral to a child and adolescent psychiatrist for non-retentive soiling—it is part of an emotional disorder.[546] NB: this demarcation is not absolute: behavioural techniques such as differential attention, contingency management, and contracting are relevant to both forms of encopresis.[547] Rarely, encopresis signifies autoeroticism or a defecation disorder or learning difficulty.[548] Whatever the cause, ☺adopt a holistic stance and set the symptom in the family context. This is important because we know that encopresis is associated with anxiety, depression, attention difficulties, and environments with less expressiveness and poor organization, and social problems (disruptive behaviour, poorer school performance etc).[549] Aim to give the family time to air feelings that encopresis engenders (anger, shame, ridicule).

Enuresis: Infrequent bedwetting (<2 nights/week) occurs in ~15% at 5yrs and 5% at 10yrs. 1–2% of >15y continue to wet the bed, usually from delayed maturation of bladder control (family history often +ve). Girls are earlier to achieve bladder control than boys; enuresis is defined as continued wetting >5yrs and in boys >6yrs. Tests for diabetes, UTI and GU abnormality (p174) can occasionally yield surprises but are by no means compulsory unless there are clinical suspicions. The term 'secondary enuresis' implies wetness after >6 months' dryness, and raises concerns about worries, illness, or abuse. *History:* Ask about nights per week he wets the bed? Does it happen more than once per night? Severe bedwetting is less likely to resolve spontaneously. Are there any daytime symptoms? Frequency/urgency may indicate an overactive bladder; diurnal wetting may respond to oxybutynin. How much does he drink during the day? Is there constipation/soiling; history of recurrent UTI (underlying urological abnormality)? If the child was dry and recently started bedwetting consider systemic illness and the possibility of child abuse. *Treatment:* Start with advice and reassure parents than many children continue to wet the bed after achieving day-time dryness. Ensure that caffeine-based drinks are avoided and the toilet is used regularly during the day (4–7 times is typical). Reassure that he is neither infantile nor dirty. A system of rewards for *agreed behaviours* (eg drinking recommended levels of fluid, using the toilet before bedtime, taking medicines, or helping change the sheets (*not for dry nights which the child can't control*) may be effective. Alarms (± vibrations) triggered by urine in the bed can make 56% dry at 1yr; relapses are preventable by continuing use after dryness. They are cheap or loanable from Child Guidance Services (or equivalent)—eg Drinite®[551] www.bedwetting.co.uk. **Desmopressin** sublingual dose (if >5yrs): 120mcg at bedtime (max 240mcg); useful for sleepovers and school trips but relapse is common. Have 1 week 3-monthly with no drugs. CI: cystic fibrosis, uraemia, BP↑.

Further reading

NICE (2014). *Clinical Knowledge Summaries: Bedwetting (Enuresis)*. http://cks.nice.org.uk/bedwetting-enuresis#!scenariorecommendation:7.

Paediatrics

Speech develops in conjunction with hearing; therefore any impairment in hearing may delay language development. ►Always test the hearing. *Ensure the result is as reliable as possible.* Delayed speech may be an isolated finding and language is divided into expressive (speech) and receptive (comprehension) language. It should be assessed by a speech and language therapist. Delayed speech may also be part of global developmental delay or neurological problems. Check other developmental milestones, examine for neurological deficit and consider autism, especially if there is regression of speech. *There is much variation in speech timing (first word between 11 and 20 months): what is 'clearly abnormal'?*

Speech and language development This dialogue portrays the mystery of language learning: *Daughter:* 'I don't want to eat my ice cream yet.' *Father:* 'Don't procrastinate!' 'Daddy, how can I understand you if you use words I don't understand?'

'If I only ever used words you understood we could never have started talking.'

Early signs that the child is hearing and vocalizing normally:
• Newborn: quietens to voice and startles to loud noises
• 6 weeks: responds to mother's voice
• 12 weeks: begins to laugh, coo and will vocalize when alone or spoken to.

Early language development:
• 6 months: uses consonant monosyllables eg ba and da
• 8 months: non-specific two-syllable babble eg mama, dada
• 13 months: two-syllable words become appropriate in their context; understands single words such as 'no'
• 18 months: vocabulary of 10 words, can demonstrate 6 parts of the body; 2-word phrases eg 'Daddy come.'
• 24 months: subject–verb–object sentences appear eg 'I want ice cream!'

Conversation development:
• Sentence development becomes increasingly complex by the second year
• By age 3, the child knows their age, name, and several colours
• At 3½yrs old... the child has mastered thought, language, abstraction, and the elements of reason, having a 1000-word vocabulary at his or her disposal, enabling sentences such as: 'I give her cake' cos she's hungry'.

Words exist to give ideas currency, and so often that currency proves counterfeit—a process which so often starts with if, eg 'If I hadn't thrown the cup on the ground, I might have got a pudding'. The uttering of 'If...', linked with an emotional response, is the most human of all constructions, opening up worlds divorced from reality, providing for the exercise of imagination, the validation of dreams, the understanding of motives, and the control of events. The rest of life holds nothing to match the intellectual and linguistic pace of these first years. Further linguistic development is devoted to seemingly conceptually minor tasks, such as expanding vocabulary.

Causes of delayed talking

• Familial: family history of language delay; parents have been late in developing speech, or have had speech therapy
• Hearing impairment: chronic otitis media is a common cause of delayed or poor clarity of speech in pre-school age children
• Environmental: deprivation; poor social interaction; abuse
• Neuropsychological: global developmental delay; autism spectrum disorder (see p372); Landau–Kleffner syndrome (epilepsy + progressive loss of language).

Vocabulary size: If <50 words at 3yrs old, suspect deafness—or:
Expressive dysphasia or speech dyspraxia (eg if there is a telegraphic quality to speech, poor clarity, and deteriorating behaviour, eg frustration).
- Audio-premotor syndrome (APM). The child cannot reflect sounds correctly heard into motor control of larynx and respiration. Instead of babbling, the child is quiet, unable to hum or sing.
- Respiro-laryngeal (RL) dysfunction (dysphonia from incorrect vocal fold vibration/air flow regulation). The voice is loud and rough.
- Congenital aphonia (thin effortful voice; it's rare).

Speech clarity: By 2½yrs, parents should understand most speech. If not, suspect deafness—or:
- Articulatory dyspraxia (easy consonants are *b* and *m* with the lips, and *d* with the tongue—the phonetic components of babbling). ♂:♀ ≈ 3:1. Tongue-tie is a possible cause (∴ poor sounds needing tongue elevation— *d* and *s*)—surgery to the frenum may be needed (+speech therapy). Distinguish from phonological causes (disordered *sound for speech processing*—may present as *sound awareness problems* (difficulty in analysing sound structure of words). Both are common.
- APM or RL dysfunction, as described in 'Vocabulary size'.

Understanding: By 2½ years a child should understand 'Get your shoes', if not suspect: • Deafness—if the hearing is impaired (eg 25-40dB loss) secretory otitis media is likely to be the cause. Worse hearing loss is probably sensorineural • Cognitive impairment • Deprivation.

Speech therapy Refer early, before school starts. NB: randomized trials have not shown any clear benefits from this strategy.[552][N=159]

Global neurodevelopmental delay

This is used to describe delay in all skill areas; it may be more pronounced in fine motor, speech, and social skills. There are many causes although in some instances it remains unknown. The more severe the delay, the more likely a cause will be found.
- *Genetic:* Chromosomal disorders eg Down's, fragile X, Duchenne muscular dystrophy, metabolic eg PKU
- *Congenital brain abnormalities:* Hydrocephalus, microcephaly
- *Prenatal cause:* Teratogens such as alcohol and drugs (including prescription), congenital infections (particularly rubella, CMV, or toxoplasmosis), hypothyroidism (rare in Westernized countries)
- *Perinatal cause:* Extreme prematurity leading to intraventricular haemorrhage or periventricular leukomalacia; birth asphyxia; metabolic disorders such as hyperbilirubinaemia or hypoglycaemia
- *Postnatal cause:* Brain injury from suffocation, drowning, head injury; CNS infection, particularly meningitis or encephalitis; hypoglycaemia.

Babies usually learn to walk by ~18 months old. If this has not occurred by then, ask: Is the child physically normal? Is development delayed in other areas? Family history of late walking? Arrange hip x-rays and check creatine kinase (CK). The commonest causes reflect chronic illness, global delay, benign immaturity, and joint hypermobility (MINIBOX). In boys consider Duchenne muscular dystrophy. Exclude cerebral palsy.

Cerebral palsy (CP) comprises chronic disorders of posture and movement caused by non-progressive CNS lesions sustained before 2yrs old, resulting in delayed motor development, evolving CNS signs, learning disability (35%), and epilepsy. Most are due to antenatal events unrelated to birth trauma. *Prevalence:* 9% if gestation 23–27wks; 6% if 28–30wks; 0.1% if term.[553] *Survival:* 20yrs if quadriplegic (much longer if less affected). ♀:♂ ≈1:1. *Signs:* Weakness, paralysis, delayed milestones, seizures, language/speech problems. *Classification:* There are four main types: spastic, dyskinetic, ataxic, and mixed CP. Spasticity suggests a pyramidal lesion; uncoordinated, involuntary movements and postures (dystonias) suggest basal ganglia involvement. Most have either a *spastic hemiplegia* (arm>leg; early development of hand preference—ie <12mth; delay in walking, increased deep reflexes of affected limb) or a *spastic diplegia* (both legs affected worse than the arms, so that the child looks normal until he is picked up, when the legs 'scissor'—hip flexion, adduction and internal rotation; with knee extension and feet plantar-flexed). *Spastic quadriplegia* is the most severe form and is associated with seizures and IQ↓. Swallowing difficulties (2° to retrobulbar palsy) may lead to aspiration pneumonia. *Dyskinetic (athetoid) cerebral palsy:* Unwanted actions; poor movement flow/posture control; spasticity; hypotonia; hearing↓; dysarthria. Association: kernicterus. *Ataxic palsies* are uncommon. There may be hypo- or hypertonia.

⁘Management teams Children's views must be taken into account in all matters concerning them.[554] [UN Convention on the Rights of the Child] ▶*Assume that all disabled children are entitled to a 'full and decent life'.* The aim is quality of life and full integration into society. Because children have grown up hand-in-hand with disability and are often uncowed by it, they often score as high as anyone else on quality of life, if pain is treated.[554] Parents may find it a comfort to know this. Physio- and occupational therapists, orthopaedic surgeons, and orthoses experts aid holistic assessment: can he roll over (both ways)? Sit? Grasp? Transfer objects from hand to hand? Good head righting? Ability to shift weight when prone with forearm support. IQ. Is continence possible? Can he hold a pen or a spoon? Muscle strengthening can help.[555] Callipers may prevent deformity (equinovarus, equinovalgus, hip dislocation from excessive flexion/adduction). Attempts to show benefits of neurophysiotherapy (to help equilibrium and righting) don't show benefit over simple motor stimulation. Some parents try the Hungarian *Petö approach:* ⁘Here the 'conductor' devotes herself to the child, using interaction with peers to reinforce successes: eg manipulation, art, writing, fine movement, and social skills.[556] Treat co-morbidities such as epilepsy (p208). *Botulinum toxin* (p417) benefits many children with spasticity. *Epidural cord electrostimulation & intrathecal or oral baclofen* (benefits uncertain).[557,558] **Prognosis** By 6yrs, 54% with quadriplegia (80% if hemiplegic or diplegic) gain urinary continence spontaneously. If IQ↓, 38% are dry at this age.[559][n=601]

Typical causes
Prenatal factors:
• APH (with hypoxia)
• x-rays
• Alcohol
• CMV; rubella; HIV
• Toxoplasmosis
• Rhesus disease
Perinatal factors:
• Birth trauma
• Fetal distress
• Hypoglycaemia
• Hyperbilirubinaemia
Postnatal factors:
• Trauma/intraventricular haemorrhage
• Hypoxia
• Meningoencephalitis
• Cerebral vein thrombosis (from dehydration)

Paediatrics

WHO definitions *Impairment* entails a pathological process, eg spina bifida, which may cause certain *disabilities*, eg walking difficulty resulting in social consequence (eg cannot walk to school).

Learning difficulties *The mother often makes the first diagnosis.* An IQ <35 constitutes a severe learning disability (p378).

►Beware equating IQ with intellect: the latter implies more than problem-solving and memory. Intellect entails the ability to speculate, to learn from mistakes, to have a view of oneself and others, to see relationships between events in different domains of experience—as well as the ability to use language either to map the world, or to weave ironic webs of truth and deceit (and, on a good day, to do both simultaneously).

Causes: Severe mental impairment usually has a definable cause, whereas mild intellectual disability is often familial, with no well-defined cause. Be prepared to refer to an expert. *Congenital disorders* are legion: chromosomal (eg Down's; fragile X, p648); metabolic (eg PKU p183). *Acquired:* Perinatal infection p34–37, birth injury and cerebral palsy, trauma, meningitis, fetal alcohol spectrum disorder.

Lead exposure: This is a leading preventable cause of mildly impaired IQ. For example in 2-yr-olds for each 0.48μmol/L plasma increment there is an associated 5–8-point fall in IQ as measured on the Wechsler Intelligence Scale for Children (revised). This defect is long-lasting.

Chemical defects associated with intellectual disability—eg *Homocystinuria:* Paraplegia, fits, friable hair, emboli, cataracts; homocystine is found in the urine. Treat with a low-methionine, cystine-supplemented diet, with large doses of pyridoxine. *Maple syrup urine disease:* Hypoglycaemia, acidosis, fits, death. Urine smells of maple syrup, due to defective metabolism of branched chain keto acids. Treatment: high-calorie amino acid controlled diet. Thiamine has been tried. *Tryptophanuria:* Rough, pigmented skin. Treat with nicotinic acid.

Management: Refer to an expert, so that no treatable cause is missed. Would the family like help from group, such as MENCAP? Other members of the family may need special support (eg normal siblings, who now feel neglected). If the IQ is >35, life in the community is the aim.

Physical disability *Sensory:* Deafness, see p548. Blindness: congenital defects are described on p442. Principal acquired causes of blindness are: retinopathy of prematurity, vitamin A deficiency, onchocerciasis (p460), eye injuries, cataract (eg Down's syndrome).

CNS & musculoskeletal problems: (Congenital or acquired) *Causes:* Accidents (eg near-drowning), cerebral palsy (p214), spina bifida (p140), after meningitis, polio, congenital infections (above), tumours, syndromes (p638).

Wheelchairs:[44] For indoors or outdoors? Patient-operated, motorized or pushed? What sort of restraints to prevent falling out? If collapsible, how small must it be to get into the car? Are the sides removable to aid transfer from chair to bed? Can the child control the brakes? Are there adjustable elevated leg rests? Liaise with the physio and occupational therapist.

Callipers will allow some patients to stand and walk. Long-leg callipers are required for those with complete leg paralysis. The top should be constructed so that it does not induce pressure sores. A knee lock supports the knee in the standing position. An internal coil spring prevents foot drop.

44 Disabled Living Foundation: www.dlf.org.uk

Checklist to guide management of disability

In hospitals or the community, we should address each of these points:
• Screening and its documentation on local disability registers.
• Communication with parents.
• Referring to/liaising with district team + community paediatrician.
• Access to specialist services, including physiotherapy, orthopaedic surgery.
• Assessing special needs for schooling and housing.
• Co-ordinating neuropsychological/neurodevelopmental assessments.
• Co-ordinating measures of severity (eg electrophysiology ± CT/MRI).
• Liaison with dietician on special foods.
• Promotion of long-term concordance with treatment/education programmes.
• Education about the consequences of the illness.
• Encourage contact with family support groups.
• Offering family planning *before* patients become unintentionally pregnant.
• Pre-conception counselling; referral to geneticist if appropriate.
• Co-ordinating prenatal diagnostic tests and fetal assessment.

Society, paediatrics in the community, and family-oriented care

Most paediatric care goes on in the community, provided by mothers, fathers, GPs, nurses, physios, community paediatricians, child-minders, special-needs teachers, sports/PE teachers, and their assistants. Inevitably if you are studying paediatrics within hospital you will have a biased view of what paediatrics is like—nowhere more at odds with reality than in the spheres of impairment and disability. ▶*If you really want to make a difference to children's lives, get out into the community at every chance.* Find out what is going on—and then start contributing.

Increasingly, this is being advocated by paediatric training programmes in the UK and abroad—eg the ***Community Paediatrics Training Initiative.***[560]

Children's health and well-being are inextricably linked to their parents' physical, emotional and social health, social circumstances, and child-rearing practices.[561] These cannot be appreciated or moulded to the child's advantage without at least one foot in the community.

No paediatrician can work well without understanding the multicultural demographics and marriage statistics of the population from which her patients come. For example, in some areas the median income of families with married parents has increased by 146% since 1970, but female-headed households have had growth of 131% (less in inner city areas). In one study, the median income of female-headed households was only 47% of that of married-couple families and only 65% of that of families with 2 married parents in which the wife was not employed. The proportion of children who live in poverty is ~5-fold greater for female-headed families than for married-couple families.[561] In the UK, 1.4 million children live in poverty despite one parent having a job.[562] This has a greater effect on children's health than all the goings on in paediatric wards and hospitals. These problems seem resistant to socialism, the minimum wage, tax credits, and benefits.

Most families with young children depend on child care, of varying quality. This causes ↑ costs (only partly mitigated by government funds), long days for children, with stress imposed by travel and exposure to infections.[561]

More and more parents are devoting time once available to their children to the care of their own parents. They won't tell you of this in brief ward encounters, but these facts become clear when working in the community.[561]

☺Paediatricians have a key role in fostering interdisciplinary collaboration between schools, hospitals, and other child-related institutions, and they must feel able to refer parents for physical, emotional, or social problems, or health risk behaviours that can adversely affect the health or emotional or social well-being of their child.

Developmental disorders are a group of conditions leading to impairment in at least one functional area—eg cognition, motor skills (gross or fine), social-emotional, or communication (speech, language, hearing or vision). Around 20-25% of children have at least one developmental delay, and as many as 50% of these will not be detected before starting primary school.[563] Conditions falling under the umbrella of developmental disorders include autism spectrum disorders, speech-language impairment, learning disabilities, and psycho-social problems. *Biological risk factors* include: prematurity, low birth weight, birth asphyxia, chronic illness and hearing/vision impairment. *Environmental risk factors* include: poverty, low parental education, parental mental illness and social isolation, maternal alcohol or other drugs.[564]

Developmental surveillance refers to an ongoing process of following a child over time with a view to contextualizing a child's development. It involves discussing concerns with parents, eliciting a perinatal history, identifying risk factors, as well as observing the child attempting different skills at different times and referring the child when appropriate to other health professionals (eg physiotherapists, speech therapists or audiometrists). Developmental surveillance can be incorporated into well-child checks, general physical examination, and routine immunization visits.

Developmental screening refers to a brief assessment aimed at identifying those children who require further investigation and assessment. It is typically carried out using a developmental screening tool. Screening should be carried out within the broader undertaking of developmental surveillance. Repeating screening at different ages increases the accuracy of the test. Parental concern about a child's development may in itself constitute a reliable screening test.[565] The *Denver Developmental Screening Test (DDST)* and its successor the *Denver II* have largely been replaced with more sensitive tests. Screening may be based on parent report alone (parent-completed tests) or through direct observation together with parent report (directly administered tests). Some of the most commonly used tests are discussed as follows—all are copyrighted products:

The *Parents' Evaluation of Developmental Status (PEDS)* tool is a parent-completed test consisting of 10 questions (8 yes/no, 2 open ended). It can be given to parents to complete prior to attending health visits and takes less than 5 minutes to complete. It has a sensitivity of 74-80% and is suitable for children up to 8 years old.[563] It identifies children as low, moderate, or high risk for various disabilities and identifies an optimal course of action. Available at www.pedtest.com.

The *Ages and Stages Questionnaire (ASQ)*, another parent completed test, consists of 21 age-specific questionnaires. It can be used to evaluate children aged 1 month to 5½ years old. It has a sensitivity of 85% and takes 10-20 minutes to complete.[563] It has a single cut-off score indicating which children need further referral. Available at: www.agesandstages.com.

The *Modified Checklist for Autism in Toddlers (M-CHAT)* is a second-stage parent-completed test that is more specific for autism spectrum disorders. It has a sensitivity of 90%. Available free online at: www.firstsigns.org.

The *Brigance Screens-II* is a directly administered test, combining parental observation and the eliciting of skills from children. It covers multiple domains of development including speech-language, motor, general knowledge, as well as reading and maths at the older age groups.
  Available at: www.curriculumassociates.com.

Whilst the American Association of Pediatrics recommends both developmental surveillance and screening,[566] the National Screening Committee (UK) doesn't recommend developmental screening.[567]

Developmental milestones		
Average age	Milestone	Red flags
6 weeks	• *smiles,* • *follow eyes past midline*	
4–6 months	• *sits with support* • *rolls* • *reaches out for objects* • *starts babbling*	At 6 months if • no smile • no grasp • not rolling • poor head control
6–9 months	• *crawls* • *sits without support* • *pulls to stand* • *gives toy on request* • *turns head to name* • *responds to 'bye-bye'* • *gestures with babbling* • *first tooth*	At 9 months if • no response to words • lack of eye contact or facial expression • no gestures • no passing of toys from hand to hand • not sitting without support or crawling
7–12 months	• *develops pincer grasp* • *plays 'peek-a-boo'* • *walks with a hand held* • *waves goodbye*	At 12 months if • unable to pick up small items • not crawling / bottom shuffling • not standing holding on to furniture • no babbled phrases
12–15 months	• *single words* • *listens to stories* • *drinks from cup*	
18 months	• *speaks 6 words* • *able to walk up steps* • *names pictures* • *walks independently* • *scribbles* • *builds with blocks*	• uninterested in playing with others • no clear words • not walking without support • not able to hold crayon • unable to stack 2 blocks
1.5–2 years	• *kicks/throws a ball* • *runs* • *2-word sentences* • *follows a 2-step command* • *stacks 5–6 blocks* • *turns pages* • *uses a spoon* • *helps with dressing*	At 2 years if • has <50 words • difficulty handling small objects • unable to climb stairs • no interest in feeding or dressing

Paediatrics

If there is regression, or loss of a previously developed skill, this should be considered a red flag requiring immediate investigation. Other red flags at any age include poor interaction with others, difference in strength between right and left sides of body, abnormal tone, and strong parental concern.

Paediatrics

Biochemistry (1mmol = 1mEq/L)

Albumin^P	36–48g/dL
Alk phos^P	see below
α1-antitrypsin^P	1.3–3.4g/dL
Ammonium^P	2–25μmol/L; 3–35mcg/dL
Amylase^P	70–300u/L
Aspartate aminotransferase^P	<40u/L
Bilirubin^P	2–16μmol/L; 0.1–0.8mg/dL
Blood gases, arterial	pH 7.36–7.42
$PaCO_2$	4.3–6.1kPa; 32–46mmHg
PaO_2	11.3–14.0kPa; 85–105mmHg
Bicarbonate^P	21–25mmol/L
Base excess	−2 to +2mmol/L
Calcium^P	2.25–2.75mmol/L; 9–11mg/dL
neonates:	1.72–2.47; 6.9–9.9mg/dL
Chloride^P	98–105mmol/L
Cholesterol^{P,F}	≤5.7mmol/L; 100–200mg/dL
Creatine kinase^P	<80u/L
Creatinine^P	25–115μmol/L; 0.3–1.3mg/dL
Glucose^F	2.5–5.3mmol/L; 45–95mg/dL
(lower in newborn; fluoride tube)	
IgA^S	0.8–4.5g/L (low at birth, Rising to adult levels slowly)
IgG^S	5–18g/L (high at birth, falls and then rises slowly to adult level)
IgM^S	0.2–2.0g/L (low at birth, rises to adult level by 1 year)
IgE^S	<500u/mL

Iron^S	9–36μmol/L; 50–200mcg/dL
Lead^{EDTA}	<1.75μmol/L; <36mcg/dL
Mg^{2+P}	0.6–1.0mmol/L
Osmolality^P	275–295mosmol/L
Phenylalanine^P	0.04–0.21mmol/L
Potassium^P mean mmol/L	3.5–5.5
Protein^P	63–81g/L; 6.3–8.1g/dL
Sodium^P	136–145mmol/L
Transferrin^S	2.5–4.5g/L
Triglyceride^{F,P}	0.34–1.92mmol/L
	(=30–170mg/dL)
Urate^P	0.12–0.36mmol/L; 2–6mg/dL
Urea^P	2.5–6.6mmol/L; 15–40mg/dL
Gamma-glutamyl transferase^P	<20u/L

Hormones—a guide ▶ Consult lab

Cortisol^P	9am 200–700nmol/L
	midnight <140nmol/L, mean
Dehydroepiandrosterone sulfate^P:	
day 5–11	0.8–2.8μmol/L (range)
5–11yrs	0.1–3.6μmol/L
17α-Hydroxyprogesterone^P:	
days 5–11	1.6–7.5nmol/L (range)
4–15yrs	0.4–4.2nmol/L
T$_4$ ^{P}	60–135nmol/L (not neonates)
TSH^P	<5mu/L (higher on day 1–4)

B=boy; ^{EDTA}=edetic acid; ^{F}=fasting
G=girl; ^{P}=plasma; ^{S}=serum.

Alk phos^P u/L: *0–½yr* 150–600; *½–2yr* 250–1000; *2–5yr* 250–850; *6–7yr* 250–1000; *8–9yr* 250–750; *10–11yr* G = 259–950, B ≤ 730; *12–13yr* G = 200–750, B ≤ 785; *14–15yr* G = 170–460, B = 170–970; *16–18yr* G = 75–270, B = 125–720; *>18yr* G = 60–250, B = 50–200.

Haematology mean ± ~1 standard deviation. Range ×10⁹/L (median in brackets)

Day	Hb *g/L*	MCV *fl*	MCHC %	Retics %	WCC	Neutrophils	Eosins	Lymphs	Monos
1	190±20	119±9	31.6±2	3.2±1	9–30	6–26	(11)	0.02–0.8	2–11	0.4–3.1
4	186±20	114±7	32.6±2	1.8±1	9–40				
5	176±10	114±9	30.9±2	1.2±0.2					
Weeks									
1–2	173±20	112±19	32.1±3	0.5±0.03	5–21	1.5–10	(5)	0.07–0.1	2–17	0.3–2.7
2–3	156±30	111±8	33.9±2	0.8±0.6	6–15	1–9.5	(4)	0.07–0.1	2–17	0.2–2.4
4–5	127±20	101±8	34.9±2	0.9±0.8	6–15		(4)		(6)	
6–7	120±20	105±12	33.8±2	1.2±0.7	6–15		(4)		(6)	
8–9	107±10	93±12	34.1±2	1.8±1	6–15		(4)		(6)	
Months—all the following Hb values are Medians/Lower limit for normal									
3	115/90	88/88			6–15		(3)		(6)	
6	115/90	77/70			6–15		(3)		(6)	
12	115/90	78/72			6–15		(3)		(5)	
Year									
2	115/90	78/74			6–15		(3)		(5)	
4	122/100	80/75			6–15		(4)		(4)	
6	130/104	82/75			5–15		(4.2)		(3.8)	
12	138/110	83/76			4–13		(4.9)		(3.1)	
14B	142/120	84/77			4–13		(5)		(3)	
14G	140/115								
16B	148/120	85/78	30–36	0.8–2	4–13	2–7.5	(5)	0.04–4	1.3–3.5	0.2–8
16G	140/115								
18B	150/130								

Note: *Basophil range:* 0–0.1×10⁹/L; B⁵₁₂; ≥150ng/L.
Red cell folate^{EDTA} 100–640ng/mL. **B = boys; G = girls.**
Platelet counts don't vary with age: 150–400×10⁹/L.

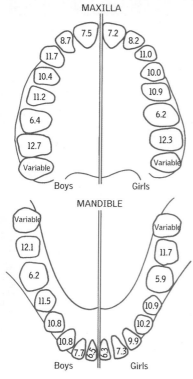

Fig 2.24 Mean times of eruption (in years) of the permanent teeth.

Deciduous teeth	Months		Months
Lower central incisors	5–9	First molars	10–16
Upper central incisors	8–12	Canines	16–20
Upper lateral incisors	10–12	Second molars	20–30
Lower lateral incisors	12–15		
A 1-year-old has ~6 teeth; 1½yrs ~12 teeth; 2yrs ~16 teeth; 2¼yrs ~20 (see fig 2.24).			

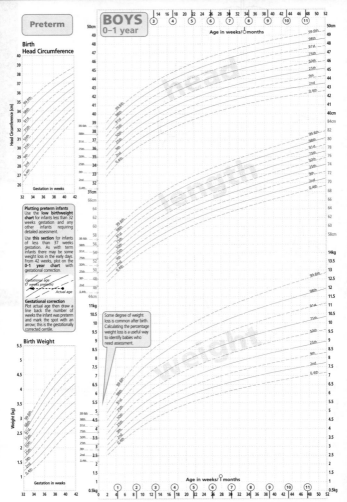

Fig **2.25** UK-WHO growth charts—boys aged 0–1 yrs

© 2009 Department of Health.

In 2006, the WHO introduced new growth standards which were adopted in the UK in 2009 (2010 in Scotland) for children 0–4y (UK-WHO charts, figs **2.25–2.28**). These growth standards were compiled from data from breast-fed babies (who grow slower than formula-fed infants)—from 6 different nations (the US, Norway, Oman, Brazil, India, and Ghana). The linear growth patterns were similar between nations—so for this age group there aren't thought to be any ethnospecific differences in rate of growth. This rate of growth is taken to be an optimal growth rate for children, as opposed to

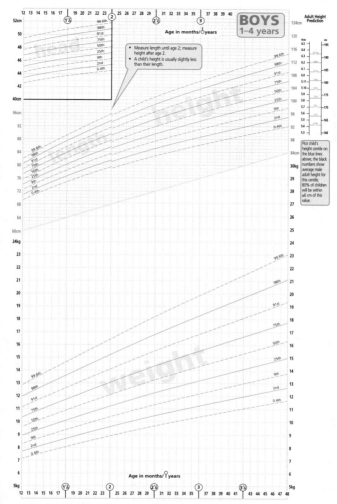

Fig 2.26 UK-WHO growth charts—boys aged 1–4 yrs.   © 2009 Department of Health.

the previous growth charts (UK90) which described the prevailing growth patterns of UK children compiled from surveys done in the 1980s. As a result the UK-WHO charts have an increased number of overweight children and fewer underweight children, when compared with the UK90 charts. For <4yrs, the UK-WHO charts replace the UK90 charts. The UK90 charts are still used for children >4 (not reproduced here)

• Separate charts exist for children with Down's syndrome, Turner's, and achondroplasia

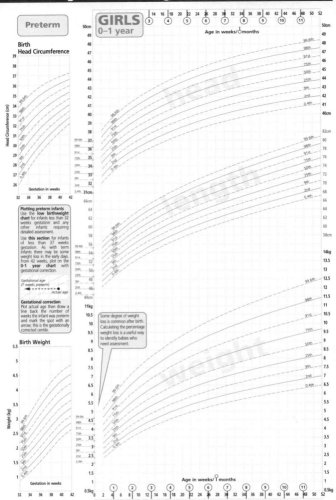

Fig 2.27 UK-WHO growth charts—girls aged 0–1 yrs. © 2009 Department of Health.

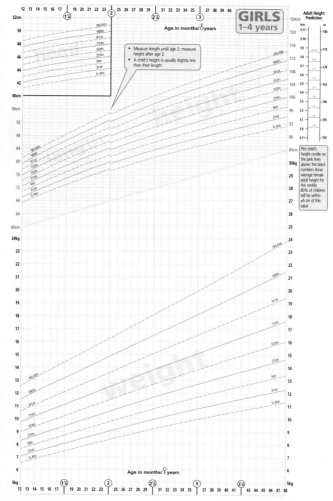

Fig 2.28 UK-WHO growth charts—girls aged 1–4 yrs.   © 2009 Department of Health.

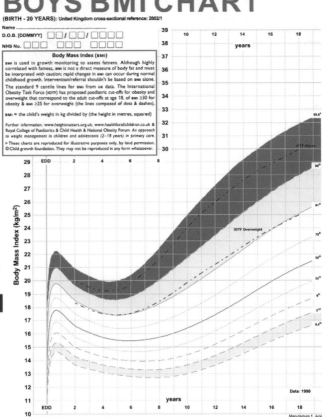

BOYS BMI CHART

(BIRTH - 20 YEARS): United Kingdom cross-sectional reference: 2002/1

Name

D.O.B. [DDMMYY]

NHS No.

Body Mass Index (BMI)

BMI is used in growth monitoring to assess fatness. Although highly correlated with fatness, BMI is not a direct measure of body fat and must be interpreted with caution: rapid changes in BMI can occur during normal childhood growth. Intervention/referral shouldn't be based on BMI alone.

The standard 9 centile lines for BMI from UK data. The International Obesity Task Force (IOTF) has proposed paediatric cut-offs for obesity and overweight that correspond to the adult cut-offs at age 18, of BMI ≥30 for obesity & BMI ≥25 for overweight (the lines composed of dots & dashes).

BMI = the child's weight in kg divided by (the height in metres, squared)

Further information: www.heightmatters.org.uk; www.healthforallchildren.co.uk & Royal College of Paediatrics & Child Health & National Obesity Forum *An approach to weight management in children and adolescents (2–18 years) in primary care.*

► These charts are reproduced for illustrative purposes only, by kind permission. © Child growth foundation. They may not be reproduced in any form whatsoever.

Designed and Published by
© CHILD GROWTH FOUNDATION 1997/1
(Charity Reg. No 274325)
2 Mayfield Avenue,
London W4 1PW

Printed and Supplied by
HARLOW PRINTING LIMITED
Maxwell Street · South Shields
Tyne & Wear · NE33 4PU

Reference

Body Mass Index reference curves for the UK, 1990 (TJ Cole, JV Freeman, MA Preece) *Arch Dis Child* 1995; **73**: 25-29 Establishing a standard definition for child overweight and obesity: international survey, (Cole TJ, Bellizi MC, Flegal KM, Dietz WH) *BMJ* 2000; **320**: 1240-3

Fig 2.29 Boys' BMI chart.

© Child Growth Foundation, reproduced with permission.

Risk factors for childhood obesity Changes in food availability and activity levels during the past 30 years are well known. Also: low socioeconomic status, maternal obesity, rapid infancy weight gain. *Obesity prevention programmes* have some success and show that changes in school and community environments can decrease childhood weight gain. In France, for example, children are weighed in school regularly, and regular exercise and healthy eating (not diets) are promoted in systematic ways. Input from a family healthy-eating coach has also been found to help.[568,569] Peer encouragement and feedback in the form of pedometer readings is one way of promoting more exercise.[570]

For methods of preventing adult consequences of childhood obesity by intervening in childhood, see p156.

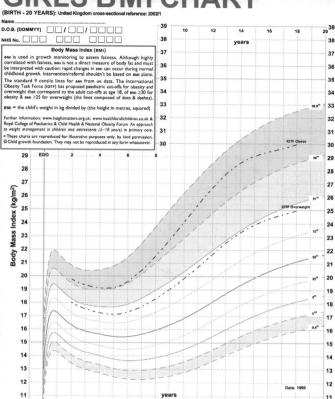

GIRLS BMI CHART

(BIRTH - 20 YEARS): United Kingdom cross-sectional reference: 2002/1

Name ....

D.O.B. [DDMMYY] ☐☐/☐☐/☐☐☐☐

NHS No. ☐☐☐☐ ☐☐☐ ☐☐☐☐

Body Mass Index (BMI)

BMI is used in growth monitoring to assess fatness. Although highly correlated with fatness, BMI is not a direct measure of body fat and must be interpreted with caution; rapid changes in BMI can occur during normal childhood growth. Intervention/referral shouldn't be based on BMI alone.

The standard 9 centile lines for BMI from UK data. The International Obesity Task Force (IOTF) has proposed paediatric cut-offs for obesity and overweight that correspond to the adult cut-offs at age 18, of BMI ≥30 for obesity & BMI ≥25 for overweight (the lines composed of dots & dashes).

BMI = the child's weight in kg divided by (the height in metres, squared)

Further information: www.heightmatters.org.uk; www.healthforallchildren.co.uk & Royal College of Paediatrics & Child Health & National Obesity Forum An approach to weight management in children and adolescents (2–18 years) in primary care.
► These charts are reproduced for illustrative purposes only, by kind permission.
© Child growth foundation. They may not be reproduced in any form whatsoever.

Body Mass Index (kg/m²)

Reference
Body Mass Index reference curves for the UK, 1990 (TJ Cole, JV Freeman, MA Preece) Arch Dis Child 1995; 73: 25-29
Establishing a standard definition for child overweight and obesity: international survey (Cole TJ, Bellizi MC Flegal KM, Dietz WH) BMJ 2000; 320: 1240-3

Designed and Published by
© CHILD GROWTH FOUNDATION 1997/1
(Charity Reg. No 274325)
2 Mayfield Avenue,
London W4 1PW

Printed and Supplied by
HARLOW PRINTING LIMITED
Maxwell Street ⬩ South Shields
Tyne & Wear ⬩ NE33 4PU

Fig 2.30 Girls' BMI chart.

© Child Growth Foundation, reproduced with permission.

z-scores for weight, height, and BMI: what do they mean? A z score (for weight-for-age) of –1 indicates that weight is 1 standard deviation (OHCM p737) below the median for that age/sex group. This means mildly underweight. z –2 (minus 2 standard deviations) is moderate, and z –3 is severe. Ditto for height. In the care of children with chronic diseases, eg HIV, monitoring and improving the BMI z-score is an important way of reducing morbidity and mortality.[571]

A BMI z-score of +2 to +2.5 counts as moderate obesity (severe if >2.5).[572,573] BMI z-score is chief determinant of metabolic syndrome in children;[574] a 1-point increase in BMI z-score yields a 2-fold increase in its prevalence (↑ from 27.6% to 60.7% if BMI z-score increases from 2.3 to 3.3). (See figs 2.29 & 2.30 for BMI charts.)

BMI z-scores also help monitoring weight-intervention programmes.[575]

Dubowitz system for assessing gestational age

See figs 2.31 & 2.32 for neurological criteria for Dubowitz scoring and assessment of gestational age.

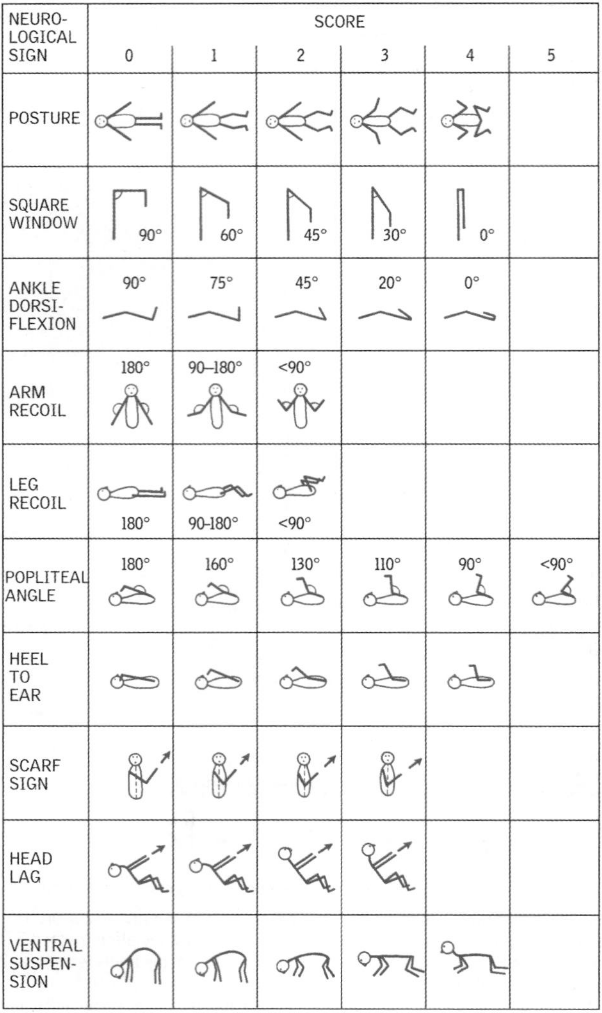

Paediatrics

NEURO-LOGICAL SIGN	SCORE					
	0	1	2	3	4	5
POSTURE						
SQUARE WINDOW	90°	60°	45°	30°	0°	
ANKLE DORSI-FLEXION	90°	75°	45°	20°	0°	
ARM RECOIL	180°	90–180°	<90°			
LEG RECOIL	180°	90–180°	<90°			
POPLITEAL ANGLE	180°	160°	130°	110°	90°	<90°
HEEL TO EAR						
SCARF SIGN						
HEAD LAG						
VENTRAL SUSPEN-SION						

Fig 2.31 Neurological criteria for Dubowitz scoring (use in conjunction with TABLE on p230–2).
Reproduced from *Archives of Disease in Childhood*, L. Dubowitz, volume 44, Issue 238, pp. 782,
Copyright © 1969 with permission from BMJ Publishing Group Ltd.

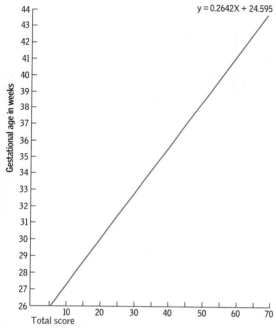

Fig 2.32 Assessment of gestational age: Dubowitz system. Graph for reading gestational age from total score.

Paediatrics

Assessment of gestational age: Dubowitz system

Physical (external) criteria (for neurological criteria, see p228)

External sign	Score				
	0	1	2	3	4
Oedema	Obvious oedema hands and feet: pitting over tibia	No obvious oedema hands and feet: pitting over tibia	No oedema		
Skin texture	Very thin, gelatinous	Thin and smooth	Smooth: medium thickness Rash or superficial peeling	Slight thickening Superficial cracking and peeling, especially hands and feet	Thick and parchment-like superficial or deep cracking
Skin colour (infant not crying)	Dark red	Uniformly pink	Pale pink: variable over body	Pale Only pink over ears, lips, palms, or soles	

Skin opacity (trunk)	Numerous veins and venules clearly seen, especially over abdomen	Veins and tributaries seen	A few large vessels clearly seen over abdomen	A few large vessels seen indistinctly over abdomen	No blood vessels seen
Lanugo (over back)	No lanugo	Abundant long and thick over whole back	Hair thinning especially over lower back	Small amount of lanugo and bald areas	At least half of back devoid of lanugo
Plantar creases	No skin creases	Faint red marks over anterior half of sole	Definite red marks over more than anterior half, indentations over less than anterior third	Indentations over more than anterior third	Definite deep indentations over more than anterior third
Nipple formation	Nipple barely visible, no areola	Nipple well defined, areola smooth and flat diameter <0.75cm	Areola stippled, edge not raised, diameter <0.75cm	Areola stippled, edge raised diameter >0.75cm	
Breast size	No breast tissue palpable	Breast tissue on one or both sides <0.5cm diameter	Breast tissue both sides, one or both 0.5–1.0cm	Breast tissue both sides: one or both >1cm	

Paediatrics

Assessment of gestational age: Dubowitz system (continued)

Physical (external) criteria (for neurological criteria, see p228)

External sign	Score				
	0	1	2	3	4
Ear form	Pinna flat and shapeless, little or no incurving of edge	Incurving of part of edge of pinna	Partial incurving whole of upper pinna	Well-defined incurving whole of upper pinna	
Ear firmness	Pinna soft, easily folded, no recoil	Pinna, soft, easily folded, slow recoil places, ready recoil	Cartilage to edge of pinna, but soft in places, ready recoil	Pinna firm, cartilage to edge, instant recoil	
Genitalia • Male	Neither testis in scrotum	At least one testis high in scrotum	At least one testis right down		
• Female (with hips half abducted)	Labia majora widely separated, labia minora protruding	Labia majora almost cover labia minora	Labia majora completely cover labia minora		

Reproduced from Dubowitz, L 'Assessment of gestational age: a practical scoring system' *Archives of Disease in Childhood* with permission from BMJ Publishing Ltd.

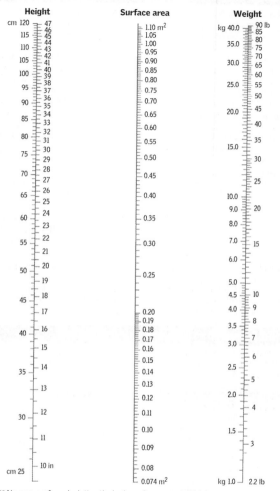

Fig 2.33 Nomogram for calculating the body surface area of children.
Reproduced from *Archives of Disease in Childhood*, L. Dubowitz, volume 44, Issue 238, pp. 782, Copyright © 1969 with permission from BMJ Publishing Group Ltd.

Paediatrics

Water See p235. An intake of 180mL/kg/day (range 150–200mL/kg/day) of human or formula milk meets the water needs of very low birthweight infants (VLBW; <1500g) under normal circumstances. In infants with heart failure water restriction is necessary (eg 130mL/kg/day).

Energy 130kcal/kg/day (range 110–165) meets the needs of the LBW infant in normal circumstances, and can be provided by formulas with similar energy density to human milk (65–70kcal/dL) in a volume of 180–200mL/kg/day. If a higher energy density is required keep it <85kcal/dL. The problems with energy densities above this are fat lactobezoars and U&E imbalance.

Protein Aim for between 2.25g/100kcal (2.9g/kg/day when fed at 130kcal/kg) and 3.1g/100kcal (4g/kg/day). Lysine should be as high as possible. Precise guidelines on taurine and whey:casein ratios cannot be given. At present LBW formulas are whey-predominant. Signs of protein deficiency: ↓urea; ↓prealbumin.

Fat Aim for 4.7–9g/kg (fat density 3.6–7.0g/100kcal). Longer-chain unsaturated fatty acids (>C12) are better absorbed than saturated fatty acids. Aim to have ≥4.5% of total calories as the essential fatty acid linoleic acid (500mg/100kcal).[576]

Carbohydrates Aim for 7–14g/100kcal, eg with lactose contributing 3.2–12g per 100kcal. Lactose is not essential; substitutes are glucose (but high osmolality may cause diarrhoea) or sucrose (± starch hydrolysates, eg corn syrup oils).

Vitamins See p122 & ESPGAN committee.[577]

Elements Na^+: 6.5–15mmol/L. K^+: 15–25.5mmol/L. Ca^{2+} 1.75–3.5mmol per 100kcal. PO_4^{3-}: 1.6–2.9mmol/100kcal. Ca^{2+}:PO_4^{3-} ratio: 1.4–2.0:1. Magnesium: 0.25–0.5mmol/ 100kcal. Iron: if breastfed, give 2–2.5mg Fe/kg/day (recommended total intake). Formula-fed infants may need a supplement to achieve this. Iodine: 10–45mcg/100kcal. Manganese: 2.1μmol/100kcal. ►1cal=4.18 joules.

Fluid regimens to correct dehydration

If tolerated, always use oral rehydration. Dioralyte® comes in sachets which contain glucose, Na^+ and K^+. Show the parent/guardian how to make it up (water is the vital ingredient!). If breastfeeding, continue.

Daily IV water, Na, and K (mmol/kg/day) MAINTENANCE needs				
Age (yr)	Weight (kg)	Water (mL/kg/day)	Na^+	K^+
<0.5	<5	150	3	3
0.5–1	5–10	120	2.5	2.5
1–3	10–15	100	2.5	2.5
3–5	15–20	80	2	2
>5	>20	45–75	1.5–2	1.5–2

Use 0.45% saline with 5% glucose for these needs (contains few calories, but prevents ketosis). 0.9% saline is used for many conditions at risk from hyponatraemia (see NICE guidance). Pre-existing deficits and continuing loss must also be made good. Reliable input–output fluid balance charts are essential.

Calculating pre-existing deficit mL≈%dehydration×weight (kg)×10; give eg as 0.45% saline over 48h (eg 750mL for a 10kg child who is 7.5% dehydrated). Add in K^+ (20mmol/500mL) once the child has passed urine. Don't forget the maintenance fluids for ongoing losses. Replace deficit over 48h if >5% dehydrated.

Estimating dehydration is difficult. In the West, dehydration >7.5% is rare, even with DKA. *Mild dehydration (0–5%):* 5% weight loss in infants; 3% in children. Dry mucous membranes; skin turgor may be ↓; may have decreased urine output. *Moderate dehydration (5–10%):* Weight loss of 10% in infants; 6% in children. Decreased skin turgor, very dry mucous membranes, oliguric, pulse↑, capillary refill time >2s, lethargy, hoarse cry. *Severe dehydration (>10%):* Weight loss of 15% in infants; 9% in children. Skin turgor ↓ with tenting, mucous membranes parched, anuric, shock, hypotension; comatose.

Fluids for the first 24h in mild dehydration This is best managed at home. Encourage parents to give little and often (ie 5mL every 5min by syringe). The patient will not need treatment until they are more dehydrated.

IV fluids for the first 24h in moderate dehydration
- Give maintenance water requirement (above) + the deficit over 48h. The most physiological method are oral rehydration salts eg Dioralyte® by NG tube, if tolerated. Some patients manage on oral fluids only. 'Rapid rehydration' involves 4h of 10mL/kg/h 0.9% NaCl then maintenance after if needed. Ensure the nurses are aware to drop the fluid rate after 4h, and change to 0.45%/5% glucose.
- Measure or estimate and replace ongoing losses (eg from the bowel).
- Monitor U&E on admission, and at least daily.

▸▸IV fluid replacement in the first 24h in severe dehydration (APLS)Treatment aims to restore any circulatory compromise, then to correct deficits over 48h. If IV access fails, use the intraosseous route, p236).
- 0.9% saline 20mL/kg IVI bolus, while calculations are performed.
- Continue with saline boluses, then use blood, until the signs of shock ease.
- Then give the daily requirement + fluid deficit as above, making good continuing loss with 0.45% or 0.9% saline depending on type of dehydration (0.45% in isotonic/hyponatraemic; 0.9% in hypernatraemic dehydration—cerebral oedema is a risk during rehydration with ↑ serum Na⁺; correct slowly).
- Measure plasma and urine creatinine and osmolality (p176), and plasma bicarbonate if renal impairment or electrolytes significantly abnormal. Metabolic acidosis usually corrects itself.

Guidelines for success: Above all be simple. Complex regimens cause errors.
1 Stay at the bedside; use clinical state + blood gas results to adapt IVI.
2 Beware sudden changes in Na⁺ (↑ or ↓); may cause seizures or central pontine demyelinolysis.
3 Beware hidden loss (oedema, ascites, GI pools), and shifts of fluid from the intravascular space to the interstitial space ('third-spacing').
4 Measure U&E and urine electrolytes every 8h.
5 Give potassium once you know that urine is flowing (apart from DKA). The ready-prepared fluid '0.45% Saline With 5% glucose With Potassium Chloride 20mmol/L' is usually a good choice. Be guided by serum K⁺.[578]

Hypernatraemic dehydration: (greater water loss than Na⁺, eg from wrongly made feeds, or rarely, if breastfed.) It causes intracellular dehydration (± fits).[579] A big danger is too rapid rehydration. *Hyponatraemic dehydration:* Most common abnormality (symptoms likely if <125mmol/L). Due to sepsis, use of hypotonic fluids, or excessive GI losses. If no symptoms, treatment depends on volume status. Hyponatraemia with seizures requires hypertonic saline—seek senior advice.

Water balance in the preterm infant Water comprises 50–70% of weight gain (eg of 15g/day) in preterm babies. *Insensible water loss (IWL)* falls with increasing body weight, gestational age, and postnatal age; it increases with ↑↑T° (ambient & body) and low humidity. In a single-walled, thermoneutral incubator with a humidity of 50–80% IWL ≈30–60mL/kg/day (may double in infants on phototherapy under a radiant heater). *Faecal water loss* ≈5–10mL/kg/day (except during diarrhoea). *Urine loss:* If ~90mL/kg/day, there is no excessive renal stress.

(APLS=advanced paediatric life support.)

Immediate vascular access is required in paediatric and neonatal practice in the following circumstances: cardiopulmonary arrest, severe burns, prolonged status epilepticus, hypovolaemic and septic shock. In many cases rapid intravenous access is not easily obtained. Intraosseous (IO) infusion is a rapid, safe, easy, and effective means of obtaining vascular access, and is recommended for life-threatening paediatric emergencies in which IV access cannot be obtained.[580] Most with easy access to IO would not attempt IV access first. It is safe to administer all intravenous medicines via the IO. Bloods can be taken and sent to the lab for crossmatch, FBC, U&E.[581] Inform the haematology lab they will see blasts. A blood gas can be sent (if no fluids given already)—but it shouldn't be used on an autoanalyser as it may clog the machine. Send it to the lab and inform them that it is a marrow sample—they may be able to test it in a cartridge analyser.[581]

Contraindications Osteoporosis, osteogenesis imperfecta, and infection or fracture at the site of insertion.

Technical aspects *Learn from an expert.* The major choice is between a manual needle or a semi-automatic device such as an intraosseous gun or drill. The two major devices available are the Bone Injection Gun® (B.I.G.®)—a spring-loaded device available for children and adults, and the EZ-IO® device a reusable drill with a 15mm needle for children <39kg, and a 25mm needle for patients >40kg. A new 45mm needle is available for those with significant tissue/oedema overlying the site of injection. The EZ-IO may be faster than both manual needles and the B.I.G., and easier to place 1st time.[582]

Preparation Set trolley: Dressing pack, povidone iodine, needles, 10mL syringe, lidocaine (=lignocaine) 1% (5mL), scalpel, intraosseous needle, paediatric infusion set, 10mL 0.9% saline, adhesive tape.

Choosing the site of insertion The proximal tibia is the best site. Other sites are, distal femur or distal tibia. Choose a point on the flat anteromedial surface of the tibia, 1–2cm medial to and 1–2cm below the tibial tuberosity. The child's leg should be restrained, with a small support placed behind the knee.

Procedure
- Sterilize the skin with antiseptic, infiltrate with lidocaine as necessary. (Puncturing the skin with the scalpel is not usually necessary.)
- Insert the intraosseous needle at an angle of 90° to the skin; advance with a boring or screwing motion into the marrow cavity. Correct location of the needle is signified by a decrease in resistance on entering the marrow cavity.
- Stabilize the needle and verify the position by aspirating marrow, or by the easy flushing of 5–10mL of 0.9% saline, without any infiltration of surrounding tissue. The needle should stand upright without support, but should be secured with tape.
- Take samples for culture, U&E, FBC, group & save!
- Connect to IV infusion via an extension: better flow rates are often got by syringing in fluid boluses (standard bolus is 20mL/kg of crystalloid or colloid).

Complications (Infrequent.) There may be extravasation of fluid, or cellulitis, fractures, osteomyelitis, pain, and fat or bone microemboli. These are more common with prolonged use—so intraosseous infusion should be discontinued as soon as conventional IV access is attained (should be within 24h).

NB: Intraosseous delivery may also be used in adults.[583] The position on the tibia in adults is 2cm medial to tibial tuberosity and 1cm above it (as opposed to below it in children).

🏥 Never blame yourself for forgetting anything, except your humanity (and the dose of adrenaline (adrenaline=epinephrine)). See www.resus.org.uk.

▸▸ Call the resuscitation/cardiac arrest team (paramedics if in the community).

▸▸ Ideally place patient on back with legs raised. If they have significant respiratory distress allow the patient to put themselves in a position of comfort. Do not let them stand or sit up rapidly. If comatose, use left-lateral position (to prevent caval compression).

▸▸ ABCDE: Airway (any swelling, hoarseness, stridor?); breathing (rate ↑, wheeze, fatigue, cyanosis, S_pO_2 <92%?); circulation (pale, clammy, BP↓, faints?); disability (conscious level, eg drowsy/coma?); exposure of skin (erythema/urticaria?).

▸▸ *The chief drug priority is adrenaline.* Give intra-muscularly (IM). Use a suitable syringe for measuring small volumes; absolute accuracy isn't essential.[584] Note strength! (1:1000 not 1:10,000.)

IM dose of 3 drugs	Adrenaline 1:1000	Chlorphenamine	Hydrocortisone
If aged <6 months	0.15mL (150mcg)[12]	25mcg/kg	25mg
If aged 6 months–6yrs	0.15mL (150mcg)	2.5mg	50mg
Dose if aged 6–12yrs	0.3mL (300mcg)	5mg	100mg
Adolescent/adult dose	0.5mL (500mcg)	10mg	200mg

▸▸ Repeat adrenaline dose after 5min if no improvement. Also: high-flow O_2 (±IPPV) & crystalloid (20mL/kg IVI). *NB:* weight (kg)≈2(age in yrs+4). OK if 1-10yrs old.

▸▸ Remove the trigger, eg bee sting; turn off any drug or colloid IVI.

• *IV route:* This can be used for hydrocortisone and chlorphenamine, although there is little evidence these help much. Don't use the IV route for adrenaline (unless on ITU with experienced user; special doses apply).

• *If bronchospasm is a feature:* give salbutamol 2.5mg nebulized too (5mg if >30kg child), every 15min as required.

• *Continuously monitor:* pulse, BP, S_pO_2, and ECG. If cardiac arrest, start CPR.

• *Differential diagnosis:* asthma; septic shock; breath-holding or panic attack.

• *After the emergency:* if reaction is due to a drug, idiopathic or due to an envenomation, take blood as soon as possible after symptoms start; ideally 1-2h, but definitely within 4h for mast cell tryptase (>0.5mL in LFT bottle, ask lab to freeze; helps confirm diagnosis of anaphylaxis but a negative test does not exclude it); admit as an in-patient; refer to an allergist. Self-use of pre-loaded pen injectors may be needed (after training).[585] There are several brands of pre-loaded pens. Patients should be prescribed the brand with which they have been trained eg EpiPen® which has 0.3mg of adrenaline (1:1000). This is suitable if weight >30kg.

This algorithm (fig 2.34) assumes no equipment and that only 1 professional rescuer is present. Remove yourself and the child from danger. Phone for help at once.

How to give the rescue breaths *to a child:*[586] Ensure head tilt and chin lift. Pinch the soft part of his nose. Open his mouth a little, but maintain chin up. Take a breath, and place your lips around his mouth (good seal). Blow steadily into his mouth over 1-1.5sec. Does his chest rise? Take your mouth away, and watch for the chest to fall. Take another breath, and repeat this sequence up to 5 times. *To an infant:* Do as above, but cover the nasal apertures and the mouth with your lips. The head should be in the neutral position. If the chest does not move, respiratory obstruction may exist ▸▸move on to *'Removing foreign body' sequence* for obstructed airway—ie:

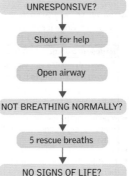

Paediatric Basic Life Support
(Healthcare professionals
with a duty to respond)

UNRESPONSIVE?

Shout for help

Open airway

NOT BREATHING NORMALLY?

5 rescue breaths

NO SIGNS OF LIFE?

15 chest compressions

2 rescue breaths
15 compressions

Call the resuscitation team

• If coughing, encourage to cough. Once unconscious or an ineffective cough:
• Remove any obvious obstructions. Recheck that there is adequate head tilt and chin lift, but do not overextend the neck.
• Do up to 5 back blows between the scapulae to dislodge hidden obstructions (hold on your lap whilst seated, positioning the head lower than chest).
• If this fails, do 5 chest thrusts: turn to supine; over 12sec, give 5 sternal thrusts (same position as for compressions, but be sharper and more vigorous. Remove any foreign bodies which have become visible.
• Tilt head upwards; lift chin to reopen the airway, and assess breathing.
• If not breathing; do 5 more rescue breaths: does the chest move now?
• If not, for a child >1 year, give 5 abdominal thrusts (directed towards diaphragm); use the upright position if the child is conscious; supine if not.
• Repeat these sequences until breathing is

Fig 2.34 Paediatric basic life support, applicable only to healthcare professionals with a duty to respond.
Reproduced with the kind permission of the Resuscitation Council (UK).

ok, alternating chest and abdominal thrusts. *Do not give abdominal thrusts to infants (risk of internal injury).*

When breathing place in the recovery position—as near to the true lateral position as possible, with mouth dependent to aid draining of secretions. The position must be stable (eg use pillows placed behind back). The degree of movement is determined by risk of spinal injury.

How to give chest compressions Compress lower half of sternum to ⅓ of the chest's depth; use the heel of one hand (or, in babies, with both your thumbs, with your hands encircling the thorax) If >8yrs, the adult 2-handed method is ok. For an infant, 2 fingers are sufficient, in the middle of a line joining the nipples. Perform resuscitation for ~1min before going for help. Remove the cause, if possible. Causes are: shock; hypoxia; drowning; pulmonary embolism; trauma; electrocution; hypercapnia; hypothermia; u&e imbalance; drugs/toxins, eg adrenaline (= epinephrine), and digoxin.[587]

Cardiac arrest: paediatric advanced life-support

Neonates: see p107.

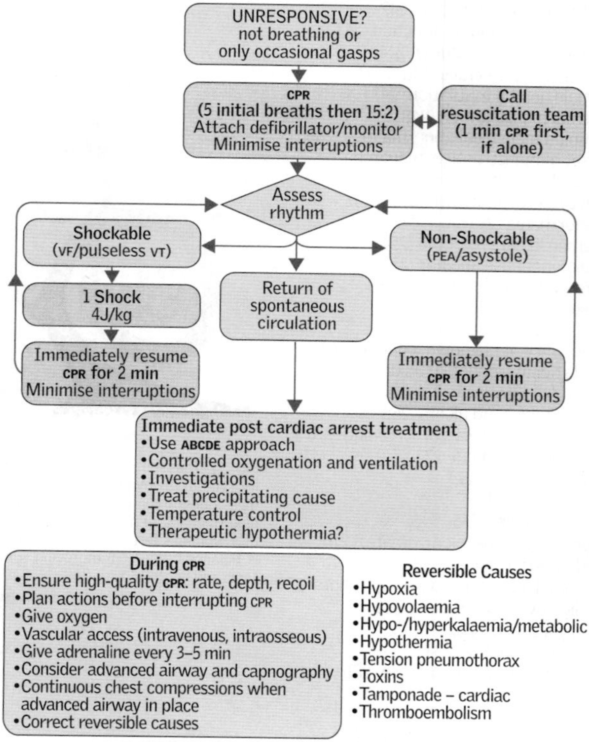

Fig 2.35 Paediatric advanced life support.

Reproduced with the kind permission of the Resuscitation Council (UK).

Fig **2.35** shows the paediatric advanced life support algorithm.[45] Order of assessment and intervention for any seriously ill or injured child follows the ABCDE principles: Airway (AC for airway and cervical spine stabilization for the injured child); Breathing; Circulation; Disability (level of consciousness and neurological status); Exposure to ensure full examination (while respecting dignity and temperature conservation). *Note:* 15:2 means 15 compressions (rate=100–120/min) to 2 ventilations.

In shockable VF/VT ►►After 3rd shock, give adrenaline (epinephrine) 10mcg/kg IV/IO + amiodarone 5mg/kg IV over 3min, once compressions resumed. ►►Repeat adrenaline on alternate cycles until spontaneous circulation returns. ►►Amiodarone (5mg/kg IV) is given after the 3rd shock and one further time after the 5th shock if still in VF/VT. ►►Continue shocks every 2min, and continue compressions during defibrillator chargings. Outcome depends on maximizing adequate and uninterrupted chest compressions. **Non-shockable rhythm** ►►Give adrenaline as soon as you have IV/IO access, and repeat on alternate cycles until spontaneous circulation returns.

45 PEA = pulseless electrical activity.

Gynaecology

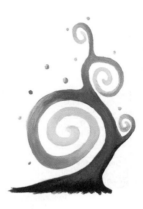

Fig 3.1 The spiral is a Pagan fertility symbol. In gynaecology, the major milestones are marked by the beginning (menarche) and end (menopause) of a woman's fertile period. Treatment is balanced between improving symptoms and her fertility wishes.

© Charlotte Goumalatsou.

We thank Mr George Goumalatsos MRCOG and Miss Sarah Flint FRCOG, our Specialist Readers, and Octavia Wilkes and Matthew Heron, our Junior Readers, for their contribution to this chapter.

A holistic approach to gynaecology: Parry's dictum

'*It is more important to know what sort of patient has the disease than what kind of disease the patient has.*'

Caleb Parry (1755–1822; fig 3.2) was a doctor in Bath who was fascinated by events in his patients' lives, and their connection with their diseases, some of which he described for the first time. These early descriptions are notable for their effortless intertwining of psychological and physical phenomena.[1]

All this suggests a serious, one-sided doctor, but this is wrong. To get away from it all, he became a keen balloonist, lending ideas and materials to Edward Jenner, who dedicated his magnum opus on smallpox to him.

His aphorism is particularly relevant to this chapter because many of its diseases are chronic, and the choices of treatment are many. Take endometriosis (p288), for example. If an examiner were to ask you 'What is the treatment for endometriosis?'—you might well look at him thoughtfully, before replying that it all depends on who has got it—where they are in their lives, how much the pain matters, what the plans are for future

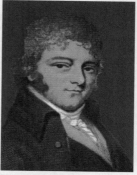

Fig 3.2 Caleb Parry, MD FRS, was a Welshman who chose to peruse his medical studies at Edinburgh as the lectures there, by William Cullen, were given in English, not Latin (for the most part, the current edition of *OHCS* follows Cullen's practice).

Caleb Hillier Parry (1755–1822).
The James Lind Library.
© Roger Rolls, by kind permission.

pregnancies, how these plans may be ambiguous and change, according to work, relationships, and the onset of friendships. What does the patient feel about long-term medication with agents that can change her sexuality, and hence the person who is suffering the disease? Some may tolerate doctor-induced hypo-oestrogenism (flushes, decreased libido, loss of bone density) thinking the price well worth paying for relief of endometriosis symptoms; others will take the opposite view; in a few, their ability to take a decision will be influenced by the drugs they are already taking.[2]

Sometimes rational choice is the hardest thing: 'How can you expect me to make a rational choice until you sort out these dreadful periods of mine: I cannot even think...'[3]

 Be optimistic; let the woman set the agenda: ►Listen to the woman's complaint and ensure she feels listened to ►Take time ►Understand your patient ►Offer all options, *then let her choose*.

History Introduce yourself. Let her tell the story and use open questions. She may be reluctant to admit some problems, particularly in front of relatives. If required, use a professional translator. A frustration for the medical student is that the story you are told is different to the one elicited by the consultant or the GP. But sometimes the first telling is the most valid. ▶It is also true that none of us (doctors and patients) can tell the same story twice.[1]

1 *Symptoms:* If she has *pain* what is it like? Uterine pain may be colicky and felt in the sacrum and groins. Ovarian pain tends to be felt in the *iliac fossa* and radiates down front of the thigh to the knee. Ask about *dyspareunia* (painful intercourse). Is it superficial (at the entrance) or deep inside? If she has *vaginal discharge* what is it like (amount, colour, smell, itch)? When does she get it? Ask about *prolapse* and *incontinence*. Is incontinence stress or urge? How does it affect quality of life? Ask about bowel symptoms (irritable bowel can cause pelvic pain), and faecal incontinence.

2 *Menstrual history:* ▶Date of last menstrual period (LMP; 1st day of bleeding) or menopause. Was the last period normal? Cycles: number of days bleeding/number of days from day 1 of one period to day 1 of next (eg 5/26). Are they regular? If heavy, are there clots or floods? Are periods painful? If so, does the pain precede the start of the period? Are there any associated bowel symptoms? Is bleeding intermenstrual (IMB), postcoital (PCB), or postmenopausal (PMB)? Age at menarche?

3 *Sex and contraception:* Is she sexually active? Are there physical or emotional problems with sex (see p243)? What contraception is she using and is she happy with it? What has she tried previously? Has she had problems conceiving? If so, has she had treatment for subfertility? What about sexually transmitted infections? Date and result of last cervical smear, and history of abnormal smears.

4 *Obstetric history:* How many children? For each pregnancy: antenatal problems, delivery, gestation, outcome; weights of babies; puerperium? Terminations/miscarriages—at *what* stage, *why*, and (terminations) *how*?

5 *Other:* General health, past medical history, profession, drug history, smoking and alcohol use. Previous gynaecological treatment or surgery.

Examination ▶Women may find pelvic examination painful, undignified, and embarrassing. Explain what you are going to do and stop if it is too painful. Be gentle. Use of a trained chaperone is mandatory; this is to support the patient but also to protect yourself medicolegally. A family member or friend cannot chaperone. Let the woman undress in privacy and provide a sheet to cover.

General: Is she well or ill? If the woman looks unwell, start with ABC.

Abdomen: Inspect the abdomen. Palpate for tenderness and peritonism. If there is a mass, could it be a pregnancy? If distended, percuss for ascites.

Vaginal examination: (p246) Inspect the vulva, and use a *speculum* to examine the vagina and cervix and your *fingers* to assess the uterus and adnexae bimanually. Examination is usually done with the patient on her back or in the left lateral position (best for detecting prolapse). *Sims' speculum* has 2 right-angle bends, and is used for inspecting the vaginal walls in left lateral position, eg for prolapse and incontinence.

Cusco's (bivalve) speculum is used for inspecting the cervix with the aid of a light. Lubricate with jelly (unless taking a smear, in which case use warm water). Insert closed, with blades parallel to the labia, usually up to the hilt and aim for the sacrum. Rotate it, open it, and usually the cervix pops into view. If it does not, do a bimanual to check the position of the cervix, and try again. Take swabs (p284) and a cervical smear (p271) if needed. Close the speculum gradually, under direct vision, as you withdraw it, to avoid trapping the cervix.

1 The first telling awakes memories which colour or transform the next telling, which itself influences the next telling in an infinite regression in which one telling becomes the audience for the next.

Sex involves the mind and body and when there is a problem, or sexual dysfunction, it often involves both. It affects 20% of women attending gynaecology clinics and may present overtly with the woman wanting help, or covertly with a different complaint (such as pelvic pain or dissatisfaction with genitalia).

What is 'normal'? The pioneers of research into sexual function were Masters and Johnson, who studied the sexual response of men and women between 1957 and the 1990s. They characterized female sexual arousal, proved that lubrication is vaginal, not cervical and that some women are capable of multiple orgasms and unlike men, have no refractory period. Importantly, they also did much to promote sex as a normal and healthy activity. They described the four-stage model of sexual response: arousal/excitement, plateau, orgasm, and resolution. However, this type of linear model is thought by some to better reflect the male sexual response. Basson proposed an intimacy-based cyclical model which reflects the importance of other factors including emotional and physical satisfaction, biological, psychological, and sexual stimuli, and sexual drive.

Hypoactive sexual desire disorder (HSDD) presents with loss of libido and decline in overall sexual desire, affecting personal relationships and causing distress. Most have a psychosexual cause but organic causes include menopause, depression, chemotherapy, and radiotherapy. When did it start? For example, does she have concerns about what is 'at the end of her vagina' after hysterectomy? What is normal sexual function to her? Is this realistic and is this at odds with her partner's beliefs? Are there any relationship problems? Testosterone supplementation may help (especially if symptoms started following oophorectomy) but psychosexual counselling is recommended.

Sexual pain *Dyspareunia* (p310) may be superficial or deep. Superficial dyspareunia can be due to infections, or skin conditions such as lichen sclerosis. Treat the underlying cause—but pain can start a cycle of fear, anticipation, and avoidance. Lubricants and local anaesthetic gel may also help break the cycle. *Vaginismus* is the difficulty of the woman to allow vaginal penetration despite wanting to; it involves involuntary contraction of the pelvic floor muscles and thigh adductors and is a symptom or sign, not a diagnosis. It is usually precipitated by another cause, be it physical or psychological, or a combination. Exclude anatomical problems such as vaginal septae. It may be so severe that vaginal penetration is not possible. Using vaginal dilators may help eliminate the pubococcygeal reflex, but encouraging the woman to use her own fingers in combination with relaxation exercises may be more useful. *Vulvodynia* is described as a burning pain, occurring in the absence of relevant visible findings or a specific, clinically identifiable neurological disorder. It can be difficult to treat; use a team-based approach with physiotherapy, psychosexual medicine, and pain management. Explain the diagnosis. First-line treatment is with pelvic floor exercises, internal and external perineal massage, and topical anaesthetic. Tricyclic antidepressants or gabapentin may help.

Treatment What does the woman want? *Motivation is important*, as is the quality of the non-sexual component of the relationship. *Lifestyle:* Diet, exercise, stress reduction, exploration of relationship problems/body image issues. *Education* about body function, encourage exploration; sexual education material, lubricants. *Hormonal:* Oestrogen replacement in menopausal women; testosterone if oophorectomy and hypoactive sexual desire disorder. *Behavioural therapy* with a range of psychotherapeutic techniques. *Devices* eg for anorgasmia or vaginismus such as dilators or clitoral stimulators.

Further reading

Cowan *et al.* (2015). The management of common disorders in psychosexual medicine. *TOG* 17 (1): 47–53.

Institute of Psychosexual Medicine: www.ipm.org.uk

The vulva (fig 3.3) comprises the entrances to the vagina and urethra, the structures which surround them (clitoris, labia minora, and fourchette), and the encircling labia majora and perineum. The hymen, when broken (by tampons or intercourse) leaves tags at the mouth of the vagina (*carunculae myrtiformes*).

Look for: Rashes; atrophy; ulcers; lumps (p266 & p268); deficient perineum (you can see the back wall of the vagina); incontinence; discharge.

The vagina is a potential space with distensible folded muscular walls. The contents of the rectum, which runs behind the posterior wall, are palpable through the vagina. The cervix projects into the vault at the top which forms a moat around it, deepest posteriorly, conventionally divided into anterior, posterior, and 2 lateral fornices. From puberty until the menopause, lactobacilli in the vagina keep it acidic (pH 3.8–4.4), discouraging infection.

Look for: Inflammation; discharge (p284); prolapse (p290).

The cervix is mostly connective tissue. It feels firm, and has a dent in the centre (the opening, or os, of the cervical canal). Mucin-secreting glands of the endocervix lubricate the vagina. The os is circular in nulliparous women, but is a slit in the parous.

Look for: Pain on moving the cervix (excitation—p262 & p286); cervical ectropion; cervicitis and discharge; polyps, carcinoma (p273).

The uterus has a thick muscular-walled *body* made from myometrium, lined internally with columnar epithelium (the endometrium) connected to the cervix or neck. It is supported by the uterosacral, cardinal, and round ligaments. The peritoneum is draped over the uterus. The valley so formed between it and the rectum is the rectovaginal pouch (of Douglas), and the fold of peritoneum in which the fallopian tubes lie is known as the broad ligament. The *size* of the uterus is by convention described by comparison with its size at different stages of pregnancy. Since that is variable, estimates are approximate, but the following is a guide: non-pregnant—plum-sized; 6 weeks—egg; 8 weeks—small orange; 10 weeks—large orange; 14 weeks—fills pelvis.

In most women the uterus is *anteverted*, ie its long axis is directed forward in relation to the vagina. The body then flops forwards on the cervix—*anteflexed* (the relation of the long axis of the uterus in relation to the cervix). An anteverted uterus can be palpated between the hands on bimanual examination (unless she is obese, or tense, or the bladder is full).

In 20% it is retroverted, retroflexed, and mobile. It rarely causes problems but is more difficult to palpate on bimanual examination and may fail to lift out of the pelvis after 12 weeks of pregnancy, presenting with discomfort and urinary retention. A fixed retroverted uterus is not normal and may be due to adhesions caused by endometriosis or previous pelvic inflammatory disease.

Look for: Position (important to know for practical procedures); mobility (especially if retroverted); size (including fibroids); tenderness (p262 & p286).

Adnexae These are the *fallopian tubes, ovaries*, and associated connective tissue (parametria). They are palpated bimanually in the lateral fornices, and if normal may not be felt. The ovaries are the size of a large grape and may lie in the rectovaginal pouch.

Look for: Masses (p280) and tenderness (p286).

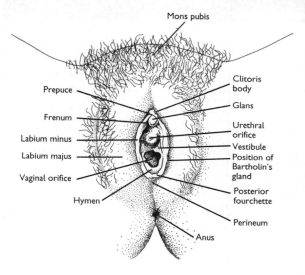

Fig 3.3 Gynaecological anatomy.

Vagina and uterus These are derived from the Müllerian duct system and urogenital sinus and formed by fusion of the right and left parts. Different degrees of failure to fuse lead to duplication of any or all parts of the system (fig 3.4).

Vaginal septae are quite common (and often missed on examination).

Duplication of the cervix and/or uterus may also be missed, eg until the woman becomes pregnant in the uterus without the IUCD!

A partially divided (*bicornuate*) uterus or a uterus where one side has failed to develop (*unicornuate*) may present as recurrent miscarriage, particularly in the second trimester, or as difficulties in labour. Such abnormalities are diagnosed by *hysterosalpingogram*.

An absent uterus or a rudimentary uterus with absent endometrium is rare. They present with primary amenorrhoea.

An absent or short vagina is uncommon but can be corrected by plastic surgery. The membrane at the mouth of the vagina where the Müllerian and urogenital systems fuse (the hymen) may be imperforate. There is apparent primary amenorrhoea, with a history of monthly lower abdominal pain and swelling, and the membrane bulging under the pressure of dammed up menstrual blood (haematocolpos). It is relieved by a cruciate incision in the membrane. NB: in some communities, female genital mutilation (p247) is still practised, and this is another cause of haematocolpos.

▶Renal system abnormalities often coexist with genital ones, so IVU and US should be considered.

Ovary Thin, rudimentary 'streak' ovaries are found in Turner's syndrome (p655). Ovaries are absent in testicular feminization syndrome, but primitive testes are present (p134). Remnants of developmental tissue (eg the Wolffian system) may result in cysts around the ovary, broad ligament, and vagina.

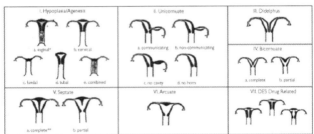

* Uterus may be normal or take a variety of abnormal forms.
** May have two distinct cervices

Fig 3.4 ASRM classification of uterine anomalies.
Reprinted by permission from the American Society for Reproductive Medicine (*Fertility and Sterility*, 1988, 49(6), pp.944-55).

Female genital mutilation

Female genital mutilation, circumcision, or cutting, is the removal or partial removal of external female genitalia or injury to other internal female genital organs, for cultural or non-therapeutic reasons. It is illegal in the UK under the 2003 Female Genital Mutilation Act and more recently has been openly recognized as a form of child abuse. 140 million women are believed to be affected (2 million/year). It is traditionally practised mainly in Africa, but also in some parts of India and Indonesia. In the UK most affected women come from Somalia, Sudan, Kenya, Eritrea, Ethiopia, and the Yemen. It is common in Mali, Guinea, and Egypt. It is not limited to any particular cultural or religious group. The type of mutilation varies between countries, with 90% types I, II, and IV and the remaining 10% type III (see BOX).

Gynaecology

When talking to women about FGM, it is important to remember that they did not choose it. It occurred in childhood when they were too young to consent, often in a society where the practice is traditional and may be viewed as normal, even by themselves. Affected women prefer the term genital cutting to FGM. Treat with dignity and respect. Where FGM is illegal, families may seek a traditional circumciser, take the girl 'on holiday', or try and approach a health-care worker. It is illegal in the UK to undertake or assist with FGM. There is also a duty of child protection and it should be reported and safeguarding advice sought. Social expectations are changing in countries that practise 'cutting' but parents believe the social harm of not cutting is greater than the physical, psychological, and legal risk of not doing so.

Acute complications include death, blood loss, sepsis, pain, urinary retention, tetanus, hepatitis, and HIV. It is carried out in unhygienic conditions, by a traditional circumciser, birth attendant, or midwife, usually using no anaesthesia and shared blades. **Long-term sequelae** include apareunia, superficial dyspareunia, anorgasmia, sexual dysfunction, chronic pain, keloid scar, very slow urination, urinary tract infections, haematocolpos, subfertility, increased susceptibility to HIV and other blood-borne diseases, as well as emotional trauma. Maternal consequences include fear of childbirth, increased risk of CS, postpartum haemorrhage, episiotomy, severe vaginal lacerations and fistula, and difficulty in examining and catheterization.

Management Defibulation may be performed before marriage, electively at 20 weeks' gestation, or in the 1st stage of labour. If not corrected antenatally, deliver in a unit with emergency obstetric care, having planned labour after expert advice. If vaginal examination is poorly tolerated, or anterior episiotomy anticipated, offer epidural. Repair post-delivery should control bleeding but re-infibulation is illegal, and must not result in a vaginal opening making intercourse difficult or impossible. In 2003–5 female genital cutting affected 1.4% of UK maternities and was implicated in 4 maternal deaths.[4]

Further reading

(2009). *Female Genital Mutilation and its Management* (Green-top Guideline No. 53). London: RCOG.

Puberty is the development of adult sexual characteristics. The sequence: breast buds→growth of pubic hair→axillary hair→menses begin (*menarche*) from ~10yrs onwards (mean ~12.7yrs and falling—earlier if low birth weight; African; short & overweight in childhood; urban environment; various fascinating pheromone-related family events mediating anti-inbreeding strategies).[2][5]

Investigate if no periods by ~16yrs (p250) or no signs of puberty by 14. A growth spurt (p184) is the 1st change in puberty and is usually completed 2yrs after menarche when the epiphyses fuse.

The menstrual cycle (fig 3.5). The cycle is controlled by the 'hypothalamic–pituitary–ovarian (HPO) axis'. Pulsatile production of gonadotrophin-releasing hormones by the hypothalamus stimulates the pituitary to produce the gonadotrophins: follicle-stimulating hormone (FSH) and luteinizing hormone (LH). These stimulate the ovary to produce oestrogen and progesterone. The ovarian hormones modulate the production of gonadotrophins by feeding back on the hypothalamus and pituitary.

Day 1 of the cycle is the first day of menstruation. Cycle lengths vary greatly (eg 20–45 days in adolescence); only 12% are 28 days. Cycles soon after menarche and before the menopause are most likely to be irregular and anovulatory. In the first 4 days of the cycle, FSH levels are high, stimulating the development of a primary follicle in the ovary. The follicle produces oestrogen, which stimulates the development of a glandular 'proliferative' endometrium and of cervical mucus which is receptive to sperm. The mucus becomes clear and stringy (like raw egg white) and if allowed to dry on a slide produces 'ferning patterns' due to its high salt content. Oestrogen also controls FSH and LH output by positive and negative feedback.

14 days before the onset of menstruation (on the 16th day of the cycle of a 30-day cycle) the oestrogen level becomes high enough to stimulate a surge of LH. This stimulates ovulation. Having released the ovum, the primary follicle then forms a corpus luteum and starts to produce progesterone. Under this influence, the endometrial lining is prepared for implantation: glands become convoluted ('secretory phase'). The cervical mucus becomes viscid and hostile to sperm and no longer ferns. If the ovum is not fertilized the corpus luteum breaks down, so hormone levels fall. This causes the spiral arteries in the uterine endothelial lining to constrict and the lining sloughs—hence menstruation.

Menstruation is the loss of blood and uterine epithelial slough; it lasts 2–7 days and is usually heaviest at the beginning. Normal loss is 20–80mL (median 28mL). In practical terms, menstrual loss is not measured unless for research purposes.

Menopause The ovaries fail to develop follicles. Without hormonal feedback from the ovary, gonadotrophin levels rise. Periods cease (menopause), usually at ~50 years of age (p256).

Postponing menstruation (eg on holiday) Try norethisterone 5mg/8h PO from 3 days before the period is due until bleeding is acceptable, or take 2 packets of combined contraceptive pills consecutively without a break.

---

2 *The socioendocrinology of family life:* Presence in the household of the biological father *delays* sexual maturation—as does having a sister at home (esp. an elder sister). Brothers have no influence, but half- or step-brothers at home are associated with an *earlier* menarche. In addition, stressful life events such as immigration for adoption is associated with early menarche (risk of precocious puberty ↑×20, p184).

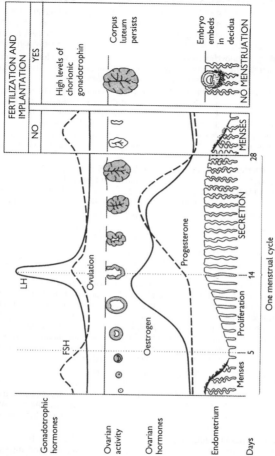

Fig 3.5 The menstrual cycle.

Primary amenorrhoea (see p251) This is failure to start menstruating. It needs investigation in a 16-year-old, or in a 14-year-old who has no breast development. For normal menstruation to occur she must be structurally normal with a functioning control mechanism (hypothalamic–pituitary–ovarian axis).

Secondary amenorrhoea (see p251) This is when periods stop for >6 months, other than due to pregnancy. Hypothalamic–pituitary–ovarian axis disorders are common, ovarian and endometrial causes are rare.

Ovarian insufficiency/failure This may be secondary to chemotherapy, radiotherapy, or surgery. Many genetic disorders can cause ovarian follicle dysfunction or depletion—especially those affecting x chromosomes. One x chromosome is needed for ovarian differentiation, but 2 are needed by oocytes. In Turner's syndrome (XO), oocyte apoptosis starts as 12 weeks and numbers deplete in the 1st 10yrs of life, mosaics 45XO/46XX may menstruate for several years after menarche.

Oligomenorrhoea This is infrequent periods. It is common at the extremes of reproductive life when regular ovulation often does not occur. Menstrual cycles in adolescents are typically <45 days, even in the 1st year. A common cause throughout the reproductive years is polycystic ovary syndrome (p252).

Menorrhagia (p253) This is excessive menstrual blood loss.

Dysmenorrhoea This is painful periods (± nausea or vomiting). 50% of British women complain of moderate pain, 12% of severe disabling pain.

Primary dysmenorrhoea is pain without organ pathology—often starting with anovulatory cycles after the menarche. It is crampy with ache in the back or groin, worse during the first day or two. Excess prostaglandins cause painful uterine contractions, producing ischaemic pain. ℞: NSAIDs inhibit prostaglandins, eg **mefenamic acid 500mg/8h PO** during menstruation so reduce contractions and hence pain. No particular preparation seems superior. **Paracetamol** is a good alternative to NSAIDs. In pain with ovulatory cycles, ovulation suppression with the **combined Pill** can help. Smooth muscle antispasmodics eg **hyoscine butylbromide** (20mg/6h PO) give unreliable results. Cervical dilatation during childbirth may relieve it but surgical dilatation may render the cervix incompetent and is no longer used as therapy.

Secondary dysmenorrhoea: Associated pathology: adenomyosis (p288), endometriosis, pelvic inflammatory disease, fibroids—and so it appears later in life. It is more constant through the period, and may be associated with deep dyspareunia. Treatment of the cause is the best plan and this may be with hormonal contraception. IUCDs increase dysmenorrhoea, except the Mirena® which usually reduces it.

Intermenstrual bleeding This may follow a midcycle fall in oestrogen production. *Other causes:* Cervical polyps; ectropion; carcinoma; cervicitis/vaginitis; hormonal contraception (spotting); IUCD; chlamydia; pregnancy-related.

Postcoital bleeding *Causes:* Cervical trauma; polyps; cervical, endometrial and vaginal carcinoma; cervicitis and vaginitis of any cause. Screen for chlamydia and treat if positive. Refer all with persistent bleeding. Risk of cervical carcinoma in those with post-coital bleeding is 1:2400 aged 45–54; 1:44,000 aged 20–24.[6]

Postmenopausal bleeding This is bleeding occurring >1yr after the last period. ►It must be considered due to endometrial carcinoma until proven otherwise (p278). *Other causes:* Vaginitis (often atrophic); foreign bodies, eg pessaries; carcinoma of cervix or vulva; endometrial or cervical polyps; oestrogen withdrawal (hormone replacement therapy or ovarian tumour). She may confuse urethral, vaginal, and rectal bleeding.

Gynaecology

►*Always ask yourself 'Could she be pregnant?'* See pregnancy tests (p6).

Primary amenorrhoea (see also p250). This may cause great anxiety. In most patients puberty is just late (often familial), and reassurance is all that is needed. In some, the cause is structural or genetic, so check:

• Has she got normal external secondary sexual characteristics? If so, are the internal genitalia normal (p246)?

• Causes can be the same as for secondary amenorrhoea: consider tests below.

• If she is not developing normally, examination and karyotyping may reveal Turner's syndrome (p655) or androgen insensitivity syndrome (p134). The aim of treatment is to help the patient to look normal, to function sexually, and, if possible, to enable her to reproduce if she wishes.

Causes of secondary amenorrhoea

• *Hypothalamic–pituitary–ovarian causes* are common (34% of cases) as control of the menstrual cycle is easily upset, eg by stress (emotions, exams), ↑exercise, weight loss. Up to 44% of competitive athletes have amenorrhoea.

• *Hyperprolactinaemia:* (14%) (30% have galactorrhoea.) Other hormonal imbalances (hypo- or hyperthyroidism). Severe systemic disease, eg renal failure. Pituitary tumours and necrosis (Sheehan's syndrome) are rare.

• *Ovarian causes:* Polycystic ovarian syndrome (p252) is common (28%); tumours; ovarian insufficiency/failure (premature menopause: the cause in 12%, it affects ~1% of women under 40, see p250).

• *Uterine causes:* Pregnancy-related, Asherman's syndrome (uterine adhesions after a D&C: consider also TB, p274). 'Post-pill amenorrhoea' is generally oligomenorrhoea/secondary amenorrhoea masked by regular withdrawal bleeds so, if need be, investigate as below.

Tests • βhCG (eg urinary) to exclude pregnancy. • Serum free androgen index (↑ in polycystic ovary syndrome) • FSH/LH (low if hypothalamic-pituitary cause but may be normal if weight loss or excessive exercise the cause: raised eg FSH>20IU/L if premature menopause, in which case, if age <30 and concerns for future fertility, refer for karyotyping). • Prolactin (↑ by stress, hypothyroidism, prolactinomas and drugs, eg phenothiazines, domperidone, metoclopramide). If level >1000IU/L do MRI scan (p294). 40% of those with hyperprolactinaemia have a pituitary tumour. • TFT (4% of women with amenorrhoea have abnormal thyroid function). • Testosterone level: levels >5nmol/L may indicate androgen secreting tumour or late-onset congenital adrenal hyperplasia so need more investigation, eg dehydroepiandrosterone sulfate level.

Treatment is related to cause. Premature ovarian failure cannot be reversed but hormone replacement (p256) is necessary to control symptoms of oestrogen deficiency and protect against osteoporosis. Pregnancy can be achieved with oocyte donation and *in vitro* fertilization techniques.

Hypothalamic–pituitary axis malfunction: If mild (eg stress, moderate weight loss) there is sufficient activity to stimulate enough ovarian oestrogen to produce an endometrium (which will be shed after a progesterone challenge, eg **medroxyprogesterone acetate 10mg/24h** for 10 days), but the timing is disordered so cycles are not initiated. If the disorder is more severe the axis shuts down (eg in anorexia). FSH and LH and hence oestrogen levels are low. Reassurance and advice on diet or stress management, or psychiatric help if appropriate (p382), and time may solve the problem. She should be advised to use contraception as ovulation may occur at any time. If she wants fertility restored now, or the reassurance of seeing a period, mild dysfunction will respond to **clomifene** but a shut-down axis will need stimulation by gonadotrophin-releasing hormone (see p294 for both).

PCOS comprises hyperandrogenism, oligomenorrhoea, and polycystic ovaries on US in the absence of other causes of polycystic ovaries, eg as seen with later-onset adrenal hyperplasia and Cushing's. The cause is unknown. It is one of the most common endocrine disorders in women of childbearing age, affecting 5-20%. Many women are obese and it is associated with metabolic syndrome (hypertension, dyslipidaemia, insulin resistance, and visceral obesity) and there is an adverse cardiovascular risk profile with higher prevalence of type 2 diabetes and sleep apnoea. Darkened skin (acanthosis nigricans) on neck and skin flexures reflects hyperinsulinaemia.

Presentation is usually with oligomenorrhoea, with or without hirsutism, acne, and subfertility.

Diagnosis is made using the Rotterdam criteria (2 out of 3 must be present):
• Polycystic ovaries (12 or more follicles or ovarian volume >10cm³ on US)
• Oligo-ovulation or anovulation
• Clinical and/or biochemical signs of hyperandrogenism.

Other causes of irregular cycles should be excluded before the diagnosis is made if there is clinical suspicion eg thyroid dysfunction, hyperprolactinaemia, congenital adrenal hyperplasia, androgen secreting tumours, and Cushing's syndrome (OHCM p217). If clinically hyperandrogenic and total testosterone >5nmol/L check 17-hydroxyprogesterone and exclude androgen secreting tumours. LH is raised in 40%, testosterone in 30%.

Management *Weight loss* and exercise are the mainstay of treatment in order to increase insulin sensitivity. Advise smoking cessation. Find and treat diabetes, hypertension, dyslipidaemia, and sleep apnoea. *Metformin* improves insulin sensitivity in the short term and may improve menstrual disturbance and ovulatory function but does not have a significant impact on hirsutism or acne (it does not cause weight loss). It is not licensed for use in treating PCOS so the risks and benefits should be fully discussed. *Clomifene citrate* induces ovulation (50-60% conceive in 1st 6 months of treatment; but it should only be used by a specialist and in conjunction with fertility investigations, in women with a BMI <35 and for no more than 6 cycles). Warn of risk of multiple pregnancy and ovarian cancer (p282). Monitor response by US in at least 1st cycle. Women with PCOS are at ↑ risk of ovarian hyperstimulation (p311) with assisted conception. *Ovarian drilling* (needlepoint diathermy in 4 places per ovary with the intent of reducing steroid production) is recommended by NICE_NICE for those not responding to clomifene (though it may be useful as primary treatment). 65% conceive. It does not increase risk of multiple pregnancy. Preterm birth, pre-eclampsia, gestational diabetes, and large babies are more common. *The COCP* (p300) will control bleeding and reduce risk of unopposed oestrogen on the endometrium (risk of endometrial carcinoma). Recommend *regular withdrawal bleeds* if not taking the pill eg 3-monthly, eg induced with norethisterone 5mg TDS PO for 7-10 days in those in whom oestrogen use is not wanted or is contraindicated. *Hirsutism* may be treated cosmetically, or with an anti-androgen, eg cyproterone 2mg/day, as in co-cyprindiol eg Dianette®. Depilatory creams, electrolysis, waxing, shaving, and laser help (but laser is not funded by the NHS). Eflornithine facial cream is anti-androgen and can also help with acne. Spironolactone 25–200mg/24h/PO (unlicensed use) is also antiandrogenic (avoid pregnancy as teratogenic).

Long-term consequences include gestational diabetes (screen in pregnancy at 24-28 weeks), type 2 diabetes (screen if overweight or other risk factors), cardiovascular disease, endometrial cancer (3-4-monthly withdrawal bleeds reduce risk). There is no increased risk of ovarian or breast cancer.

Further reading

(2014). *Long-term Consequences of Polycystic Ovarian Syndrome* (Green-Top Guideline No. 33). London: RCOG.

This is heavy menstrual bleeding that interferes with quality of life. Historically it had been defined as menstrual blood loss >80mL/cycle but this is meaningless as it is impossible to measure unless in a research setting. What makes a woman consult may be a change in volume (clots, floods, etc.), or a worsening impact on her life. Ask about both. It is the most common gynaecological symptom.

Causes Most is due to dysfunctional uterine bleeding (DUB), which is heavy and/or irregular bleeding in the absence of recognizable pelvic pathology—this is a diagnosis of exclusion. With increasing age, think also of IUCD, fibroids, endometriosis and adenomyosis, pelvic infection, polyps, hypothyroidism, and coagulation disorders. In women >45 years with failed medical management, consider endometrial carcinoma.

Symptoms and signs Heavy, prolonged vaginal bleeding, often worse at the extremes of reproductive life, dysmenorrhoea, symptoms of anaemia, pallor. IMB and PCB are abnormal therefore need investigation—check smear history. An enlarged uterus suggests fibroids or adenomyosis, and speculum examination may reveal a cervical polyp.

Investigations Exclude pregnancy. FBC, haematinics if indicated, TSH if clinically hypothyroid, cervical smear if due, STI screen. If <45yrs no further investigation required; treatment should be started. If >45yrs with risk factors or failed medical therapy, TVUS (looking for fibroids, polyps, endometrial thickness), endometrial biopsy, and out-patient hysteroscopy and endometrial biopsy if scan shows abnormality or bleeding still persists.

Treatment drugs *Mirena®* IUS should be considered 1st-line treatment. It reduces bleeding (by up to 86% at 3 months, 97% at 1yr) and 30% are amenorrhoeic at 12 months. It releases levonorgestrel into the endometrial cavity, leading to atrophy. Side effects include irregular bleeding for the 1st 4–6 months and progestogenic effects. *Antifibrinolytics* Taken during bleeding, they reduce loss (by 49%)—eg **tranexamic acid** 1g/6–8h PO (for up to 4 days). CI: thromboembolic disease—but this is no more common in those on tranexamic acid. Useful in those trying to conceive as non-hormonal. *NSAIDs,* eg **mefenamic acid** 500mg/8h PO pc (CI: peptic ulceration) taken during days of bleeding particularly help if there is also dysmenorrhoea. They reduce bleeding by 29%. *The COCP* is effective (20–30% reduction in blood loss and improvement in dysmenorrhoea) but see contraindications (p300).

3rd-line recommendation is *progestogens* IM (p304). Norethisterone 5mg/8h PO for 7–10 days is used to stop heavy bleeding in the short term.

Rarely *gonadotrophin (LHRH)-releasing hormones* are used in treating very anaemic women quickly but induce a temporary menopausal state (p276).

Surgery should be reserved for the small number of women who do not respond to medical management. *Endometrial ablation* (p308) is now commoner than hysterectomy in the UK for menorrhagia. It involves destruction of the endometrium by microwave, thermal balloon, or electrical impedance. About 30% become amenorrhoeic and 80–90% of the remainder have reduced flow. Contraception is still required. If not used, pregnancy is commoner in those who bleed (3.2% vs 0.3%).[8] Treat as with uterus for HRT (p256).

For women wishing to retain fertility who have fibroids >3cm consider *uterine artery embolization* or *myomectomy* (p276).

Women not wishing to retain fertility and fibroids >3cm may benefit from *hysterectomy* (p308), vaginal hysterectomy being the preferred route, but if fibroids or uterus are large, abdominal hysterectomy may be the best option.

Further reading

NICE (2010). *Heavy Menstrual Bleeding* (CG44). London: NICE.

Most women notice that their mood or physical state may be worse premenstrually. Symptoms tend to be worse in those who are obese, perform less exercise, and have lower academic achievement. Incidence is lower in those on hormonal contraception. 5% of women regularly have cyclical symptoms so severe that they cause major disruption to their lives: premenstrual syndrome (PMS) or tension (PMT). Causes: See BOX.

Definition A condition which manifests with distressing physical, behavioural, and psychological symptoms in the absence of organic or psychiatric disease, regularly occurring during the luteal phase of the menstrual cycle and with significant improvement by the end of menstruation.

Symptoms Mood swings, irritability, depression; bloating and breast tenderness; headache; reduced visuospatial ability, increase in accidents. Almost any symptom may feature.

Diagnosis Use symptom diary filled in over 2 prospective cycles (eg Daily Record of Severity of Problems)—recall of symptoms retrospectively is unreliable.

Treatment
* General health measures regarding increasing exercise, improving diet, stress reduction, smoking cessation and weight loss should be addressed prior to starting pharmacological treatment
* Women with psychopathology exacerbated by PMS should be referred to a psychiatrist
* Symptom diaries should be used to assess the effect of treatment
* When simple measures have failed, consider referral to a gynaecologist.

First line: Exercise, cognitive behavioural therapy, vitamin B₆ 10mg/24h (unlicensed use) PO; combined pill such as Yasmin®, Cilest® either cyclically or continuously; continuous or luteal-phase low-dose SSRIs. Cognitive behavioural therapy has been shown to be as effective at fluoxetine, effects possibly lasting longer when assessed at 12 months.

Second line: Estradiol patches (100mcg) + progestogen (eg dydrogesterone 10mg PO day 17–28 or Mirena®); higher dose SSRIs continuously or luteal-phase eg fluoxetine 20mg/day PO. Newer SSRIs such as sertraline may work where fluoxetine has failed, and can also be tried first line.

Third line: GnRH analogues + addback HRT (eg goserelin 3.6mg sc every 28 days with tibolone 2.5mg PO daily). Goserelin (p276) may help severe PMS but symptoms return when ovarian activity recommences and after 6 months' use bone thinning can be detected. Adding tibolone can ameliorate this effect. Goserelin is better used to predict the severely affected women who may benefit from hysterectomy with oophorectomy (results in 96% satisfaction rates⁹—these women can then have oestrogen replacement).

Fourth line: Total hysterectomy plus bilateral salpingo-oophorectomy (if possible, laparoscopic-assisted vaginal hysterectomy or total laparoscopic hysterectomy and BSO because recovery is quicker than with abdominal hysterectomy) with HRT, including testosterone replacement.

Complementary therapies may be of benefit, but studies are often small and under-powered and remedies are not licensed for use in treating PMS. Having said that, most women benefit from an integrated approach, but access to alternative therapies is usually not funded on the NHS. The best evidence exists for calcium with vitamin D, magnesium, and Agnus castus. Interestingly, there is no evidence for the benefit of vitamin B₆. Evening primrose oil may benefit those with mastalgia but not for other PMS symptoms.

Further reading

(2007). *Management of Premenstrual Syndrome* (Green-top Guideline No. 48). London: RCOG.

Some physiological and pharmacological observations.[10,11]

- There is no evidence that ovarian events cause premenstrual syndrome: models presupposing progesterone deficiency have not been confirmed (and progesterone suppositories are no panacea for the condition).
- Artificially altering circulating progesterone and estradiol (oestradiol) does not induce premenstrual symptoms in previously well women—only in those already prone to PMS.
- Studies with psychoactive compounds suggest that the key events are occurring in the brain, not the ovary—eg an abnormal CNS response to normal progesterone excursions occurring in the luteal phase.
- Allopregnanolone and pregnenolone (metabolites of progesterone) are psychoactive, interacting with γ-aminobutyric acid A (GABA-A) receptors.
- Allopregnanolone is anxiolytic, so lower levels may be associated with anxiety.

Putative conclusion: Neurons or glia in those with PMS preferentially metabolize progesterone to pregnenolone (which heightens anxiety) rather than allopregnanolone (which is anxiolytic and up-regulates serotonin receptors, so ameliorating depression). On this view, alprazolam, by augmenting GABA-A-receptor function, is a substitute for allopregnanolone.

Gynaecology

The menopause is the time of waning fertility leading up to the last period. It is a retrospective diagnosis, having said to have occurred 12 months after the last period. Average age in the UK is 52yrs. Although it causes symptoms, it is not a disease, and part of a natural process. Problems are related to falling oestrogen levels:

• Menstrual irregularity as cycles become anovulatory, before stopping.
• Vasomotor disturbance—sweats, palpitations, and flushes (brief, nasty, and may occur every few minutes for >10yrs, disrupting life and sleep).
• Atrophy of oestrogen-dependent tissues (genitalia, breasts) and skin. Vaginal dryness can lead to vaginal and urinary infection, dyspareunia, traumatic bleeding, stress incontinence, and prolapse.
• Osteoporosis: the menopause accelerates bone loss which predisposes to fracture of femur neck, radius, and vertebrae in later life.

Management ≥20% of women seek medical help.

• Is it the menopause? Thyroid and psychiatric problems may present similarly. 2 consecutive FSH levels >30IU/L is suggestive of menopause but NICE does not recommend testing—levels vary and it is unreliable if taking hormones.
• Diet and exercise can help relieve symptoms.
• Menorrhagia responds to Mirena® coil (p253). An endometrial biopsy is required if irregular bleeding is very heavy or could be postmenopausal.
• Use contraception until >1y amenorrhoea if >50y; 2y if <50y.
• Vaginal dryness responds to **oestrogen** (eg oestrogen cream 0.1% PV every night for 2 weeks, and twice per week thereafter as required (may be indefinitely).

Hormone replacement therapy (HRT)

There are many preparations of HRT, consisting of different strengths, hormones, routes of administration, and combinations. It can be given systemically (eg tablets or patches) or locally (oestrogen creams). The first thing to establish is presence or absence of a uterus: those with a uterus should be given combined HRT; those without can have oestrogen-only. Use of unopposed oestrogens is a major risk factor for developing endometrial cancer and should therefore be avoided.

• Use oestrogen-only HRT in women without a uterus:
• Use oestrogen plus progestogen HRT in women with a uterus:
  •Use oestrogen and cyclical progestogen in women who are still having periods, or who are within 12 months of a period. This usually results in regular withdrawal bleeding.
  •Use continuous-combined HRT in post-menopausal women eg Kliofem®, oestradiol 2mg and norethisterone 1mg. Oestrogen can be administered orally, transdermally (patch or gel), subcutaneously, and vaginally.
• Progestogens can be administered orally, transdermally and via the intrauterine system (Mirena®).

►HRT does not provide contraception and a woman is considered potentially fertile until 2y after her LMP if <50y, and for 1yr if >50y. If any potentially fertile woman needs HRT, non-hormonal contraception is required (eg condoms).

HRT contraindications: • Oestrogen-dependent cancer • Past pulmonary embolus • Undiagnosed PV bleeding • LFT↑ • Pregnancy • Breastfeeding • Phlebitis.

Avoid or monitor closely in Dubin–Johnson/Rotor syndromes (*OHCM* p712). If past spontaneous DVT/PE: *is there thrombophilia (OHCM p368)?*

Side effects: Fluid retention, bloating breast tenderness, nausea, headaches, leg cramps, and dyspepsia. Mood swings, depression, acne, and backache are thought to be due to progestogens. Irregular breakthrough bleeding on combined HRT may need further investigation.

Annual check-up: Breasts; BP (stop if BP >160/100mmHg pending investigation and treatment). Weight; any abnormal bleeding?

Alternatives to HRT SSRIs can help treat vasomotor symptoms (clonidine used to be the mainstay for this but its effect is limited). Osteoporosis should be treated with calcium and vitamin D, bisphosphonates or strontium, or selective oestrogen receptor modulators (SERMs); HRT should not be used first-line for osteoporosis unless menopausal symptoms need to be treated. If vaginal dryness is the most prominent symptom, local treatment with vaginal oestrogen helps and does not require systemic progestogens; if local treatment with vaginal oestogens is contraindicated or the woman wishes to avoid hormones, try lubricants (eg Replens®; for improvement in dryness; for sexual intercourse, use a lubricant containing silicone eg Yes® or Astraglide® (water-based lubricants are absorbed too quickly).

Benefits of HRT
- Reduction of vasomotor symptoms is brought about by oestrogen, and improvement is usually evident by 4 weeks and maximum effect by 3 months. HRT should be continued for at least 1 year to minimize symptom recurrence.
- Improvement in urogenital symptoms and sexual function via systemic or vaginal oestrogens may take several months and need to be long term.
- Osteoporotic fractures are reduced but studies suggest that treatment needs to be lifelong and sustained for HRT to be an effective method.
- Reduced risk of colorectal cancer by about a third (but prevention of colorectal cancer is not an indication for HRT).

Risks of HRT
- Breast cancer risk is increased by 2.3% per year and risk is dependent on duration of HRT. 5 years after stopping, risk returns to that of a woman who has never had HRT. The risk is also dependent on the regimen used and is greatest with combined oestrogen-progestogen therapy. Combined HRT probably leads to 3 extra cases of breast cancer per 1000 women who start at age 50 and continue for 5 years. This effect is not seen in those who start HRT for premature menopause.
- Unopposed oestrogens increase risk of endometrial cancer (RR 2.3); this remains for 5 or more years after stopping.
- HRT more than doubles risk of VTE, but the absolute risk remains small. It is most likely to occur in the first year of taking HRT and risk is lower with transdermal preparations compared with oral. Risk also increases with age; the number of additional VTE events in healthy women on HRT >5 years is 4:1000 women aged 50–59 years, and 9:1000 women aged 60–69 years.
- Gallbladder disease appears to be increased, but risk also increases with age and obesity.

Uncertainties concerning HRT include its role in cardiovascular disease, dementia, and ovarian cancer. Women in the Women's Health Initiative study who started HRT within 10 years of the menopause had a lower risk of coronary heart disease than those starting later. Oestrogen may delay or reduce onset of Alzheimer's disease, but has no effect once the disease has become apparent. Unopposed oestrogens seem to increase the risk of ovarian cancer in the long term, but this is unresolved and not seen with continuous combined therapy.

Recommendations for use
- Consider diet, exercise, and local treatments before systemic therapy
- Starting HRT closer to the menopause may be safer than waiting 5 or 10 years post-menopause
- Discuss the benefits and risks of HRT with each patient
- Encourage breast awareness and to report breast change. Attend breast screening
- Use the lowest effective dose, for the shortest time possible
- Be wary about HRT in those with a family history of breast cancer.

Further reading
NICE (2015). *Clinical Knowledge Summaries: Menopause.* http://cks.nice.org.uk/menopause

Gynaecology

Incidence Worldwide, >20% of pregnancies are terminated and in the UK ⅓ of women have had a TOP by age 45. >200,000 TOP/yr in Great Britain (GB).

Legal (GB) constraints The Abortion Act 1967 (amended 2002) and Human Fertilisation and Embryology Act 1990 allow termination if:

A There is risk to mother's life if pregnancy continues.

B Termination is necessary to prevent permanent grave injury to physical/ mental health of the woman.

C Continuance risks injury to the physical or mental health of the woman greater than if terminated (and fetus not >24 weeks).

D Continuance risks injury to physical/mental health of existing children of the woman greater than if terminated (and fetus not >24 weeks).

E There is substantial risk that if the child were born he/she would suffer such physical or mental abnormalities as to be seriously handicapped.

At present, two doctors must sign certificate HSA1. If <16yrs try to get patient's consent to involve her parents or other adult.[3] 97% are for ground C; 1% for D. <1% of TOPs are done after 20 weeks, usually after amniocentesis, or when very young or menopausal mothers have concealed, or not recognized, pregnancy. TOPs after 24 weeks may only be carried out in NHS hospitals. Clauses A, B, and E have no time limit; C and D have time limit of 24 weeks. Evidence suggests that women undergoing TOP are no more or less likely to suffer psychological sequelae than if they continued the pregnancy.

Before TOP

• Offer counselling and support with both verbal and written information.

• US to confirm gestation and identify non-viable or ectopic pregnancies.

• Screen for chlamydia: ± other STIs.

• Give antibiotic prophylaxis to reduce post-op infection rate (10% without) eg **metronidazole** 1g PR/800mg PO at TOP and **azithromycin** 1g PO same day.

• Discuss contraception (IUCD or sterilization at operation speeds planning).

• If RhD-ve she needs anti-D (all gestations, whatever method see BOX, p11). Bloods for Hb, ABO + RhD group and antibodies; ± HIV, hepatitis B & C, and haemoglobinopathies, if relevant.

Methods Depends on gestation of pregnancy and the woman's choice, as well as which resources are available locally.

Medical termination uses an antiprogestagen, eg **mifepristone** to prime the cervix followed by a prostaglandin eg **misoprostol**. It is highly effective from ≥6 weeks (98% effective at ≤7 weeks, 95% for weeks 7–9) and is also used for 2nd-trimester terminations. Misoprostol can be used orally or vaginally. For early TOP arrange follow-up (and scan) 2 weeks after procedure to confirm it is complete. 5% will need surgical evacuation. Give NSAID pain relief; narcotic analgesia may also be needed, especially if gestation >13 weeks.

Surgical termination (suction or dilatation and evacuation): Consider need for preoperative cervical preparation to reduce difficulty with cervical dilatation (particularly gestation >10 weeks, women <18 years of age) in all women eg with misoprostol 400mcg PV 3h or PO 2–3h pre-op. Osmotic dilators provide superior dilatation from 14 weeks, but misoprostol can be used up to 18 weeks. Surgical TOP >13 weeks requires skilled practitioners; there is a greater risk of bleeding, incomplete evacuation, and perforation. Offer NSAID pain relief during TOP (paracetamol is ineffective). Bleeding and pain is less than with medical termination. *Vacuum aspiration:* Used from 7 to 14 weeks. Local anaesthesia or GA. If <7 weeks check for gestational sac in aspirate, follow-up with βhCG if not seen. Access to US is desirable. *Dilatation & evacuation:* Surgical forceps may be used at 13+0–24+0wks after cervical priming. Real-time US reduces uterine perforation rates and is recommended.

---

3 If the girl is a ward of court, the court has to approve abortion.[12]

Early medical terminations ≤9 weeks' gestation
At ≤ 49 days' gestation use mifepristone 200mg PO + misoprostol 400mcg orally 24–48h later. At ≤ 63 days' gestation mifepristone 200mg PO + misoprostol 800mcg (4×200mcg tablets) PV/buccal or sublingual 24–48h later. For women at 50–63 days' gestation, if not successful 4h after misoprostol give a further 400mcg PO/PV (route depending on preference and amount of bleeding).

Medical terminations 9–13 weeks' gestation
Check local guidelines. Mifepristone 200mg PO + misoprostol 800mcg vaginally 36–48h later. A maximum of 4 further doses of misoprostol 400mcg may then be given 3-hourly PV/PO.

Medical terminations 13–24 weeks' gestation
Check local guidelines. Mifepristone 200mg PO followed 36–48h later by misoprostol 800mcg PV then misoprostol 400mcg PV/PO every 3h to a maximum of 4 further doses. If abortion does not occur mifepristone can be repeated 3h after the last dose of misoprostol and 12h later misoprostol recommenced. If there is clinical evidence that TOP is incomplete, surgical evacuation of the uterus will be needed.

Feticide
In terminations later than 21 weeks + 6 days (eg for abnormality) it is essential that the fetus is born dead (unless it is a lethal fetal abnormality). This may be achieved by use of 3mL intracardiac 15% potassium chloride (± anaesthetic and/or muscle relaxant) instillation beforehand to abolish fetal movement. Confirm asystole with US. (Intra-amniotic digoxin is a less effective alternative requiring less expertise.) If born after 24 weeks the dead fetus is a stillbirth and needs registering (p83). If there are signs of life then a death certificate is required.[14]

Complications of termination (terminology of risk)[4]
• Failed TOP (<1:100 medical TOP failure rate is higher than surgical)
• Infection (~ 2:100); see 'Before TOP', p258
• Haemorrhage (<1:1000), (4:1000 if at ≥20 weeks)
• Uterine perforation (1–4:1000), surgical terminations only
• Uterine rupture (mid-trimester medical TOP): < 4:1000
• Cervical trauma (1:100). Risk less if early abortion: if experienced operator
• Retained products of conception (1:100).

After termination Has she had anti-D (p11)? (250iu if <20 weeks; 500iu +Kleihauer if later.) Is contraception arranged? (Can start Pill same day. Advise that long-acting methods are more effective.) Give letter with sufficient information for practitioners elsewhere to manage complications. Give written and verbal information on symptoms to be expected, those requiring emergency care, and of symptoms of ongoing pregnancy. Give 24h telephone helpline number. Offer follow-up. Refer women requiring emotional support/ at mental health risk. Women having medical terminations not confirmed as successful at time of procedure need follow-up to ensure no ongoing pregnancy (rate 0.5–1%). Misoprostol risks teratogenicity. Decision to arrange uterine surgical evacuation is made on clinical signs and symptoms.

Worldwide it is estimated there are 210 million pregnancies at any one time, and 1 in 5 are terminated. Over three-quarters of women live in developing countries, where 97% of the estimated 20 million unsafe terminations are carried out. 68,000 women die annually after unsafe termination. Accessible contraception reduces need for termination. Legalization of termination reduces the number of unsafe terminations and subsequent maternal death.

Gynaecology

4 *The language of risk*: 1:1–1:10 is very common; 1:10–1:100 is common; 1:100–1:1000 uncommon; 1:1000–1:10,000 is rare; <1:10,000 is very rare (modified from Calman *et al*).[15]

Miscarriage is the loss of a pregnancy before 24 weeks' gestation. 15–20% of pregnancies miscarry, mostly in the 1st trimester. Most present with bleeding PV. Diagnosis may not be straightforward (consider ectopics p262): have a low threshold for doing an US. Pregnancy tests remain +ve for several days after pregnancy loss.

Management of early pregnancy bleeding Consider the following:

►Is she haemodynamically shocked? There may be blood loss, or products of conception in the cervical canal (remove them with sponge forceps).

• Has pain and bleeding been worse than a period? Have products of conception been seen? (Clots may be mistaken for products.)

• Is uterine size appropriate for dates?

• Is she bleeding from a cervical lesion and not from within the uterus?

If symptoms are mild and the cervical os is closed it is a *threatened miscarriage*. 75% will settle. If symptoms are severe and the os is open it is likely to be an *inevitable miscarriage* or, if most of the products have already been passed, an *incomplete miscarriage*. If bleeding is profuse, consider **ergometrine** 0.5mg IM. If there is unacceptable pain or bleeding, or significant retained products on US, arrange surgical management of miscarriage (SMM, previously called evacuation of retained products of conception, ERPC).

Missed miscarriage: The fetus dies but remains *in utero*. There may have been bleeding and/or pain or no symptoms, and the cervix is closed. Confirm with US: fetal pole >7mm with no fetal heart activity, or mean gestation sac diameter >25mm with no fetal pole or yolk sac. Mifepristone and misoprostol may be used as medical management of miscarriage.

Pregnancy of uncertain viability: Intrauterine gestation sac <25mm with no fetal pole or yolk sac, or crown-rump length <7mm with no fetal heart activity. Arrange rescan in 10–14 days.

Expectant management: Appropriate if the woman is not bleeding heavily; effective for incomplete miscarriage but less so for missed miscarriage. Offer rescan in 2 weeks to ensure complete if there has been no significant bleeding.

Medical management: Uses mifepristone (an antiprogestagen) to prime, and then 24–48h later misoprostol either orally or vaginally. Bleeding may continue for 3 weeks following medical management. 80–90% successful in those <9 weeks gestation. Risk of heavy bleeding requiring urgent SMM.

Surgical management: If heavy or persistent bleeding >2 weeks or patient choice. Suction evacuation is used, usually under GA and <13 weeks.

Mid-trimester miscarriage This may be due to mechanical causes, eg cervical weakness (rapid, painless delivery of a fetus), uterine abnormalities, chronic maternal disease (eg DM, SLE), infection or no cause identified. Cervical cerclage[16] at ~14 weeks of pregnancy (eg if 3+ premature deliveries/mid-trimester losses, or previous loss/preterm delivery and US proven cervical shortening) may help. It is removed prior to labour. Mid-trimester loss should be investigated to ensure that any treatable factors are identified to reduce risk in the next pregnancy.

After a miscarriage ►Miscarriage is a bereavement and is usually very distressing. Give the parents space to grieve, to ask why it happened, and if it will recur.[5] Offer follow-up.[17] Fetal products should be incinerated but if the mother requests alternative disposal (to bury herself) respect her wishes. Give in opaque container.[18] Most early pregnancy losses are due to aneuploidy and abnormal fetal development; 10% to maternal illness, eg pyrexia. 2nd-trimester loss may be due to infection, eg CMV (p34). Bacterial vaginosis has been implicated. Most subsequent pregnancies are normal although at increased risk.

5 The Miscarriage Association can provide extra support: http://www.miscarriageassociation.org.uk

Gynaecology

This is the loss of 3 or more consecutive pregnancies before 24 weeks' gestation with the same biological father. It affects 1% of women. Prognosis for future successful pregnancy is affected by the previous number of miscarriages, and maternal age. (Rates of miscarriage are greatest when maternal age is ≥35 years, and paternal age ≥ 40 years.) They may follow a successful birth and approximately half are unexplained.

Possible causes

Endocrine: Well-controlled endocrine disease (eg thyroid or DM) does not increase miscarriage risk, and neither does PCOS.

Infection: Bacterial vaginosis (p284) is associated with 2nd-trimester loss. Screening (and treatment) was previously recommended for those with previous mid-trimester miscarriage or pre-term birth (benefit unproven).

Parental chromosome abnormality: 2–5%. It is usually a balanced reciprocal or Robertsonian translocation (p152). The parent is phenotypically normal but 50–75% of gametes will be unbalanced. Refer to a clinical geneticist. Genetic counselling offers prognosis for future pregnancy, familial chromosome studies, and appropriate advice for subsequent pregnancy. Pre-implantation genetic diagnosis (BOX, p15—involving *in vitro* fertilization) has lower rates of achieving healthy pregnancy outcome compared to natural conception (30% vs 50%).

Uterine abnormality: It is uncertain how much abnormality is associated with recurrent miscarriage or if hysteroscopic correction of abnormality contributes to successful pregnancy outcome, though septum division may help.[19] Open uterine surgery increases chance of uterine rupture.

Antiphospholipid syndrome (lupus anticoagulant, phospholipid, and anti-cardiolipin antibodies): These are present in 15% of women with recurrent miscarriage. Defined as presence of antibodies on 2 occasions plus 3 or more consecutive miscarriages <10 weeks, 1 fetal loss 10 weeks or older, or 1 or more births of a normal fetus >34/40 with severe pre-eclampsia or growth restriction. Give aspirin eg 75mg/24h PO from the day of positive pregnancy test + LMWH, eg enoxaparin 40mg/24h SC)[20] as soon as the fetal heart is seen (eg at 5 weeks on vaginal US) until delivery.[21] Get expert advice. Resulting pregnancies are at high risk of repeated miscarriage, pre-eclampsia, fetal growth restriction, and pre-term birth so need special surveillance. Live birth rate is approximately 80%.

Thrombophilia: In those with inherited thrombophilia (eg factor V Leiden and prothrombin gene mutations, and protein C and S deficiency), heparin helps reduce risk of miscarriage.

Alloimmune causes: The theory is that these women share human leucocyte antigen (HLA) alleles with their partners and do not mount the satisfactory protective response to the fetus. Immunotherapy has not been found to increase live birth rate, is potentially dangerous, and should not be offered.

Recommendation

- Offer referral to specialist recurrent miscarriage clinic.
- Test all women for antiphospholipid antibodies: positive if 2 tests +ve, taken 12 weeks apart.
- Thrombophilia screening.
- Pelvic US to assess uterus; further tests eg 3-D US/laparoscopy/hysteroscopy if anatomy abnormal.
- Karyotype fetal products (3rd and subsequent fetal losses). If an unbalanced chromosome abnormality is identified in the products of conception then karyotype the peripheral blood of both parents.

The fertilized ovum implants outside the uterine cavity. The UK incidence is 11.1:1000 pregnancies and rising; worldwide rates are higher. ~7% of maternal deaths are due to ectopics (1.8 deaths/1000 ectopic pregnancies).

Predisposing factors Anything slowing the ovum's passage to the uterus increases risk: damage to the tubes (pelvic inflammatory disease; previous surgery); previous ectopic; endometriosis; IUCD; the POP (p304), subfertility and IVF (p293), smoking. Pregnancy after tubal ligation is 9 times more likely to be ectopic.

Site 97% are tubal, mostly in ampulla; 25% in the narrow inextensible isthmus (presents early; risk of rupture↑). 3% implant on ovary, cervix, or peritoneum.

Symptoms and signs ►Always think of an ectopic in a sexually active woman with abdominal pain; bleeding; fainting; or diarrhoea and vomiting.
• Often no symptoms or signs; uncertain LMP
• Amenorrhoea 6–8 weeks
• Pain; may be non-specific lower abdominal pain, but classically unilateral
• Vaginal bleeding
• Diarrhoea, loose stools, and/or vomiting
• Dizziness
• Shoulder tip pain from diaphragmatic irritation from haemoperitoneum
• Collapse
• Normal sized uterus
• Cervical excitation with or without adnexal tenderness
• Rarely an adnexal mass
• Peritonism.
Vaginal and speculum examinations do not rupture ectopic pregnancies! Failure to examine a woman with a suspected ectopic is indefensible.

Investigations should include FBC, group and save (cross match 6 units of blood, insert 2 large-bore IV cannulas, give IV fluids, and call senior help if unstable), serum progesterone to help identify a failing pregnancy and hCG for when a normal pregnancy should be visible on TVS (hCG >1500IU). These hormones, contrary to popular belief, do not distinguish where the pregnancy is—only TVS can do that. In a pregnancy of unknown location (p263) where a diagnosis cannot be made, laparoscopy may be necessary.

Management As long as the woman is stable, the woman should be offered the options of expectant and medical management according to strict selection criteria:
• Asymptomatic or mild symptoms
• hCG <3000IU
• Ectopic pregnancy <3cm on scan with no fetal heart activity
• No haemoperitoneum on TVS
• The woman must understand the diagnosis and risks of an ectopic pregnancy and must be willing to undertake regular follow-up and live close to the hospital with support at home

Expectant: Falling hCG and the above criteria; take serum hCG every 48h until confirmed fall, then weekly until <15IU. Plateauing or slowly rising hCG needs senior clinician involvement in the management plan.

Medical: Methotrexate (unlicensed use) is used (50mg/m² IM) as a single dose with the criteria above, followed by hCG levels on days 4 and 7. If hCG has fallen by <15% a repeat dose is given (up to 25% cases). Methotrexate is teratogenic and the woman should use reliable contraception for 3 months afterwards. Side effects include conjunctivitis, stomatitis, diarrhoea, and abdominal pain. If the pain does not improve with simple analgesia she should come to hospital immediately. hCG level is not predictive of rupture, which may occur at any time.

Surgical: Laparoscopy is the preferred surgical treatment option due to reduced operating time, reduced length of hospital stay, reduced analgesia requirements and less blood loss with a quicker recovery. However, in women who are haemodynamically unstable, laparotomy may be quicker but this partly depends on the experience of the operating surgeon. Do not delay seeking senior help (registrar, consultant and anaesthetist plus the senior ward nurse) in an unstable patient with a suspected ruptured ectopic pregnancy.

Salpingotomy vs salpingectomy: If the contralateral tube is healthy, RCOG guidelines recommend salpingectomy (removal of the tube) over salpingotomy (removal of the ectopic through a tubal incision). Subsequent intrauterine pregnancy rates are no different after salpingectomy, and salpingotomy has higher rates of persistent trophoblast (8% vs 4%) and subsequent ectopic pregnancy (18% vs 8%). Salpingotomy should be primary treatment if the other tube is not healthy to preserve chance of future intrauterine pregnancy (49%), but warn of risk of future ectopic pregnancy.[23,RCOG] Women with salpingotomy should be followed up with serum hCG to detect and treat persistent trophoblast early (methotrexate may be considered if the woman is stable).

Pregnancy of unknown location (PUL)

Definition There is no sign of intrauterine or ectopic pregnancy or retained products of conception in the presence of a positive pregnancy test, or serum hCG >5IU. Approximately 10% of attendances to the early pregnancy clinic are given this as their first diagnosis. The outcomes are as follows:
• Early intrauterine pregnancy (too early to see on scan)
• Complete miscarriage (no previous scan to prove that it was intrauterine)
• Failing PUL which will never be seen on scan but will resolve on its own
• Ectopic pregnancy (10% of PULs)
• Persistent PUL
• Extremely rarely, from an hCG-secreting tumour.

History is unreliable in diagnosing location of pregnancy, and even if the history suggests complete miscarriage, classify it as a PUL until there is proof that it isn't.

Management is primarily according to symptoms because the most dangerous option for diagnosis is ectopic pregnancy. If the woman has significant pain and haemoperitoneum then laparoscopy is appropriate. If she is well with no haemoperitoneum, hCG and progesterone on the day of the first scan, followed by repeat 48h later and follow-up is appropriate. Check local guidelines but the following plan is reasonable:
• Progesterone <20nmol/L suggests failing pregnancy. If asymptomatic, repeat hCG in 7 days' time
• hCG rise >66% in 48h: hCG should double every 48h in a normal pregnancy; arrange a rescan when it is likely to be >1500IU or in 10-14 days' time
• hCG rise <66% in 48h or plateau: monitor until <15IU, or consider rescan with more senior clinician to make diagnosis
• hCG plateauing or fluctuating: senior advice after 2-3 serial hCGs. If asymptomatic can continue expectant management or offer methotrexate.

hCG levels and their use in early pregnancy

In a normal intrauterine pregnancy, hCG rises >66% every 48h. There is no hCG level that will correspond to weeks' gestation. The 'discriminatory zone' (the level at which a normal pregnancy should be visible on TVS) is not absolute and also relies upon experienced sonographers and quality of equipment. hCG should not be used in following up intrauterine pregnancies or women who are symptomatic—they should be managed clinically. It is unreliable in those who have multiple pregnancies and after assisted conception with hCG support.

This comprises premalignant hydatidiform mole, and the malignant conditions of choriocarcinoma and the rare (0.23%) placental site trophoblastic tumour. Complete moles are diploid and androgenic, 75–80% following duplication of a single sperm after fertilization of an 'empty ovum', 20–25% after dispermic fertilization of an 'empty' ovum so no maternal nuclear DNA although mitochondrial DNA is maternal. Partial moles usually follow dispermic fertilization of an ovum and are triploid (2 sets paternal haploid genes, 1 haploid maternal set) but 10% are tetraploid or mosaic conceptions. Partial moles usually have evidence of fetal parts or red cells. They are 3 × commoner, grow slower (so present later), and are less often malignant (1% vs 15%).

Hydatidiform moles (see fig 3.6) Tumours consist of proliferating chorionic villi which have swollen and degenerated. Derived from chorion, it makes lots of hCG, giving rise to exaggerated pregnancy symptoms and strongly +ve pregnancy tests. *Incidence:* 1.54:1000 pregnancies (UK). It is commoner at extremes of child-bearing age, after a previous mole, and in Asian women. A woman who has had a past mole is at ↑risk for future pregnancies; 0.8–2.9% after one mole, and 15–28% after 2 moles. <1% have familial recurrent moles (recessive) with <1:50 chance of normal pregnancy.[24] *Signs:* Most present with early pregnancy failure, eg failed miscarriage or signs on US. Bleeding may be heavy; molar tissue may look like frogspawn. *US* may show 'snowstorm' effect'. Severe morning sickness or 1st trimester pre-eclampsia are rarer presentations. If twin pregnancy, proceed, if wished (40% viable baby outcome without ↑ persisting neoplasia or adverse treatment results).

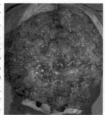

Fig 3.6 Hydatidiform mole.
Courtesy of Prof. J. Carter.

Abdominal pain may be due to huge theca-lutein cysts in both ovaries. These may rupture or tort. They take ~4 months to resolve after molar evacuation. hCG resembles TSH, and may cause hyperthyroidism. ▶Tell the anaesthetist as thyrotoxic storm can occur at evacuation. *Treatment:* Molar tissue is removed from the soft, easily perforated uterus by gentle suction. Send to histology for confirmation of diagnosis. Give anti-D if rhesus –ve (BOX, p11). Pregnancy should be avoided until hCG normal for 6 months. Register the woman at specialist centre (below) for hCG monitoring. Levels should return to normal within 6 months. If levels drop rapidly to normal, oral contraceptives may be used after 6 months. If they do not, either the mole was invasive (myometrium penetrated) or has given rise to choriocarcinoma (10%). Invasive moles may metastasize, eg to lung, vagina, brain, liver, and skin. Both conditions respond to chemotherapy. See BOX p265.

Choriocarcinoma ▶*Investigate all persistent post-pregnancy PV bleeding to exclude choriocarcinoma.* This highly malignant tumour occurs in 1:40,000 deliveries. The chief contexts are following a benign mole (50%), miscarriage (20%), or a normal pregnancy (10%). *Presentation: May be years after pregnancy,* with general malaise (due to 'malignancy' and ↑hCG) or uterine bleeding; signs and symptoms from metastases (may be very haemorrhagic, eg haematoperitoneum); nodules on CXR. Pulmonary artery obstruction via tumour emboli may cause pulmonary artery hypertension (haemoptysis; dyspnoea). *Treatment:* Choriocarcinoma in the UK is treated at 3 specialist centres; it is extremely responsive to combination chemotherapy based on **methotrexate**. Outlook is good if non-metastatic and fertility is usually retained.

Placental site trophoblastic tumour These grow slower, present later, produce less hCG. Post chemotherapy residual disease is excised (eg womb and nodes).

Indications for chemotherapy[25]

- hCG ≥ 20,000 IU/L 4 weeks post evacuation
- Static or rising hCG after evacuation in absence of new pregnancy
- ↑ hCG 6 months post evacuation, even if levels dropping
- Heavy vaginal bleeding, or gastrointestinal or intraperitoneal bleeding
- Evidence of brain, liver, or gastrointestinal metastases, or lung opacities >2cm (smaller lesions may regress spontaneously)
- Histology of choriocarcinoma.

Further reading

RCOG (2010). *The Management of Gestational Trophoblastic Neoplasia* (Guideline No. 38). London: RCOG.

Pruritus vulvae Vaginal itch is distressing and embarrassing. *Causes:* There may be a disorder causing general pruritus (p586) or skin disease (eg psoriasis, lichen planus). The cause may be local: infection and vaginal discharge (eg candida); allergy eg to washing powder, fabric dyes; infestation (eg scabies, pubic lice, threadworms); or vulval dystrophy (lichen sclerosis, leukoplakia, carcinoma). Psychosexual sequelae may ensue. Obesity and incontinence exacerbate symptoms. Postmenopausal atrophy does not cause itch.

The history may suggest the cause. Ask about autoimmune disorders and atopy. Examine general health and look for wider spread skin conditions. Examine the vulva and genital tract, under magnification if possible, and take a cervical smear, if due. Consider taking vaginal and vulval swabs and tests for diabetes and thyroid disease. If vulval dermatitis check serum ferritin and dermatology patch tests. Biopsy if diagnosis in doubt, if there is no response to treatment, or vulval intraepithelial neoplasia or carcinoma are suspected.

▶Scratching and self-medication may have changed the appearance.

Treatment is often unsatisfactory. Treat the cause if possible. Avoid sensitizers (patch testing may reveal sensitizing agents eg 26–80% in vulval dermatitis studies). Reassurance can be very important. Vulval care advice (BOX, p267), may help. A short course of topical steroids, eg **betamethasone valerate** cream 0.1% may help. Avoid any topical preparation which may sensitize the skin.

Lichen sclerosis Thought to be an autoimmune disorder (40% develop other autoimmune disorders), elastic tissue turns to collagen (usually after middle age—or, occasionally, before puberty). The 'bruised' red, purpuric signs may appear, to the unknowing, to suggest abuse—particularly if there are bullae, erosions, and ulcerations. The vulva gradually becomes white, flat, and shiny. There may be an hourglass shape around the vulva and anus. It is intensely itchy. It may be pre-malignant and long-term surveillance is desirable if unresponsive to treatment. *Treatment:* **Clobetasol propionate** cream daily for 28 days, then alternate days for 4 weeks, then twice weekly for 8 weeks, then as needed. The 4–10% who are steroid unresponsive may respond to topical **tacrolimus** (off licence, use in specialist clinic only, for <2 years). In children, 50% resolve by menarche.

Leukoplakia (white vulval patches due to skin thickening and hypertrophy). It is itchy. It should be biopsied as it may be a pre-malignant lesion. *Treatment:* **Topical corticosteroids** (problems: mucosal thinning, absorption); **psoralens** with ultraviolet **phototherapy**; **methotrexate**; **ciclosporin**.

Lichen planus Of unknown cause, this is more likely to present with pain than pruritus. In mouth & genital area it can be erosive, appearing with a well demarcated glazed appearance around the introitus. It can affect all ages.

Lichen simplex This presents with chronic intractable itching, especially at night, in those with sensitive skin or eczema. There is non-specific inflammation of vulva, (±mons pubis and inner thighs). Stress, sensitizing chemicals an low body iron stores can exacerbate symptoms. Treatment is with vulval care (BOX, p267), using steroids to break the itch/scratch cycle, if needed. Antihistamines or antipruritics (above) can help.

Vulvovaginitis Think of fixed drug reactions (NSAIDs, statins); stop for 2 weeks. Desquamative inflammatory vaginitis, of unknown cause, characterized by shiny erythematous patches ± petechiae. It responds to 2-4 weeks of intravaginal **clindamycin** cream with hydrocortisone to the vulva.

Vulval intraepithelial neoplasia

Vulval malignancy has a pre-invasive phase, vulval intra-epithelial neoplasia (VIN, fig 3.7, note white areas with surrounding inflammation). It may be itchy. **Cause** Often HPV, p269 (esp. HPV16); there may not be visible warts but 5% acetic acid stains affected areas white. If VIN is found on biopsy, examine cervix, anal canal if within 1.5cm, natal cleft skin and breasts (>10% have coexistent neoplasia elsewhere, most commonly cervical).

Treating VIN Surveillance is the key with biopsy of suspicious lesions. Painful or irritating lesions can be removed but vulvectomy or laser ablation is not recommended as a general rule due to high recurrence rate and poor functional outcome. Histology reveals 12–17% unrecognized invasion in wide excision samples. Medical treatments have used 5% imiquimod cream with re-

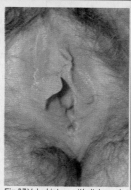

Fig 3.7 Vulval intra-epithelial neoplasia (VIN).

gression of grade 2–3 disease in 77% (it is also used in the treatment of genital warts). It stimulates monocytes and macrophages, which secrete cytokines resulting in T-helper cell coordination of a cell-mediated immune response. Apply the cream 2–3 times per week for 12 weeks. Therapeutic use of human papilloma virus vaccine, photodynamic therapy, interferon use, and cavitron ultrasonic surgical aspiration techniques have been tried but none are currently recommended treatments. Recurrence is common so follow-up regularly.

Vulval care for those with vulval disorders

- Use soap substitute with water for washing (less drying than water alone).
- Shower, bath (with emollient), or clean vulva once daily only.
- Wash vulva with hand (not sponge/flannel); dab dry or blow dry with hair-dryer on cool setting held well away from the skin.
- Wear loose fitting silk or cotton white or light coloured underwear (blue/black dyes can be irritant). Sleep without underwear.
- Avoid tight jeans/cycling trousers but wear loose trousers, dresses, or skirts. At home, wearing skirts without underwear may be more comfortable.
- Avoid soap, bubble bath, shower gels, biological washing powders, fabric conditioners, vulval creams or douches, antiseptics, regular sanitary towel or panty liner wear, baby wipe use, coloured toilet paper, nail varnish.
- Regular emollient use (throughout day) can soothe and reduce flare ups.
- For irritated skin, dabbings of aqueous cream kept in the fridge can soothe.

Gynaecology

Gynaecology

Causes of vulval lumps Local varicose veins; boils; sebaceous cysts; keratoacanthomata (rare); viral warts (condylomata acuminata); condylomata lata (syphilis); primary chancre; molluscum contagiosum; Bartholin's cyst or abscess; uterine prolapse or polyp; inguinal hernia; varicocele; carcinoma.

Vulval warts Human papilloma virus (HPV)—is usually spread by sexual contact. *Incubation:* weeks. Her partner may not have obvious penile warts. The vulva, perineum, anus, vagina, or cervix may be affected. Warts may be very florid in the pregnant and immunosuppressed. HPV types 6 and 11 cause vulval warts and 16, 18, and 33 can cause vulval and cervical intra-epithelial neoplasia. Warts may also cause anal carcinoma (*OHCM* p633). Treat both partners. Exclude other genital infections. Warts may be destroyed in the clinic by cryotherapy, trichloroacetic acid or electrocautery/excision/laser. Vulval and anal warts (condylomata acuminata) may be treated at home with podophyllotoxin cream for 4–6 weeks, washed off after 30min (CI: pregnancy). Only treat a few warts at once, to avoid toxicity. Self-application with 0.15% **podophyllotoxin cream** (Warticon® 5g tubes—enough for 4 treatment courses—is supplied with a mirror): use every 12h for 3 days, repeated up to 4 times at weekly intervals if the area covered is <4cm². Relapse is common. In pregnancy, warts may grow rapidly and usually regress after delivery. Problematic warts can be treated with cryotherapy. It is not an indication for delivery by CS. *HPV immunization and cervical cancer:* See p272. NB: HPV types 6 and 11 may cause laryngeal or respiratory papillomas in the offspring of affected mothers (risk 1:50–1:1500; 50% present at <5yrs old). Any warty lesion in a post-menopausal woman should be biopsied to exclude vulval cancer.[28]

Urethral caruncle This is a small red swelling at the urethral orifice. It is caused by meatal prolapse. It may be tender and give pain on micturition. *Treatment:* Excision or diathermy.

Bartholin's cyst and abscess (fig 3.9) The Bartholin's glands and ducts lie under the labia minora. They secrete thin lubricating mucus during sexual excitation. If the duct blocks, a painless cyst forms; if this becomes infected the resulting abscess is extremely painful (she cannot sit down) and a hugely swollen, hot red labium is seen. *Treatment:* The abscess should be incised, and permanent drainage ensured by marsupialization, ie inner cyst wall is folded back and stitched to the skin, or by balloon catheter insertion.[29] *Tests:* Exclude gonococcus.

Vulvitis Vulval inflammation may be due to infections, eg candida (p284), herpes simplex; chemicals (bubble-baths, detergents). It is often associated with, or may be due to, vaginal discharge.

Vulval ulcers (fig 3.10) *Causes* Always consider syphilis. *Herpes simplex* is common in the young. Others: carcinoma; chancroid; lymphogranuloma venereum; granuloma inguinale; TB; Behçet's syndrome; aphthous ulcers; Crohn's disease.

Herpes simplex (fig 3.8) Herpes type II classically causes genital infection, but either type can be the cause (30% type I). It is the third most common STI in the UK. The primary infection is usually the most severe, starting with the prodrome (itching/tingling of affected skin) and flu-like illness, progressing to vulvitis, pain, and small vesicles on the vulva. Urinary retention may occur due to autonomic nerve dysfunction. Recurrent attacks are usually less severe and may be triggered by illness, stress, sexual intercourse and menstruation. *Treatment:* Strong **analgesia**, **lidocaine gel 2%**, **salt baths** (and micturating in the bath) help. Exclude coexistent infections. **Aciclovir** orally shortens symptoms. Oral dose: 200mg 5 times daily or 400mg/8h for 5 days (longer if new lesions appear during treatment or if healing is incomplete). If immunocompromised/HIV+ve: 400mg 5 times daily for 7–10 days during 1st episode or 400mg/8h for 5–10 days during recurrent infection. If >6 outbreaks/year consider suppressive aciclovir for 6–12 months. Topical aciclovir is not beneficial. HSV can be transmitted during asymptomatic phases of viral shedding, and from areas of the genitals not protected by barrier contraception. Men are usually less symptomatic and may never have been aware of the infection, thereby unknowningly infecting their partners months or even years later, so don't assume infidelity.

For herpes in pregnancy, see p36.

Carcinoma of the vulva ► Refer unexplained vulval lumps urgently.

90% are squamous. Others are melanoma, basal cell carcinomas or carcinoma of Bartholin's glands. They are rare and usually occur in the elderly (age 70–80).

Presentation may be as a lump; as an indurated ulcer which may not be noticed unless it causes pain and bleeding hence often presenting late (50% already have inguinal lymph node involvement). There may be a pre-invasive phase as VIN (for explanation and treatment see p267).

Treatment🔬 If tumour <2cm width and <1mm deep, lymph node excision is not needed. If >1mm deep do 'triple incision surgery' =wide (>15mm margin) local excision + ipsilateral groin node biopsy (and, if affected, sample contralateral side too). More advanced disease may need radical vulvectomy (wide excision of the vulva + removal of inguinal glands). Skin grafts may be needed. Radiotherapy may be used pre-op to shrink tumours if sphincters may be affected. Chemoradiation is used if unsuitable for surgery, to shrink large tumours preoperatively and for relapses. 5-yr survival is >80% for lesions <2cm with no node involvement; otherwise <50%.

Gynaecology

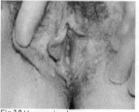

Fig 3.8 Herpes simplex.
Reproduced from Pattman et al., *OH of Genitourinary Medicine, HIV, and Sexual Health* (2010) with permission from Oxford University Press.

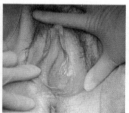

Fig 3.9 Bartholin's abscess.
Reproduced from Sarris, Bewley, & Agnihotri, *Training in Obstetrics and Gynaecology* (2009) with permission from Oxford University Press.

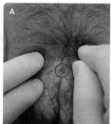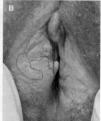

Fig 3.10 Vulval cancer.
Reprinted from *American Journal of Obstetrics and Gynecology*, Volume 203, issue 2, Michiel Simons et al, A patient with lichen sclerosis, Langerhans cell histiocytosis, and invasive squamous cell carcinoma of the vulva, pp. e7–e10, (2010), with permission from Elsevier.

This is the part of the uterus below the internal os. The endocervical canal is lined with mucous columnar epithelium, the vaginal cervix with squamous epithelium. The transitional zone between them—the squamo–columnar junction—is the area which is predisposed to malignant change.

Cervical ectropion/erosion (see fig 3.11) There is a red ring around the os because the endocervical epithelium has extended its territory over the paler epithelium of the ectocervix. Ectropions extend temporarily under hormonal influence during puberty, with the combined pill, and during pregnancy. As columnar epithelium is soft and glandular, ectropion is prone to bleeding, to excess mucus production, and to infection. *Treatment:* No treatment if asymptomatic, pregnant or pubertal. If taking hormonal contraception consider changing to non-hormonal methods; cautery with diathermy as an out-patient if the woman wishes.

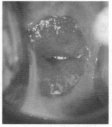
Fig 3.11 Cervical ectropion.
Courtesy of Mike Hughey.

Nabothian cysts These mucus retention cysts found on the cervix are harmless.

Cervical polyps These pedunculated benign tumours of endocervical epithelium may cause increased mucus discharge or postcoital bleeding. *Treatment:* In young women they may be simply avulsed, but in peri- and postmenopausial women includes TVS ± hysteroscopy to exclude intrauterine polyps.

Cervicitis This may be follicular or mucopuru-lent, presenting with discharge. *Causes:* Chlamydia (up to 50%), gonococci, or herpes (look for vesicles). Chronic cervicitis (see fig 3.12) is usually a mixed infection. Cervicitis may mask neoplasia on a smear.

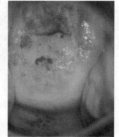
Fig 3.12 Chronic cervicitis.
Courtesy of Mike Hughey.

Cervical screening (cytology)

Cervical cancer has a pre-invasive phase: cervical intra-epithelial neoplasia (CIN). CIN 1 affects the lower basal third of cervical epithelium and will regress to normal in 60% within 2 years. CIN is associated with oncogenic human papilloma viruses (HPV) 16, 18, 31, and 33. CIN II and CIN III affect <⅔ and >⅔ or full thickness of epithelium respectively, and are less likely to regress (43%, 32% respectively) with a significant number developing into invasive squamous carcinoma of the cervix. Smears collect cervical cells for microscopy for dyskaryosis (abnormalities which reflect CIN). Women with borderline or mild changes are tested for high-risk HPV and if positive, referred for colposcopy (HPV triage). Moderate and severe changes require colposcopy regardless of HPV status. The degree of dyskaryosis approximates to the severity of CIN (TABLE, p271). CIN III lesions are more likely to progress to invasive carcinoma. This may take ~10yrs, but may happen much faster in young women. In women following LLETZ (p272) for CIN, if cytology is normal and HPV –ve at 6 months, 3-yearly smears are appropriate. Abnormal cytology or HPV +ve smears require referral back to colposcopy (HPV test of cure).

HIV +ve women should have annual smears. 83% of the eligible UK population is now screened, and mortality is 50% that of 1988 (the year screening started).

Taking a smear

- Explain the nature and purpose of the test, and how results will be conveyed. Warn that results are not always unequivocal.
- The cervix is visualized with a speculum (p242). Are there any suspicious areas? If so, carry on with the smear and indicate this on the referral form, and refer immediately for colposcopy under the 2-week rule.
- Cells are scraped from the squamo-columnar transformation zone with a special brush which is agitated in a liquid, ready for analysis (liquid-based cytology). This has advantages over fixing immediately onto a slide: it is quicker and easier to read and inadequate cytology is cut by 80%.
- Suspensions can also be tested for human papilloma virus (see p273) and chlamydia.
- Ensure regular training and supervision, and audit of numbers of 'inadequate sample' reports. Don't do smears on a one-off basis (in the UK NHS, professionalism mandates formal methods of quality control, and specifies an acceptable number of smears per year, etc).

Risk factors for CIN
- Persistent high-risk HPV infection
- Exposure to HPV is increased by multiple partners
- Smoking
- Immunocompromise (HIV, transplant patients, immunosuppressants)
- The oral contraceptive pill is associated with CIN but probably due to reduced use of barrier contraception, thereby increasing exposure to HPV.

English cervical screening criteria
- Sexually active women aged 25–64
- 3-yearly for woman 25–50 years, and 5-yearly until 64 (if normal)
- 95% of abnormalities are identified by 3-yearly screening
- In Scotland, screening begins at 20 years, and worldwide screening intervals vary considerably.

Management of abnormal smears		
Papanicoulao class	**Histology**	**Management**
Normal	0.1% CIN II–III	Repeat in 3 years
Inflammatory	6% CIN II–III	Repeat in 6 months Swabs Colposcopy after 3 abnormal
Borderline changes	20–30% CIN II–III	High-risk HPV test; if +ve refer for colposcopy; if -ve repeat in 3 years
Mild dyskaryosis	30% CIN II–III	High-risk HPV test; if +ve refer for colposcopy; if -ve repeat in 3 years
Moderate dyskaryosis	50–75% CIN II–III	Refer to colposcopy
Severe dyskaryosis	80–90% CIN II–III	Refer to colposcopy
Suspected invasion	50% invasion	Urgent colposcopy
Abnormal glandular cells	Adenocarcinoma of the cervix	Urgent colposcopy

Further reading

NHSCSP (2010). *Colposcopy and programme management: guidelines for the NHS cervical screening programme*. http://www.cancerscreening.nhs.uk/cervical/publications/nhscsp2-.html

NHSCSP (2011). *HPV triage and test of cure protocol*. http://www.cancerscreening.nhs.uk/cervical/hpv-tirage-test-flowchart.pdf

Gynaecology

Aim to detect pre-invasive disease by attendance at cervical screening. ~1900 women die yearly of cervical cancer in the UK. The main cause is human papilloma virus (eg HPV 16, 18, 31, 33, 35, 39, 45, 51, 52, 56, 58, 59, 68). Vaccines work only against a subset, eg Gardasil® covers HPV 6, 11, 16 & 18, the cause in 70% of cases. 99.7% of cervical cancers contain HPV DNA.

Dyskaryosis is a cytological term used to describe cervical smears. There are high false positive (10-15%) and false negative rates (5-15%), hence the need for further assessment by colposcopy.

Colposcopy

This is the examination of the cervix by a colposcope—a binocular micro-scope which magnifies by 6–40×. The woman is in the lithotomy position and a bivalve speculum is inserted into the vagina. Once the cervix is visualized, the transformation zone is identified and painted with 5% acetic acid. This is preferentially taken up by neoplastic cells (fig 3.13 on p275). Lugol's iodine is also used, which is not taken up by neoplastic cells. Aceto-white areas identify abnormal areas and this enables a punch biopsy to be taken in order to gain a histological diagnosis (CIN or malignancy). If there is strong uptake of acetic acid (termed high-grade colposcopy), CIN II-III is more likely and the option is to 'see and treat'—perform definitive treatment in the same appointment without waiting for a biopsy result. CIN is also associated with vascular ab-normalities. Very abnormal-looking vessels are associated with micro-invasive carcinoma. Colposcopy does not detect adenocarcinoma (it usually lies within endocervical canal). A pregnant woman can have colposcopy but not a LLETZ, and should wait until she is 12 weeks postpartum for definitive treatment.

Large loop excision of the transformation zone (LLETZ)

CIN is managed according to grade of abnormality and patient preference, either conservatively or by excision. A LLETZ is usually performed in the col-poscopy clinic under local anaesthesia, using loop diathermy. It is safe, easy to perform (all those treating CIN should be qualified to do so) and tissue is avail-able for histology and confirmation of clear excision margins. It gives ~90% cure rates with one treatment.

Low-grade CIN (CIN I) regresses spontaneously in 60% with no treatment. If HPV +ve offer 6-monthly colposcopy, and LLETZ if persistent.

High-grade CIN (>CIN I) progresses to cervical cancer in 3–5% of those with CIN II and 20–30% with CIN III within 10 years if left untreated. Spontaneous regres-sion is possible but much less likely. It is therefore recommended for excision with LLETZ.

After LLETZ, the woman should have a smear at 6 months with high-risk HPV testing. If negative, she can return to 3-yearly smears. An abnormal smear result and/or positive HR-HPV test requires repeat assessment with colposcopy.

Complications of LLETZ include haemorrhage, infection, vaso-vagal symptoms and signs, anxiety, cervical stenosis and a small risk of cervical incompetence and premature delivery (risk is thought to be increased with repeated LLETZ or biopsy depth >1cm).

CGIN is cervical glandular intraepithelial neoplasia, and can co-exist with CIN or be a sole finding. It is also associated with high-risk HPV and can be difficult to manage, because the endocervical epithelium extends into the cervical canal and is therefore not completely visible at colposcopy, has no specific colposcopic appearances and is associated with higher 'skip lesions'. It is managed with a cylindrical LLETZ or cone biopsy, or if family is complete, hysterectomy.

HPV vaccination

HPV is a key player in the development of cervical cancer, and schoolchildren in the UK (girls primarily, but it is likely that boys will be offered vaccination in the future because they also spread the virus) are offered the HPV vaccine at 12 years, before their sexual debut. They offer no protection once HPV infection has occurred and are therefore not recommended in the management of CIN. The vaccines are primarily against HPV subtypes 6 and 11 (anogenital warts) and 16 and 18 (HR-HPV). They do not prevent all cancers (there are 15 HR-HPVS) and the long-term antibody response is at present unknown.

Cervical cancer

83% of cervical cancer occurs in developing countries and is the second most common cancer in women worldwide. Incidence has two peaks: the first at 30–39 years and the second in the over 70s. Screening in the UK has increased the proportion of micro-invasive disease and adenocarcinomas (most are squamous carcinomas). High risk HPV is strongly associated with cervical cancer. Risk factors are the same as for CIN (p271). See figs 3.14 on p275.

Symptoms and signs
• Cervical smear showing ?invasion (unreliable)
• Incidental finding on treatment of CIN
• Post-coital and/or post-menopausal bleeding; watery vaginal discharge
• Features of advanced disease include heavy vaginal bleeding, ureteric obstruction, weight loss, bowel disturbance, vesicovaginal fistula, and pain.

Examination on colposcopy shows an irregular cervical surface, abnormal vessels and dense uptake of acetic acid. On bimanual examination, the cervix feels roughened and hard, and if disease is advanced, there is loss of the fornices and the cervix is fixed. Speculum examination shows an irregular mass that often will bleed on contact.

Investigations should include FBC, U&E, LFTS, punch biopsy for histology (LLETZ is contraindicated as it will bleed heavily and is not definitive treatment), CT abdomen and pelvis (staging), MRI pelvis (very accurate for staging and identifying suspicious lymph nodes). Examination under anaesthetic helps staging, and includes cystoscopy, hysteroscopy, PV/PR examination and sometimes sigmoidoscopy. MRI is so accurate that EUA is now performed less often.
Stage I tumours are confined to the cervix; *Ia* microscopic; *Ib* macroscopic
Stage II have extended locally to upper ⅔ of the vagina; *IIb* if to parametria
Stage III have spread to lower ⅓ of vagina *IIIa*; or pelvic wall *IIIb*
Stage IV have spread to bladder or rectum. *IVb* if spread to distant organs
Most present in stages I or II. Up to stage 1b, 5 year survival is 90–95%.

Treatment depends on stage and functional status:
• *Stage 1a1* (<3mm depth): Local excision (fertility-sparing) or hysterectomy
• *Stage 1a2* (<5mm depth) and *1b1* (<4cm diameter): Lymphadenectomy and if node negative, proceed to Wertheim's hysterectomy
• *Stage 1b2* (>4cm diameter) and early IIa: Chemoradiotherapy. If negative lymph nodes, consider Wertheim's hysterectomy
• >*Stage IIb*: Combination chemoradiotherapy
• *Stage IVb*: Chemoradiotherapy; palliative radiotherapy to control bleeding
Laparoscopic lymphadenectomy is being used increasingly prior to hysterectomy; some units are now doing Wertheim's hysterectomy laparoscopically. Cisplatin is the main chemotherapy agent used.

Complications of treatment for Wertheim's (radical) hysterectomy and lymphadenectomy include bleeding, infection, VTE, ureteric fistula, bladder dysfunction, and lymphoedema. Radiotherapy can cause acute bladder and bowel dysfunction with tenesmus, mucositis, bleeding, ulceration, strictures and fistula formation, vaginal stenosis, shortening, and dryness.

Gynaecology

Endometritis Uterine infection is uncommon unless the barrier to ascending infection (acid vaginal pH and cervical mucus) is broken, eg after miscarriage, TOP and childbirth, IUCD insertion, or surgery. Infection may ascend further to involve fallopian tubes and ovaries. *Presentation:* Lower abdominal pain and fever; uterine tenderness on bimanual palpation, offensive vaginal discharge. *Tests:* Take high vaginal swabs and blood cultures if septic. Remove IUCD if not responding to antibiotics. *Treatment:* Give antibiotics (eg **cefalexin 500mg/8h** PO with **metronidazole 400mg/8h** PO for 7 days).

Endometrial proliferation Oestrogen stimulates endometrial proliferation in the first half of the menstrual cycle; it is then influenced by progesterone and is shed at menstruation. A particularly exuberant proliferation is associated with heavy menstrual bleeding and polyps.

Continuous high oestrogen levels (eg with obesity) make the endometrium hyperplastic ('cystic glandular hyperplasia'—a histological diagnosis after endometrial biopsy). It eventually breaks down, causing irregular heavy bleeding. *Treatment:* Address the cause; if no atypia on histology, treat with progestagens eg Mirena coil and re-biopsy in 6-12 months. In older women proliferation may contain foci of atypical cells which may lead to endometrial carcinoma (p278).

Pyometra This is a uterus distended by pus eg associated with salpingitis or secondary to outflow blockage. *Treatment:* Drain the uterus, treat the cause.

Haematometra This is a uterus filled with blood due to outflow obstruction. It is rare. The blockage may be an imperforate hymen in the young (p246); carcinoma; or iatrogenic cervical stenosis, eg after LLETZ.

Endometrial tuberculosis Genital tract tuberculosis is rare in Britain, except among high-risk groups (eg immigrants). It is blood-borne and usually affects first the fallopian tubes, then the endometrium.

It may present with acute salpingitis if disease is very active, or with subfertility, pelvic pain, and menstrual disorders (40%) eg amenorrhoea, oligomenorrhoea. There may be pyosalpinx. Send peritoneal fluid at laparoscopy, and/or endometrial curettings for culture and histology. Exclude lung disease by CXR. *Treatment* is medical with antituberculous therapy (OHCM p398–9). Repeat endometrial histology after 1 year. Total abdominal hysterectomy with bilateral salpingo-oophorectomy is treatment of choice if there are adnexal masses and the woman is >40yrs.

Pelvic US Transvaginal US gives better resolution than transabdominal. Homogeneity, echoes of low intensity and presence of a linear central shadow are associated with absence of endometrial abnormality.

Normal cycle thickness: <5mm early cycle, 11mm in proliferative phase; 7-16mm late cycle. Endometrial cancer should be ruled out by endometrial biopsy ±hysteroscopy if endometrial thickness >20mm (4mm if postmenopausal), heterogeneous appearance, and hypoechoic areas. Polyps have cystic appearance (also with hyperechoic endometrium) and are most clearly seen in the early days of the cycle.

If postmenopausal and not on HRT, double-layer endometrial thickness should be <5mm. Sequential hormone replacement ↑endometrial thickness (average 5–8.5mm); if on continuous combined replacement HRT thicknesses are ~4.5–7mm; tibolone treated endometrium <5mm; but tamoxifen thickens it to ~13mm (also associated with endometrial polyps, often large, usually benign). It thins down by 6 months after stopping tamoxifen, then stays thin.

US is useful for detecting fibroids, assessing ovaries and adnexal masses. It is operator dependent, and obesity can hinder the view. It is unable to detect endometriotic deposits (unless ovarian endometrioma).

Primary vaginal cancers are extremely rare, accounting for <1% gynaecological malignancies. Vaginal tumours are most commonly due to metastatic spread from cervical, uterine, or vulval cancers. Of the true primary vaginal cancers, most are squamous in origin and present on older women. There is an association with previous CIN, pelvic radiotherapy and long-term vaginal inflammation from pessaries or a procidentia (complete uterine prolapse). It is commonly HPV-related.

They are commonest in the upper third of the vagina. Presentation is usually with bleeding. Clear cell adenocarcinoma is associated with intrauterine exposure to diethylstilboestrol before 18 weeks' gestation but risk is low (0.1–1:1000). (Note: risk of invasive cervical carcinoma is also increased 3-fold, and structural abnormalities of the genital tract—uterine 69% and cervical 44%—are problems following past exposure).[30, RCOG] Spread is local and by lymphatics. Treatment is usually radiotherapy. Prognosis is poor eg 58% 5-yr survival for squamous vaginal carcinoma; 34% for adenocarcinoma.

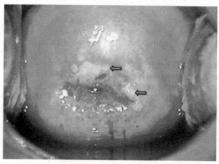

Fig 3.13 Colposcopic view of CIN-III.
Reproduced from Sarris, Bewley & Agnihotri, *Training in Obstetrics and Gynaecology* (2009) with permission from Oxford University Press.

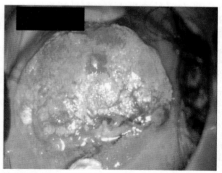

Fig 3.14 Exophytic cervical carcinoma.
Reproduced from Sarris, Bewley & Agnihotri, *Training in Obstetrics and Gynaecology* (2009) with permission from Oxford University Press.

Gynaecology

Fibroids are benign smooth muscle tumours of the uterus (leiomyomas) (fig 3.15). They are often multiple, and vary in size from seedlings to tumours occupying a large part of the abdomen. They start as lumps in the wall of the uterus but may grow to bulge out of the wall so that they lie under the visceral peritoneum (subserosal, 20%), intramurally, under the endometrium (submucosal, 5%), or become pedunculated. Fibroids are common (20–40% of women of reproductive age have fibroids), increasing in frequency with age, in Afro-Caribbean women and those with a family history of fibroids.

Associations Mutation in the gene for fumarate hydratase can cause fibroids and a rare association with skin & uterine leiomyomata, and renal cell cancer.[6] [31]

Natural history Fibroids are oestrogen dependent. Consequently they enlarge in pregnancy and on the combined pill and atrophy after the menopause. They may degenerate gradually or suddenly (red degeneration, see BOX on p277). Occasionally they calcify ('womb stones'). Rarely, they undergo sarcomatous change—usually causing pain, malaise, bleeding, and increase in size in a postmenopausal woman.

Presentation Many are asymptomatic:
- *Menorrhagia:* Fibroids often produce heavy and prolonged periods (± anaemia. They do not generally cause intermenstrual or postmenopausal bleeding.
- *Fertility problems:* Submucosal fibroids may interfere with implantation. Large or multiple tumours which distort the uterine cavity may cause miscarriage should pregnancy occur but this is unproven.
- *Pain:* This may be due to torsion of a pedunculated fibroid, producing symptoms similar to that of a torted ovarian cyst. 'Red degeneration' following thrombosis of the fibroid blood supply: see BOX, p277.
- *Mass:* Large fibroids may be felt abdominally. They may press on the bladder, causing frequency, or on the veins, causing oedematous legs and varicose veins. Pelvic fibroids may obstruct labour or cause retention of urine.

Treatment If symptoms are minimal, no treatment is needed.
- *GnRH analogues* eg goserelin 3.6mg sc monthly, for 3–6 months prior to surgery can be used to shrink the fibroids but it is not a long-term option due to demineralization of bone.
- *Ulipristal acetate* is a selective progesterone receptor modulator, and can be taken daily for 3–6 months to specifically shrink fibroids and induce amenorrhoea and is licensed for this purpose prior to surgery. In some women the reduction in fibroid size (up to 40%) extends beyond that of the treatment and they may then decline surgery.
- *Myomectomy* can be hysteroscopic, laparoscopic or open, depending on size and location. Submucosal fibroids are better removed hysteroscopically, and laparoscopic myomectomy demands advanced minimal access skills as well as an isolated, subserous fibroid. Open myomectomy has a 10% risk of hysterectomy due to bleeding, and is less straightforward. If the endometrial cavity is breached at laparoscopic or open myomectomy, resulting pregnancies require elective cs for delivery to prevent uterine rupture in labour.
- *Uterine artery embolization (UAE)* is undertaken by an interventional radiologist after assessment by MRI. The uterine artery is catheterized and then embolized. It avoids a general anaesthetic but can be extremely painful in the recovery period, and may lead to a necrotic, infected uterus. Pregnancy outcomes are better after myomectomy than UAE, and UAE is not recommended by fertility specialists for women wishing to retain fertility.
- *Hysterectomy* is the only cure for fibroids and is reserved for women who have completed their family or have no wish for preserving fertility.

6 Gene location: 1q42.3–q43.

5:1000 Caucasian women have fibroids in pregnancy. They are commoner in Afro-Caribbean women. They increase in size in pregnancy—especially in the 2nd trimester. US aids diagnosis. Colour flow Doppler distinguishes fibroids from myometrium. If pedunculated they may tort. Red degeneration is when thrombosis of capsular vessels is followed by venous engorgement and inflammation, causing abdominal pain (± vomiting & low-grade fever), and localized peritoneal tenderness—usually in the last half of pregnancy or the puerperium. 'Here, a certain feverishness leads them to their final degeneration', and imitating the course of all grand passions, 'they grow big and tender, and then die'. D.H. Lawrence *Sons & Lovers*

Treatment is expectant (bed rest, analgesia) with resolution over 4–7 days.

Most fibroids arise from the body of the uterus and do not therefore obstruct labour, as they tend to rise away from the pelvis throughout pregnancy. If large pelvic masses of fibroids are noted prior to labour, caesarean section should be planned. Obstruction of labour also needs cs.

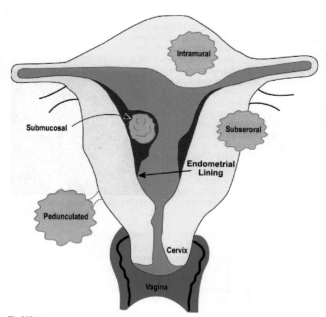

Fig 3.15 Diagram demonstrating the potential locations of uterine fibroids: pedunculated, subserosal, intramural, and submucosal.

Reproduced from Sarris, Bewley, & Agnihotri, *Training in Obstetrics and Gynaecology* (2009) with permission from Oxford University Press.

▶ *Investigate postmenopausal vaginal bleeding **promptly** as the cause may be endometrial cancer.* Cancer of the endometrium is less common than cancer of the cervix. 91% of cases occur in postmenopausal women. Most are adenocarcinomas, and are related to excessive exposure to oestrogen unopposed by progesterone. There is marked geographical variation: North American:Chinese ratio ≈7:1, reflecting differences in risk factors, which are as follows:

• Obesity, type 2 diabetes, hypertension (increased peripheral oestrogens)
• Nulliparity (pregnancy associated with high progesterone levels)
• Anovulatory cycles, such as PCOS (absence of corpus luteum and therefore progesterone)
• Early/late menopause
• Genetic predisposition: HNPCC (Lynch II syndrome) confers a high risk of colorectal, endometrial and ovarian cancers
• Breast cancer (similar lifestyle factors, and tamoxifen use)
• Oestrogen-only HRT
• Protective factors are parity, and the combined oral contraceptive pill.

Presentation is usually as postmenopausal bleeding (PMB). A woman with PMB has a 10% risk of gynaecological cancer. Premenopausal women have heavy or irregular periods,and 1% are detected on routine smear. PV discharge and pyometra can also occur—50% with pyometra have underlying cancer.

Diagnosis PMB is an early sign, and generally leads a woman to see her doctor, but examination is usually normal. TVS shows endometrial thickness >4mm. ET <4mm on scan has 96% negative predictive value with no requirement for biopsy, unless symptoms are recurrent. Biopsy can be performed either in out-patients (p279) or with hysteroscopy. Hysteroscopy enables visualization of abnormal endometrium to improve accuracy of sampling. Once diagnosis has been made, CT/MRI are used to help preoperatively stage. **Histology** Major prognostic indicators are grade of differentiation and FIGO stage of disease. It may metastasize to the vagina (5%), ovary (5%), or any of the pelvic lymph nodes (7%).

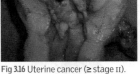

Fig 3.16 Uterine cancer (≥ stage II).
Courtesy of Prof. J. Carter.

Staging (fig 3.16) The tumour is...
  I   in the body of the uterus only
  II in the body and cervix only
  III advancing beyond the uterus, but not beyond the pelvis
  IV extending outside the pelvis (eg to bowel and bladder).

Treatment depends on stage and functional status of the patient.

Total hysterectomy with bilateral salpingo-oophorectomy and peritoneal washings can be performed open or laparoscopically. Pelvic lymphadenectomy is controversial in early stage disease with Cochrane suggesting no survival benefit. Adjuvant radiotherapy is used in low-grade disease with deep myometrial invasion, and high-grade disease with superficial invasion. Radiotherapy has been shown to reduce pelvic recurrences but confers no survival benefit to late stage I disease, because those recurrences are responsive to radiotherapy if it has not previously been used. In advanced disease, high-dose progesterone helps with palliation of symptoms, and external beam radiotherapy can be used to control bleeding. Stage I disease has 85% 5-year survival, dropping to 25% by stage IV.

This bedside investigation is used for postmenopausal bleeding, women >45 years with abnormal menstrual symptoms, and unexpected bleeding patterns in women on HRT. It is cheap, reliable, and gives quick results without the need for anaesthesia. If transvaginal uterine US precedes the procedure, sample if endometrium >4mm thick. It is less useful in menorrhagia in women <45 years with regular cycles, as pathology is less common.

A sample is obtained using a side-opening plastic cannula in which a vacuum is created by withdrawal of a stopped central plunger mechanism. As the cannula is withdrawn and rotated in each quadrant of the uterine cavity, endometrial tissue is sucked into its interior, through the hole in its side (fig 3.17). Successful insertion is possible in 90–99% of women (hysteroscopy and biopsy possible in 99%). Adequate samples will be obtained in 91% of these, and in 84% of those for whom PMB was the indication. Abandon the procedure if it is impossible to enter the uterus, or if it causes too much pain.

Technique
1 Bimanual examination to assess size and position of uterus (p242).
2 Bend cervical cannula to follow the curve of the uterus.
3 Insert device, watching the centimetre scale on the side; observe resistance on entering the internal os (at 3–4cm) and then as the tip reaches the fundus.
4 When the tip is in the fundus, create a vacuum by withdrawing plunger until the stopper prevents further withdrawal. Then move sampler up and down in the uterus, rotate and repeat to sample whole cavity.
5 Remove cannula, and expel tissue into formalin. Send for histology. Vabra vacuum aspiration samples a greater area of tissue, and has higher cancer detection rates, but is more uncomfortable.[32]

Management Reassure those in whom the results show normal or atrophic endometrium and those in whom tissue was sufficient for diagnosis. If those with PMB re-bleed, refer for hysteroscopy (polyps or a fibroid will be present in 20%). Those with simple hyperplasia on histology can be treated with progesterones. Refer those with polyps or necrotic tissue on histology for hysteroscopy and biopsy, and those with atypical hyperplasia or carcinoma for hysterectomy and bilateral salpingo-oophorectomy. If transvaginal uterine US is not already done, perform in those on whom the procedure was impossible or abandoned to establish endometrial thickness (<4mm normal in the postmenopausal; refer if >4mm thick or if polyps seen, for hysteroscopy, biopsy, and polypectomy).

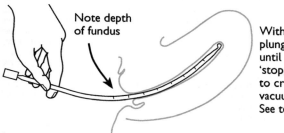

Note depth of fundus

Withdraw plunger until 'stopped' to create vacuum. See text

Fig 3.17 Endometrial sampling.   Redrawn from information supplied by Genesis Medical.

Ovarian cysts are extremely common, and most often physiological due to either follicular cysts or corpus luteal cysts. In a woman of reproductive age, cysts <5cm should not cause concern unless imaging shows complex or suspicious features, or if she is symptomatic (most frequently pain). Whilst most ovarian cysts are benign, one of the cornerstones of management is to identify cysts with a high risk of cancer so that the woman can be treated in a cancer centre.

Presentation
• Asymptomatic; an incidental finding on imaging for a different indication
• Chronic pain with dull ache, dyspareunia, cyclical pain, or pressure effects
• Acute pain due to bleeding into the cyst, ovarian torsion (the ovary does not tort unless a mass disturbs the balance), or rupture
• Irregular vaginal bleeding
• Hormonal effects eg sudden development of androgenic features
• Abdominal swelling or mass; ascites suggests malignancy.

Cyclical pain and deep dyspareunia are features of endometriosis, which may be evident as an endometrioma on tvs (small deposits are poorly identified by us). *Ovarian torsion* is uncommon, classically presenting with severe lower abdominal pain and vomiting. The pain may then start to improve after 24h after the ovary starts to die. During torsion, the venous return from the ovary is occluded, causing the ovary to become oedematous, eventually leading to interruption of arterial blood supply. wbc and crp may be normal or raised. Cyst rupture presents similarly to ovarian torsion but the woman may have additional features of haemorrhagic shock.

Examination may be normal if the cyst is small or the woman obese. If this is an acute presentation, be systematic and check observations and treat signs of shock first. Abdominal examination may reveal a mass arising from the pelvis, tenderness, peritonism, or ascites. Vaginal examination may show vaginal discharge or bleeding, cervical excitation, adnexal mass or tenderness. Nodular uterosacral ligaments and a fixed retroverted uterus are features of endometriosis.

Investigations Check fbc; tumour markers depend on the age of the patient. ca125 is less sensitive in women <40 years but should be checked in anyone >40. In a woman <40 years check afp, ca19-9, ldh, hcg, and cea.

Imaging tvs is the most appropriate modality to start with. It is useful in distinguishing benign from malignant masses (concerning features: multilocular cyst, large papillary cyst wall projections, solid areas, metastases, ascites and bilateral lesions). A cyst extending out of the pelvis will need transabdominal imaging with us, and in cysts >7cm consider mri (superior for distinguishing benign from malignant disease; endometriomas and dermoid cysts have particular features on mri). mri and ct are used in staging malignancy.

Management Acute onset of symptoms with severe pain requires admission to hospital. If she is stable, arrange urgent tvs. If she is unstable, arrange urgent laparoscopy. *Pre-menopausal women* Aim to preserve fertility and exclude malignancy. Rescan in 6 weeks. If no features of malignancy and she is asymptomatic with a cyst <5cm, no surgical intervention is required. If the cyst is >5cm, she is symptomatic or it has features of a dermoid or endometriosis, arrange laparoscopic ovarian cystectomy. Avoid spilling cyst contents (if dermoid can lead to chemical peritonitis and if malignant can up-stage the disease). *Post-menopasual women* Calculate Risk of Malignancy Index (uses menopausal status, ca125 and us features). Low-risk cysts <5cm can be managed conservatively with repeat tvs and ca125 every 4 months and the woman discharged if there is no change after 1 year. Moderate-risk cysts require (usually) bilateral oophorectomy; high-risk cysts require referral to a cancer centre for staging laparotomy (see box).

Functional cysts These are enlarged or persistent follicular or corpus luteum cysts. They are so common that they may be considered normal if they are small (<5cm). They may cause pain by rupture, failing to rupture at ovulation, or bleeding. If <5cm they usually resolve over 2-3 cycles.

Endometriomas Ovarian cysts filled with old blood; also known as chocolate cyst (see p288).

Serous cystadenomas These develop papillary growths that may be so prolific that the cyst appears solid. They are commonest in women aged 30–40 years. About 30% are bilateral and about 30% are malignant.

Mucinous cystadenomas The commonest large ovarian tumours; these may become enormous. They are filled with mucinous material and rupture may rarely cause pseudomyxoma peritonei (p283). They may be multilocular. They are commonest in the 30–50yrs age group. About 5% will be malignant. Remove the appendix at operation in those with suspected mucinous cystadenoma and send for histology. (Interestingly men can get pseudomyxoma from intestinal or appendicular neoplasms; most women with pseudomyxoma peritonei do not have overt rupture of ovarian tumours and 90% have concurrent intestinal or appendicular tumours and it is now thought that the ovarian tumours may be secondary to GI tumours.)

Fibromas These are small, solid, benign, fibrous tissue tumours. They are associated with *Meigs' syndrome:* pleural effusion, often right sided + benign ovarian fibroma (or thecoma, cystadenoma, granulosa cell tumour) + ascites.

Teratomas These arise from primitive germ cells. A benign mature teratoma (dermoid cyst) may contain well-differentiated tissue, eg hair, teeth. 20% are bilateral. They are most common in young women. Poorly differentiated malignant teratomas are rare.

Other germ cell tumours (all malignant and all rare) Non-gestational choriocarcinomas (secrete hCG); ectodermal sinus tumours (yolk sac tumours—secrete α-fetoprotein); dysgerminomas.

Sex-cord tumours (rare; usually of low-grade malignancy) These arise from cortical mesenchyme. Granulosa-cell and theca-cell tumours produce oestrogen and may present with precocious puberty, menstrual problems, or postmenopausal bleeding. Arrhenoblastomas secrete androgens.

Calculating Risk of Malignancy Index (RMI)

RMI = U × M × CA125
• U = US score (0, 1 or 3)
• M = menopausal status (1 = premenopausal, 3 = postmenopausal)
• CA125 = serum CA125 level (U/L)
US scoring system: 1 point for each of the following:
• Mulitlocularity
• Solid areas
• Metastases
• Ascites
• Bilaterality of lesions.
Score 0 for no features, 1 if 1 feature and 2 if there are 3 or more present.

Overall risk
• Low; RMI <25 with <3% risk of cancer
• Moderate; RMI 25–250 with 20% risk of cancer
• High; RMI >250 with 75% risk of cancer.

Further reading

The Management of Ovarian Masses in Pre- and Post-Menopausal Women (Green-top Guidelines No. 34 & 62) London: RCOG.

Ovarian cancer is the leading cause of death from gynaecological malignancy in the UK, and the majority are epithelial in origin. The peak incidence is in women aged 75–84 years. It causes more deaths than endometrial or cervical cancer because it often presents late, due to vague symptoms with an insidious onset.

Aetiology Originally thought to be related to irritation of the ovarian surface from ovulation. However, recent evidence suggests a role for the fallopian tubes in the development of ovarian cancer. It was found that in women with BRCA mutations, more had microscopic evidence of fallopian tube cancer than ovarian cancer at the time of salpingo-oophorectomy.

• Nulliparity increases risk
• Early menarche and/or late menopause increases risk
• Gene mutations in BRCA 1 and 2 increase risk of ovarian and breast cancer:
  • BRCA 1 has risk of 46% by age 70
  • BRCA 2 has risk of 12% by age 70
• HNPCC (Lynch II syndrome) gives a lifetime risk of ovarian cancer of 11%
• Pregnancy, breastfeeding, and COCP are protective
• Tubal ligation (female sterilization) is protective.

Refer for clinical genetics counselling and testing if there are two primary cancers in one 1st or 2nd degree relative; three 1st- or 2nd-degree relatives with breast, ovary, colorectal, stomach, or endometrial cancers; two 1st- or 2nd-degree relatives, one of whom has ovarian cancer at any age, and the other with breast cancer <50 years; two 1st- or 2nd-degree relatives with ovarian cancer at any age.

The role for screening Yet to be proven (there are studies underway). If a gene mutation is identified, consider yearly TVS with CA125. If BRCA +ve offer BSO and warn of risk of finding incidental disease at the time of surgery.

Presentation
• Often vague symptoms which may be misinterpreted as irritable bowel syndrome or diverticular disease and 50% present to a non-gynaecological specialty; 75% present once disease has reached FIGO stage III (see BOX, p283)
• Bloating
• Unexplained weight loss; loss of appetite; early satiety
• Fatigue
• Urinary symptoms eg frequency or urgency
• Change in bowel habit
• Abdominal or pelvic pain
• Vaginal bleeding
• Pelvic mass palpable by the woman or her GP.

Examination may reveal a fixed abdominal/pelvic mass, ascites, omental mass, pleural effusion, and/or supraclavicular lymph node enlargement.

Investigations
• FBC, U&E, LFTs
• Tumour markers: CA125 (raised in 80% of epithelial cancers and used to work out RMI, see TABLE on p281). CEA is raised in colorectal cancers and normal in ovarian cancer. CA19.9 may be raised in mucinous tumours. If the woman is <40 years, check AFP, LDH and hCG.
• TVS
• CXR (looking for pleural effusion or lung metastases; needed for staging)
• CT abdomen/pelvis (to detect peritoneal disease, omental metastases, liver metastases and para-aortic lymph nodes)
• MRI is useful to further evaluate the ovarian mass and help distinguish benign from malignant disease
• Ascites or pleural effusion can be sampled and sent for cytology.

FIGO staging for ovarian cancer		
Stage	**Extent of disease**	**5-yr survival**
I	Limited to one or both ovaries; IC if the capsule is breached, tumour is present on the ovarian surface or peritoneal washings are positive. Rupture of the cyst at time of surgery is IC.	75–90%
II	Limited to the pelvis	45–60%
III	Limited to the abdomen, including regional lymph node metastases	30–40%
IV	Distant metastases outside abdominal cavity	<20%

Treatment Best carried out in specialist centres; this depends on tumour stage.

Surgery consists of a full staging laparotomy through a midline incision by a cancer specialist (improves prognosis). As much tumour as possible should be removed. Stage III or IV cancers may benefit from neoadjuvant chemotherapy (chemotherapy prior to debulking surgery). A full staging laparotomy involves the following:
• Midline laparotomy
• Hysterectomy
• Bilateral salpingo-oophorectomy
• Omentectomy
• Para-aortic and pelvic lymph node sampling
• Peritoneal washings and biopsies.

In a young woman with early disease, the uterus and other ovary may be left for fertility. Ensure optimal surgical staging. NICE says low-risk stage Ia or b disease may not need chemotherapy.🏵️NICE

Chemotherapy is recommended in everyone following surgery, unless disease is low-grade and stage Ia or b. Platinum agents are superior—carboplatin with **paclitaxel** (from Pacific yew trees) produces higher response rates and longer survival both when used for initial treatment and for treatment of recurrences compared to use of carboplatin alone. Advanced or relapsed ovarian cancer: see NICE guidance. Options include **paclitaxel**, pegylated liposomal **doxorubicin**, and **topotecan**. Palliative care involves relief of symptoms, which are generally due to extensive peritoneal disease.

Borderline ovarian tumours are epithelial in origin and are not benign. They are more common in younger women and are staged as for ovarian cancer. Characteristics include confinement to one ovary, pre-menopausal age group, metastatic implants, difficulty in diagnosing histologically and with a much better prognosis than ovarian cancer. In young women, conservative surgery is appropriate with unilateral oophorectomy and staging biopsies. Relapse can occur any time up to 25 years after initial diagnosis.

Pseudomyxoma peritonei is extremely rare and can arise from primary tumour of the appendix, but may be associated with mucinous cystadenoma (p281). There are thick, jelly-like deposits throughout the abdomen. Two specialist centres exist in the UK and treatment involves extensive abdominal surgery and intraperitoneal chemotherapy. It is difficult to treat and the prognosis is poor.

Discharge may be physiological (eg pregnancy; sexual arousal; puberty; COCP). Most discharges are smelly, itchy, and due to infection. Foul discharge may be due to a foreign body (eg forgotten tampons, or beads in children). Note the details of the discharge. Could it be a sexually transmitted disease (STD)? See *OHCM* p404. If so, refer to a genitourinary clinic. Do a speculum examination and take swabs: vulvovaginal/endocervical samples for chlamydia and gonorrhoea (p285; *OHCM* p416). ► Discharges rarely resemble their classical descriptions.

Thrush *(Candida)* The 2nd commonest cause of discharge (1st is bacterial vaginosis), 95% is due to *C. albicans*, 5% *C. glabrata* (harder to treat). Vulva and vagina may be red, fissured, and sore, especially if allergic component; discharge is non-offensive, classically white curds. Her partner may be a carrier who is asymptomatic. Pregnancy, contraceptive and other steroids, immunodeficiencies, antibiotics, and diabetes are risk factors—check glucose. *Candida* elsewhere (eg mouth, natal cleft) in both partners may cause reinfection. Thrush is not necessarily sexually transmitted. *Diagnosis:* Microscopy (shows mycelia or spores) and culture. *Treatment:* Topical treatment (eg clotrimazole 500mg pessary + cream for the vulva) gives similar cure rates to oral **fluconazole** 150mg PO as a single dose. *C. glabrata* may require topical **nystatin** or 7–14-day course of an **imidazole**. Use topical regimen alone if pregnant or breastfeeding. Very recurrent infection may be treated by weekly maintenance doses of treatment (unlicensed).

Trichomoniasis *Trichomonas vaginalis* (TV; fig 3.18; sexually transmitted) produces vaginitis and a bubbly, thin, fish-smelling discharge. Cervix may have 'strawberry' appearance. Exclude gonorrhoea (often coexists). Motile flagellates are seen on wet films (×400), or cultured. *R̵:* (treat partner too) **metronidazole** 2g PO stat or 400mg/ 12h PO for 5 days (eg if pregnant).

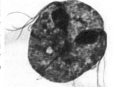

Fig 3.18 TV. © Prof S Upton; Kansas Univ.

Bacterial vaginosis Prevalence ~10% mostly asymptomatic. Any discharge has fishy odour, from cadaverine & putrescine. Vaginal pH is >4.5. The vagina is not inflamed and pruritus is uncommon. Mixed with 10% potassium hydroxide on a slide, a whiff of ammonia may be detected. Stippled vaginal epithelial 'clue cells' may be seen on wet microscopy (fig 3.19, top). There is altered bacterial flora—overgrowth, eg of *Gardnerella vaginalis*, *Mycoplasma hominis*, peptostreptococci, *Mobiluncus*, and anaerobes, eg *Bacteroides* species—with too few lactobacillae. There is ↑ risk of preterm labour, intra-amniotic infection in pregnancy, susceptibility to HIV,[34] and post-termination sepsis. *Δ·* By culture. *R̵:* **Metronidazole** 2g PO once, gel PV, or **clindamycin** 2% vaginal cream, 1 applicator full/night PV 7 times. If recurrent, treating the partner may help. If pregnant, use metronidazole 400mg/12h PO for 5 days. Balance Activ® vaginal acidic gel can be a useful (more natural) alternative.

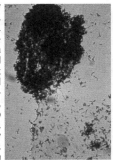

Fig 3.19 Clue cells.

Reproduced from Warrell, Cox, Firth, *The Oxford Textbook of Medicine* (2010) with permission from Oxford University Press.

Gynaecology

Discharge in children may reflect infection from *faecal flora*, associated with alkalinity from lack of vaginal oestrogen (prepubertal atrophic vaginitis). *Staphs* and *streps* may cause pus. *Threadworms* cause pruritus. Always consider *sexual abuse*. Gentle rectal examination may exclude a *foreign body*.

Tests: Vulval ± vaginal swab (hard to know if result is normal flora). MSU: *is there glycosuria?* For prolonged or bloody discharge, examine under anaesthesia (paediatric laryngoscopes can serve as specula) ± US or x-rays.

Management: Discuss hygiene. If an antibiotic is needed, **erythromycin** is a good choice. An **oestrogen cream** may be tried (≤1cm strip).

Chlamydia

Chlamydia is the most common bacterial STI in the UK and is an important cause of tubal infertility. 70% cases are asymptomatic, but symptoms may include dysuria, vaginal discharge, and/or intermenstrual or postcoital bleeding. In the UK, the National Chlamydia Screening Programme tests over a million people per year, and has caused an estimated 20% drop in prevalence in those <25 years. *Complications* include pelvic inflammatory disease (p286) in 10–40% of those infected, perihepatitis (Fitz-Hugh–Curtis syndrome), Reiter's syndrome (arthritis, conjunctivitis, and urethritis, more common in men), tubal infertility and increased risk of ectopic pregnancy. *Diagnosis* is by vulvo-vaginal or endocervical swab for nucleic acid amplification test (NAAT) using a special medium. Swabs may be self-taken. *Treatment:* Azithromycin 1g single dose or doxycycline 100mg BD for 7 days (>95% cure). It is essential to treat partners and abstain from intercourse until this happens. Chlamydia in pregnancy is treated with erythromycin 500mg BD for 10–14 days; untreated, there is an increased risk of preterm rupture of membranes and premature delivery, and neonatal conjunctivitis and pneumonia.

Gonorrhoea

Full name *Neisseria gonorrhoeae*, a Gram –ve diplococcus. It is the fourth most common STI in the UK, and there is increasing antibiotic resistance. There are often no symptoms, but may present with lower abdominal pain, vaginal discharge, intermenstrual or postcoital bleeding. *Complications* include PID (10% of those infected), Bartholin's or Skene's abscess, tubal infertility and increased risk of ectopic pregnancy. Disseminated gonorrhoea leads to fever, pustular rash, migratory polyarthralgia, and septic arthritis. *Diagnosis* is by vulvovaginal or endocervical swab for NAAT using a special medium. Swabs may be self-taken. Urethral, pharyngeal, and rectal swabs should be taken if appropriate. If NAAT +ve, take further swabs for culture for sensitivities prior to treatment due to high rates of antibiotic resistance (35% strains resistant to ciprofloxacin and 70% to tetracyclines). *Treatment* is with ceftriaxone 500mg IM stat, plus azithromycin 1g PO stat. If severely penicillin-allergic, spectinomycin 2g IM plus azithromycin 1g PO stat. Treat partners and contact trace. Treatment is the same in pregnancy (untreated, gonorrhoea in pregnancy is associated with preterm rupture of membranes, preterm delivery, and chorioamnionitis, and to the baby, ophthalmia neonatarum).

Further reading

National Chlamydia Screening Programme: http://www.chlamydiascreening.nhs.uk

Pelvic inflammatory disease (PID) is defined as infection of the upper genital tract. Many cases probably go undetected due to lack of symptoms, so prevalence is difficult to ascertain.

Causes
- Usually from ascending infection from the endocervix:
  - STIs
  - Uterine instrumentation eg hysteroscopy, insertion of IUCD, TOP
  - Post-partum
- Can descend from other infected organs, eg with appendicitis
- 25% due to chlamydia and gonorrhoea
- Remainder may be due to anaerobes and endogenous bacteria.

Age <25 years, previous history of STIs and new or multiple sexual partners increase risk. Protective factors are use of barrier contraception, Mirena® IUS and the COCP.

History and examination The woman may give a history of lower abdominal pain which may be uni- or bilateral, which is constant or intermittent. There may be deep dyspareunia, vaginal discharge, intermenstrual or postcoital bleeding, dysmenorrhoea, and/or fever. On examination, vaginal discharge may be evident. There is cervical motion tenderness (cervical excitation) on vaginal examination, with or without adnexal tenderness. In mild or chronic PID she will be afebrile.

Investigations Take vulvovaginal/endocervical swabs for chlamydia and gonorrhoea, and MC&S. If the woman is acutely unwell, check FBC (elevated WCC) and CRP and take blood cultures if sepsis. If tubo-ovarian abscess is suspected, arrange TVS. Laparoscopy is not indicated unless diagnosis is uncertain, for example right iliac fossa pain and possible appendicitis or drainage of tubo-ovarian abscess is required.

Complications
- Tubo-ovarian abscess
- Fitz-Hugh–Curtis syndrome (liver capsule inflammation with perihepatic adhesions)
- Recurrent PID (can be instigated by gynaecological procedures)
- Ectopic pregnancy
- Subfertility from tubal blockage (8% after 1 episode; 40% after 3 episodes).

Management ►Prompt treatment and contact-tracing minimizes complications. Start treating with antibiotics before culture results are available. Well patients can be treated as outpatients and should be reviewed 72h later to check response. Admit for IV antibiotics if symptoms severe, there is sepsis or symptoms fail to respond.

Outpatient management
- Ceftriaxone 500mg IM stat or azithromycin 1g PO plus doxycycline 100mg PO BD for 14 days and metronidazole 400mg PO BD for 14 days.
- If gonorrhoea suspected, discuss with microbiologist due to high rates of antibiotic resistance.

Inpatient management
- Ceftriaxone 2g IV OD plus doxycycline 100mg IV BD, followed by oral doxycycline 100mg BD for 14 days + metronidazole 400mg PO BD for 14 days.

Chronic PID Unresolved, unrecognized, or inadequately treated infection. Inflammation leads to fibrosis, so adhesions develop between pelvic organs. The tubes may be distended with pus (pyosalpinx) or fluid (hydrosalpinx).

Pelvic pain, menorrhagia, secondary dysmenorrhoea, discharge, and deep dyspareunia are some of the symptoms. Look for tubal masses, tenderness, and fixed retroverted uterus. Laparoscopy differentiates infection from endometriosis. Difficult to manage pain; antibiotics are generally not helpful.

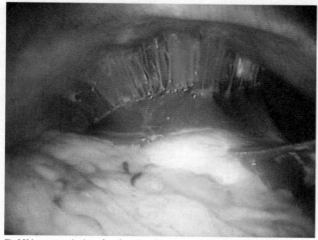

Fig 3.20 Laparoscopic view of perihepatic adhesions seen in Fitz-Hugh–Curtis syndrome.
Reproduced from Sarris, Bewley, & Agnihotri, *Training in Obstetrics and Gynaecology* (2009) with permission from Oxford University Press.

Endometriosis is defined as the presence of endometriotic tissue outside the uterus (figs 3.21 & 3.22). It is hormonally driven, principally by oestrogen, and therefore affects women of reproductive age. Adenomyosis refers to the presence of endometrial tissue within the myometrium. There is wide variation in severity of disease and its impact on pain. Some women are relatively asymptomatic with extensive disease, whilst others have only superficial endometriotic deposits with debilitating symptoms.

Cause Unknown. Three main theories exist: the first is retrograde menstruation, leading to adherence, invasion, and growth of tissue; the second is metaplasia of mesothelial cells (which may explain how it can develop in unusual places such as the lung and nasal cavity); the third, impaired immunity, suggests that endometrial cells from retrograde menstruation fail to be destroyed by the immune response. 10–12% of the general female population are estimated to have the disease, 20–50% of those undergoing fertility or chronic pain investigation and 40–60% of those with dysmenorrhoea.

Presentation
• Pain:
  • Cyclical due to endometrial tissue responding to the menstrual cycle
  • Constant due to formation of adhesions from chronic inflammation
  • Severe dysmenorrhoea leading to time off work or school
  • Deep dyspareunia from involvement of uterosacral ligaments
  • Dysuria
  • Dyschezia (pain on defaecation) and /or cyclical rectal bleeding (rectovaginal nodules with invasion of rectal mucosa
• Subfertility
• No symptoms; incidental finding.

Examination may be normal if there is minimal disease. Speculum examination may show visible lesions in the vagina or cervix, but this is rare and a sign of deep infiltrating endometriosis. On bimanual vaginal examination, a fixed retroverted uterus is a classic sign. There may be adnexal masses or tenderness, and tender nodules palpable over the uterosacral ligaments.

Investigations TVS is useful for diagnosis of ovarian endometriotic cysts but poor at identifying other parameters of disease. If bowel involvement is suspected, MRI is being used increasingly to map the extent of the endometriosis. CA125 may be raised but should not be used as a screening test. The gold standard for diagnosis is laparoscopy with biopsy for histological confirmation. It is especially important for diagnosis of deep infiltrating lesions and should be avoided within 3 months of hormonal therapy, as this leads to under-diagnosis. The extent of disease should be documented with photographs.

Treatment depends on severity of symptoms and whether the main symptom is pain or subfertility. It is acceptable to treat empirically with COCP or progestagens without a laparoscopic diagnosis if fertility is not the issue. NSAIDs are also effective. Suspected severe endometriosis should be managed and treated by a centre with expertise in advanced laparoscopic surgery. *Medical treatment:* COCP cyclically or continuous; progestagens orally, IM or SC; Mirena® IUS (can be inserted at laparoscopy); GnRH analogues eg goserelin can be used short-term <6m and should be used with add-back HRT eg tibolone. Goserelin can be used in subfertility patients prior to IVF to increase success rates. *Surgical treatment:* Indicated once medical treatment has failed. Laparoscopy is the mainstay of management using ablation, excision, or co-agulative techniques to destroy endometriosis. Nodules should be excised and endometriomas removed rather than drained (otherwise high recurrence). In mild–moderate disease, spontaneous pregnancy rates are increased after surgical removal of endometriotic lesions. Hysterectomy is a last resort.

Endometriosis and chronic pelvic pain

There are high rates of relapse after stopping treatment such as COCP, and some patients with deep or superficial endometriosis, and those with adenomyosis (endometriotic tissue is largely inaccessible by surgery) will be left with chronic pain. This can be difficult to treat and ideally should be undertaken by an endometriosis specialist, in a centre where there is access to other support such as a clinical specialist nurse and a chronic pain team. Multiple repeat laparoscopies are not usually the answer unless there is evidence of recurrence. Consider other non-gynaecological causes which may coexist, eg irritable bowel syndrome, constipation, neuropathic pain from previous surgery or endometriosis, and fibromyalgia. Manage with analgesia (opiates may be required but if needed regularly should be managed with the help of a pain clinic), neuropathic treatments such as gabapentin, and hormonal treatments. If she is requesting a hysterectomy, a successful trial of GnRH analogues predicts successful pain relief. Also consider support groups (www.endo.org.uk) and if depression is also present, it should be treated.

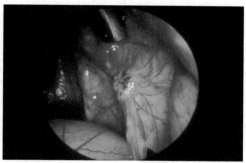

Fig 3.21 Endometriotic nodule. Note raised appearance with scarred peritoneum. Deep infiltrating endometriosis is more commonly found in the pouch of Douglas and the uterosacral ligaments, but may also involve the bladder, bowel and ureters.

Reproduced with permission from Dan Martin, www.danmartinmd.com.

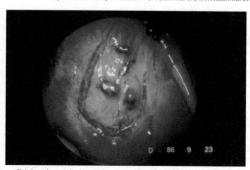

Fig 3.22 Superficial endometriosis most commonly affects the ovaries and pelvic peritoneum (particularly the pouch of Douglas and uterosacral ligaments).

Reproduced with permission from Dan Martin, www.danmartinmd.com.

Further reading

ESHRE (2013). *Guideline on the Management of Women with Endometriosis.*

ESHRE (2013). *Management of Women with Endometriosis.* www.eshre.eu/Guidelines-and-Legal/Guidelines/Endometriosis-guideline/Guideline-on-the-management-of-women-with-endometriosis.aspx

Gynaecology

A prolapse occurs when weakness of the supporting structures allows the pelvic organs to protrude within the vagina. The weakness may be congenital, and is associated with prolonged labour, trauma from instrumental delivery, lack of postnatal pelvic floor exercise, obesity, chronic cough and constipation. Poor perineal repair reduces support. Prolapse is exacerbated by the menopause and is not a danger to health—except for third-degree uterine prolapse with cystocele when ureteric obstruction can occur.

Types of prolapse are named according to structure affected. Several types may coexist in the same patient. *Cystocele* The anterior wall of the vagina, and the bladder attached to it, bulge. Residual urine within the cystocele may cause frequency and dysuria. It is associated with urethral prolapse (cystourethrocoele). *Rectocele* The lower posterior wall, which is attached to rectum, may bulge through weak levator ani. It is often symptomless, but she may have to reduce herniation prior to defecation by putting a finger in the vagina, or pressing on the perineum. *Enterocele* Bulges of the upper posterior vaginal wall may contain loops of intestine from the pouch of Douglas. *Uterine prolapse* Protrusion of the uterus downwards into the vagina, taking with it the cervix and upper vagina. If the woman has had a total hysterectomy, the vaginal vault is left and may also prolapse.

Grading of prolapse *First degree:* The lowest part of the prolapse descends halfway down the vaginal axis to the introitus. *Second degree:* The lowest part of the prolapse extends to the level of the introitus, and through the introitus on straining. *Third degree:* The lowest part of the prolapse extends through the introitus and outside the vagina. *Procidentia* refers to fourth-degree uterine prolapse—the uterus lies outside the vagina.

Symptoms May be asymptomatic. Dragging sensation, discomfort, feeling of a lump 'coming down,' dyspareunia, backache. With cystocele, urinary urgency and frequency, incomplete bladder emptying, urinary retention if the urethra is kinked. With rectocele, constipation and difficulty with defecation. How do the symptoms affect her quality of life? *Prevention:* Lower parity; better obstetric practices, pelvic floor exercises.

Examination Bimanual to exclude pelvic masses. Examine for prolapse with the woman in left lateral position using a Sims speculum. Inspect anterior and posterior walls for atrophy and descent. If no obvious prolapse, ask the woman to strain or stand. Arrange urodynamic studies if urinary incontinence.

Management *Conservative:* Mild disease may improve with reduction in intra-abdominal pressure, so encourage her to lose weight, stop smoking, and stop straining. Improve muscle tone with exercises or physiotherapy. *Pessaries* are useful in those who decline surgery, are unfit for surgery, or if surgery is contraindicated. They affect sexual function. They should be changed every 6 months and if the woman is post-menopausal, topical oestrogen is useful to prevent vaginal erosion. Ring pessaries are the most common and come in many different sizes. It is placed between the posterior aspect of the symphysis pubis and posterior fornix of the vagina. The Gelhorn® pessary is similar in principle but is shaped like a mushroom. Shelves, cubes, and doughnuts are less commonly used. *Surgery* is useful if symptoms are severe, the woman is sexually active, and pessaries have failed. The type of prolapse repair depends on type of prolapse. Repair operations (p308) excise redundant tissue and strengthen supports, but may reduce vaginal width. Marked uterine prolapse is treated by hysterectomy with or without sacrospinous fixation, or by laparoscopic sacrohysteropexy. Post-hysterectomy vault prolapse may be treated by sacrocolpopexy (eg with mesh).[32] Primary anterior or posterior pelvic floor repair should not use mesh due to the high complication rate.

Gynaecology

▶ *This can be devastating to both partners* and its investigation a great strain. Sympathetic management is crucial. 84% of couples having regular intercourse conceive within a year (92% by 2 years). Offer investigation after 1yr of trying (earlier if ♀ aged ≥35 years, amenorrhoea, oligomenorrhoea, or past PID, undescended testes or cancer treatments which may affect fertility). Fertility decreases with age: girls are born with ~300,000 potential eggs; by 30yrs, only 12% are left (by 40yrs, just 3%).

Causes
• Anovulation: 21%
• Male factor: 25%
• Tubal factor: 15–20%
• Unexplained: 28%
• Endometriosis: 6–8%.

Anovulation may be caused by premature ovarian failure, Turner's syndrome, surgery or chemotherapy, as well as PCOS, excessive weight loss or exercise, hypopituitarism, Kallman's syndrome, and hyperprolactinaemia.

History It takes 2 to be infertile (♀ causes ≈67%); see both partners. Note age and duration of subfertility. Have they had any previous pregnancies and does either partner have children? Menstrual history, regularity, pelvic pain, history of STIs, previous surgery (tubal or for ectopic pregnancy) are all important. Smoking reduces fertility, as does drinking more than the recommended amount of alcohol per week—in both partners. Check the medical history and drugs to optimize both. Ask about frequency of sexual intercourse and any problems during sex including erectile dysfunction. Ask the man about history of undescended testes or mumps as an adult, and check his medical, drug history, and smoking and alcohol use.

Examination BMI (obesity has an adverse effect on fertility, and there are BMI ranges above which treatment cannot be started). Are there signs of endocrine disorder eg PCOS? Exclude pelvic pathology eg endometriosis or fibroids, take a cervical smear if due, and high vaginal and chlamydia swabs. Surgical treatment of a varicocele has no effect on pregnancy rate.

Investigations
Primary care
• Chlamydia screening
• Baseline hormonal profile (day 2–5 FSH (should be <10IU/L) and LH
• TSH, prolactin, and testosterone and rubella status (vaccinate if non-immune)
• Mid-luteal progesterone level to confirm ovulation (7 days before expected period eg day 21 if 28-day cycle, >30nmol/L is indicative of ovulation)
• Semen analysis (p295). Repeat in 3 months if abnormal, after making lifestyle changes and starting a multivitamin containing selenium, zinc and vitamin C.

Secondary care
• TVS to rule out adnexal masses, submucosal fibroids or endometrial polyps, or help confirm PCOS.
• Hysterosalpingogram (HSG) uses x-ray and contrast injected through a small cannula in the cervix to demonstrate uterine anatomy and tubal patency. May cause period-like cramps and tubal spasm, giving false positive. Only perform once chlamydia swabs negative and give *azithromycin* 1g PO stat.
• Hysterosalpingo-contrast sonograph (HyCoSy) is similar to the above, but using US contrast and TVS.
• Laparoscopy and dye test is a day-case procedure and the gold standard for assessing tubal patency. Methylene blue dye is injected thought the cervix whilst the tubes are visualized with a laparoscope. Used first line if strong clinical suspicion of tubal abnormality or needs a laparoscopy for other reasons. Used second line if HSG or HyCoSy abnormal. Pelvic pathology can be treated at the same time.

DI	Donor insemination is used when the male partner has azoospermia with failed surgical sperm retrieval, in those at high risk of transmitting a genetic disorder and those at high risk of transmitting HIV. It is also used for women with no (male) partner.
ICSI	Intracytoplasmic sperm injection (directly into an egg). Sperm may be taken from the ejaculate, or surgically from the testis or epididymis. This technique is used when the semen parameters are severely abnormal or failed fertilization has occurred with IVF cycles. There is some concern that genetic mutations (especially Y chromosome deletions) will be propagated by transmission to the offspring.
IUI	Intrauterine insemination: useful in mild male factor subfertility, coital difficulties, unexplained subfertility, and same-sex couples. It can be combined with ovarian stimulation, but if >3 follicles develop, the treatment cycle should be cancelled due to a high chance of multiple pregnancy (>25%).
IVF	*In vitro* fertilization: see p69 and p294.
IVM	*In vitro* maturation: immature eggs are collected from the ovaries, matured in the lab before sperm injection (ISCI). Avoids expensive ovulation-inducing drugs and risk of ovarian hyperstimulation, it may be especially suitable for women with polycystic ovaries.
OT/NT(P)	Ooplasmic transfer/nuclear transfer procedure: the baby has 2 mothers: one (too old to conceive normally) gives a nucleus; the other gives fresher cytoplasm (+mitochondrial DNA) for the ovum. This is an example of human germline modification. 15 babies were born using this technique in the USA (2 had Turner's syndrome).
PESA	Percutaneous epididymal sperm aspiration (uses a needle inserted into the epididymis, so scrotal exploration is not needed).
POT	Pregnancy by ovary transplant has been reported (autologous transplant, 1 between identical twin sisters, another between sisters).

Various national embryology authorities exist and pronounce on the ethics of fertility options, and their edicts can appear to be set in stone (although being mutually contradictory with those from other countries). One problem with this approach is that fertility options are constantly changing, as are society's views on what is acceptable. It is not clear whether these views should lead, or simply be taken into account (an opaque phrase) or be trumped by appeal to some higher authority (God, or the conscience of a quango).

The above methods allow embryos to be sexed and screened for genetic diseases with implantation only for those with the desired characteristics, eg offering a perfect match for stem-cell transplantation to an older sibling, with Fanconi's anaemia. Controversies surrounding creating an individual expressly for the purposes of another might seem to be new, but mythology has, since before the dawn of time,[7] acclimatized us to this activity—which is why it is gaining acceptance.

Further reading

NICE (2013). *Fertility: Assessment and Treatment of People with Fertility Problems* (cg156). London: NICE.

www.nice.org.uk/guidance/cg156

7 According to *Paradise Lost*, the First Operator, in a controversial act of vivisection, 'opened my left side, and took from thence a rib, with cordial spirits warm, and life-blood streaming fresh: wide was the wound, but suddenly with flesh filled up and healed: the rib he formed and fashioned with his hands; under his forming hands a creature grew, manlike, but different sex, so lovely fair, that what seemed fair in all the world, seemed now mean, or in her summed up.' Thus was Eve made, not for herself, but simply to delight Adam and keep him company.[36]

Gynaecology

Lifestyle modification Treatment of subfertility is directed at the cause. The couple should lose weight if necessary, eat a healthy diet, stop smoking ± recreational drugs, reduce alcohol consumption to less than the recommended limits, take regular exercise, folic acid (the woman), aim to have regular intercourse every 2–3 days (avoid timed intercourse), and avoid ovulation monitors (they increase stress and there is no evidence of benefit). Couples who time intercourse for the day of ovulation may be too late—ideally there should be some sperm available for fertilization whenever ovulation occurs.

Ovulation induction There are several methods by which to induce ovulation. PCOS is the most common cause of anovulatory subfertility, accounting for 80%.

• *Weight loss or gain*
• *Clomifene citrate:* 50mg days 2–6 of cycle
  • Anti-oestrogen, which increases endogenous FSH via negative feedback to the pituitary
  • 10% multiple pregnancy rate (higher if used inappropriately)
  • Can cause hot flushes, labile mood. If severe headache or visual disturbance, stop immediately
  • Should only be used for 6–12 cycles (possible link with ovarian cancer)
  • Needs follicular monitoring by US (risk of hyperstimulation)
  • Should be prescribed by a specialist, ideally after tubal patency confirmed and semen count normal or near-normal and BMI <30–35.
• *Laparoscopic ovarian drilling:*
  • Used in patients with PCOS only
  • Small holes are drilled into each ovary using needlepoint diathermy with the aim of reducing LH and restoring feedback mechanisms
  • Successful in 50% and effects last for 12–18 months.
• *Gonadotrophins:* Used in specialist fertility units for clomifene-resistant PCOS or low oestrogen with normal FSH. Injected, expensive, and needs US monitoring.
• *Metformin* is controversial and is used in women with PCOS. There is a possible small increase in ovulation rates but it is not licensed and weight loss is more effective.

Surgical techniques *Tubal disease:* Proximal blocks may respond to tubal catheterization or hysteroscopic cannulation. High rates of ectopic pregnancy. *Endometriosis:* p288. *Intrauterine adhesions:* Use hysteroscopic adhesiolysis.

In vitro fertilization *Indications* include tubal disease, male factor subfertility, endometriosis, anovulation not responding to clomifene, subfertility due to maternal age, unexplained subfertility >2yrs. *Success* depends on many factors including age, duration of subfertility, previous pregnancy (higher success rate), smoking, and high BMI (lower success). Low anti-Mullerian hormone (AMH) levels predict poorer response. Women with hydrosalpinges should have salpingectomy prior to IVF to ↑chance of live birth. Screen couple for HIV, hepatitis B & C. Ovaries are stimulated (see 'Ovarian hyperstimulation syndrome', p311), ova collected (by transvaginal aspiration under transvaginal US guidance), fertilized, and 3–5 days later, 1–2 embryos returned under US guidance to the uterus as an outpatient procedure. Luteal support is given in the form of progestagens, and 2 weeks later the woman should do a pregnancy test. *NHS-funded assisted conception:* Inclusion criteria varies between regions but generally is limited to couples with no children, non-smokers, BMI <30, under 42yrs of age (35 in some counties) and who do not require gamete donation. *Egg donation* can offer women a chance of pregnancy when previous IVF attempts have failed, in ovarian failure and in women >45yrs. Adoption and fostering are also options and this can be arranged locally.

Gynaecology

Spermatogenesis takes place in the seminiferous tubules. Undifferentiated diploid germ cells (spermatogonia) multiply and are then transformed into haploid spermatozoa, a process taking 74 days. FSH and LH are both important for initiation of spermatogenesis at puberty. LH stimulates Leydig cells to produce testosterone. Testosterone and FSH stimulate Sertoli cells to produce essential substances for metabolic support of germ cells and spermatogenesis.

Spermatozoa A spermatozoon has a dense oval head (containing the haploid chromosome complement) capped by an acrosome granule (contains enzymes essential for fertilization), and is propelled by the motile tail. Seminal fluid forms 90% of ejaculate volume and is alkaline to buffer vaginal acidity.

Normal semen analysis (WHO criteria 2009)
- Volume >1.5mL
- Concentration >15 × 10⁶/mL
- Progressive motility >32%
- Total motility >40%
- Normal forms >4%.

Male factors Male factors are the cause of subfertility in ~25% of subfertile couples. Only a small number of men have an identifiable treatable cause.
- Semen abnormality (85%):
  - Idiopathic oligoasthenoteratozoospermia, testicular cancer, drugs such as alcohol and nicotine, varicocele
- Azoospermia (5%):
  - Pre-testicular, eg anabolic steroid use, hypogonadotrophic hypogonadism, Kalmann's syndrome
  - Non-obstructive: cryptorchidism, orchitis, 47XXY (Klinefelter's syndrome), chemotherapy
  - Obstructive: congenital bilateral absence of the vas deferens (CBAVD), vasectomy, chlamydia, gonorrhoea
- Immunological (5%):
  - Anti-sperm antibodies, idiopathic, infective
- Coital dysfunction (5%):
  - Erectile dysfunction with normal sperm function (remember drug causes such as beta-blockers, antidepressants)
  - Hypospadias, phimosis, disability
  - Retrograde ejaculation
  - Failure in ejaculation (multiple sclerosis, spinal cord injury).

Examination Look at body form and secondary sexual characteristics. Any gynaecomastia? Normal testicular volume is 15–35mL (compare with Prader orchidometer). Rectal examination may reveal prostatitis.

Tests *Plasma FSH* is raised in testicular failure. *Testosterone and LH* levels are indicated if you suspect androgen deficiency. *Karyotype* to exclude 47XXY and *cystic fibrosis screen* (associated with CBAVD).

Treatment Address lifestyle issues, such as alcohol and smoking. Optimize underlying medical conditions and consider stopping or changing medication. Consider starting a multivitamin containing zinc, selenium, and vitamin C. Repeat the semen analysis 3 months after making changes. *ICSI=intracytoplasmic sperm injection* (direct into egg), the main tool for most male subfertility. The source of sperm is the epididymis or testis in men with obstructive azoospermia; even if the problem is non-obstructive, sperm can be retrieved in ~50%.

▶ *Any method, even coitus interruptus, is better than none.* Without contraception about 85 of every 100 premenopausal sexually active women will become pregnant each year, and 1 in 3 pregnancies are unplanned. Properly used, contraception reduces this rate (see 'The ideal contraceptive' BOX, p297). When dealing with under-16s use Fraser guidelines (BOX). After the menopause, stop contraception 2y after amenorrhoea if <50y, after 1y if >50y.

Barrier methods ▶ The main reason for failure is not using them. Condoms reduce transmission of most STDs but not those affecting the perineum. When failure has occurred (eg 'split condom'), remember post-coital emergency contraception (p299).

- *Condoms* Effective when properly used, unroll onto the erect penis with the teat or end (if teatless) pinched to expel air. This prevents bursting at ejaculation. Use a new condom with each episode of sexual intercourse. Do not use with oil-based lubricants—this destroys the latex. Method failure rate 5%, typical user failure rate 15%/yr.
- *Caps* come in several forms.[8] Diaphragms stretch from pubic bone to posterior fornix. Check after insertion that the cervix is covered. Cervical caps fit over the cervix (so need a prominent cervix). Insert <2h before intercourse (keep in place >6h after sex). Use with a spermicide.* Problems: UTIs, rubber sensitivity. They need professional fitting. 92–99% effective if perfect use.**
- *Cervical sponges* Simple to use: spermicide* impregnated: unavailable in UK.
- *The female condom* (eg Femidom®) Prescription and fitting are not needed. It has not proved popular. One reason for failure is that the penis goes alongside it, rather than in it; another, that it gets pushed up in the vagina or may fall out. They can be noisy. Uses lubricant, not spermicide. 95% effective.‡
- *Spermicide* Unreliable unless used with a barrier. Nonoxinol-9, the only spermicide available in UK is not recommended for those with or at high risk of HIV as it irritates vaginal epithelium and ↑ chance of HIV transmission.

Fertility awareness ('natural') methods involve physiological monitoring to find fertile times (6 days prior to ovulation; the life of a sperm) to 2 days afterwards (the life of the ovum). Cervical mucus becomes clear and slippery prior to ovulation, and then abruptly thicker and tacky. No intercourse from the day mucus becomes slippery to 3d after if becomes tacky. Basal body temperature ↑~0.3°c after ovulation (affected by fevers, drugs, recent food, or drink). Additional observations (mittelschmerz, p310 ± cervix changes) improve accuracy. Success is common if: • Regular cycles • Dedication • Self-control.

Lactational amenorrhoea See p95.

High-technology natural methods Devices eg Persona® use urine test sticks to measure *oestrone-3-glucuronide* (E3G—peaks 24h pre-ovulation) and luteinizing hormone (LH—ovulation occurs within 36h of LH surge and sperm penetration of cervical mucus drops after surge). Microtechnology builds a database of the woman's natural variability over time, to give her a green light (almost infertile), a red light (fertile—typically days 6–10), or an orange light (test early-morning urine for E3G and LH). Usually, only 8 urine tests are needed per cycle. She purchases sticks and monitor. A button is pressed the morning her period starts: she checks the monitor lights before passing urine each morning, in case a test is needed. *Reliability:* 93–95% (manufacturer's data, in motivated patients; it may be less in practice; results should be regarded as only preliminary; explain uncertainty). *CI:* Cycle <23 or >35 days or variation >10 days; breastfeeding; if already on hormones or tetracycline (minocycline is OK); menopausal; liver or kidney disease; polycystic ovaries, or if pregnancy is definitely undesired.

8 RCOG 2007 FFPRHC *Guidance* Female Barrier Methods.³⁷ₖₒₗ This paper gives great detail of all caps, diaphragms etc available. ** but typical use failure rate (TUFR; user+method failure) = 16% in 1st year use of diaphragm, (TUFR) for cervical caps: 9% nullips, 20% parous ♀. ‡ (TUFR) 21%.

Gynaecology (side margin)

The ideal contraceptive—and the realities

An ideal contraceptive is: *100% effective*, with only desirable side effects (eg protection from sexually transmitted disease), and it must be *readily reversible*, and be usable *unsupervised by professionals*. Find the best compromise for each person depending on age, health, and beliefs. Methods available:

- 'Natural methods' (no intercourse near time of ovulation): acceptable to Catholic Church; also, the simplest are free, requiring no 'pollution of the body' with drugs: see p296
- Barrier methods (low health risk but need high user motivation & some protection from HIV). See p296
- Hormonal (complex health interactions, but highly effective, p300–3)
- IUCD/IUS (convenient and effective—if not contraindicated—p298)
- Sterilization (very effective but effectively 'irreversible', p305).

Failure rates % in 1st year with typical (T) and perfect (P) use[38]		
• No method	85(T)	85(P)
• Cervical cap	16–32	9–20
• Natural methods	25	1–9
• Female condom	21	5
• Withdrawal	27	4
• Diaphragm +spermicide	16	6
• Male condom	15	2
• Pills (CoC+PoP)	8	0.3
• Copper coil (for T-safe® Cu380A)	0.8	0.6
• Depo Provera®	3	0.3
• Tubal ligation	0.5	0.5
• Vasectomy	0.15	0.1
• Levonorgestrel IUS (Mirena®)	0.1	0.1

'Is she pregnant already?'

This is a frequent question in family planning and other clinics. If a pregnancy test is not available, women who could be pregnant already will often be denied the contraception they need. Here, consider using this checklist to see if the patient may be pregnant. If she answers Yes to *any* of these questions, and she is free from signs or symptoms of pregnancy, then pregnancy is very unlikely (negative predictive value >99%):

- Have you given birth in the past 4 weeks?
- Are you <6 months postpartum and fully breastfeeding, and free from menstrual bleeding since you had your child?
- Did your last menstrual period start within the last 7 days?
- Have you been using a reliable contraceptive consistently and correctly?
- Have you not had sex since your last period?[39]

Fraser guidelines

Those <16yrs may be prescribed contraception without parental consent if:
- They understand the doctor's advice.
- The young person cannot be persuaded to inform their parents that they are seeking contraceptive advice.
- They are likely to begin or continue intercourse with or without contraceptive treatment.
- Unless the young person receives contraceptive treatment their physical or mental health is likely to suffer.
- The young person's best interests require that the doctor gives advice and/or treatment without parental consent.
- Fraser guidelines and Gillick competence are not interchangeable terms. Fraser guidelines are narrower than 'Gillick competence' as they relate only to contraception, whereas Gillick competence relates to children aged <16 who have the legal capacity to consent to medical examination and treatment.

IUCDs (coils) are plastic shapes ~3cm long with copper winding, and a plastic thread for a tail. They inhibit fertilization, implantation, and sperm penetration of cervical mucus. Most need changing every 5–10 years. Use those with ≥300mm² copper eg T-safe® copper T380A (the most effective),for which pregnancy rate is 2.2 per 100 woman-years. Most of those who choose the IUCD (5%) are older, parous women in stable relationships, in whom the problem rate is low. They can be used for emergency contraception (p299).

Problems with IUCDs 1 They may be expelled (5%) by a uterus which is nulliparous or distorted (eg by fibroids). **2** They are associated with pelvic inflammatory disease up to 21d following insertion. **3** They may cause dysmenorrhoea and menorrhagia (most common reason for discontinuation). **4** Risk of ectopic pregnancy is 1:20 should she become pregnant. *Contraindications:* Pregnancy; current pelvic infection/STD (including TB); allergy to copper; Wilson's disease; heavy/painful periods; trophoblastic disease or gynaecological malignancy; undiagnosed abnormal uterine bleeding; distorted cavity. Use with caution if anticoagulated.

Insertion Screen for STD prior to insertion or use prophylactic antibiotics eg azithromycin 1g PO stat following insertion. Specialist training is required.

An IUCD can be inserted any time (and as emergency contraception), as long as she's not pregnant. Insert immediately after TOP/miscarriage or >4 weeks after birth. Advise taking simple analgesia prior to insertion and warn her that this may cause cramps. Uterine perforation rate is <1:1000. Teach her to feel the threads: ask her to check after each period. ►Insertion of IUCDs may provoke 'cervical shock' (from increased vagal tone). Tip the woman head down with legs raised. Have IV **atropine** (and anti-epileptics if patient epileptic) and resuscitation equipment to hand.

Follow-up Most expulsions are in the first 3 months. Follow-up after 1st period. Threads may be easier to feel than to see. Expulsion rate <1:20 in 5 years.

Lost threads The IUCD may have been expelled, so advise extra contraception and exclude pregnancy. Seek coil on US; if missing arrange x-ray to exclude extra-uterine coils (surgical retrieval advised). If present and not due to be changed, leave *in situ*.

Infection Treat with the device in place, but if removed do not replace for 3 months. With symptomatic *Actinomyces*, remove coil, cut off threads, and send for culture. If positive, seek expert advice on treatment.

Pregnancy >90% are intrauterine. Remove coil, if you can as soon as pregnancy is diagnosed to reduce risk of miscarriage (20% if removed early, 50% if left), and to prevent miscarriage with infection. Exclude ectopic.

Removal Alternative contraception should be started (if desired) prior to removal, or abstinence for >7d. At the menopause, remove after 2 years' amenorrhoea if age <50yrs (1 year's amenorrhoea if age >50yrs).

IUS, intrauterine systems—eg Mirena® or Jaydess® (carries levonorgestrel). Local effect (reversible endometrial atrophy) makes implantation less likely, and periods lighter and less painful. 20% may experience reversible amenorrhoea (reliability equals sterilization, see p305). It lasts ~5 years (Jaydess® lasts 3 years). Risk of ectopic pregnancy and PID is reduced compared with copper IUCD. Can be used in breastfeeding, obesity, cardiovascular disease, and in women taking hepatic enzyme-inducing drugs. Warn about spotting ± heavy bleeding for the first few weeks following insertion; this usually settles within 3–6mo. Pregnancy rate <1:1000 over 5 years. It may benefit women with endometriosis, adenomyosis, or simple endometrial hyperplasia without atypia. It cannot be used as emergency contraception.

Gynaecology

This is for use after isolated episodes of unprotected intercourse (UPSI), eg 'the split condom', and should not be used regularly.[40] Tablets cover that UPSI only. Although usually given after UPSI, advance issue does not increase use and it may be sensible to 'be prepared'. ('Carrying an umbrella in the British climate is considered sensible, not a wish for rain.')[41] However, advance issue has not been shown to reduce pregnancy rates.

Management History of LMP; normal cycle; number of hours since unprotected intercourse. Any CI to later COCP use (p300)? Check BP. Explain that teratogenicity has not been demonstrated. Discuss future contraception. Give supply of oral contraceptives if day 1 start at next period is planned; if started immediately advise extra precautions as below. Offer infection screen and to cover HIV. Offer follow-up at 3–6 weeks if coil inserted; or if pregnancy or STI tests desired, or if she has contraceptive concerns.

Emergency IUCD More effective than tablet contraception (prevents 99% of expected pregnancies); a copper IUCD can be inserted within 120h of unprotected sex. If exposure was >5 days previously it can be inserted up to 5 days after likely ovulation, so is useful in women who present later. Screen for infection. Insert under antibiotic cover, eg azithromycin 1g PO if screening results unavailable. It is thought to inhibit fertilization by toxic effects and to inhibit implantation. If for long-term use, coils with 380mm² Cu have the lowest failure rates so should be used. Unaffected by enzyme inducers (p300), it is the method of choice for those taking them (but see below).

Ulliprostal acetate (eg EllaOne®) Initiate within 120h of unprotected sex. Failure rate is ≤1.6% in non-inferiority (with levonorgestrel) trials. Efficacy is not reduced by obesity (levonorgestrel may be). It is thought to inhibit or delay ovulation. If vomiting ≤3h of taking the tablet, advise another (30mg). A progesterone receptor moderator, it is unsuitable for use if on, or within 28 days of taking, an enzyme inducer (p300), if on antacids or drugs raising gastric pH, for those with severe asthma uncontrolled by oral corticosteroids. Use with caution if liver dysfunction, hereditary galactose intolerance, Lapp lactase deficiency, glucose-galactose malabsorption. Avoid breastfeeding for 36h after use. Use only once per menstrual cycle. Periods average 2 days' delay (7 days in ≤20%). Advise extra contraceptive precautions for 14 days for combined pills, 16 days for Qlaira®, 9 days for progesterone only pills , if started or continued. Starting oral contraceptive immediately after ulipristal acetate is off licence. Should pregnancy occur, though no harm known, register via manufacturer.

Levonorgestrel Initiate within 72h of unprotected sex. Failure rates are ≤2.6%. Suitable for those with focal migraine and past thromboembolism, there are no medical contraindications to its use. Levonorgestrel 1.5mg preferably within 12h and no later than 72h after unprotected sex. If on, or within 28 days of, taking an enzyme inducer (p300), or with post-sexual exposure HIV prophylaxis, the dose is 3mg. If vomiting occurs within 2h of taking the dose, take another immediately. The earlier taken after UPSI, the fewer the pregnancies which occur. It is believed to inhibit ovulation. It can be used more than once in 1 cycle; and can be used (but may be less effective) in same cycle after ulipristal acetate.

Warn that effective contraception should be used until the next period; and that she should return if she suffers any lower abdominal pain or the next period is abnormal. Advise pregnancy test if period >7 days late or unusually light, or after 21 days if 'quick start' contraception started. If immediate ('quick start') oral contraception started, or continuing, extra contraceptive precautions are needed for 7 days for combined pills (avoid immediate co-cyprindiol start), 9 days for Qlaira®, 2 days for progesterone-only pills.

Combined hormonal contraception (CHC) as vaginal ring, transdermal patch (p304), or pills (COCP) contain oestrogen with a progestogen, either in fixed ratio or varying through the month (phased). Standard-dose pills (30mcg oestrogen) are the norm. The combined pill is taken daily for 21d followed by a 7d break. This inhibits ovulation, giving a withdrawal bleed in the pill-free week.

COCP *Oestrogen content:* Most contain ethinylestradiol, but alternatives are estradiol valerate (Qlaira®) or mestranol (Norinyl-1®). Low-strength preparations contain 20mcg ethinylestradiol and are used if there are risk factors for circulatory disease, or oestrogenic side effects from a higher dose. The standard strength is 30–35mcg ethinylestradiol and is used for most women. Use phased preparations for women who have bleeding problems with monophasic products. *Progestogen type:* Most commonly, levonorgestrel and norethisterone are used. Consider using pills containing desogestrel, norgestimate, drosperidone or gestodene if symptoms such as acne, headache, breakthrough bleeding. Cyproterone acetate is licensed for the treatment of acne and does provide contraception. Use for 3–4 months after resolution of symptoms. Higher risk of VTE compared with levonorgestrel.

Contraceptive patch (eg Evra®) Transdermal patch containing 20mcg ethinylestradiol and norelgestromin. Useful if compliance with taking daily tablets a problem. Apply patch on day 1 of cycle, change on days 8 and 15, and remove on day 22. Apply a new patch after 7d patch-free interval to start the cycle again.

Contraceptive vaginal ring (eg NuvaRing®) Flexible ring which releases 15mcg/24h ethinylestradiol and etonogestrel. The woman inserts the ring into the vagina on day 1 of cycle, and leaves it in for 3 weeks. It is removed on day 22 for a 7d ring-free interval.

Reasons to avoid combined hormonal contraception[9].

- *Venous disease:* Avoid if current/past VTE or sclerosing treatment to varicose veins. Use with caution if 1 risk factor, avoid if >1 of: age >35y, smoker (avoid if >35y and smokes >15/day), BMI >30kg/m² (avoid if BMI >35kg/m²), family history of VTE in 1st-degree relative <45y (avoid if known thrombophilia), immobility (avoid if bed-bound or in plaster), superficial thrombophlebitis.
- *Arterial disease:* Avoid if valvular or congenital heart disease with complications, or history of cardiovascular disease including stroke, TIA, IHD, peripheral vascular disease, hypertensive retinopathy. Risk factors for CVD (use with caution if 1, avoid if >1: age >35y, smoker (avoid if smokes >40/day), family history of arterial disease in first-degree relative <45y (avoid if atherogenic lipid profile), diabetes mellitus (avoid if vascular, renal, neurological, or eye complications), hypertension with BP >140/90mmHg (avoid if >160/95mmHg), migraine without aura (avoid if migraine with aura, migraine treated with ergot derivatives and those lasting >72h).
- *Liver disease:* Avoid if active or flare of viral hepatitis, liver tumours, severe cirrhosis, active gallbladder disease, and seek advice if history of contraceptive-associated cholestasis and avoid if previous obstetric cholestasis.
- *Cancer:* Avoid if current history of breast cancer. If no alternative and breast cancer >5y ago with no known gene mutation, seek specialist advice.
- *Previous pregnancy complications:* Avoid if pruritis in pregnancy, obstetric cholestasis, chorea, pemphigoid gestationis. Avoid if postpartum and breastfeeding (can be used from 6 weeks if other methods unacceptable).
- *Hepatic enzyme-inducing drugs:* Avoid if taking rifampicin or rifabutin. For others, increase the dose to 50mcg ethinylestradiol and shorten pill/patch/ring-free interval to 4d. There is no evidence that broad-spectrum antibiotics decrease efficacy of combined contraceptives.

9 UKMEC4 category denotes that use poses unacceptable health risk: UKMEC3=risk from use outweighs advantage; UKMEC2=advantage of use outweighs risk; UKMEC1=no restriction to use. UKMEC 2009.[42]

The problem is ischaemic stroke. The background annual incidence is 2 per 100,000 women aged 20, and 20 per 100,000 for those aged 40. Migraine itself is a risk factor. For those with migraine and CHC use, incidence of ischaemic stroke becomes 8:100,000 if aged 20; and 80:100,000 in those aged 40. Low-dose COCPs only should be used. Those with migraine with aura are known to be at special risk precluding use of combined Pills in these women (however, there is no problem with them using progesterone only or non-hormonal contraception). Other risk factors for ischaemic stroke include smoking, age >35yrs, ↑BP, obesity (BMI >30), diabetes mellitus, dyslipidaemia, and family history of arterial disease <45yrs. Women known to have migraine should be warned to stop CHC immediately if they develop aura or worsening of migraine. If a woman has 1st migraine attack on CHC, stop it, observe closely: restart cautiously only if there are no sequelae and if migraine attack was without aura and there are no other risk factors (above).[43]

Diagnosing migraine with aura (formerly called *classical/focal migraine*)
1 Slow evolution of symptoms (see below) over several minutes.
2 Duration of aura usually 10–30min, resolving within 1h, and typically before onset of headache.
3 Visual symptoms (99% of auras), eg:
   •Bilateral homonymous hemianopia.
   •Teichopsia and fortification spectra, eg a gradually enlarging C C with scintillating edges.
   •Positive (bright) scotomata.
4 Sensory disturbance (31% of auras):
   •Usually associated with visual symptoms.
   •Usually in one arm spreading from fingers to face (leg rarely affected).
5 Speech disturbance (18% of auras): dysphasia; dysarthria; paraphasia.
6 Motor disturbances (6% of auras).

Both motor and speech disturbances are usually accompanied by visual and/or sensory disturbances.

Migraine without aura (formerly called *simple* or *common* migraine) includes symptoms of blurred vision, photophobia, phonophobia, generalized flashing lights affecting the whole visual field in both eyes, associated with headache.

Absolute contraindications to COC use
• Migraine with aura.
• Migraine without aura in women with >1 risk factor for stroke (above).
• Severe migraine or migraine lasting >72h (status migrainosus).
• Migraine treated with ergot derivatives.

Short-term side effects usually resolve within 2–3 cycles.

- *Oestrogenic:* Commonly include breast tenderness, nausea, cyclical weight gain, bloating, and vaginal discharge. Due to relative oestrogen excess.
- *Progestogenic:* Side effects include mood swings, PMT, vaginal dryness, sustained weight gain, decreased libido, and acne.
- *Headache* affects 2.9% of those taking CHC, and women should report increase in headache frequency or the development of focal symptoms. Discontinue immediately if focal symptoms occur and if not typical of migraine and last >1h, admit to hospital.
- *Breakthrough bleeding* is most common in the first 6 months of use. If it persists >3 months, check compliance, exclude persistent diarrhoea/vomiting, and check for gynaecological causes. Screen for chlamydia, check cervix, check smear is up to date, exclude pregnancy and if >45y consider US and referral to gynaecologist for endometrial biopsy. Increase oestrogen content of COCP if on low-dose pill, if not change progestogen.

Risks and benefits of combined hormonal contraception	
Risks	**Benefits**
VTE risk doubled (absolute risk low)	Improvement in acne
Ischaemic stroke (small ↑ risk)	↓ menorrhagia/dysmenorrhoea
Breast and cervical cancer (↑ risk small and disappears <10y after stopping)	↓ risk ovarian, endometrial and bowel cancer (persists after stopping CHC)
Mood changes (no ↑ risk depression)	↓ menopausal symptoms

Start CHCs/PoPs on day 1 of cycle, on day of TOP, ≥21 days postpartum (>6 weeks if CHC and breastfeeding), or ≥2wks after fully mobile post major surgery. If starting CHC on day 1–5, cover is immediate, no other precautions (condoms) are needed. If later start (and not pregnant, p297), use condoms for 1wk. Qlaira®: start on day 1 (condoms for 9 days).

Stopping the Pill Tell to stop at once if she develops: • Sudden severe chest pain • Sudden breathlessness (±cough/bloody sputum) • Severe calf pain • Unexplained leg swelling • Severe stomach pain • Unusual severe prolonged headache; sudden visual loss; collapse; dysphasia; hemi-motor/sensory loss; 1st seizure • Hepatitis, jaundice, liver enlargement • BP ≥160/95 • 4 weeks before leg or major surgery (p300) • Any CI (p300). On stopping, 66% menstruate by 6 weeks, 98% by 6 months; women amenorrhoeic post-CHC usually were before.

Missed Pills (or severe diarrhoea): Consult package inserts; advice varies. In general, if the start delay is ≥48h, or >48h since last Pill continue Pills but use condoms too for 7 days (+ days of diarrhoea); if this includes Pill-free days, start next pack *without break* (omit inactive Pills in 'ED' formulations). If 2 pills of 1st 7 days in pack forgotten, use emergency contraception if unprotected intercourse since end of last pack. Vomiting <2h post-Pill: take another. Non-enzyme-inducing (p300) broad-spectrum antibiotics need extra precautions only if causing diarrhoea or vomiting. Postcoital options: p299. Diarrhoea and vomiting does not affect the contraceptive patch or ring.

Postnatal Start 21 days after birth: eg CHC if not breastfeeding; PoP, Depo-Provera® (or Nexplanon®) if breastfeeding. IUCD: fit ~4 weeks postpartum.

Flying and high altitude Avoid immobility if flight ≥3h. If trekking higher than 4500 metres for ≥1 week consider alternative.

Further reading
Family Planning Association: www.fpa.org.uk
Faculty of Sexual & Reproductive Healthcare: www.fsrh.org

1st-generation Pills are the original Pills containing 50mcg oestrogen. *2nd-generation Pills* are those containing ≤35mcg oestrogen and levonorgestrel, norethisterone, norgestimate, or cyproterone acetate. *3rd generation Pills* contain desogestrel or gestodene as the progesterone. Although designed to be more lipid friendly 3rd generation Pills have not been proven to be better in those with cardiac risk factors and are more thrombogenic.[44]

Risk of venous thromboembolism

Risk of thromboembolism is increased by combined hormonal preparations, whether pill, ring or patch. Figures are not well known for progesterone-only preparations but they do not appear to be thrombogenic. Carriage of factor V Leiden mutation particularly increases risk of thrombosis (↑ risk

EURAS study 2007[46]	
Not on Pill	44:100,000
Levornorgestrel	80:100,000
Drospirenone	91:100,000
Others	91:100,000
Pregnant	291:100,000

×35). 3rd-generation Pills particularly increase resistance to our natural anticoagulant (activated protein c, APC), so increasing thrombosis. With antithrombin 3, protein c or s deficiency have thrombosis rates ↑ ×5. Counsel those starting the Pill that it does increase the risk of thrombosis, particularly in 1st year of use, but it is still a rare event.

The Pill and travel If immobile for >3h, the *BNF* recommends mid-journey exercises ± support stockings.

The Pill and surgery Stop oestrogen containing contraception 4wks pre-op when immobilization expected and arrange alternative contraception.

When to use emergency contraception (eg missed-Pill)[47]

- coc: if 3 or more 30–35mcg pills or 2 or more 20mcg pills forgotten in 1st 7 days of pack and unprotected sexual intercourse (UPSI) occurred in those 1st 7 days or pill-free week.
- PoP: if 1 or more PoPs have been missed or taken >3h late (>12h if desogestrel 75mcg eg Cerazette®) and UPSI has occurred in the 2 days following this.
- IUCD IUS: if complete or partial expulsion identified or midcycle removal has been necessary and UPSI in the 7 days preceding this.
- Progesterone injection: if >12 weeks 5 days from last Depo-Provera® or >8 weeks from Noristerat® injection and UPSI occurred.
- Barrier method: failure of method (eg splitting, slippage).

Progestogen-only contraceptives thicken cervical mucus, reduce receptivity of the endometrium to implantation, and in some women, also inhibit ovulation. They have the advantage of reducing pelvic infection and are used where oestrogen-containing contraceptives are contraindicated.

Reasons to avoid progestogen-only contraception
• Current breast cancer but may be used if >5y disease free, no other alternative, and after specialist advice
• Trophoblastic disease
• Liver disease; active viral hepatitis, severe decompensated cirrhosis, benign or malignant liver tumour
• New symptoms or diagnosis of migraine with aura, IHD, stroke/TIA when taking progestogen-only contraception
• Avoid if SLE with antiphospholipid antibodies
• Any undiagnosed vaginal bleeding should be investigated before starting progestogen-only contraception.

Progestogen-only pill (POP) There are several brands available in the UK containing differing progestogens. Pills containing etynodiol, norethisterone, or levonorgestrel have a 3h window. Desogestrel-containing POPs (desogestrel 75mcg eg Cerazette®) have a 12h window, and have a stronger ovarian suppressive effect than the others. *Side effects:* Higher failure rate than COCP, menstrual irregularities, increased risk of ectopic pregnancy and functional ovarian cysts, breast tenderness, depression, acne, reduced libido and weight change. *Start* on day 1-5 of the cycle (effective immediately) or any other time (use condoms for 2d), or >3 weeks postpartum. Efficacy is affected by hepatic enzyme-inducing drugs- use alternative.

Depot progestogen ('the injection') 2 preparations are available: medroxy-progesterone acetate 150mg given deep IM 12-weekly; start during the 1st 5 days of a cycle (postpartum see p95) or norethisterone enantate (Noristerat®) 200mg into gluteus maximus 8-weekly—licensed for short-term use only. Exclude pregnancy and use condoms for 7 days after late injections >2 weeks late. *Advantages:* Can be used up to age 50y if no other risk factors for osteoporosis reduced risk of ectopic pregnancy, functional cysts and sickle cell crises, reduced risk of endometrial cancer; may help PMS and menorrhagia. *Problems:* Menstrual disturbance usually settles with time, and amenorrhoea then supervenes. 33% amenorrhoeic after 6 months' use; 60% after 18 months (14% and 33% respectively for Noristerat®). If very heavy bleeding occurs, exclude pregnancy; give injection early (but >8 weeks from previous dose) and give oestrogen if not CI. Fears of osteoporosis in users; recommend review after 2 years' use and avoidance in adolescents unless the only acceptable method. Bone mass density increases when stopped. Other problems include weight gain (up to 2kg in 70% of women). There may be some delay in return of ovulation on stopping injections (median delay 10 months).

Implants Progesterone implants give up to 3 years' contraception with one implantation. Nexplanon® is a radiopaque flexible rod containing etonogestrel 68mg which is implanted subdermally into the medial surface of the upper arm. Insert on day 1-5 of cycle (immediately effective), or any other time but use condoms for 7d. Contraceptive effect stops when the implant is removed. It has no impact on bone density. <23% of users become amenorrhoeic after 12 months' use. Infrequent bleeding occurs in 50% in the 1st 3 months' use; 30% at 6 months. Prolonged bleeding affects up to 33% in 1st 3 months; frequent bleeding affects <10%. Effective contraception may not occur in overweight women (BMI >35kg/m^2) in the 3rd year, so consider earlier changing of implant. There is reduced efficacy with hepatic enzyme-inducing drugs.

Sterilization is permanent, irreversible contraception. There are no absolute contraindications provided that they make the request themselves, are of sound mind, and are not acting under external duress. In the UK, funding on the NHS may depend on location; it is a 'low-priority procedure' and in some regions special funding needs to be agreed first and after alternative methods have failed or are contraindicated.

Ideally see both partners and consider the following:

- *Alternative methods:* Do they know about depot progesterone injections, coils, and implants? Give written information (in relevant language) about alternative contraception and ♂ and ♀ sterilization.
- *Consent:* Is it the wish of both partners? Legally only the consent of the patient is required but the agreement of both is desirable. Those lacking mental capacity to consent require High Court judgment.
- *Who should be sterilized?* Does he fear loss of femininity? Does he see it as being neutered? Does the ♀ really want or need hysterectomy? Examine the one to be sterilized.
- *Irreversibility:* Reversal is only 50% successful in either sex and **never** funded by the NHS. Sterilization should be seen as an irreversible step. Sterilizations most regretted (3–10%) are those in the young (<30yrs), childless, at times of stress (especially relationship problems), or immediately after pregnancy (termination or delivery). For sterilization at CS, it should be discussed at least twice in the pregnancy (excluding the day of CS).
- *Warn of failure rates*—1:200 for women (1:100 at CS), 1:2000 for men. In women, it is no better than the Mirena® coil. Advise seeking medical confirmation if future pregnancy suspected or abnormal vaginal bleeding or abdominal pain. If pregnancy occurs there is ↑ risk of ectopic (4.3–76%).
- *Side effect:* A women who has been on the COCP for many years may find her periods unacceptably heavy after sterilization. ▶Record in the notes: *Knows it's irreversible; lifetime failure rate discussed*, eg 1:2000 for vasectomy, and 1:200 for ♀ sterilization.

Female sterilization The more the tubes are damaged, the lower the failure rate and the more difficult reversal becomes. In the UK, most sterilizations are carried out laparoscopically with general anaesthesia. Filshie clip occlusion is recommended with local anaesthetic applied to tubes (or modified Pomeroy operation at mini-laparotomy if postpartum or at caesarean). Do pregnancy test pre-op. Advise use of effective contraception until the operation and next period. Remove IUCD after the next period in case an already fertilized ovum is present. Alternatively, hysteroscopic sterilization using fallopian implants under local anaesthetic or IV sedation is endorsed by NICE.[48][NICE]

Vasectomy This is a simpler and safer procedure than female sterilization and can be performed as an outpatient under local anaesthetic. The vas deferens is identified at the top of the scrotum and is ligated and excised or the lumen cauterized. Fascial interposition improves effectiveness.[49] Bruising and haematoma are complications. No-scalpel techniques reduce these complications.[50] Late pain affects 3% from sperm granulomata, which are less common if thermal cautery (rather than electrical cautery) is used. Warn of risk of chronic testicular pain.

The major disadvantage of vasectomy is that it takes up to 3 months before sperm stores are used up. Obtain 2 ejaculates 'negative' for sperm (the first 8 weeks post-op; 2nd 2–4 weeks later) before stopping other methods of contraception. Reversal is most successful if within 10 years of initial operation.

Control of bladder function Continence in women is maintained in the urethra by the external sphincter and pelvic floor muscles maintaining a urethral pressure higher than bladder pressure. Micturition occurs when these muscles relax and the bladder detrusor muscle contracts.

Urinary history Incontinence is involuntary leakage of urine, which is divided into urge, stress, and mixed urinary incontinence. The woman may have waited for over 10y to seek help. Continuous urinary leakage is most commonly associated with a vesicovaginal fistula or congenital abnormality such as ectopic ureter. Ask about daytime voids (normal 4–7), nocturia (up to 70y, >1 night-time void is abnormal), nocturnal enuresis, urgency (most frequently due to detrusor overactivity), and voiding difficulties (hesitancy, straining, and slow or intermittent stream, most commonly seen with neurological conditions). Ask about the feeling of incomplete emptying, bladder pain (seen with interstitial cystitis), dysuria, haematuria, and recurrent UTI. Are there any symptoms of prolapse or bowel symptoms? It is important to check PMH, and record current drug treatment. How is the urinary incontinence affecting her quality of life? Does it affect her relationship? *Frequency/volume charts* are a simple, objective way of obtaining information about fluid intake and voiding problems and should be filled in for a 72h period.

Examination Check weight, BMI, BP, and signs of systemic disease. Note manual dexterity and mobility as this can affect which treatment options are available to the woman. If symptoms suggest a neurological cause, perform a neurological examination (the most common cause of a neurogenic bladder in a woman is MS). Exclude an abdominal or pelvic mass, including a full bladder. Is the vulval/vaginal skin atrophic? Record any prolapse. Is there any urinary leakage on coughing?

Investigations
• *Urinalysis* and MSU for MC&S to exclude UTI; OGTT if diabetes is suspected
• Check residual volume post-micturition to exclude incomplete emptying
• *Imaging* is not routinely used but may include US to exclude incomplete bladder emptying and define any pelvic mass.
• *Cystoscopy* is used to visualize the urethra, bladder mucosa, trigone, and ureteric orifices. Biopsies can be taken. Indicated if recurrent UTI, haematuria, bladder pain, suspected fistula, tumour, or interstitial cystitis.
• *Urodynamics* are a combination of tests which look at the ability of the bladder to store and void urine. Uroflowmetry screens for voiding difficulties and the patient voids in private onto a commode with a urinary flow meter, measuring voided volume over time and plotting it on a graph. Cystometry is more invasive and involves measuring pressure and volume within the bladder during filling and voiding, and is a test of bladder function. The bladder is filled with saline via a catheter, and an intravesical and rectal probe measure differences in pressure, to give the detrusor pressure. The patient is asked for first desire to void, strong desire to void, and to cough. The results are printed onto a graph and any detrusor contractions and/or leakage noted.

Classification *Stress urinary incontinence* is the involuntary leakage of urine on effort or exertion, or on sneezing or coughing. Commonly due to urethral sphincter weakness. *Urge urinary incontinence* is the involuntary leakage of urine with a strong desire to pass urine. Commonly coexists with frequency and nocturia and forms overactive bladder syndrome. *Mixed urinary incontinence* is the combination of stress and urge incontinence and usually one symptom will predominate (treat that first). *Overflow incontinence* is usually due to injury or insult eg post-partum. Treat with catheter.

Further reading

NICE (2013). *Urinary Incontinence in Women: Management* (CG171). London: NICE. https://www.nice.org.uk/guidance/cg171

Stress urinary incontinence (SUI)

This is the most common urinary reason for which a woman will seek help. It affects up to 1 in 10, and in 50% will be pure stress incontinence. It occurs when detrusor pressure exceeds the closing pressure of the urethra. Pregnancy itself is a risk factor (mode of delivery much less so). At the menopause, oestrogen deficiency leads to weakening of pelvic support and thinning of the urothelium. Other causes include radiotherapy, congenital weakness and trauma from radical pelvic surgery (eg for gynaecological cancer).

Investigations: Exclude UTI (this will worsen symptoms). A frequency/volume chart shows normal frequency and functional bladder capacity. Urodynamics are indicated when surgery is being considered, in order to confirm the diagnosis, check for detrusor overactivity (which can be worsened irreversibly by surgical procedures) and check for voiding dysfunction (a woman with a poor flow rate is at risk of long-term urinary retention).

Management
- *Conservative measures* should be tried first. These include optimizing control of other medical problems such as diabetes, weight loss, smoking cessation, treatment of chronic cough, and constipation. *Pelvic floor exercises* for at least 3 months and continued long-term (refer to a pelvic floor physiotherapist for optimal results). Biofeedback uses a device to convert the effect of pelvic floor contraction into a visual or auditory signal.
- *Pharmacological agents* are not recommended as first-line treatment by NICE. Duloxetine is the only licensed drug for this but it is rarely used.
- *Surgery* is considered after other measures have failed. *Peri-urethral injections* of bulking agents are successful in 20–40% and have lower morbidity than other procedures. May be better for frail, older women or younger women yet to complete their family. The *tension-free vaginal tape* (TVT) is the most common surgical procedure for SUI in the UK. A polypropylene mesh tape is placed under the mid-urethra via a small vaginal incision. The mean cure rate is 94%. Risks include bladder injury, voiding difficulty, and tape erosion. The *transobturator tape* is an alternative to this and has a lower incidence of bladder injury but higher risk of groin pain. The *Burch colposuspension* is now rarely performed due to the success of the TVT.

Overactive bladder syndrome (OAB)

OAB is a chronic condition affecting up to 1 in 6 women, and implies underlying detrusor overactivity (DO). DO is a diagnosis made on urodynamic testing. Incidence increases with age. It is mostly idiopathic, but may be found with MS, spina bifida, or secondary to pelvic or incontinence surgery. Symptoms may be provoked by cold weather, opening the front door, or by coughing or sneezing leading to confusion with symptoms of stress incontinence. It is unpredictable and the urine leakage may be significant, having a huge impact on the woman's quality of life.

Investigations: Exclude UTI. A frequency/volume chart typically shows increased diurnal frequency and nocturia. Urodynamics show involuntary detrusor contractions during filling and should be performed if there is doubt about the diagnosis, complex symptoms, or drug treatment has failed.

Management: Avoid excessive fluid intake, caffeinated and carbonated drinks and alcohol. Bladder retraining aims to suppress the urinary urge and extend the intervals between voiding. *Anticholingerics* are the mainstay of pharmacological treatment, blocking the parasympathetic nerves and relaxing detrusor. Try oxybutynin 2.5–5mg 1–4 times/day. Alternatives are solifenacin 5–10mg daily, or tolterodine 2mg bd. Side effects include dry mouth, constipation and nausea. *Intravaginal oestrogen cream* can help in those with vaginal atrophy. Other measures include *botulinum toxin A* injected cystoscopically into detrusor (90% effective). Neuromodulation can help. Surgery is a last resort.

Gynaecology

Hysterectomy is performed less commonly now due to the success of the Mirena® IUS in treating menorrhagia and ablative procedures of the endometrium. It may be:
• *Total* (including the cervix) or
• *Subtotal* (leaving the cervix behind; she will continue to need smears)
• *Approach* may be open, laparoscopic, laparoscopic-assisted or vaginal
• *Removal of the tubes and ovaries* may be carried out at the same time and this depends on the woman's wishes, her menopausal status, and why she needs a hysterectomy. Due to the recent research suggesting that some ovarian cancer originates from the fallopian tubes, it is increasingly common to perform a salpingectomy if the woman wants to keep her ovaries.

A subtotal hysterectomy is an option if all smears have been normal, and if pelvic adhesions or disease make it impossible to remove the cervix. There is no link between better sexual function with or without a cervix, and a woman's sex life often improves after hysterectomy due to cessation of pain and heavy bleeding. 10% of women continue to have cyclical bleeding after a subtotal hysterectomy and should be warned of this. A *Wertheim's* (extended to include local lymph nodes and a cuff of vagina) is used for malignancy and has a higher rate of complications (particularly ureteric injury) due to the more extensive nature of the surgery. Patients who have had laparoscopic or vaginal hysterectomy have less post-operative pain and shorter recovery time. *Risks* include bleeding, infection, injury to bladder, bowel, vessels or ureters, scarring (low transverse, midline or laparoscopic scars), VTE, earlier menopause if ovaries retained (due to sharing of blood supply with uterine arteries). In a laparoscopic or vaginal procedure, there is a risk of converting to an open operation.

Hysteroscopy is one of the most common gynaecological procedures and can be carried out under no, local, or general anaesthesia. A fine scope (3–12mm) is inserted through the cervix into the uterus to visualize the endometrium. Visualization of both ostia (where the fallopian tubes join the uterus) confirms that the hysteroscope is in the correct cavity. It is mainly used in the diagnosis of abnormal uterine bleeding. A curette is used after removal of the hysteroscope to take endometrial biopsies. Depending on the findings, the surgeon may then proceed to transcervical removal of fibroid (TCRF), which uses an operating hysteroscope and monopolar or bipolar diathermy to shave off submucosal fibroids or polyps, or the endometrium (TCRE). *Out-patient hysteroscopy* is used for diagnosis of postmenopausal or abnormal uterine bleeding, as well as: endometrial polypectomy, removal of small submucosal fibroids, endometrial ablation, removal of lost IUCDs, and transcervical sterilization. Use of saline distension medium gives better views, reduced vasovagal episodes, reduced procedure time, and the ability to use cautery. *Risks* include bleeding (usually spotting), infection, perforation of the uterus or damage to the cervix, and if hysteroscopic surgery is being carried out and a perforation occurs, injury to surrounding organs. If the cervix is stenosed, it may be impossible to gain access to the uterus.

Endometrial ablation by diathermy, microwave, electrical impedance (Novasure®), or thermal balloon (Thermachoice®) (under GA or spinal ± paracervical block) reduces bleeding by destruction of the endometrium down to the basalis layer. It is most commonly performed with hysteroscopy immediately prior to the ablation. It is less effective if the endometrial cavity is >10cm. 90% of women have a reduction in bleeding by 9 months and 30% are amenorrhoeic. It has no effect on pain and should not be offered if dysmenorrhoea is significant. The woman should have completed her family and have reliable contraception. *Risks* include bleeding, infection, uterine perforation with or without surrounding organ damage, failed procedure (eg if cavity too large or the ablative system used fails its safety checks), haematometra. Some endometrium remains in most (so give progesterone-containing HRT later, if needed).

Laparoscopy may be diagnostic or operative and allows direct visualization of the pelvic organs. Minimal access surgery has the advantage of shorter hospital stays with minimal abdominal scarring. Many gynaecological procedures are carried out using this approach, including ovarian cystectomy, salpingectomy (for ectopic pregnancy), diathermy or excision of endometriosis, myomectomy, hysterectomy (total or subtotal), and some prolapse surgery. The abdomen is insufflated via a Verres needle in the umbilicus with carbon dioxide gas to create a pneumoperitoneum. Ports are introduced and instruments are inserted through the ports in the iliac fossae or suprapubically. *Risks* include bleeding (potential for large vessel injury on laparoscopic entry which is thankfully rare, and reduced with safe technique), infection, injury to bladder, bowel, vessels and ureters, failed entry, scarring, VTE, laparotomy and any risks specific to the operation being performed.

Colporrhaphy or 'repair' The lack of support from the anterior or posterior vaginal wall in cases of prolapse is rectified by excising redundant mucosa and doing a fascial repair. It is *not* an operation to correct urinary incontinence. The operation may be combined with a vaginal hysterectomy. The more mucosa is removed, the tighter the vagina. Enquire before surgery if she is sexually active. An anterior repair may be performed as a day-case procedure, but posterior repairs are at higher risk of haematoma formation and many surgeons insert a vaginal pack and catheter overnight. It is approximately 90% curative. Vaginal mesh is never used in a primary repair. *Risks* are bleeding, infection, injury to bladder, bowel or ureters, dyspareunia, recurrence, and VTE.

Surgical management of miscarriage used to be known as 'evacuation of retained products of conception.' It is a day-case procedure that can be carried out under local, or most commonly, general anaesthetic. For miscarriage, gestational age should be <13 weeks (otherwise higher risk of complications, and medical management is safer). Prostaglandin administered PV prior to the procedure reduces the risk of uterine and cervical trauma. Once the woman is anaesthetized, the cervix is grasped and dilated to between 1 and 2cm. A rigid or flexible curette in the appropriate size is used to remove the products of conception under suction. *Risks* are bleeding, infection, uterine perforation (rarely intraperitoneal injury), retained products of conception, intrauterine adhesions, and cervical tears.

Enhanced recovery This looks at patient pathways with a view to optimizing preoperative and postoperative care, to minimize inpatient length of stay. Measures adopted include admission on the day of operation, early removal of drips and catheters, and early postoperative feeding. Daily ward rounds and good pain management are an integral part of care.

This is a symptom, not a diagnosis, and describes intermittent or constant lower abdominal pain of >6 months' duration not associated exclusively with menstruation, intercourse, or pregnancy. Pain may cause, or be exacerbated by, emotional problems. She may be depressed. Adequate time needs to be given to allow the woman to tell her story and express her views as to the cause of pain, and explore psychological aspects. A past history of abuse is more common. A multidisciplinary approach effects most all round improvement.

Laparoscopy may reveal a likely cause: chronic pelvic infection, endometriosis, adenomyosis, adhesions (eg residual ovary syndrome and trapped ovarian syndrome).[52][RCOG] Consider also irritable bowel syndrome (*OHCM* p268), and interstitial cystitis (p306).

If pain is cyclical, ovarian suppression (COCP/GnRH analogues) may help.

Pelvic congestion Controversial diagnosis. Congested lax pelvic veins (seen at laparoscopy) cause pain worse on standing, walking, and premenstrually. Typically variable in site and intensity, there may be unpleasant postcoital ache. Deep palpation reveals maximal tenderness over ovaries. Vagina and cervix may look blue from congestion. Look for associated posterior leg varicosities.

Remedies include explanation ('pelvic migraine'), ovarian suppression, migraine remedies (*OHCM* p450), and relaxation techniques. For severe symptoms bilateral ovarian vein ligation, radiological embolization, or hysterectomy with salpingo-oophorectomy (±HRT) may cure.

Mittelschmerz This is mid-cycle menstrual pain which may occur in teenagers and older women around the time of ovulation—from the German *mittel* (=middle) and *Schmerz* (=pain).

Further reading

RCOG (2012). *Chronic Pelvic Pain, Initial Management* (Green-top Guideline No. 41). London: RCOG.

Dyspareunia

This means pain during intercourse. There may be a vicious circle in which anticipation of pain leads to tense muscles and lack of lubrication, and so to further pain. ▶*The patient may not volunteer the problem so ask about intercourse*. Her attitude to pelvic examination may tell you as much as the examination itself. Ask her to show you where the problem is. If the problem is actually vaginismus do not insist on examination and consider counselling and psychosexual therapy (p243). Was there female genital mutilation (p247)?

Dyspareunia may be superficial (introital), eg from infection, so look for ulceration and discharge. Vaginal dryness may be caused by oestrogen deficiency (p256) or lack of sexual stimulation (p243). Has she had a recent postpartum perineal repair? A suture or scar can cause well-localized pain which is cured by massage or by removing the suture and injection of local anaesthetic. If the introitus has been rendered too narrow, she may need surgery.

Deep dyspareunia is felt internally (deep inside). It is associated with endometriosis and pelvic infection; treat the cause if possible.

Dermatographism is a rare cause of dyspareunia: look for itchy vulval wheals some minutes after calibrated dermatographometer application. It can occur on any surface. It is the commonest physical cause of urticaria, and the clue to its presence is linear wheals with a surrounding bright red flare (but no angio-oedema) elsewhere on the skin, in response to a firm stroke. Cause is unknown. Relief of dyspareunia in these cases has been achieved by 2% **adrenaline** (epinephrine) cream, and **cetirizine** 10mg/24h PO.

Gynaecology

Ovarian hyperstimulation syndrome (OHSS) is a complication of ovulation induction or superovulation. This is a systemic disease and vasoactive products (particularly vascular endoethelial growth factor, VEGF) are central to its pathophysiology. It has an incidence of up to 33% in mild forms, and in 1:200 it is severe, requiring hospitalization.

Characteristics
• Ovarian enlargement
• Fluid shift from intravascular to extravascular space:
   • This leads to the accumulation of fluid in peritoneal and pleural spaces
   • Intravascular volume depletion causes haemoconcentration and hypercoagulability.

Risk factors
• Young age
• Low BMI
• Polycystic ovaries
• Previous OHSS.

Presentation Abdominal discomfort, nausea, vomiting, and abdominal distension ± dyspnoea. Presentation is usually 3–7 days after hCG administration, or 12–17 days, if pregnancy has ensued.

Prevention Prediction and prevention are the key. Women should be given the lowest effective regimen of gonadotrophins. Cycle cancellation may be necessary, or elective embryo cryopreservation, for use in a further frozen-thawed cycle. In women with PCOS, *in vitro* maturation (IVM, p293), where immature eggs are collected, avoids ovarian stimulation and the risk of OHSS.

Management
Mild and moderate OHSS (Abdominal bloating, mild to moderate pain, US evidence of ascites, and ovarian size usually 8–12cm):
• Outpatient management
• Analgesia (paracetamol and/or codeine)
• Avoid NSAIDs (CI in pregnancy; will worsen fluid shift and renal impairment)
• Drink to thirst, not to excess
• Avoid strenuous activities and intercourse due to risk of ovarian torsion
• Continue with progesterone luteal support, and avoid hCG.
• Review by the assisted conception unit every 2–3 days.

Severe OHSS (Clinical ascites, oliguria, haematocrit is >45%, hypoproteinaemia, ovarian size >12cm):
• Admit to hospital
• Analgesia and anti-emetics (avoid NSAIDs)
• Daily FBC, U&E, LFTS, albumin
• Strict fluid balance
• Daily assessment of girth (ascites), weight, and legs (thrombosis)
• Thromboprophylaxis with compression stockings and LMWH
• Paracentesis for symptomatic relief (± IV replacement albumin)
• Urinary catheter.

Critical OHSS (Tense ascites, haematocrit >55%, WCC >25×10⁹/L, oligo- or anuria, thromboembolism, acute respiratory distress syndrome; OHCM p178):
• Get senior help early. Admit to ITU. Symptomatic pleural effusions may need drainage. Use antiembolic measures as above. Pay meticulous attention to fluid balance. Aim to maintain intake at 3L/24h using normal saline if unable to tolerate oral fluids. Beware hyponatraemia.

Further reading
RCOG (2006). *The Management of Ovarian Hyperstimulation Syndrome* (Green-top Guideline No. 5). London: RCOG.

We thank Dr Dane Rayment, our Specialist Reader, for his significant contribution to this chapter and to Suzanne Dash and Robert Jennings, our Junior Readers, for their hard work.

Stare at the image in the centre of the page (fig 4.1) and let your mind go blank. If you aren't already asleep (or checking your phone to make sure you haven't missed something important), you will start to see the spiral spin downwards to infinity. Your brain is tricking you into believing that this two-dimensional image has genuine depth and movement. You know that this isn't the case—turn the page over and confirm your hypothesis—but you can still see the lines moving. The Fraser spiral illusion is an optical illusion that was first described by the British psychologist Sir James Fraser in 1908, and like all optical illusions it causes your brain to confuse its subjective experience (seeing the spiral move) with an objective reality (a black and white image in a high-quality textbook). This happens because your brain is working as it should do. So what would it mean if the images on p329 also started to move? Or meow? Or tell that you were 'never going to pass your exams because you are just bluffing your way through revision and are really a failure'?

You might initially discount this as a single odd experience and put it down to tiredness, stress, or too much caffeine. You know that these things should not, in fact cannot, happen. But they keep happening. Do you become upset? Anxious? It may start to play on your thoughts disrupting your concentration in lectures and affecting your sleep. Friends start to check if you are ok. So what will you tell them? If you say what is really happening then they may react badly, call your GP, or worse, the police. People may think that you are going mad. It's hard to know what to do or who to trust (worse still when the voices you hear say to trust no one). You isolate yourself. These experiences for some mark the start of their journey through the world of mental illness and of psychiatry.

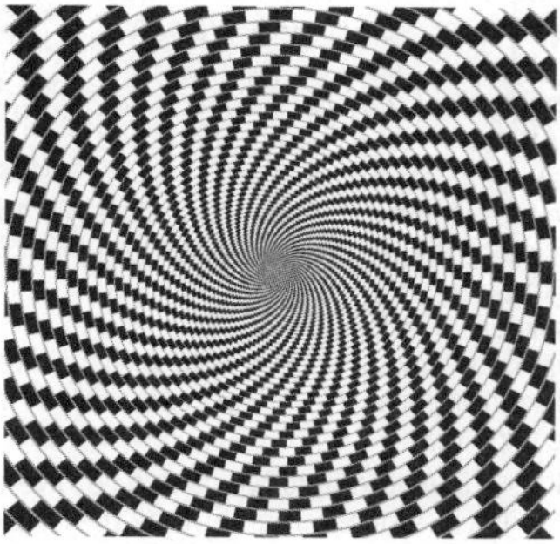

Fig 4.1 An example of a Fraser spiral illusion.

Reading the last few sentences, you were forced to flick between either side of the image. Aware of it, perhaps even slightly irritated (sorry!), but your brain probably filtered it out. Having a mental illness isn't so easy. For some it can define who they are (an 'anorexic', a 'schizophrenic', a 'druggie') in a way that many physical illnesses do not. The stigma attached to having a mental illness diagnosis is embedded in society, despite the fact that 1 in 4 people in the UK will experience mental illness each year. Even in recovery, there can remain background checking to make sure that there aren't signs of relapse—'I've been dumped. I'm sad. Is this another episode...'.

Psychiatry isn't hopeless. People with previous experiences of mental illness live 'normal' lives—full of happiness, sadness, worry, but mostly just day-to-day living like most of us. This chapter hopes to guide you through understanding, recognizing, and treating people who are having experiences which are stopping them living their lives the way they would like.

At its best, psychiatry combines a knowledge and understanding of biology (basic medical sciences, organic conditions), psychology (therapies, personality, emotions) and social concepts (culture, society, environment) to engage with a person who needs our help. To be a good psychiatrist (doctor, friend, or human) you need to listen to the person telling you about their experiences. So listen...if you listen, you may be able to help.

Mental illness In the 1400s, people held the impression that physical illnesses were natural and mental illnesses were supernatural. As this became entrenched in society, it was found necessary to legally define what comprised witchcraft, possession, and insanity. The book, *Malleus Maleficarum* (or the *Witches' Hammer*) was written in 1489 and quickly became the authority for witch identification. It was so popular that ten editions were produced over the next 150 years. Thomas Szasz[1] describes this as the 'scapegoat theory of witchcraft'—the human tendency to try to master human problems and social conflicts, often through organized persecution (fig 4.2).

It was Johann Weyer, a Dutch doctor, occultist, and demonologist who challenged this belief. Born in 1515 (2015 marks his 500th anniversary), he described 'melancholy' in women accused of practising witchcraft and became the 'founder of modern psychiatry'. It wasn't well received. The political philosopher Jean Bodin wrote that he 'should stick to examining urine rather than intruding into the lofty territories of theology and jurisprudence'.

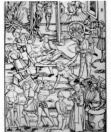

Fig 4.2 Punishments for witchcraft in 16th century Germany. Woodcut from Tengler's *Laienspiegel*, 1508.

Weyer, in his book *De Praestigiis Daemonum*, said that these 'witches'—shunned and punished by society—actually had 'disorders of the senses'. From this approach, he illustrated several different 'melancholies', including those *melancholics* who 'fear death, and yet sometimes they choose death by committing suicide'. He theorized that when the 'melancholic humour seizes control of the brain it alters the mind'. Where society saw a supernatural evil, Weyer saw suffering. It is this legacy that we should continue to explore.

Empathy As well as showing empathy, we should give our patients respect and protect their dignity—not the dignity that they deserve but the dignity that confirms to our patients that, mad, bad, or rambling, they are just as human as their doctors despite their suffering. Let patients:
• Decide on modes of address, 'Mr Pettifer' may be preferred to 'John, dear'. Dignity entails giving choices, and then respecting them.
• Know who we are (eg wear a name badge). But don't label patients ('Go and see the new schizophrenic on Amber ward'). If you put a patient in a box the next thing you'll do is put a lid on it and stop thinking.
• Participate in their treatment plans; explain about common side effects.
• Choose whether to see students or take part in research.
• Have personal and private space to keep their belongings, and to have a space to be in whether alone, or with visitors.
• Wear their own clothes. Clothe them decently if they have none.
• Know what to do if a crisis develops. It's a great help to know that you will be seen in four hours rather than be left to stagnate all weekend.

People claimed that Weyer 'must be a wizard in league with the devil to have shown such sympathy with witches'. But these seven points are congruent with NICE and Human Rights law which lay out the right to life, freedom from inhuman or degrading treatment and torture, respect for privacy, the right to a fair hearing, and freedom of expression. Some of these rights are inalienable and irrevocable. Hopefully things have moved forward in the last 500 years.

---

1 Thomas Szasz is a psychiatrist who is best known as a strong critic of the moral and scientific foundations of psychiatry (often called an anti-psychiatrist). He has described Weyer as the founder of a system which 'confines and silences troublesome individuals'. It is interesting to read Szasz's arguments regarding psychiatry and its place in the modern world, but perhaps wait until after you have finished the chapter...

Suspending judgement We want our patients to achieve insight. Our judging does not help this. Judgement turns patients away from us. We cannot expect them to be honest with us if they know we are judging them.

- The good listener is not silent, but reflective—a mirror not a message. Mirrors do not judge but they enable self-judgement. If a mirror is a reflective listener, a silent listener would be a void rather than a message. This is about 'active listening'.
- Unless some criminal act is underway, it really does not matter what we think about our patients. What matters is how the patient thinks about him- or herself and their near-ones—and how these thoughts can be transformed.
- If we judge people they will not trust us. No trust $\approx$ no therapeutic alliance.
- If we judge, patients will leave us for others perhaps less well qualified.
- There is no evidence that judging improves outcomes. Worse outcomes are likely if the patient feels alienated.
- Patients know if we think negatively of them. They may internalize this, and assume that things will always be bad because they themselves are bad.

Despite these bullets, there is a problem that won't go away. If we find ourselves talking to perpetrators rather than victims, we may not be wise to suspend judgement forever. If a crime is afoot putting others at risk, you may need to break confidentiality. Discuss this with a colleague.

Whenever you think the time may have come to judge, check with yourself that it is not from outrage or disgust, and not through the exercise of pride or from a position of power that you are judging—but reluctantly, and from duty. Unless we exercise judgement, it might be thought, we may be condoning evil. 'For evil to flourish in the world, all that is required is for the good to remain silent.' What human duties do doctors have which trump anything that goes on in the consulting room? We must be human first, and physician-scientists second. Or as Weyer pleaded 'let the judgement of the physicians be consulted—physicians are renowned for their understanding of natural objects and the properties thereof'.

Recovery Quite a few doctors hope to *make* patients better by taking re-sponsibility for ordering their internal world and the credit when things go well. In psychiatry this approach is wrong. Mental health is about people (not patients) taking responsibility for themselves and their programme of change. The psychiatrist knows that their job is done, not when the patient is cured but when he becomes self-actuating, insightful, and interacting with the world in creative (not necessarily satisfactory) ways.

'Why am I as I am? To understand that of any person, his whole life, from Birth must be reviewed. All of our experiences fuse into our personality. Everything that ever happened to us is an ingredient.'

Malcolm X, *The Autobiography Of Malcolm X*

On starting psychiatry you may feel unskilled. A medical problem will come as a relief—you know what to do. Do not be discouraged: you already have plenty of skills (which you will take for granted) to build on. Anyone who has sat an important exam knows what anxiety is like, and anyone who has passed one knows how to master anxiety, at least to some extent. We have all survived periods of being 'down'. While not the same as clinical anxiety or depression, these experiences allow us to develop the psychiatric skills of respect and empathy and a curiosity to ask how we have recovered and how others might too.

The first element is *time*. Simply waiting for time to go by is an important psychotherapeutic principle. (Voltaire teasingly remarked that the role of the doctor is to amuse the patient until nature effects a cure.) Of course, there are instances when waiting for time to go by leads to fatal consequences. But this does not prevent the principle from being useful.

Another skill with which we are all able to use is *listening*. One of the central tenets of psychiatry is that it helps our patients just to be listened to. Just as we all are helped by talking and sharing our problems, so this may in itself be of immense help to our patients, especially if they have been isolated, and feel alone—which is a very common experience.

Both spontaneous improvement and relapse are common occurrences in psychiatry as many mental disorders go through a relapsing-remitting course. To understand this we need to understand *humility*, an essential psychiatric skill. Our current understanding of mental illness and the mind (not the brain) remains limited. While psychopharmacology and therapy can significantly benefit some patients, to consider them a 'cure' is naive. Often the best management is to support each individual through a difficult time, reducing the duration of their illness while trying to minimize the harm done to their health, relationships, and life. Every management plan should be *holistic*, including psychological therapy and social support alongside biological therapy. Looking through the admissions register of any acute psychiatric ward is likely to show that the same people keep on being re-admitted. In one sense this is a failure of the processes of psychiatry, but in another sense each (carefully planned) discharge is a success, and a complex infrastructure often exists for maintaining the patient in the community. These include group support meetings, group therapy sessions, and social trips out of the hospital. For those with a chronic condition, the concept of 'recovery' is important—rather than removing symptoms this can mean living well, with purpose and meaning, in spite of their symptoms.

So taking time, listening, and thinking holistically are our chief skills, and with these simple devices much can be done to rebuild the bridges between the patient and her outside world. These skills are simple compared with highly elaborate skills such as psychoanalysis and psychopharmacology for which psychiatry is famous. The point of bringing them to the fore is so that the newcomer to psychiatry need not feel that there is a great weight of theoretical work to get through before she starts doing psychiatry. You can engage in the central process of psychiatry from day one. In fact, with the exception of specific knowledge about conditions and treatments, the skills that make a good psychiatrist are not specific to psychiatry. Rather they are they skills that define a good communicator, and a caring, empathic, and effective doctor.

Taking a history sounds like an active, inquisitorial process, with lists of questions, and the tone of our page on this process (see p318) and mental state examination, (see p320) seems to perpetuate this error. It isn't a question of *taking* anything. It's more about *receiving* the history, and allowing it to unfold. If you only ask questions, you will get only answers as replies.

As the history unfolds, sit back and listen. This sounds easy, but during a busy or difficult day you will find your mind wandering (or galloping away)—over the last patient, the next patient, or some aspect of your own life. You may find yourself worrying about having to 'section' this patient or see the relatives afterwards. By an act of Zen, banish extraneous thought, and concentrate totally on the person in front of you—as if your life depended on it. Concentrate on the whole person—the language, the words, the non-verbal cues, and get drawn into their world. Initially don't even think of applying diagnostic labels. Open your mind and let everything flood in. Listening is hard. We wish we did it better. We all need to practise it more. Listening enables patients to start to trust us. Depressed patients often believe they will never get better. To believe that they can get better, patients need to trust us, and this trust often starts the therapeutic process. In general, the more we listen, the more we are trusted. Our patients' trust can be one of our chief motivations, at best inspiring us to pursue their benefit with all vigour.

Avoid interruptions and seeming to be too purposeful, at least for the first few minutes. Expect periods of silence. If prompts are needed try 'and then how did you feel?' or just 'and then...'; or repeat the last words the patient spoke. Don't be anxious if the patient is not covering major areas in the history. Lead on to these later, as the interview unfolds. Early in your career you will have to ask the relevant questions (p318) in a rather bald way (if the information is not forthcoming during the initial unstructured minutes), but it is important to go through this stage as a prelude to gaining information by less intrusive methods. Always keep in mind the chief aims of making a diagnosis, defining problems, and establishing a therapeutic relationship.

Even if we all listen the same way, what we will hear will depend on our own expectations, anxieties, and past experience. Listening, not judging. So often when we listen the fact that we are also judging leaks out in an unconscious disapproving gaze—and our patient clams up.

The first meeting...

The mnemonic FIRST can help when you meet a new patient:

Frank conversation about why they came in today. What changed? Let the patient tell you about their problems in their own word—validate their concerns. Consider the sense of fear and isolation they may feel in this new environment.

Individualize your care for every patient through active listening, empathy, and appropriate questioning. Everyone should have a say in their own treatment.

Reach out to the patient's family and friends for collateral information and support; get them to think about the strengths and skills in your patient.

Use **S**omatic symptoms to engage that person—many find it easier to talk about physical symptoms than emotional ones (partly due to the stigma attached to mental health).

Tease out which psychiatric symptoms are important. Keep a high index of suspicion to rule out medical conditions without medicalizing the situation.

Psychiatry

Introduce yourself; explain how long the interview may take. Describe its aim; emphasize that 'this is a safe place to talk'. Find out how they came to be referred, and what their expectations are. If they deny any problems or are reluctant to start talking, don't hurry. It is important to take what they say seriously and include the content that they bring to the consultation. Try asking 'How are you?', 'What has been happening to you?' 'Does anyone else think there is a problem?' These are beautiful questions because they don't impose categories. Hearing what your patient brings unprompted, will often tell you plenty. Listen, without interrupting, noting relevant information but also give eye contact and establish a rapport. Don't make judgements, challenges, or interpretations at this point, just gather information.

Presenting symptoms Agree a problem list with the patient early on, and check it is comprehensive, eg by asking 'If we were able to deal with all these, would things then be all right?' Then take each problem in turn and find out about onset, duration, effects on life and family; events coinciding with onset; solutions tried; reasons why they failed. Next enquire about mood and beliefs during the last weeks (this differs from the mental state examination (p320), which is the mental state at the time of interview). Specifically check for suicidal thoughts, plans, or actions—the more specific these are, the greater the danger. Discussing suicide does not increase the danger. Once you have a thorough understanding of the patient's perspective of their problems, you might need to ask specific questions about particular symptoms to help you reach a diagnosis. At this point 'soft' skills are no longer adequate and a structured approach to history taking is needed, requiring specific knowledge about which symptoms support a particular diagnosis. Specific examples are given in the BOX.

The present Find out about their current situation. Housing, finance, work, relationships: Where do they live? With whom? Do they work? How is their home and work life? Are they facing any danger, threat, police action? How do they spend their time? Has this changed because of their symptoms? Relationships are often very important in mental disorder and changes in these can result in a presentation to mental health services.

Birth and development Particularly for younger patients, but helpful for everyone to consider how they have developed. Ask about school, further education, and employment history. What were their significant relationships (sexual and friendships) and relationship style(s)? Think about social life: play and hobbies. Have they always been shy and lonely, or do they make friends easily? In life, what stress have they had and how have they coped with it?

Premorbid personality Before all this happened, how were they? Happy-go-lucky or driven, tense or laid-back, social or antisocial? How would others describe them? Impulsive, fussy, irritable, shy? Talk to whoever accompanies them, to illumine premorbid personality and their view of current problems.

Relevant past history including *psychiatric* admissions, treatments and previous psychiatry contact; *medical* particularly anything that might have a neurological impact, eg opiate analgesia, or cause stress, eg illness; *family* members with mental illness, consider making a genogram going back to grandparents; *forensic* contact; and *substance (mis)use* including alcohol.

Lastly examine the *mental state* (p320). At this point you may have enough information to make a confident diagnosis, or decide that labelling is unwise. Often, the patient's problems are complex and do not fit neatly into a diagnostic category at this point. A differential diagnosis, impression, or formulation may be a more appropriate way to summarize the case.

Ask yourself '*Why did they get ill in this way, at this time?*' and '*What are the consequences of the illness?*'.

Some direct questions to try:

- *Depression:* Are you low/depressed? Is life worth living? Can anything give you pleasure? Energy levels? Sleep and appetite? Can you concentrate? Are you feeling guilty? Is your confidence low? Have you lost your libido? Are you preoccupied with guilt, regret, and/or hopelessness? Suicidal thoughts?
- *Mania:* Have you felt you have more energy than normal (despite not sleeping)? Is it too much? Can you focus on things? Are you having difficulty settling? Are you spending more than usual? Are you more interested in sex (with different, inappropriate people)?
- *Psychosis* (persecutory beliefs, delusions, hallucinations): Has anything odd or unusual been happening recently? If they have odd ideas ask how did these occur? What actions do you feel you need to take? Ask about thoughts: Might your thoughts be being interfered with? Do you feel anyone is controlling you? Is anyone putting thoughts into your head? Do other people access or hear your thoughts? Is anyone harming you? Any plots against you? Do you hear voices when there's no one nearby? What do they say? Telling you off? Do you see things that others cannot see?
- *Drug and alcohol use:* What do you take? How much, how often, and for how long? How much do you spend on all this? Is it impacting on you the next day? Has your use changed recently (up or down)? Withdrawal signs?
- *Obsessions:* Any odd thoughts? Recurring, intrusive worries? Note compulsive behaviour, eg excessive hand-washing.
- *Anxiety:* Any worries/anxieties? Are you always worried or does it happen in discrete episodes ('attacks')? What causes this? What physical symptoms do you get? How do you manage your anxiety?
- *Eating disorders* (often not volunteered, and important): What are you currently eating? How do you feel about your weight? Are you dieting?
- *Suicide:* Have you ever felt so low that you have considered harming yourself? Have you ever actually harmed yourself? What stopped you harming yourself any more than this? Have you made any detailed suicide plans? Have you bought tablets for that purpose?
- *Risk:* Are you wanting to harm anyone? Yourself? Have you stopped caring about yourself (dressing, washing, eating, drinking)?

Differential diagnosis vs formulation

Differential diagnosis A limited list of three or four possible diagnoses with one selected as the most relevant (or likely) working diagnosis. It is sometimes helpful to mention other less likely possibilities you have considered and excluded if this has been brought up by the patient or referrer, eg 'The patient reported feeling "psychotic" but she did not have any first rank symptoms and her presentation was more in keeping with a diagnosis of PTSD'.

Formulation aims to contextualize the patient's symptoms in a broader, personalized way by identifying the '3 P's' (**P**redisposing, **P**recipitating, and **P**erpetuating factors) for the current presentation. Every formulation should include a statement on why that person has become ill at this point in time.

After an assessment, psychiatrists will often write a formulation and/or a differential diagnosis list. While both can contain similar information—summarized assessment, key symptoms and relevant background information—the formulation focuses on a prediction of how a patient might react to a new situation or psychotherapy whereas the differential diagnosis is aimed at categorizing the illness into a diagnostic label. Together both of these are important in guiding us towards a suitable management plan which will include investigations and treatment options.

Psychiatry

The mental state examination (MSE) is a structured and formalized approach to describing someone's state of mind at the time of interview and recording these under standard headings. It is obtained through a doctor's observation of a patient's mental processes, communication, and behaviour. Data is collected by a combination of direct and indirect means: unstructured observation during history taking, focused systematic questioning, and formalized testing. The MSE and psychiatric history together should provide evidence regarding current mental health, and if mental illness is present, judgement about its type, severity, and any risks to patient and others. The MSE should be recorded and presented in a standardized format under the following headings:

Appearance The majority of the MSE is focused on the patient's internal experiences; however, direct observation of the appearance, behaviour, and manner yields important information regarding mental state. For example, a patient may deny psychotic symptoms but appear to react to internal stimuli.
• Overall impression • Physical condition • Suitability of dress • Cleanliness.

Behaviour A general observation of activity and arousal levels and specific observations of the patient's eye contact, gait, and any abnormal movements.
• Appropriateness of behaviour, eg aggressive, agitated, over-familiar • Eye contact • Distractibility • Abnormal involuntary movement • Rapport.

Speech Content of speech (what the patient says) is the main source of our history and MSE. The form of speech (how they say it) can reveal abnormal thinking processes. It is helpful to record a patient's description of significant symptoms exactly and any abnormal phrases or sentences verbatim.
• Rate, rhythm, volume and tone • Coherence • Relevance • Quantity and fluency • Abnormal associations, clang, and punning • Flight of ideas.

Mood There is a distinction between mood (the emotional state over a long period) and affect (our emotional state at a certain point). The common analogy is: 'affect is the weather, whereas mood is a climate'. Any disturbance should be probed for severity, duration, and ubiquity and for associations with other pathological (biological or psychotic) features.
• Subjective (patient's) and objective (doctor's) assessment of mood in full • Anxiety and panic symptoms • Obsessional thoughts ('ruminations').

Perception Perceptual experiences can be a distorted internal perception of a real external object (altered perception, eg illusions) or without an external object (false perceptions, eg hallucinations).
• (Pseudo) Hallucinations in any modality • Depersonalization.

Thought As in speech form describes the structure and process of thought and content is the meaning and experience.
• Formal thought disorder • Delusions • Over-valued ideas • Preoccupations • Obsessive thoughts, ideas, and impulses.

Risk and suicidal ideation Thoughts of suicide, deliberate self-harm, or harm to others are included to stress their importance and act as a reminder to ask:
• Intent • Plan (active and imagined) • Lethality of plan • Urge to act upon these • Reasons for/against • Other dangers (to themselves or others).

Cognition Consciousness ranges from fully alert to clouded for a variety of reasons (organic, iatrogenic, psychiatric) and may fluctuate.
• Attention and concentration • Orientation to time, place, and person • Level of comprehension • Short-term memory (memory can also be tested formally).

Insight In physical illness, patients recognize their symptoms as 'anomalous' and seek a diagnosis and treatment. In contrast, many psychiatric illnesses impair insight so a patient reacts differently to their difficulties and cause (denial or failure to recognize problem). This reduces help-seeking behaviour.

Asking a patient whether they think they have a mental disorder, and what they think should be done, often establishes the divergence between the patient's and the clinician's perspective, if there is one.

What is a mental state?

Drugs, psychotherapy, and behavioural methods are the main tools available to the clinician for significantly improving a person's mental state. However, we cannot tell if these methods are actually helping when we can't access a patient's mental state, which is why the MSE on p320 is so important.

If you think you can access mental states just by applying the formulaic regimen on p320, you will often fail, as any trip into the mind of another is not just a voyage without maps, it is ultimately a creative and metaphysical enterprise. A true description of mental state entails valid knowledge about current emotions plus reactions to those emotions. So often it's non-verbal behaviour that allows valid judgement about mental state: don't rely on words alone—those capricious (but indispensable) tokens of disguise and deception.

Non-verbal behaviour

Why are we annoyed when we blush, yet love it when our friends do so? Part of the answer to this question is that non-verbal communication is less well controlled than verbal behaviour. This is why its study can yield valuable insights into our patients' minds, particularly when analysis of their spoken words has been not particularly revealing. For example, if a patient who consistently denies being depressed sits hugging himself in an attitude of self-pity, remaining in a glum silence for long periods of the interview, and when he does speak, using a monotonous slow whisper unadorned even by a flicker of a gesticulation or eye contact—we are likely to believe what we see and not what our patient would seem to be telling us.

All of these aspects of behaviour can be commented on as part of the MSE:

Items of non-verbal behaviour
- Gaze and mutual gaze
- Facial expression
- Smiling, blushing
- Body attitude (eg 'defensive').

Signs of auditory hallucinations
- Inexplicable laughter
- Silent and distracted while listening to 'voices' (but could be an 'absence' seizure, p206)
- Random, meaningless gestures.

Signs of a depressed mood
- Hunched, self-hugging posture
- Little eye contact.

Dress
('The apparel oft proclaims the man')[1]
- Hairstyle
- Make-up
- Ornament (ear-rings, tattoos, piercings).

Anxious behaviour
- Fidgeting, trembling
- Nail-biting
- Shuffling feet
- Squirming in the chair
- Sits on edge of chair.

- Downcast eyes; tears
- Slow thought, speech, and movement.

Predicting the future Surely we should be able to predict what will happen. In draughts (chequers) games are won or lost by using rules of thumb (heuristics). In 2007, for the first time, there was sufficient computing power to replace these rules of thumb by *perfect knowledge*. In draughts, there are >500 billion billion play-positions (500,995,484,682,338,672,639), and each has been analysed to decide what the next best move is. Well-programmed computers are right every time. When we ask psychiatrists to do a risk assessment we want them to be right every time too. It is vital that they are. We blame them if they are wrong. But this isn't rational. Psychiatrists do best using rules of thumb combined with validated risk assessment tools (*imperfect knowledge*), such as the *violence risk appraisal guide*.[2] Forensic risk-assessment models all stress risk factors, but often disregard the other side of the equation: protective factors. Mediating and moderating effects must also be considered.[3] We need to involve patients in risk assessment and management. This may increase validity,[4] but it also adds unpredictability

This is a common problem: the courts, the GP, or the relatives want to know 'Will he be violent again if he takes the medication?' A great deal—a person's freedom, no less, may depend on our answers. But risk is not dichotomous despite often being treated as such and nor is it fixed—within any individual, it will change over time, circumstance, and intervention. Every assessment of risk has two parts. The initial part can be weighed up using an objective (actuarial) approach, whilst the second is a more subjective decision based on pragmatic pressures. We consider the extent of the risk then we estimate the tolerability of that risk. Often professionals within a team cannot reach a consensus about the overall risk, reflecting the different priorities, biases, and experience each individual has.

Approaches to risk assessment have broadly been grouped into 'clinical' versus 'actuarial' approaches. The *actuarial approach* provides us with clues to broad populations at risk, but informs us inadequately on the individual. The *clinical approach* has been characterized as providing an individualized and contextualized assessment, but purely clinical perspective are vulnerable to poor inter-rater reliability and influence of political considerations. Defensive psychiatry will always prefer false positives over false negatives.

Risk assessment provides useful information regarding management but can also impact on our relationship with a patient and their engagement and concordance with treatment. Several key principles underpin risk assessment:
- *Risk cannot be eliminated*. A more achievable aim is risk minimization: anticipating problems, lowering stress, and reducing or stopping harm.
- *A patient's risk fluctuates:* It is perpetually influenced by their perception, experience, and interaction with the world. Risk assessment is a dynamic process; risk management plans should be continually evaluated and amended.
- The best way to reduce risk is to *engage a patient* in a positive therapeutic relationship. This is strengthened with support, engagement, and listening.
- *Continued skills development* through ongoing training, reflection, and clinical supervision will increase the effectiveness of clinical work and practice.

Risk factors Regression analysis shows that four factors are paramount: **1** Previous violence **2** Substance abuse **3** Lack of empathy and **4** Stress.[5] But risk factors are based on population studies and do not necessarily allow practitioners to identify risks in a particular individual. When in doubt, use a formal risk assessment tool. Some of the advantages of these tools derive simply from having a well-structured approach, others from combining specific kinds of risk factors (static and dynamic).[6]

Focusing on risk The emphasis on extreme but fortunately rare events such as suicide or murder, takes attention away from the much more common risks of self neglect, discrimination and abuse, and disenfranchisement from society.

Psychiatry

'And about whatever I may see or hear in treatment, or even without treatment, in the life of human beings, I will remain silent, holding such things to be unutterable.'
                                                                    Hippocratic Oath

As today, patients in ancient times shared deeply personal information with doctors on the assumption that their details would not be revealed to others. Without this trust, patients may withhold facts that would help the doctor make an accurate diagnosis. Patients have a right to expect that all material about their assessment, symptoms, and mental state will be kept confidential. This must be genuine if we expect patients to speak freely and establish a trusting therapeutic alliance between them and their doctor. In the absence of this assurance, patients will be reluctant to disclose their inner world which limits the care they can receive.

Being clear from the start about the nature of the confidentiality, its scope, and its limits is essential. For every encounter, but most importantly the first, you should be prepared to spend a few minutes explaining:
- Who you will share the information with: the multidisciplinary team, referrer, GP, patient's family
- Who you will approach for collateral and what you will say for this request
- In what circumstances you will break confidentiality.

Breaking confidentiality Information should not be disclosed to a relative, solicitor, or police officer without express consent being given by the patient, except in exceptional circumstances. If the risk to someone is so serious that it outweighs the patient's privacy then you must inform the appropriate person or authority without delay. If you make this decision you should always document your judgement and reasons. You should feel able to justify this decision to whoever asks (patient, relative, or court).

Examples of this include:
- Where disclosure will prevent a serious crime (risk of serious harm or death)
- A patient who continues to drive, against medical advice. There is a duty to inform the medical adviser of the Driver and Vehicle Licensing Agency (DVLA).

If you are unsure whether a disclosure is justified, consult with a professional body (BMA or your protection organization) and/or seek advice from a senior colleague. Do this without delay; don't avoid a decision.

Tarasoff vs Regents of the University of California (1976)

NB: Although this case has no legal bearing in the UK, it is often quoted when considering when to break confidentiality.

Prosenjit Poddar attended the University of California as a graduate where he met Tatiana Tarasoff. After she rebuffed his advances, he stalked her, developing a wish for revenge. Poddar sought help from Dr Lawrence Moore, a psychologist, and confided his intent to kill Tarasoff. Poddar was diagnosed with paranoid schizophrenia but not detained. Neither Tarasoff nor her parents received any warning of the threat. Poddar befriended Tarasoff's brother, even moving in with him, and over six months later he killed Tarasoff.

The Supreme Court of California decided all mental health professionals have a 'duty to protect' anyone being threatened with physical harm by a patient. The professional may perform this duty by notifying the police, warning the individual, and/or taking other reasonable steps to protect the intended target. This decision was reached despite one member of the Supreme Court, Justice Clark dissenting 'the very practice of psychiatry depends upon the reputation in the community that the psychiatrist will not tell'. As a final statement, the Court stated 'protective privilege ends where public peril begins'.

'Good psychiatry begins with a responsible Doctor undressing the patient and carrying out a proper physical examination.'

Donald Winnicott, paediatrician and psychoanalyst

A thorough physical examination is a fundamental part of the psychiatric assessment to identify physical illness: • Due to an existing mental disorder or its treatment • Imitating a mental disorder • Alongside a mental disorder.

If a physical disorder is present it may be the primary cause of, or a contributing factor to, the psychiatric symptoms. For example, a treatable UTI in an elderly patient may result in disinhibited behaviour. Physical symptoms can be a direct result of a mental health problem, eg bradycardia in anorexia nervosa. Deterioration may result from self-neglect in severe mental illness such as depression or due to psychiatric drug side effects, eg antipsychotic-induced parkinsonism. Poor mental health can increase the risk of physical health problems just as poor physical health can negatively affect mental health. A baseline set of physical findings allows medication to be commenced safely and quickly, and allows for early detection of new physical conditions.

But often the physical examination is brief in order to 'medically clear' the patient before the real assessment is started or deferred and never completed. If a patient is acutely unwell, labile in mood or expressing conflicting delusions, it makes sense to avoid causing unnecessary distress, but minimal investigations can be completed and properly documented.

As in all of medicine, a routine physical examination should document any abnormal signs, or their absence if important, record the baseline physical state, and make plans for anything which needs further investigation.

'Psychiatric' symptom	Examples of physical causes
Mood changes (depression/mania)	Multiple sclerosis, stroke, diabetes mellitus, brain tumour, hypothyroidism
Insomnia	Sleep apnoea, hyperthyroidism, gastro-oesophageal reflux disease (GORD), pain
Confusion/disorientation	Renal failure, cerebral arteritis, sepsis
Personality change	Multiple sclerosis, mass lesion, SLE
Hallucinations	Migraine, substance misuse, encephalitis, seizures
Behavioural change	Lyme disease, vascular infarct, Parkinson disease, subdural haematoma, mass lesion
Psychosis	Sensory loss, syphilis, dementia, Wilson's disease
Irritability	Vitamin B_{12} deficiency, drug withdrawal (eg analgesics), substance misuse/withdrawal

Medically unexplained symptoms (p489) need careful management. All new symptoms need an initial assessment which will include a focused history, examination and investigation. However, this needs to be balanced with 'over investigating' physical symptoms without considering a psychological component. For example, a patient may have real unexplained pain, which they focus on. This attention (to the exclusion of other alleviating factors such as work, hobbies, etc.) amplifies their experience, increasing their subjective pain and leading to low mood and further focus on the pain. A vicious circle can result which may also trigger other symptoms (physical and psychological).

Occasionally a patient may 'cry wolf' so often (eg with central chest pain) that it becomes necessary to reduce unnecessary repeated investigations and prevent behavioural reinforcement. This should be done in a thoughtful, holistic, and safe manner—not in the middle of the night with a new patient!

Psychiatry

Some physical signs in psychiatric illness and possible cause	
General appearance	
Parkinsonian facies	Antipsychotic drug treatment
	Depression (psychomotor retardation)
Abnormal pupil size	Opiate use
Argyll–Robertson pupil	Neurosyphilis
Enlarged parotids ('hamster face')	Bulimia nervosa (secondary to vomiting)
Hypersalivation	Clozapine treatment
Goitre	Thyroid disease
Multiple forearm scars	Borderline personality disorder
Needle tracks/phlebitis	IV drug use
Gynaecomastia	Antipsychotic drug treatment
	Alcoholic liver disease
Russell's sign (knuckle callus)	Bulimia nervosa (secondary to inducing vomiting)
Lanugo hair	Anorexia nervosa
Piloerection ('goose flesh')	Opiate withdrawal
Excessive thinness	Anorexia nervosa
Cardiovascular	
Rapid/irregular pulse	Anxiety disorder
	Drug/alcohol withdrawal
	Hyperthyroidism
Slow pulse	Hypothyroidism, anorexia nervosa
Abdominal	
Enlarged liver	Alcoholic liver disease
	Hepatitis
Multiple surgical scars ('chequer-board' abdomen)	Somatization disorder
Multiple self-inflicted scars	Borderline personality disorder
Neurological	
Resting tremor	Increased sympathetic drive (anxiety, drug/alcohol misuse)
	Antipsychotic drug treatment
	Lithium treatment
Involuntary movements	Antipsychotic drug treatment
	Tic disorder
	Huntingtons's/Sydenham's chorea
Abnormal posturing	Antipsychotic-induced dystonia
	Catatonia
Broad-based gait	Cerebellar disease (alcohol, lithium toxicity)
Festinant (shuffling) gait	Parkinsonism (Parkinson's disease or drug-induced parkinsonism)

Psychiatry

Reproduced from Semple and Smyth, *Oxford Handbook of Psychiatry*, 3rd edition (2013) with permission from Oxford University Press.

'And I said, "You're not seein' things like how I'm seein' things. I'm seein' things that I don't wanna see. I see the devil sit right before me. Fire in his eyes as he spoke to me.' 'Awfully Deep', Roots Manuva

It is important to decide if a patient has delusions, hallucinations (*that the patient believes are real*), or a major thought disorder, because if present the diagnosis must be schizophrenia, an affective disorder, an organic disorder, or a paranoid state (or a culturally determined visionary or spiritual experience), and not a neurosis or a personality disorder.

Patients may be reluctant to reveal odd ideas. Ask gently: 'Have you ever had any thoughts which might now seem odd; perhaps that there is a conspiracy against you, or that you are controlled by outside voices or the radio?'

Delusions are beliefs held unshakably, irrespective of counter-argument, that are unexpected and out of keeping with the patient's cultural background. If the belief arrives fully formed, and with no antecedent events or experiences to account for it, it is said to be *primary*, and is suggestive of schizophrenia. Such delusions appear 'out of the blue' as a fully formed idea (delusional intuition) or form around a real perception given a delusional interpretation (delusional perception), as illustrated by the patient who, on seeing the traffic lights go green knew that he had been sent to rid his town of capitalism. Especially relevant if these involve persecution and loss of control.[7] A careful history may reveal the delusions are *secondary* based on the patient's current affect or preoccupations (eg fear, hope, stress) in an understandable manner.

Delusions can be **mood congruent** in affective psychosis, eg a depressed person who believes that he is literally rotting away (nihilistic delusion), or the manic patient who believes she is the Queen of England (grandiose delusion). In schizophrenia, delusions are often **mood incongruent**, with horrific beliefs discussed without commensurate distress.

Specific delusions most associated with psychosis (eg mania, schizophrenia):
- **Persecution:** the most common type of delusions. A theme of being followed, spied on, and conspired against with a belief that the persecutors intend to cause harm. Often described by patients as a feeling of 'paranoia'[2]
- **Infestation:** a belief that the skin is infested with parasites causing itching (formication), eg in organic states and cocaine use (*Ekbom's syndrome*)
- **Religious:** eg on visiting Jerusalem, a person becomes overwhelmed and develops religious themed delusions. Shown to affect people of all backgrounds: Jews, Christians, and Muslims (*Jerusalem syndrome*)
- **Delusional misidentification:** a person believes that those close to them have been replaced by an exact double (*Capgras syndrome*) or that a single person is impersonating multiple familiar people (*Fregoli syndrome*)
- **Jealousy:** firm belief that a sexual partner is unfaithful made without proof; whether actual infidelity occurred is immaterial (*Othello syndrome*)
- **Love:** belief that a celebrity, high-status individual or stranger is in love with them, and secretly sending messages or signs (*de Clérambault's syndrome*)
- **Communicated:** an already psychotic person transmits their beliefs to another, usually subservient close relative, who now shares them (*folie à deux*)

Ideas of reference Coincidental or innocuous events which are interpreted to have great personal significance, eg a TV news broadcast making direct references to the patient, or other people on the train talking (or thinking) about them. Associated with social phobia, psychosis, or stress. Often accompanied by *delusions of reference*—with bizarre, unfeasible interpretations, eg a dog's bark carries coded message. Differ from overvalued ideas: understandable and reasonable beliefs which dominate a patient's life to detriment of functioning.

(left margin) Psychiatry

2 Paranoia really means: mental illness where a delusional belief of any variety is the most prominent feature.

Psychopatholgy is the *'systematic study of abnormal experience, cognition and behaviour; the study of the products of a disordered mind'*[8]. Descriptive psychopathology attempts to describe, and in so doing understand, the experiences in mental illness. It does this through observation of behaviour, empathic exploration of subjective experience, and classification of these into categorical symptoms. This forms the basis of all clinical psychiatry. These general qualifiers describe terms used in this chapter:

• *Subjective and objective:* Subjective signs are reported by the patient; Objective signs are seen by an external observer.
• *Primary and secondary:* Primary symptoms arise directly from disordered mental states, and cannot be not fully understood (although we can still empathize with the subjective experience); secondary symptoms occur as an understandable reaction to another condition, eg depression, drug use.
• *Congruent and incongruent:* A subjective impression regarding the 'appropriateness' of a patient's experience, affect, or behaviour. If this fits with the apparent mental state, it is congruent; if not, it is incongruent, eg a patient talking pleasantly whilst describing a traumatic experience has an incongruent affect.
• *Form and content:* Every abnormal symptom has both form—the type of experience (eg primary delusion, hallucination) attributable to the underlying mental illness, and content—the composition of the symptom which is richly illustrative of the patient's internal world.
• *Structural and functional:* Often used in neurology/neuropsychiatry to distinguish syndromes which have abnormal investigation findings (eg Huntington's) from those without (eg conversion paralysis). In the past, brain disorders with observable structural abnormalities on post-mortem (eg dementia) were compared to those without (eg schizophrenia); however, modern imaging has shown observable brain changes in many disorders formerly called functional.
• *Endogenous and reactive:* Rarely used today, it was thought that some conditions arose spontaneously from within (endogenous) whereas others arose in response to external events.

Psychiatry

What's it like having hallucinations? Try virtual reality to find out

Doctors often get hung up on hallucinations, without acquiring any real knowledge of what it's like to have them. For doctors who have never experienced hallucinations, Professor Yellowlees has devised a virtual reality experience on *Second Life*[3]: a complex, unruly 3D world where people get sucked into virtual clinics... Floors can fall away, leaving us walking riskily on stones above clouds. The eyes of a portrait flash 'shitface' as we pass, and a politician on an in-world TV might move in a single breath from platitudes to shouting 'Go and kill yourself, you wretch!'. When it gets to the stage of our reflection in a mirror bleeding its eyes out before expiring, most of us switch off.[9] But our patients cannot quit so easily. Virtual reality is just one way of sensitizing us to their difficulties: other ways include blogs, painting (figs 4.3–4.5 p329), and arts (eg Shakespeare's Ophelia effect).[10] Consideration of the 'patient experience' is an essential part of medicine and nevermore so than in psychiatry where there is often a stigma attached to the diagnosis and discrimination to those having to manage their symptoms.

Hallucinations occur in any sensory modality (visual, auditory, olfactory, proprioceptive) without any external stimulus. The main characteristics of a hallucination are that they are felt to occur in the external world along other objects, have the same qualities as everything else (eg colouring, density), and cannot be consciously manipulated or stopped. To the person experiencing them, these experiences are real. fMRI imaging studies show similar areas of brain activity are seen when 'hearing' an auditory hallucination or real voices.

Most hallucinations start as simple, brief experiences in a single modality, with only some going on to change over time into a more complex, multiple sensory experience. A patient reporting hearing a sudden voice giving them a specific instruction should be followed up carefully—with consideration to any secondary gain given from a mental health diagnosis (eg avoiding blame).

Auditory hallucinations can be elementary (eg hissing, whistling) or complex (eg voices, music). The subjective experience can vary depending on the hallucination: a pleasant, friendly, known voice offering support or an aggressive, unfamiliar voice (or voices) criticizing. Patients can experience both. These hallucinations must be felt to originate from outside the body and out of conscious control. Experiences include: *Thoughts spoken aloud,* heard either as they are thought (*gedankenlautwerden*) or just after (écho de la penseé); *Second-person hallucinations,* a voice talking directly to the person or giving them instructions (eg 'you are being followed; run away'); *Third-person hallucinations,* voices heard arguing or giving a running commentary (eg 'He is going off to sleep') just before, simultaneously or after the person's actions.

Visual hallucinations are much more common in eye pathology and epilepsy than psychosis. Not to be confused with an illusion, an involuntary misperception of a real stimulus transformed or distorted (p313) often brought on by tiredness or emotion; affective component, eg fearful mood = scary images.

Non-pathological hallucinations are experiences we all have, eg feeling your leg vibrate with a text message before remembering the phone is plugged in elsewhere. These are common and do not indicate pathology: 2-4% of the general population experience auditory hallucinations, but only ~30% of these have a mental illness (more likely if associated with distressing delusions).[7] *Hypnagogic and hypnopompic hallucinations*—eg hearing a voice calling our name when going (hypnagogic = going) to sleep or waking up. A *pseudohallucination* is one in which the person knows the stimulus is in the mind (eg a voice heard within themselves, rather than over the left shoulder)— these may also be a sign that a genuine hallucination is waning. *Panoramic memories* are seen with near-death and out-of-body experiences alongside complex hallucinatory phenomena (all have proved to be unsubstantiated, so far...[4]). *Extracampine hallucinations* or 'concrete awareness' occur outside the sensory field (eg 'right behind me') as a non-specific feeling which can be associated with epilepsy, psychosis, but also when anxious (eg at home, alone). *Pareidolia* where an ill-defined, random stimulus is given significance, occurring without conscious effort (eg seeing a rabbit shape in clouds).

Organic disorders present as tactile or visual hallucinations without any auditory input. Seen in alcohol withdrawal or Charles Bonnet syndrome (p451).

Obsessional thoughts are sometimes hard to distinguish from hallucinations. Often both are 'odd' and cause distress. If a person recognizes a 'voice' or their unusual thoughts as their own, then they more likely have obsessive thoughts or pseudohallucinations. If they experience a voice as external to themselves (auditory hallucination) or a thought as being 'put into their head' by an external agency (thought insertion) they may have a psychotic illness.

---

4 AWARE II study (AWAreness during REsuscitation) uses hidden targets on shelves only visible from above to test this. It is a multicenter observational study of ~1500 cardiac arrests due to report in mid-2016.

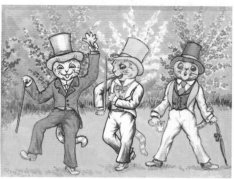

Fig 4.3 Three cats performing a song and dance act. Gouache by Louis Wain, 1925/1939.
Wellcome Library, London.

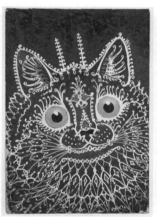

Fig 4.4 A cat in 'gothic' style. Gouache by
Louis Wain, 1925/1939.

Wellcome Library, London.

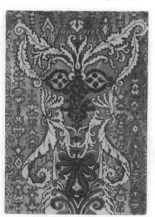

Fig 4.5 A cat standing on its hind legs,
formed by patterns supposed to be in the
'Early Greek' style. Gouache by Louis Wain,
1925/1939.

Wellcome Library, London.

Figs 4.3–4.5 Wain's cat paintings. Thought to show a progressive schizophrenic illness.

Louis Wain (5 August 1860–4 July 1939) was an English artist known for his drawings of anthropo-
morphized cats. He developed schizophrenia (perhaps related to the parasite *Toxoplasma gondii*
found in cats' faeces) and, in 1924, he was committed to a pauper ward. Later after appeals from
the rich and famous, including H.G. Wells, and the personal intervention of Prime Minister Ramsey
MacDonald he was transferred to the Bethlem Royal Hospital. He remained in hospital for the
rest of his life.

These paintings, arranged by Dr Walter Maclay a psychiatrist treating Wain, show a series of
different styles thought by Maclay to demonstrate Wain's deteriorating mental state. This is a
controversial claim, as it is unclear of the chronological order of the paintings, however it is clear
that Wain's paintings move between charming and psychedelic and aptly illustrate the different
views of the world as seen by an artist with schizophrenia.

For the full range of Wain's cat variations see:
bristolunipsychiatrysoc.wordpress.com/2014/08/18/psychiatry-in-public-louis-wain/

Conventional thought processes have four broad characteristics: 1 *Thought stream:* Speed, quality, and quantity of thinking; how is something being thought about? 2 *Thought content:* Substance of thinking: what is being thought about? 3 *Thought form:* Formation and coherence of thinking: how are separate thoughts linked to one another? 4 *Thought possession:* Who created thoughts: are these considered by the person to be their own thoughts?

Major thought disorder Most healthy thinking shows constancy, organization, and continuity—a thought (or speech) begins, continues, and reaches a goal in a logical manner without veering off track or leaping between disconnected points. Without this there entails bizarre thoughts, or incongruent transition from one idea to another (*mania*—flight of ideas, p348; *schizophrenia*, p336).

Disorders of thought stream Flight of ideas is subjective quickening of thoughts so most are not carried to completion before being overtaken. Meaningful connections between ideas are kept although often linked by distracting environmental cues or from words themselves spoken aloud (eg puns, rhymes, and clang associations). Retardation of thinking is a slowing of the train of thought although it remains goal directed. The opposite is pressure of speech.

Disorders of thought content Delusions and overvalued ideas (p328).

Disorders of thought form Main features of a formal thought disorder (FTD) include: •Derailment: a break in the linked association of sequential thoughts or change in track of thoughts—neither patient nor observer understands the connection •Omission: all or part of a thought is absent without a reason •Fusion: thoughts are fused together •Substitution: an inappropriate or illogical thought replaces another as though slotted into a space.

'Loosening of association' occurs where normal thought structure breaks down resulting in confused, illogical answers which no exploration can explain. The more questions asked, the less clear things become. Here, answers show: • Circumstantiality: laborious detail given no matter how inconsequential or insignificant it is but without losing track of the question • Overinclusion: inability to maintain the boundaries of a topic or restrict thoughts to the limits of a topic • Tangential thinking: talking past or around the point as thoughts diverge from the topic. Also called *Knight's move thinking*—the pattern of movement a knight in chess makes • Talking past the point: getting close to the discussion point, but then skirting around it and never actually reaching it •Verbigeration (also called *word salad* or *schizophasia*) speech is reduced to a senseless repetition of sounds and phrases. Different to neologisms (made up words/phrases or normal words used in idiosyncratic ways eg *foothat* to mean *shoe*) and metonyms (word approximations, eg *menu* to mean *meal*).

Disorders of thought possession Most of us never question the belief that 1 We have ultimate control of our thoughts 2 Our thoughts are our own or 3 These thoughts are not being externally manipulated. An *obsession* (or rumination) is a thought which endures and dominates thinking even though the person knows that it is unhelpful and irrelevant. These cannot be dismissed or controlled which often results in anxiety and distress (see OCD, p352). *Thought alienation* (or thought interference) is the subjective experience of one's own thoughts being under the control of an outside agency. Often described as 1 Thought insertion: foreign thoughts placed into one's mind, 2 Thought withdrawal: thoughts suddenly disappearing—having been taken by an external force and 3 Thought broadcast: thoughts being transmitted to everyone around—as though being played on a radio. These are considered to be a first-rank symptom of schizophrenia (p336)—pathological when present.

Classification of disorders

Diagnostic classification systems are used throughout medicine to categorize and collate conditions. The purpose of this classification: • Enhance reliability • Facilitate communication (and reduce confusion) • Aid research • Formulate management plan • Medico-legal issues. Having a universally recognized 'depression' diagnosis means that a patient can move from China to France to the UK and all clinicians involved would reach the same diagnosis and treatment.

Unfortunately, there is no single handbook for diagnosing mental illness. There are two classification systems used today: the American Psychiatric Association's *Diagnostic and Statistical Manual of Mental Disorder* (DSM-5, as it's in its 5th edition), and the WHO's *International Statistical Classification of Diseases and Related Health Problems* (ICD-10, for the 10th edition). Why are there these two separate, but similar, systems? The ICD is global, multidisciplinary, and multilingual. It is written by authors from 193 WHO countries, distributed at low cost (free online: www.who.int/classifications/icd/en/), and aims to help countries reduce the disease burden of mental disorders. The DSM is approved and produced by an American professional association for American psychiatrists. It generates money for that association through book sales, related products, and copyright.

Hierarchical categories used in ICD-10	
F00–F09	Organic, including symptomatic mental disorders
F10–F19	Mental and behavioural disorders due to psychoactive substance abuse
F20–F29	Schizophrenia, schizotypal, and delusional disorders
F30–F39	Mood [affective] disorders
F40–F48	Neurotic, stress-related, and somatoform disorders
F50–F59	Behavioural syndromes associated with physiological disturbances and physical factors
F60–F69	Disorders of adult personality and behaviour
F70–F79	Mental retardation
F80–F89	Disorders of psychological development
F90–F98	Behavioural and emotional disorders with onset usually occurring in childhood and adolescence

Multiaxial classification The DSM previously used this (dropped in DSM-5)
• *Axis I: clinical disorder* with acute symptoms which require immediate intervention, eg major depressive episode, anorexia nervosa
• *Axis II: personality disorders and mental retardation:* Lifelong and permanent difficulties arising in childhood, which may affect treatment (ICD multiaxial version splits this into two axes (making the total axes into six)
• *Axis III: general medical conditions* which may influence or impact on a mental health problem, eg diabetes can exacerbate depression by causing fatigue and altering which antidepressant is initially prescribed
• *Axis IV: psychosocial and environmental problems:* Life problems and acute psychosocial stressors affecting well-being, eg homelessness, bereavement
• *Axis V: global assessment of functioning (GAF):* Using an established scale of 0–100 to quantify a patient's ability to socially, occupationally, and psychologically function in daily life. 100 is superior functioning; generally <50 indicates severe symptoms. (Google 'GAF+scale' for full copy.)

Strengths and weaknesses Both manuals allow for common and universal diagnosis. Through revisions they remain relevant and clinically useful. Critics argue they promote a medicalization of living (eg patients have anorexia so they are 'ill' and need 'treatment'). Categories reflect societal norms—so homosexuality was considered a 'deviant sexual behaviour' in DSM until 1973.

'Quis custodiet ipsos custodes?' (Who watches the watchmen?) Juvenal

Doctors have a higher than average incidence of suicide and alcoholism, and we must all be prepared to face, and try to prevent, these and other health risks of our professional and private lives. Our own illnesses are invaluable in allowing us to understand our patients, what makes people go to the doctor (or avoid going to the doctor), and the barriers we may erect to resist advice.

If the time comes when our mental health seriously reduces our ability to work, we must be able to recognize this and take appropriate action. The following may indicate that this point is approaching:
• Drinking alcohol before ward rounds, surgeries, or patient contact.
• The minimizing of every contact with patients, so that the doctor does the bare minimum which will suffice.
• Inability to concentrate on the matter in hand. Your thoughts are entirely taken up with the workload ahead or with other problems in your life.
• Excessive irritability with those around you at work or outside work.
• Inability to take time off without feeling guilty.
• Feelings of excessive shame or anger when reviewing past débâcles. To avoid mistakes it would be necessary for us all to give up medicine.
• Emotional exhaustion—eg knowing that you should be feeling pleased or cross with yourself or others, but on consulting your heart you draw a blank.
• Prospective studies suggest that introversion, masochism, and isolation are important risk factors for doctors' impairment.

The first step in countering these unfavourable states of mind is to recognize that one is present. The next step is to confide in someone you trust (fig 4.6). Give your mind time to rejuvenate itself.

If these steps fail, various psychotherapeutic approaches may be relevant, eg cognitive behavioural therapy (p390), or you might try prescribing the symptom. For example, if you are plagued by recurring thoughts about how poorly you treated a patient, set time aside to deliberately ruminate on the affair, avoiding distractions. This is the first step in gaining control. You initiate the thought, rather than the thought initiating itself. The next step is to interpose some neutral topic, once the 'bad' series of thoughts is under way. After repeated practice, the mind automatically flows into the neutral channel once the bad thoughts begin, and the cycle of shame and rumination is broken. ▶In addition...learn from the experience!

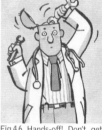

Fig 4.6 Hands-off! Don't get too drawn into treating your own mental illness without consulting a colleague.

If no progress is made, the time has come to consult an expert, such as your GP or the *Practitioner Health Programme* (www.php.nhs.uk) a confidential, NHS treatment service for doctors and dentists who have a mental health, addiction, or physical health problem affecting their work. If you think you need to consult a doctor, then do so, in privacy. Avoid 'corridor consultations' with colleagues. Other than for minor ailments, avoid self-diagnosis and management. Treat yourself as you would expect a patient with the same condition to be treated—and have a confidential consultation with a trusted health professional.

If you are the expert that another doctor has approached, do not be deceived by this honour into thinking that you must treat your new patient in any special way. Special treatment leads to special mistakes, and it is far better for doctor-patients to tread well-worn paths of referral, investigation, and treatment than to try illusory short cuts.

☼ Burnout (running beyond empty)

Definition Falling performance and personal accomplishments, emotional exhaustion, negative affect, poor leadership, and depersonalization brought on by months or years of overexposure to emotionally demanding situations at work, on the battlefield, or at home (see MINIBOX and fig 4.7).

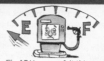

Fig 4.7 Have you felt this way?

Measurement The Five minute speech sample and the Maslach burnout inventory.[12]

Risk factors *For doctors:* Lack of hobbies, lack of physical activity, and lack of enough time for vacations and religious activities are all important.[13] Pressure of work, conflict with colleagues,[14] less personal relationships with patients, overly formal hierarchies, and suboptimal income are put forward to explain the fact that some doctors (eg urologists) in the public sector are more at risk of burnout compared with private-service urologists.[15] Factors associated with emotional exhaustion: 'having to deaden one's conscience', lack of time to provide needed care, work being so demanding that it influences one's home life, and not being able to live up to others' expectations.[16]

Signs of burnout
• Stress and depression
• Fatigue
• Non-restorative sleep[11]
• Emotional exhaustion
• Motivation↓; apathy↑
• Libido↓
• Insomnia
• Guilt or denial
• Paranoia/isolated
• Demoralization
• Amnesia
• Indecision
• Temper tantrums
• Low personal accomplishment
• Depersonalization
• Irritability/impatience

Risk factors for psychiatric nurses: Unreciprocated giving, violent client population[17] leading to vicarious traumatization,[18] frequency of on-calls.[19] High expressed emotion (evidenced by critical comments ± negative relationships) predicts depersonalization elements of burnout.[12]

For medical students: Impulsivity, depression, & money worries are predictive.[20]

For military personnel: Past history of physical trauma is predictive.

Management (Difficult.) Some may respond to plans such as these:
• Diagnose and treat any depression (p334-9).
• Allow time for the person to recognize that there is a problem.
• More hobbies, and more nice holidays.
• Advice from wise colleagues in the specialty (regular follow-up). Mentoring consists in forming a supportive relationship with an independent colleague for the sole purpose of support.
• Return meaning and purpose to life via dialogue, self-transcendence, and a sense of connectedness with others (meaning-centred psychotherapy).[21]
• Learn new professional skills—or consider early retirement.
• Set achievable goals in work and leisure (eg protected time with family).

Prevention Strategies such as career counselling are said to be effective but really do no more than point a lollipop at a furnace.[22, n=171] *Reducing stress* is one (unproven) way of avoiding burnout. Psychiatrists have found their own 'stress busting' groups helpful—these entail problem-solving with airing of stresses—ideally accompanied by talking to colleagues for support and catharsis. Having outside interests helps, as does getting support from family and friends, time management, and exercise.[23] On a more universal plane, ►*we are all responsible for each other's burnout*. By being attentive to our own and others' feelings of troubled conscience we all have a role in preventing the burnout of our colleagues. We need opportunities to reflect on our troubled consciences. Appraisals (p526) and less formal routes to this awareness are becoming more accepted by professionals.[16]

Psychiatry

Since the 1980s, most UK inpatients with psychosis have had the focus of their care moved from hospital to the community. The aim has been to save money and improve care. But has community care failed, or have there been successes? Five questions keep recurring, each (ominously) prefixed by a 'surely...'

1 *Surely hospitals will always be needed for severely mentally ill people?* In general, the problem is not the severity of the mental illness but its social context which determines if community care is appropriate. Patients aren't always admitted to hospital because they aren't able to manage life in the community, sometimes a community is unable to manage the person. Clinic appointments are inadequate for chaotic, disorganized individuals. Assertive community management is demonstrated to reduce hospital admissions.

2 *Surely community care, if it is done properly, will be more expensive than hospital care, where resources can be concentrated?* Not so—at least not necessarily so. Some concentration of resources *can* take place in the community in day hospitals and mental illness hostels. It is also true that the 'bed and breakfast' element of inpatient care is expensive, if the running and maintenance costs associated with deploying inpatient psychiatric services are taken into account. In most studies, costs of each type of service doesn't differ much, and sometimes good community care turns out cheaper.[24,25]

3 *Surely there will be more homicides and suicides if disturbed patients are not kept in hospital?* Offending by the mentally ill is of great public concern (60 homicides/year in England). A cohort study, however, found rates of violent offending are low and the strongest association with offending was previous offending. Psychiatric variables were less important, with diagnosis and number of previous admissions showing no significant association. Substance misuse and sexual abuse are associated with increased offending risk.[26]

4 *Surely if inpatient psychiatric beds are not available, however good the daytime team is in the community, some patients will still need somewhere to go at night?* The implication is that the skills available in bed-and-breakfast accommodation may be inadequate at times of day when there is no other support, other than the ED. Studies that have looked at this have certainly found an increase in non-hospital residential care in those selected for community care, and this increase may be as much as 280% over 5 years. In the UK, new proposals guarantee 24-hour open access to skilled help, but it is not known what pressures this will put services under.

5 *Surely community care will involve a huge bureaucracy in pursuit of the unattainable goal of 100% safety?* This will be so if every patient has a lengthy care plan and repeated risk assessments. Concern for safety may also spawn a non-therapeutic custodial relationship.

Advantages reported for community care are: better social functioning, satisfaction with life, employment, and drug compliance—but in randomized studies in the UK these advantages are not always manifest. Furthermore, trends have been repeatedly found indicating that the longer studies go on for, the harder it is to maintain the initial advantages of community care. If teams and patients don't keep up their enthusiasm during a trial, it will be even harder once the trial period ends and regular life sets in.

Assertive community care and case management is one way out of this impasse (here a key-worker has direct responsibility for care plans). This set-up helps ensure more people remain in contact with psychiatric services; this inevitably increases hospital admission rates.[27,28] When combined with family therapy and social skills training results are good.[29]

Current UK community psychiatric services can be categorized as follows:
• Intensivist teams: Crisis and Home Treatment, eg with 24-h phone helpline.
• Support and recovery teams—community mental health teams (CMHT); assertive outreach; rehabilitation.
• Drug and alcohol teams: part of a wide range of substance abuse services.
• Inreach mental health services—residential care, acute hospital liaison, primary care liaison teams (PCL)—integrated CPNs/psychiatrists with GP practices/hospitals with good links into secondary community services.
• IAPT services (improved access to psychological therapies)—offer a wide range of community-based therapies eg, CBT (p390), group therapy, etc.

Typically all these services are multidisciplinary (to a varying degree) with nurses, OTs, physios, psychologists, psychiatrists, and social workers.

Many of these community services are supported by 3rd-sector (voluntary) organizations, eg MIND, Alzheimer's society, and other local organizations and charities that provide drop-in centres, group or individual therapy, homecare, advocacy, educational information, etc.

PWD (patients with dementia) use more or less specialist residential or nursing homes; social services input is very important as is close working with local councils, and health authorities. *Integrated care* has theoretical advantages—eg for a schizophrenic patient who is a substance abuser.[30,31]

Psychiatry

Schizophrenia is a common chronic relapsing condition often presenting in early adulthood with *psychotic symptoms* (hallucinations, delusions); *disorganization symptoms* (incongruous mood, abnormal speech and thought); *negative symptoms* (apathy, ↓motivation, withdrawal, self neglect, blunted mood); and, sometimes, *cognitive impairment*.[32,33] It has major implications for patients, work and families. *Incidence:* ~0.15:1000/yr. *Prevalence:* ~1%.

Psychosis, distorted thinking, and perception, eg delusions and hallucinations, is a common symptom: 1 Affective psychoses (depression, bipolar disorder) 2 Transient psychotic disorders (usually substance misuse) 3 Psychosis due to a medical disorders (eg brain tumour) and 4 Schizophrenia-like non-affective disorders (brief psychotic disorder; delusional disorder; schizophreniform disorder).[34] When diagnosing schizophrenia look for:

1 *Thought insertion:* 'He's is putting ideas into my head' *Thought broadcasting:* 'People overhear my thoughts'. *Thought withdrawal:* 'Thoughts are being taken out of my head' (seen objectively as a patient suddenly stopping mid-sentence), or repeating of thoughts.

2 Delusions that thoughts, feelings, impulses, or actions are influenced or even controlled by external forces. Also includes delusional perceptions (p326).

3 Hallucinatory voices giving a running commentary on a patient's behaviour, or discussing the patient among themselves.

4 Persistent delusions of other kinds that are culturally inappropriate and completely impossible ('Ryan Reynolds has put a transmitter in my brain').

5 Persistent hallucinations in any modality (somatic, visual, tactile) which occur every day for weeks on end.

6 Breaks or interpolations in the train of thought, resulting in incoherence or irrelevant speech—*knight's move thoughts* that change direction, flying off at tangents, with odd logic, or neologisms (made-up words).

7 Catatonic behaviour described as 'strange, purposeless behaviour', such as sudden excitement, posturing, or waxy flexibility, negativism, mutism, echopraxia (involuntary imitation of the movements).

8 Negative symptoms (apathy, paucity of speech, blunting or incongruity of affect, eg laughing at bad news) usually resulting in social withdrawal.

(1-5 are co-extensive with Schneider's 1st-rank symptoms of schizophrenia.)

Diagnostic guidelines for schizophrenia The main criterion is at least one very clear symptom (and usually two or more if less clear-cut) belonging to any of the groups 1-4 above, or symptoms from at least two of groups 5-8. Because many people have brief psychosis-like symptoms, *do not* diagnose schizophrenia unless symptoms last for ≥6 months *and* symptoms are present much of the time for at least 1 month, *and* there is marked impairment in work or home functioning. Also, 'rule out' other causes of psychosis (eg bipolar disorder, drugs/alcohol, CNS tumours, head injury).

ICD-10 distinguishes the following subtypes of schizophrenia: *Paranoid* (commonest subtype, here hallucinations and/or delusions are prominent). *Hebephrenic* (age of onset 15-25yrs, poor prognosis, fluctuating affect prominent with fleeting fragmented delusions and hallucinations). *Catatonic* (characterized by stupor, posturing, waxy flexibility, and negativism). In *simple* and *residual* types, negative symptoms predominate.

Prodromal symptoms precedes most first episodes of psychosis by up to 18 months (sometimes just a few days). It is characterized by a gradual deterioration in functioning—sometimes conceptualized as 'altered life trajectory'.

Changes include: • Transient and/or attenuated (lower intensity) psychotic symptoms • Odd (out of character) thoughts, beliefs and behaviours • Concentration problems • Altered affect • Social withdrawal • Reduced interest in daily activities.

Other 'schizophrenia' disorders *Schizoaffective* causes confusion as its neither (or both) a variant of schizophrenia and affective (mood) disorders. It is given when a patient experiences both symptoms of a mood disorder (mania or depression) and schizophrenia at the same time (within days) and of the same intensity without another medical disorder or substance misuse cause. Treatment is managing both conditions: often an antipsychotic and mood stabilizer. Lifetime prevalence is ~0.5%.

Schizotypal is a personality disorder (see p380) which may represent a partial expression of schizophrenia. Usually treated without medication.

Schizophreniform is given to those disorders that fail to meet threshold for schizophrenia (usually duration of psychosis) but have some symptoms of schizophrenia and deterioration in functioning. Treated with antipsychotics.

Genes and environment

Many genes implicated in schizophrenia also increase risk of bipolar disorder.[35-47 International Schizo-phrenia Consortium] Some are susceptibility genes (needing environmental triggers). Genome-wide studies point to a gene coding for myosin on chromosome 22 and a region of >450 gene variants, in the major histocompatibility complex (MHC) region on 6p. The dysbindin gene on chromosome 6 is important too. Early use of cannabis is a trigger: those with vv homozygosity of the catechol-o-methyl-transferase gene (COMT; risk ↑×10 compared with mm variants). The timing of triggers is important.[48] Those starting cannabis at 15yrs old are 3× more likely to develop schizophreniform psychosis.[49,50]

Is schizophrenia a neurodevelopmental disorder?

People with schizophrenia may suffer unusual neurodevelopment either through inheriting genes and/or some insult to the brain that impairs its development. This leads to subtle cognitive and behavioural effects in childhood[51] and then psychosis at or just after adolescence. Relevant prenatal/obstetric events: early rupture of membranes, gestational age <37 weeks, incubator use, winter births.[52]

MRI shows differences in the brains of those with schizophrenia (and their 1st degree relatives[53]): eg larger lateral ventricles, reduced frontal lobe and parahippocampal gyrus. Reduced (particularly on left) temporal lobe, hippocampus (subserves memory/emotion) and amygdala (involved in expression of emotion). MRI has shown diffuse reduction in cortical grey matter associated with poor premorbid function.[54] NB: use of psychotics may also cause brain shrinkage—eg up to 20%.[55] However, schizophrenia also has an onset later in life, particularly women over 30.[56] It has been estimated that about 40% of people who develop schizophrenia have a developmental problem, but the majority are not remarkably different from the general population and have no cognitive deficits. So what are the other pathways that lead to psychosis?

Social factors Being brought up in cities increases the risk of schizophrenia (UK incidence is particularly high in London), and there are higher levels of schizophrenia in migrant groups such as Asians and African-Caribbeans (possible mechanisms through social adversity, racial discrimination, social isolation).[57] The associated 'stress' on the brain has been suggested to affect the morphology of the brain via hormonal influences as well as the stress of being psychotic resulting in high cortisol levels causing further brain changes.

Psychosis and schizophrenia Some believe that the term 'schizophrenia' has outlived its usefulness as it implies that everyone with schizophrenia has the same pathology and all need antipsychotics. A more nuanced approach is to avoid diagnostic labels, and treat the first episode as 'psychosis' (see p339).

Patients require a range of management interventions but the first step is to determine what it is that you, and the patient, want to focus on treating (and the methods used to do this). *Frequent symptoms:* Lack of insight,[97%] auditory hallucinations,[74%] ideas of reference,[70%] paranoia,[66%] flat affect,[66%] persecutory delusions.[62%] *Frequent behaviours:* Social withdrawal,[74%] anhedonia (inability to feel pleasure),[50%] apathy,[56%] lack of conversation,[54%] psychomotor retardation,[48%] over activity,[41%] self neglect,[30%] posturing ± odd movements.[25%]

Medication once a diagnosis is made of psychosis (or schizophrenia), then antipsychotic medication should be commenced (see p340-1). Don't dawdle! Delaying antipsychotics worsens negative symptoms.[58] but managing schizophrenia is much more than drugs; it requires an individualized *care plan* that includes psychosocial interventions and *support for families*.[59] If concordance with medication is an issue, depots (long-lasting injections) are useful.

Psychological interventions Given the adverse effects of antipsychotic drugs, psychological interventions should be recommended in all management plans to promote *quick recovery* and *relapse prevention*. There is strong evidence to support early use of CBT, general or targeted on auditory hallucinations ('hearing voices'), and other interventions aimed at reducing the impact of symptoms on the patient's life, limit relapses, and promote early detection of another episode. Towards end of acute episode focus on treating residual symptoms, eg difficult thoughts, voices, negative symptoms. If there is concurrent substance misuse (high prevalence) abstinence improves overall prognosis—in fact, better prognosis at 18 months than if a patient had never had substance misuse problem at all.

Other interventions include *working with family:* Address carers' issues (embarrassment, self-blame, and shame are prevalent).[60] Family therapy may have a role.[61] and support groups.[5] *Social support:* Particular social circumstances may result in alterations in dopamine that ↑relapse likelihood. Addressing housing, benefits, and social skills training are just as important as being concordant with medication. Supported employment can be helpful.

Referral to an Early Intervention Service (see BOX) should be considered. They offer these interventions under a single dynamic team.

Aftercare Coordinated via an allocated key worker and a multidisciplinary team (to look at biological, psychological, social, and risk issues). It is performed through the Care Programme Approach (CPA).

Prognosis is better if: sudden onset; no negative symptoms; supportive home; ♀ sex (better social integration[62]); later onset of illness; no CNS ventricular enlargement; no family history.

Overall, only 10% ever have one episode. With treatment, ≤7% need intensive input/hospital admission for more than 2 years after *first* admission. 28% go over 2 years without needing further hospital admission. Recovery at 15 years (measured by global assessment of function >60) in 40% of patients. *Suicide rates:* incidence of 10% during acute phase, then 4% in chronic phase.

Psychiatry

---

5 eg Rethink (http://www.rethink.org/) and Mind (http://www.mind.org.uk/) are UK mental health charities.

Psychosis: 'a break from reality'

Psychosis is a mental disorder causing a person to perceive, believe, or interpret things differently. In its florid form, it is the archetype of the layman's 'madness' But, the *usual* picture is less obvious: the patient may be sitting alone, quietly attending to his or her voices. Psychosis interferes with the ability to function and can be very debilitating. If hallucinations, delusions, or a thought disorder (defined on p326–8) are present, the cause could be schizophrenia (or related disorders), a disorder of affect (mania, p348, or depression, p342, or both), or be organic (eg head injury drug-induced—a transient psychosis).

So the term psychosis is not in itself a diagnosis, but is a useful term to employ, while the underlying diagnosis is being formulated. Beware labelling people; remember that even during the best of times, only a thin veil separates us from insanity.

Early Intervention Services (EIS)

The principal aim of an EIS is to provide a service to identify, assess, treat, and support people experiencing their first psychotic episode. Their aim during the formative stages of the condition is: **1** Reduction of an individual's duration of untreated psychosis **2** Provision of the most effective possible care at an early stage to maximize the chance of recovery **3** Increase likelihood of return to education or employment **4** Prevent loss of life trajectory.

The EIS model has clinicians with a small caseload working with patients in a proactive manner, meeting in a patient's home, workplace (or school), and local community rather than clinic. EIS provide holistic care to reflect patients' needs and priorities using a multidisciplinary team. Dates and times of these appointments are often not fixed in frequency or duration. Because of this flexibility EIS are better able to reflect the needs of this complex group and react quickly to changes in their mental state or acute difficulties. EIS will often receive referral from psychiatric services, other statutory and non-statutory services (eg housing providers, probation, drug services).

EIS model is of low-threshold for discussion, referral, and acceptance of patients. Usual exception criteria are limited to location, organic (including substance-induced) psychosis, and previous EIS care of over 2 years. Most teams offer an initial assessment period (eg up to 8 weeks) to engage the person and ascertain suitability for the service with liaison with the referrer, and other services as required. If accepted, EIS work intensively with the patient, and their support network, for 3 years, even if they are admitted.

This is a model which has been shown to have good outcomes: halving likelihood of admission (especially detention under the Mental Health Act), lowering rates of negative symptoms, reducing suicide risk (from 15% to 1%), limiting duration of episode, and increasing early relapse detection. Employment rate for 18–35s in an EIS is 35% (12% for people in standard mental health care) with social functioning has been shown to improve.

EIS is not without critics. Accusations include selectively cited findings to support early intervention, focus on short-term improvements without longer-term follow-up, and more 'spin' than research in published literature. An analysis of published abstracts showed implied positive results in 75%, whereas examination of primary measures found only 13% positive results[63].

Advice and monitoring Before starting an antipsychotic ask about personal/family history of diabetes, hypertension, and cardiovascular disease. Give advice on diet, weight control, and exercise. Perform BP, weight, fasting blood glucose, lipid profile, FBC, ECG if on clozapine. Additional 6-monthly monitoring of LFT, U&E, prolactin, weight, HbA_{1c} is recommended.[64]

Antipsychotic medication all show a degree of D2 antagonism—responsible for antipsychotic efficacy. Historically divided into typical (neuroleptic) or atypical based on side effect profile. However, a more helpful way to consider these is into 'generations' based on when they were first commonly used.

First generation (FGA) are D2 agonists which also causes the extrapyramidal side effects (EPSE). Side effects are often what make people stop their tablets. Examples include: chlorpromazine, haloperidol. *Second generation* (SGA) are 5HT2A and D2 antagonists; associated with lower risk of EPSE but more metabolic side effects: weight gain, hyperglycemia, and dyslipidemia. Examples include amisulpride, olanzapine, quetiapine, risperidone, zotepine. *Third generation* (TGA) are dopamine partial agonists. Only licensed TGA is aripiprazole.

Comparing efficacy SGA relieve psychotic symptoms as effectively as FGA[65,66] and may lower relapse rates. NICE considers oral SGA 'the choice of first line treatment for those with newly diagnosed schizophrenia'●※ However, CATIE and CUTLASS trials suggest there is not enough evidence to favour either. SGA and TGA are much more costly than FGA—with additional pressure from pharmaceutical companies promoting non-generic medication and funding research designed to produce biased findings. Risperidone was top when psychiatrists were asked 'If you become psychotic, what would you want?'[67,n=543] Except for clozapine (see next paragraph) there is no clear advantage within any generation of one medication over another, so side effects, and long-term compliance are important in tailoring treatment to the individual patient. Most unwanted effects are dose related, so 'start low increase slow'.

Clozapine remains the most popular medication of treatment-resistant schizophrenia with clear utility despite its risks (agranulocytosis risk ≤0.8% in 1st year of treatment: specialist monitoring is needed). Associated ↓ suicide risk.

Treating EPSE: Above all else, try to reach the lowest tolerated dose of antipsychotic to encourage concordance • Parkinsonism: ↓dose, change to SGA, or try procyclidine • Acute dystonia can occur within hours of starting antipsychotics. Treat with procyclidine IM/IV—may take up to 30 minutes to work; discouraged due to anticholinergic side effects • Akathisia (subjective sense of psychomotor restlessness) occurs within hours to weeks of starting antipsychotics, it may be very distressing; so use lowest possible dose or change to SGA—treatment may be needed with propranolol ± cyproheptadine • Tardive dyskinesia (chewing, grimaces, choreoathetosis) may be irreversible; but try tetrabenazine.

Main lifestyle issues • Hunger after taking medication (~3 hours): consider bedtime dose • Increased thirst: suggest water or sugar-free alternatives • Smoking induces metabolism and thus reduces antipsychotic plasma levels: higher doses and review dose if they quit smoking • Include targeted health promotion: three key areas are diet, physical exercise, and smoking cessation.

Failure to respond A number of interventions, not limited to medication, should have been completed before 'treatment failure' is confirmed. Within this, all medication must have been given at an adequate dose with verified compliance, cross-tapered to a new drug;[68] and clozapine considered and/or attempted. At this stage, combination therapy[69] is often tried, eg olanzapine with either amisulpride or risperidone, or quetiapine with risperidone. In theory, by acting on different receptors benefit may occur.[70] But often it doesn't go according to plan, and safety issues are opaque.

Psychiatry

Common side effects of antipsychotic medication

Extrapyramidal side effects are drug-induced movement disorders which include: tremor, slurred speech, akathesia (motor restlessness), dystonia (continuous spasms and muscle contractions). These are rare with quetiapine[71] and clozapine, uncommon with aripiprazole and zotepine but can occur at high doses with amisulpride, olanzapine, and risperidone.

Hyperprolactinaemia Aripiprazole, clozapine, and quetiapine have no or minimal effect on serum prolactin, olanzapine does at higher doses.[72]

Sexual dysfunction All SGA can cause sexual dysfunction, eg erectile dysfunction, ↓libido, ↓arousal, anorgasmia, eg from ↑prolactin (check level)[73] and ↓semen volume/viscosity;[74] retrograde ejaculation (α_1-receptor antagonism, eg with risperidone).[75] In one study, ~30% had stopped their drugs at some point owing to sexual side effects.[76] So ask about sex (p385); few will volunteer this information. Even drug-free patients with schizophrenia have reduced libido so its not a dose-related side effect.[77]

Weight gain is common. This causes ↓compliance, ↑risk of cardiovascular events and diabetes (greatest with olanzapine and clozapine, moderate with risperidone and zotepine; least with amisulpride and aripiprazole).[78]

Diabetes mellitus Prevalence in schizophrenia is twice the expected rate;[79] antipsychotics further increase risk (esp. clozapine and olanzapine).

Cardiovascular effects Olanzapine and risperidone ↑risk of stroke in the elderly when used to treat behavioural symptoms of dementia.[80] Postural hypotension is common (α_1 adrenoreceptor blockade), especially in the first 3 months of starting. Long QTc on ECG; fatal myocarditis and cardiomyopathy (clozapine).

Daytime drowsiness ~40% of those on clozapine (30% if on olanzapine or risperidone; 15% if on amisulpride or quetiapine).

Seizure threshold All antipsychotic medications decrease seizure threshold.

Special patient groups Elderly, children, and adolescents may get more side effects. In breast-feeding, most SGA enter breast milk. Trials of use in pregnancy are few; weigh up potential benefits against harm to mother, fetus and neonate. Advise against breast-feeding.

'I don't want to go on with the tablets...'

Take the time to talk with your patient and understand their reasoning for stopping. There are lots of reasons why people want to stop and some may be due to misunderstanding or incomplete information. Relapse is not always a disaster, and drug side effects can be difficult to deal with (or embarrassing to talk about). We tend to be over-impressed by positive symptoms (eg hallucinations) which respond better to drugs than negative symptoms.[81]

Ultimately, respect the patient's decision (unless there is genuine risk of stopping medication and an admission needs to be considered). It is better to work with a patient to safely withdraw medication with careful monitoring than refuse to discuss it and have them manage their own stopping in secret. If they feel listened to and understood, the therapeutic relationship can be strengthened.

In any year, 40% of us experience intense feelings of low mood, unhappiness, and disappointment which resolve without clinical intervention. But clinical depression is different from depressive symptoms. Worldwide, 5.8% of men and 9.5% of women will experience a depressive episode in a 12-month period, around 121 million people. It ranks fourth as a cause of disability worldwide and accounts for 5–10% of consultations in primary care in the UK.

Diagnosis Symptoms must be present, every or nearly every day without significant changes throughout the day, for over 2 weeks and represent a change from normal personality without alcohol/drugs, medical disorders, or bereavement. There must be at least two *core symptoms*:

- Depressed mood for most of the day, every day. Little variation in mood despite changes in time, circumstances, or activity. There may be diurnal mood variation (worse in mornings and improving as day proceeds).
- Anhedonia: Loss of interest or pleasure in daily life especially in things previously enjoyed; this change can be a subjective or observed change.
- Fatigue: a lack of energy which goes beyond poor sleep and pervades life.

Plus two or more *typical symptoms* (the first five are 'biological' symptoms):

- Poor appetite with marked weight loss (>5% of body weight in the past month) without dieting. Rarely, there is increased appetite and weight gain.
- Disrupted sleep: initial insomnia or early waking (3+ hours earlier than usual).
- Psychomotor retardation (limited spontaneous movement or sluggish thought processes) or agitation (subjective feeling of restlessness).
- Decreased libido (sexual drive) and other appetites.
- Evidence of (or subjective feelings of) reduced ability to concentrate.
- Feelings of worthlessness, inappropriate guilt (which may be delusional), or self-reproach. Not just about current illness but also past decisions or events.
- Recurrent thoughts of death, suicide ideation, or suicide attempts. These may be passive 'I wish I could disappear' or active 'My plan to overdose is...'.

Classification of a depressive episode is based on number and severity of these features; helps to determine management, treatment, and prognosis.

Aetiology is likely due to the interaction between biological, psychological, and social factors in an individual with risk factors for these. *Biological* • Point estimate of heritability for major depression is 37%. • Twin studies show 60% more concordance for depression in monozygotic twins than dizygotic twins • Monoamine theory of depression ↓monoamine (eg 5-HT, noradrenaline, dopamine) function may cause depression. Antidepressants ↑monoamines • Endocrinology ♀:♂ >1:1; dexamethasone suppression test is abnormal in ⅓ • Structural brain change ventricular enlargement and raised sucal prominence. *Psychological* • Personality traits neuroticism (high 'N' in Five Factor Model[6]) suggests mood lability, autonomic hyperarousal, and negative biases in attention and processing • Low self-esteem is considered a risk factor but is debatable if cause or symptom • Childhood experiences may ↑sensitivity to events. *Social* • Disruption due to life events (births, job loss, divorce, illness) in 60% of cases • Stress associated with poor social environment and social isolation can precipitate and perpetuate depression; social drift to lower social class.

Differentials • Psychiatric disorders: bipolar disorder, schizophrenia, anorexia nervosa, anxiety • Dysthymia • Substance misuse • Dementia • Sleep disorders • Neurological disorders • Physical illness • Medication SEs (eg β-blockers).

Depression is often missed or ignored when patients (♂>♀) dismiss depressive symptoms as temporary or due to a physical illness. An avoidance of psychiatric labels (often due to the stigma attached to these diagnosis) obstructs help-seeking behaviour. If professionals and patients collude to ignore depression or focus on physical causes then serious symptoms are untreated.

6 Collectively known as OCEAN: openness, conscientiousness, extraversion, agreeableness, and neuroticism.

Criteria for severity in depression (ICD-10)

These categories should really only be used for a single (first) depressive episode. Further depressive episodes should be classified as a recurrent depressive disorder. Categorization guides management and prognosis.

	Typical symptoms	Other core symptoms
Mild	2	2
Moderate	2	3+
Severe	3	4+

Additional classification includes with/without:
• Somatic symptoms (biological features of depression)
• Psychotic symptoms (mood-congruent delusions or hallucinations)
• Manic episodes (suggestive of bipolar not unipolar depression).

'Normal depression': adjustment disorder and bereavement

It is important to differentiate reactions to stress, life events, and bereavement from a depressive episode, in order to determine prognosis and treatment. Adjustment disorders are proof that stress can cause psychopathology (also: extraordinarily severe responses such as acute stress reaction and post-traumatic stress disorder, see p353). In adjustment disorder there is 'subjective distress and emotional disturbance, usually interfering with social functioning and performance...would not have arisen without the stressor' (ICD-10). For example, abnormally excessive reactions to a life stressors such as a fire or flood, divorce, financial difficulties, or physical illness. In normal adaptive reactions to stress, functioning is less impaired. If there is an adjustment disorder without criteria met for major depression then antidepressants are not useful.

In bereavement there is an assumed period of grief, low mood, and adaptation, which has been summarized in the Kubler–Ross model below (see also OHCM p7). These 'stages' are no longer considered to occur in a defined order—so someone can start in, and move to, any stage (or revisit a stage multiple times) during the bereavement process.

Denial: shutting out reality to cope with overwhelming difficult feelings

Anger: can be angry with themselves, or with others, or at a higher power

Bargaining: hoping to avoid or undo grief through negotiation or promises

Depression: disconnect from people in an attempt to avoid further trauma

Acceptance: coming to terms with inevitable situation; create calm mind-set.

If someone becomes stuck in a stage and unable to resolve their grief then additional support is needed from GP or psychiatrist. If mood symptoms deepen and affect appetite, energy and sleep then it may be depression.

NB: grief can be about many things, not just death, eg divorce or incarceration and can be experienced by the patient given a terminal prognosis.

Medication improves mood and ↑synaptic availability of noradrenaline or serotonin (5HT). So, medication and therapy (p388) should be part of a holistic approach. Think about how you manage your own mood. Increasing activity is important: exercising, engaging in productive activity, socializing. Improve sleep, relaxation, and 'self soothing' (being kind to oneself) techniques. Work out what each patient wants and support them to move in that direction. Inactivity, drugs, alcohol, daytime TV and isolation will perpetuate a problem.

Mild depression suggest low-intensity psychological interventions focused on sleep hygiene, anxiety management (mindfulness), and problem-solving techniques. These include individual guided self-help (books, websites and apps, eg Headspace), computerized CBT, and structured group-based physical activity programmes. Unless the symptoms persist beyond 8 weeks or previous history of depression, antidepressants should not be routinely used.

Moderate depression Use a combination of an antidepressant and a high-intensity psychological intervention (8–12 sessions CBT or interpersonal therapy). The Improving Access to Psychological Therapies (IAPT) programme has been created to meet this need—it offers a realistic and routine first-line treatment across the NHS.[7] For a first episode of depression, a generic selective serotonin reuptake inhibitor (SSRI) is recommended (see p346).

Severe depression includes psychotic depression, high risk of suicide, and atypical depression. These need a rapid specialist mental health assessment with a consideration of inpatient admission (using the MHA if necessary) or ECT (see BOX).

Recurrent depression 50–85% of people who have had one episode of moderate or severe depression will have further episodes and may require maintenance treatment to reduce relapse risk. Intervene quickly and early for any recurrence. If a medication has worked before it has a very good chance of working again, so this should always be first line. Continuing antidepressants lowers the odds of relapse by ~65%, halving absolute risk.[82] CBT can be offered to manage residual symptoms. Psychoeducation around the relapsing nature of the condition is essential. Normalize reoccurrence—many conditions carry a risk of this (eg basal cell carcinoma, p590).

Lifestyle changes Many people want to avoid medication or therapy. If safe to do so, positive suggestions should include: exercise (in wild nature), tai chi, yoga, social interaction, psychotherapy, reading clubs, meditation, poetry (reading/writing). For some, rest from work—always plan a phased return.

Follow-up All patients should be reviewed regularly, frequently at first and then less often, to consider their current symptomatology and level of functioning. Investigate their response to any interventions, adherence to treatments, and adverse effects—direct questioning and probing may be required to elicit 'embarrassing' or assumed unconnected complaints. Alongside this, consider: co-morbid conditions associated with depression (eg alcohol or drug misuse), suicide risk and safeguarding concerns (children or vulnerable adults). Include psychoeducation on depression and recovery—promotion of lifestyle changes (using identified stressors and supports) with ongoing reviews and reflection to highlight gains and maintain positive changes.

St John's wort or *Hypericum perforatum* is widely available as a (non-prescribed) herbal remedy for depression. A Cochrane review states superiority to placebo and equivalent to antidepressants in major depression with fewer side effects (½ that of SSRIS). However, use should not be encouraged: it upregulates the CYP3A4 cytochrome (within liver's P450 system), affecting drug metabolism, eg reducing efficiency of oral contraceptive pill. In addition, different preparations have varying amounts of active ingredient. Always ask if its being taken.

7 Also developed for under 18s: Children and Young People's IAPT (or CYP-IAPT).

Severe depression

When there is persistent low mood or anhedonia for >2 weeks, and ≥4 of the following seven markers of severe depression, there is a high risk of suicide:

Suicide plan or ideas of self-harm.

Unexplained guilt or worthlessness.

Inability to function (eg psycho-motor retardation or agitation).

Concentration impaired.

Impaired appetite.

Decreased sleep/early waking.

Energy low/unaccountable fatigue.

Enquire about these whenever depression is possible. Ask the patient sensitively but directly whether they think about suicide and how often.

Sometimes, in severe depression, antidepressants need to be prescribed as a matter of urgency, eg if suicide is likely or if a parent's functioning is so impaired they cannot look after their family.

Over-diagnosing severe depression is undesirable. Patients' lives can become medicalized and drugs, with significant SEs, are needlessly given. In some areas of the UK prescriptions for antidepressants tripled from 1993 to 2007 without clear benefits for patients. In primary care there isn't the luxury of an hour-long assessment to differentiate clinical depression from its alternatives. NICE and QOF recommend using the PHQ-9 diagnostic tool to help prevent this.

Electroconvulsive therapy (ECT)

ECT is a very effective treatment for depression, particularly severe depressive episodes which have not responded to medication. However, the public perception of it as barbaric, coercive, or dangerous makes it controversial. Sadly, there is often a gross misunderstanding of ECT based on a belief that treatment hasn't changed since 1950s or films ('One Flew Over the Cuckoo's Nest' shows a lobotomy not ECT).

Reality (fig 4.9) is less scary than the perception (fig 4.8) of ECT.

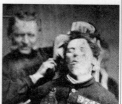

Mechanism There is MRI evidence for the idea that ECT interrupts the hyperconnectivity between the various areas of the brain that maintain depression[83]

Indications NICE recommends ECT is used to gain rapid improvement of severe symptoms after an adequate trial of other treatments has proven ineffective and/or when the condition is considered to be potentially life-threatening, in patients with: • A prolonged or severe manic episode • Severe depression • Catatonia.

Fig 4.8 Patients at the West Riding Lunatic Asylum, Wakefield, Yorkshire; attributed to Henry Clarke. Number 17, young man restrained by two warders.

Wellcome Library, London.

Emergency ECT is possible, but rarely used—the success rate is good (80%)[84] Carry on antidepressants when ECT ends: this *may* prevent recurrences.[85] *Typical course length:* 6-12 sessions (2 per week).

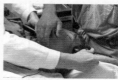

Contraindications Mainly to the general anaesthesia; There are no absolute contraindications to ECT itself; no consent (p408; involve relatives, but they cannot consent for an adult). **Cautions** Recent subdural/subarachnoid bleed, stroke, MI, arrhythmia, CNS vascular anomalies.

Fig 4.9 Modern ECT.
Courtesy of University of Michigan.

Side effects memory loss: short term reterograde amnesia (usually resolves completely), confusion, headaches, and clumsiness; common anaesthetic SEs.

There is good evidence that antidepressants are helpful in major depression and in particular preventing relapse, but their limitations shouldn't be ignored. It can feel perplexing prescribing antidepressants; often more like trial and error to work out what works well in one person but may not help another. In this context, the basic approach to prescription should be:

- Discuss choice of drug and non-pharmacological therapy. CBT is known to be as effective as antidepressants in mild to moderate depression.[86] Combined use is better than either treatment alone.[87,88]
- Discuss side effects. Warn patient that there may be an initial worsening of symptoms in the first weeks so persevere before therapeutic effects are seen. Remember to monitor closely during this time for increased suicidality. Not all side effects are undesirable (SSRI may help premature ejaculation).
- Assess formally after (at least) 4 weeks. If effective continue for at least 6 months after recovery; if stopped too soon 50% of patients relapse.[89]
- If there is a minor/low response, titrate the dose up looking for additional response. Switching is better than augmenting although commonly doctors will combine medication if there has been a partial recovery on one drug.
- If no response after 4 weeks or poor tolerability, switch to an alternative class of antidepressant. Do not continue to increase the dose; there is little evidence for dose response except tricyclics, venlafaxine, and escitalopram.[8]

NICE guidance Full guideline on depression concluded that antidepressants have largely equal efficacy and that choice should mainly depend on: • Side-effect profile • People's preference • Previous experience of treatments • Propensity of discontinuation symptoms • Safety in overdose • Interactions • Cost. SSRIs are recommended as first choice due to favourable risk–benefit ratios. Neither escitalopram nor the 'dual action' antidepressants (eg venlafaxine, duloxetine), were judged to have any clinically important advantages.

First line: A generic SSRI should be commenced with low starting dose which can be titrated up. Advise that full effect may take up to 6 weeks (initial positive effects most likely due to placebo) and effective dose will be continued for at least 6 months after recovery. Fluoxetine (only antidepressant licensed for <18s), citalopram (or escitalopram), or sertraline (best in IHD) are all good choices in terms of safety, efficacy, and tolerability. Monitor FBC (anaemia due to GI bleeding and avoid concurrent NSAIDs) and U&E (hyponatraemia) in any SSRI. With citalopram there may be dose-dependent prolongation of QTc interval (if unnoticed, Torsades de Pointes). Discuss potential adverse effects and risks of discontinuation/withdrawal symptoms—including sexual side effects (often an unspoken reason why medication is stopped).

Second line: An alternate SSRI from above (all are very different molecules).

Third line: In no particular order, mirtazapine (noradrenergic and specific serotonergic antidepressant: NaSSA), or venlafaxine (serotonin and noradrenaline reuptake inhibitor: SNRI) are all acceptable. Mirtazapine can cause drowsiness at low doses, which may be helpful to aid sleep when given as an evening dose, and can lead to weight gain. Venlafaxine may be more effective for patients who are anxious, but requires a baseline BP and ECG and monitoring for any cardiovascular side effects.

Fourth line: The Star* D trial essentially showed that if a medication is ineffective, keep switching until you find one that works. Lithium is effective as an adjunctive therapy but has significant toxicity problems. Consider older antidepressants •Tricyclics (TCA): nortriptyline, clomipramine • Monoamine oxidase inhibitors (MAOIs): moclobemide, phenelzine • Serotonin agonist and reuptake inhibitor (SARI): trazodone. Whatever is used, review regularly.

---

8 Escitalopram is the active enatiomer of citalopram. While some studies show an increased efficacy, others question if there is any appreciable difference—and if this was a means to repatent, and therefore sell at a high price, an older drug (citalopram) which was about to become available in a cheaper generic form.

Swapping antidepressants: how to cross-taper

When an antidepressant has failed to work at an adequate dose, or is poorly tolerated, changing the drug is appropriate. Avoid abrupt withdrawal when swapping antidepressants; cross-tapering is preferred. Speed of cross-tapering is best judged by patient tolerability. NB: co-administration of some antidepressants is absolutely contraindicated, see 'Cautions'—dangers include precipitating the *serotonin syndrome*[90] (restlessness; diaphoresis, ie excessive sweating); tremor; shivering; myoclonus; confusion; convulsions; death).

Example of cross-tapering based on the Maudsley regimen[91]

	Week 1	Week 2	Week 3	Week 4
Withdrawing amitriptyline from 150mg/24h	100mg/24h	50mg/24h	25mg/24h	Nil
Introducing sertraline	25mg/24h	50mg/24h	75mg/24h	100mg/24h

Cautions When swapping from MAOIs to any other antidepressant, withdraw and wait for 2 weeks (the time taken for monoamine oxidase to be replenished); for moclobemide wait 24h. Do not co-administer clomipramine and SS-RIs or venlafaxine. Beware fluoxetine interactions (may still occur for 5 weeks after stopping, due to long half-life).

Antidepressant medication effects and side effects

Eight pharmacological actions are known, and over 20 antidepressants exist. How do all they lead to a similar response? Why is there a delay? Two theories: The *neurotransmitter receptor hypothesis:* Postulates that a change in receptor sensitivity by desensitization and down-regulation of different receptors (not just ↑neurotransmitter at the synapse) leads to clinical effects after a few weeks. The *monoamine hypothesis of antidepressants on gene expression:* This suggests the effect of increased neurotransmitter at the synapse initiates a sequence of events to give the antidepressant response. This includes up- and down-regulation of various genes with subsequent varying expression of receptors and critical proteins.[92]

The associated side effects, cautions and contraindications for all antidepressant medications are too numerous to list here. Use the *British National Formulary* (BNF) or Maudsley Prescription Guidelines (http://maudsley-prescribing-guidelines.co.uk/) for up-to-date information and current recommendations regarding prescribing dosages.

Prevalence Lifetime: 1.5% ♀=♂; peak prevalence is between 15–19♀ and 20–24♂.

Signs of mania *Mood:* Irritability[80%], euphoria[71%], lability[69%]. *Cognition:* Grandiosity[78%], distractibility/poor concentration[71%], flight of ideas/racing thoughts[71%], confusion[25%], lack of insight. *Behaviour:* Rapid speech[98%], hyperactivity[87%], ↓sleep[81%], hypersexuality[57%], extravagance[55%]. *Psychotic symptoms:* Delusions[48%], hallucinations[15%]. This elevated mood must be present for at least a week (or shorter but requiring admission) to be considered mania. Any impairment must be severe enough to limit function.

Less severe states are termed *hypomania:* many of the characteristic symptoms of mania, without psychotic symptoms, impairment in daily functioning, or need for inpatient treatment. If depression alternates with mania, the term *bipolar affective disorder* is used (the term 'manic-depressive' is still used colloquially but not clinically). During mood swings, risk of suicide is high. Cyclical mood swings with subclinical features are termed *cyclothymia.* A patient's ability to manage their symptoms (ie degree of 'impairment') is partially socially defined—a single mother of twin toddlers may have a harder time 'coping' than a wealthy, childless married woman.

Causes *Medication:* Steroids, illicit substances (amphetamines, cocaine), antidepressants. *Physical:* Infection, stroke, neoplasm, epilepsy, multiple sclerosis, and metabolic disturbances (esp. hyperthyroidism).

Assessment *Ask* about: Infections, drug use, and past or family history of psychiatric disorders. *Do:* CT of the head, EEG, and screen for drugs/toxins.[93]

Treating acute mania[NICE] *Assess:* Psychotic symptoms (p369); cycling speed; suicide risk. For acute moderate/severe mania: any SGA (SE: weight↑; glucose↑), or **valproate semisodium** (eg Depakote®). NB: some people are most fulfilled and creative when manic[9] and don't want to change; others recognize, in retrospect, that use of mental health law (a last resort) was a turning point.

Prophylaxis Those who have bipolar affective disorder after successful treatment of the manic or depressive episode should have a mood stabilizer for longer-term control. If compliance is good, and U&E, ECG, and T₄ normal, give **lithium carbonate**. Adjust dose to give a plasma level of ~0.6-1mmol/L Li⁺, by day 7, ~12h post-dose. Elderly show ↑sensitivity to Li⁺ neurotoxicity.[94]
• Check Li⁺ levels weekly (~12h post-dose) until the dose has been constant for 4 weeks; then check monthly for 6 months; then 3-monthly, if stable; more often if on diuretic, NSAIDs, ACE-i (all ↑Li⁺), a low-salt diet, or if pregnant.
• If Li⁺ levels are progressively rising, suspect progressive nephrotoxicity.
• U&E + TSH 6-monthly; Li⁺ SE: hypothyroidism; nephrogenic diabetes insipidus).
▶Avoid changing brands [Li⁺↓↑]. ▶Ensure you can reach them urgently if Li⁺ >1.4mmol/L. ▶Toxic effects: vision↓; D&V; K⁺↓; ataxia; tremor; dysarthria; coma.

Psychosocial interventions Target the emotional consequences of having a cycling disorder with periods of acute illness, stigma, fear of recurrence ('I'm having a good time but am I happy, or *too* happy?') and other problems arising from illness (eg manic overspending, hypersexualized behaviour, etc). Key elements include psychoeducation, CBT, and support groups.

Risk of suicide is higher if: •Previous suicide attempt •Family history of suicide •Early onset of bipolar disorder •Extent of depressive symptoms (eg hopelessness) •Increasingly bad affective signs •Mixed affective states •Rapid cycling •Abuse of alcohol or drugs.[95] Lithium reduces risk of suicide[95] if contraindicated, olanzapine and fluoxetine may be better than lamotrigine. ▶But don't only rely on medication: CBT (p390) is of great value in helping people (who retain some insight) to ride their cycles without falling off.[96]

---

9 A counter argument from the periodically depressed poet Thomas Krampf: 'one can have a vision but no vision is worth anything if one is too sick to implement it'—and many writers have found their creativity flourish more when treatment is underway. M Berlin 2008 *Poets on Prozac*, Baltimore.

There is an increased risk of perinatal psychiatric illness in women with bipolar disorder so regular discussions about contraception and the importance of seeking advice early if she is thinking about pregnancy (or unexpectedly pregnant) are essential. >50% of pregnancies are unplanned. Remember this, when considering medication in any women of childbearing potential. NICE recommends that sodium valproate should not be used in this group if avoidable, due to its particular teratogenic and developmental effects.

Lithium is considered to be the most teterogenic medication in bipolar disorder with an increased risk to lithium-exposed babies being up to 12% (compared to 4% in control group). Particular concerns about Ebstein's anomaly (see p342), floppy baby syndrome, and thyroid abnormalities.

For these women, frequent reviews and close contact is essential during the perinatal period. Stopping medication when pregnant carries a risk of relapse, with studies showing women who stop medication are over twice as likely to have symptom recurrence compared to those who continue. If a woman decides to stop (and there is no strong evidence for either choice) immediately commencing prophylactic medication postpartum should be considered—with advice about breast-feeding. Other interventions include reducing stress, and promoting good sleep (especially in late pregnancy and first months after birth).

When lithium does not give good control

Note that abrupt cessation of lithium precipitates acute mania in up to 50% of patients. Discontinuation should be gradual over 2-4 weeks.

Anticonvulsants Consider semisodium valproate or carbamazepine as 2nd line. The most specific indication may be in rapid cyclers (≥4 acute mood swings/year). Lamotrigine is a mood stablizer and as good as citalopram in bipolar depressive states.[97] Gabapentin and topiramate are potential mood stabilizers. **Antipsychotics** Olanzapine has a role.[98] In one meta-analysis, there was no difference in overall efficacy of treatment between haloperidol and olanzapine or risperidone. Some evidence suggests that haloperidol could be less effective than aripiprazole.[99]

Combination treatments (Often tried.) Lithium plus carbamazepine may be synergistic.[100] If mania persists despite long-term treatment with lithium, adding in another antimanic such as an antipsychotic or valproate is a rational strategy. Lithium (or valpoate) plus an 2nd-generation antipsychotic, eg risperidone or olanzapine, may help if unresponsive to monotherapy.[101,102]

Antidepressants with lithium Lithium (or an alternative mood stabilizer) reduces risk of mood fluctuations from mania to depression in people with bipolar affective disorder. For depression occurring during lithium treatment, antidepressants can be used: SSRIs and venlafaxine are considered the most effective. Avoid tricyclics as they seem most likely to cause iatrogenic mania. Also consider antipsychotics such as quetiapine. Taper from 2 to 6 months after remission to minimize manic relapse.[103]

Consider **monoamine oxidase inhibitors** for anergic (=lacking in energy) bipolar depression.[104] ECT also has a role (p345),[105] and meta-analyses support use of omega 3 oils (only for when mood is low).[106]

Psychiatry

Anxiety is a normal response to threat or danger and part of the usual human experience, but it can become a mental health problem if the response is exaggerated, lasts more than 3 weeks, and interferes with daily life. Anxiety disorders (♀:♂ ≈2:1) can cause suffering and cost the UK ≥£5 billion/yr. **Neurosis** refers to *maladaptive psychological symptoms not due to organic causes or psychosis, and usually precipitated by stress.* Apart from generalized anxiety and depression, symptoms include: fatigue[27%], insomnia[25%], irritability[22%], worry[20%], obsessions, compulsions, and somatization—all more intense than the stress precipitating them would warrant. Symptoms are not just part of a patient's normal personality, but they may be an exaggeration of personality: a 'worrier' may become even more so, ie develop an anxiety neurosis, as a result of job loss. The *type* of neurosis is defined by the chief symptom (eg anxiety, obsessional, depressive). Before diagnosing anxiety, consider carefully if there is underlying depression needing antidepressants.[107]

Symptoms of anxiety *Cognitive:* Agitation; feelings of impending doom; poor concentration; difficulty in getting to sleep (insomnia); excessive concern about self and bodily functions; repetitive thoughts and activities (p352). *Somatic:* Tension; trembling; a sense of collapse; 'goose flesh'; 'butterflies in the stomach'; hyperventilation (so tinnitus, tetany, tingling, chest pains); headaches; sweating; palpitations; nausea; 'lump in the throat' unrelated to swallowing (globus hystericus). *Behaviours:* (not strictly symptoms but these actions in response to anxiety state) reassurance seeking (from partner, doctor, etc.); avoidance; dependence on person or object. *Children's symptoms:* Thumb-sucking; nail-biting; bed-wetting.

Causes Genetic predisposition; stress (work, noise, hostile home), events (losing or gaining a spouse or job; moving house). *Others: Faulty learning* or *secondary gain* (a husband 'forced' to stay at home with agoraphobic wife).

Treatment *Symptom control:* Listening is a good way to ↓anxiety. Explain that headaches are not from a tumour, and that palpitations are harmless. Anything done to enrich patients' relationship with others may well help. Anxiety management teaches that anxiety feels bad (even life-threatening) but it does not cause physical damage and that if left, it will resolve with time.
- *Regular (non-obsessive!) exercise:* Beneficial effects appear to equal meditation or relaxation. Acute anxiety responds better than chronic anxiety.
- *Meditation:* Intensive but time-limited group stress reduction intervention based on 'mindfulness meditation' can have long-term beneficial effects.[108]
- *Progressive relaxation training:* A type of behavioural therapy (see: p390). Teach deep breathing using the diaphragm (see BOX), and relaxation of muscle groups (see p391). Practise is essential. CDs aid learning; in some contexts, eg stress, relaxation is not as good as cognitive restructuring.
- *Cognitive behavioural therapy* (p390) and *relaxation* appear to be the best specific measures[109] with 50-60% recovering over 6 months.[110][N=404]
- *Behavioural therapy* with a *graded exposure* to anxiety-provoking stimuli.
- *Hypnosis* Initially the therapist induces progressively deeper trances eg using guided fantasy and concentration on bodily sensations, eg breathing. Later, some patients will be able to induce their own trances. It can strongly reduce anxiety, and is useful, eg medical contexts (eg post-op).[111]
- *Medication:* NICE recommend one or the other—equal efficacy but no evidence of synergy (strangely): see BOX.

Prognosis General anxiety disorder (GAD) often gets better by ~50yrs although is often replaced by somatization.[112]

Deep breathing exercise

▶Try this yourself. You never know when an ability to calm yourself down and avoid becoming overwhelmed with stress may come in use.

We all tend to breathe faster and/or too deeply than normal when stressed or anxious. This can make us feel light headed, which in turn, increases our anxiety, so we breathe even faster, feel dizzier and become more anxious...

This exercise should take around 5 minutes. It is recommend you practise this every day at a time when not anxious. In a stressful situation, or when you feel your stress rising, having a well-rehearsed technique is very helpful.

1 Breathe slowly and deeply in through your nose, and out through your mouth in a steady rhythm
2 Try to make your breath out twice as long as your breath in. It is often helpful to count slowly 'one, two' as you breathe in, and 'one, two, three, four' as you breathe out
3 Fill up the whole of your lungs with air, without forcing. Imagine you're filling up a bottle, so that your lungs fill from the bottom
4 Focus on mainly using your diaphragm ('lower chest muscles') to breathe. When we become anxious we tend to forget to use this muscle and favour the muscles at the top of the chest and shoulders. These create shorter, shallow breathes. Diaphragmatic breathing pulls the lungs downwards which expands the airways to allow air to flow in
5 Relax your shoulders and upper chest muscles when you breathe. With each breath out, consciously try to relax those muscles until you are mainly using your diaphragm to breathe.

(If this is unclear, you can check if you are using your diaphragm by feeling just below your sternum at the top of your abdomen. If you cough, you can feel the diaphragm push out here. When you hold your hand here you should feel it move in and out as you breathe using your diaphragm).

Treating anxiety with medication

Based on NICE guidelines, published in January 2011:
• Consider first-line treatment with a SSRI (as best tolerated). Use the ones you are familiar with, the evidence doesn't strongly favour one over another. Also consider SNRI (venlafaxine or duloxetine) or tricyclic antidepressants, MAOI (phenelzine) as second- or third-line treatments.
• Benzodiazepines are often used first line (especially in general practice) but patients can build up a tolerance to them, and they can be hard to stop. People with a history of harmful drug and alcohol use are likely to over-rely on them. Generally they are not a long-term solution to an anxiety disorder and are best used sparingly and infrequently for acute distress and agitation. If trials of several other medications have failed then long-term use of a benzodiazepine isn't unreasonable.
• Pregabalin can be used as a monotherapy or in conjunction with an antidepressant.
• Antipsychotics (eg quetiapine) are generally reserved for acute distress or sometimes used to augment antidepressant therapy, eg in OCD.
• β-blockers can improve the somatic symptoms of anxiety such as tremulousness, sweating, etc. and can be useful, eg for those who give public speeches. However, they do not improve cognitive anxiety—and can in fact be detrimental as people feel anxious but do not look it—which can affect relationships adversely.

Obsessive-compulsive disorder (ocd) Compulsions are senseless, repeated rituals. Obsessions are stereotyped, purposeless words, ideas, or phrases that come into the mind. They are perceived by the patient as intrusive, nonsensical (unlike delusional beliefs) and, although out of character, as originating from themselves (unlike hallucinations or thought insertion). The compulsions are normally a way to reduce the distress of the obsession. They are often resisted by the patient, but if chronic, the patient may have given up resisting them.

2–3% of people will experience ocd during their lifetime with 7% of British adults reporting 'obsessions' in any week and 4% reporting 'compulsions'. However, it often takes 10–15 years for people to seek professional help.

An example of non-verbal compulsive behaviour is the rambler who can never do a long walk because every few paces he wonders if he has really locked the car, and has to return repeatedly to ensure that this has, in fact, been done. Cleaning (eg hand-washing), counting, and dressing rituals are other examples. *Pathophysiology:* cns imaging implicates the orbitofrontal cortex[113] and the caudate nucleus. Successful treatment is reflected by some normalization of metabolism in these areas.[114] *Treatment:* cbt (p372). **Clomipramine** (start with 25mg/day po) or ssris (eg **fluoxetine**, start with 20mg/day po) really can help (even if patients are not depressed): see p340.

What's it like to have ocd? 'That afternoon, I found that when I got home from school, I couldn't get around the house or do normal things without performing rituals to cancel out bad thoughts over and over again. It was weird and I didn't want to do it, but if I didn't I would feel a lot of anxiety and panic like something was very wrong. I kept having to enter and re-enter through the front door. I ended up spending about three or four hours in the bathroom because I couldn't get out of there because every time I tried to do the perfect ritual, my body would itch or something else would go wrong and I had to redo the rituals over again. After a few hours, I wanted to get out of there so bad, I felt like a prisoner in my own bathroom!'[115]

Phobic disorders Phobias describe a group of disorders in which anxiety is experienced only, or predominantly, in certain well-defined situations that are not dangerous. As a result, these situations are avoided or endured with dread. They become a disorder when they cause marked distress and/or significantly impair a person's ability to function. Phobias are much more common in women than men, affecting about 22 in 1000(♀) compared with 13 in 1000 (♂) in Britain. Phobias are labelled according to specific circumstance.
• Agoraphobia (*agora*, Greek for market place): cluster of phobias: fear of crowds, travel (usually alone on trains or buses) or events away from home.
• Social phobias: where we might be minutely observed, eg small dinner parties; characterized by a fear of scrutiny by other people. Symptoms may include blushing, shaking hands, nausea, or the urgent need to go to the toilet.
• Simple phobia: numerous phobias restricted to specific situations eg dentists (odontophobia), spiders (arachnophobia, p392), clowns (coulrophobia).[10]
• There may also be a free-floating 'fear of fear', or fear of disgracing oneself by uncontrollable screaming.

Elicit the *exact* phobic stimulus. It may be specific, eg travelling by car, not bicycle. Why are some situations avoided? If deluded ('I'm being followed/ persecuted'), paranoia rather than phobia is likely. For panic attacks, try cbt[116] (p373), ± ssri, tca, pregabalin, clonazepam (paroxetine has a short half life and the worst discontinuation symptoms of ssri).[117,118]

---

10 For an exhaustive list of phobias see: http://phobialist.com/. It includes every phobia from Agateophobia (fear of insanity) to Zemmiphobia (fear of the great mole rat).

Psychiatry

'There are some experiences and intimations which scar too deeply to permit of healing, and leave only such an added sensitiveness that memory reinspires all the original horror.'   H.P. Lovecraft; *At the Mountains of Madness*

A reaction to a stressful event is to be expected (and worrying if absent). An *acute stress reaction* is a transient condition (lasting hours to days). There is an immediate dissociation ('daze'), followed by mixed emotions including anxiety, anger, and confusion. These usually resolve without psychiatric intervention (although talking to friends and family often helps). If these symptoms become *chronic*, adjustment disorder (within 1 month) or PTSD (within 6 months) should be considered; symptoms may be delayed for years in some.

Post-traumatic stress disorder (PTSD) develops after an exceptionally stressful, life-threatening, or catastrophic event or situation. Common symptoms include re-experiencing the event in vivid nightmares or flashbacks (often with autonomic arousal: ↑pulse; ↑BP; ↑sweating) often precipitating anxiety or panic attacks, avoidance of things associated with the event, hypervigilance (increased startle reaction), sleep disturbance, and poor concentration. Depression, emotional numbing, drug or alcohol misuse, and anger are also common comorbid conditions. In children, re-experiencing symptoms may take the form of re-enacting the experience, repetitive play, or frightening dreams without recognizable content. There is often denial or suppression of memory for the traumatic event. Intentional acts of violence are more likely than natural events or accidents to result in PTSD. The risk of developing PTSD after a traumatic event is 8% for men and 20% for women.

Pathophysiology: MRI implicates the anterior cingulate area, with failure to inhibit amygdala activation ± ↓amygdala threshold to fearful stimuli.[119,120]

Treatment: Immediate debriefing does more harm than good. Evidence strongly supports trauma-focused treatments, specifically CBT and *Eye movement desensitization and reprocessing* (EMDR). EMDR uses a patient's voluntary rapid, rhythmic eye movements to reduce the anxiety associated with traumatic thoughts/images thereby process the emotions attached to these experiences. While this approach is 'unique', there is enough evidence to suggest that it is effective (and NICE approved). That said, the mechanism for EMDR has not been explained and it has been shown that eye movements are not actually an essential part of the intervention. Other interventions include hypnotherapy (to help control arousal) and stress management. After the 2004 Indian Ocean tsunamis, psychopathology was as common as physical injury: WHO advised practical outreach help, and to avoid mental health labels (different culture to NICE's medicalizing approach to PTSD).[121]

Medication is second line to therapy, however it can be used in combination or if a patient is too distressed to use psychological therapy. If used, SSRIs (paroxetine) are licensed; also consider TCAs (amitriptyline), mirtazapine, MAOIs (phenelzine) and second-generation antipsychotics (p340); warn of SEs and discontinuation phenomena (p356).[122–124]

Prognosis: Dependant on initial symptoms and their severity; usually 50% will recover within 1 year. Recovery improved by lack of maladaptive coping strategies (eg denial), single traumatic event, and no on-going secondary problems (eg disfigurement, legal action, acquired disability).

Prevention: Rehearse teamwork—and techniques of stress inoculation (by exposure), and desensitization (by helping real casualties, eg if preparing for war). Keeping combatants in tight-knit groups cemented by the ties of mutual interdependency is recommended by military strategists. NB: morphine use at the time of injury may be protective. www.killology.com

Psychiatry

Depersonalization This is an unpleasant state of disturbed perception in which people, or the self, or parts of the body are experienced as being changed ('as if made of cotton wool'), becoming unreal, remote, or automatized ('replaced by robots'). There is insight into its subjective nature, so it is not a psychosis, but the patient may think he is going mad. Depersonalization may be primary, or part of another neurosis. CNS imaging shows that it is associated with functional abnormalities in the sensory cortex in areas where visual, auditory, and somatosensory (cross-modal) data integrate.[125]

Derealization These are psychosensory feelings (akin to depersonalization) of detachment or estrangement from our surroundings. Objects appear altered: buildings may metamorphose in size and colour. The patient acknowledges the unreality of these ideas, but is made uneasy by them.

Dissociation (formerly *hysteria*) *Example of mass hysteria spread by TV—Pokeman induced 'seizures': see 'the Pokeman contagion'*[126]
R: Behavioural therapy (p372 ± antidepressants) if he really wants to change.

Types of dissociation Amnesia is the commonest type: see box. *Depersonalization:* Feeling of being detached from one's body or ideas, as if one were an outsider, observing the self; '*I'm in a dream*' or '*I'm an automaton*' (unrelated to drugs/alcohol) eg from stress.

Dissociative identity disorder: The patient has multiple personalities which interact in complex ways. It is present in 3% of acute psychiatric inpatients.

Fugue: Inability to recall one's past ± loss of identity or formation of a new identity, associated with unexpected, purposeful travel (lasts hours to months, and for which there is no 'me' ie the person is no longer themselves).

Follow-up (~6yrs) shows that ~5% of those referred to a CNS hospital who had hysteria/dissociation diagnosed turned out to have organic illness.

Treatment Exploring life stresses may help. Be ready to recognize psychological components of physical illness, and get expert psychiatric help, while leaving the door open for new diagnoses.

Seeking a physical cause Why do some doctors preferentially diagnose somatic illness? Why, when confronted by unexplained symptoms, do we often subconsciously try to fit them to a physical ailment? The reason is usually that prescribing a pill is easier than changing, or regulating, intrapsychic events. The patient and the doctor may collude with this approach, and then get angry when it yields nothing. Alternatively, some doctors are so used to diagnosing psychopathology that they are all too prone to launch into treating someone's depression and malaise, rather than their endocarditis or brucellosis. There is no single correct approach. We all make errors: the point is to find out in which direction you tend to make errors, then allow for this in your work.

Some patients are naively keen to name their condition, eg 'fibromyalgia', or 'somatization disorder'. Being able to name a disease or a condition is to start to control it. But it's only a start. In time, having named a condition may not prove all that helpful—and neither may seeing a string of experts. This paves the way for a cognitive shift that may allow progress—even healing—to come about. As one patient said: 'I stopped focusing on the specific diagnoses years ago, and switched to finding the best ways to increase my overall wellness. I use what I learned about my fibromyalgia to inform my choices, and have figured out what works best for me...Experts are just people, and are sometimes wrong...'

Hypnotic phenomena share features with conversion (hysterical) symptoms, eg lack of concern, involuntariness with implicit knowledge, and a compliant tone (la belle indifférence—a relative lack of concern about the nature or implications of symptoms). Theories of consciousness postulate an altered relationship between self-awareness and the supervisory attentional system in both conditions (frontal and cingulate cortices are implicated).[127] Most subside spontaneously, but if they do not it is important to refer early to a psychiatrist, before associated behaviour becomes habitual.

Things to consider with a dissociative experience include:
• Has a physical cause been carefully discounted? (Drugs, epilepsy, etc.)
• Is the patient young? Beware making the first diagnosis if >40yrs old.
• Have the symptoms been provoked by stress? Ask the family.
• Do related symptoms 'make sense' (eg aphonia in a news-reader)?
• What is the pattern of amnesia? If for distant *and* near memories, then dissociation is more likely (vs organic causes) than if the amnesia is for shorter-term memory.
• Indifference to major handicap is of little diagnostic use.
• Is malingering likely? The answer is usually 'No', except in prisons and the military (when secondary gain is easy to identify).
• Is there a dissociative personality?

The dissociative experiences scale (DES) screens for this: a 28-item visual analogue scale about the proportion of time spent on dissociative experiences (not those from drugs/alcohol) going from the normal, eg being so absorbed in TV that we are unaware of events around us, to severe forms, eg of having no memory of cardinal personal events, or feeling that our body belongs to another. In dissociative disorders, typical DES scores are ≥30; most others score nearer 0.[128]

Withdrawing benzodiazepines ▶*The withdrawal syndrome may well be worse than the condition for which the drug was originally prescribed.* So try to avoid benzodiazepine use, eg relaxation techniques for anxiety, or, for insomnia, a dull (text)book, sexual intercourse, and avoiding night-time coffee may facilitate sleep (see p371). If not, limit hypnotics to alternate nights.

The 'Z' drugs: zaleplon, zolpidem, and zopiclone are commonly prescribed, although this is not advised because tolerance develops with long-term use. Of those on benzodiazepines for 6 months, 30% experience withdrawal symptoms when treatment is stopped, and some will do so after only a few weeks of treatment. Symptoms appear sooner with rapidly eliminated benzodiazepines (eg lorazepam vs diazepam or chlordiazepoxide). It is not possible to predict which patients will become dependent, but 'passive dependent' or neurotic personality is partly predictive. Symptoms often start with anxiety or psychotic symptoms 1-2 weeks after withdrawal, followed by many months of gradually decreasing symptoms, such as insomnia, panic, and depression. Irritability and feelings of unreality and depersonalization (p355) are common; hallucinations less so. Multiple sclerosis may be misdiagnosed as there may be diplopia, paraesthesiae, fasciculation, and ataxia. Gut symptoms include D&V, abdominal pain, and dysphagia. There may also be palpitations, flushing, and hyperventilation symptoms. The problem being not so much how to stop benzodiazepine treatment, but how to avoid being manipulated into prescribing them unnecessarily. This is addressed in the BOX.

How to withdraw • Augment the patient's will to give up (stress disadvantages of continuous treatment) • Withdrawal is harder for short-acting benzodiazepines, so change to diazepam • Agree a contract to prescribe a weekly supply, and not to add to this if it is used up early • Withdraw by ~2mg/week of diazepam. Warn to expect withdrawal symptoms, and not to be alarmed.

Withdrawing antidepressants: All antidepressants may cause a *discontinuation syndrome*. Distinguish between this and *withdrawal symptoms* (implies addiction). Patients often worry that they will get hooked on medication which can affect compliance. Discontinuation symptoms are explained by the theory of *receptor rebound*, eg an antidepressant with potent anticholinergic effects may be associated with diarrhoea on withdrawal,[129] ~30% get the syndrome and it may mimic the original symptoms of the illness (don't confuse withdrawal for relapse.).[130] Withdrawal is best over ≥4 weeks unless fluoxetine is co-prescribed (it has a long t½, so no withdrawal regimen is needed, and it also helps reduce symptoms). For antidepressant cross-tapering, see p349.

Discontinuation symptoms • Onset is within ~5 days of stopping, sometimes after cross-tapering or missing doses. Usually mild and self-limiting but can be prolonged and severe. Some symptoms are more likely with certain drugs. ▶Consider stopping alcohol before starting withdrawal, and starting meditation and an exercise programme.[131,132] *SSRIs: Common:* •'Flu-like symptoms; headaches; nasty shock-like sensations;[133] dizziness; insomnia; tears, irritability, vivid dreams. *Rare:* • Movement disorders; poor concentration/memory; delirium. *The most troublesome is:* paroxetine (short half-life). *MAOIs: Common:* • Agitation, irritability, ataxia, movement disorders, insomnia, ↓cognition, altered speech. *Rare:* • Hallucinations, paranoid delusions. *The most troublesome:* tranylcypromine (metabolized it has amphetamine-like properties so may have real withdrawal). *TCAs: Common:* •'Flu symptoms; insomnia *Rare:* • Movement disorders; mania; arrhythmias. *The most troublesome:* imipramine.

▶Warn the patient about these symptoms. If they expect to feel worse before they feel better, then their reaction will be more measured. They will also tell you if there is something unexpected happening. Ask them to tell family and friends 'I won't be myself for a while.' but assure them this is transient.

We have all been manipulated by our patients, and it is wrong to encourage in ourselves such stiffness of character and inflexibility of mind that all attempts by our patients to manipulate us inevitably fail. Nevertheless, a patient's manipulative behaviour is often counter-productive, and reinforces maladaptive behaviour. A small minority of patients are *very* manipulative, and take a disproportionate toll on your resources, and those of their family, friends, and colleagues. We are all familiar with these patients whom Madox Ford describes as being 'like fireships on a crowded lagoon, causing conflagration in their wake'.[134] After destroying their family and their home we watch these people cruise down the ward or into our surgeries with some trepidation. Can we stop them losing control, and causing meltdown of our own and our staff's equanimity? The first thing to appreciate is that these people *can* be communicated with, and you *can* help them

Setting limits One way of avoiding becoming caught up in this web of maladaptive behaviour is to set limits, as soon as this behaviour starts. In a small minority of patients, the doctor may recognize that their needs for time, attention, sedation, and protection are, for all practical purposes, insatiable. Whatever a doctor gives, such patients come back for more and more, and yet in spite of all this 'input' they don't get any better. The next step is to realize that if inappropriate demands are not met, the patient will not become sicker (there may be vociferous complaints!). This realization paves the way for setting limits to behaviour, specifying just what is and is not allowed.

Take, for example, the patient who demands sedation, threatening to 'lose control' if it is not given immediately, stating that he cannot bear living another day without sedation, and that the doctor will be responsible for any damage which ensues. If it is decided that drugs do not have a part to play in treatment, and that the long-term aim is for the patient to learn to be responsible for himself, then it can be simply stated to the patient that medication will not be given, and that he is free to engage in destructive acts, and that if he does so this is his responsibility.

The doctor explains that in demanding instant sedation he undermines her professional role, which is to decide these matters according to her own expert judgement, and that this is not beneficial to anyone. If there is serious risk of real harm, admission to hospital may be indicated, where further limits may be set. If necessary, he is told that if he insists on 'going crazy' he will be put in a seclusion room, to protect others. Every person is responsible for the decisions they make, and if necessary, security can be asked to escort a patient out of the hospital, in line with hospital policies on abusive behaviour.

Suicide can be simply defined as an intentional self-inflicted death. It is the most common cause of death in men under 35 (in 2014, 78% of deaths by suicide were men <45). In the UK, it is the third ranked category to 'years of potential life lost' after coronary heart disease and cancer. The most common method of suicide in the UK was 'hanging' (56% and 40% of all 6233 suicides)—previously the most common method by women was overdose ('poisoning').

Understanding suicide For some, suicide may feel like the only solution to a life of unyielding mental distress or unbearable social situations—the only viable way to end torment. It can be a form of protest, a way of avoiding shame, ameliorating physical pain (assisted suicide) whilst keeping honour/autonomy.

Risk Increased with mental illness: bipolar disorder, depression, borderline personality disorder, anorexia, substance abuse, and with past self-harm and suicide attempts. See BOX for further suicide risk demographics.

Assessment[11] Think of a target with three concentric rings.

The inner ring is the circumstances of the act: what happened that day; were things normal to start with? When did the feelings and events leading up to the act start? Get descriptions of these in detail. Was there any last act (eg a suicide note)? What happened after the act? Who called for help? Was what followed what they expected? How do they feel about it now? Embarrassed, guilty, regretful (because they attempted suicide or because it didn't succeed).
The middle ring is the background to the act: how things have been over the preceding months. Might the attempt have been made at any time over the last months? What relationships were important over this time? Have they planned for these? Hoarding tablets (by not taking medication they may precipitate mood changes), researching methods, looking at pro-suicide websites.
The outer ring is the relevant family and personal history (p318). Remember to include strengths and positives as well as negatives. Use the patient's own words and descriptions—it is much more powerful to use these later to suggest coping strategies and demonstrates that you really did listen.

Now...come to the *bullseye*, the intention lying behind the act, and the present feelings and intentions. Does the attempt reflect a wish to die (a grave, not-to-be-ignored sign); was it sending a message or to change circumstances? Ask: 'If you were to leave hospital today, how would you cope?' Examine the mental state (p320): is there any mental illness? Ask 'what has changed?'
Summary: • Any plans? What? When? Where? • Are means available? • Other attempts? Seriousness? • Preparations (writing a will, giving things away).

Before arranging hospital admission, ask what this is *for*. Is it only to make you feel less anxious or to gain something that cannot be gained outside hospital. Ask: *Why will discharge be safer in a few weeks rather than now?*

After the assessment, there are four stages in trying to help survivors
• Agree a contract offering help, by negotiation. Discuss confidentiality, then if possible, talk with the support network (ie family, friends) as to how problems are to be tackled. Patients may want to 'go it alone' but is this helpful?
• Treat any co-morbid conditions: depression, anxiety, substance misuse.
• Problem-solving therapy helps by pointing out how the patient coped with past problems.[135]N=1094 The aim is to engender a greater ability to cope in the future and to help with immediate personal or social problems.
• Follow-up, either alone or with the family, with *preventive strategies:*[136] *Promote access to:* Samaritans and doctors; online help (Facebook is addressing this). *Limit access* to lethal means (guns, stored tablets, rope for a noose). *Shift position* from an unstable position (drugs, alcohol, abuse, violence, criminal action) to a stable one (job, community support, caring relationships etc.). Social support if needed.

11 Use clinical judgement and assessment tools: www.medscape.com/viewarticle/730857

A knowledge of risks associated with certain demographics helps inform decisions made about service planning and public health interventions. However, these are based on general trends, treat each individual on their own terms:

• *Gender:* In Britain, completed suicides have a ratio of 3♂:1♀ (between 25-34 this increases 4♂:1♀). These differences are less marked in Asia. Attempted ('unsuccessful') suicides have a ratio of 1♂:3♀ suggesting overall rates are equal. The WHO noted men tend to choose more violent mechanisms, eg hanging and firearms, whereas women favour less violent acts, eg poison.

• *Age:* Highest rates (20% of all suicides) are in the elderly with 2♂:1♀.

• *Marital status:* Risks highest in widow > divorced > single > married.

• *Occupation:* Higher in unemployed and retired, within employment highest rates in unskilled workers, followed by professionals (access to lethal drugs or guns: vets four times expected rate, pharmacists and farmers two times). High rates among prisoners, especially those on remand. Students, contrary to assumption, show risk similar to general population age group.

• *Ethnicity:* Rates among immigrants closely reflect those of their countries of origin, although added pressure from other factors (eg occupation, refugee status). In the UK, place of birth rather than ethnicity is recorded so research is harder. In a London study those of African–Caribbean origin had relatively low suicide rates and young Indian women relatively high rates.

• *Seasonal:* Worldwide, suicide rates are highest in spring and summer.

NB: Comparing global suicide trends is complex as economic and political changes impact differently. In many countries until recently unexplained deaths were not classified as suicide due to cultural pressures and stigma. Changes over time (ie ↑suicide rates) may reflect societal acceptance.

Managing threats of suicide

A psychiatrist can become enmeshed in a web of suicide threats, and may wrongly assume that because someone threatens suicide, they should be admitted to hospital (compulsorily if necessary) so that they can be kept under surveillance, and suicide prevented. This reasoning has three faults. The first is the idea that it is possible to prevent suicide by admission. There is no such thing as constant surveillance. Second, admission may achieve nothing if it removes the person from the circumstances they need to learn to cope with. Third, we must distinguish between suicide gestures, which have the object of influencing others' behaviour, and a genuine wish to die.

Before death, many suicide victims see a GP, and it is wise to be alert to undercurrents of suicide which only sometimes surface during consultations. Ask *unambiguously* about suicide plans (p322). On deciding that a threat is more manipulative than genuine, very experienced therapists may influence the person's use of suicide behaviour by forcing him to face the reality of his suicide talk, eg by asking: 'When will you kill yourself?' 'How will you do it?' 'Who will discover the corpse?' 'What sort of funeral do you want? Cremation, burial, with or without flowers?' 'Who will come?'

See the BOX for risk factors for suicide; they may be of no help in individual cases, so aim to think dynamically of risks and protective factors (eg family support), with suicide occurring after key events that accumulate risk.

▶*Take all suicide threats seriously*—but emphasis differs depending into which group the patient falls. Aim to form a *contract* with the patient, eg:

• The therapist will listen and help if the patient agrees to be frank, and to tell the therapist of any suicide thoughts or plans.

• Agreement about which problems are to be tackled is made explicit.

• Agree the type of change to aim for and who will be involved in treatment (eg family, friends, GP). Agree the timing and place of sessions.

• An agreement to collaborate with the therapist, and to do any homework.

Psychiatry

Suicide and deliberate self-harm (DSH) are not on a continuum. DSH is 'self-poisoning or injury, irrespective of the apparent purpose of the act' whereas suicide is 'intentionally taking of one's life'. NICE state 'DSH is an expression of personal distress, not an illness, and there are many varied reasons for it'.

▶DSH may be 'a cry for help' but *every non-fatal event may be fatal next time*.

Prevalence The UK has one of the highest rates of self-harm in Europe: 0.4%. Of those who have engaged in DSH, 15% repeat the act within 1 year and 25% within 4 years. In a school survey of 15–16-year-olds[137]: DSH lifetime act was 10%, with 7% in previous year. 4♀:1♂ (thoughts of DSH 2.5♀:1♂). WHO estimates 50% of 13–19-year-olds experience suicidal ideation at some point in adolescence. Overdose makes up 90% of referred cases (although it is estimated only 50% of overdoses present to hospital) followed by laceration (8%).

Why do people self-harm? Communicating a message, or gaining power by escalating conflict, often after an argument with a partner. Emotional immaturity, inability to cope with stress, weak religious ties, and availability of drugs (psychotropics and alcohol are popular poisons) are important. For many, DSH offers a release from psychological pain (emotions and worries), replacing these feelings with physical pain. A maladaptive coping strategy with long-term consequences—but in the short term often feels effective (patients report feeling 'alive') and can become addictive due to its immediate effect.

Risk factors *Witnessed DSH:* Family history of DSH (likely environmental and genetic factors), learned behaviour/'copycat' DSH from friends or celebrities—exacerbated by social media (eg tumblr #dsh); *Biological:* reduced endorphin response to emotional arousal (eg traumatic brain damage), abnormalities in serotonin release (mechanism unknown); *Developmental:* poor early care (neglect), physical, emotional and sexual abuse, parental separation; *Peer relations:* conflicts, bullying, poor interpersonal skills; *Psychological:* identity problems (eg cultural, sexual orientation, poor body image), low self-esteem; *Antisocial behaviour:* conduct disorder, impulsivity, substance misuse.

DSH occurs equally across all socioeconomic groups in adolescence. In adults higher rates occur in lower socioeconomic groups.

Management before a psychiatric intervention, prioritize treating physical effects of DSH. NICE include a telling statement 'adequate anaesthesia and/or analgesia should be offered to people who have self-injured throughout the process of suturing or other painful treatments.' During this, issues of capacity (p409), informed consent and when to override this should be considered.

All patients need a psychiatric assessment. Most hospitals will offer a specialist approach in <18s (eg admission and assessment by a CAMHS professional trained to engage this group); some offer this for >65s (increased risk of completed suicide). Waiting for a specialist should be balanced with delay.

Focus assessment on 1 initial risk management—immediate risk of suicide; need for admission 2 on-going risks with subsequent DSH 3 relevant psychiatric, medical and social issues. Try to create a positive therapeutic relationship.

Discharge against medical advice If a person with DSH states a desire to leave before this assessment has been completed, decide if there is diminished capacity and/or the presence of a significant mental illness. If so, referral for urgent mental health assessment is needed. Take time to explain the situation and discuss their options, try to understand why they wish to leave (ie do they have a child home from school?). Offer food/drink (never underestimate what 'a nice of tea' can accomplish). If that fails, you may have to take appropriate measures to prevent a person leaving this 'safe' environment.

Prognosis ~10% of DSH patients require psychiatric admission (mainly depression or alcohol misuse), 1/3 need psychiatric follow-up in community; remainder need help to understand and cope with their psychosocial stressors.

Psychiatry

Occupying the interval between the spilling of our lives and their congealing into history, crisis intervention recognizes that moments of maximum change are times of greatest therapeutic opportunity (fig 4.10).[138] Debate these questions:

• What events have led to these difficulties? Thoughts/actions in the last days.
• What is his mental state *now* (p320)? Depressed? Suicidal? Psychotic?
• In the past how has he been able to combat stress and to resolve crises?
• What solutions to this crisis have been tried? How have they failed?
• Who are the significant people in his life? Can you rely on any of them?

Therapeutic strategy

• If he has been very badly affected by the crisis, you may insist on postponing all normal obligations/ responsibilities to allow concentrated contact ('intensive care') in a therapeutic environment (eg a hospital or crisis unit).

• Take practical steps to safeguard patient's commitments (eg transport of children to other family).

• Choose the best way of lowering arousal (time spent talking is often preferable to administering anxiolytics, which

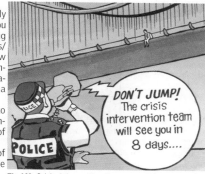

Fig 4.10 Crisis intervention teams must be responsive, immediate, accessible, and available 24/7—anywhere.

may only delay the natural process of adaptation). If the patient is shocked, stunned, or mute, take time to establish normal channels of communication.

• As soon as the person is receptive, promote a sense of hope about the outcome of the crisis. If there is no hope (a mother, consumed by grief, after losing all her children in a fire), then this too must be addressed.

• The next step is to encourage creative thinking about ways whereby the patient might solve the problems. Start by helping him think through the consequences of all options open to him. Then help compartmentalize his proposed solutions into small, easily executed items of behaviour.

As the immediate crisis passes, and the patient has reasonable psychological functioning, it will be necessary to put him back in charge of his own life. A period of counselling is likely to be appropriate (p398). Making a contract about therapy is important in encouraging the patient to transfer from the 'sick role' to a self-dependent, adult role.

Crisis intervention often focuses on loss of face, loss of identity, or loss of faith—in oneself, in one's religion, one's goals, or one's roots.

Meta-analyses suggest that crisis intervention is a viable part of home-care, and can be used during the acute phase of any mental illness.[139]

▶All home-care packages for severe mental illness need crisis management plans. Where implemented, this keeps the vulnerable in contact with staff (NNT≈13 over 1 year) *and* reduces family burden (NNT≈3), *and* is a more satisfying form of care for patients and families. It is also said to be cheaper. In one trial,[140] availability of a crisis-resolution team reduced admission rates from 59% to 22% at 8 weeks—and was highly cost-effective.

There is a widespread misconception that psychiatry has no *genuine* emergencies. Its true that psychiatrists won't descend onto a ward in a flurry of bleeps blaring, ABGs rushing off and everyone shouting 'Stat!'. Psychiatrists often work without a larger team as immediate back-up, expected to make decisions, start treatments, and manage problems alone. Help is often available over a telephone or via discussion the next day so 'holding the anxiety' of the patient, family, and your own is a skill that is often developed through training. That said, overnight on-calls can be lonely and, even in quieter periods, sleep can be prevented as past choices are considered, self-checked, and doubted.

When there are acute situations, a psychiatrist should act as doctor first. That means keeping up-to-date and confident in essential examination techniques and basic life support. Knowing their limits is equally important: when to call for help and how to do this—familiarize yourself with local protocols, crash team contact numbers, and where important equipment is kept (and if it's missing then follow this up and request a replacement—better to ask early than need something on a dark and lonely 2am call out and discover it absent).

> *'At a cardiac arrest, the first procedure is to take your own pulse.'*
> Laws of the House of God, House of God, Samuel Shem

When arriving at a crisis, don't forget first principles: find out who requested you attend, ask them what has happened, what their main concerns are, what they have already done, and what they expect you to do (ie what's your role?).
▶ Whatever else is happening, keep safety a priority: yours, staff and patient's

Severe behavioural disturbances can be due to a variety of causes: *Organic:* delirium (p364), brain injury, intellectual disability (p378); *Intoxication:* drugs and alcohol; *Psychiatric:* psychosis, anxiety, mania; *Personality:* antisocial personality disorder (p380), frustration—or a combination of any of these. If there are concerns about safety then manage the danger first (see p363) before attempting an assessment. When safe to do so, consider triggers, diagnosis, and management. If there is no psychiatric or physical reason for the behaviour then have a low threshold to involve hospital security and/or police.

Intoxication It is unhelpful to try to engage a patient in a meaningful assessment while they are intoxicated. If you have ever had a conversation with a very drunk friend you will have experienced slurred speech, unfinished sentences, and misplaced melancholy. Better to allow them to 'sober up' before assessing. However, it is important to ensure their medical needs are still cared for and not ignored. Agree a plan with ED staff and a time you will return.

Self-harming behaviour It is tempting to not respond to these behaviours in a effort to avoid reinforcing them, however it is essential that appropriate medical care is given promptly. Try to manage your frustrations in these cases. If in doubt, liaise with medical colleagues, eg consult Toxbase: www.toxbase.org/ in overdose, and delay a full assessment until medically safe to do so.

Safeguarding Everyone working with vulnerable patients has a duty to keep them safe. Safeguarding is often applied to <18s but can equally relate to older adults or those who lack capacity. Concerns can be direct (ie reported abuse, domestic violence) or indirect (admitting a single father means children will need to have someone to look after them). Ask about risks and dependants. Discuss any concerns with nominated safeguarding team. A safeguarding lead should always be available.

Neuroleptic malignant syndrome Uncommon life-threatening neuroleptic (antipsychotic)-induced disorder which requires immediate treatment. *Symptoms:* Fever, muscle rigidity, delirium and autonomic instability. Markedly raised serum creatine kinase. *Management:* Stop the causative factor, use supportive measures, treat rhabdomyolysis and admit. *Mortality:* 10–20%

A person can be violent as a result of psychiatric illness, substance misuse, personality disorder, or physical illness. Or it may be the result of adverse ward environments: overcrowding, noise, alienation, and nowhere to go (no blue skies or green fields). This is the danger if sequestration on the ward is the result of withdrawal of privileges for 'bad behaviour'.

- Recognize early warning signs: tachypnoea, clenched fists, shouting, chanting, restlessness, repetitive movements, pacing, gesticulations. Your own intuition may be helpful here. At the first hint of violence, get help. If alone, make sure you are nearer the door than the patient.
- Do not be alone with a patient you do not feel safe with; have a low tolerance to request security/police if needed (although be aware that this can intimidate a patient or cause them to become more aggressive).
- Try and take them out of a crowded area if that is appropriate and possible—consider the other patients and bystanders.
- Try calming and talking with the patient. Do not touch him. Use your body language to reassure: sitting back (closer to door than the patient), open palms, attentive. Listen to their concerns without judgement:

▸▸De-escalation ▸▸Time-out ▸▸Placement, as appropriate

- Get his or her consent. If he does not consent to treatment, emergency treatment can still be given to save life, or if serious deterioration.
- Use minimum force possible.

(After the Maudsley *Prescribing Guidelines*.)

Rapid tranquillization

This is the use of medication in controlling behaviour. It should only be used as a last resort when non-pharmacological methods of behaviour control have failed.

- Offer *oral* treatment. If the patient is prescribed a regular antipsychotic, *lorazepam* 1-2mg or *promethazine* 25-50mg avoids risks associated with combining antipsychotics. Oral options if not already on regular oral or depot antipsychotic: (*olanzapine* 10mg, *quetiapine* 100-200mg, *risperidone* 1-2mg or *haloperidol* 5mg). Avoid using more than one antipsychotic to avoid QT prolongation (rapid tranquillization predisposes to arrhythmias).
- Repeat after 45-60min. Monotherapy with buccal *midazolam* 10-20mg may avoid the need for IM drugs (unlicensed).

If 2 doses fail or sooner if the patient is placing themselves or others at significant risk—consider IM treatment. Consider the patient's legal status and consider consulting a senior colleague. Options:

- *Lorazepam* 1-2mg IM (dilute with equal volume of water for injections). Have flumazenil to hand ∴ respiratory depression. Be cautious if very young or elderly, and those with pre-existing brain damage or impulse control problems, as disinhibition reactions are more likely.
- *Promethazine* 50mg IM is useful in a benzodiazepine-tolerant patient. Promethazine has slow onset, but is often effective. Dilution is not needed before IM injection. It may be repeated up to 100mg/day. Wait 1–2h to assess response. It is an extremely weak dopamine antagonist.
- *Olanzapine* 10mg IM; don't combine olanzapine with IM benzodiazepine.
- *Haloperidol* 5mg is last-choice as incidence of acute dystonia is high; ensure IM procyclidine is to hand. Repeat after 30–60min if insufficient effect.

Seek expert advice from consultant or senior clinical pharmacist on call.

▸▸Monitor vital signs every 5–10min for 1h, and then half-hourly until ambulatory (if he refuses, observe for signs of pyrexia, hypotension, oversedation and well-being). If unconscious, monitor oximetry. A nurse must accompany until ambulatory. Monitor ECG, U&E, & FBC if high-dose IM antipsychotics used.

Acute confusion state (ACS) or delirium is an organic reaction which can be differentiated from chronic conditions, such as dementia. Patients in ACS have a fluctuating, impaired consciousness with onset over hours or days, or a rapid deterioration in preexisting cognitive function, with associated behavioural changes which include:

• *Cognitive function:* Worsened concentration, slow responses, confusion and disorientation in time (doesn't know day or year).
• *Perception:* Visual or auditory hallucinations.
• *Physical function:* Reduced mobility, reduced movement, restlessness, agitation, changes in appetite, sleep disturbance. Often these behaviours are fluctuating: varying between quiet or drowsy with occasional agitated outbursts so that you are called when he is 'disrupting the ward'.
• *Social behaviour:* Lack of cooperation with reasonable requests, withdrawal, or alterations in communication, mood and/or attitude. As part of their ACS, patients may become delusional (usually poorly developed delusions), for example accusing staff of plotting against them.

ACS can be hyperactive (agitated and upset), hypoactive (drowsy and withdrawn), or mixed. On a busy ward, it is the hyperactive ACS patients who cause disruption and gain attention while those hypoactive ACS are not noticed.

It is most often seen in those patients with prior vulnerabilities such as post-operative patients, the elderly, and the very young, and therefore common on surgical and medical wards (10–20%). ACS can have serious consequences (such as increased risk of dementia and/or death) and, for people in hospital, may increase their length of stay in hospital and their risk of new admission to long-term care. If there is no past psychiatric history, and in the setting of a physical illness or post-surgery, an ACS is particularly likely.

Differential diagnosis Withdrawal from alcohol/drugs, mania, post-ictal or if agitated, consider psychosis or anxiety. All are readily distinguished on history-taking. Always consider dementia (which usually has an insidious onset and occurs in clear consciousness ie without drowsiness, etc.)

Causes See TABLE; almost anything with a neurological/systemic effect can result in an ACS. Most often the cause is: infection; drugs (benzodiazepines, opiates, anticonvulsants, digoxin, L-dopa); U&E↑↓; hypoglycaemia; ↓P_aO_2; alcohol withdrawal; trauma; surgery (esp. if pre-op Na+↓ or sensory loss).

Investigations U&E, FBC, blood gases, glucose, cultures (blood, MSU), LFT, ECG, CT, CXR, LP. If a cause is not identified, consult a neurologist urgently.

Management should consider a holistic approach:
• Find the precipitating cause and treat this, and other exacerbating factors.
• Optimize supportive surroundings and nursing care (see BOX).
• Avoid sedation unless there is extreme agitation, risk, or needed for investigations to take place. Give antipsychotics in first instance as benzodiazepine tend to worsen delirium with exception of alcohol withdrawal.
• If needed, consider haloperidol 1–10mg/24h or olanzapine 2.5–10mg/24h (smallest dose possible, esp. if elderly). Monitor BP. Wait 20min to judge IM effects (side effects: BP↑↓, stroke, insomnia, dyspepsia).
• Regular clinical review and follow-up.

Interventions to limit acute confusional states

Because ACS is a common occurrence, it is often thought of as an unavoidable adverse effect to admission. However, preemptive steps can be taken:
- Avoid moving people within and between wards unless absolutely necessary.
- Manage disorientation by providing appropriate lighting, clear signage, and a clock (consider providing a 24-hour clock in critical care) and a calendar.
- Talk to the person to re-orientate them by explaining where they are, who they are, and what your role is; explanation of what is happening and why.
- Introduce cognitively stimulating activities: talking, reminiscence work and facilitating regular visits from family and friends.
- Address dehydration and nutritional needs by ensuring adequate fluid intake to prevent dehydration and by encouraging the person to drink and eat.
- Address infection by looking for and treating infection, avoiding unnecessary catheterization, and implementing infection control procedures.
- Address immobility or limited mobility by encouraging people to mobilize soon after surgery.
- Carry out a medication review for people taking multiple drugs, taking into account both the type and number of medications.
- Address sensory impairment by resolving any reversible cause, eg impacted ear wax, and ensuring hearing and visual aids are available to and used by people who need them, and that they are in good working order.
- Promote good sleep patterns and sleep hygiene by avoiding nursing or medical procedures during sleeping hours, if possible scheduling medication rounds to avoid disturbing sleep.

Causes of organic reactions		
	Acute (delirium)	**Chronic (dementia)**
Degenerative		*Alzheimer's; Huntington's (OHCM p694); *Lewy-body (OHCM p478), CJD & Pick's (p650)
Other CNS	Cerebral tumour or abscess; subdural haematoma; epilepsy; acute post-trauma psychosis	Tumours; subdural haematoma; multiple sclerosis; Parkinson's; normal pressure hydrocephalus
Infective★	Many, eg meningoencephalitis; septicaemia; cerebral malaria; trypanosomiasis	Late syphilis; chronic or sub-acute encephalitis; CNS cysticercosis; cryptococcosis; HIV
Vascular	Stroke (or TIA); hypertensive encephalopathy; SLE	Thromboembolic multi-infarct (arteriosclerotic) dementia
Metabolic	*U&E↑↓; *hypoxia; *liver and kidney failure; non-metastatic cancer; porphyria; *alcohol withdrawal	Liver and kidney failure non-metastatic or metastatic cancer
Endocrine	Addisonian or hyperthyroid crisis; diabetic pre-coma; hypoglycaemia; hypo/hyperparathyroidism	T_4↓; Addison's; hypoglycaemia hypopituitarism; hypo-/hyper-parathyroidism[141]
Toxic	*Alcohol; many drugs (check datasheet/statement of product characteristics); lead; arsenic; mercury	*'Alcohol dementia'; barbiturate abuse; too much manganese or carbon disulfide
Deficiency	Thiamine; B_{12}; folate; nicotinic acid	Thiamine; B_{12}; folate; nicotinic acid

★ denotes a leading cause.

Dementia is a syndrome of progressive and global intellectual deterioration without impairment of consciousness. Memory loss is often the first symptom noted although progression to other deficits will continue including:

• *Behaviour:* restless, repetitive and purposeless activity; rigid, fixed routines.
• *Personality changes:* sexual disinhibition; social gaffes; shoplifting; blunting.
• *Speech:* syntax errors; dysphasia; mutism.
• *Thinking:* slow, muddled; poor memory (with confabulation); no insight.
• *Perception:* illusions, hallucinations (often visual).
• *Mood:* irritable, depressed, emotional incontinence (labile mood and crying).
Remember the **4A's** *of Alzheimer's*: **A**mnesia, **A**phasia, **A**gnosia, **A**praxia.

Dementia incidence is 6% of those ≥65 years old. For a diagnosis to be made, there should be significant impairment of normal function with other differentials, in particular normal ageing, delirium, and depression, ruled out.

Irreversible causes of dementia include: Alzheimer's disease[62%], vascular[15%], mixed[10%], Lewy body[4%], fronto-temporal[2%]. Reversible causes[15%] include: subdural haematoma, hydrocephalus, hypothyroidism.

Investigations Full history of function and decline; a collateral history from friends/relatives FBC; B_{12}; folate (MCV↑ suggests alcoholism, or ↓B_{12} or folate); ESR (malignancy); U&E, LFT, γGT, Ca^{2+} (renal/hepatic failure, alcoholism, malignancy, endocrinopathy (Ca^{2+} ↑ or↓). TSH (hypothyroidism); serology: syphilis (*OHCM* p419) ±HIV (only if suspected by history); CT/MRI excludes tumours, hydrocephalus, subdural, stroke, etc.

Management ► *Involve the patient in her own therapy.*
• Full assessment, including functional and social needs for the patient and consider the needs of carers and any risk factors
• Exclude the treatable and manage exacerbating factors eg medical illness, depression (SSRI), insomnia (hypnotics), agitation (antipsychotics)
• Psychological work: patient and carer; there may be a time when patient no longer recognizes those closest to them and may need institutionalized care
• Cognitive enhancement: acetylcholinesterase inhibitors and/or antioxidants
• Supportive work: promote independence; help with functional (mobility, self-care) and social (financial, accommodation) issues
• Relative support: carer's allowance, holiday, admissions, and support groups.

Alzeimer's disease (as an example of dementia)

Presentation: In *mild Alzheimer's disease* there is amnesia and spatial disorientation. In *moderate Alzheimer's disease* (some years later): personality disintegration, eg with aggression or depression, and focal parietal signs, eg dysphasia and apraxia. Parkinsonism may occur. She may use her mouth to examine objects (hyperorality). *Severe Alzheimer's disease* Neurovegetative changes with apathy (or ceaselessly active—akathisia), wasting, incontinence, ±seizures/spasticity.

Mean survival: 7 years from clinical (overt) onset; 5–15 years from diagnosis.

Pharmacological treatment: Increase CNS acetylcholine by inhibiting the enzyme causing its breakdown (donepezil; rivastigmine; galantamine). Memantine, a NMDA (N-methyl-D-aspartate) receptor antagonist, may help moderate to severe Alzheimer's disease. Cautions: creatinine↑; epilepsy; bradycardia with ACEI. SE: confusion, headache, hallucinations, and tiredness; rarer: vomiting, anxiety, hypertonia, and cystitis, ↑libido. Dose: initially 5mg each morning, ↑in steps of 5mg at intervals of 1 week to 10mg/12h.

Prevention/protection: Looking after cardiovascular health, attaining higher educational level before the illness ('cognitive reserve'), statins (relative risk 0.29); antioxidants.[142][n=1364]

Cognitive function tests

For mild memory impairment the TYM test (Test Your Memory, *OHCM* p85) is widely available The most commonly known measure for cognitive impairment is the mini mental state examination. It is a sensitive, valid, and reliable 30-point questionnaire which includes checks for registration, attention and calculation, recall, language, ability to follow simple commands, and orientation. However, it cannot be freely used in clinical settings for copyright reasons. This has led to researchers looking for alternative strategies in assessing cognition for example, the abbreviated mental test:

The following questions are put to the patient. Each question correctly answered scores one point. A score of 7–8 or less suggests cognitive impairment at the time of testing, although further and more formal tests are necessary to confirm a diagnosis of dementia

 1 Patient's age?
 2 Time (to the nearest hour)?
 3 Address for recall at end of test (eg 42 West Street)
 4 Current year?
 5 Identification of this place (eg hospital)
 6 Identification of two persons (doctor, nurse, etc.)
 7 Date of birth?
 8 Year of First World War?
 9 Name of present monarch?
10 Count backwards from 20 to 1.

Clearly this test is very culturally specific, and while it can be updated (for example, changing monarch to prime minister) this will impact on its validity.

The MOCA (Montreal Cognitive Assessment: 30-points) and the Addenbrookes Cognitive Examination revised (ACE-R: 100-points) are also widely used. The AMT is a screening tool mostly used in acute medical settings.

Frontal lobe function tests

The frontal assessment battery (FAB) is a bedside test to help discriminate fronto-temporal type dementia from others. The maximum score is 18, higher scores indicating better performance.

 1 Similarities (conceptualization)
 2 Lexical fluency (mental flexibility)
 3 Motor series 'Luria' test (programming)
 4 Conflicting instructions (sensitivity to interference)
 5 Go–No-Go (inhibitory control)
 6 Prehension behaviour (environmental autonomy).

For full instructions for the FAB see:
www.dementia-assessment.com.au/frontotemporal/frontal_fab_scale.pdf

Many issues in child psychiatry overlap with aspects of adult psychiatry, and also with paediatrics. The psychiatry of intentional overdose is a good example. Many of these patients will be in the last phases of childhood, and it is unclear which service will suit them best. As ever, take a holistic view of the young person and tailor a care plan which takes these facets into account.

Child and Adolescent Mental Health (CAMH) services are organized into four tiers to provide help to children, young people and their support network
- T_1: professionals whose main training and role is not CAMH eg GP, teacher
- T_2: CAMH specialists working in teams in community eg psychologist
- T_3: multidisciplinary CAMH team in a specialized service for more severe, complex or persistent disorders eg CAMH psychiatrist, nurse, OT
- T_4: essential tertiary services such as intensive community treatment services, day units and inpatient units eg eating disorders or secure ward.

Depression in children and adolescents Remembering back to our own teenage years, it's no surprise that many adolescences face major mental health challenges as they change and start to develop their adult identity: body, dress, responsibilities, and sexuality. Add to this pressure from school (exams!), peers (sex, drugs, and socializing), parents, urban stress, and the media ('fizzy drinks make teenagers more violent'[12]) . Its a lot to manage.

Depression affects around 3% of children and 5.6% of adolescents. The stress-vulnerability model is helpful to consider aetiology: vulnerability (genes, endocrine) interact with stress to cause depression at times of life stress.

Clinical features are often more subtle and less constant than in adults:
- Mood changes: grumpy or irritable rather than very 'sad'; anhedonia
- Thought changes: loss of self-esteem, confidence, and concentration
- Physical changes: reduced energy, sleep, appetite; self-harming behaviour.

But the result is an impairment of functioning: missing school and social life.

Assessment One-to-one interviewing is often difficult as adolescents are not very talkative so it's important to pick up on non-verbal communication, use silences to give space, and non-judgemental language. Collateral from parents and school is helpful, as are objective rating scales. Always ask the patient directly about alcohol and drug use, bullying, abuse, and suicidal thoughts. Offer them the opportunity to discuss these issues initially in private.

Treatment Mild depression is best managed in tier 1/2 services with up to 4 weeks of 'watchful waiting' followed by simple non-directive supportive therapy or guided self-help; if unresponsive then refer to CAMH specialists. For moderate/severe depression, newest NICE guidance suggests an antidepressant (only fluoxetine is licensed for under 18s) and psychological therapy may be started concurrently, without an initial trial of psychological therapy (previously NICE suggested therapy alone for at least 3 months). There is little clear evidence to favour one psychological therapy over another. Antidepressant use should be 'cautiously' in children aged 5-11. If combined treatment is not effective within a further six sessions, review the formulation in a MDT.

Also consider addressing sources of distress (eg bullying) and removing opportunities for self-harm (eg no paracetamol at home). Improve sense of belongingness, especially if they feel like an outsider (eg sexuality, substance abuse).[143] If criminality and gang culture invovled, peer mentorship may help.[144]

Specific drugs to avoid if <18yrs old, if possible (BNF): Citalopram, paroxetine, sertraline. Also tricyclics, venlafaxine, and fluvoxamine.[145,146]

Recovery is 10% at 3 months, 50% at 1 year, and 80% at 2 years. Treatment shortens the illness duration. Even after recovery 3% risk of completed suicide over next 10 years. Follow-up monitoring is essential.

12 Chris Smyth, *The Times*, asks (www.thetimes.co.uk/tto/health/news/article3204986.ece) and NHS choices answers (www.nhs.uk/news/2011/10October/Pages/fizzy-drinks-teenage-violence.aspx). Spoiler: 'no.'

Child and Adolescent Psychiatry: Psychosis

Psychotic symptoms do not mean psychosis or 'schizophrenia'. In fact, around 3 out of every 100 young people will experience a psychotic episode and many more will have transient psychotic symptoms. There can be many reasons for this: sleeplessness, drugs, music ('earworms') or cultural norms (ie ghosts[147]). In young children, fantasy play involving imaginary friends and a blurring of reality and fact is an important stage of neurotypical development. However, 5% of adults with schizophrenia report onset of psychosis before 16 years and 20% before the age of 20, so all new symptoms should be fully assessed.

In many centres, early-onset schizophrenia is diagnosed with the same criteria as adults as it seems to be continuous with later-onset forms (eg more males affected). A sustained psychosis is considered to be >4 weeks.

Assessment As with any new patient, take a full history to understand that individual's difficulties at that time. Obtain collateral information from carers and school—especially about recent changes. Complete a MSE (p320) and physical examination and consider screening investigations (urine drug screen).

Symptoms Adolescents occasionally present with non-specific psychotic symptoms, such as odd beliefs, mistrust of others, and magical thinking. These overvalued ideas lead to a decline in interpersonal and school functioning. Whether this represents the prodromal phase of a severe psychotic disorder is difficult to answer prospectively. However, frank psychosis develops in up to 40% of affected patients within 12 months of symptom onset. A positive family history of psychosis and marked impairment of functioning with evolving psychosis-like symptoms are considered to be risk factors for psychotic illness.

▶ Some hallucinations are more serious and should receive urgent attention:
• Those which are imperative ('kill your sister') or exciting strong emotions.
• Those heard unambiguously outside the head.
• Those referring to ideas that the person feels are not their own.
• Multiple voices talking at once, and especially voices talking to each other.

Sometimes hallucinations resist diagnosis. This is not in itself a problem as the diagnosis will sooner or later become clear. Check whether these odd ideas are likely to indicate an increased risk of serious outcome, eg suicide.[148,149]

Causes of odd ideas • Substance abuse • Psychosis (schizophrenia) • Anxiety • Depression • Hypomania • Head injury • Epileptic aura • SLE • Anti-NMDA receptor antibody encephalitis • Alice-in-Wonderland syndrome (OHCM p708).

Management Early intervention (see p393) helps, and may reduce chances of later chronic illness, so prompt referral is essential.[150] Every treatment plan should include a named worker and incorporate antipsychotics (if indicated) in conjunction with psychoeducational work, psychotherapy (individual CBT and family interventions), and social components. Newer antipsychotics (p340) are rarely specifically licensed for children, but their use in well-monitored environments is encouraging.[151] If a clear diagnosis of psychosis cannot be made, NICE advise regular monitoring for changes in symptoms and functioning for up to three years in CAMH or by the patient's GP.

Compliance is especially challenging in adolescents. Keep the young person engaged in their treatment by establishing a good rapport, encouraging insight, and education about relapse prevention. Even with the best of care, adolescents want to experiment with non-compliance. It may be better to shift from optimal care to harm minimization in order to keep engagement.

Prognosis Spontaneous improvement of psychotic-like symptoms occurs in the majority of children. In one follow-up study, many developed chronic mood disorders; <50% met diagnostic criteria for a major disorder (schizoaffective, bipolar, depression). In those not developing a mood or psychotic disorder, disruptive behaviour disorders are very common.[152]

Psychiatry

Attachment is the powerful emotional bond between baby and caregiver. Babies need someone to protect, care, and look after their emotional and physical needs. Sensitive care giving helps a child learn to understand the world and their place in it. They establish a fundamental understanding of love and trust, which allows a child to develop emotional regulation, awareness of others' feelings, and promotes healthy relationships. Attachment fails if a child is abused, neglected (eg drug addiction), or abandoned physically or psychologically (primary care-giver with severe mental illness, eg postnatal depression, psychosis). Without secure attachment, a child is at risk of forming emotional, social, and behavioural problems lasting into adulthood.

Reactive attachment disorders can be diagnosed before 5 years old. These fall into two categories: a child is *inhibited* (extremely withdrawn, emotionally detached, and hypervigilant) or *disinhibited* (seeking comfort from anyone, even strangers, and extremely dependent and immature). Most have anger, an undeveloped conscience, and control issues. Treatment combines psychological therapy (family and play therapy) and parenting skills education.

Behavioural disorders 30–40% of all CAMH referrals will be for a disruptive <18-year-old; within these referrals oppositional defiant disorder (ODD): 5–10% children and conduct disorder: 2–9%. Many behaviours, eg changing appearance, withdrawing (a little) from family, emotional lability, experimentation (drugs, alcohol), and selfies might seem bizarre to parents but are a normal part of adolescence. Even fighting, lying, and stealing are seen in varying degrees in most 'normal' children over the course of development.

Conduct disorder (CD) costs £100,000 more per person aged 10–28 than average. The lifetime cost of a 1-year cohort of CD children is £5.2 billion. The overriding feature is an intense, repetitive, and persistent pattern which significantly deviate from age-related, socially acceptable norms. These cause significant impairment of the child as judged by parents, teachers, or others. Isolated acts of aggression, destruction, theft, or fire setting may be sufficiently severe to warrant concern in their own right. *Diagnosis:* CD core symptoms are: 1 Defiance of will of authority (usually police) 2 Aggression 3 Antisocial behaviour (eg property damage, vandalism, theft, truancy). Three acts must have been exhibited in the last 12 months with at least one present in the last 6 months in multiple places (school, home, community). *Oppositional defiant disorder* is considered a subsection of CD with a enduring pattern of negative, hostile, and defiant behaviour without serious violation of societal norms or rights of others. It may only be present in one environment and is more evident in interactions with familiar adults or peers. *Treatment:* Three empirically supported treatments: 1 Parent Training Programs (eg 'Triple P' or Webster Stratton courses) 2 Individual cognitive therapy for older children 3 Multisystemic therapy (eg with young person, family, criminal justice system). *Prognosis:* Most children with CD will not progress to antisocial personality disorder (although 40% of those with an adult PD met criteria for childhood CD). CD infers higher risk of other mental health problems, substance misuse, criminal activity, and early death often by violent and sudden means.

School refusal is different from truancy (intentional non-attendance at school). It is a severe difficulty in attending school, often amounting to prolonged absence with parental knowledge, due to emotional upset and excessive fearfulness, and somatic complaints. *Setting:* Emotional overprotection; high social class; neurotic parents; schoolwork of high standard. In truancy, the reverse is true. *Treatment:* Liaise with head teacher, parents, and an educational psychologist. Escort by an education welfare officer aids prompt return. Other methods: educational-support therapy, CBT, and parent-teacher interventions.[153] In the past, hypnosis has been used. Often anxiety (eg separation-anxiety or phobias) ± depression need treatment too.[154]

Not falling asleep Try plenty of daytime activity (each hour of sitting ↑sleep latency by 3min).[155] Insist on a routine wind-down one hour before bed→warm bath for 10min→a story→then straight into a darkened bedroom.^{Gurney method}

Waking at 3am *(ready to play or wanting entry to parent's bed)* Most don't appreciate these visitations, refuse to play, and buy earplugs to lessen the impact of tantrum (or let the child into the bed). Try extinguishing the behaviour by attending to the child ever more distantly: cuddle in bed→cuddle on bed→sitting on child's bed→voice from doorway→distant voice. Some accept this as part of normal development (I was awake today at 6:20am thanks to my 3-year-old!). In any case, avoid hypnotics (unless there is extreme concern).

Other sleep disturbances Hunger/colic (infants); poor routines (preschool); worry (adolescence). Bedroom TV may be to blame. Try behavioural therapy before hypnotics. Day-time sleepiness: *Causes:* night sleep↓; depression; sleep apnoea (OHCM p186); narcolepsy;[13] encephalitis lethargicans (rare in children): suspect this whenever sleepiness occurs with extrapyramidal effects, oculogyric crises, myoclonus, inversion of diurnal rhythms, obsessions, and mood change. *Possible causes:* influenza; flu vaccination;♣ measles; Q fever; mycoplasma. MRI: subcortical involvement.

Sleepwalking & parasomnias[14] The young are by far the best somnambulists (sleepwalkers) although the old may emulate them, eg if stress is augmented by excess alcohol or caffeine use, and lack of stage IV sleep—our deepest sleep. Any psychic event associated with sleep may be termed a parasomnia. *Parasomnias comprise:* •*Arousal disorders* (sleepwalking; night terrors; 'confusional arousal') •*Sleep-wake transition disorders* (rhythmic head-banging disorder) • *REM sleep parasomnias* (REM sleep-associated nightmares, sleep paralysis, hallucinations, and REM sleep behaviour disorder. •*Others.*[13]

It is common to observe movement in children during sleep: it is their *repetitive* nature which allows the diagnosis of rhythmic movement disorder. The movement may be body-rocking, leg-rolling, or head-banging (this 'jactatio capitis' may lead to subdurals, fractures, eye injuries, and false accusations of abuse). Tongue-biting may suggest epilepsy. But do not try to be too obsessive in differentiating parasomnias from nocturnal epilepsy. EEG: rhythmic slow anterior activity; video polysomnography: sleep-related violent behaviour, sudden awakening and dyskinetic or dystonic movements, and complex behaviours ± enuresis.[156] *Antiparasomniacs:* Bedtime clonazepam; amitriptyline; carbamazepine. Self-hypnosis or waking ½h before the expected event.[157]

Sleep hygiene teaches patients to sleep without medication. SLEEP summarizes the non-pharmacologic treatment of uncomplicated sleep disturbances: •schedule—consider a patient's sleep-wake schedule. Consistency is key to normalizing sleep. Keep sleep to night-times only • Limit caffeinated or alcoholic drinks and nicotine (nocturnal withdrawal) well before bedtime • Eliminate factors that create a 'hostile' sleep environment: noise, excessive light, and poor ventilation and temperature control (cooler is better) • Exercise performed during the day (but not immediately before going to bed) is an effective antidote to the psychic stress and physical tension that often contribute to insomnia. Helpful exercise routines enhances overall health and restrict daytime sleeping • Psychotherapy (CBT) for insomnia has demonstrated efficacy and may simultaneously improve associated anxiety and/or depression.

13 In narcolepsy we succumb to irresistible attacks of inappropriate sleep ± vivid hallucinations, cataplexy (sudden hypotonia), and sleep paralysis (BOX). Mutations lead to loss of hypothalamic hypocretin-containing neurons, via autoimmune destruction. HLA DR2+ve. R̃: 1 Methylphenidate, 10–15mg PO after breakfast and lunch) may cause dependence and psychosis 2 Modafinil (~200mg/d PO, before noon; SE: anxiety, aggression, dry mouth, euphoria, insomnia, BP↑, dyskinesia, alk phos↑ 3 Gamma-hydroxybutyrate (GHB).[158]

14 Sleep-related dissociative disorder, sleep enuresis, exploding head syndrome, hypnagogic or hypnopompic hallucinations, catathrenia (end-inspiratory apnoea + groaning), sleep-related eating disorders, drug-induced parasomnias, myoclonus nocturnus; nocturnal bruxism, ie teeth grinding.

Psychiatry

Psychiatry

ASDs are *the* lifelong pervasive developmental disorders of our times. *Prevalence:* ≥1:200[159] ♂:♀ ≈4:1. Managing autism is challenging, however ASDs are a range of conditions along a severity spectrum. The core symptoms are:

1 Persistent deficits in social communication and social interaction across multiple contexts (NB: previously split into language and social interaction)
2 Restricted, repetitive patterns of behaviour, interests, or activities.

These must have been present in the early developmental period, although may not have become problematic until social demands exceed limited capacities. When manifested, these symptoms cause clinically significant impairment in functioning (social, occupational, etc.). These difficulties are not due to another condition, intellectual disability, or global developmental delay.

Cause Unknown; genes (on chromosome 11p12 ± neurexin) play a part.[160] If one child is affected, risk of next sibling being affected is ~5-10%. There is associated epilepsy in 30%. No association with MMR vaccine (p151).[161]

Diagnosis requires a specialist team often made up of doctor (psychiatrist/ paediatrician), psychologist, and speech and language therapist. There is no individual test so assessment includes a detailed history, collateral from school, and observation across different settings. Often a team will be trained to use diagnostic instruments such as the Autism Diagnostic Observation Schedule (ADOS) or developmental, dimensional, and diagnostic interview (3di) to produce a formalized framework for diagnosis, including severity.

Clinical features of ASDs fall into three broad areas. These are usually observed by the child's carers or teachers prior to referral as being 'different' than others.

1. Impaired reciprocal social interaction
• Unawareness of the existence and feelings of others (treating people as furniture; being oblivious to others' distress or need for privacy).
• Abnormal response to being hurt: he doesn't come for comfort; or makes a stereotyped response, eg just saying 'Kiss it better, kiss it better, kiss it...'
• Impaired imitation (eg does not wave 'bye-bye' or copies/echoes without understanding, eg waves on passing a door when no one is in fact leaving).
• Repetitive play: eg solitary, or using others as mechanical aids.
• Bad at making friends (lack of empathy). If he tries at all, the effort will lack the social conventions, eg reading the phone directory to uninterested peers.

2. Impaired imagination *(part of abnormal communication)*
• Little babbling, few facial expressions or no gestures in infancy.
• Avoids mutual gaze; no smiles when making a social approach; does not greet his parents; stiffens when held.
• Does not act adult roles; no interest in stories; no fantasy/pretend play.
• Odd speech, eg echolalia (repetitions); odd use of words and pronouns.
• Difficulty in initiating or sustaining reciprocal roles in conversations.

3. Poor range of activities and interests
• Stereotyped movements (hand-flicking, spinning, head-banging).
• Preoccupation with parts of objects (sniffing or repetitive feeling of a textured object, spinning wheels of toys) or unusual attachments (eg to coal).
• Marked distress over minor or trivial changes (eg a vase's place).
• Insists on following routines in precise detail.
• Narrow fixations, eg lining up objects, or amassing facts about weather.

Management *Early intensive behavioural intervention* ± *speech therapy*[162] ± *special schooling* starting at 3 can ↑IQ in >60% and enhance motor, social, and living skills.[163] *Parent training:* ↑ ASD knowledge, enhances parent-child interaction, and ↓parental maternal depression.[159] *Support:* eg National Autism Society. *Social skills training* can help. *Drugs* have a small role: risperidone (agression), melatonin (sleep), and SSRIs (repetitive behaviour).[164] *Diet:* Eliminating gluten is popular but unproven.[165] *Benefits:* eg Disability Living Allowance.

Attention deficit hyperactivity disorder (ADHD)

Attention deficit hyperactivity disorder (ADHD) is the most common neurobehavioural disorder of childhood. It has prevalence of 3–5% in Western nations.[166] 80% of cases are genetically inherited. The core diagnostic criteria are: *impulsivity*, *inattention*, and *hyperactivity* (see MINIBOX) across settings. *There is no diagnostic test* (but positron emission tomography may show ↓function of frontal lobes and nearby connections). Most parents first note hyperactivity at the toddler stage, but most locomotor hyperactivity at this stage abates with time, so the diagnosis is usually delayed until school entry or later. *Differentials* include: age-appropriate behaviour, low (or high) IQ, hearing impairment and behavioural disorders. *Associations:* Conduct disorder (p370) or other disruptive behaviour disorders (eg ODD p370).[167] Young people with ADHD are at risk of being victims of assaults, as well as suicide and self-harm.[168] Signs often attenuate during adolescence, but may persist into mid-adulthood—evidence suggests by 18 years ⅓ have no symptoms, ⅓ have symptoms which don't need medication and ⅓ still need medication.

Inattention
Often unable to:
• Listen/attend closely to detail (∴ carelessness)
• To sustain attention in play activities
• Follow instructions
• Finish homework (when not due to defiance)
• Organize tasks needing sustained application
• Loses/forgets things
Hyperactivity
• Squirming/fidgeting
• 'On the go all the time'
• Talks incessantly
• Climbs over everything
• Restless
• No quiet hobbies
Impulsivity
• Blurts out answers
• Interrupts others
• Cannot take turns
• Intrudes on others
• Poor road safety

Diagnosis is made through careful history taking from young person and collateral from parent and teachers, observation at school and clinic, rating scales (eg Conner's), and screen for comorbidity and organic causes.

Treatment:[169 NICE] Diagnosis and treatment ought to be initiated by a specialist (eg psychiatrist/paediatrician). Following diagnosis, time for explanation is required; offer a booklet to parents, give advice on *positive parenting* and *behavioural techniques*. In moderate ADHD impairment, parent training/education programmes are recommended. Older children may also benefit from CBT. If non-drug treatments fail, the 1st-line treatment is *methylphenidate* available as immediate release (eg Ritalin®) lasting 4 hours or modified release lasting up to 12 hours. Longer-lasting medications are better tolerated and allow a child to last an entire school day. It is recommended that medication is not given at weekends/holidays as it reduces appetite and therefore can suppress growth. *Atomoxetine*, an alternative drug, takes up to 6 weeks to reach full efficacy but appears to show lasting effect even on withdrawal (maybe due to its gradual effect rather than the on/off effect in methylphenidate). Severe ADHD in school age children: methylphenidate and atomoxetine are 1st-line treatments so ensure referral. Evidence for long-term use is uncertain.[170,171] but 70% of young people show symptomatic improvement on medication. Caution is required when prescribing methylphenidate (a controlled drug) due to its street value as a drug of misuse (as it is an amphetamine, similar to speed). Check for substance misuse.

Does ADHD exist?

ADHD 'overdiagnosis' is a controversial topic with some claiming that doctors are medicalizing normal childhood activity and undermining parents in order to increase pharmaceutical profits (mainly in the US). However those who have treated a child who is initially unable to sit still and focus in school before treatment and then, on medication, has improved grades and demonstrably social functioning feel justified in continuing to use the label ADHD.

Psychiatry

'I hurt myself today. To see if I still feel. I focus on the pain. The only thing that's real. The needle tears a hole. The old familiar sting. Try to kill it all away. But I remember everything.' 'Hurt', Johnny Cash (originally by Nine Inch Nails)

Epidemiology of drug addiction Cannabis is commonly used by young people (♂: 33% ♀: 22%), ecstasy is the commonest class A drug (♂: 9% ♀: 4% aged 16-24).[172] Heroin users account for ~70% of Home Office[uk] notified addicts. Naming all drugs is too numerous.[15] NB see p513 (nicotine) and p376 (alcohol).

Causes Individual factors (age, gender, family) interact with external factors (culture, price, availability, advertising).[173] Being a novelty seeker and impulsive greatly increases risk. Inherited vulnerability is equally important.[174]

Suspect drug addiction if: • Arrests for theft, to buy drugs • Odd transient behaviour, eg visual hallucinations, elation, mania • Unexplained nasal discharge (cocaine sniffing or opiate withdrawal) • Withdrawal symptoms (eg red eyes, shaking) • Injection stigmata: marked veins; abscesses; hepatitis; HIV • Repeated requests for analgesics, only opiates acceptable, or sedatives.

Clinical presentation[175] *Acute intoxication:* Administration of a psychoactive substances resulting in disturbances of level of consciousness, cognition, perception, affect, or behaviour. *Harmful use:* A pattern of psychoactive substance use that is causing actual damage to mental or physical health or social functioning. *Dependence syndrome* (see BOX) is a cluster of physiological, behavioural, and cognitive phenomena where the use of a substance takes on a much higher priority than other behaviours which once had greater value. There is evidence that returning to a substance after abstinence leads to a more rapid dependance than occurs with non-dependent individuals.

Opiate detoxification and methadone maintenance is ideally as part of a regimen in which a contract is made with the patient (p357), eg in a special clinic or in primary care, provided GP has an interest and commitment.[rcgp.org.uk]

Methadone prescribing should be used as part of the transition to abstinence. Physiologically, methadone use is still opiate addiction—the difference being it is free (eliminating a need for crime/prostitution to fund the next fix) and taken orally (no injection-related issues). In reality, many patients cannot commit to abstinence so methadone maintenance is used as an alternative which is safer to both addict and society. *Daily observed methadone dosing* is the norm (NB: monthly supplies are not necessarily abused).[176] Cocaine use by patients on methadone is a big problem, and is associated with a poorer prognosis. **Disulfiram** has a role here.[177,N=67] A non-addictive alternative is **lofexidine** (α_2-noradrenergic agonist like clonidine) SE: drowsiness, BP↓, pulse↓, dry mouth, rebound hypertension on withdrawal.[178] **Buprenorphine** is a synthetic partial agonist at μ-opioid receptors. It may be safer then methadone;[179] Cautions: liver dysfunction; intoxication with other drugs (eg CNS depressants). **Naltrexone** is an opioid antagonist (blocks euphoria—useful in former addicts to prevent relapse). Warn patient of possible withdrawal reactions and monitor for 4h after 1st dose; monitor LFT.
Psychological support: Tailor to specific needs (residential or outpatient care, in groups or 1-to-1). Counselling, motivational therapy, cognitive therapy (p390), Alcoholics Anonymous, '12 steps programme', family therapy (p396) are all valuable ways to address triggers, motivation to change, and relapse prevention. Counsel about HIV & hepatitis C risk, needle exchange, and safe sex.

Relapse prevention As strong cravings precede relapse, anti-craving drugs seem to be a promising but unvalidated approach. See acamprosate, p376.

Barbiturate withdrawal may cause seizures ±death; withdraw as an inpatient (⅛ of the previous daily dose as phenobarbital over 2 weeks).

15 Hydrocarbons/glue sniffing, barbiturates, opiates, LSD, ecstasy, amphetamine, MDMA, cocaine, salvia divinorum, mephedrone, 'legal highs', magic mushrooms (psilocybin), nitrous oxide, Meow-Meow, cake...

Dependence syndrome

A central descriptive characteristic of the dependence syndrome is the desire (often strong, sometimes overpowering) to take a substance (which may or may not have been medically prescribed). Requires 3 or more of the following:
1 A strong desire or sense of compulsion to take the substance (craving)
2 Difficulty in controlling substance use (onset, termination, level of use)
3 A physiological withdrawal state when reducing or ceasing substance use (or using the same (or closely related) substance to avoid withdrawal)
4 Tolerance: increased doses are required to produce the original effect
5 Progressive neglect of alternative pleasures or interests
6 Persisting use despite clear evidence of harmful consequences.

Drug-induced psychosis

A typical problem is trying to diagnose a young man presenting with hallucinations and/or delusions. The question often is: *Are these odd ideas due to schizophrenia, drug abuse, or physical illness?*
7 Most auditory hallucinations not associated with falling asleep or waking up are caused by schizophrenia or depression.
8 In 90% of those with non-auditory hallucinations (eg seeing things), the cause is substance abuse, drug withdrawal, or physical disease.
9 Evidence that substance abuse is to blame includes:
  •*The history:* Ask the patient, the family, and friends about abuse. Be precise about timing. If ≥4 weeks elapse between abuse and starting of odd ideas, substance abuse is an unlikely cause (but substance abuse may be an enabling factor promoting later psychosis).
  •*Severity of symptoms:* If symptoms are severe, and the quantity of drug ingested is trivial, the drug is unlikely to be causative.
  •*Drug-seeking behaviour:* Be on the lookout for this.
  •*Physical examination:* This may reveal signs of drug abuse (eg injection marks ± cellulitis), chronic alcohol abuse (eg spider naevi, liver palms, atrophic testes), or a physical medical illness (eg brain tumour).
  •*Blood or urine tests* may disclose the substance abused or give a hint of abuse (MCV↑ and γ GT↑ in alcohol abuse).
  •*Imaging:* Consider CNS imaging if the patient is elderly with nothing to suggest substance abuse, or if there are CNS signs.
NB: middle-age is not a typical time for schizophrenia to present: alcohol abuse or a primary CNS condition is more likely.

Diagnosing a *substance-induced psychotic disorder* implies that the patient responds to the hallucinations or delusions as if they were real. If the patient recognizes the hallucinatory nature of the experience, then consider diagnosing *substance intoxication, substance withdrawal,* or, if there is past but no current exposure to hallucinogens, the diagnosis may be 'flashbacks'—ie *hallucinogen persisting perception disorder*. This condition presents episodically up to 5 years after exposure to an hallucinogen, with flashback hallucinations—or phenomena such as geometric visual hallucinations, seeing coloured flashes, or intensified colours, dots, spots, or flashes, seeing trailing images or after-images, seeing complementary coloured images of objects gone from view, seeing halos, seeing things too small (micropsia), or seeing things too big (macropsia). These phenomena may be self-induced or triggered by darkness, stress, or fatigue. DSM-5 175

Psychiatry

In medical students, alcohol correlates with missing study, sexual escapades, fisticuffs, etc.[180] In Britain it is estimated that 26% of adults (♂: 38% ♀: 15%) were assessed as being 'hazardous drinkers' ie showing a pattern of drinking which risked physical or psychosocial harm. Alcohol *abuse* implies that repeated drinking harms a person's work or social life. *Addiction* implies:

- *Increased tolerance* to alcohol
- *Withdrawal:* sweats, nausea, or tremor
- Narrowing of drinking repertoire
- Priority is to maintain alcohol intake
- Difficulty or failure of abstinence
- Often aware of compulsion to drink.

Assessment History usually shows a gradual deterioration in function, as alcohol dependence overtakes work, relationships, financial stability, and health as the patient's primary concern. An early warning sign is that the patient's drinking habits are excessive within their own social context. Are they always the last one at the bar or finding new contexts in which to drink (at a cinema, immediately on return from work, etc.)?

Screening questions Two simple, short tools to highlight at-risk drinking are the CAGE and TWEAK questions. Remember, these do not assess dependence or abuse—often a mistake made is to ask about drinking first, then use these.

Withdrawal signs (Delirium tremens) Pulse↑; BP↓; tremor; fits; visual or tactile hallucinations, eg of insects crawling under the skin (formication). **℞** *treatment:* • Admit; monitor vital signs (beware BP↓). • For the 1st 3 days give diazepam generously, eg 10mg/6h PO or PR if vomiting—or IVI during fits; chlordiazepoxide is an alternative. After a few days, ↓diazepam (eg 10mg/8h PO from day 4-6, then 5mg/12h PO for 2 more days).

Management Does the patient want to change? If so, be optimistic, and augment his will to do so. Should *abstinence* or *controlled intake* be the aim? If the former, remarkable recovery of organs (eg hippocampus) is possible.[181]

Treat coexisting depression (p344). Refer to specialists. Self-help/group therapy (Alcoholics Anonymous) help, ± drugs which produce a nasty reaction if alcohol is taken (disulfiram 200mg/24h PO). Reducing the pleasure that alcohol brings (and craving on withdrawal) with naltrexone 25-50mg/24h PO (an opioid receptor antagonist) can halve relapse rates.[182] N=111 SE: vomiting, drowsiness, dizziness, joint pain. CI: hepatitis; liver failure; monitor LFT. Get expert help. Acamprosate (OHCM p445) can improve abstinence rates. CI: pregnancy, severe liver failure, creatinine >120μmol/L; SE: D&V, libido ↑ or ↓; dose example: 666mg/8h PO if >60kg and <65yrs old. Economic analysis supports its use, at least in some communities.[183] N=448

Alcohol & organ damage *Liver:* (normal in 50% of alcoholics). *Fatty liver:* Acute, reversible; hepatitis; 80% progress to cirrhosis (*liver failure* in 10%) *Cirrhosis:* 5yr survival 48% if alcohol intake continues (if it stops, 77%).

CNS: Poor memory/cognition; cortical/cerebellar atrophy; retrobulbar neuropathy; fits; falls; accidents; neuropathy; Korsakoff's/Wernicke's encephalopathy (SEE BOX and OHCM p728); ⇒Urgent parenteral vitamins are needed.

Gut: D&V; peptic ulcer; erosions; varices; pancreatitis.

Heart: Arrhythmias; BP↑; cardiomyopathy; *fewer* MIs (?benefit only if ≥55yrs).

Skeleton: Heavy drinking disrupts calcium metabolism (osteoporosis risk↑).[184]

Sperm: Fertility↓; sperm motility↓ *Malignancy:* GI & breast. *Marrow:* Hb↓, MCV↑

Social: Alcohol is related to violent crime and suicide.

Alcohol and drug levels Regular heavy drinking *induces* hepatic enzymes; binging *inhibits* enzymes. Be alert with phenytoin, warfarin, tolbutamide, etc. NB: paracetamol may cause ↑N-acetyl-*p*-benzoquinoneimine (it is hepatotoxic). **Homelessness** is common; help with housing & rent, problem-solving, communication, drink refusal, and goal setting *can* help this desperate problem.[185]

See also 'Managing alcohol misuse' p512.

Alcohol screening tools

CAGE **questionnaire**

1 Have you ever felt you should **C**ut down on your drinking?
2 Have people **A**nnoyed you by criticizing your drinking?
3 Have you ever felt bad or **G**uilty about your drinking?
4 Have you ever had a drink first thing in the morning to steady your nerves or to get rid of a hangover (**E**ye opener)?

A total score of *2 or greater* is considered clinically significant (sensitivity of 93% and a specificity of 76% for the identification of problem drinking). However, CAGE is less sensitive for identifying those not alcohol-dependent but still at-risk drinkers. A patient's demographics have been found to limit its performance. Some studies show a sensitivity as low as 50% in adult white women and just 40% in at risk groups aged 60+.

The TWEAK is a modification of the CAGE and includes a question about tolerance; it has a sensitivity of 87% for harmful drinking and 84% for dependence. It has also been found to be better than the CAGE for screening pregnant patients

1 **T**olerance: How many drinks can you hold? or How many drinks does it take to make you feel high? (not both)
2 **W**orried: Have close friends or relatives worried or complained about your drinking in the past year?
3 **E**ye-opener: Do you take a drink in the morning when you first get up?
4 **A**mnesia (blackouts): Has someone ever told you about things you said or did while you were drinking that you could not remember?
5 **C**ut down: Do you sometimes feel the need to cut down on your drinking?

Scoring: Q1: two points if ≥6 drinks, Q2: two points if 'yes' and Q3–5: one point for each positive answer. An answer of *>6 to either part of Q1* or a *total score of ≥3* denotes a problem with alcohol use.

Wernicke's encephalopathy and Korsakoff's syndrome

Wernicke's encephalopathy resulting from thiamine (vitamin B_1) deficiency, usually related to alcohol abuse. *Symptoms:* A classical triad of 1 confusion 2 wide-based gait ataxia 3 ophthalmoplegia (nystagmus, conjugate gaze, and bilateral lateral rectus palsies). Also with clouding of consciousness, memory disturbance, peripheral neuropathy, hypotension, hypothermia, and ptosis.

Causes: Chronic alcohol consumption can cause ↓ nutritional thiamine intake, ↓ absorption from GI tract and ↓ utilization in cells resulting in inadequate dietary intake. Always consider this complication in alcoholics, although also occurs due to brain tumor, malabsorption, and to prolonged vomiting: hyperemesis gravidarum, chemotherapy. *Treatment:* This is a medical (not just psychiatric) emergency. Give high-dose IV/IM thiamine (Pabrinex®) over 1 week, then oral supplementation until no longer 'at risk' (also consider if other vitamin deficiencies). NB: if there is coexisting hypoglycaemia (often seen in this group), ensure thiamine is given before glucose, to prevent Wernicke's being precipitated by glucose administration (in a thiamine-deficient patient).

Prognosis: Failure to appropriate treatment results in death in ~20% of patients, and 85% remaining left with Korsakoff's syndrome.

Korsakoff's syndrome Hypothalamic damage and cerebral atrophy due to thiamine deficiency. There is an inability to acquire new memories, confabulation (invented memory, owing to retrograde amnesia), lack of insight and apathy. ¼ of cases are reversible but ¼ will require long-term institutional care. Even if successful, recovery is slow and often incomplete.

Definition Below-average general intellectual functioning which originated during the development period and is associated with impairment in adaptive behaviour (Heber 1981). Be aware: *people with an intellectual disability are at an increased risk of developing physical and mental illnesses.*

Four subtypes: *Mild* (IQ 50-70): accounts for 80% of people with intellectual disabilities. There is useful development of language, and intellectual difficulty only emerges as schooling gets under way. Most can lead an independent life. *Moderate* (IQ 35-49): most can talk and find their way about. *Severe* (IQ 20-34): limited social activity is possible. *Profound* (IQ <20): simple speech may be un-achievable. Special schooling and medical services are needed, as is adequate care and counselling for the families involved. In the UK, lack of resources and ambiguous community responsibilities are big problems.[186] *Further information:* ask MENCAP (www.mencap.org.uk).[187]

Epidemiology 27 per 1000 (80% have IQ 50-70). People with intellectual difficulties are at ↑risk for mental illness compared to the general population.

The patient *Physical:* Sensory and motor disabilities, epilepsy, incontinence. *Psychiatric:* All psychiatric disorders can occur but the *presentation* is modified by low intelligence. In the *diagnosis* of psychiatric disorder, emphasis is given to the behavioural manifestation of the disorder.

Causes *Physical causes* are found in 55-75% of severely intellectually disabled individuals. *Chromosomal abnormalities:* Down's syndrome, fragile x syndrome (Martin–Bell syndrome, p648). *Antenatal causes:* Infections, alcohol, hypoxia, nutritional growth retardation, hypothyroidism. *Perinatal causes:* Cerebral palsy. *Post-natal causes:* Injury, infections, impoverished environment.

Forensic issues Arson and sexual offences, eg exhibitionism (♂) or, more rarely, 'public disrobing' (♀).[188] Care is needed in questioning a person with an intellectual disability about an alleged offence, due to increased suggestibility and risk of making false confessions. Treatment may centre on issues of accepting that the offence took place, the taking responsibility for offences, accepting the intention of the offending behaviour, and on victim awareness.[189] Behavioural approaches might focus on masturbatory satiation, covert sensitization, and stimulus control procedures.[190]

Assessing a person with an intellectual disability •Cause(s) of the intellectual disability •Associated medical conditions •Intellectual and social skills development •Psychological and social functioning •Dialogue with and support for carers.

Care of people with an intellectual disability •Prevention and early detection is the aim—as is care in generic (eg NHS) services (minimized specialist care) unless there are complex physical, emotional, and behavioural issues.[191] •Regular assessment of attainments and disabilities •Advice, support, and help for families—eg teaching parents how to be better 'tutors' can help[192] •Arrange special needs teaching at school and training/occupation •Housing and social support to enable self-care •Medical, nursing, and other services, as outpatients, day patients, or inpatients •Psychiatric and psychological services usually from a community-based multidisciplinary team.

Treatment of psychiatric disorders •Side effects of medication may not be apparent as a person with a intellectual disability may not be able to draw attention to them •Antipsychotics can lower seizure threshold and patients with intellectual disability are more likely to get seizures •Behavioural therapy is widely used.

The following 14 *specific* rights must be taken in the context of *general* psychiatric rights: • To have a professional skilled in dealing with your condition • To receive treatment based on sound evidence • To have treatment in a setting which is decent, humane, and non-abusive • regimens must promote a fulfilling social life • Active participation in all decisions taken about care.

1 Ensure full assessment within the context of joint strategic needs assessment by Social Services, GPs, and other professionals fully trained in 'partnership working'.

2 Include the person in all decisions affecting him or her.

3 Promote enriching activity to counter idle humdrum impoverished living.

4 Listen to concerns of both the person and their carer.

5 Derive personalized care plans via dialogue with the person and carer(s).

6 Explain what the options are, ideally in terms that he/she understands.

7 Help him or her decide from a defined list of genuine choices.

8 Don't hurry through consultations 'to get back to normal people'; spend *more* time; go *slowly*. Not being able to give a good history doesn't mean you can skip this bit: it means you must use other methods to get the information. For example, discussions with carers eg 'The Cardiff Healthcheck for People with a Learning Disability' a questionnaire looking at all aspects of health completed by carers prior to annual review, or by your own direct observation of the patient.

9 Don't be pleased because they are not complaining of anything. No reported symptoms and no complaints about circumstances does not let you off the hook! You may need to insist to carers that a nasty but apparently painless ulcer be treated—or that a fire-escape be unblocked.

10 Check for physical illnesses which may otherwise go unreported.

11 Watch for neglect/abuse from well-meaning, under-trained, over-worked staff (who may desperately crave your support and encouragement).[193]

12 Don't reach too readily for drugs to curb behaviour. Consider all options.

13 Be aware of local authority *Protection of Vulnerable Adults* protocols.

14 No tokenism! (paying lip service to the above without intending change)

Psychiatry

'There's such a lot of different Annes in me. I sometimes think that is why I'm such a troublesome person. If I was just the one Anne it would be ever so much more comfortable, but then it wouldn't be half so interesting.'

L.M. Montgomery, Anne of Green Gables

Personality is a mix of lasting characteristics which make us who we are: easy-going or anxious; optimistic or pessimistic; placid or histrionic. This spectrum of distinct traits overlap and are describable in terms of a few independent dimensions (eg introvert/extrovert). Those with abnormal personalities occupy an extreme in the spectrum. Abnormal personality only matters if it is maladaptive, causing suffering either to its possessor or his associates—called a *personality disorder*. In general, psychological symptoms which are part of a personality disorder are harder to treat than those arising from other causes.

But personality can change and develop as we learn and adapt (consider the naïve medical student morphing into confident consultant) so is it really fixed? Many consider this a controversial diagnosis. Critics claim it is used to medicalize anyone having difficulties coping with life or as a final resort when symptoms do not easily fit any other diagnosis. At worst, a diagnosis of blame.

Personality disorders are characterized by long-lasting rigid patterns of thought, affect, and behaviour. The attitudes of people with a disorder usually exaggerate part of their personality and result in behaviour at odds with 'normal' expectations. These conditions must not be attributable to brain damage or another psychiatric disorder. They all meet the following criteria:

1 Markedly disharmonious attitudes and behaviour, involving usually several areas of functioning, eg affectivity, arousal, impulse control, relationships
2 Prevailing, chronic, abnormal behaviour patterns, not limited to discrete episodes, which are pervasive and clearly maladaptive
3 Present in a broad range of personal and social situations
4 Manifestations appear <18 years old and continue into adulthood
5 There is considerable personal distress caused by these patterns of behaviour (although this may only become apparent later in the course)
6 Associated (usually but not invariably) with significant problems in occupational and social performance.

Classification of personality disorders is categorical whereas personality is dimensional. A TABLE (see p381) is provided to give a summary and should be used to understand features rather than form a diagnosis.

▶ Remember everyone has a personality but not every personality, no matter how distinct it may be, is disordered. Avoid labels and engage with the person.

Management Scant evidence that psychiatry helps those with a personality disorder diagnosis—essentially treating someone with a problem integrating into society not a mental illness. However, these disorders are associated with higher rates of premature death (including suicide) and other mental illnesses. In general: • Treat the individual • Reflect their goals • Help manage crises • Treat comorbid conditions • Consider patient/professional relationship.

Medication plays no part in treating a personality disorder (can be used for comorbid condition) so talking therapies are recommended: • Dialectical behavioural therapy (DBT) combines individual and group therapy using mindfullness, CBT and Eastern philosophy • Therapeutic communities • Mentalization.

Prognosis is generally poor. As mentioned, people diagnosed with a personality disorder have higher rates of morbidity and mortality, worse outcomes for associated mental and physically illnesses, and lowered quality of life markers. Taking this in account, the prevalence of personality disorders (particularly borderline and antisocial) declines with age. This may be as older adults tend to be less impulsive and aggressive or maybe just better at hiding these traits.

Psychiatry

Personality disorder clusters Research suggests that personality disorders tend to fall into three groups, according to their emotional 'flavour' (historically and anecdotally labelled as 'mad, bad, and sad'):
• Cluster A: *Odd or Eccentric*
• Cluster B: *Dramatic or Emotional*
• Cluster C: *Anxious or Avoidant*.

	ICD-10	Gender bias	Description
A	Paranoid	Male	Suspicious, preoccupied with conspiratorial explanations, distrusts others, holds grudges
	Schizoid	Male	Emotionally 'cold', lacks interest in others, rich fantasy world, excessive introspection
	Dissocial (*In DSM-5*: Antisocial)	Male	Aggressive, easily frustrated, callous lack of concern for others, irresponsible, impulsive, unable to maintain relationships, criminal activity, lack of guilt, conduct disorder (<18yrs)
B	Emotionally unstable (two types)	Female	*Borderline:* Feeling of 'emptiness', unclear identity, intense and unstable relationships, unpredictable affect, threats or acts of self-harm, impulsivity, pseudohallucinations *Impulsive:* Inability to control anger or plan, unpredictable affect and behaviour
	Histrionic	Male	Over-dramatize, self-centred, shallow affect, labile mood, seeks attention and excitement, manipulative behaviour, seductive
	(*DSM-5 only*) Narcissistic	Male	High self-importance, lacks empathy, takes advantage, grandiose, needs admiration
	Anankastic (obsessive–compulsive)	Male	Worries and doubts, orderliness and control, perfectionism, sensitive to criticism, rigidity, indecisiveness, pedantry, judgemental
C	Anxious	Equal	Extremely anxious, self-conscious, self-conscious, insecure, fearful of negative evaluation by others, timid, desires to be liked
	Dependent	Female	Passive, clingy, submissive, excess need for care, feels helpless when not in relationship, feels hopeless and incompetent

Psychiatry

► You may well recognize some aspects of your own personality in these descriptions. This doesn't (necessarily) mean a personality disorder. Some of these characteristics may even be helpful in some areas of your life (eg anakastic renal physicians triple check U&Es and narcissistic surgeons operate successfully where others might waver). Disorder arises when there is disruption to the person's life (whether they see it or not).

Anorexia nervosa ►The most fatal of all mental illnesses (~20%, if severe). There is a compulsive need to control eating and body shape. Weight loss becomes an over valued idea, ie belief in being 'fat' even when weight is very low. Males with anorexia tend to want high muscle mass rather than thinness. In both of these, ideal body shapes are 'achieved' by food refusal (initially diet restriction) combined with over-exercising, induced vomiting, laxative abuse. Many also have episodes of binge eating, followed by remorse, vomiting, and concealment. Low self-worth is common in all. *Diagnostic criteria:* 1 Weight <85% of predicted (taking into account height, sex, and ethnicity, p181), or BMI ≤17.5kg/m². 2 Intense fear of gaining weight, or becoming fat, with persistent behaviour that interferes with weight gain 3 Feeling fat when thin.

NB Endocrine change (♀: amenorrhoea, ♂: ↓libido) have been removed in DSM-5

Epidemiology: ♀:♂≥4:1[194] Men are likely to be undiagnosed as anorexia isn't investigated. Typical age of onset is mid-adolescence—but can start at any age. *Prevalence:* 0.7% in teenage girls and no restriction to a particular ethnic group. *Incidence in primary care:* 20:100,000♀ aged 10-39.

Cause: The exact cause of eating disorders is unknown.[195] The evidence for risk factors includes *biological:* genetics (55% concordance in MZ twin studies), serotonin dysregulation; *psychological:* depression; anxiety; obsessive compulsive features; perfectionism;[196] low self-esteem; absent sense of identity; *developmental:* adverse life events and difficulties (most commonly in close family/friend relationships), dietary/feeding problems in early life; parents preoccupied with food (ie parent with own eating disorder). There is scant evidence that the chief problem is psychosexual immaturity (antecedent sexual abuse is not a *specific* risk factor); *sociocultural:* substance abuse; negative body images due to media exposure; image-aware activities (eg ballet);[197] past teasing or criticism for fatness.[198]

Signs: Most due to starvation or vomiting. *General:* fatigue, ↓cognition, altered sleep cycle, sensitivity to cold, dizziness. *Gastrointestinal:* constipation, fullness after eating. *Reproductive:* psychosexual problems, subfertility, amenorrhoea. *Haematologic:* ↓WCC, anaemia, ↓platelets. *Endocrine/metabolic:* glucose↑↓, ↓K⁺, ↓PO₄³⁻, ↑bicarbonate, ↑LFT, ↑amylase, ↑T₃/T₄, ↓TSH, ↓LH/oestrogen, ↑GH, ↑cortisol, ↑CCK, ↓renal function, osteoporosis. *Cardiovascular:* ↓BP; prolonged QT, arrhythmias. *Neurological:* ↓visuo-spatial ability, ↓visual memory, ↑speed of information processing, peripheral neuropathy. *Dental:* caries. *Dermatological:* dry skin, brittle hair, lanugo hair (fine downy hair all over body).

SCOFF questionnaire: (Can be used for screening.) Do you ever make yourself sick because you feel too full? Do you worry you've lost control over eating? Have you recently lost more than one stone in 3 months? Do you believe you are fat when others say you are thin? Does food dominate your life? One point for every 'yes'; >2 indicates a likely anorexia nervosa or bulimia

ΔΔ: Depression, Crohn's/coeliac disease, hypothalamic tumours.

Red flags—risk↑↑ if: ⚬ BMI <13 or below 2nd centile ⚬ Wt loss >1kg/wk ⚬ T°: <34.5°⚬ Vascular: BP <80/50; pulse <40; S₃O₂ <92%; limbs blue and cold ⚬ Muscles: unable to get up without using arms for leverage. ⚬ Skin: purpura ⚬ Blood (mmol/L): K⁺ <2.5; Na⁺ <130; ↓PO₄³⁻ <0.5. ⚬ ECG: long QT; flat T waves.

Treatment: Aim to restore nutritional balance eg weight gain of 0.5-1kg (~3500-7000 extra calories/week); final BMI 20-25). Treat complications of starvation. Explore comorbidity. Involve family/carers: difficult family dynamics are often a prominent feature; address this appropriately (avoiding blame) and include family in treatment and as a resource needed to help manage the condition. Address factors maintaining the illness. Patients initially coming into services will often be in denial—do not allow them to disengage.

Severe anorexia (BMI <15kg/m², rapid weight loss + evidence of system failure) requires urgent referral to eating disorder unit (EDU), medical unit (MU), or paediatric medical wards (P). Re-feeding is considered 'treatment' under the Mental Health Act 1983/Children Act 1989, and it may be needed if insight is lacking. In *moderate anorexia* (BMI 15-17.5, no evidence of system failure) routine referral to local eating disorder service or EDU if available. In *mild anorexia* (BMI >17.5) focus on building a trusting relationship, acknowledging problem and change. If no response in 8 weeks, consider referral to secondary care. Psychological interventions include CBT (p390), interpersonal, supportive, or family therapy (±parent-to-parent consultations[16]). In <18s consider family therapy.[199] Limited evidence base for the pharmacological treatment; mainly to treat comorbid conditions. **Olanzapine** may help stimulate appetite (unlicensed use). **Fluoxetine** has been used (need to monitor QT interval).

Prognosis: ⅓ recover completely, ⅓ improve, and ⅓ develop a chronic eating disorder. 5% die (mostly from suicide or direct medical complications, eg ↓K⁺ and prolonged QT interval predisposing to arrhythmias). Median time between diagnosis and death is ~11 years.[200] Mortality is higher if: aged 20-29 at presentation, delayed access to treatment, bingeing, and vomiting.

Re-feeding syndrome Potentially fatal condition from ↓PO₄³⁻, due to rapid initiation of food after >10 days of undernutrition. *Signs:* Rhabdomyolysis, respiratory or cardiac failure, ↓BP, arrhythmias, seizures, and sudden death. *Treatment:* Consult a dietician to develop a plan of slow refeeding with careful increase in calories. Monitor serum PO₄³⁻ (stop re-feeding if falling), also glucose↑, K⁺↓, and Mg²⁺↑. Milk is often used initially (high in PO₄³⁻ and well tolerated); correct metabolic imbalances (PO route). Prescribe thiamine, vitamin B complex (strong), and multivitamin. Over 4-7 days increase dietary intake.

Bulimia (binge eating disorder)

Definition 1 Recurrent episodes of binge eating characterized by uncontrolled overeating 2 Preoccupation with control of body weight 3 Regular use of mechanisms to overcome the fattening effects of binges, eg starvation, vomit-induction, laxatives, overexercise 4 BMI >17.5.[201]

Epidemiology ♀:♂≈9:1. Prevalence (↑ in developed countries) ≈ 0.5-1.0% in young women. No social class differences. In Britain, young Asian women are at ↑risk.[202] Homosexuality/bisexuality may be a specific risk factor for bulimia in males (asexuality is more typical in ♂ anorexia nervosa).[203]

Cause/associations Urbanization (*not* a risk factor for anorexia); premorbid obesity. Commoner in female relatives of anorexics (?shared familial liability). Genetic contribution of 54-83%. **Natural history** *Age of onset:* ~18yrs.

Symptoms Fatigue, lethargy, feeling bloated, constipation, abdominal pain, oesophagitis, gastric dilatation with risk of gastric rupture, heart conduction abnormalities, cardiomyopathy (if laxative use), tetany, occasional swelling of hands and feet, irregular menstruation, erosion of dental enamel, enlarged parotid glands, calluses on the back of the hands (Russell's sign, from tooth marks during induction of vomiting), oedema (use of laxatives and diuretics), metabolic alkalosis, hypochloraemia, ↓K⁺, metabolic acidosis (if laxative use), less commonly: ↓Na⁺, ↓Ca²⁺, ↓PO₄³⁻, ↓Mg²⁺, abnormal EEG, abnormal menstrual cycle, blunted response of TSH and GH to thyroid-releasing hormone.

Treatment Mild symptoms: support, self-help books and food diary (similar to anorexia). Referral to EDU in case of no response, moderate/severe symptoms, and to a medical unit if medical complications.[204] Antidepressants are recommended to ↓binges and purging. First line: SSRIs—specifically fluoxetine (effective dose higher than for depression: 60mg); CBT can help (p390).[205]

Prognosis In 2-10yrs, 50% improve, 20% show no change.[206]

---

16 Parents describe parent-to-parent consultations as an intense emotional experience that helps them to feel less alone, to feel empowered to progress, and to reflect on changes in family interactions.

Sexual dysfunction is hard to define because defining what is 'normal' is complex and has changed over time. As always, if there are persistent impairments in functioning, response, or enjoyment then this should be considered an area to explore by questioning.

Sexual history Early experiences; present practices; any hints pointing towards transexualism, commercial sex work, or drug abuse? Orientation to either or both sexes. Difficulties with other partners? When did you meet? What attracted you to each other?

Common triggers for sexual problems *Psychological:* Relationship problems; life stressors; anxiety/depression; low self-esteem; sexual performance anxiety; excessive self-monitoring of arousal; feelings of guilt about sex; fear of pregnancy or sexually transmitted infections (STIs); body changes, eg following surgery, lack of knowledge about sexuality/'normal' sexual responses; previous significant negative sexual experience (especially rape or childhood sexual abuse issues). *Environmental:* (Fear of) interruptions (eg from children, parents); physical discomfort. *Physical:* Use of drugs or alcohol; medication side effects; pain or discomfort due to illness or injury; feeling tired or 'run down'; recent childbirth. *Factors related to the partner:* Sexual attractiveness (gender, physical characteristics); evidence of disinterest, constant criticism, inconsideration, and inability to cope with difficulties (esp. sexual); sexual inexperience/poor technique; preference for sexual activities that are unappealing to the partner.

Prescribed medication Hypotensives (erectile dysfunction, ED); SSRIs (delayed ejaculation); β-blockers, finasteride, OCP (see p304), and phenothiazines (loss of libido).

Other causes of ED (OHCM p222): diabetes, cord pathology, ↑prolactin, drugs, and alcohol.

Psychosexual therapeutic interventions There is much more to helping people with sexual difficulties than *couple therapy.* Often the problem is not specifically sexual, and sexual difficulties may recede once other aspects of the relationship improve. Specific sexual dysfunctions are considered using a modernized *Masters & Johnson* approach with a model of sexual response entailing excitation, plateau, orgasm, and resolution. But this is just one approach to one problem, behavioural therapy is not suited to dealing with forbidden or disturbing sexual feelings, fantasies, and urges. For this, experiential psychotherapy and psychodynamic approaches are valid alternatives.[207] Also, we should not focus on performance of acts at the expense of promoting the quality of erotic connection.

In any therapy the following concepts need to be understood:
- Never assume that a patient is too old or too ill for sexual issues to be relevant. ►Assume that everyone has a sex life, perhaps in fantasy only (fantasy is always found to be an important component of sexuality).[208]
- Treat sexual problems holistically—eg there may be relevant medical, drug, or other psychopathologies (depression is common).
- Psychological approaches are always important, whatever is offered by way of physical props or drugs such as sildenafil. Men randomized to receive group therapy *plus* sildenafil had more successful intercourse than those receiving only sildenafil. Group psychotherapy also significantly improves erectile dysfunction compared to sildenafil alone.[209]
- Psychological events have physical sequelae, and physical events have psychological sequelae.

Psychiatry

Sexual issues are easier to talk about when an overt part of consultations (contraception, fertility, and sexual diseases). More commonly they are a covert part of other emotional or behavioural problems. We may find sexual dialogue embarrassing and avoid it—with unpredictable or fatal consequences, eg distress caused by abuse[210] or confusion from emotions relating to sexuality.

Language is important. It may be medical ('coitus'); slang ('screwing'); or socially acceptable ('having sex'). It is not advisable to use slang—it's unprofessional, makes some people confused or uncomfortable, and can make you appear very out dated. Most will expect socially acceptable language; slang may shock and may put up barriers. Occasional mirroring of patient's words can gain rapport but use verbal or non-verbal cues to check if words are acceptable. If in doubt, ask. If you aren't afraid to talk about sex they won't be.

Psychiatry

- Ambiguity is a frequent pitfall. Make sure that you both know what the other is talking about! If a new phrase or ambiguous euphemism crops up (slang changes all the time), ask for an explanation right away (a little gentle helping on your part usually overcomes any embarrassment).
- Don't assume sexual knowledge. People are often exposed to graphic sexual content on the internet at a young age, however don't confuse this with understanding. Sex can be confusing and mysterious. There are still many myths, and it is just as hard as it ever was for someone to admit that they don't know something. Sex education in schools is uneven, and may be useless or non-existent (teachers may be too embarrassed to do it).[211]
- Don't assume a sexual orientation. It may be best to let these issues surface gradually rather than asking directly early on. Imply that it is safe to reveal feelings that are confused or non-standard. Your patient may be boxed in by societal, religious, or family views of what sexuality should be, so that suicide can seem the only way out.[212] Through your dialogue you may be able to show that there are other options, and that 'there is no straight way through this world for any of us'.[213] If orientation is causing distress, point out that there is more to a person than sexuality—roles they are good at may include being a friend, colleague, parent, or child—as well as lover, now or in the future. 'You don't need to have sex just to settle the issue of sexuality; feelings can be explored without sex acts, which can be left until you feel ready'. In helping gay people decide when to 'come out', eg to parents, explain that reactions can be unpredictable.[214] 'How well do you know your parents?' 'How have they dealt with religious or sexual issues with your brothers and sisters?'; 'Are you economically dependent on them?'; 'Do you have a social support outside the home?'[215]
- Don't appear embarrassed. It is easier for people to open up if they think that you aren't going to blush, tell them off, or, worst of all, laugh. Don't act shocked and don't judge; give the wrong impression and they will stop being honest with you—see p315 for further discussion of this vital point.
- Act as if you have plenty of time to listen—this is hard conversation for anyone to have, don't make them finish prematurely or feel rushed.

The more you practise talking about sex, the easier it gets. If you avoid it, it will remain a problem to you. Also, your patients may learn communication techniques, helpful in their lives as a whole, augmenting self-esteem, enabling sexual negotiation (useful in negotiating safer sexual practices with partners).[216] Also, you may lay the foundation for honest sexual dialogue between this person and their family, improving everyone's communication.

Asking about sexual abuse Have you been in any relationships that made you feel uncomfortable? Has anyone touched you in a way that made you feel embarrassed? I am wondering if anyone has hurt you in a sexual way.

Confidentiality People need to know that you will only ever breach this if they, or someone else, is in serious danger[217] (see p323).

Baby blues are a transient, self-limiting condition seen in up to 75% of new mothers, most often 3–5 days after delivery. She is tearful, anxious, and irritable, commonly lasting for 1–2 days, but may persist for up to 2 weeks. Reassurance from midwifery with increased social/family support is normally enough. If symptoms fail to resolve, psychiatric review should be completed.

Postnatal depression The risk of major depression after pregnancy is greater in those with a history of postpartum depression (50%) or unipolar/bipolar depression (25%) compared to 10% without psychiatric history. Other factors include unplanned pregnancy, lack of support, marital problems, social circumstances, sleep deprivation, and hormonal changes.[218]

Natural history Although most postnatal depression resolves in ≤6 months, don't put off treatment, and just hope for the best. *Consider these facts:*
• For the patient, 6 months is a long, long time.
• For the infant, 6 months is more than a long time: it's literally an age.
• Suicide is always awful but the worst outcomes in postpartum mental health are universally devastating.
• Postnatal depression impairs infant cognitive and social skills.[219,220]

Management of postnatal depression ▶*Have a low threshold for referring to multidisciplinary teams in mother-and-baby units.* Screen for depression (see TABLE) to avoid missing major depression. Pregnancy and motherhood are often reported as a time of unclouded joy. But what if *she* is not delighted? Instead she is unaccountably sad, spends the nights crying, and that her exhausted days are filled with a sense of foreboding. The place to start to pre-empt these feelings is in the antenatal clinic. ▶Involve fathers;[221] explain: 'When the baby comes you'll need help and rest—don't think you can do it all yourself: become a team—eg taking turns in getting the baby off to sleep'.[222] In the puerperium give permission for the new mother to tell her woe. When this is revealed, counselling, and input from a health visitor and a psychiatrist/GP is wise, as is close follow-up. You may need to arrange emergency admission under the Mental Health Act: but the point of being prepared for postnatal depression is to avoid things getting this bad. *Pharmacology* Short-term, antidepressant medication is as good as CBT. All antidepressants are excreted in breast milk, but tricyclics and SSRIs are rarely detectable by standard tests, *except for fluoxetine which shows significantly higher levels.* Observe babies for possible SEs; it may be best to stop breast-feeding if large doses are used. In severe cases, where the patient is not eating/drinking or strongly suicidal, ECT should be considered. The quicker the mother's symptoms can be brought under control, the less the disruption to the mother and baby bond.

Postpartum psychosis ▶*Any suspicion of postpartum psychosis should trigger an emergency referral to a specialist team.* Peak onset at 2 weeks postpartum, this is a psychotic episode with prominent affective symptoms (depression or mania) occurring with rapidly fluctuating symptoms, mood lability, insomnia, and disorientation. Previous postpartum psychosis has 30% recurrence risk (~40% risk of postnatal depression). Other factors include single parenthood, reduced social support, and previous mental illness.

Prevention: High-risk patients need an individualized care plan with antenatal specialist perinatal mental health input. *New cases:* Early detection is essential. Due to the risks to self and baby—infanticide is a rare (1 in 50,000) but serious risk—hospitalization is often necessary. A combination of medication to target affective symptoms (mood stabilizer, antidepressant, or ECT) and psychotic symptoms (second-generation antipsychotic and long-acting benzodiazepine) combined with therapy, reassurance, and emotional support (with and for family) is best practice. At discharge, a referral to local mental health services and health visitors will be needed.

Edinburgh postnatal depression scale (EPDS)

1 *I've been able to laugh & see the funny side of things:*	As much as always could
	Not quite so much now
	Definitely not so much
	Now not at all
2 *I've looked forward with enjoyment to things:*	As much as I ever did
	Rather less than before
	Definitely less than before
	Hardly at all
3 ★*I've blamed myself unnecessarily when things went wrong:*	Yes, most of the time
	Yes, some of the time
	Not very often
	No, never
4 *I've been anxious or worried for no good reason:*	No, not at all
	Hardly ever
	Yes, sometimes
	Yes, very often
5 *I've felt scared/panicky for no very good reason:*	Yes, quite a lot
	Yes, sometimes
	No, not much
	No, not at all
6 ★*Things have been getting on top of me:*	Yes, most of the time I haven't been able to cope at all
	Yes, sometimes I haven't been coping as well as usual
	No, most of the time I have coped quite well
	No, I have been coping as well as ever
7 ★*I've been so unhappy that it is difficult to sleep:*	Yes, most of the time
	Yes, sometimes
	Not very often
	No, not at all
8 ★*I've felt sad or miserable:*	Yes, most of the time
	Yes, quite often
	Not very often
	No, not at all
9 ★*I've been so unhappy that I've been crying:*	Yes, most of the time
	Yes, quite often
	Only occasionally
	No, never
10 ★*Thoughts of harming myself have occurred to me:*	Yes, quite often
	Sometimes
	Hardly ever
Instructions *Underline what comes closest to how you have felt in the last 7 days.*	Never

Ask to score answers 0, 1, 2, or 3 according to increased severity; some (★above) are reverse scored (3, 2, 1, 0). Add scores for 1–10 for the total. Let her complete the scale herself, eg at the 6-week check-up, unless literary difficulty. ►A score of 12/30 has a sensitivity of 77% for postnatal depression (specificity: 93%).

Validity for the EPDS is limited with a suggestion that face-to-face detection is still the best determinant of postnatal depression.

When Hollywood wants to show psychotherapy (or psychiatry), they show an older, bearded, white man (Freud, fig 4.11), with a patient on his couch, asking 'how was the relationship with your mother?'—this is not modern psychotherapy.

Psychotherapy denotes treatment of mental disorders and behavioural disturbances using...support, suggestion, persuasion, re-education, reassurance, and insight in order to alter maladaptive patterns of coping, and to encourage personality growth. Dorland's Medical Dictionary

Today's psychotherapy can be active, dynamic, and used to treat a range of different conditions. It has a strong evidence base and hardly ever uses a chaise lounge.

Therapy is of great importance in psychiatry—and of great importance in therapy is communication. The first step in communication is to open a channel. The vital role that listening plays has already been highlighted (p316). So is 'just being nice to patients' in the course of one's medical activities an example of therapy at work? The answer is 'no'—not because being nice is therapeutically neutral, but because one's attention is not focused on planning change through the systematic use of interpersonal techniques.

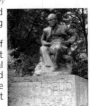
Fig 4.11 Sigmund Freud. Pictured as an older, bearded, white man.
© Gil Myers.

This section is a highly selective glimpse at different types of therapy, in an attempt to show the range of skills needed, and to whet your appetite. Its unlikely you will be given an opportunity, and it would be unsafe, to try out the more advanced techniques without appropriate supervision.

Medicine has three great branches: prevention, curing by technical means, and healing—and psychotherapy is the embodiment of healing: a holistic approach in which systematic human dialogue becomes a humanizing enterprise for the relief of suffering and the advancement of self-esteem. Questions such as 'What is the meaning of my life' and 'what is significant?' are answered in a different way after exposure to a gifted therapist. Changes occur in cognition, feelings, and behaviour. This is why therapy is dangerous and exciting: it changes people. Hence the need for supervision and ongoing training and self-awareness on the part of the therapist.

The *types of psychotherapies* may be classified first in terms of *who is involved* in the treatment sessions: an individual, a couple, a family, or a whole group; and secondly they may be classified by their *content and methods* used: analytic, interpersonal, cognitive, behavioural.

Cognitive therapies (p390) focuses on thoughts and assumptions, promoting the theory that we respond to our interpretation of events, not to raw events alone. If this is the case, cognitive change is required to produce emotional and behavioural change.

Behavioural therapies (p392) aim to alter behaviour first, with the theory that if these change then our thoughts and emotions will also evolve.

Psychodynamic therapies (p394), also called psychoanalytical therapies, are concerned with the origin and meaning of symptoms not necessarily the 'presenting complaint'. They are based on the view that vulnerability comes from early experiences and unresolved issues, often from childhood.

Group therapies (p400) as the name suggests, are delivered to a group rather than an individual. Group interactions change the therapeutic environment and provide an alternative space to explore interpersonal relationships.

Play and art therapies (p402) demonstrate the variety of approaches to therapist-patient communication within the field of psychotherapy.

Which psychotherapy is most successful? See p389.

Psychiatry

Westen's dictum Beware making false dichotomies into supported and unsupported therapies. Randomized trial methodologies don't suit all therapies.[224, 225] What follows does not entirely avoid the trap Westen alludes to. Also be aware of many different variations on a theme, eg CAT (cognitive and analytic therapy) and DBT (dialectical behaviour therapy).[17]

Principal recommendations and levels of evidence[18]

• Psychological therapy should be routinely considered as an option when assessing mental health problems.[B] Evidence shows benefits over no treatment for a wide range of mental health difficulties.

• Patients who are adjusting to life events, illnesses, disabilities, or losses may benefit from brief therapies such as counselling.[B] Evidence of counselling effectiveness in mixed anxiety/depression, most effective when used with specified client groups, eg postnatal mothers, bereaved groups.

• Post-traumatic stress symptoms (p354) are helped by psychological therapy, with most evidence for trauma-focused cognitive behavioural methods. Routine debriefing following traumatic events is not recommended.[A] Studies have shown that playing *Tetris* reduces likelihood of developing on-going stress sequale.

• Depression (p344) may be helped (but is often not cured) by cognitive therapy or interpersonal therapy. A number of other brief structured therapies for depression may be of benefit, eg psychodynamic therapy and counselling.[A]

• Anxiety disorders (p350–3) including agoraphobia, panic disorder, social phobia, obsessive–compulsive disorders, generalized anxiety disorders are likely to benefit from cognitive behaviour therapy (CBT).[A]

• Psychological intervention should be considered for somatic complaints with a psychological component, including gastrointestinal and gynaecological problems, with most evidence for CBT for improving functioning in the treatment of chronic pain and chronic fatigue.[C]

• Eating disorders (p382) can be treated with psychological therapy. Best evidence in bulimia nervosa is for CBT, interpersonal therapy (IPT) and family therapy for teenagers. Treatment usually includes psycho-educational methods. There is little strong evidence on the best therapy type for anorexia nervosa.[C] Early onset of anorexia may indicate family therapy, and later onset, broadly based individual therapy but the evidence is weak.

• Structured psychological therapies delivered by skilled practitioners can contribute to the longer-term treatment of personality disorders (p380). A number of therapy approaches have shown some success with personality disorders, including DBT, psychoanalytic day hospital programme, and thera-peutic communities.

---

17 CAT is a collaborative programme for looking at the way a person thinks, feels, and acts, and the events and relationships that underlie these experiences (often from childhood or earlier in life). It combines under-standings from cognitive psychotherapies and psychoanalytic approaches into an integrated whole.
18 A Based on a consistent finding in a majority of studies in high-quality systematic reviews or evidence from high-quality studies. B Based on ≥1 high-quality trial, a weak or inconsistent finding in high-quality reviews, or a consistent finding in reviews that don't meet all the high-quality criteria. C Based on evidence from single studies that don't meet all the criteria of 'high-quality'. D Based on evidence from structured expert consensus.

CBT helps change unhelpful thoughts (cognitions) and actions (behaviours) which can occur during times of distress. Altering these changes how we feel about the world, other people, and ourself. It focuses on the here-and-now problems, tackling the current state of mind rather than exploring past causes of distress or developmental experiences. It is not a quick fix. A therapist is like a personal trainer who can advise and encourage—but cannot 'do' it for the patient. CBT needs a patient to actively participate in their own recovery.

Key concepts The 'hot cross bun' model (fig 4.12) illustrates the many interactions between thoughts, feelings, behaviours, and body sensations. Any situation will trigger a set of internal and external reactions. These can result in a negative experience creating a vicious cycle which maintains or increases avoidant or negative patterns.

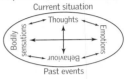
Fig 4.12 Hot cross bun diagram.

Beck suggests that a person who habitually uses depressed or anxious *cognitive distortions* (see BOX) will be more likely to become distressed when faced with minor problems. These mechanisms lead to distortions within the cognitive triad of the self, the world, and the future.

- In CBT, the patient first learns to identify cognitive distortions from present or recent experiences with the guided use of daily diaries and questioning.
- The patient records such ideas and then learns to examine the evidence for and against them and experiment, testing out these beliefs in real life.
- The patient is encouraged to restart the pleasurable activities that were given up at the onset of difficulties (even if they don't enjoy them... yet!).
- In this way, cognitive restructuring takes place when the patient is able to identify, evaluate, and change the distorted thoughts and associated behaviour.

Technique • Grounded history of the nature of the difficulties • Assessment tools or questionnaires used • Treatment usually takes place on a weekly basis for 5–20 sessions, each lasting 30–60 minutes • A *treatment plan* is formulated with clear goals and objectives and progress is monitored • Each session breaks difficulties into different areas of thoughts, feelings, and behaviours, and helps the patient analyse these to determine effect and consider change • Between sessions, the patient is expected to do 'homework' (practise these changes in their everyday life) and report back the effect in the next session.

Refresher courses CBT teaches skills which can be applied straightaway to a current problem and later to new issues. There is always a risk that these skills will need updating or encouraging (especially if they haven't been practised recently). A short refresher course of a few sessions is encouraged and efficient.

Indications[226] *General:* • The patient prefers a psychological intervention, either alone or in addition to medication • The target problems for CBT (extreme, unhelpful thinking; reduced activity; avoidant or unhelpful behaviours) are present • No improvement or only partial improvement has occurred on medication • Side effects prevent a sufficient dose of medication from being taken over an adequate period. *Specific:* • Depression • Generalized anxiety or panic disorder • Phobias • OCD • PTSD • Hypochondriasis • Bulimia.

Caution • Severe depression • Poor concentration • Difficulties talking about feelings • Patient focused on childhood events • Poor motivation to change.

Modalities CBT is efficient in a variety of different forms • Individual therapy with one-to-one therapy sessions • Group CBT (see p400) • Bibliotherapy self-help books as recommended by 'Reading Well Books on Prescription' scheme • Computerized CBT (CCBT) with (free) online resources such as MoodGym, an interactive website to prevent depression and FearFighter, an online program treating panic/phobia (Trusts must pay a fee, then doctors can 'prescribe' it).

The main cognitive distortions in cognitive theory are:
- *All-or-nothing thinking:* Seeing everything as binary: black/white, true/false, good/bad, etc. Thinking in these terms is called dichotomous reasoning and often forces negativity as things are rarely wholly positive.
- *Arbitrary inference:* Quickly drawing conclusions (usually negative or of failure) with little or no evidence to support them.
- *Disqualifying the positive:* Ignoring or undermining any positive statements/events/relationships.
- *Emotional reasoning:* Assuming that (negative) emotions reflect the way things truly are: 'I feel it, therefore it must be true.'
- *Jumping to conclusions:* Reaching a negative conclusion from insufficient (if any) evidence. This utilizes *mind reading*, concluding that someone is thinking negatively from their behaviour and then reacting to this assumption without checking with them and *fortune telling*, predicting a negative outcome and acting as though this prediction was an established fact.
- *Magnification and minimization:* Exaggerating any perceived failure/weakness and diminishing any success/strength. Also called the 'binocular trick'. An extreme example of this is *catastrophizing*, assigning the greatest emphasis to the most terrible possible outcome, however unlikely.
- *Mental filtering:* Concentrating on a negative element in a situation to the exclusion of everything else.
- *Overgeneralization:* Drawing global conclusions about worth/performance on the basis of insufficient (often only a single) negative experience. In its extreme form, this is *(mis)labelling*—attributing a person's whole character based on a single action/behaviour which may have been due to error.
- *Personalization:* Attaching personal responsibility, and usually guilt, for an event over which there was no control. Also *blaming* (opposite of personalization) is holding other people responsible for distress (often emotional) caused even if was out of their control.
- *Selective abstraction:* Dwelling on insignificant (negative) detail while ignoring more important features or stimuli.

CHANGE VIEW: 10 key facts about CBT

Change: your thoughts and actions
Homework: practice makes perfect
Action: don't just talk, do!
Need: pinpoint the problem
Goals: move towards them
Evidence: shows CBT can work
View: events from another angle
I can do it: self-help approach
Experience: test out your beliefs
write it down: to remember progress.

▶From the Royal College of Psychiatrists' excellent leaflet on CBT (Google: RCPSYCH+CBT). This is a very useful resource for patient information leaflets on many different therapies, disorders, and treatments. Highly recommended.

Behavioural therapy aims to change a person's behaviour using one of several techniques depending on the condition. It is most often used as part of CBT (see p390) but can be used independently.

Relaxation training *Indication:* Mild/moderate anxiety. *Technique:* • A system of exercises (p393) and regular breathing (p351) to progressively relax individual muscle groups • Link the relaxed state with pleasant, imagined scenes so that relaxation can be induced by recalling the imagined scene.

Systematic desensitization *Indications:* Phobic disorders. *Technique:* Patients form a hierarchy of fears about the phobic stimulus. Therapy uses graded exposure (least fearsome first) to real or imagined stimuli,[Joseph 227][Wolpe] while patients perform relaxation techniques until anxiety is extinguished. It is ethically less controversial than flooding[228] as progress up the hierarchy is only when patients are completely comfortable with the current level; eg fig 4.13 can be preceded by an almost neutral image, such as ψ.[229]

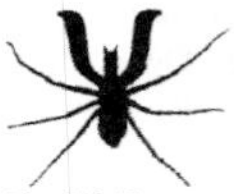

Fig 4.13 (See text.) ©JML.

Response prevention *Indications:* Obsessions. *Technique:* • Involves exposure to an anxiety-provoking stimulus (eg a toilet seat for patients fearing contamination). • The patient is subsequently prevented from carrying out the usual compulsive behaviour or ritual until the urge to do so has passed.

Exposure/flooding/implosion *Indication:* Phobias. *Technique:* • The anxiety-provoking object or situation is presented *in vivo* or in imagination (prolonged *in vivo* in flooding) • Implosion involves imagined exposure to stimuli in a non-graded manner • The patient then stays with the anxiety-provoking stimuli until there is habituation (ie she becomes accustomed to the anxiety by frequent exposure), and the avoidance response is extinguished.

Thought stopping *Indications:* • Obsessional thoughts occurring without compulsive rituals • Undesired sexually deviant thoughts. *Technique:* The patient is asked to ruminate and then taught to stop negative anticipatory thoughts or obsessional thoughts before they gather enough momentum by arranging a sudden intrusion, eg snapping an elastic band on the wrist.

Aversion therapy/covert sensitization *Indications:* • Alcohol dependence syndrome (disulfiram used to induce nausea if alcohol is consumed). • Sexual deviations. *Technique:* • Aversive therapy involves producing an unpleasant sensation in the patient in association with an aversive or noxious stimulus (eg electric shocks, chemically induced nausea, pain) with the aim of eliminating unwanted behaviour. • Covert sensitization involves the use of aversive stimuli in imagination (eg the approach of a policeman to arrest him/her for his/her undesirable behaviour). *Cautions:* • Punishment procedures are generally ineffective unless patients are taught more appropriate behaviours.

Social skills training *Indications:* Patients with social deficits due to a psychiatric disorder. *Technique:* • Aims to modify a patient's social behaviour in order to help overcome difficulties in forming/maintaining relationships • Video is used to define and rate elements of a patient's behaviour in standard social encounters • The patient is then taught more appropriate behaviour by a combination of direct instruction, modelling, video-feedback, and role play.

Token economy *Indications:* • Children (p210) • Intellectual disability • Addictive disorders • Chronic psychiatric disorders. *Technique:* Positive reinforcement improves behaviour: tokens are given when desirable behaviour is displayed. These can later be exchanged for goods or privileges. *Problems:* • Patients become mercenary as they only behave well in exchange for tokens. • Poorly prepares people for a world where rewards are subtle and delayed.

Modelling and role play *Technique:* The acquisition of new behaviours by the process of imitation. *Indications:* Lack of social skills and assertiveness.

▶Try this yourself. Experimental learning or 'learning through reflection on doing' helps us to remember things more efficiently than just reading it.

Preparation In a quiet, comfortable place, sit down (a reclining chair is great for this), loosen any tight clothing, close your eyes, and let your whole body go loose. Some people like to lie down—the danger with this is that this will precipitate sleep (which is nice but not the point of the exercise). Assume a passive attitude: tune out all other thoughts and focus on yourself and on achieving relaxation in specific body muscles.

Tension Apply muscle tension to a specific part of the body. Focus on just the target muscle group, eg left hand. Practice allows you to isolate just that group rather than surrounding muscles (eg shoulder or arm). Take a slow, deep breath and squeeze the muscles as hard as you can, eg make a fist, for the count of 5 seconds. Make the muscle tension deliberate, yet gentle. This may cause slight shaking or discomfort but should never cause pain. The intention is to really feel the tension in that muscle group.

Relaxation After the count of 5, quickly relax the tensed muscles, allowing it to become limp and loose. Exhale slowly as the tightness dissipates. Make a conscious effort to notice the difference between states; observe the feelings of relaxation compared to tension in that muscle group.

Systematic order To avoid confusion, start at your toes and work up (or vice versa). Focus on each muscle group in turn and repeat the exercise, at each group deliberately focus on those muscles and the difference between tension and relaxation.

Example muscle group exercises
For each limb complete the three muscle groups and then repeat, starting at the distal point, on the other limb.

Foot	Curl toes downward
Lower leg & foot	Tighten calf muscle by pulling toes towards body
Entire leg	Squeeze thigh muscles while doing above
Hand	Clench fist
Entire arm	Tighten biceps by drawing forearm up towards shoulder and 'make a muscle', while clenching fist
Buttocks	Tighten by pulling your buttocks together
Stomach	Suck your stomach in
Chest	Tighten by taking a deep breath
Neck & shoulders	Raise shoulders up to touch bottom of ears
Mouth	Open mouth wide enough to stretch the jaw hinges
Eyes	Clench eyelids tightly shut
Forehead	Raise eyebrows as far as possible

Psychiatry

Key concepts 1 *The unconscious:* Individual dynamic psychotherapy is based on the premise that a person's behaviour is influenced by unconscious factors (thoughts, feelings, fantasies). Evidence for the existence of unconscious activity include •Dreams •Artistic and scientific creativity •Hysterical symptoms (p354) •Abreaction[19] •Parapraxes, a 'slip of the tongue' (often called a Freudian slip: 'saying one thing, but meaning your mother').

2 *Psychological defences:* Our immune system protects our physical integrity, and our psychological vulnerabilities are shielded by psychological defences. In both cases, overactive defences can lead to trouble, eg: *Psychotic defences:* •Delusional projection/paranoia •Denial •Distortion. *Immature defences:* •Projection[20] •Schizoid/autistic fantasy •Dissociation •Acting out •Hypochondriasis •Passive aggression. *Neurotic defences:* •Repression •Displacement[21] •Reaction formation[22] •Intellectualization. *Mature defences:* •Altruism •Humour •Suppression •Anticipation •Sublimation.[23][230]

3 *Transference and countertransference:* The past patterns (transfers) our present reactions to people. If we have trusted our parents, we will be likely to trust our doctors, teachers, and friends. The intense psychotherapeutic relationship brings these assumptions to the fore where they can be examined, understood, and learned from. We in turn have unconscious reactions to patients based on our past, ie countertransference. Errors from this arise when we react as though our patient were a significant person in our early life[231] (if our mother was an alcoholic we may be oversolicitous or rejecting with alcoholics). *Our reactions are also a key to our patient's feelings:* if a patient makes us feel rejected (as alcoholics often do), perhaps that person himself was rejected as a child and turned to the bottle in compensation.

Assessing suitability *Psychological understandibility:* The patient's difficulties must be understandable in psychological terms. *Psychological mindedness:* The capacity to think about problems in psychological terms. *Motivation:* There must be motivation for insight and change. *Intelligence and verbal fluency:* The ability to communicate thoughts and feelings through talking. *Introspectiveness:* The ability to reflect and think about their feelings. *Dreams:* The capacity to remember dreams. *Ego strength:* The ability to tolerate frustrating or distressful feelings without engaging in impulsive behaviour. *Capacity to form relationships:* There should be a history of at least one sustained relationship in the past or present.

Specific indications •Dissociative/conversion disorders •Depression •Psychosomatic disorders •Relationship problems •Grief.

Technique The therapist provides a secure *frame*—a regular time and place and her own consistency and acceptingness. The patient *narrates* vignettes about himself and his life (~3/session). The therapist *listens* carefully, to the stories and to her reactions to them. She then makes *linking hypotheses*, or *interpretations* that offer *meaning*. Previously inexplicable behaviour begins to make sense. Meanwhile, the patient forms a close relationship with the therapist based on *empathy*, *genuineness*, and *non-possessive warmth* (shown experimentally to be key factors) and sometimes *challenge*. These may be novel experiences for the patient that can be *internalized* as he *works through* difficulties safely. Reactions to *ending* will bring up past unprocessed losses.

Psychodynamic therapy can be *time-limited* (brief dynamic psychotherapy)—suitable for circumscribed problems, eg unmourned grief, or *open-ended* (p394) eg if there are severe personality disorders or complex needs.[232] $_{N=1053}$ In depression, 16 sessions seem to be no better than eight.[233]

19 *Abreaction:* cathartic reliving of buried traumas; repressed terrors are made conscious and *tamed*.[232]
20 *Projecting* our own undesirable impulses to another, so pretending that the subjective is objective.
21 *Displacement:* redirection of an undesired intense emotion towards someone neutral and harmless.
22 *Reaction formation:* doing the opposite of true desires (eg training to be a pilot to cover up fear of flying).
23 In sport, for example, we *sublimate* (and make safe) brutal urges into rituals of formal competition.

Psychiatry

Cautions: when dynamic psychotherapy might not be right

1 Repeated admissions, many suicide attempts, repeated risk-taking, and severe somatization suggest insufficient ego strength for psychotherapy.
2 A history of repeated failed ventures or dropping out of relationships.
3 In general, patients with acute psychosis are less amenable.
4 Severely depressed patients may be too slowed up and too unresponsive.
5 Over-sedation may hinder capacity to access feelings (?reduce doses).
6 Patients who are actively abusing alcohol or illicit drugs are problematic.
7 No real motivation to change or grossly unreal expectations of therapy.

Acknowledging and using our own feelings

▶Are you afraid of uncomfortable questions? Here are some asked by a very experienced psychotherapist.[24]

? Are you a saint? or have you ever...

? Felt so bored and irritated by certain patients you want to quit?

? Longed for the consultation to end, at any price?

? Can you say you have *never* felt a flicker of sexual interest in a patient?

? Have you never imagined the death of certain patients and the relief that would bring, not just to them but to us, their impotent carers?

? Have you never resented the demands of people for whom illness seems to have become a way of life?

? Whose thoughts have not sometimes drifted off towards their own concerns—to the need for sleep, food, or distraction or to some family, career, or future plans?

▶The key to good doctoring is not regulation or revalidation, but fostering the ability to put ourselves in our patients' shoes. And we can use the feeling patients engender in us to understand how the patient's nearest and dearest are frustrated, perplexed, and deluded. For example, excessive worry about a patient may be the result of being infected by the patient's anxiety—beyond what is reasonable. This is know as *projective identification*.

Why does bad or harmful practice continue, despite GMC guidelines? It is because we are motivated by forces of which we are unaware.

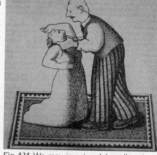

Fig 4.14 We may imagine doing all sorts of things to our patients. The crime is not the thought but the deed. The vital thing is to not bury these things but to know that they are just that: imaginings. Perhaps we can use them in the service of our work? If the stressed, isolated doctor had been aware of and able to voice his fantasies maybe he would not have ended up in custody or in bed with his sexually abused, vulnerable, and depressed patient.

24 See Good doctor, bad doctor—a psychodynamic approach. *BMJ* 2002; 325: 722 by Jeremy Holmes (whom we thank for permission to quote from his excellent article).

What used to be called family therapy is now better known as systemic practice, which is an evolving body of ideas and techniques focusing on a person's difficulties within the context of the people and culture that surround them. Therapy is based on the assumption that most people have the resources and potential for resolving life's difficulties.

A family can be described in terms of dimensions. Research interviews have given rise to a measure of '*expressed emotion*' (EE) which is associated with severity of chronic illness in many disorders (eg schizophrenia, anorexia nervosa, cystic fibrosis). Therapists work in partnership with families and others, not on them. Family therapy practice is sensitive to diverse family forms and relationships, beliefs, and cultures. Families do not necessarily mean just those related by genetics and can include step-parents, half-siblings, etc.

Family therapy sessions Family therapists tend to adopt an approach which does not blame individuals, favour adults over children, or take sides. Family therapists tend to be more interested in the maintenance and/or solving of problems rather than in trying to identify a single cause. The therapist should be inclusive and considerate of the needs of each member of the family (not putting anyone above or below the others). The focus is on getting the family to discuss the problems that are putting a strain on their relationships. The therapists help the family recognize and build on each person's strengths and relational resources in ways that respect their experiences, invite engagement, and support recovery. Everyone is given an opportunity to contribute so that the family explores ways forward which will work for them as a unit.

Deciding which family members attend each session will vary depending on a family's therapy goals and availability (eg elder sibling away at university may join during holidays). A family therapist may offer supplemental individual sessions before or between regular family sessions. This is particularly helpful for those wanting to consider how best to express their thoughts and feelings with the wider family. When parents and children are involved, the therapists may meet with parents separately to work on themes or topics they feel are inappropriate to discuss in front of their children (eg sex, drugs, and death).

Although some family therapists work individually, most will collaborate with a co-therapist or a larger team. Often co-therapists observe family interactions during therapy via a one-way screen ('team behind the screen'). They can observe how the family therapist and family interact. They will then be in a position to share reflections and explore possibilities to help resolve issues. Many families find this approach to complex issues very helpful.

Family therapy models
- Systemic—focus on family beliefs, patterns, and meanings with no objective truth—everyone has their own 'truth' which is subjective.
- Structural—focus on a family's hierarchies and rules; if these are broken a 'problem' individual is blamed. Family structure is viewed by Minuchin[234] as an invisible set of functional demands that organize family interactions. These patterns are self-regulating in a way that attempts to return a family to its habitual mode and minimize anxiety. The therapist actively tries to highlight behaviours and re-organize structures within the family.
- Solution focused—focus on the family, setting, the task, and their goals; the therapist helps the family to collaborate to reach these.
- Narrative—focus on family 'scripts' which are ways to live; problems emerge when individuals deviate from the 'dominant family narrative'; the therapist helps the family to develop a new encompassing narrative.
- Transactional—focus on the problem actually serving a purpose (eg difficult child prevents parents divorcing) and interplay between family members ('transactions'); family given tasks by therapist to challenge these roles.

Dimensions of family functioning

The McMaster Model of Family Functioning has six dimensions of family life. A family therapist can observe and consider all of these, and their relation to each other, in order to understand how a family behaves:[35,36]

• *Problem-solving:* Can the family act together to solve everyday emotional and practical problems? Can they identify a problem, develop, agree, and enact solutions, and evaluate their performance? Success may be dependent upon functioning in other dimensions.

• *Congruence of verbal and non-verbal communications:* Are communications clear and direct or are there hidden agendas or hidden meanings? Do people listen to one another?

• *Roles:* Who is in charge and how are executive decisions made? Who provides for the family? Who is concerned for the child's education and emotional development? Families may function most effectively when roles are appropriately allocated and responsibilities explicit.

• *Affective involvement:* Relationships in families tend to exist on a continuum from over-involved (enmeshed) to disinvolved (disengaged). Empathic involvement is ideal. This depends on development, as greater involvement is needed for babies than adolescents. Enmeshment may lead a child to be so anxious about a parent that they feel unable to leave them, and avoid school as a consequence.

• *Affective responsiveness:* How do individual family members respond emotionally to one another both by degree and quality? Welfare feelings would include love, tenderness, and sympathy. Emergency feelings would include fear, anger, and disappointment.

• *Behavioural control:* How is discipline maintained? Is there negotiation? Is it flexible? Chaotic? Absent? (depends on quality of communication).

Dysfunctional family patterns

• *Triangulation:* When parents are in conflict, each demands the child sides with them. When the child sides with one, they are automatically considered to be attacking the other. The child is paralysed in a no-win state where every movement is a perceived attack on a parent.

• *Scape goating:* When an individual is singled out by the family as the sole cause of the family troubles. This serves to temporarily bury conflicts that the family fear will overwhelm them.

• *High expressed emotion:* Derived from a family interview: reflects hostility, emotional over-involvement, critical comments, and contact time.

'A problem shared is a problem halved.' Old English proverb

Counselling is defined as 'provision of professional assistance and guidance in resolving personal or psychological problems'; counselling is, in essence, two people talking together in order to find a solution to a stressful situation or problem. It has existed in many forms for years (family, priests, teachers) but more recently has been professionalized, diversified, and accepted into modern medicine as a legitimate management option for treating psychological needs.

There are a myriad of different modalities of counselling, those focused on career, bereavement, or pre-conception, and in a variety of approaches: email, telephone, or face-to-face. Counselling remains distinct from other types of therapy and should never be considered to be psychotherapy-lite or diet-CBT. As with all therapies, counselling is not advice-giving or persuasion orientated to the therapist's point of view. Proper counsellors are trained, registered (for example, www.bacp.co.uk) and self-reflective.

Indications • Current problems and stresses (eg experiencing acute psychological distress in response to life events or relationship problems) • Brief anxiety disorders, especially when anxiolytic drugs not required.

Technique Aim for adult relationships between patient, family, and therapist, eg with a contract vis-à-vis duties, frequency, and duration of therapy, and what is expected of the client (homework) • Listening, understanding, and reflecting • Note how past stress has been coped with • Producing an agreed full list of problems • Redefining problems in terms of attainable goals • Use of therapeutic contracts to negotiate small behaviour changes, eg learning anxiety-reducing techniques, and carrying out rewards • Talking out (not acting out) anger in safe but cathartic ways • Reassurance: the therapist must give overt reassurance and also, by demeanour, reassure the patient that whatever he reveals (eg incest or baby battering), he will not be condemned.

Not all counselling is non-directive: problem-solving models of counselling are sometimes directive, and may be appropriate if you know the client well.

Caution • 'Giving expert advice': patients may need medical, legal, or financial advice. It may be best if this comes from a specialist agency not involved in the counselling • Patients with personality disorder, where the problems are too deep seated to be changed by counselling. Here there must be an awareness of the need to refer such patients for more formal psychotherapy.

Counselling has long been a central activity in primary care. Many UK general practices employ or have access to counsellors. This huge growth reflects the fact that people love to be listened to, and that a GP may not have the time or inclination to satisfy this need. It is hard to prove the effectiveness of counselling, especially as skills and training vary markedly. This does not mean it is ineffective. Some psychiatrists also offer an 'advisory' service for counsellors.

There are three facets to **counselling in general practice**:

1 In some patients, problem-solving strategies are used, with the counsellor using a non-directive approach.

2 In fostering coping strategies, the therapist helps the patient to make the most of the position they are in (eg afflicted by a chronic disease).

3 In cognitive therapy, we concentrate on elucidating negative thinking, and help patients learn how to intervene in negative cycles of thinking.

Randomized trial evidence Counselling and CBT within primary care are both more effective in treating depression than usual GP care in the short term. But in one study, there was no difference[25] in outcome after 1 year.[237] [238] [·N=197]

---

25 'No difference' may indicate that too few counselling sessions were offered, that GPs involved were already effective counsellors, or maybe more focused counselling would be more effective.[239]

Supportive psychotherapy

Supportive psychotherapy is an attempt by a therapist to help patients deal with their emotional distress and reinforce health patterns of behaviour through a pragmatic combination of psychodynamic, interpersonal and CBT approaches. Unlike some therapies, the therapist engages in an encouraging and supportive relationship (not a passive conduit) who comforts, reassures, and listens attentively and sympathetically.

Techniques include:
• Listening to what the patient is saying, picking up verbal and non-verbal cues. Ensure a reasonably full account of the situation and problems
• Reassurance: relieve fears, boost self-confidence, and promote hope
• Explain to a patient why they are experiencing certain symptoms
• Guidance and suggestion with regard to a particular problem
• Expression of feelings, eg anger and despair within a supportive setting.

Although supportive psychotherapy is not currently included in NICE guidance as the primary therapy for most conditions, it can be useful in engaging patients and introducing therapeutic modalities, eg CBT. It also has been shown to be beneficial in crisis intervention and in bulimia nervosa.

Brief solution-focused therapy

Brief solution-focused therapy[240] makes use of a structured approach to draw on people's resilience, and motivate problem solving. It centres conversations on solutions, not problems. 'If it works, do more of it. If it doesn't work do something different. No problem happens all the time.' In this therapy the therapist may use various questioning techniques:

'Miracle' question: Help the patient think about how the future will be different without the problem and set positive goals: 'If you woke up and a miracle had occurred overnight, how would you know? How would life be different?'

Exception question: Search with the patient for possible times when the identified problem is less severe or absent. Then encourage them to identify these occurrences and ask 'What happened that was different?'

Spectograms: These allow a patient to quantify, measure, and track their own experience, in a non-threatening way. 'On a scale of 0 to 10, how much would you like your miracle to happen?' 'What would have to happen/What would you have to do to make your score move from 3 to 4?'

Coping questions: Elicit information about a patient's positive approach that may have gone unnoticed. Even the most hopeless story can have examples of coping which can be shown: 'Things have been really difficult for you, yet you get up each morning and get organized for work. How do you do that?'

Problem-free talk: Create a judgement-free zone where patients can discuss what is going well and what areas of their life are problem-free, without minimizing the real problems they have.

Psychiatry

Group psychotherapy

Groups are interactive microcosms in which the patient can be confronted by the effect his behaviour and beliefs have on others, and be protected during his first attempts to change. Group therapy involves one or more therapists working with several people at the same time. The therapy delivered can be of any type (CBT, interpersonal, etc.) however usually this name is given to psychodynamic therapy where the group itself and communication within the group are used to explore interpersonal relationships and develop new ways of interacting thus promoting change through observation and experimenting.

General indications We know that the most suitable patients are:

1 Those who enter into the group voluntarily, not as a result of pressure from relatives or therapists

2 Those who have a high expectation from the group, and do not view it as inferior to individual therapy

3 Those who have adequate verbal and conceptual skills. See also psychodynamic psychotherapy (see p394).

Specific indications • Personality disorders • Addictions,[241] drug and alcohol dependence (12-step models are all group therapies) • Victims of childhood sexual abuse • People with difficulties in socialization • Major medical illnesses—eg breast cancer.[242] N=50

Contraindications Those who are unlikely to benefit include those with severe depression, acute schizophrenia, hypochondriacs, or extreme schizoid personality (cold, aloof, hypersensitive introverts). Group therapy is contraindicated for extreme antisocial behaviour and perpetrators of abuse (especially paedophilia) as the group itself can condone or normalize past thoughts or actions rather than weaken them.

Technique The group selection procedure should be completed by an experienced psychotherapist. Each group is limited to 6–8 members, balanced for sex, and avoiding mixing extremes of age. A decision is made beforehand if the group is to be 'closed', or whether it will accept new patients during its life. The therapist will usually take on a co-therapist of the opposite gender.

The life of the group (~18 months) will develop through a number of phases ('forming → storming → norming → performing'). First there is a settling-in period when members are on their best behaviour, seeking to be loved by the therapist, and looking to them for directive counselling (which is rarely provided). Next is the stage of conflict, as each person strives to find their place in the group other than through dependency on the leader. Frustration, anger, and other negative feelings are helpful by testing the group's trustworthiness. Learning that expressing negative feelings need not lead to rejection is a vital prelude to the next stage: intimacy, in which the group starts working together.

Typically the therapist steers the group away from outside crises and searches for antecedent causes towards the here and now—eg asking 'Who do you feel closest to in the group?' or 'Who in the group is most like you?' The therapist avoids sacrificing spontaneity, and learns to use what the group gives, eg 'You seem very angry that John stormed out just now'. Unanswerable questions, especially those beginning 'Why?' are ignored in favour of interaction, observation, and learning. Special methods used to augment this process include written summaries of group activities, video, and psychodrama.

Psychiatry

Irvin Yalom, an American existential psychiatrist developed a number of therapeutic factors essential to positive group work and group therapy:

• *Universality:* Recognition of shared experiences and feelings among group members to remove individual sense of isolation, validate experiences, and raise self-esteem.

• *Altruism:* Group members help each other. By doing this an individual will experience giving something to another person which helps develop own self esteem, adaptive coping styles, and interpersonal skills.

• *Instillation of hope:* In a mixed group with members at various stages of development or recovery, members are inspired and encouraged by another member who has overcome the problems with which they are still struggling.

• *Imparting information:* Not a true psychotherapeutic process, however members usefully learn factual or practical information from other members in the group (but not the therapist).

• *Corrective recapitulation of the primary family experience:* Members often unconsciously identify the therapist and other members with their own parents and family. Group interpretations help group gain an understanding of the impact of their experiences on their personality, and learn to avoid unconsciously repeat unhelpful past behaviour patterns in current relationships.

• *Development of socializing techniques:* The group setting provides a safe and supportive environment for members to take risks by extending their repertoire of interpersonal behaviour and improving their social skills.

• *Imitative behaviour:* Group members develop social skills through a modeling process, observing and imitating the therapist and other members.

• *Cohesiveness:* All members feel a sense of belonging, acceptance, and validation from being in the group.

• *Existential factors:* Learning that one has to take responsibility for one's own life and the consequences of one's decisions.

• *Catharsis:* Relief from emotional distress through the free and uninhibited expression of emotion. When members tell their story to a supportive audience, they can obtain relief from chronic feelings of shame and guilt.

• *Interpersonal learning:* Self-awareness through feedback given by the group on the member's behaviour and impact on others.

Therapeutic communities, and the example of substance misuse

Therapeutic communities (TCs) are a popular treatment for the rehabilitation of IV drug users and dealing with personality disorders—in both the USA and Europe. The rationale is that the benefits of peer-feedback (group therapy) can be magnified in the microcosm of a therapeutic community. Also these communities provide a safe environment for those with complex needs.

In trials of residential therapy vs therapeutic communities the latter can come out better vis à vis staying off drugs and not reoffending (eg if the 'residential' arm of the trial is prison).[243] Life in a community is more beneficial (vis à vis reoffending or reusing drugs) if it is for 12 months compared with 6 months. After the time in the community, aim to give continuing aftercare.[244] However, there is little evidence that TCs offer major benefits compared with other residential treatment, or that one type of TC is better than another.

European TCs adapt the early harsh behaviourism found in the USA by concentrating more on milieu-therapy and social learning emphasizing dialogue and understanding. Either professionals or ex-addicts can provide input.[245]

Psychiatry

▶Never underestimate a child's capacity for insight: *don't expect children's methods of communicating insight to mesh with adults'*.

Play therapy Children often communicate their experiences and reactions to events through their actions (fig 4.15). This therapy allows them to express emotions through play and also to develop an understanding of themselves and others, resolve psychosocial challenges, and gain acceptance of their experiences and feelings. This builds toward social integration and emotional regulation.

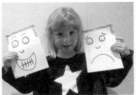

Fig 4.15 A child with an emotion.
© Gil Myers.

Play therapy is often divided into directive or non-directive play. In directive play, the therapist offers more structure and guidance in order to lead the play toward an identified difficulty to work through. Non-directive play therapy encourages a child to play freely without intrusion and in so doing recognize and solve problems. Non-directive play is more comparable to psychodynamic therapy than the behaviouralist/CBT approach offered by directive play.

Technique (non-directive) Play, rather than talk, may be the medium for communication between child and therapist.[246]

The basic 10 rules are:

1 Take time early on to make friends with the child. *Don't rush.*
2 Accept the child on his own terms—*exactly as he or she is.*
3 Avoid questioning, praising, or blaming. Be *totally permissive.*
4 *Don't say 'Don't',* and only restrain to prevent serious imminent harm.
5 Show the child that he or she is free to express *any* feeling openly.
6 The responsibility for making choices is *always* the child's *alone.*
7 Follow *wherever* the child leads: avoid directing the conversation.
8 Use *whatever he/she gives you.* Reflect his or her feelings back to him.
9 Encourage the child to move from acting-out his feelings in the real world, to *expressing them freely* in words and play.
10 Prepare the parents for change in the child.

Play therapy is usually used with children aged 3–11 although more frequently with those children who are less verbal or who use play more. Compared to control groups, play therapy treatment groups show an improvement by 0.8 standard deviations.[247] Play therapy appeared equally effective across age and gender. Using parents in play therapy produced the largest effects.

Evidence on 'activity-based interventions' (broader than play therapy) is mixed: no effect on war-torn children,[248] but good effects on social functioning after sexual abuse,[249] neglect,[250] and in autism.[251]

Play as a diagnostic tool Play can be used in diagnosis, however this is separate from play therapy. Here, the therapist observes the child's play: choice of toys, situations and actions, and their interactions with others, and considers the underlying reasons for these behaviours and their impact on the child's life. Rich evidence can be drawn from seeing a child explore an environment at their own rate, even when they know they are being watched. For example, school observations in ADHD assessments can highlight differences in playtime routines: does she play football with the rest of the class or sit alone in the corner? And if she does play can she take turns in goal (waiting for the ball to come) or is she always chasing after it impulsively? These are observations which are missed in a foreign, clinical environment.

Psychiatry

Art therapy is the use of art materials for self-expression and reflection in the presence of a trained art therapist. No previous experience or skill in art is needed as the art therapist is not primarily concerned with making an aesthetic or diagnostic assessment of the client's work. It is not an art lesson or recreational activity. The chief aim is to effect change and growth in self-esteem through use of art materials in a safe and facilitating environment. Patients stop being patients, and take the initiative in externalizing pain and problems through self-expression.[252]

As ever, the relationship between therapist and client is vital, but art therapy differs from other psychotherapies as it is a three-way process between client, therapist, and artefact. The therapist's evaluating of the art establishes the intellectual, spiritual, cultural, and emotional status of clients in ways that are helpful to those who find it hard to express thoughts and feelings verbally.[253] It can be a mistake for therapists to interpret the art: leave this to the client.[254]

Art therapists have a good understanding of art processes with sound therapeutic knowledge. They work with individuals and groups of all ages across a range of issues: mental health (in anorexia and dementia, art therapy can improve interactive and coping skills[255]), learning disabilities, palliative care (coping with a cancer diagnosis), disaster zones[254] and in prisons.

NICE says to always consider non-drug treatments for depression. In a trial with artists-in-residence (a ceramicist, a poet, and a painter) there was a reduction in anxiety, an increase in self-esteem, and fewer consultations from 'heartsink' patients.[256] Art therapy also helps coping in the context of cancer.[257]

Art therapy myths

Edited list from: *Top 10 Art Therapy Myths* on Art Therapy Spot blog:[258]

Art therapy is only for children and not for adults. Children are usually receptive to art therapy because it appeals to their innate curiosity and desire to create. But art therapy can be beneficial to adults of all ages. Art has the ability to express what (even adults) do not always have the words for. Art may bypass purely intellectual thought, and shed light onto the unconscious.

The art therapist know patients' secrets just by looking at their art work. Art therapists do have a foundation training in interpreting art. However, this understanding helps them ask questions, rather than supply answers. The meaning of the artwork is always derived directly from the patient.

Art therapy is like going to an art class. During art therapy you learn to draw, paint, or sculpt. The goal of art therapy is not to 'teach' art skills. Some art therapists may instruct clients in how to use various art materials so that the client has the freedom to then create whatever they desire.

An art therapist cannot be your primary therapist, but must be an adjunct therapist. An art therapist can be the primary therapist or be part of a treatment team, made up of psychiatrists, psychologists, social workers, etc.

Sessions are awkward for patients because the art therapist just stares at them in silence as they draw. Most art therapists are directly engaged during sessions. Everyone will have thier own personal style within the therapeutic relationship. Some create art alongside their clients or some ask clients to create art outside of sessions and bring this in to share and discuss.

Patients have to make art during every art therapy session. There may be sessions when the client decides to just talk or engage in a different type of therapy experience—eg guided meditations, dream work, or more body-centred work such as breathing exercises. Some sessions may be devoted to 'problem-solving' skills such as creating daily schedules.

AC	approved clinician	LSSA	local social services authority
AMHP	approved mental health professional	MCA	Mental Capacity Act 2005
CPA	care programme approach	MHAC	Mental Health Act Commission
CTO	community treatment order	MHRT	Mental Health Review Tribunal
ECHR	European Convention on Human Rights	NHSFT	NHS foundation trust
ECT	electroconvulsive therapy	PCT	primary care trust
GSCC	General Social Care Council	RC	responsible clinician
IMCA	independent mental capacity advocate	RMO	responsible medical officer
IMHA	independent mental health advocate	SCT	supervised community treatment
LHB	local health board	SOAD	Second Opinion Appointed Doctor

'I want freedom for the full expression of my personality.'   Mahatma Gandhi

The Mental Health Act (MHA), enacted in 1983 and amended in 2007, is the law which allows people with a 'mental disorder' to be admitted to hospital, detained, and treated without their consent. A person is detained in the interests of their own health or safety or with a view to the protection of other persons. The law only applies in England and Wales; Scotland and Ireland have their own laws about compulsory treatment with mental disorders.

Under this Act, there are a set of guiding principles to be considered when making decisions:

- Purpose principle: the MHA must be used to minimize the undesirable effects of mental disorder by maximizing their safety and well-being (mental and physical) of patients, promoting recovery, and protecting others from harm.
- Least restrictive principle: people taking action without a patient's consent must attempt to keep to a minimum the restrictions they impose on the patient's liberty.
- Respect principle: people taking decisions under the MHA must recognize and respect each patient including their race, religion, culture, age, etc.
- Participation principle: patients must be involved in their care as much as is practicable. The involvement of family and friends is encouraged.
- Effectiveness, efficiency, and equity principle: this refers to the most appropriate use of resources to meet the needs of patients.

Procedures governing use of compulsory powers (2007)

Stage 1—preliminary examination: Decisions to begin assessment and initial treatment of a patient under compulsory powers must be based on a preliminary opinion by two doctors and an AMHP that a patient needs further assessment or urgent treatment by specialist mental health services and, without this, might be at risk of serious harm or pose a risk of serious harm to others.

Stage 2—formal assessment/initial treatment under compulsory powers: A patient will be given a full assessment of his or her health and social care needs and receive a formal care plan; the initial period of assessment and treatment under compulsory powers is up to 28 days; after that, continuing use of compulsory powers must be authorized by a new independent decision making body, the Mental Health Tribunal, which gets advice from independent experts as well as taking evidence from the clinical team, the patient ± his or her representatives, and other agencies, as appropriate.

Stage 3—care and treatment order: The Tribunal (or the Court in the case of mentally disordered offenders) can make a care and treatment order to authorize the care and treatment specified in a care plan recommended by the clinical team. This must be designed to give therapeutic benefit to the patient, or to manage behaviour associated with the mental disorder that might lead to serious harm to other people. The first two orders can be up to 6 months each; subsequent orders may be for periods of up to 12 months.

Significant amendments were made in 2007 to the Mental Health Act (1983):

- A single definition of 'mental disorder' is used throughout, replacing the previous four subcategories, which included mental impairment and psychopathic disorder. Dependence on alcohol or drugs is not considered to be a disorder in the amended MHA.
- Community treatment orders were introduced (see BOX).
- A new 'treatability' test to ensure that compulsory treatment is of therapeutic benefit. So any prolonged detention should include 'medical treatment the purpose of which is to alleviate, or prevent a worsening of, the disorder or one or more of its symptoms or manifestations'.
- People diagnosed with severe antisocial personality disorders are now within the scope of mental health law and can be detained even if they have committed no crime, if they are deemed a danger to themselves or others.
- Age-appropriate services are expected: children protected from admission to adult wards (section 140) and under 18s treated in a suitable environment for their age.
- Widening professional roles to allow non-medical staff (such as psychologists, nurses, etc.) to be Responsible Clinicians and non-social workers to be approved mental health professionals (AMHPs).
- ECT (see p345) cannot be given when there is capacitous refusal, other than in emergency, ie if immediately necessary to save life or immediately necessary to prevent a serious deterioration.
- Patients may be transferred from one place of safety to another. The hope is that patients detained by police on section 136 will be quickly transferred from a police cell to a more therapeutic environment (see p407).

Community treatment orders

In the 2007 amendment, community treatment orders (CTOs) were introduced which allow for compulsory treatment in the community. A patient under section 3 can be discharged from hospital to receive treatment which can be provided outside hospital but they remain subject to a power of recall if specific conditions are not met (outlined when CTO is made) or the risk of harm to patient or others necessitates immediate return to hospital.

CTOs are authorized by the Responsible Clinician and AMHP using the same criteria as for a section 3 application. CTOs have a similar duration and renewal period as section 3 orders.

Psychiatry

A patient who makes the capacious choice to come into hospital cannot be held under the Mental Health Act (MHA). They are a 'voluntary' patient. If they are held using the MHA they are called 'involuntary' or, more colloquially, 'sectioned' as a section of the MHA is used (for 2007 law, see p404).

▶ If voluntary means have failed, before compulsion may be used, it must be demonstrated that: **1** A patient has a mental disorder and **2** Needs detention for assessment/treatment of it, or **3** admission is to protect himself or others.

The main sections used for compulsory detention in hospital are section 2: admission for assessment, section 3: admission for treatment, section 4: emergency admission, and section 5(2): emergency detention of an inpatient.

Section 2: admission for assessment (for ≤28 days)
• The period of assessment (and treatment) is up to 28 days.
• The AMHP makes the application on the recommendation of two doctors, one of whom is 'section 12 approved' under the MHA (in practice a psychiatric consultant or registrar). The other doctor should be from a different Trust and ideally know the patient in a professional capacity. If not possible, the Code of Practice recommends the second doctor should be an 'approved' doctor.
• Patient's appeals must be sent within 14 days to the Mental Health Tribunal (composed of a doctor, lay person, and lawyer).

Section 3: admission for treatment (for ≤6 months)
• The exact mental disorder must be stated and the appropriate treatment should be available and specified. A patient can be compelled to have certain treatments under a section 3.
• Two doctors must sign the appropriate forms and know why treatment in the community is contraindicated. They must have seen the patient within 24 hours. They must state that treatment is likely to benefit the patient, or prevent deterioration; or that it is necessary for the health or safety of the patient or the protection of others.
• Detention is renewable for a further 6 months (annually thereafter).

Section 4: emergency treatment (for ≤72 hours)
• Admission to hospital must be an urgent necessity.
• May be used if admission under section 2 would cause undesirable delay (admission must follow the recommendation rapidly).
• An AMHP, or the nearest relative although this is rare, makes the application after recommendation from one doctor (usually here the patient's GP).
• The patient must be seen within 72 hours by a second doctor, usually on arrival in hospital by the duty psychiatrist, at which point the decision is made: conversion to a section 2 (or 3), voluntary admission or discharge. This section should not be allowed to lapse.

Section 5(2): detention of a patient already in hospital (≤72 hours)
• Any doctor looking after the patient (although officially only the doctor in charge or their delegated deputy can complete this section).
• Plan where the patient is to go before the 72 hours has elapsed, eg by liaising with psychiatrists for a formal MHA assessment.
• A patient in an ED is not in a ward, so cannot be detained under this section. Common law is all that is available, to provide temporary restraint 'on a lunatic who has run amok and is a manifest danger either to himself or to others' while awaiting an assessment by a psychiatrist.

Nurses' holding powers: section 5(4) (for ≤6 hours)

- Any authorized psychiatric nurse may forcibly detain a voluntary 'mental' patient who is taking his own discharge against advice, if such a discharge would be likely to involve serious harm to the patient (eg suicide) or others.
- During the 6 hours the nurse must find the necessary personnel to sign a section 5(2) application or allow the patient's discharge.

Sections 7 and 8: guardianship (for 6 months)

- A guardian, usually a social worker, acts in the best interest of someone with a 'mental disorder', to ensure their welfare or protect other people. They help someone live as independently as possible within the community.
- Application is made by an AMHP or 'nearest relative' and also needs two medical recommendations. It can be renewed after 6 months.
- Under section 8, a guardian can require the patient to live in a specified place, to attend for treatment and allow authorized persons access to the residence. Guardianship does not allow treatment to be given without a person's consent.

Section 17: leave of absence from hospital

- While detained in hospital, it is against the law for a patient to leave without permission.
- Under section 17, the responsible clinician agrees to a time-limited leave of absence. Often for family visits or a trial visit home prior to discharge. Sometimes, a member of staff might escort a patient on leave.

Section 117: aftercare & the Care Programme Approach (CPA)

- Section 117 requires provision of after-care for patients who have been detained on the 'long sections' (3, 37, 47, or 48).
- The CPA is not part of the Act but stipulates that no patient should be discharged without planned aftercare: the systematic assessment of health and social needs, an agreed care plan, the allocation of a keyworker, and regular reviews of progress.

Police powers—'place of safety' orders

A 'place of safety' is a nominated safe space where a person can be kept safe and assessed. Every ED should have a designated room for this as well as every police station and the police will have a list of these. Colloquially these spaces are called a '136 suite' in the ED, as this is their main function, although often all 'psychiatric referrals' are assessed there as they offer more privacy.

Section 135 allows the police to force entry into someone's premises to allow an assessment under the MHA to be made, or to bring them to a 'place of safety'. A warrant from a Magistrates' Court is required before this power can be used. The police must be accompanied by an AMHP and/or a doctor.

Section 136 allows police to arrest a person 'in a place to which the public have access' who they believe to be suffering from a mental disorder in order to convey them directly to a 'place of safety'. People can be held under section 136 for up to 72 hours, during which time they should be seen by a doctor and by an AMHP who can choose to complete a MHA assessment, admit them informally or discharge them from the section.

Consent to treatment comes in Part 4 of the MHA; it applies to:
• Treatments for mental disorders.
• All formal patients unless detained under sections 4, 5, 35, 135, and 136. The Act doesn't apply to those subject to Guardianship or Supervised Discharge, who have the right to refuse treatment, except in emergencies.

Where a person is deemed to have given their consent to treatment under section 57 or section 58, the person can withdraw that consent at any time. The treatment must then stop and the appropriate procedures followed, unless discontinuing treatment would cause 'serious suffering' to the patient, in which case continued treatment *may* be justified.

Section 57: treatments requiring consent *and* a 2nd opinion

Some treatments are deemed so restricting that patients cannot automatically have them even if they do consent. Also:
• Three people (one doctor and two others who cannot be doctors) must certify that the person concerned is capable of understanding the nature, purpose and likely effects of the treatment and has consented to it (*competence*). They are appointed by the Mental Health Act Commission.
• Treatments falling into this category are destruction of brain tissue, or functioning and implantation of hormones to reduce male sex drive.

Section 58: treatments requiring consent *or* a 2nd opinion

Applies to people who are detained under certain sections without consent, or where the person is not able to consent, eg to ECT or drugs for a mental disorder if 3 months since the person first had the drugs during their current period of detention under the Act.
• In the first three months the treatment can be given without consent. The 3-month period starts from when drugs are first given.
• If the person is capable of understanding the nature, purpose, and effects of the treatment and consents to it, the Responsible Medical Officer (RMO) must certify that understanding and consent are present. If the person is capable of understanding the nature, purpose, and likely effects of the treatment and doesn't consent to it, or has ↓capacity so cannot consent, then a doctor is appointed by the Mental Health Act Commission to give a 2nd opinion. She must consult two professionals involved in the patient's treatment; one must be a nurse.
• The certificates must state the treatment plan in precise terms, eg the number of ECT treatments. If the plan changes, new certificates are required.
• The provisions of section 58 don't prevent urgent treatment (section 62).

Section 62: urgent treatment

The requirements of section 57 and section 58 need not be followed for urgent treatment to save the patient's life or to:
• Prevent serious deterioration, so long as the treatment is not irreversible.
• Alleviate serious suffering (if the treatment isn't irreversible or hazardous).
• Prevent the patient behaving violently or endangering self or others, so long as the treatment is neither irreversible nor hazardous, and is not excessive.

Psychiatry

Capacity

Capacity entails being able to grasp and retain information relevant to a decision, and to weigh it as part of a process of making that decision.[259] Mental Capacity Act 2005

Mental Capacity Act (2005) has five statutory principles:

1 A person must be assumed to have capacity unless it is established that they lack capacity.
2 A person is not to be treated as unable to make a decision unless all practicable steps to help him to do so have been taken without success.
3 A person is not to be treated as unable to make a decision merely because he makes an unwise decision.
4 An act done, or decision made, under this Act for or on behalf of a person who lacks capacity must be done, or made, in his best interests.
5 Before the act is done, or the decision is made, regard must be had to whether the purpose for which it is needed can be as effectively achieved in a way that is less restrictive of the person's rights and freedom of action.

In order to decide that someone lacks capacity they must be unable to do any (or all) of the following, in regards to a particular decision at that point in time:

- Understand the information given to them, ensuring it is appropriately presented (eg in a language they understand) about the decision
- Weigh up the information, considering both pros and cons of any decision in an environment free from inappropriate external influence, eg a relative pressuring them to chose one decision through emotional or physical force
- Retain that information while they make the decision
- Communicate their decision (in any means possible: talking, sign language, written, or by any other means).

We mustn't assume that because a patient lacks capacity today for one issue that she will lack capacity on all issues. We must plan for changes in capacity.[260]

However old the person is, it is capacity which matters not age. Parents' wishes are *not* supreme so long as that young person has capacity. If we make a decision on behalf of a patient, we must have a 'reasonable belief' that capacity is lacking and that the act is in their best interests.

Medicolegal issues: use of common law in clinical situations

Deliberate self-harm Adapted from Feldman 2000:[261] *'A 30-year-old man is brought to ED after an overdose. There is no history available and the patient refuses to say anything, other than he wants to be left alone to die. He refuses to give blood for a drug level and is refusing any treatment.* What should we do?' Should we assume he has full capacity? If so, he may die—but autonomy is maintained. Or should the clinician act in the patient's best interests (the doctrine of necessity) as part of their duty of care?

Most people who self-harm are depressed—but this does not prove incapacity. However, in the acute setting, Feldman asserts that 'there are usually good grounds for reasonable doubt with respect to the patient's capacity to make a fully informed and reasoned choice, and to proceed with whatever action is necessary to save his life under the common law'.

Restraint The MHA is an *enabling act* (it needn't be used in all valid situations). Its use gives certain legal safeguards for patients and staff. *'A 40-year-old woman with alcohol problems was admitted two days ago with a head injury. She has fluctuating levels of confusion, agitation. She is now trying to leave the ward.'*

Here, due to refusal or lack of capacity, the transient nature of the disturbance, and the need for intervention, common law is applicable. If stronger measures are needed, or the situation persists, it is wise to use the MHA to detain a patient with delirium; however, it is not commonly used.

*D*octors assume that our eyes are passive organs whose sole job is receiving and organizing photons. Philosophers and physiologists are less sure. Ludwig Wittgenstein said 'we do not see the human eye as a receiver, it appears not to let anything in, but to send something out. The ear receives; the eye looks. (It casts glances, it flashes, radiates, gleams.) One can terrify with one's eyes, not with one's ear or nose. When you see the eye, you see something going out from it. You see the look in the eye. If you only shake free from your physiological prejudices, you will find nothing queer about the fact that the glance of the eye can be seen too. For I also say that I see the look that you cast at someone else.'[1]

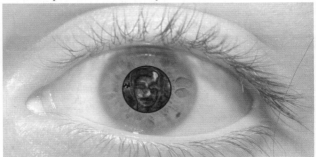

Fig 5.1 Between blinks.   Derived from image of an eye, ©Ken Banks.

If you were Wittgenstein's pupil[1] (fig 5.1[2]) and he cast you one of his notorious glances in a tutorial, would you meet his gaze? Choosing where to look can be perplexing. You might toy with the idea of looking him in the eye, but then back off. MRI shows different parts of the medial frontal cortex are active when we choose to make eye movements of our own free will, compared with when we face duress and conflicting choices.[2]

So studying eye movements teaches us about the seat of the soul, if we accept that appreciating and resolving ambiguities is the essence of consciousness.

1 *Pupilla* is Latin for doll. Pupils are named after our own doll-like reflections, seen on gazing into an eye, which perfectly mirror our movements. (Wittgenstein's pupils were never so obedient.)

We thank Mr Arun Brahma, our Specialist Reader, Ciara Hennesey, Mr Kenneth Yau, and Jins Kallampallil for their kind help. We also thank Gillian Bennerson and the imaging department at the Bristol Eye Hospital for permission to reproduce images.

Accommodation Changing of lens shape to focus near objects, using the ciliary muscle. Young lenses can go from furthest (a star) to nearest in 0.35 seconds (approaching kisses go out of focus at ~7cm).

Acuity A measure of how well the eye sees a small or distant object (p414).

Amblyopia ↓Acuity uncorrectable by lenses, with no anatomic defect.

Amsler grid Test chart of intersecting lines used for screening for macular disease. If present, lines may appear wavy and squares distorted.

Anisocoria Unequal pupil size (p425).

Anisometropia Having different refractive errors in each eye.

Aphakia The state of having no lens (eg removed because of cataract).

Blepharitis Inflamed lids.

Canthus The medial or lateral angle made by the open lids.

Chemosis Oedema of the conjunctiva.

Choroid Vascular coat between the retina and the outer scleral coat.

Ciliary body Portion of uvea (uveal tract) between iris and choroid, containing ciliary processes and ciliary muscle (for accommodation).

Conjunctiva Mucous membrane on anterior sclera and posterior lid aspect.

Cycloplegia Ciliary muscle paralysis preventing accommodation.

Dacryocystitis Inflammation of the lacrimal sac.

Dioptre Units for measuring refractive power of lenses.

Ectropion The lids evert (especially lower lid).

Entropion The lids invert (so that the lashes may irritate the eyeball).

Epiphora Passive overflow of tears on to the cheek.

Fornix Where bulbar (scleral) and palpebral (lid) conjunctivae meet.

Fovea Cone-rich area of macula capable of 6/6 vision, p450. Foveola: p450.

Fundus That part of retina normally visible through the ophthalmoscope.

Keratoconus The cornea is shaped like a cone.

Keratomalacia The cornea is softened.

Limbus The annular border between clear cornea and opaque sclera.

Macula Retinal area ~5mm across, lateral to optic disc (surrounds fovea), p450.

Miotic An agent causing pupil constriction (eg pilocarpine).

Mydriatic An agent causing pupil dilatation (eg tropicamide).

Near point Where the eye is looking when maximally accommodated.

Optic cup The cup-like depression in the centre of the optic disc (p445).

Optic disc That part of optic nerve seen ophthalmoscopically in the fundus.

Papillitis Inflammation of the optic nerve head.

Presbyopia Age-related reduced near-acuity from failing accommodation.

Pterygium Wing-shaped degenerative conjunctival condition (p416).

Ptosis Drooping lids.

Refraction Ray deviation on passing through media of different density; or determining refractive errors and correcting them with lenses.

Retinal detachment The sensory retina separates from the pigmented epithelial layer of retina.

Sclera The whites of the eyes starting from the corneal perimeter.

Scotoma A defect causing a part of the field of view to go missing.

Slit lamp A device which illuminates and magnifies structures in the eye (p414).

Strabismus (squint) Eyes deviate (they are not looking at the same thing).

Tarsorrhaphy A surgical procedure for uniting upper and lower lids.

Tonometer A device for measuring intraocular pressure.

Uvea Iris, ciliary body, and choroid.

Vitrectomy Surgical removal of the vitreous.

Vitreous Jelly-like substance filling the globe behind the lens.

Our eyes are the windows to the world around us. The eyes are a complex optical system. The most important components of the eye are in the MINIBOX. They function very similiarily to a car in that multiple complex parts work together (fig 5.2).

History Focused questions—trauma, smoker, contact lens wearer p463 (dailies vs extended wear), previous eye surgeries/injections, current correction if known. ►Eye disease is a common presenting issue for inflammatory conditions p452.

Components of the eye (fig 5.3)
• Cornea
• Sclera
• Iris and pupils
• Posterior and anterior chambers
• Lens of the eye
• Ciliary body
• Vitreous body (corpus vitreum)
• Retina
• Choroid(chorioidea)
• Optic nerve (nervis opticus)
• Fovea (fovea centralis)

Symptoms: Pain on movement, irritation 'gritty sensation/sand in the eye sensation', (consider all corneal pathologies, not just conjunctivitis), loss of vision (onset, pattern), discharge (unilateral/bilateral; purulent/watery).

Divide the eye into a car to examine it Stand back and look at the car (eyes) for any obvious abnormality. Use this stage to examine the visual acuity before the bright light and drops can affect it (see p413). Using the widest full circle illumination, examine the *eye lids*; anterior and posterior borders. Symmetrical? Normal retraction on upward gaze (abnormal in thyroid disease), ptosis (p416), spasm, inflammation, or

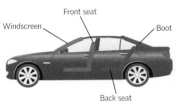

Fig 5.2 Windscreen = cornea, conjuctiva
Front seat = anterior chamber
Back seat = posterior chamber (lens, pupils)
Boot = retina, vitreous, choroid.

swellings (p416)? The anterior margin—2–3 rows of eyelashes, look for scaling, lacrimal papilla. The posterior border rests against the eye. Make sure to flip the eyelids;[2] it is common for foreign bodies to get stuck up there. On the palpebral side, yellowish ducts are clearly seen.

Windscreen components *The conjunctiva* lines the inner eyelids and sclera. What colour is it? Get the patient to look up, down, left and right to examine all the bulbar conjunctivia. It attaches to the corneascleral junction . It is a highly vascular region of the eye. Look for inflammation (if circumcorneal, suspect anterior uveitis; injection of the bulbar, fornix, and the tarsal surfaces suggests conjunctivitis; focal injection adjacent to cornea means a problem on the cornea). Is there discharge, follicles, or upper lid cobblestone patterning, or any sub-conjunctival haemorrhage?(p432).

The cornea is a transparent cover for the anterior chamber, iris and pupil. When the beam from the slit lamp passes through the cornea, you can see the anterior and posterior surfaces (the cornea is 5 layers thick). The clear aqueous humor can be cloudy in anterior uveitis (p430), may have sterile pus (*hypopyon*) with corneal ulcer, or blood (*hyphaema*) after injury (fig 5.4). If you angle the slit lamp, light reflects from both these surfaces and you can appreciate the depth of a foreign body in the cornea and if it has penetrated through the posterior surface. The cornea must always be smooth and translucent to ensure optimal clarity of the images it sees (fig 5.5). Fluorscein testing is the next step. By turning on the blue light, it helps demarcate irregularities on the corneal surface and assesses for leaks (seidal test).

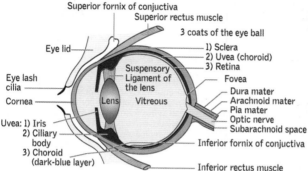

Fig 5.3 Anatomy of the eye. The average human eye has a diameter of 24 millimetres and weighs just about 7.5 grams. It is composed of 6 grams of water.

Front seat components *Anterior chamber:* A small cavity lying behind the cornea and in front of the iris. It is 0.2mL. At its peripheral margin, the corner is created by the cornea, sclera, ciliary body, and the iris. The angle is the space between this and the trabecular meshwork (see fig 5.27).

Fig 5.4 Hyphaema. Courtesy of Prof J Trobe.

Get the patient to move the eye in all four directions and then straight ahead. If there are inflammatory cells in the anterior chamber (eg in anterior uveitis p432) the appearance can be like a snow globe ('cell flare'). Use the pupil as a canvas to help visualize any cells.

Lens: With a normal lens a pupil is black; cataract may make it white. *Pupils* should be equal and react to light and accommodation (written 'PERLA'). They are small and irregular in anterior uveitis (p432), and dilated, oval and fixed in acute glaucoma (p430). For other pupil signs, see p424.

Backseat components *The posterior chamber* is bounded anteriorly by the iris, peripherally by the ciliary processes and posteriorly by the lens and the zonules. It holds 0.06mL of aqueous humor.

Boot components *Retina, vitreous, and choroid:* See p448.

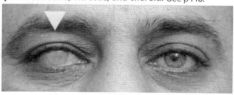

Fig 5.5 Corneal opacity in the right eye makes the pupil look hazy. The aetiology of corneal opacities include genetic, metabolic, and idiopathic. The most common cause of corneal opacity is scarring secondary to corneal infections. When looking for a cataract, only the lens (seen in front of the pupil) will look hazy.

Reproduced with permission from Zahid H Sheikh and Wasif Hafeez, The unknown source of communicable Diseases: A New Discovery, *Pakistan Journal of Ophthalmology*, Copyright © 2001 Pakistan Journal of Ophthalmology.

2 Everting the eyelid: gently grasp the eye lashes and edge of eye lid with your fingers, and with the other hand place a cotton wool bud in the centre of the eyelid which you then use as a lever to evert the eye lid over. This should reveal the inner aspect of the eye lid; look for foreign bodies.

Further reading

International Council of Ophthalmology (2009). *Handbook for Medical Students Learning Ophthalmology.* http://www.icoph.org/downloads/ICOMedicalStudentEnglish.pdf.

Examining eyes 2

Acuity is a measure of the clarity or sharpness of vision. Record it accurately, especially in eye injury. Sit the patient 6m from the Snellen chart; to get 6m in a small room, place a reversed (mirror-image) chart just above the patient, pointing towards a mirror 3m away. Obscure the left eye to occlude the visual axis (cards are more reliable than fingers). Ask the patient to read the chart from the top using the right eye, then the left. Use glasses if worn. The last line completed indicates the acuity for distant vision. An objective test of vision? Not quite.[3] The chart is designed so that the top line can be read by someone with normal vision at 60m etc. Indicate the last line accurately read as 6 over m at which a normal person would read at (6/6 vision is normal). For acuities <6/60 patients can be brought forward to 5, 4, 3, 2 and 1m from the chart to read the top line. Acuity is expressed as that distance, eg 5/60. If vision is below 1/60 ask the patient to count your fingers at 50cm distance; recorded as CF (count fingers). If he can only detect hand movement, record HM (hand movement). If only light is perceived, record PL. No perception; the eye is blind. *If the patient sees less than 6/6* with or without glasses, examine with a *pinhole* in front of the eye: a narrow beam removes the need for focus. In simple refractive errors, acuity will improve through the pinhole. This test can prove that refractive errors are the likely cause of reduced acuity.

Visual field The area seen with both eyes without shifting gaze. See p428.

Extraocular movements (see p422) Always examine in those with diplopia. Ask the patient to watch a pen move and ask which movement provokes most diplopia, and when looking in that direction, block each eye in turn and ask which one sees the *outer* image: that is the eye with pathology.

Ophthalmoscopy This helps detect pathology in the lens, vitreous, and retina. Start with high + numbers (often marked in colour on the dial). To examine the lens and the vitreous focus the beam of the ophthalmoscope at the pupil at ~1m from the eye. In the normal eye there is a red glow from the choroid (the red reflex). Red reflexes are absent with dense cataract and intraocular bleeding. Any lens opacity (cataract) will be seen as a black pattern obstructing the red reflex. Blood or loose floaters in the vitreous are seen as black floaters. When the retina is in focus, ask the patient to look right ahead into the distance. This may bring the optic disc into view. It should have precise boundaries (p456) and a central cup (p445). Examine radiating vessels and the macula (ask the patient to look at the light).

Slit lamp examination This instrument has a bright light source and a horizontally mounted microscope to examine the structures of the living eye. The light source can be converted to a slit (hence the name). Tonometric attachments allow intraocular pressure measurement. When you are working in the ED, ask someone to show you how to use it; the basics are within your grasp.

Colour vision and colour blindness

A disorder characterized by a deficiency in colour detection or processing. In order for light rays to make the images we see, the rays need to pass through photoreceptors. We require all three cones, red, green, and blue, to perceive colour. If any are missing or not functioning, one can be colour blind in that spectrum of colour. There are at least 19 different chromosomes involved in colour vision deficiencies. However, the condition is mostly inherited on the x chromosome.[4] 8% ♂ and 0.5% ♀ affected—so those with Turner's syndrome have ♂ incidence and those with Klinefelter's have ♀ incidence. **Diagnosis** This is by use of coloured pattern discrimination charts (eg Ishihara plates, see endpapers). Depressed colour vision may be a sensitive indicator of acquired macular or optic nerve disease.[5]

---

3 Mood affects Snellen reading. If we feel 'strong , active and proud' we perform better.[4] Children may give inconsistent answers, eg 'unable' to read big type (hoping for spectacles, or a spectacle case all of their own) while correctly reading very small type (unable to resist a challenge!).

4 This is due to the fact that males have only one x chromosome. Women inherit two copies of the x chromosome. For the deficiency to be present, women need 2 mutations present which is highly unlikely.

1 *Always test visual acuity* in each eye separately and wearing glasses (if worn). A 1mm pinhole will improve acuity in refractive errors.

2 *More mistakes in medicine are made by not looking than not knowing.* Optimize illumination and magnification (slit lamp optimal) for examination of the fundus. Use tropicamide 0.5% (if no head injury) to dilate the pupil.

3 *Examine the pupil reflexes* if visual acuity is abnormal (p424).

4 *Visual field examination* can differentiate an ocular cause from central cause of vision loss. Horizontal defect in glaucoma, branch retinal artery, or vein occlusion; bitemporal vertical defect in pituitary tumour; homonymous vertical defect in intracranial lesion or cva (p436).

5 *No child is too young for an eye exam.* Check the red-reflex of every newborn (p419) and refer any suspected squint immediately.

6 *Sudden loss or blurring of vision is an emergency.* Always exclude temporal arteritis because of immediate risk to other eye. Other causes are retinal artery or vein occlusion (p436), vitreous and macular haemorrhage, retinal detachment (vision loss preceded by floaters and flashes) and optic nerve ischaemia. Distortion of vision may indicate macular disease (p449).

7 *Never ignore new-onset diplopia* Binocular diplopia can be the first sign of temporal arteritis or posterior communicating artery aneurysm.

8 *Orbital cellulitis* is a life-threatening infection pain on eye movement is often the first sign of orbital involvement in a patient with lid swelling and redness (p421).

9 *Headaches are rarely due to a refractive cause.* Ocular causes include acute closed-angle glaucoma and anterior uveitis.

10 *Always irrigate chemical burns immediately.* Irrigate copiously with water for 15 minutes (instill local anaesthetic eye drops to assist).

11 *A corneal abrasion* should improve in 24 hours if the cause is removed. Evert the eyelid to check all foreign bodies have been removed and check conjunctival fornices. Exclude corneal ulcer (p434).

12 *Irritable eyes* are either dry eyes if they burn and sting. Consider blepharitis (p416) if lids are red and raw, and allergy if itchy.

13 *Viral conjunctivitis* is almost always bilateral, usually self-limiting, and will resolve without antibiotics.

14 *Topical steroid use* should be limited and supervised. Do not allow prolonged use without ophthalmic supervision. Topical steroids can promote herpes simplex corneal ulceration and fungal infection. Systemic steroids can induce cataract (p446).

15 *Blindness in diabetes mellitus* is largely preventable with tight glycaemic control, reducing lipid and blood pressure. Refer all patients with diabetes for retinopathy screening and concurrent management of hypertension is critical. Refer as soon as diagnosed (see p446).

16 *Age-related macular degeneration* may be treatable. Suspect age-related macular degeneration if gradual vision loss and distortion on Amsler grid. Sudden changes need urgent assessment (p440).

17 *Simple lifestyle advice can improve ophthalmic health.* Regular eye exam every 2 years. Use eye protection (sports, industry, and sunglasses). uv exposure is related to pterygium, cataract, macular health, and lid tumours (most are basal cell carcinomas). Eat fish and green vegetables (macular health). Smoking cessation (macula health, diabetic, cataract risk).

Adapted from Dr John Colvin's 'Golden eye rules', The Royal Victorian Eye and Ear Hospital. www.eyeandear.org.au

Styes 'Stye' is a word used more by patients than doctors for referring to inflammatory lid swellings. *Hordeolum externum* is an abscess or infection, usually staphylococcal, in a lash follicle; these may also involve the glands of Moll (sweat glands) and of Zeis (sebum-producing glands attached directly to lash follicles). They 'point' outwards and may cause much inflammation. Treat by applying a warm compress for 5–10 minutes several times each day until the stye resolves. Less common is

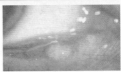

Fig 5.6 Chalazion (meaning hailstone in Greek) A granular mass to palpation.

Courtesy of Bristol Eye Hospital.

the *hordeolum internum*, an abscess of the Meibomiam glands (hordeolum is Latin for *barleycorn*). These 'point' inwards, opening on to conjunctiva, cause less local reaction but leave a residual swelling called a *chalazion* (fig 5.6) or a *Meibomian cyst* (tarsal cyst) when they subside. Vision may be ↓ if corneal flattening occurs (rare).[7] Treat residual swellings by incision & curettage under local anaesthesia.

Blepharitis (Lid inflammation eg from staphs, seborrhoeic dermatitis, or rosacea.) Eyes have 'burning' itching red margins, with scales on the lashes. *Treatment:* Good eyelid hygiene is the mainstay of treatment. Use a cotton bud and baby shampoo diluted 1:10 with warm water and clean along the lid margins twice each day. In children with blepharokeratitis, consider oral erythromycin too.[8]

Pinguecula (fig 5.7) Degenerative vascular yellow-grey nodules on the conjunctiva either side of the cornea (esp. nasal side). *Typical patient:* Adult male. *Associations:* ↑Hair and skin pigment; sun-related skin damage.[9] If inflamed (pingueculitis) topical steroids are tried. If invading the cornea, as it may in dusty, wind-blown life-styles, the word *pterygium* (fig 5.10) is used; surgery may be needed.

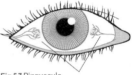

Fig 5.7 Pinguecula.

Entropion (fig 5.8) Lid inturning is typically due to degeneration of lower (rarely upper) lid fascial attachments and their muscles. It is rare if <40yrs old. The inturned eyelashes irritate the cornea. Taping the (lower) eyelids to the cheek, or botulinum toxin injection to the lower lid gives temporary relief; more lasting relief needs surgery.

Ectropion (fig 5.9) Lower lid eversion causes eye irritation, watering (drainage punctum malaligned) ± exposure keratitis. *Associations:* Old age; facial palsy. Plastic surgery may correct the deformity. If facial palsy is the cause, consider surgical correction with an implant in upper lid to aid closure.

Upper lid malposition results from the globe's hypotropic position (→'*pseudoptosis*') or intrinsic levator weakness (→*true ptosis*) from: •Congenital (absent nerve to levator muscle; poorly developed levator) •Mechanical (oedema, xanthelasma, or upper lid tumour) •Myogenic (muscular dystrophy, myasthenia) •CNS (III nerve palsy, p422; Horner's, p424). Congenital ptosis is corrected surgically early if the pupil, ie the visual axis is covered (risk of amblyopia, p422). Dermatochalasis denotes excess lid tissue (may obstruct sight).

Lagophthalmos is difficulty in lid closure. *Causes:* Exophthalmos; mechanical impairment of lid movement (eg injury or lid burns); leprosy; paralysed orbicularis oculi giving sagging lower lid. Corneal ulcers & keratitis may follow. *R*: Lubricate eyes with liquid paraffin ointment. If corneal ulcers develop, temporary tarsorrhaphy (stitching lids together) may be needed.

Xanthelasma (fig 5.11) are lipid depositions seen in hyperlipidaemia.

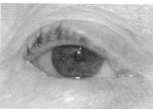

Fig 5.8 Entropion.
Courtesy of Bristol Eye Hospital.

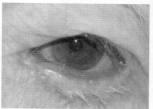

Fig 5.9 Ectropion.
Courtesy of Bristol Eye Hospital.

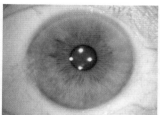

Fig 5.10 Pterygium. Note the new vessels crossing over the boundary between the sclera and the cornea.   Courtesy of Jon Miles.

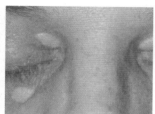

Fig 5.11 Xanthelasma.
Courtesy of Jon Miles.

Ophthalmology

Blepharospasm

Blepharospasm is involuntary contraction of orbicularis oculi. It commonly occurs in response to ocular pain. Repetitive blepharospasm, which may have a serious impact on quality of life, or make the patient effectively blind, is a *focal dystonia* (*OHCM* p473). If the condition is not recognized, it is all too easy to dismiss the patient as hysterical and to think that screwing up of the eyes is deliberate—especially, the more the sceptical doctor questions and probes the afflicted patient, the worse the blepharospasm may become (stress is an important exacerbating factor). It is important to understand that it may have a serious negative impact on patients' lives.[7]

Presentation ♀:♂ ×1.8:1. Blepharospasm is often preceded by exaggerated blinking. Other dystonias may be present (eg oro-mandibular). It usually starts unilaterally, becoming bilateral. Patients may develop tricks to reduce it such as touching or pulling the eyelids—a variation of '*geste antagoniste*' seen in other forms of dystonia. *Causes:* (Mostly unknown.) Neuroleptic drugs, Parkinson's disease, progressive supranuclear palsy, paraneoplastic (eg from lung ca).

Treatment *Drugs—Botulinum neurotoxin:* Palliation is achieved with small doses injected to orbicularis oculi; here it produces a temporary flaccid paralysis. It can help some people recover effective vision. It binds to peripheral nerve terminals and inhibits release of acetylcholine. 3-monthly treatments are needed. Response is variable; good effects may wear off. *Other options:* anticholinergics (**trihexyphenidyl**, eg 1mg/day PO, max 5mg/6h; tablets are 2mg or 5mg). Dopamine agonists (levodopa, bromocriptine) may help.[8] *Supportive treatment:* If the cause is compensation for apraxia of lid opening, wearing goggles may help.[9]

Further reading

Defazio G *et al.* (2013). Development and validation of a clinical guideline for diagnosing blepharospasm. *Neurology* 81(3):236–40. The Dystonia Society: www.dystonia.org.uk

Tears play a very important role in refraction. The lacrimal apparatus consists of the lacrimal gland which produces most tears, the lacrimal lake, the lacrimal canaliculi; the lacrimal sac and the nasolacrimal duct carry the tears into the nasal cavity (fig 5.12). **Components of tears** Lipid layer, aqueous layer, mucin layer. The volume of tears normally in the eye is 6μL, the turnover rate being 1.2μL/min. Tears are similar in electrolyte concentration to plasma, but rich in proteins, especially IgA. They also contain lysozyme and beta-lysin which have antibacterial properties. Meibomian glands, conjunctival glands, goblet cells, and lacrimal glands produce tear fluid. Reflex secretion is from the lacrimal gland alone via parasympathetic fibres of the trigeminal n.[5][10][11]

Dry eyes *(keratoconjunctivitis sicca)* may be due to ↓tear production by lacrimal glands in old age, or rarely in: Sjögren's syndrome (associated with connective tissue disorders, esp. RA); mumps; sarcoidosis; amyloidosis; lymphoma; leukaemia; haemochromatosis. Other causes: excess evaporation of tears (post-exposure keratitis); or mucin deficiency in tears (avitaminosis A, Stevens–Johnson syndrome, pemphigoid, chemical burns). Schirmer's test (strip of filter paper put overlapping lower lid; tears should soak >15mm in 5min) reveals ↓production. Artificial tears give symptomatic relief. The outflow of tears in dry eyes can be restricted by using lubricating drops or by reducing the size of the punctum lacrimale by plugs, by cautery or by laser. ▶▶Consider blepharitis and chronic allergy (p462).

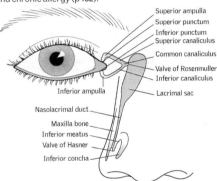

Superior ampulla
Superior punctum
Inferior punctum
Superior canaliculus
Common canaliculus
Valve of Rosenmuller
Inferior canaliculus
Lacrimal sac
Inferior ampulla
Nasolacrimal duct
Maxilla bone
Inferior meatus
Valve of Hasner
Inferior concha

Fig 5.12 Three categories of watery eyes.   © D P Austin.

1. Decreased drainage eg from punctal stenosis/obstruction or canaliculitis? Use the ophthalmoscope as a magnifier to see if the punctum is stenosed. Surgery may help.[12]

2. Increased lacrimation. Are both eyes affected? Is the environment dust- or irritant-laden? Corneal injury/FB (these tears contain ↑nerve growth factor, which aids healing, which is rather clever). Lubricating drops will help here.

3. Pump failure. On blinking, positive and negative pressure is created in the lacrimal sac which accordingly sucks tears into it. This is the tear pump. Gravity helps keep the sac empty. If the cause if *pump failure* look for causes such as *entropion*, *ectropion*, or *CNS causes* (myasthenia, VII palsy). Refer for consideration of corrective surgery.

NB: the lacrimal glands are in the upper outer area of the orbit (lacrimal fossa of the frontal bone) and have autonomic innervation. Parasympathetics start in the lacrimal nucleus of the facial nerve in the pons. Sympathetic postganglionic fibres start in the superior cervical ganglion and travel as a periarteriolar plexus with the middle meningeal artery.

5 Emotional tears were a breakthrough in the evolution of the human face as a platform for emotional signalling. Faces with tears removed by doctoring the image seem to others to be of neutral emotional valence: without tears we tend to misinterpret these faces as expressions of awe, concern, or puzzlement.[13] NB: sceptics argue that tears of joy don't exist. Sandor Feldman claims they are really tears of anticipated loss.[14] In support of this, the 'fact' is cited that children do not cry with tears of joy. Were such psychoanalysts too absorbed to have noticed infant tears of joy at family reunions?

This is the most common primary intraocular tumour in children.[15]

Signs Strabismus and leukocoria (ie a white pupil). Always suspect retinoblastoma when the red reflex is absent (fig 5.13; the mother may come with a photo showing only one eye reddened during flash photography). NB: multiple tumours may be present.

Inheritance Retinoblastomas were the first tumours to highlight the genetic aetiology of cancer. Hereditary retinoblastoma is different from the non-hereditary type: there is a mutation of the RB gene located at 13q14. Inheritance is autosomal dominant with 80% penetrance. The RB gene is present in everyone, and is normally a suppressor gene or anti-oncogene. Those with hereditable retinoblastomas typically have one altered allele in every cell. If a developing retinal cell undergoes mutation in the other allele, a retinoblastoma results. The retinoblastoma gene is the best characterized tumour suppressor gene. Its product is a nuclear phosphoprotein which helps regulate DNA synthesis. **Incidence** 1 in 15,000 live births.

Associations 5% occur with a pineal or other tumour (=trilateral retinoblastoma). Secondary malignancies such as osteosarcoma and rhabdomyosarcoma are more frequent, and they are the main causes of death of patients with hereditary retinoblastoma.

Treatment There is a trend away from enucleation (eye removal). Aim towards focal procedures to preserve eye and sight, if possible.

Chemotherapy: Useful in bilateral tumours. Combination of carboplatin, etoposide, and vincristine. Ciclosporin helps reduce multidrug resistance.

Enucleation may be needed with large tumours, long-standing retinal detachments, and optic nerve invasion or extrascleral extension.

External beam radiotherapy has a role (may *cause* secondary non-ocular cancers in the radiation field, esp. if carrying the RB-1 germline mutation).

Ophthalmic plaque brachytherapy has a more focal and shielded radiation field, and may carry less risk, but is limited to small–medium retinoblastomas in accessible locations.

Cryotherapy and transpupillary thermotherapy (TTT) can give control of selected small tumours. 'Chemoreduction' is achieved by IV or subconjunctival chemotherapy to allow TTT, cryotherapy, and radiotherapy.

Screening parents and siblings This is needed for accurate genetic counselling and to allow presymptomatic treatment. Germ-line mosaicism must be considered as a genetic transmission pattern. If a parent is germ-line mosaic, the possibility of bearing more babies with retinoblastoma is higher than conventionally believed.[16]

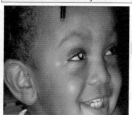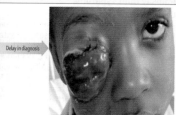

Delay in diagnosis

Fig 5.13 Absent red reflex during flash photography is a worrying sign; if untreated retinoblastomas have a high risk of local metastasis and death within 2 years. Early recognition and treatment can be life and vision saving.

Reprinted with permission from Elsevier (*The Lancet*, 2012, Volume 379(9824), pp. 1436–1446).

Further reading

Dimaras H (2012). Retinoblastoma. *Lancet* 379:1436–46.

Ophthalmology

Ophthalmology

(Herpes zoster ophthalmicus, HZO; also see BOX, p599). Varicella zoster infection has two distinct forms: It tends to first occur in childhood as chickenpox (varicella), it then lies dormant within the sensory ganglia for years until in 20% of individuals it reactivates and spreads across a dermatome as shingles (zoster).[17] **Shingles** typically affects those >50 years old. Most common site of shingles (55%) is the thoracic nerves, followed by the 1st (ophthalmic) branch of the trigeminal nerve (20%). *Risk factors:* Increasing age is the leading risk factor (esp after 50yrs old), trauma to the area, immunocompromised patients (especially HIV, transplant patients, and Hodgkin's lymphoma).[18] *Presentation:* Pain and neuralgia in the distribution of cranial nerve V_1 dermatome (p746–7) precedes a blistering inflamed rash (fig 5.14). The most common complication is post-herpetic neuralgia. *Predictors of ocular involvement:* In 50% of those with HZO the globe is affected (corneal signs ± iritis in >40%—sectoral iris atrophy, p425, fig 5.18). Nose-tip involvement (Hutchinson's sign) makes it likely that the eye will be affected (since it indicates involvement of the nasociliary branch of the trigeminal nerve which also supplies the globe). The eye can be seriously affected with little rash else-where; so age and severity of rash are not reliable predictors.[17] Beware dissemination if immunocompromised. Varicella zoster virus (VZV) may persist in the eye. *Assesment:* Visual acuity and normal corneal appearance is reassuring. Refer for more detailed examination if pain, redness, or altered vision is reported. Look carefully for Hutchinson's sign! ℞ Oral antivirals improve symptoms if given within 72 hours of rash onset or if new vesicles still forming (additional antiviral drops are not needed) but cannot be relied on to prevent post-herpetic neuralgia.[6] **Famciclovir** offers the best dose schedule (750mg once daily for 1wk; SE vomiting; headache) but is much more expensive than **aciclovir** (800mg 5 times daily PO for 7 days—it has more serious SE such as hepatitis and renal failure). Other options are aciclovir and valaciclovir. Start within 4 days of onset. It is wise for all to see a specialist if the nose-tip is involved, or the eye turns red within 3 days, to exclude anterior uveitis with a slit lamp. Prolonged steroid eyedrops may be needed. Advise isolation from pregnant ladies with no immunity to chickenpox until several days after the vesicles dry up.

Ocular involvement
• Purulent conjunc- tivitis
• Visual loss/keratitis
• Episcleritis/scleritis
• Iritis (±atrophy)
• Cranial nerve palsy
• Pupillary distortion
• Limbal lesions
• Pre-auricular node tenderness
• Optic atrophy

Ramsay Hunt syndrome See p652.

Carotico-cavernous fistula may follow carotid aneurysm rupture with reflux of blood into the cavernous sinus. *Causes:* Spontaneous; trauma; post-septorhinoplasty. There is engorgement of eye vessels + lid & conjunctival oedema. Exophthalmos may be pulsatile, with a loud bruit over the eye ± tinnitus. Arterial ligation or embolization may occasionally be tried. Read a short case study with images here.[19]

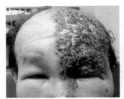

Fig 5.14 Ophthalmic shingles. Read about the case study here: http://www.nejm.org/doi/full/10.1056/NE-JMicm0803343

From The *New England Journal of Medicine,* Charlotte Page Wills, Gerin River: Herpes Zoster, Volume 362, Copyright © (2010) Massachusetts Medical Society. Reprinted with permission from Massachusetts Medical Society.

Further reading

BMJ Best Practice (2015). *Herpes Zoster Infection.* http://bestpractice.bmj.com/best-practice/monograph/23.html

NICE (2015). *Clinical Knowledge Summaries: Cellulitis –* Acute. http://cks.nice.org.uk/cellulitis-acute

Wareham DW *et al.* (2007). Herpes zoster. *BMJ* 334:1211.

6 Incidence of neuralgia is 16% if >65yrs (risk↑ if rash is extensive). It causes insomnia, and depression—even suicide. Amitriptyline 25mg at night may help—or gabapentin (max 3.6g/day;[24] see BNF).[25]

Lesions in the bony orbit typically present with proptosis (ie exophthalmos), whatever the pathological origin. Proptosis (protrusion of orbital contents) is also a cardinal sign of intraorbital problems. If pressure is eccentric within the orbit there will be deviation of the eyeball ± diplopia.

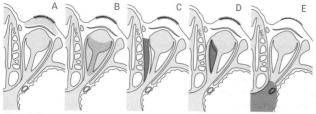

Fig 5.15 Patterns of infection within the orbit. Both orbital and preseptal cellulitis cause ocular pain and eyelid swelling, but preseptal cellulitis is confined to structures anterior to the orbital septum. Orbital cellulitis affects the extraocular muscles and fatty tissues within the orbit; infection can subsequently spread systemically through the valveless venous drainage of the orbit into the cavernous sinuses. Neither infection involves the eye globe. Both conditions are more common in children and both are typically caused by *Staphylococcus aeureus* and *Streptoccus pneumoniae*.

Orbital cellulitis ➤➤ Severe sight- and life-threatening emergency. Infection of soft tissues posterior to the orbital septum (fig 5.15). Spread is typically via paranasal sinus infection (or eyelid, dental injury/infection, or external ocular infection). *Typical patient:* A child with inflammation in the orbit, fever, lid swelling, and ↓eye mobility ±diplopia; eye movements will be painful. Conjuctival swelling (chemosis) and proptosis may be present. *Associated complications:* Subperiosteal and orbital abscesses are common and may develop rapidly, they can be difficult to identify at first so monitor patients closely. Confirmation of abscess is made by surgery or CT. Extra-orbital extension is rare but devastating. Visual loss can arise from optic neuritis or central retinal vein or artery occlusion (see p436). Intracranial involvement can result in meningitis, brain abscesses and thrombosis in the dural or cavernous sinuses.[20]
R: Admit for prompt CT, ENT, and ophthalmic opinion + antibiotics.[7] The decision to CT scan is difficult as there is significant radiation exposure involved in a young patient population, but clinically difficult to correlate the severity of infection or presence of abscesses; which if present need surgical drainage to prevent extension to meninges or cavernous sinus. Paranasal sinus surgery is not advised. Rule out underlying rhabdomyosarcoma, Grave's disease or cavernous sinus thrombosis (p484 OHCM).[21]

Indications for CT[21]
• Central signs
• Unable to assess vision
• Gross proptosis
• Bilateral oedema
• Ophthalmoplegia
• Deteriorating visual acuity or colour vision
• No improvement at 24hr/pyrexic at 36h

Preseptal (periorbital) cellulitis Infection of soft tissues anterior to the orbital septum (fig 5.15). Commonly caused by sinusitis or facial skin lesions (insect bites, trauma, etc.). Characterized by acute erythematous swelling of the eyelid. The absence of painful eye movements, diplopia, and visual impairment are key features which distinguish this from orbital cellulitis; they can present in a similar fashion but have drastically different clinical implications. If in doubt, treat as for orbital cellulitis. *R:* is based on empirical treatment for cellulitis eg amoxicillin 1g TDS 7–10-day course. Compared to orbital cellulitis, it is much more common, has a better response to treatment, no long-term sequelae, and a minimal risk of recurrence.[22]

7 Adults: **cefotaxime** 2g/6h IVI + **metronidazole** 500mg/8h IVI ± **vancomycin**. Check with local protocol.

To maintain single vision, fine co-ordination of eye movement of both eyes is necessary. Abnormality of the co-ordinated movement is called squint. *Other names for squint: strabismus; tropia.* Consider the impact on quality of life; children with squints are invited to less birthday parties.[23] Exotropia is divergent (one eye turned out) squint; esotropia is (one eye turned in) convergent squint. Prominent epicanthic folds (fig 5.17) may produce pseudosquint. There are two broad categories of squint: paralytic and non-paralytic, either can be convergent or divergent.

Convergent squint (esotropia) This is the commonest type in children. There may be no cause, or it may be due to hypermetropia (p426). In strabismic amblyopia, the brain suppresses the deviated image, and the visual pathway does not develop normally.[8]

Divergent squint (exotropia) Occur in older children, often intermittent.

Non-paralytic squints These usually start in childhood. Squints may be constant or not. All squints need ophthalmological assessment as vision may be damaged if not treated.

Diagnosis Difficult, eg in uncooperative children. Screening tests:

1 Corneal reflection: reflection from a bright light falls centrally and symmetrically on each cornea if no squint, asymmetrically if squint present.
2 Cover test: movement of the uncovered eye to take up fixation as the other eye is covered demonstrates manifest squint; latent squint is revealed by movement of the covered eye as the cover is removed (see fig 5.17).

Management Remember 3 'O's: Optical; Orthoptic; Operation. Treatment starts as soon as the squint is noticed. *Optical:* Assess the refractive state after cyclopentolate 1% drops; the cycloplegia allows objective determination of the refractive state; the mydriasis allows a good view into the eye to exclude abnormality, eg cataract, macular scarring, retinoblastoma, optic atrophy. Spectacles are then provided to correct refractive errors.

Orthoptic: Patching the good eye encourages use of the one which squints. Orthoptic review charts progress.

Operations (eg resection and recession of rectus muscles): These help alignment and give good cosmetic results. NB: use of **botulinum toxin** in some patients is reasonable and preferable to surgery(see p460).[24]

Paralytic squint Diplopia is most on looking in the direction of pull of the paralysed muscle. When the separation between the two images is greatest the image from the paralysed eye is furthest from the midline and faintest.

Third nerve palsy (oculomotor) Ptosis, proptosis (as recti tone ↓), fixed pupil dilatation, with the eye looking down and out. *Causes:* p424.

Fourth nerve palsy (trochlear) There is diplopia and the patient may hold his head tilted (ocular torticollis). The eye looks upward, in adduction and cannot look down and in (superior oblique paralysed).[9] *Causes:* Trauma 30%, diabetes 30%, tumour, idiopathic.

Sixth nerve palsy (abducens) There is diplopia in the horizontal plane. The eye is medially deviated and cannot move *laterally* from midline, as the *lateral* rectus is paralysed. *Causes:* Tumour causing ↑intracranial pressure (compresses the nerve on the edge of the petrous temporal bone), trauma to base of skull, vascular, or multiple sclerosis. Diabetes is a risk factor.[25]

Medial rectus: 'Look at your nose' (adduction).

Lateral rectus: 'Look away from your nose'.

---

8 In anisometropic amblyopia, each eye has different refractive powers. The brain favours the eye with the clearer image, ignoring the other. Other types of amblyopia: congenital cataract; uncorrected myopia or hypermetropia in one or both eyes; severe ptosis. *Amblyopia ex anopsia* means ↓acuity from failure of development of visual pathways due to lack of a sharp image on the macula at a critical stage of development.

Superior rectus (fig 5.16) primarily moves the gaze upward and secondarily rotates the *top* of the eye towards the nose (intorsion). Note its eccentric attachment.

Superior oblique primarily rotates the top of the globe towards the nose, secondarily depresses gaze.[7] Note its eccentric attachment.

Inferior rectus primarily moves the gaze down. (Secondary action: rotation of the *bottom* of the globe towards the nose.)

Inferior oblique primarily rotates the bottom of the globe towards the nose[10] & secondarily moves gaze upward.

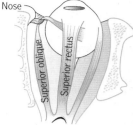

Right orbit seen from above

Fig 5.16 Superior oblique.

Ophthalmology

Best results are achieved in childhood strabismus by:
• Early detection; if >7yrs old, amblyopia may be permanent.
• Conscientious and disciplined amblyopia treatment.
• Optimal glasses (especially full plus in esotropia).[28]

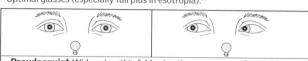

Pseudosquint Wide epicanthic folds give the appearance of a squint in the eye looking towards the nose. That the eyes are correctly aligned is confirmed by the corneal reflection.

Normal Corneal reflection shows correct alignment. Neither eye moves as they are alternately covered.

Left convergent squint Corneal reflection shows malalignment. As the right eye is covered the left moves out to take up fixation.

Left divergent squint Corneal reflection shows malalignment. As right eye is covered the left moves in to take up fixation.

Fig 5.17 The *cover test* relies on the ability to fixate. If there is *eccentric fixation* (ie foveal vision is so poor that it is not used for fixation), the deviating eye will not move to take up fixation. Corneal reflection shows that malalignment is present.

Further reading

Montgomery TM (2015). *The Extraocular Muscles.* http://www.tedmontgomery.com/the_eye/eom.html
Nield LS *et al.* (2011). Strabismus: *A Close-Up Look.* http://www.pediatricsconsultant360.com/content/strabismus-close-look

9 Superior oblique and inferior oblique aid eye abduction (ie lateral rotation), while superior and inferior recti adduct the eye. The superior oblique also lowers the gaze while the inferior oblique elevates it.[26, 27]
10 The primary muscle moving an eye in a given direction is the *agonist*. A muscle in that eye that moves it in the same direction as the agonist is a *synergist*—eg in abducting the left eye, the left lateral rectus is the agonist, the left superior and inferior obliques are synergists; the left medial, superior, and inferior recti are *antagonists*.[29] Superior & inferior obliques are the primary muscles of torsion.

Pupil reflexes Light detection by the retina is passed to the brain via the optic nerve (afferent pathway) and pupil constriction is mediated by the oculomotor (third) cranial nerve (efferent pathway). The sympathetic nervous system is responsible for pupil dilatation via the ciliary nerves.

Afferent defects (Absent direct response.) The pupil won't respond to light, but constricts to a beam in the other eye (consensual response). Constriction to accommodation still occurs. *Causes:* optic neuritis, optic atrophy, retinal disease. The pupils are the same size (consensual response unaffected). *Swinging flashlight test:* On beaming light to the normal eye, both pupils constrict (direct & consensual response); if, on swinging the light to the affected eye, the pupil *dilates* it is a *relative afferent pupillary defect* (RAPD).

Efferent defects The 3rd nerve also mediates eye movement and eyelid retraction. With complete palsy there is complete ptosis, a fixed dilated pupil, and the eye looks down (superior oblique still acts) and out (lateral rectus acting). *Causes:* cavernous sinus lesions, superior orbital fissure syndrome, diabetes, posterior communicating artery aneurysm. The pupil is often spared in vascular causes (diabetes; hypertension). Pupillary fibres are peripheral and are the first affected by compressive lesions eg tumour; aneurysm.

Other causes of a fixed dilated pupil Mydriatics, trauma (blow to iris), acute glaucoma, coning et uncal herniation (OHCM p840).

Tonic (Adie) pupil *A lack of parasympathetic innervation results in poor constriction to light.* Initially monolateral, then bilateral, pupil dilatation with delayed responses to near vision effort, with delayed redilation. *Typical patient:* A young woman, with sudden blurring of near vision, and a dilated pupil, with slow responses to accommodation, and, especially, to light (looks unreactive, unless an intense light is used for >15min). *Slit lamp exam:* Iris shows spontaneous wormy movements (*iris streaming*). Can be caused by damage to local structures, but most are idiopathic. *Holmes-Adie syndrome:* Tonic pupil, absent knee/ankle jerks and impaired sweating.[11] The pupil's size may fluctuate, and get smaller than the other (if both pupils are involved they may be confused with Argyll Robertson pupils). See below for other tonic pupils.[12]

Horner's syndrome occurs on disrupting sympathetic fibres, so the pupil is miotic (smaller) with no dilation in the dark and there is partial ptosis. Unilateral facial anhydrosis (sweating↓) may indicate a lesion proximal to the carotid plexus—if distal, the sudomotor (*sudor* = sweat) fibres will have separated, so sweating is intact. Congenital Horner's: iris heterochromia (see fig 5.18 & 5.19).

Causes of Horner's
• Posterior inferior cerebellar artery or basilar artery occlusion
• Multiple sclerosis
• Cavernous sinus thrombosis
• Pancoast's tumour
• Hypothalamic lesions
• Cervical adenopathy
• Mediastinal masses
• Pontine syringomyelia
• Klumpke's palsy, p750
• Aortic aneurysm

Argyll Robertson pupil occurs in neurosyphilis and diabetes; there is bilateral miosis, poor pupillary dilation, pupil irregularity and light-near dissociation (LND, -ve to light +ve to accommodation). 'Prostitute's pupil' accommodates but does not react.

Other causes of light-near dissociation Argyll Robertson pupil; Holmes-Adie and Parinaud syndromes;[13] meningitis; alcoholism; tectal lesions, eg pinealoma; mesencephalic or thalamic lesions.[14]

---

11 Selective impairment of monosynaptic connections of 1a afferents ± ↑presynaptic inhibition on afferent 1a input to ventral horn motor neurons ∴ absent deep reflexes persist despite cord pathology. There is autonomic dysfunction too with disturbed vasomotor and sweating functions.[30]
12 Migraine; syphilis; diabetes; chickenpox; arteritis; sarcoid; myasthenia; hamartoma; anti-Hu autoantibodies to neural nuclei; Sjögren's; Meige's syndrome; botulism; dermatomyositis; amyloidosis; paraneoplasia.
13 LND + nystagmus, upward gaze palsy and eyelid retraction (Collier's sign).
14 The path from the optic tract to the Edinger-Westphal nucleus is disrupted but deeper cortical connections remain intact, so accommodation is spared.

What colour are your eyes?

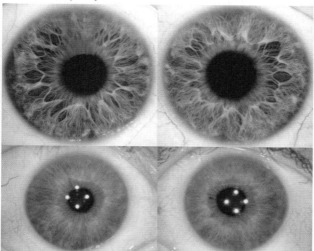

Fig 5.18 Heterochromia (sectoral above, central below). Both may be a normal variant; sectoral heterochromia may be a feature of Waardenburg syndrome (WS, p548). Type 1 WS is an autosomal dominant disorder whose other signs are hearing loss, pigmental abnormalities of the hair and skin, and dystopia canthorum (wide nasal bridge due to sideways displacement of the inner angles of the eyes).

Courtesy of Jon Miles.

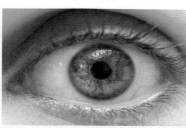

Fig 5.19 Sectoral heterochromia iridium. Different coloured irises can look very striking. Search online for a picture of David Bowie's eyes, he also had unequal pupils (apparently from an injury in his youth).

© Heather Smyth, with thanks to Megan Hale.

Anisocoria: an emergency?

A descriptive term of unequal pupils.[31] If noticed in the acute setting, it can prompt frantic searches for a cerebrovascular event, but may just be normal for that patient. Look at old photos and ask about previous eye disease/ surgery. Identification of the 'normal' side is the first step; is it the small (impaired dilation) or large pupil (impaired constriction) which is abnormal? Physiological anisocoria is present in 20% of people. Sympathetic lesions tend to cause a small pupil, often associated with Horner's syndrome. Parasympathetic causes include CN III palsy, drugs, and trauma.

Further reading

Broadway DC (2012). How to test for a relative afferent pupillary defect (RAPD) *Community Eye Health* 25:58–9.

Snell R *et al.* (1998). The visual pathway. *In Clinical Anatomy of the Eye* (2e), pp379–90. Oxford: Blackwell Science.

Refractive errors arise from disorders of the size and shape of the eye. Correct refraction depends upon the distance between the cornea and the retina, and the curvatures of the lens and cornea (see fig **5.20**).

Myopia (short sight) The eyeball is too long. In any eye, the nearer objects come to the eye, the further back their image falls. With myopia, only close objects focus on the retina (short sightedness) unless concave spectacle (or contact) lenses are used. *Causes:* Genetic (chromosome 18p & 12q).[32] Very close work in the early decades (not just at school) may lead to changes in the synthesis of mRNA and the concentration of matrix metalloproteinase, resulting in myopia. Acetylcholine, dopamine, and glucagon are triggers for eye growth.[33]

In normal growth, changes in eyeball and lens curvature compensate for the eye getting longer as it grows, but in myopic children, such compensations may not be occurring, so myopia worsens with age. Most do not become myopic until the age of ~6yrs (a few are born myopic). Myopia will then usually continue to worsen until the late teens, when changes stop below 6 dioptres in most people. It is important, therefore, for children with myopia to have their eyes regularly checked, as spectacle changes are to be expected, perhaps every 6 months. Avoid over-correction as this can make myopia worse. In later life, increasing myopia may indicate developing cataracts. Due to the short longitudinal axes, myopes are at higher risk of posterior vitreous detachment and retinal detachment (p450).

NB: when aboriginal people are exposed to Western education, rates of myopia rise from ~0 to Western levels (eg 50%) and there appears to be a dose–response curve relating hours spent indoors to degree of myopia. But before we all instantly put down this book and go out to play, remember that this relationship has only been proven in children.[34]

Pathological myopia: Rarely (≤3%), myopia progresses above 6 dioptres (sometimes up to >20 dioptres). This has serious consequences later in life because secondary degeneration of the vitreous and retina can lead to retinal detachment, choroidoretinal atrophy and macular bleeding.

Management: Spectacles, contact lenses, or LASIK, p464.

Astigmatism a common eye condition that occurs when the cornea does not have the same degree of curvature. In the not perfectly curved, the cornea becomes an irregular surface. Usually, one half is flatter or steeper than the other half. This means when light rays strike the cornea, they do not focus together in one point and produce a blurred image either longitudinally or vertically. Correcting lenses compensate accordingly. It can occur alone or is associated with myopia or hypermetropia.

Hypermetropia (long sight) The eye is too short. Distant objects, when the eye is at rest, are focused behind the retina. The ciliary muscles contract, and the lens gets more convex to focus the object on the retina. This can produce tiredness of gaze, and sometimes, convergent squint in children. It is corrected by convex lenses to bring the image forward to focus on the retina.

Presbyopia The ciliary muscle reduces tension in the lens, allowing it to get more convex, for close focusing. Young lenses can go from far to near in 0.4sec (but an approaching kiss still goes out of focus at ~7cm). With age, the lens stiffens and (presbyopia), hence the need for glasses for reading (but which do not make that approaching kiss any easier either in its appreciation or execution).[c] These changes start in the lens at ~40yrs and are complete by 60. Laser surgery to the cornea attempts to correct refraction, but this process of ageing means that glasses may still be required as ageing continues.

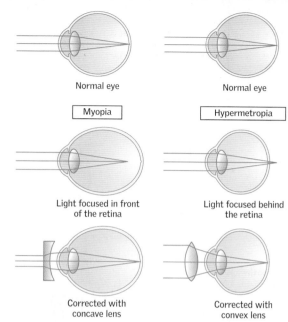

Fig 5.20 Myopia and hypermetropia.

Understanding the error and type of lens used to correct it is key to refractive errors making sense. Corrective lenses aim to help the endogenous lens focus the light rays onto the back of the retina; if the rays are not focussed accurately the image becomes blurry.

A convex lens is sometimes called a positive lens; it helps converge light rays. Convex lenses are used by hypertropic patients who struggle to converge rays approaching from nearby images. The convex lens helps move the image further forward to accurately hit the retina.

A concave lens will diverge the incoming light rays and is typically used for myopic eyes to help diverge the light rays so that they meet further back onto the elongated eyeball of a myope.

Further reading

Powell C (2005). Screening for correctable visual acuity deficits in school-age children and adolescents. *Cochrane Database Syst Rev* 1:CD005023.

Wojciechowski R (2011). Nature and nurture: the complex genetics of myopia and refractive error. *Clin Genet* 79(4):301–20.

When assessing for visual field defects, it is important to ask focused questions to correctly classify the defect: ►*Because of CNS plasticity, people often think that the area of defect (scotoma) is smaller than it is.*

1 Is the defect unilateral or bilateral?
2 Does the defect have sharp bounderies or blurred?
3 Does the defect lie in the vertical or horizontal meridians?
4 What is the current acuity?
5 Onset? Lesions of sudden onset are often due to vascular cause.

Scotomata

Arcuate scotoma—moderate glaucoma

Unilateral defect found with:
arterial occlusion
branch retinal vein
thrombosis
inferior retinal
detachment

Central scotoma
macular
degeneration or
macular oedema

The visual pathways

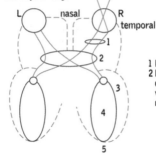

1 R optic nerve lesion
2 Lesion of chiasm—complicated defects depending upon which of the fibres are most affected

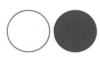

3 Left superior quadrantanopia due to R temporal lobe lesion

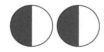

4 Homonymous hemianopia from lesions affecting all R optic radiation or visual cortex

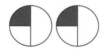

5 L homonymous scotoma due to lesion at tip of R occipital lobe

Fig 5.21 The retina, the optic nerve, the optic chiasma, the optic tracts, the lateral geniculate bodies, the optic radiations, and the visual cortical areas make up the visual pathway. They are all part of the central nervous system. Lesions of many pathologic causes in these areas can cause visual impairment.

Optic nerve (fig 5.21) Having a complete lesion on the optic nerve causes total blindness of that eye. Direct pupillary reflex is absent, indirect remains intact. Lesions tend to occur in the horizontal meridian when in the optic nerve. When the lesions are behind the optic chiasma, the boundaries are in the vertical meridian. Acuity tends to be affected .

Optic chiasma Lesions in the chiasma will produce a bitemporal hemianopia. This is due to the fact that the fibres coming from the nasal halves of both retinas are involved. There is a normal direct, consensual light reflex and accommodation reflex.

Optic tracts A lesion on the optic tract causes a contralateral homonymous hemianopia. For example, a right-sided optic tract lesion causes a left temporal hemianopia and a right nasal hemianopia. There is a normal direct light reflex, consensual light reflex and accommodation reflex.

Optic radiation Optic radiation lesions produce a contralateral homonymous hemianopia. Lesions over the lateral portions of the lateral geniculate body which received impulses from the inferior rental quadrants (superior visual field). Lesions in the nerve fibres passing more directly posterior to the cortex cause an inferior quadrantic hemianopia.

Visual cortex Destruction of the the primary visual cortex produces contralateral homonymous hemianopia and the pupils react normally to reflex stimulation. The macula is often spared because in some people there is an anastomosis between the posterior and middle cerebral arteries.[36]

Tests *Finger confrontation:* The patient closes one eye, fixes on your eye and notes the presence of a finger in all fields mapped, against your vision. It is used for testing peripheral fields. *Hat-pin confrontation:* The patient fixons on your eye (sit ~1 metre away). Red (central vision) or white (peripheral vision) hat-pins are used to define any vertical meridian, the size of the blindspot, and the boundaries of any scotomas.

Amsler grids detect distortion in central vision, eg from macular disease. The chart is 10×10cm square with 5mm squares drawn on it and a dot in the centre. With the chart held at 30cm the patient is instructed to look at the dot and report any distorted squares or wavy lines (metamorphopsia) (see fig 5.41, p451).

Diagnosing the lesion's site Superior parts of the visual field fall inferiorly on the retina, temporal fields on the nasal retina, and vice versa. Fibres from the nasal retina of both eyes cross in the optic chiasm to join uncrossed temporal retinal fibres. A pituitary tumour may disrupt the chiasm, affecting fibres crossing from nasal retinas, so causing bitemporal field defects. If it grows more to one side than the other, it can superimpose a central optic nerve defect as well. As fibres cross they maintain position (superior fibres stay superior). From the optic chiasma fibres pass in the optic tract to the lateral geniculate body, then as the optic radiation to the visual cortex.

A contralateral upper homonymous quadrantanopia may be caused by temporal lobe tumours. Posterior visual cortex lesions cause non-peripheral homonymous hemianopic scotomas (anterior visual cortex deals with peripheral vision)—with macular sparing, if the cause is posterior cerebral artery ischaemia (central areas have overlap flow via the middle cerebral artery, which is why acuity may be preserved).

Causes of visual cortex field defects: • Ischaemia (TIA, migraine, stroke) • Glioma • Meningioma • Abscess • AV malformation • Drugs, eg ciclosporin.[37] NB: cortical visual defects may be fundamentally capricious—in that when an object is presented to the affected field of view, the patient announces that he cannot see it—yet 'guesses' correctly that it is there (non-cortical visual pathways): there are some things we know we can see; other things we see without knowing (blindsight[15]); and others that we know without seeing (eg that a table has 4 legs when we can only see 3 at any one time).

15 Blindsight lesion patients respond to visual fear signals independently from conscious experience—ie these signals reach the amygdala bypassing the visual cortex.[38]

Ophthalmology

Subconjunctival haemorrhage (fig 5.22) This harmless but alarming pool of blood behind the conjunctiva is from a small bleed ('Are you on warfarin?etc'; your INR is...?'); check BP. It often occurs in frail old ladies who you can make laugh by asking 'Have you been white-water rafting recently?' (leptospira in sewage).[48]

Inflammation of the sclera manifests as episcleritis and scleritis. The former is common, frequently self-limiting, and usually benign. In contrast, scleritis is much rarer, very painful with sight-threatening sequelae, and a strong association to systemic disease (see below).

▶**Clinical distinction between scleritis and episcleritis**. The episclera lies superficially and subsequently the episcleral vessels will move when probed with a cotton bud and blanch with the application of 10% phenylephrine. The deeper scleral vessls will neither move nor blanch.

Episcleritis (fig 5.23) Inflammation below the conjunctiva in the episclera is often seen with an inflammatory nodule. 70% of patients are women. Bilateral in 30%. Acute onset. The sclera may look blue below a focal, cone-shaped wedge (thin end towards pupil) of engorged vessels that can be moved over the area, unlike in scleritis, where engorged vessels run deeper. The eye aches dully and is tender (esp. over inflamed area). Acuity is usually OK. No cause is found in 70%,[49] but in a small proportion it may complicate rheumatic fever, PAN or SLE. *R:* Symptomatic relief is the mainstay with artificial tears and topical or systemic NSAIDs.

Scleritis[50] (fig 5.24) Generalized inflammation of the sclera itself with oedema of the conjunctiva, scleral thinning, and vasculitic changes. Two subtypes: anterior (90%) and posterior scleritis. The necrotizing variety can cause globe perforation. 50% of patients have associated systemic disease (typically rheumatoid arthritis or granulomatosis with polyangitis).[51] Patients describe a constant, severe dull ache which 'bores' into the eye. Ocular movements are painful since the muscles insert into the sclera. May present with headache and photophobia. *R:* ▶Urgent referral. Management is guided by subtype: non-necrotizing anterior scleritis may only require oral NSAIDs ± oral high-dose prednisolone. Posterior scleritis or if there is evidence of necrotizing changes require more aggressive therapy. Systemic immunosuppression is influenced by underlying systemic disease; typically cyclophosphamide or rituximab and a course of methylprednisolone. Recalcitrant disease may benefit from infliximab.[51] Imminent globe perforation requires surgical intervention. Prognosis tends to follow that of the underlying systemic disorder. Visual loss is common in those with the necrotizing form.

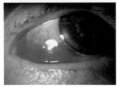

Fig 5.22 Subconjuctival haemorrhage.

Reprinted by permission from Macmillan Publishers Ltd: *Eye*, Wells et al, Spontaneous inferior subconjunctival haemorrhages in association with circumferential drainage blebs, Volume 19, issue 3, copyright (2004).

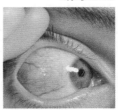

Fig 5.23 Episcleritis.

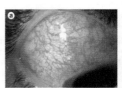

Fig 5.24 Scleritis.

Reprinted by permission from Macmillan Publishers Ltd: *Nature Reviews Rheumatology*, Artifoni et al, Ocular inflammatory diseases associated with rheumatoid arthritis, volume 10, issue 2, p.108–116, copyright (2013).

Further reading

Mahmood AR *et al.* (2008). Diagnosis and management of the acute red eye. *Emerg Med Clin North Am* 26(1):35–55.

NICE (2012). *Clinical Knowledge Summaries: Red Eye*. http://cks.nice.org.uk/red-eye

Carefully examine all red eyes to assess acuity, cornea (use fluorescein drops p432), and pupillary reflexes.

The key questions to ask are as follows:

1 *Is acuity affected?* A quick but sensitive test is the ability to read news-print with refractive errors corrected with glasses or a pin-hole. ↓ acuity suggests dangerous pathology.

2 *Is the globe painful?* Pain is potentially sinister, foreign body sensation may be so, irritation rarely is.

3 *Does the pupil respond to light?* Absent or sluggish response is sinister.

4 *Is the cornea intact?* Use fluorescein eyedrops, p432. Corneal damage may be due to trauma or ulcers.

Ask about trauma and discharge, general health and drugs; remember to check for raised pressure. Use of contact lenses? (risk of bacterial infections and corneal ulcers). Past history of eye disease? Any systemic features?

	Conjunctivitis	Episcleritis	Scleritis	Anterior uveitis	Acute glaucoma
Hyperaemia	Diffuse	Focal, may be nodular			
Pain	Mild irritation	Mild irritation	++ Dull aching Painful ocular movements	++	++ to +++
Photophobia	+	±	±	++	−
Visual acuity (VA)	Patients can describe blurring. VA testing is normal.	Normal	Normal initially	↓	↓
Discharge	+	−	−	No discharge but lacrimation ++	−
Cornea	Normal			Normal	Steamy or hazy
Pupil	Normal	Normal		Small	Large
Intraocular pressure	Normal	Normal	Normal		↑
Referral?	No	Only if very painful	Within 24 hours	Within 24 hours	Immediately

Easily treated
Episcleritis
Conjunctivitis
Conjunctival haemorrhage

Urgent referral
Acute glaucoma
Acute iritis
Corneal ulcers
Scleritis

Common causes
Conjunctivitis
Foreign Bodies
Corneal ulceration
Subconjunctival haemorrhage

Uncommon causes
Acute glaucoma
Acute iritis
Scleritis
Episcleritis

Ophthalmology

Uveitis The uvea is the pigmented part of the eye (iris, ciliary body, choroid). The anterior uvea comprises of the iris and ciliary body, subsequently inflammatory processes in this anterior chamber are termed *anterior uveitis (iritis)*. The posterior uvea comprises of the choroid, inflammation here is termed *posterior uveitis (choroiditis)*. *Intermediate uveitis* affects the vitrous and *panuveitis* is as the name suggests. There are multiple causes of uveitis; a significant proportion are due to underlying systemic disease (inc. autoimmune causes). Traditionally it was largely considered idiopathic, although this number is dwindling as research delves deeper into autoimmune causes; HLA seems to play a role.

Types & causes of uveitis
Anterior uveitis:[40]
• Ank.spond.;Still's,[17] p654
• Sarcoid; Behçet's, etc[18]
• IBD; reactive arthritis
• Herpes, TB, syphilis, HIV
Intermediate uveitis:
• MS; lymphoma; sarcoid
Posterior & panuveitis:
• Herpes simplex + zoster
toxoplasmosis; TB; CMV;
endophthalmitis
• Lymphoma; sarcoidosis
• Behçet's

'*Great philosophers dream of a day when war will be no more. Uveitis physicians merely dream of a day when idiopathic uveitis will be no more.*'[39] Uveitis is an important cause of visual impairment in people of working age. Acute anterior uveitis tends to have a good visual prognosis whilst other forms can lead to significant visual impairment.[40]

Anterior uveitis is the most common form of uveitis in the UK and also the form most likely to present with a red eye.[16] Affects adults of working age. *Presentation* is classically with pain, blurred vision, & photophobia. The red eye starts with conjuctival injection around the junction of the cornea and sclera and increased lacrimation (no sticky discharge, unlike in conjunctivitis). The pupil may be small, initially from iris spasm; later it may be irregular or dilate irregularly due to adhesions between lens and iris (synechiae) (fig 5.25). Onset is over hours/days. Ask about associated headaches and features of systemic disease. *Diagnosis*[19] is by slit lamp with a dilated pupil to visualize the location of inflammatory cells (in anterior uveitis you see leucocytes in the anterior chamber); if no cells visualized then consider posterior uveitis. Ocular imaging such as fundus fluorescein and indocyanide green-angiography are used to further examine for retinal and choroidal disease. ℞.»» Urgent eye clinic. Treatment is guided by cause. »» Involve multidisciplinary care in systemic disease as controlling the underlying disease is key. Use the slit lamp to monitor inflammation; it may relapse so regular eye clinic care and follow-up is vital. Aim

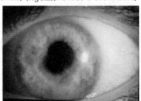

Fig 5.25 Posterior synechiae in acute anteior uveitis. The iris adheres to the lens and when inflamed causes an irregular pupillary border.

Reproduced from Sundaram et al, *Oxford Specialty Training: Training in Ophthalmology* (2009) with permission from Oxford University Press.

to prevent damage from prolonged inflammation (disrupts flow of aqueous →glaucoma ± adhesions between iris & lens). Drops: 0.5–1% **prednisolone/2h**, to ↓ inflammation (hence pain, redness, and exudate). To prevent adhesions between lens and iris (synechiae) and to relieve spasm of ciliary body keep pupil dilated with **cyclopentolate** 1%/8h, unless very mild. Biological agents (eg infliximab, adalimumab) are showing promise but currently none are licensed just for uveitis in the absence of a systemic disease.[40] *Prolonged visual loss* was present in ⅔ of patients attending a tertiary uveitis centre (UK), 22% of patients met the criteria for blindness. Panuveitis had the highest risk of visual loss. Cystoid macular oedema and cataracts were the main causes. Others: chorioretinal scarring, glaucoma, retinal detachment and vitreous opacities.[41]

16 Posterior uveitis is much less common. It can be painless with blurred vision or floaters. The eye is typically *not* red. In contrast to anterior uveitis, posterior inflammation does not respond as well to topical treatment and may need peri-ocular or intra-ocular glucocorticoids.

Acute closed-angle glaucoma (figs 5.26 & 5.27) (see p444) A form of glaucoma where the angle of anterior chamber narrows acutely causing a sudden rise in intraocular pressure (IOP) to ≥30mmHg (normal 15–20), the pupil becomes fixed and dilated and axonal death occurs. IOP↑ may make the eye feel hard. *Primary angle-closure* occurs in patients with anatomical predisposition. *Secondary angle-closure* arises from pathological processes (eg traumatic haemorrhage pushing the posterior chamber forwards).

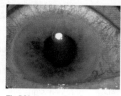

Fig 5.26 Acute closed-angle glaucoma.
Courtesy of Prof J Trob.

Peak incidence in ages 40–60 and more common in Asia. *Presentation:* Patients are often generally unwell with nausea and vomiting; they can easily present to the acute medical team with no visual complaints. In 25%, acute uniocular attacks occur with headache and a painful red eye, often preceded by blurred vision or haloes around lights, at night. Onset is over hours–days (see p444 when IOP rise is slow and asymptomatic). Ask about precipitating factors; is the patient on topical cyclopentolate for uveitis?[20] ►►Send to eye unit *now* for gonioscopy (see p444). Avoid eye patches or dark rooms which will worsen the angle closure by pupillary dilatation. *R̆:* Start a triad of β-blockers to suppress aqueous humour production (eg timolol 0.5%), pilocarpine 2–4% drops/2h (miosis opens a blocked, 'closed' drainage angle, fig 5.27) + 500mg IV **acetazolamide** stat then 250mg/8h PO/IV (it ↓ aqueous formation). Analgesia and antiemetics may be used. Admit to monitor IOP. **Peripheral iridectomy** (laser or surgery) is done once IOP is controlled (rarely as an emergency if IOP uncontrollable). A piece of iris is removed (at '12 o'clock') in *both eyes* to allow aqueous to flow.[42] *Complications* include visual loss, central retinal artery or vein occlusions and repeated episodes in either eye.[43]

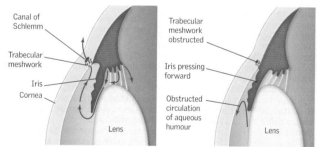

Canal of Schlemm
Trabecular meshwork
Iris
Cornea
Lens
Trabecular meshwork obstructed
Iris pressing forward
Obstructed circulation of aqueous humour
Lens

Fig 5.27 Normally, aqueous humour is produced by the ciliary body and flows through the pupil and empties out at the drainage angle through the canal of Schlemm. Any structural changes to this angle will block the flow and raise intra-ocular pressure. Predisposing factors include: shallow anterior chamber, thick lens, thin iris or ciliary bodies (eg pupil dilation at night) and hypermetropic eye (short axial eye length).

Further reading

Guly CM *et al.* (2010). Investigation and management of uveitis. *BMJ* 341:c4976.

Kent C (2013). Managing narrow angles and glaucoma. http://www.reviewofophthalmology.com/content/i/2417/c/41056/

Wittenberg S (2008). *10 Clinical Pearls for Treating Uveitis*. http://www.aao.org/young-ophthalmologists/yo-info/article/10-clinical-pearls-treating-uveitis

17 In juvenile arthritis, screen the child every 4 months until they are old enough to report symptoms.
18 This is one of the few occasions when the Sherlock Holmes's among us can properly ask 'Have you been handling tarantulas recently?' (Their hairs cause uveitis.)
19 Talbot's test is +ve: pain increases on convergence (and pupils constrict) as patients watch a finger approach their nose.
20 Topical mydriatics will dilate the pupil and push the iris forwards.

Ophthalmology

Ophthalmology

Conjunctivitis[44] The conjunctiva is red and inflamed, and the hyperaemic vessels may be moved over the sclera, by gentle pressure on the globe. It can only be diagnosed by ruling out sight-threatening features. Acuity,[21] pupillary responses, and corneal lustre are unaffected. Eyes itch, burn, and lacrimate. It is often bilateral with discharge sticking lids together. (Type of discharge depends on the cause; however, a large meta-analysis demonstrated no correlation between signs and symptoms of conjuctivitis with the underlying cause[45]). *Non-infectious causes:* Allergic conjunctivitis is the most frequent cause of all conjuctivitis cases, affecting 15–40% of the population but not many seek medical attention. Other causes: toxic,[22] auto-immune, neoplastic. Contact lens wearers may develop a reaction to the presence of a foreign substance (fig 5.28). (see also p463) *Infectious causes:* Non-herpetic viral (serous discharge) is the most common infectious cause; ~80% are adenoviruses (small lymphoid aggregates appear as follicles on conjunctiva). Bacterial (purulent discharge more prominent, especially in gonococcal infection). *Investigations:* Conjuctival cultures are only needed if you suspect gonococcal/chlamydial infection, neonatal conjunctivitis, or recurrent disease not responding to therapy. *Treatment:* Most cases are viral and only need symptomatic relief with artificial tears and topical anti-histamines. Topical anti-viral treatment does not help. Viral conjunctivitis is highly contagious so educate patients on hand and face washing. See p435 for her-

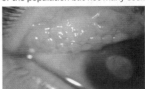

Fig 5.28 Giant papillary conjunctivitis is characterized by the formation of papillae (>1mm) on the inner aspect of the upper eye lid (to examine, evert the upper eye lid). See the grey, oval corneal ulcer ('shield' ulcer) due to corneal erosion. Contact lenses (see p463) are the typical culprits but in their absence, look for other foreign bodies. Symptoms include intense itching and mucoid discharge. Treat by abstaining from wearing lenses for a week, reduce time wearing lenses and replace lenses frequently. Ensure correct lens hygiene maintained.[46]

Courtesy of Mr D Tole **FRCO**.

pes infection. Bacterial conjuctivitis also tends to be self-limiting (60%) within 1-2 weeks but topical antibiotics can reduce duration of symptoms and reduce transmission risk. Antibiotic drops are especially useful in culture-proven conjuctivitis. Start antiobiotics immediately if sexual disease is suspected, contact lens wearers or immunocompromised patients. **Chloramphenicol** 0.5% drops/4-6h is often used (or **fusidic acid** drops). Staphs are common causes. In prolonged conjunctivitis, esp. in young adults or those with sexual diseases, consider chlamydial infection (get expert help; see ophthalmia neonatorum, p37). For allergic conjunctivitis: Try antihistamine drops, eg **emedastine** or **olopatadine** refer if not settling in a few days. **Sodium cromoglicate** and **steroid drops** (after advice from an ophthalmologist) may help.

Corneal problems

Accurate, rapid diagnosis is vital!

Keratitis is corneal inflammation (identified by a white area on the cornea—indicating a collection of white cells in corneal tissue). Keratoconjunctivitis refers to conjunctivitis with associated corneal involvement.

Corneal abrasion is an epithelial breach causing pain, photophobia, ± ↓vision. Non-infective corneal ulcers may result from accidental scratches from sharp objects, contact lenses, trauma, chemical injury, or previous corneal disease. Use fluorescein drops and the blue light on a slit lamp to aid diagnosis. Corneal lesions stain green (drops are orange and become more yellow on contact with the eye). Always invert the eye lid to look for foreign bodies. Ask contact wearers if they sleep with lenses in and how they are changed. See p742 for management.

Corneal ulcers may be bacterial (beware pseudomonas: may progress rapidly), herpetic (see BOX), fungal (candida; aspergillus), protozoal (acanthamoeba) or from vasculitis, eg in rheumatoid arthritis. Don't try treating ulcerative keratitis on your own: scarring and visual loss may occur. Except for a simple abrasion (*R̟*: chloramphenical ointment ± cyloplegia) get help *today* for urgent diagnostic smear/Gram stain and scrape. Liaise with microbiologist. *R̟*: p433. In early stages of ophthalmic shingles, use oral **aciclovir** (p420). Cycloplegics (p456) ease photophobia.

Management of corneal ulcers: Refer to a specialist today. Remove contact lenses. Test cranial nerve v. HIV +ve? Until cultures are known, alternate **chloramphenicol** drops (for Gram +ve bacteria) with **ofloxacin drops** (for Gram -ve bacteria) or 0.3% **cefuroxime** drops with **gentamicin drops**. Adapt in the light of cultures. Admit, eg if diabetes, immunosuppression, or if the patient won't manage the drops. Ofloxacin is given up to a drop every 15min to start with, (check the local protocol). Steroid drops can be added once recovery starts. ► see BOX p459 for the dangers of steroid drops.

Herpes simplex (dendritic) corneal ulcers

Herpes simplex virus (HSV) type 1 has multiple ocular manifestations, keratitis is the most common and is a major cause of corneal blindness through corneal scarring. Acute presentation with pain, photophobia, and watering. Ask about past eye, mouth, or genital ulcers.[23] Use a slitlamp and appy fluorescein 1% staining to look for dendritic ulcers which suggest active virus replication (fig 5.29). Further laboratory testing is often not necessary. If steroid drops are used without aciclovir cover, corneal invasion and scarring may occur, risking blindness. *R̟*: Aciclovir 3% eye ointment 5× daily. Corneal transplants are considered for those with significant visual impairment due to scarring.[47]

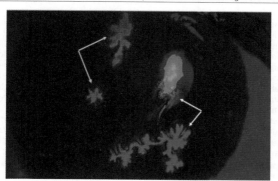

Fig 5.29 Dendritic ulcers (short arrows) are pathognomonic for HSV keratitis. The long arrows demonstrate the more developed geographic ulcers. Read about this patient's case study here: http://qjmed.oxfordjournals.org/content/early/2014/12/22/qjmed.hcu250

Further reading

Azari AA *et al.* (2013). Conjunctivitis: a systematic review of diagnosis and treatment. *JAMA* 310:1721-9.
Teng CC (2008). Corneal dendritic ulcer from herpes simplex virus infection. *NEJM* 359:e22.

21 Vision can be described as blurred, but this is not constant and visual acuity testing using a snellen chart should be normal.
22 Typically occurs in patients with prolonged use of topical ocular medications (such as in glaucoma).
23 Don't bother asking about shingles and chickenpox, it's a different virus! See p420. The *Herpesviridae* are DNA viruses which include herpes simplex, varicella-zoster (which cause chicken pox and shingles), Epstein–Barr virus and *Cytomegalovirus*. Latent infections are classic in this family, which is why the name is derived from the Greek Herpein; 'to creep'.

Ophthalmology

▸▸Urgent help is needed in: retinal artery occlusion of <6h; any sudden visual loss of <6h if the cause is unknown, or giant cell arteritis (GCA). *5 questions will* HELLP: •Headache associated? ►Do an ESR urgently in all cases ≥50yrs old for ?GCA (see below) •Eye movements hurt? (optic neuritis) (see below) •Lights/flashes preceding visual loss? (detached retina, p450) •Like a curtain descending? Amaurosis fugax may precede permanent visual loss, eg from emboli/GCA. •Poorly controlled DM and vitreous haemorrhage (p438).

Optic neuropathies Damage to the optic nerve typically produces •Monocular vision loss with a central scotoma •Afferent pupillary defects (unilateral lesions) •Dyschromatopsia (colour blindness) •Papillitis on fundoscopy which eventually progresses to optic atrophy (pale disc, indicates long-term damage). There are many causes of optic neuropathies beyond this page.[24]

Anterior ischaemic optic neuropathy (AION) The most common cause of optic neuropathy in older patients. The optic nerve is damaged if posterior vascular supply to the optic nerve is blocked by inflammation or atheroma. *Fundoscopy:* pale/swollen optic disc due to the optic nerve being damaged. There are two main types: *non-arteritic AION* and *arteritic AION*. Despite the differing pathophysiology between the types of AION, both result in ischaemic damage to vision.

Giant cell (temporal) arteritis (GCA) (p558 OHCM) is the most common arteritic AION. It is described as a medium to large vessel systemic vasculitis. Typically seen in patients >70 years old; rarely occuring before the age of 50. Lifetime risk is 1% in women and 0.5% in men.[52] *Symptoms:* New-onset headache, malaise, jaw claudication (chewing pain) ± tender scalp and temporal arteries (thickened ± absent pulses), neck pain. Visual loss is typically monocular (rarely bilateral, this is a more worrying sign), it may be transient (=amaurosis fugax[25]). Permanent vision loss tends to be preceeded by multiple episodes of amaurosis fugax, but can occur at the first presentation.[53] There is a strong association with polymyalgia rheumatica (PMR), hip and shoulder girdle aching, and morning stiffness. Onset of symptoms tend to be subacute, but in some the onset can be sudden. Not all patients experience this constellation of symptoms so retain a high index of suspicion and request the following *Tests:* ESR (>47) & CRP (>2.5mg/dL) preferably before steroids; temporal artery biopsy within 1 week of starting prednisolone; may miss affected sections of artery (skip lesions). *R:* ▸▸ *The other eye is at risk* until steroids are given. Start **prednisolone** 60mg/24h PO promptly (some advocate higher IV doses if visual failure is occurring). Tailing off steroids as ESR and symptoms settle may take >1yr.[54] Despite this, ~20% of patients are left with partial or complete visual loss.[53]

Non-arteritic AION Visual loss is typically painless and noticed upon awakening, affects patients <50 years. Associations: BP↑; lipids↑; DM, smoking. Treating these protects vision in the other eye.

Optic neuritis *Subacute loss of vision* (fig 5.31): Unilateral loss of acuity occurs over hours or days. Colour vision is affected (dyschromatopsia): reds appear less red—'red desaturation'—and eye movements hurt. The pupil shows an afferent defect (p424). Full recovery is usually over 2-6 weeks, but 45–80% develop multiple sclerosis (MS) in the next 15yrs (p500 OHCM).[55] Other causes: syphilis, Leber's optic atrophy, diabetes, vitamin deficiency. *R:* High-dose **methylprednisolone**•※ for 72h (1000mg/24h IV), then **prednisolone** (1mg/kg/d PO) for 11 days.[56]

---

24 Other causes of optic neuropathy not listed on this page: infective (eg meningitis), inflammatory (eg systemic autoimmune diseases), genetic, compressive (eg neoplasm, abscess), trauma, toxic (eg alcohol excess, radiation).
25 Amaurosis fugax is the transient, painless loss of vision in one eye. Described as a 'curtain passing across the eye'. Typical cause: atheroma (listen to carotids). Other causes include TIAs, GCA, Takayasu's arteritis, and sickle cell disease.

Transient vision loss

▶Always think of vascular causes, such as microemboli from atherosclerotic plaques in the heart or carotid arteries (any stenosis or bruit?). Be cautious in diagnosing migraine for the 1st time if aged >50yrs.

Typical causes
• Vascular; TIA; migraine
• Multiple sclerosis
• Subacute glaucoma (not always painful)
• Papilloedema

Central retinal artery occlusion

Much less common than retinal vein occlusion (p438). There is dramatic visual loss within seconds of occlusion[26] (in 90%, acuity is finger counting or worse). ▶▶This is considered a form of stroke and should be managed according to local stroke protocols. Occlusion is often thromboembolic (eg carotid artery atherosclerosis in the elderly) but consider all causes of stroke (p474 *OHCM*). Look for signs of atherosclerosis (bruits; BP↑), atrial fibrillation, heart valve disease, diabetes, smoking, or lipids↑. An afferent pupil defect (p424) appears within seconds and may precede retinal changes by 1h. The retina appears white, with a cherry red spot at the macula (figs **5.30** & **5.31**). Exclude temporal arteritis (p558 *OHCM*). **Management** ▶▶If seen within 100min of onset, attempt to increase retinal blood flow even though chances of recovering vision are poor. Emergency treatment aims to reduce intraocular pressure by ocular massage, surgical removal of aqueous from the anterior chamber or the use of intraocular hypotensive treatment. There is no universally accepted emergency treatment and one analysis failed to show a difference between the aforementioned interventions and observation.[57] Long-term management involves primary prevention of *CVS* risk factors to minimize further events.

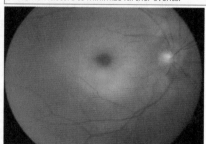

Fig 5.30 Central retinal artery occlusion. With arterial occlusion note retinal pallor and the cherry-red macula.

We thank Dr R K Reddy, Dr Badrinath, and Dr Ravishankar (Sankara Nethralya, Chennai, India) for their help with this page, and for permission to reproduce this image.

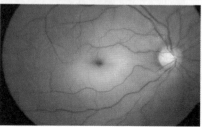

Fig 5.31 Another example of central retinal artery occlusion. Note the retinal pallor and cherry-red macula.

We thank Dr R K Reddy, Dr Badrinath, and Dr Ravishankar (Sankara Nethralya, Chennai, India) for their help with this page, and for permission to reproduce this image.

Ophthalmology (side tab)

Further reading

Balcer LJ (2006). Optic neuritis. *NEJM* 354:1273–80.

Rucker JC *et al.* (2004). Ischaemic optic neuropathies. *Current Opin Neurol* 17:27–35.

Unwin B *et al.* (2006). Polymyalgia rheumatica and giant cell arteritis. *Am Fam Physician* 74:1547–54.

26 In comparison, branch retinal artery occlusion presents with monocular vision loss and visual acuity may not be affected. Prognosis tends to be much better and >80% have normal vision restored.[58]

Ophthalmology

Retinal vein occlusion (RVO) Incidence increases with age. Much more common than arterial occlusion; it is the 2nd most common cause of blindness from retinal vascular disease (diabetic neuropathy is first).[59] *Causes/associations*: arteriosclerosis, BP↑, diabetes, and polycythaemia; glaucoma (all types). If the whole central retinal vein is thrombosed, there is visual loss (eg acuity reduced to finger counting). It is less sudden than central retinal artery occlusion. Visual loss may be perceived as sudden by the patient but the mechanism of visual loss is due to the development of ischaemia and macular oedema. RVO is classified according to anatomical location of occlusion along the central retinal vein. **Central retinal vein occlusion (CRVO)** (fig 5.33c) occurs at the level of the optic nerve and will subsequenetly present with sudden-onset painless blurred vision in one eye. CVRO is never asymptomatic. **Branch retinal vein occlusion** can be asymptomatic if the macula is not affected, but most complain of visual defects corresponding to the area of occlusion (fig 5.33a & b). CRVO is further divided into *non-ischaemic* and *ischaemic* (with cotton wool spots, swollen optic nerve, macular oedema, and risk of neovascularization; hence need for follow-up).[60] Non-ischaemic forms are more common and have better acuity (even 6/6) and prognosis (signs are less dramatic too). But this can convert to the ischaemic form in 30%; hence the need for follow-up. A fundus fluorescein angiogram is used to determine the degree of ischaemia and panretinal photocoagulation is given to prevent or treat neovascularization. Unfortunately even if the macular oedema resolves anatomically, visual prognosis is poor. *Management:* ▸▸ Refer to the oncall ophthalmologist who will initiate treatment aimed at ameliorating secondary complications which threaten vision such as retinal neovascularization (new vasculature has a high risk of haemorrhaging; see below) and chronic macular oedema. Monitor those with no secondary complications carefully. If visual loss has occured, intravitreal anti-VEGF therapy (p441) is 1st line followed by dexamethasone implants or intravitreal triamcinolone acetonide. Photocoagulation is used if retinal neovascularization has started to develop.[60] Aim to prevent rubeotic glaucoma and a painful eye (bevacizumab and ranibizumab (eg Lucentis® (p439) can treat the macular oedema) as can lasers and dexamethasone intravitreal implants.[NICE 2011]

Vitreous haemorrhage (VH) Arise from retinal neovascularization (DM, BRVO, or CRVO), retinal tears, retinal detachment, or trauma. Small extravasations of blood produce vitreous floaters (fig 5.32), (seen by the patient as small black dots or tiny ring-like forms with clear centres) which may not greatly obscure vision. *Check:* Acuity, pupil reaction, fundi. Then refer. With a large enough bleed to obscure vision, there is no red reflex and the retina may not be seen; then B-scan US can be used to identify a cause. VH normally undergoes spontaneous absorption. In dense VH a vitrectomy is done to remove the blood in the vitreous if the retina is torn/detached or the patient needs treatment

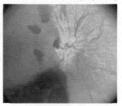

Fig 5.32 Vitreous haemorrhage (bottom left) from new vessels (top right).

for new vessels. In DM patients with previous photocoagulation for new vessels and recurrent VH, it is acceptable to wait 3 months for resolution.

Other causes of sudden loss of monocular vision: • Retinal detachment (p444) • Acute glaucoma (painful, p430) • Migraine. Stroke patients may complain of monocular blindness but visual field testing will usually reveal a homonymous hemianopia. Sudden bilateral visual loss is unusual (may be CMV infection in HIV patients, p448).

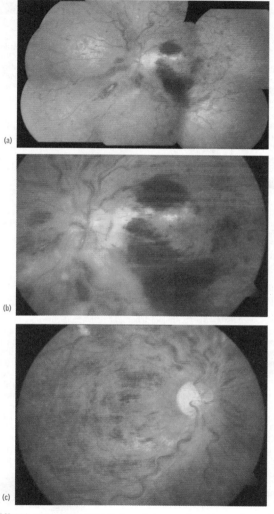

Figs 5.33 With central retinal vein occlusion note hyperaemia and haemorrhages—known as the stormy sunset appearance (c). (a) and (b) show haemarroragic changes in segments corresponding to the retinal branches.

We thank Dr R K Reddy, Dr Badrinath, and Dr Ravishankar (Sankara Nethralya, Chennai, India) for their help with this page, and for permission to reproduce these images.

Further reading

Chong V (2012). Branch retinal vein occlusion. *BMJ* 345:e8373.

Phillpotts BA (2013). *Vitreous Haemorrhage*. Medscape. http://emedicine.medscape.com/article/1230216

Wong TY *et al.* (2010). Retinal vein occlusion. *NEJM* 363:2135–44.

Be aware that for many, the chief question is likely to be 'Will I go blind?': be optimistic where possible. Patients may *not* tell you that they also fear they are going mad, having experienced complex visual hallucinations (often of faces). These occur without psychiatric signs and are often related to failing vision in the elderly: the Charles Bonnet syndrome (see BOX, p451).[62]

See p442 for causes of blindness.

Typical causes
• Cataract
• Macular degeneration
• Glaucoma (p440)
• Diabetic retinopathy
• Hypertension (p448)
• Optic atrophy (p456)
• Slow retinal detachment

Age-related macular degeneration (ARMD) is the chief cause of registrable blindness,[UK] and most common cause of irreversible vision loss in the developed world. It occurs in the elderly who present with deteriorating central vision. *Pathogenesis:* There is pigment, drusen (BOX & fig 5.34), and sometimes bleeding at the macula. Over time it progresses to retinal atrophy and central retinal degeneration which causes a loss of central vision.

Symptoms: (see fig 5.41 p451)
• Initally there is no deterioration in visual acuity testing, but difficulty making out images due to failing contrast sensitivity
• Difficulty with reading and making out faces
• Difficulty with night vision and with changing light conditions (specifically, changes in Amsler grid self-evaluation and trouble with reading)

Risk factors for ARMD
• Increasing age
• Smoking
• Cardiovascular disease
• Family history
• Cataract surgery

• Visual fluctuation (ie, some days vision is poor; other days, vision appears improved)
• Metamorphopsia (distortion of visual images): not a major patient complaint, but it may be present as the atrophy slowly progresses.

1 *Wet ARMD (exudative)* pathologic choroidal neovascular membranes (CNVM) develop under the retina. The CNVM can leak fluid and blood and cause a central disciform scar. Vision deteriorates rapidly and distortion is a key feature. Ophthalmoscopy shows fluid exudation, localized detachment of the pigment. Treatment is available for wet ARMD (BOX). Be prompt as substantial visual loss may occur while the patient waits.[64] Patients are advised to stop smoking and have a diet rich in green vegetables. Animal & clinical studies have established vascular endothelial growth factor (VEGF) as a key mediator in ocular angiogenesis. Particular attention has been focused on the development of pharmaceutical agents to block or neutralize VEGF expression.[65]

2 *Dry ARMD (non-exudative)* has a much slower (over decades), progressive visual loss relative to wet ARMD (over months). Its aetiology is not as well known. It shows mainly drusen and changes at the macula. Prevention is the best treatment for nonexudative ARMD, because no satisfactory method exists to treat this condition. Accumulated evidence suggests that ARMD is a genetic disease. Antioxidant vitamin and mineral supplements (vitamin A, vitamin E, zinc, and lutein) are recommended.[66]

Optic atrophy (fig 5.34) Discs are pale (degree doesn't correlate with visual loss). It may be from ↑intraocular pressure (glaucoma), or retinal damage (choroiditis, retinitis pigmentosa, cerebromacular degeneration), or be due to ischaemia (retinal artery occlusion).

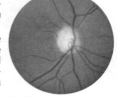

Fig 5.34 Optic atrophy.

Other causes: Leber's optic atrophy (p648), multiple sclerosis (MS), syphilis, external pressure on the nerve (intraorbital or intracranial tumours), Paget's disease affecting the skull).

Ophthalmology

Optic nerve drusen

Drusen signify optic nerve-head axonal degeneration. Abnormal axonal metabolism leads to intracellular mitochondrial calcification. Some axons rupture and mitochondria are extruded into the extra-cellular space. Calcium is deposited here, and drusen form (fig 5.35). The optic disc edge is made irregular by the lumpy, yellow matter. The optic cup is absent and vessels show abnormal branching patterns.[67]

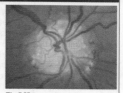

Fig 5.35 Optic drusen.
©Mr C Chau.

Managing wet age-related macular degeneration (ARMD)

Arrange a fluorescein angiogram at the outset and then 4–6-weekly reviews with a photograph and an OCT (optical coherence tomography).

Intravitreal vascular endothelial growth factor (VEGF) inhibitors Benefits: ↑acuity; ↓cell proliferation, ↓formation of new blood vessels, ↓vascular leaks.[68] Monthly bevacizumab (Avastin®) and ranibizumab (Lucentis®; NICE approved) injections for 1yr give the same acuity benefit.[69] Although Avastin® is not licensed for wet ARMD in the UK, it is often used as a cheaper alternative to Lucentis® which is NICE approved; there are no records of any doctor being penalized for prescribing Avastin® in preference.[70]

Laser photocoagulation May be used in eyes with specific signs on fluorescein angiography and juxtafoveal or extrafoveal lesions only. Persistent or recurrent CNV occurs in ~50% of treated eyes within 3 years of therapy.

Photodyamic therapy (PDT) IV verteporfin (photosensitive dye) releases free radicals that disrupt neovascular tissue when photo-active laser is applied. Less common now that anti-vGF is becoming more popular.

Intravitreal steroids Triamcinolone is an adjunct to PDT & VEGF inhibitors.[71]

Screening Once signs of ARMD are seen, ask patients to report any new signs of neovascularization: a good self-test is 'do straight lines on graph paper appear straight?'. Refer if distortions or sudden blank spots.

If these measures are inapplicable Most must rely on visual aids (eg magnifiers) to read. Advise a diet rich in fruit & leafy green vegetables.[72]

Antioxidants/vitamins AREDS (Age-Related Eye Disease Study) 'established' that supplementing diets with zinc, β-carotene, and vitamin C & E slowed AMD progression.[26] AREDS2 recently demonstrated that oral supplementation with macular xanthophylls (lutein & zeaxanthin) in place of beta-carotene decreased risk of progression but omega-3 made no difference.[73]

Choroiditis (choroidoretinitis) The choroid is part of the uvea (iris, ciliary body, and choroid), and inflammatory disorders affecting the uvea may also affect the choroid. The retina may be invaded by organisms which set up a granulomatous reaction (which can be mistaken for a retinoblastoma). Toxoplasmosis, TB, and sarcoidosis are causes. Treat the cause.

In young teenagers, think of Stargardt macular degeneration in young patients with gradual-onset visual loss. This condition was the first to be treated with embryonal stem cells.

Further reading

Chakravarthy U *et al.* (2013). Alternative treatments to inhibit vEGF in age-related choroidal neovascularisation: 2-year findings of the IVAN randomised controlled trial. *Lancet* 382(9900):1258–67.

Weir E (2004). Age-related macular degeneration; armed against ARMD. *CMAJ* 170(4):463–4.

26 Studies of monozygotic AMD-discordant twins: the twin with more advanced AMD, larger drusen, and pigment area tended to be the heavier smoker. The twin with the earlier stage tended to have ↑dietary vitamin D, betaine, and methionine intake.[74]

Ophthalmology

Registration Approximately 360,000 people are registered partially sighted or blind in the UK. It is estimated that a total of 2 million people are living with visual impairment.[75] Blindness may be voluntarily registered in England, making one eligible for certain concessions. *Criteria for partial sighted registration:* Acuity is <6/60 (or >6/60 with visual field restrictions). *Severe visual impairment (blind) registration:* Although the word blind suggests inability to perceive light, a person is eligible for registration if their acuity is less than 3/60, or if >3/60 (p412) but with substantial visual field loss (as in glaucoma).

Why register? In England, responsibility for blind registration lies with the local authority. Application is made by a consultant ophthalmologist and is voluntary, not statutory. The register is confidential. Registration as blind entitles one to extra tax allowances, 50% reduction in TV licence fees, some travel concessions, and access to audio books. It does not automatically entitle patients to welfare benefits, but it does make it easier for them to claim. Special certification from an ophthalmologist is necessary for the partially sighted to receive talking books. At one time it was statutory that the registered blind should receive a visit from a social worker but this is no longer the case, although the social services employ social workers who specialize in care of the blind. The Royal National Institute of Blind People[28] will advise on aids, such as guide dogs (available if required for employment). It sells talking mobile phones and other helpful gadgets on its website.

Special educational facilities These provide for visually impaired children. Special schools have a higher staff/pupil ratio, specialized equipment, and many have a visiting ophthalmologist. The disadvantage is that the children may not mix much with other children—especially if they board.

Living with blindness and partial sight can be socially isolating and challenging, yet people adapt remarkably.[29] Getting back to work and finding suitable employment and education requires a lot of motivation and support. The elderly are at high risk of falls. There is great value placed on having intact vision. One review has suggested that people with 6/9–6/12 vision would be willing to pay 19% of their lifetime to get back normal visual acuity. Patients with 6/60 visual acuity will give up 48% of their lifetime, and blind people would release an impressive 60%. DVLA: see p527.[76]

Use of services by older patients with failing vision

There is good evidence in the UK of under-use of services by older people. Population-based cross-sectional studies in primary care show that prevalence of bilateral visual impairment (acuity <6/12) is ~30%. Most of these are not in touch with ophthalmic services. ▶*Three-quarters of these have remediable problems.* In one study, 20% had acuity in one or both eyes of <6/60 ('blind'). Typical causes were found to be cataract (30%), macular degeneration (8%), and undiagnosed chronic glaucoma.[77]=1547 Despite the good availability of NHS-funded eye examinations for those >60 years with a personal or family history of eye disease (eg diabetes or glaucoma), many of these patients in the UK do not engage in these free services. Efforts need to focus on raising public understanding regarding the purpose of eye examinations in terms of other causes of preventable sight loss (such as diabetes or glaucoma)[30].[78]

Further reading

Read about Helen Keller—a remarkable story about deafness and blindness.

International Council of Ophthalmology: *Childhood Blindness.* http://www.icoph.org/dynamic/attachments/resources/childhood-blindness.pdf

28 Royal National Institute of Blind People: www.rnib.org.uk .
29 Read this short account of a 25-year-old woman who started to go blind at the age of 21.[78]
30 In the past, smallpox, gonorrhoea, syphilis, and leprosy (10% of those affected were blind) were also common causes of blindness.

'An eye for an eye only ends up making the whole world blind.' Mahatma Gandhi

Rates of blindness are higher than 10:1000 in some parts of Africa and Asia, but in the UK and the USA rates are 2:1000. The pattern of blindness around the world differs considerably, depending on local nutrition and economic factors. 90% of the world's blind live in developing countries—and 80% would not be blind if trained eye personnel, medicines, ophthalmic equipment, and patient referral systems were optimized. The global distribution of avoidable blindness is as follows: South East Asian (28%), Western Pacific (26%), African (16.6%), Eastern Mediterranean (10%), American (9.6%) and European (9.6%) (based on the population in each of the WHO regions).[80] www.WHO.int

Worldwide causes of *avoidable* blindness

1 Cataract
2 Glaucoma
3 Age-related macular degeneration
4 Corneal opacities
5 Trachoma
6 Childhood blindess (eg vitamin A deficiency; see p460).
7 Onchocerciasis (see p461)
8 Uncorrected refractive errors (myopia, hyperopia or astigmtism) are also a major cause and the prevalance is thought to be underestimated.

Causes of *avoidable* blindness in the least developed countries[28]

1 Cataract
2 Glaucoma
3 Corneal opacities
4 Trachoma
5 Childhood blindness
6 Onchocerciasis.

Causes of blindness in developed countries

1 Cataract
2 Age-related macular degeneration
3 Glaucoma
4 Diabetic retinopathy.

The most common cause of irreversible blindness and partial sight in developed countries is age-related macular degeneration. In patients of working age, diabetic retinopathy is the leading cause in the West.

The WHO Global Initiative to Eliminate Avoidable Blindness 'VISION 2020: The Right to Sight' aims to elimite these six groups of diseases as a public health problem by 2020. The principal diseases worked on so far are cataracts, trachoma, and onchocerciasis. Programmes are still undergoing for glaucoma, diabetic retinopathy, uncorrected refractive errors, and childhood blindness. Over the past 20 years there have been significant efforts to decrease visual impairment worldwide; especially in reducing the disease burden of onchocerciasis and trachoma related blindness.

Causes of blindness in the UK

These have changed considerably over the last 70 years. Whereas in the 1920s ophthalmia neonatorum (p37) was responsible for 30% of blindness in English blind schools, this is now a rare but treatable disease. Retrolental fibroplasia was common in the 1950s, mostly affecting premature infants: monitoring of intra-arterial oxygen in premature babies tries to prevent this. With an ever-ageing population, the diseases particularly afflicting this population are the common causes of blindness. Nearly two-thirds of the blind population are over 65 years of age, and nearly half over 75. Macular degeneration, cataract, and glaucoma are the three commonest causes of blindness. Almost ⅔ of sight loss in older people is caused by refractive error and cataract.[75]

~10% of blind registrations in the UK are attributed to glaucoma. It affects ~2% of the population >40 years old. Glaucoma is defined as optic neuropathy with death of many retinal ganglion cells and their optic nerve axons. IOP may be raised, *but this is not part of the definition*. (See fig 5.27 on p433 for a diagram of the circulation of aqueous humour.) It is asymptomatic until visual fields are badly impaired; hence the need for screening. If ↑intraocular pressure (IOP) is found, life-long follow-up is needed (≥yearly; more often early on). It accounts for 7% of new blind registrations. Visual field loss may manifest as dangerous difficulty dodging cars while crossing busy roads.[82] Risk factors include ↑ IOP, black race, family history, ↑age and maybe hypertension and diabetes.[83]

Diagnosis requires •IOP measurement using tonometry •Central corneal thickness measurement •Peripheral anterior chamber configuration and depth assessments using gonioscopy •Visual field measurement •Optic nerve assessment using a slit lamp with fundus examination.

Screen if at high risk >35yrs old (typical age at detection: 60yrs), +ve family history (esp. siblings); African-Caribbean; myopia; diabetic/thyroid eye disease. NHS offers free screening to high-risk groups, but uptake is poor (see BOX on p442). Screening is especially important in glaucoma as patients are asymptomatic until the visual field changes become very advanced at which point little can be done. Screening involves tonometry, visual fields, and optic disc examination.

Follow-up: Once diagnosed, lifelong monitoring is required to ensure visual damage is detected and treated. Once lost, sight cannot be restored. Equipment and regimens are complex, and must conform to NICE advice; 4–6-monthly visits may be needed if IOP is off target and risk of developing chronic open-angle glaucoma is high (take into account age, IOP, corneal thickness, appearance and size of the optic nerve head). If favourable, monitor every 1–2yrs.

Drug treatment Chronic glaucoma is such a heterogeneous disease process which may or may not progress to symptomatic vision loss. One study suggested that 12 patients with ↑IOP would need to be treated to prevent one case of glaucoma.[84] Compliance with eye drops is difficult when IOP is ↑ in an asymptomatic patient. Aim to reduce IOP by 30% of baseline. Surgery is used if drugs fail.

• *Prostaglandin analogues* (latanoprost 50mcg/mL; travoprost) ↑uveoscleral outflow. *Dose:* once daily (evenings). SE: red eye, iris colour change, periocular skin pigmentation, eyelash growth.

• *β-blockers* (timolol 0.25–0.5% or betaxolol 0.5%) use twice daily (once daily for Timoptol LA®) to ↓production of aqueous. They are β-blockers. (∴ caution in asthma or heart failure; systemic absorption occurs with no 1st-pass liver metabolism.) SE: dry eyes, corneal anaesthesia, ↓exercise tolerance.

• *α-adrenergic agonists* (brimonidine, apraclonidine) ↓production of aqueous and ↑uveoscleral outflow. SE: lethargy dry mouth.

• *Carbonic anhydrase inhibitors* (dorzolamide & brinzolamide drops, acetazolamide PO) ↓production of aqueous. SE of acetazolamide: lassitude, dyspepsia, K+↓, paraesthesiae. Avoid if pregnant.

• *Miotics* (pilocarpine 0.5–4% drops) ↓resistance to aqueous outflow. It causes miosis, acuity↓, and brow ache from ciliary muscle spasm. Use 4 times daily.

• *Sympathomimetic* (dipivefrine 0.1% drops). Caution if heart disease, BP↑, and closed-angle glaucoma. SE: sore, smarting, red eyes/vision↓. Use 12-hourly.

• *Fixed-dose combination drops:* Can give the best 24h efficacy NB: dorzolamide + timolol is better than brimonidine + timolol.[85]

Laser therapy (trabeculoplasty) ↑ aqueous outflow = ↓ IOP. Long-term efficacy is comparable to medical treatment and may be more cost-effective.[86]

Surgery: Trabeculectomy is a filtration surgery that establishes a pressure valve at the limbus so aqueous can flow into a conjunctival bleb. Problems include early failure, hypotony, bleb leakage, infection (normal healing can cause bleb failure, but this can be delayed by topical cytotoxics).

Optic disc cupping is characterized by loss of disc substance which makes the cup look larger. Normal cups are similar in shape and occupy <50% of the disc. Normal cup:disc ratio 0.4-0.7 but this depends on the size of the disc: ►a large cup in a small disc is probably pathological.[31] As damage progresses, the disc pales (atrophies), and the cup widens and deepens, so vessels emerging from the disc appear to have breaks as they disappear into the cup and are then seen at the base again (fig 5.36). Notching of the cup and haemorrhage at the disc may occur. As cupping develops, the disc vessels are displaced nasally. Nasal and superior fields are lost first (temporal last) and central vision tends to be maintained. Asymmetric cupping suggests glaucoma. Notching at the neuroretinal rim is usually inferior, and best seen where the vessels enter the disc. Glaucomatous optic nerve damage affects the anterior visual pathway up to the optic chiasm. To further understand the optic disc in glaucoma read the online link.[87]

Pathogenesis Glaucoma is present when, on field testing, 3 or more locations are outside normal limits, and the cup-to-disc ratio[29] (see 'Optic disc cupping') is greater than that seen in 97.5% of the population. Susceptibility of a patient's retina and optic nerve to IOP-related damage is very variable. IOP ≥21mmHg may or may not correlate with cupping, nerve damage, with scotomata (sausage-shaped field defects near the blind spot, which may coalesce to form big defects). Since the central field is intact, good acuity is maintained, so presentation is often delayed until irreversible optic nerve damage. Control of IOP *does* stop visual field loss but does not reverse it.[88] The visual defects tend to be bilateral, although are not always symmetrical. Some get glaucoma with *normal* IOP (eg if retrobulbar blood flow↓).[89]

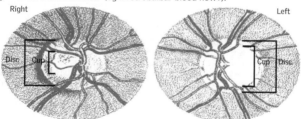

Right   Left

Disc   Cup   Cup   Disc

Fig 5.36 The right disc has been unaffected by the open angle glaucoma, the left disc is grossly cupped and atrophic.

Reproduced from Parr, *Introduction to Ophthalmology*, with permission from University of Otago Press.

Educating people about their glaucoma

It is common for people to be seen regularly for years in the glaucoma clinic and yet understand almost nothing about their condition. 'This is their fault—if they asked, we'd be delighted to tell...' But it's really our fault and we should do better, as lack of knowledge is dangerous and demoralizing. In one study, 80% thought that glaucoma drops could have no systemic effects, and 48% believed symptoms would warn them of disease progression. 30% of new patients believe that blindness is likely.[90]

So try to explain what happens in glaucoma, and give printed details (check that the patient can read them!), and stress that they should let their doctors know that they are on glaucoma treatment.

Further reading

NICE (2009). *Glaucoma: Diagnosis and Management* (CG85). London: NICE.

Quigley HA (2009). Glaucoma. *Lancet* 377(9774):1367-77.

Vas C et al. (2007). Medical interventions for primary open angle glaucoma and ocular hypertension. *Cochrane Database Syst Rev* 4:CD003167.

31 Normal small discs (1.0-1.3mm) have small cups and normal big discs (>1.8) have large cups, so large normal discs may be misnamed glaucomatous. Mean disc diameter: 1.5mm. Mean cup:disc ratio is ~0.35, 0.45, & 0.55 for small, medium and big discs (95th centiles for upper limit of normal are 0.59, 0.66, & 0.74).

Any opacity in the lens is called a cataract. The leading cause of blindness (p442). Cataracts are found in 75% of >65s but in only 20% of 45-65-year-olds.

Risk factors Most cataracts are age related. In children, many are genetic (?some genetic influence in adults too). Cataracts occur early in: diabetes mellitus ► When a cataract is found, measure fasting plasma glucose; steroid use; high myopia; dystrophia myotonica. Other associations include smoking, alcohol excess, sunlight exposure, trauma, radiotherapy, HIV +ve.[91]

Ophthalmoscopic classification is by lens appearance. With immature cataracts the red reflex still occurs; in dense cataracts there is no red reflex, or visible fundus. *Nuclear cataracts* change the refractive index and noticeably dulls colours, they are common in old age. *Cortical cataracts* are spoke-like wedge-shaped opacities which have milder effects on vision. *Posterior subcapsular cataracts* typically progress faster and cause the classic glare from bright sunlight and lights whilst driving at night, even when visual acuity is only mildly affected. Subcapsular opacities (eg from steroid use) are just deep to the lens capsule—in the visual axis. Dot opacities are common in normal lenses but are also seen in fast-developing cataracts in diabetes or dystrophia myotonica.

Presentation Blurred vision. Unilateral cataracts are often unnoticed, but loss of stereopsis affects distance judgement. Bilateral cataracts cause gradual painless loss of vision (frequent spectacle changes as refraction changes) ± dazzle (esp. in sunlight) ± monocular diplopia. Patients describe difficulties driving at night and haloes around street lights. In children they may present as squint, or a white pupil, or as nystagmus (infants)/amblyopia.

Surgery Mydriatic drops, sunshades/sunglasses help a bit, but if symptoms are troubling, lifestyle is restricted, or if unable to read a number-plate at 20 metres (and they need to drive) offer surgery. Explain risks: 2% get serious complications; even if surgery may vastly improve vision, eyes may not be entirely normal afterwards (dazzle/glare often remains). Distant spectacles are often needed too. >30% have co-existing macular degeneration,[et al] which limits outcome.

The ideal is day-case surgery using local anaesthesia with small-incision surgery and phacoemulsion + intraocular lens (IOL) implant. This applies to the vast majority. Younger people, high myopes, and the squeamish may prefer general anaesthesia. An incision of ~3mm is made, and the lens is removed by phacoemulsion (US breaks it up: it is then aspirated into a cannula). The incision is fractionally enlarged and an artificial lens (eg of Perspex®, acrylic, or silicon) implanted. Lenses are foldable so they can be put through a smaller incision. The patient can usually return home immediately afterwards with a dressing for a few hours. With phacoemulsification, full activities can be resumed next day. With complicated surgery or extracapsular extraction, a larger incision is needed and there may be more limitations. Patients use antibiotic & anti-inflammatory drops for 3-6 weeks post-op. Then they need to change spectacles to get the full benefit of surgery. Multifocal IOLs exist and in appropriately selected patients they can be helpful.

Post-op complications: Post-op posterior *capsule thickening* is common. It is deliberately left at surgery to make surgery safer. It opacifies in ~20%, over months or years post-op; it seems 'like my cataract returning' or 'I'm looking through frosted glass'. It is easily treated by capsulotomy with a Yag laser as an outpatient. As refraction is corrected, *astigmatism* is more noticed. This can be corrected during surgery (eg by toric intraocular lens or eyeball shape change by placing the incision in the exact right place) in the light of pre-op biometry. Enophthalmitis is a potential serious complication.

Prevention/photoprotection✷ **1** Use sunglasses (UV-B↓).[92] **2** ↓Oxidative stress (with antioxidants, eg vitamin C and caffeine[etc]).[93] **3** Stop smoking!

Pre- and post-operative care

Prior to surgery, *ocular biometry* must be done. This is a measurement of the curvature of the cornea and the length of the eye which enables prediction of the suitable intraocular lens implant (fig 5.37). In most cases it aims to leave the patient emmetropic (in focus for distance), or just slightly myopic, but this may vary considerably depending on patient preference and pre-existing refraction. It is not an exact science as the clinical measurements vary and many people do continue to wear spectacles post-operatively for a remaining refractive error—but heightened patient expectations for precise postoperative refractive results make biometry vital. [94]

On obtaining new spectacles many experience symptoms of imbalance; these should settle in 2-3 weeks.

▶If patients develop a painful red eye or loss of vision post-operatively, refer back to the ophthalmologist urgently. Some *eye irritation* needing additional or altered drops post-op is common. Many experience awareness of the eye or dry, or gritty sensations and lubricants such as carbomer gel eg Viscotears® may help. Some may have *anterior uveitis* requiring new medication. Rarely, there may be vitreous haemorrhage, retinal detachment, or glaucoma (± permanent visual loss), and endophthalmitis (<3/10,000; but pseudomonal clusters may occur). If vision deteriorates with time they should initially see if they need a new prescription change; and thereafter the ophthalmologist to consider Yag laser capsulotomy or exclusion of other problems.

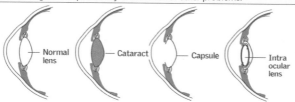

Normal lens — Cataract — Capsule — Intra ocular lens

Fig 5.37 Position of the intraocular lens after cataract surgery.

Cataracts at birth: ▶act within 4 weeks!

If there is a congenital cataract the patient needs to be referred urgently to ophthalmology for surgical consideration. Intervention needs to be done within the latent period of visual development (1st 6 weeks of life) to prevent significant deprivation amblyopia. Do a TORCH screen too (p34). [95]

Claude Monet

'Halo' refers to a circle of light, white or coloured, seen around *any* luminous body (not just saints). Also call to mind Monet, his cataracts (a cause of haloes) and his paintings and their 'investments in light' (another meaning of halo). In the poem, Monet refuses surgery

> *D*octor, you say there are no haloes around the streetlights in Paris and what I see is an aberration caused by old age, an affliction. I tell you it has taken me all my life to arrive at the vision of gas lamps as angels.
>
> Lisel Mueller: Monet Refuses the Operation
> M Faith McLellan 1996. *Lancet* 1996 348: 1641.

for his cataracts: how differently doctors and artists see the world (BOX)! So before we advise surgery it's wise to get to know our patients, and to keep a eye on posterity. Visual changes are also thought to have influenced other painters including Vincent Van Gogh and Rembrandt van Rijn. [96]

Further reading

Asbell PA *et al.* (2005). Age-related cataract. *Lancet* 365:599–609.

Keay L *et al.* (2011). Routine preoperative medical testing for cataract surgery. *Cochrane Database Syst Rev* 3:CD007293.

NICE (2015). *Clinical Knowledge Summaries*: Cataracts. http://cks.nice.org.uk/cataracts

The retina consists of an outer pigmented layer (in contact with the choroid), and an inner sensory layer (in contact with the vitreous). At the centre of the posterior part lies the macula (see p450). **Optic disc**. See p456.

Retinal detachment (RD, fig 5.38) Holes/tears in the retina allow fluid to separate the sensory retina from the retinal pigment epithelium. If a retinal break is identified before a detachment occurs, cryo/laser retinopexy may be preventive. *Types:*
1 *Rhegmatogenous retinal detachment*—a tear in the retina causes fluid to pass from the vitreous space into the subretinal space between the sensory retina and the retinal pigment epithelium. Typically caused by trauma. 2 *Exudative retinal detachment*—The retina detaches without a tear, eg hypertension, vasculitis, macular degenerative conditions, tumours.

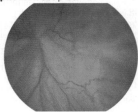
Fig 5.38 RD; note retinal folds (1–3 o'clock) & distorted disc. © Bristol Eye Hospital.

3 *Tractional retinal detachments*—pulling on the retina, eg proliferative retinapathy. Myopic eyes are more prone to detachment, the higher the myopia, the greater the risk. Cataract surgery for myopia carries ↑risk of detachment.[97]

Presents with the 4 'F's: floaters, flashes (in ~50%), field loss, and fall in acuity—painless and may be as a curtain falling over the vision (eg the curtain falls down as the lower half of the retina detaches upwards). Field defects indicate position and extent of the detachment (in superior detachments field loss is inferior). Ophthalmoscopy: grey opalescent retina, ballooning forward. Extensive detachment of the retina will pull off the macular. If it does detach, central vision is lost and doesn't always recover completely even if the retina is successfully fixed. Rate of detachment varies: upper halves are quicker. *Prognosis* depends on: •Site and extent of detachment •Time to definitive treatment •Nature of underlying pathology.

Differential diagnosis: Migraine: be very cautious to diagnosis this in an older person with no pre-existing history of it. Retinal artery occlusion (p436), posterior vitreous detachment (p450), vitreous haemorrhage.

Mangement: Rest is key—if detachment is superior, nurse flat. If the detachment is inferior, lie 30 degrees head up. Laser photocoagulation theapy. ⇥Refer urgently, for surgery: vitrectomy and gas tamponade (or silicone oil), scleral silicone implants. Cryotherapy or laser coagulation is used to secure the retina. Post-op re-detachment occurs in 5–10%.

Retinitis pigmentosa This is the most prevalent inherited degeneration in the retina. Primarily affects males presenting with night blindness followed by peripheral and central daytime vision loss. On the cellular level, this correlates with rod photoreceptor problems. The disease progresses to affect the cone photoreceptors, eventually causing complete blindness in the late stages. More than 300 mutations in the RPGR gene have been linked to retinitis pigmentosa. Its inheritancy can be autosomal dominant, autosomal recessive, or x-linked manner. Although x-linked recessive retinitis pigmentosa is thought to affect male subjects only, some documented cases of RP RPGR GR mutations have been shown in carrier female subjects, thus giving an impression of occurance in sequential generations simulating mendelian dominant transmission. Through life, 25% retain ability to read, with reduced visual fields. Only a few have acuity ≤6/60 at aged 20yrs; but by 50, many are reduced to this level.[98] Novel non-standard therapies: neural prosthetics (artificial vision by stimulating retinal ganglion cells electrically) (p465).

Lots of flashes may indicate the moment of a retinal tear or detachment; lots of floaters suggest blood or pigment released into the vitreous. Detachment of a shrinking vitreous from the retina gives flashes and floaters. 5% go on to retinal tears and detachment. Retinal damage is usually peripheral and hard to see—refer immediately for specialist help.

Floaters are a very common visual symptom. To ascertain its aetiology requires a very detailed history. *Common causes:* Often caused by RBCs (anything that causes new vessels to form on the retina can lead to vitreous haemorrhage and perceived floaters, eg diabetic retinopathy; vein occlusions), trauma/retinal detachment (often with blood in the vitreous). A showering effect of hundreds of tiny black specks in the visual fields may be indicative of a vitreous hemorrhage, resulting from disruption of a retinal vessel caused by a retinal tear or mechanical traction of a vitreoretinal adhesion. The sudden onset of large floaters in the center of the visual axis may indicate posterior vitreous detachment (PVD; see below). WBCs are the other main cause, eg from inflammatory/infective causes, posterior choroiditis (p438). *Sinister causes* are secondary to tumour seeding—either primary as in melanoma or retinoblastoma (patients often too young to complain of symptoms) or secondary metastasis. Also think of endophthalmitis (eg fungal). *Degenerative causes* include opacities in the vitreous: asteroid hyalosis (like stars in the night sky) and syneresis; these floaters are caused by shadows of mobile vitreous lakes that occur in the ageing of the eye. When they eye comes to a rest, the floaters continue to move. They are a more common in myopia, after cataract surgery, or trauma.

Management: Floaters present as small dark spots in the visual field, particularly noticeable against a bright background (fig **5.39**). Often, they are just annoying, but harmless, and may settle with time. Examine the vitreous and retina, and treat the cause before reassuring. *Sudden showers* of floaters in one eye (±flashing lights) may be due to blood. ▶*Refer immediately* (specialist assessment within 48h or sooner): the cause may be retinal detachment (below).

Flashing lights (photopsia) Either from intraocular or cerebral pathology (migraine). Is there headache, nausea, or previous migraine? Retinal tissue is stimulated by light but also responds to mechcanical disturbances. As the retinal tissues gets disturbed, it produces phosphenes (phenomenon characterized by the experience of seeing light without light entering the eye).

Posterior vitreous detachment (PVD) Degenerative changes in the vitreous lead to its eventual separation from the retina. This is part of normal ageing. Patients describe monochromatic photopsia in the peripheral temporal field. This is more obvious in dim light and with eye movements. There is an increase in floaters but vision remains unchanged and there are no field defects. Refer for fundus check as retinal tears can happen as a consequence of a PVD.

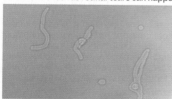

Fig **5.39** A simulated image of the appearance of floaters whilst looking at blue sky. You may notice floaters yourself eg when staring at a white wall.

Further reading

Hartong DT *et al.* (2006). Retinitis pigmentosa. *Lancet* 368(9549):1795–809.

Hollands H *et al.* (2009). Acute onset floaters and flashes: is this patient at risk for retinal detachment? *JAMA* 302:2243–9.

Kahawita S *et al.* (2014). Flashes and floaters - a practical approach to assessment and management. *Aust Fam Physician* 43:201–3.

Ophthalmology

The *macula* (fig 5.40) is an area 5.5mm across, just lateral to the optic disc. In the middle of the macula is a 1.5mm pit, the *fovea* (fovea centralis; no ganglion cells). In the middle of the fovea is the *foveola* where the cones are narrow, long and densely packed (300,000mm²). This cone gradient correlates with acuity. Any disturbance in this region can impact vision greatly. Assessment of macular function must involve documenting visual acuity. Use the Amsler grid (see fig 5.41, p451) to asses visual distortion.

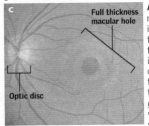

Fig 5.40 The macula lies lateral to the optic nerve and contains the structures enabling high visual acuity.

Reproduced from Sundaram *et al.*, *Oxford Specialty Training: Training in Ophthalmology* (2009) with permission from Oxford University Press.

A macular hole is a small break in the macular region of the retinal tissue. It involves the fovea therefore affecting the visual acuity causing blurred and distorted central vision. *Prevalance:* 3.3/1000 in persons >55yrs old. There is a 10–15% chance of developing a macular hole in the other eye in your lifetime and the patient must undergo surveillance. *Pathogenesis:* Usually idiopathic aetiology; with ageing, the vitreous starts to lose some of the 80% water content, which causes it to shrink causing traction on the retinal tissue. Other risk factors include high myopia, injury to the eye, and retinal detachment. *Presentation:* Distorted vision with visual loss. The effect on visual acuity is dependant on the site of macular damage. On examination, look for a tiny punched-out area in the centre of the macula; there may be yellow-white deposits at the base. Slit lamp exam with a convex lens shows a round excavation with well-defined borders interrupting the slit lamp beam. The hole is typically surrounded by a grey halo of detached retina.

Tests Amsler grids (see p429 and fig 5.41) reveal visual distortion; optical coherence tomography diagnoses and stages macular holes. Fluorescein angiography (FA) helps differentiate macular holes from cystoid macular oedema and choroidal neovascularization (CNV) **Treatment** ►Refer urgently to a specialist vitreo-retinal surgeon. In stage 1 (impending hole seen as a yellow spot on the fovea), see what happens (no treatment if there is spontaneous resolution or no progression). ~50% of holes progress to stage 2—when treatment is needed. *Surgery:* A vitrectomy is done to remove the vitreous and the internal limiting membrane over the hole is peeled. An air bubble is introduced to nudge (tamponade) the macula back into position. The patient spends 1–2 post-op weeks face down. Success is also possible if the hole is long-standing (>6 months).

However, in some patients, more than one operation is needed to close the hole, and adverse effects may occur: macular retinal pigment epithelium changes, retinal detachments, iatrogenic retinal tears, enlargement of the hole, macular light toxicity, postoperative intraocular pressure spikes. Many patients develop cataracts (76% of cases requiring extraction within 2 years). Patients not suitable or not wishing for this need visual aids (eg to read).[99]

►Refer urgently to a specialist vitreo-retinal surgeon.

Dispelling the myths There is no association between macular holes and age-related macular degeneration (p440); they have similar symptoms and both involve the macula but the pathophysiology is vastly different.

'The greatest thing a human soul ever does in this world is to see something, and tell what it saw in a plain way. Hundreds of people can talk for one who can think, but thousands can think for one who can see.' ^{John Ruskin *Modern Painters*; vol. III}

Interpreting but not over-interpreting our visual sensations entails the almost impossible task of seeing the indifferent pixels as well their patterns. When a classicist, revising for her exams, says 'I'm preparing for my Unseen' she means 'I'm preparing for a surprise. I'm going to have to translate, without warning, some unknown ancient passage (our primordial unconscious) into modern parlance (current sensations).' To do well, she (and we) have to expect the unexpected, or else the snake will bite us. More deeply, all visual experience is ambiguous, yet we believe and act on it all the time. Seers, philosophers, and, above all, poets know that the issue here is the role our imagination plays in seeing. *'I have seen sometimes what men imagine they see.'* (J'ai vu quelquefois ce que l'homme a cru voir!) ^{*The Drunken Boat* Arthur Rimbaud}

How is this important clinically? Just as we are born expecting to hear each other's voices, so we are born expecting to see each other's faces. If in later life we lose our vision, then the brain, with exaggerated zeal, compensates by creating fictive visual percepts, almost always involving faces—a surprisingly common non-psychotic hallucination named after Charles Bonnet, who first described it in his 89-year-old grandfather in 1769.

Charles Bonnet's grandfather might say with insight: *'I have imagined sometimes what other men know they see'*—ie the mirror-image of Arthur Rimbaud's formulation. The point is that neither Rimbaud nor Bonnet can pinch themselves to see if their hallucinatory state is real. By their systematic derangement of their senses they teach us something universal about our place in our external and internal worlds, namely that we can never fully disentangle what we see from what we expect to see. It is as if our propensity for illusions validates and authenticates our experience of being us.

So don't get too annoyed with your patients when they give ambiguous answers to your questions about floaters, flashes and more complex fictive visual percepts. Just smile to yourself and to Rimbaud in his embodiment as a drunken, waterlogged boat (*Le bateau ivre*) and remember that *the boat is in the drink and the drink is in the boat.*

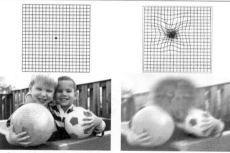

Fig 5.41 Use of Amsler grids: As wet ARMD (p440) progresses, the patient experiences distortion of straight lines (metamorphopsia); this is detected using an Amsler grid. Central vision is distorted when the fovea is involved. These images demonstrate the visual deterioration the patient experiences.

'Eye disease simulation, age-related macular degeneration' by National Eye Institute, National Institutes of Health: http://www.nei.nih.gov/photo/keyword.asp?narrow=Eye+Disease+Simulation&match=all (TIFF image). Licensed under Public Domain via Commons

Further reading

http://www.macularholesupport.org.uk/

Systemic disease often manifests itself in the eye and, in some cases, eye examination will first suggest the diagnosis. (See also p459 and *онсм* p562.)

Vascular retinopathy This may be *arteriopathic* (*arteriovenous nipping:* arteries nip veins where they cross—they share the same connective tissue sheath) or *hypertensive* (arteriolar vasoconstriction and leakage) producing *hard exudates, macular oedema, haemorrhages,* and, rarely, *papilloedema.* Thick, shiny arterial walls appear like wiring (called 'silver' or 'copper'). Narrowing of arterioles leads to infarction of the superficial retina seen as cotton wool spots and flame haemorrhages. Leaks from these appear as hard exudates ± macular oedema/papilloedema (rare).

Retinal haemorrhages are seen in leukaemia; retinal new vessel formation and comma-shaped conjunctival haemorrhages may occur in sickle-cell disease; optic atrophy in pernicious anaemia.

Note also Roth spots (retinal infarcts) of infective endocarditis (*онсм* p144).

Metabolic disease Diabetes: p454. Wilson's disease (Kayser–Fleischer ring, fig 5.42). Hyperthyroidism, and exophthalmos: *онсм* p211. In myxoedema, eyelid and periorbital oedema is quite common. Lens opacities may occur in hypoparathyroidism. Conjunctival and corneal calcification may occur in hyperparathyroidism. In gout, monosodium urate deposited in the conjunctiva may give sore eyes.

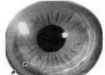

Fig 5.42 Kayser–Fleischer ring.
Courtesy of Jon Miles.

Granulomatous disorders (TB, sarcoid, leprosy, brucellosis, toxoplasmosis) all produce inflammation in the eye (uveitis). TB, congenital syphilis, sarcoid, CMV, and toxoplasmosis may all produce chorioretinitis. In sarcoid there may be cranial nerve palsies and lacrimal gland swelling.

Collagen and vasculitic diseases These also cause inflammation. Conjunctivitis is found in SLE and reactive arthritis; episcleritis in polyarteritis nodosa and SLE; scleritis in rheumatoid arthritis; and uveitis in ankylosing spondylitis and reactive arthritis (*онсм* p552). In dermatomyositis there is orbital oedema & heliotrope rash with retinal haemorrhages. Behçet's syndrome causes uveitis & retinopathies. Temporal arteritis leads to ischaemic damage to the optic nerve.

Keratoconjunctivitis sicca/Sjögren's syndrome (*онсм* p724). There is reduced tear formation (Schirmer filter paper test), producing a gritty feeling in the eyes. Decreased salivation also gives a dry mouth (xerostomia). It occurs in association with collagen diseases. Pilocarpine and cevimeline help sicca features and topical ciclosporin helps moderate or severe dry eye. Silicone nasolacrimal punctal plugs help maintain tears on the eye surface for longer. All these named treatments are specialist use only.

HIV/AIDS Those who are HIV +ve may get *CMV retinitis* and it causes 40% of vision loss in AIDS patients (often despite highly active antiretroviral R_x), with retinal spots ('pizza pie' fundus, signifying superficial retinal infarction) + flame haemorrhages involving ever more of the retina. This may be asymptomatic or cause blindness; it is an AIDS-defining illness; (CD4 count is ↓). IV ganciclovir or its prodrug (oral valganciclovir) are used. Cotton wool spots may indicate HIV retinopathy; it is a microvasculopathy, not a retinitis. Candidiasis of the aqueous and vitreous is hard to treat. Kaposi's sarcoma (fig 8.44 p607) may affect the lids or conjunctiva.[100]

Other causes of retinopathy (*haemorrhages, microaneurysms, hard exudates*)[101] Radiation; carotid artery disease; central or branch retinal vein occlusion; retinal telangiectasia/Coats' disease; Leber's miliary aneurysms and drugs (p459).

Pregnancy presents significant physiological changes to the mother which enable her body to cope with the increased demands from the foetus (p6). These changes are usually transient and benign, but can become damaging in the presence of pre-existing pathology.

Physiological changes in the eye

Eyelids don the 'mask of pregnancy'; increased pigmentation, due to hormonal changes, around the eye called cholasma. This is reversible and fades post partum. Eyes become drier in 80% of women as *tear production* is affected. Women previously unable to tolerate contact lenses may now be able to as *corneal sensitivity* decreases towards the end of pregnancy, but advise them to wait 6 weeks post partum to get new glasses as corneal refraction may also have changed. On the same note, *lens refraction* may also change subtly. *Intraocular pressure* decreases; which benefits glaucoma patients. Women with autoimmune eye disease may experience temporary relief as the *immune system* is depressed to facilitate embryo implantation. *Visual field* changes may not always be physiological and warrant further investigation.

Pre-existing ocular diseases

Glaucoma patients may show improvement due to the reduction in intraocular pressure—do involve an ophthalmologist in their care though as evidence on safety of glaucoma medication in pregnancy is lacking. Avoid beta-blockers (eg timolol eye drops) in the first trimester and days before the delivery to avoid affecting the baby. Carbonic anhydrase inhibitors are contraindicated because of teratogenic effects. Surgical trabeculoplasty can be offered to minimize reliance on medication.[102]

Diabetic retinopathy (DR) (see also p454) Pregnancy is a notorious risk factor in worsening the progression of DR, especially for type 1 DM. Other influences include degree of retinopathy at time of conception, glycaemic control, and co-existing hypertension. The pathogenesis is unclear, but likely related to the altered retinal haemodynamics and circulating growth factors/hormones. Proliferative changes develop in ~20% of women; those with pre-existing non-proliferative retinopathy are especially at risk.[103] Laser photocoagulation prior to conception protects against DR progression; counsel patients to pursue this prior to pregnancy if possible. If DR first develops during pregnancy it tends to be less severe; 50% undergo complete regression and 30% partial regression of DR after delivery.[102] NICE guidelines state that all women seeking preconception care should be offered annual retinal assessment. During pregnancy, further assessment should be at the booking clinic, 16–20 weeks (if DR was present at booking clinic) and at 28 weeks. DR is not a contraindication to rapid optimization of glycaemic control.[104]

Ocular involvement in pregnancy-related complications

Pre-eclampsia and eclampsia: (p48) Ocular sequelae occur in up to ⅓ of pre-eclampsia and half of women with eclampsia. Visual blurring is most common, but scotoma, photopsia, and diplopia are also reported.[105] The majority of women experience complete resolution after delivery, cortical blindness is a rare complication.

Occlusive vascular disorders: Pregnancy is associated with changes to platelets, clotting factors, and haemodynamics generating a hypercoagulable state. Subsequently women are at higher risk retinal vein/artery occlusion (p440), DIC (p346 OHCM), TTC (p308 OHCM), amniotic fluid embolism (p89), and ceberal venous thrombosis (p484 OHCM).

Ophthalmology

Further reading

Schultz KL *et al.* (2005). Ocular disease in pregnancy. *Curr Opin Ophthalmol* 16(5):308–14.

Somani S (2015). *Pregnancy Special Considerations*. Medscape. http://emedicine.medscape.com/article/1229740

DM is the leading cause of blindness in those aged 20–65 (UK). Almost any part of the eye can be affected: mainly cataract and retinopathy. 30% of adults have ocular problems when diabetes presents but the vast majority of patients remain asymptomatic until advanced disease takes hold; at which point there is little that can be done. This is why regular screening for progression of diabetic retinopathy (DR) is essential for targetting treatment.

Structural changes DM causes ocular ischaemia, which can cause new blood vessel forming on the iris (rubeosis), and, if these block the drainage of aqueous fluid, glaucoma may result. The formation of age-related cataract is accelerated in DM; typically this is premature senile cataract, but young diabetics can also be affected at presentation (the lens has taken up a lot of glucose which is converted by aldolase reductase to sorbitol).

Pathogenesis Microangiopathy in capillaries causes: 1 Vascular occlusion causes ischaemia ± new vessel formation (ie proliferative retinopathy) which bleed (vitreous haemorrhage). Retraction of fibrous tissue running with new vessels heightens risk of retinal detachment. Occlusion also causes cotton wool spots (ischaemic nerve fibres). 2 Vascular leakage: as pericytes are lost, capillaries bulge (microaneurysms) and there is oedema & hard exudates (lipoprotein & lipid-filled macrophages). Rupture of microaneurysms at the nerve fibre level causes flame-shaped haemorrhages; when deep in the retina, blot haemorrhages form.

Classification There are two types of DR: non-proliferative retinopathy and proliferative retinopathy; the latter is distinguished by the presence of new vessels on the retina (neovascularization). *Non-proliferative diabetic retinopathy (NPDR)* is rated as mild, moderate, or severe depending on the degree of ischaemia. Signs comprise microaneurysms (seen as 'dots'), haemorrhages (flame shaped or 'blots'), hard exudates (yellow patches), engorged tortuous veins, cotton wool spots, large blot haemorrhages (the latter 3 are signs of significant ischaemia). NPDR can progress to sight-threatening proliferative retinopathy. *Proliferative diabetic retinopathy (PDR):* Fine new vessels appear on the optic disc, retina, and can cause vitreous haemorrhage. *Maculopathy:* Leakage from the vessels close to the macula cause oedema and can significantly threaten vision (clinically significant macular oedema). It can exist with otherwise mild retinopathy. ►Refer those with maculopathy, severe NPDR, or proliferative retinopathy *urgently* for assessment[32] and treatment (eg photocoagulation) to protect vision.

►**Presymptomatic screening** enables timely laser photocoagulation. DM type 1 & 2 should have their eyes screened at time of diagnosis and at least annually thereafter.[106] Screening is by dilated fundus photography. Referrals are then made accordingly (see BOX on p455). Lesions are mostly at the posterior pole and can be easily seen by ophthalmoscope.

Management ►Ensure target BP is <140/80 (or <130/80 if end-organ damage).[33] At presentation, the lens may have a higher refractive index producing relative myopia. On treatment, the refractive index reduces, and vision is more hypermetropic, so don't correct refractive errors until diabetes is controlled. Good control of diabetes prevents new vessels forming. 'Metabolic memory' effects mean that early good glycaemic control reduces future macro-and microvascular complications.[107] Pregnancy, dyslipidaemia, BP↑, renal disease, smoking, and anaemia may accelerate retinopathy. Photocoagulation by laser is used to treat both maculopathy (focal or grid) and proliferative retinopathy (panretinal). Intravitreal **triamcinolone** & anti-VEGF drugs (p439) are used with laser to treat macular oedema. See figs 5.44 & 5.4.

32 Fluorescein angiography and optical coherence tomography OCT imaging are important tools here.
33 UKPDS data: N=1148. Absolute risk for blindness was 3.1 per 1000 patient-years if control was tight vs 4.1 for others.[108]

Ophthalmology

CNS effects Ocular palsies may occur, typically nerves III and VI. In diabetic third nerve palsy the pupil may be spared as fibres to the pupil run peripherally in the nerve, receiving blood supply from the pial vessels. Argyll Robertson pupils and Horner's syndrome may also occur (p424).

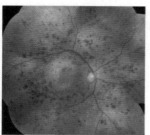

Fig 5.43 Severe non-proliferative diabetic retinopathy.

Reproduced from Sundaram et al, *Oxford Specialty Training: Training in Ophthalmology* (2009) with permission from Oxford University Press.

Ophthalmology

Results of retinal screening: when to refer to the surgeon?

Results of retinal screening in diabetes: when to refer to a surgeon:
1 Maculopathy:
   - If screening shows exudate or retinal thickening within one optic disc diameter of the centre of the fovea
   - Circinate or other group of exudates within the macula
   - Any microaneurysm or haemorrhage within 1 disc-diameter of the centre of the fovea, if best visual acuity is <6/12.
2 There are features of pre-proliferative retinopathy (venous beading; venous loops); multiple deep, round or blot haemorrhages.
3 *Proliferative diabetic retinopathy* This should be treated within 2 weeks with panretinal (scatter) laser photo-coagulation (PRP). This involves treating the peripheral retina which is not receiving adequate blood flow in order to remove the stimulus driving the neovascular process. As this treatment involves many laser applications (eg >1000) it may be divided into ≥2 sessions. NB: panretinal photocoagulation does not improve vision. It is intended to help prevent blindness. It may cause some loss of peripheral, colour, and night vision. Some patients get generalized blurring of vision which is usually transient but may persist.

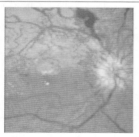

Fig 5.44 Retinopathy before the laser.
© Prof J Trobe.

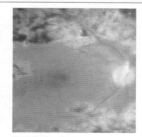

Fig 5.45 After the laser.
© Prof J Trobe.

Further reading

Free ebook on diabetic retinopathy: www.drcobook.com

Mohamed Q *et al.* (2007). Management of diabetic retinopathy: a systematic review. *JAMA* 298(8):902–16.

Ockrim Z *et al.* (2010). Managing diabetic retinopathy. *BMJ* 341:c5400.

The optic disc (fig 5.46) represents the head of the optic nerve which can be seen clinically; the rest of the optic nerve extends proximally towards the optic chiasm. The optic nerve is shorter in hypermetropic eyes and longer in myopic. Examinination of the optic disc aims to describe the *Contour* (borders should be well defined, the disc may appear oval in astigmatic eyes, and appear abnormally large in myopic eyes), *Colour* (should be pink-yellow with a pale centre, the disc colour is more pallid in optic atrophy; p438), and *Cup* (see p445)[110] the disc has a physiological cup which lies centrally and should occupy ~⅓ of the disc diameter. Cup widening and deepening occurs in glaucoma. Blood vessels radiate away from the disc. The normal arterial/venous width ratio is 2:3. Venous engorgement appears in retinal vein thrombosis; abnormal retinal pallor with artery occlusion; and haemorrhages + exudates in hypertension and DM (p440).

Causes of disc swelling
• Papilloedema
• Malignant hypertension (p132 *OHCM*)
• Cavernous sinus thrombosis
• Optic neuritis
• Cranial space-occupying lesion (SOL)
• Optic neuropathy
• Central vein occlusion
• Opaque myelinated nerve fibres (fig 5.49)
• Disorders of the nerve sheath (fig 5.50)

Papilloedema (fig 5.47) is swelling of the optic disc caused by raised intracranial pressure (ICP);[34] always bilateral, but not neccessarily symmetrical. ▶Papilloedema should be your main differential for optic disc swelling until proven otherwise. *Presentation* is usually due to symptoms of raised ICP. Nausea/vomiting. Headaches worse in the mornings, centred in the frontal region, and are aggravated by bending down? CN XI palsy. Transient visual obscurations (late stages have reduced peripheral vision). *Investigations:* An intracranial SOL must be ruled out; MRI with gadolinium contrast is gold standard, but CT head is often quicker to obtain. Measure the BP; any hypertensive changes or haemorrhages? Any signs of CRVO? (p435). In young obese women, think of idiopathic intra-cranial hypertension (p502 *OHCM*). If neuro-imaging is normal (= no risk of coning) then do a lumbar puncture to establish opening pressures and facilitate CSF analysis.[111]

Pseudopapilloedema (see fig 5.48) may mimic papilloedema; the disc margins are blurred and the disc appears elevated. Usually benign and associated with hypermetropia ± astigmatism or tilted discs. Its cup may be absent but there is no true oedema and veins are of normal size and pulsate (transmitted from a nearby artery). It is usually bilateral and symmetrical and does not change over time. Treat as papilleodema until otherwise proven; fluorescence angiography (FA) and US can distinguish it from disease states.

Diabetic papillopathy is rare but can affect both type 1 and 2 DM irrespective of glycaemic control. Presents with progressive mild visual impairment and optic disc swelling ± features of diabetic retinopathy. 30% of patients develop non-arteritic ischaemic optic neuropathy.[112]

Optic nerve head drusen (fig 5.51) (see p441) are multiple hyaline bodies extending beyond the disc margins. Abnormal branching of the retinal vessels is often present. The nerve head is usually small (bilateral 'crowded disc'). If the hyaline material is buried in the disc substance, diagnosis is confusing, especially if a field defect is also present. *NB:* optic atrophy in the contralateral eye is the Foster-Kennedy syndrome (eg from meningioma of the optic canal (fig 5.50) in the eye with optic atrophy; in practice, the usual cause is consequential ischaemic optic neuropathy).[113]

Nystagmus suggests a lesion in the posterior fossa; *Sixth nerve palsy* may be a false localizing sign.

---

34 Causes of raised ICP: intracranial mass, increased CSF production/decreased CSF resorption, head injury, idiopathic intracranial hypertension, status epilepticus. See p840 *OHCM*.

Is the optic disc swollen?

Fig 5.46 The normal optic disc has a pink neuroretinal outside with a central pale depression called the optic cup (see p445 for cupping). The neuroretinal rim should be well defined and pink; if it looks pale then consider optic atrophy, if the border looks fuzzy then the disc may be swollen.

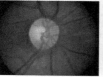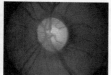

Image reprinted with permission from Medscape Drugs & Diseases (http://emedicine.medscape.com/), 2015, available at: http://emedicine.medscape.com/article/1217760-overview.

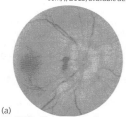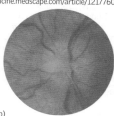

(a)   (b)

Fig 5.47 Papilloedema: the discs are swollen forwards and also outwards into the surrounding retina. Disc margins are hidden and in places retinal vessels are concealed, because oedema has impaired the translucency of the disc tissues. (a) The retinal veins are congested and there are a few haemorrhages at 9 o'clock. ►Whenever you see these appearances, get help.

We thank Mr J F Cullen FRCS for permission to use the image.

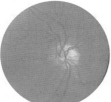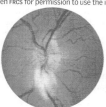

Fig 5.48 Pseudopapilloedema.
Reproduced from *Brain's Diseases of the Nervous System*, OUP.

Fig 5.49 Nerve fibres mimicking papilloedema.
We thank Mr J F Cullen FRCS for permission to use the image.

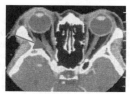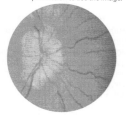

Fig 5.50 Meningioma of left optic nerve sheath.
We thank Mr J F Cullen FRCS for permission to use the image.

Fig 5.51 Optic drusen.
We thank Mr J F Cullen FRCS for permission to use the image.

Further reading

Ong HS *et al.* (2014). Acute visual loss in papilloedema: the diagnostic pitfalls. *Int Ophthalmol* 34(3):607–12. [2 interesting case reports.]

Optic-disc.org: www.optic-disc.org

Ophthalmology

The eye does not retain drops for as long as ointments and 2-hourly applications may be needed. Eye ointments are well suited for use at night. Allow 5min between doses of drops to prevent overspill. All eye preparations have warnings not to use for more than 1 month. Always consider the manual dexterity of your patients—the elderly may struggle to accurately apply topical medication (eye dropper applicators/applicators are available—speak to a pharmacist).

Common topical eye drops used in ophthalmology

Antibiotics: Chloramphenicol, fusidic acid, neomycin.

Mydriatics: (=Cycloplegics.) They dilate the pupil. They also cause cycloplegia (paralysis of ciliary muscles), hence blurred vision. ►Warn the patient not to drive. 0.5% or 1% tropcamide is used to dilate the eye before the examination and lasts 3 hours. These drugs may be used to prevent synechiae formation in anterior uveitis. *Dispelling myths* Mydriatics are typically avoided in over-60s with shallow anterior chambers (especially if a family history of glaucoma) for fear of triggering an acute glaucoma attack. See the 'Golden Eye Rules' on p415. The risk of precipitating an attack is low, the risk of missing pathology because you haven't looked is high.

Miotics: These constrict the pupil and increase drainage of aqueous. They are used in the treatment of acute glaucoma (p430).

Local anaesthetics: Tetracaine 0.5% drops are commonly used to allow examination of a painful eye when blepharospasm is an issue. An eye pad applied to the healthy side helps prevent tender consensual eye movements. Oral analgesia also helps.

Steroids and NSAID drops: they are used with care in ophthalmic inflammation and under ophthalmologist guidance for treatment in allergy, episcleritis, scleritis, or iritis. ►Care is needed when using these drops as they increase the IOP precipitating glaucoma or inducing catastrophic progression of dendritic ulcers (see p433). Ophthalmoscopy may miss dendritic ulcers, and slit lamp inspection is essential if steroid drops are being considered. Newer drops have less effect on IOP (eg **rimexolone**, comparable to **fluorometholone** and less than **dexamethasone** & **prednisolone** acetate). NSAID drops, eg **ketorolac**, may obviate the need for some steroid drops.

Systemic drugs that cause ophthalmological issues

Dry eyes: β-blockers, anticholinergics, any eye drop (can affect the tear film).

Corneal deposits: amiodarone, chloroquine, chlorpromazine.

Lens opacities: steroids (including high-dose inhaled).

Glaucoma: steroid drops, mydriatics, & anticholinergics (tricyclics and some parkinson's drugs).

Pailloedema: tetrecyclines, steroids, oral contraceptive pill.

Retinopathy: The following drugs are culprits if used chronically. *Vigabatrin*. *Ethambutol:* Warn patients to report *any* visual side-effects (loss of acuity, colour blindness). ~10% report new visual problems, and in 10% of these the cause is optic neuropathy (which may be irreversible).[35] *Isoniazid:* ↓Red-green perception; pyridoxine co-administration prevents this. *Chloroquine (cq)/hydroxychloroquine (HCQ)* can cause (untreatable) retinopathy if high doses are used. Risk of toxicity increases sharply towards 1% after 6yrs of use, or a cumulative dose of 1000g of HCQ. Risk increases with continued use. *Screening schedule:* Baseline exam on starting (maculopathy would be a contraindication). Start annual screening 5yrs (or sooner if there are unusual risk factors). Newer objective tests, such as multifocal electroretinogram, spectral domain optical coherence tomography, and fundus autofluorescence, can be more sensitive than visual fields (which remain useful).[114]

Eyedrops as a cause of systemic symptoms

Drugs applied to the eye may be absorbed through the cornea and produce systemic side effects—eg bronchospasm or bradycardia in susceptible individuals using antiglaucoma β-blocking drops, eg **timolol**, **carteolol**, **betaxolol**—which are cardioselective. ►Symptoms may be subtle and insidious—eg gradually decreasing exercise tolerance, or falls from arrhythmias. Serious problems are more likely if there is co-morbidity (eg respiratory infection).

Other anti-glaucoma drops (p440) cause headaches, and a bitter taste in the mouth; urolithiasis is reported with **dorzolamide**.

Pilocarpine may cause parasympathetic sweating. Accommodation spasm may lead to brow-ache (worse if <40 years old, or just starting treatment). Other SE: 'flu-like syndrome, sweating, urinary frequency; more rarely: urinary urgency, D&V (or constipation ±flatulence), dyspepsia, flushes, BP↑, palpitations, rhinitis, dizziness, lacrimation, conjunctivitis, visual disturbances, ocular pain, rash, pruritus.

Even highly selective α_2-receptor agonists used in glaucoma, eg **brimonidine**, can cause effects such as dry mouth (in 33% of patients), headache, hypertension, fatigue, and drowsiness.

Steroid eye drops

Be careful when initiating steroid eye drops (p458); they can be used for allergic eye disease but are associated with increasing ocular pressure (risky in glaucoma patients) and cataract formation. Steroids can potentially prolong the course of viral conjuctivitis by increasing the latency of adenovirus. ►There are disasterous consequences if a corneal ulcer is missed as steroids can propagate the ulcer causing corneal melt and blindness.

Contact lenses: Hygiene and wear tips See also p463

►Pay attention to contact lens containers, as well as lenses.

Can I reuse my daily disposable contact lenses (DDCL)? No! Overnight storage in blister-pack saline results in contaminated lenses and infections (esp. staphs and esp. in men). We *must* educate patients in correct use of DDCL.

►Do not assume that because a person uses disposable lenses there can be no nasty acanthamoebae infections. These free-living protozoa (found in soil and water, including bathroom tap water) may cause devastating keratitis even with disposable lenses.

• Scrub container's inside with cotton wool bud moistened with lens fluid.
• Disinfect the container with hot water (≥80°c); leave to dry in open air.
• Wash your hands before handling the contact lens container.
• Replace the container at least every year.
• Protozoa may survive new '1-step' solutions of 3% hydrogen peroxide. Amoebae are difficult to treat, and there is current interest in salicylate's potential to reduce microbial attachment when used in contact lens care solutions.[115]
• Follow instructions about getting used to extended wear. Most corneal ulcers from contact lenses are in people who are not used to extended wear and sleep overnight with their contact lenses in, or napped with them on a plane, or elsewhere for as little as 2-3 hours.
• Losing the lens within the eye. Hard lenses may be lost in any fornix, soft lenses are usually in upper outer fornix.
• Corneal abrasion is common early while adjusting to wear. Pain ± lacrimation occurs some hours after removing the lens.

---

35 Ethambutol eye problems: ↓acuity (65%), ↓ visual fields (65%), abnormal colour vision (61%), optic disc pallor (38%), ↑latency on visual evoked potential (65%). ~30% showed improved vision on stopping ethambutol in one Korean study; latency for recovery: 5.4±1.7 months. No one with optic disc pallor at the time of diagnosis of optic neuropathy showed visual function improvement.[116]

Xerophthalmia is dry eyes secondary to deficient tear production. If left untreated can progress to **keratomalacia** where the cornea softens, thins, and eventually ulcerates. Blindness can occur. These indicate lack of vitamin A. Peak incidence: 2-5yrs; 40 million children worldwide. *Signs:* Night blindness (nyctalopia), tunnel vision, poor acuity, and dry conjunctivae (xerosis). The cornea is unwettable and loses transparency. Small foamy plaques (fig 5.52) occur, raised from interpalpebral conjunctiva. Vitamin A reverses these changes. *Tests:* Visual fields; dark-adapted electroretinography, plasma vitamin A↓*R:* Just hand out the vitamins? It's not so simple. ☼Every Bitôt spot is a stain on the soul of politics, and as each represents a failure of education and aid, we are all implicated. Examine the cultural web that led to the deficiency, and try to take *whatever* steps are needed to correct it. Improve diet & address associated causes: alcoholism, nutrition, poverty.

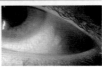

Fig 5.52 Bitôt spot.
Read a case study here: http://www.nejm.org/doi/full/10.1056/NEJMicm1205309

From The *New England Journal of Medicine*, Giulio Ferrari, Maurizia Viganó, Bitot's Spot in Vitamin A Deficiency, Volume 368, © (2013) Massachusetts Medical Society. Reprinted with permission from Massachusetts Medical Society.

Trachoma Caused by *Chlamydia trachomatis* (serotypes A, B, or C). It is spread mainly by flies, where it is hot, dry, and dusty and the people are poor, living near cattle. The most common infectious cause of blindness (onchocerciasis is the 2nd, see p443), 229 million people live in endemic areas, 1.2 million are irreversibly blind.[117] It causes scarring on the inner eye lids which directly damages the cornea, and in later stages the eye lid is distorted causing entropion; eyelashes scratch the cornea, which ulcerates. *Management:* The who have developed the SAFE strategy (Surgical, Antibiotics, Facial cleanliness, Enviromental improvement) and are aiming to eradicate trachoma by 2020. Antibiotics: PO azithromycin (20mg/kg stat) and tetracycline 1% eye ointment 12-hrly for 5 days each month for 6 months. In active disease use 8-hrly for 6 weeks + **tetracycline** 250mg/6h PO for 14 days. Initiate mass anti-trachoma in communities where prevelance of follicular trachoma is >10%, there is no point in just treating individuals as reinfection between family members is high. Azithromycin is especially useful as clinics can observe the ingestion of a stat dose, ensuring compliance with eye drops is not as easy. Facial cleanliness and improved sanitation ↓ transmission. *Lid surgery* can ↓ progression of corneal scarring and entropion. The who train local health workers to perform bilamellar tarsal rotation operations.

Onchocerciasis (river blindness) (OHCM p443.) This is caused by nematode microfilariae (*Onchocerca volvulus*), transmitted by black flies of the *Simulium* species. Of the 20-50 million people affected, 99% live in Africa. It may cause blindness in 40% of some populations. Unless the eye is affected, problems are mostly in the skin. Fly bites result in nodules from which microfilariae are released, to invade conjunctiva, cornea, ciliary body, and iris (rarely retina or optic nerve, fig 5.53). Sometimes they may be seen swimming in the aqueous or dying in the anterior chamber. Microfilariae initially excite inflammation; fibrosis then occurs around them; if in the cornea, corneal opacities (nummular keratitis) occurs. Chronic iritis causes synechiae ± cataracts and a fixed pupil. *R:* See BOX, p461 for the Mectizan Donation Program. **Ivermectin** is the chief microfilaricide but has no effect on adult worms. Give ~150mcg/kg PO stat every 6-12 months for 10–15 years, until adult worms die. Give a 3-day course of steroids prior to ivermectin in severe eye involvement. Macrofilariae are adults living in lymphatics. Macrofilaricides: **doxycycline** 200mg/day for 4wks when combined with ivermectin has promising results but doxycyline is a daily dose and compliance is an issue.[118] Recent reports have started to question the rise of resistance to ivermectin.[119]

As you learn about ophthalmology in the developing world, you may skip over this section since tropical eye disease seems so far fetched from your daily clinical encounters. Your tropical repertoire will most likely be limited to HIV, TB, and malaria as these are the disease processes which have crept into the Western world. However, ignorance of tropical diseases is not restricted to medical students, in 2005 the WHO identifed a list of NTDs which principally impacted the poorest populations and caused significant morbidity and mortality; in sub-saharan Africa the disease burden may be comparable to TB and malaria in addition to making HIV infection more dangerous![120] The economic and health impact of ignoring these diseases is huge. These are often debilitating, chronic disease processes with associated stigma (eg leprosy). They are of particular importance in ophthalmology, since four key NTDs affect the eyes; Chagas disease, cysticercosis, onchocerisasis, and trachoma; improving education and school attendance is impossible if students and workers are going blind.... Research funding and treatment has been overshadowed by the international focus on the big three named above, it simply wasn't financially viable for pharmacy companies to invest in long trials for medication unlikely to generate financial gain. In recent years, awareness has risen and schemes set in place to encourage treatment for the five NTDs where mass drug administration is possible (trachoma, onchocerciasis, lymphatic filariasis (p443 *OHCM*), soil-transmitted helminths and schistosomiasis), although drug resistance may be becoming a problem. Many of the drugs can be given together, as stat doses, which makes distribution more efficient. Combine praziquantel, ivermectin and albendazole to treat schistosomiasis, onchocerciasis, and soil-transmitted helminths respectively. Delivery of drugs to a rural community is challenging, not only is infrastructure and funding lacking, but locals may be mistrusting of 'free drugs' and there are significant compliance issues. The leading example of mass drug administration is for onchocerciasis; in 1987 Merck started a remarkable donation programme of ivermectin with a view to eradicate this disease (Mectizan Donation Program[121]). This unprecedented move by a pharmaceutical company has revealed how successful simple targeted treatments can be.

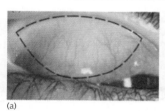
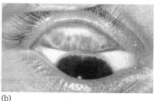

(a)   (b)

Fig 5.53 Trachoma: (a) dots outline the area to be examined; (b) follicular trachomatous inflammation causes intense inflammation and trachomatous scars (white bands or sheets in the tarsal conjunctiva).

Reproduced from the *Oxford Textbook of Medicine*, with permission from OUP.

Further reading

Utzinger J *et al.* (2012). Neglected tropical diseases: diagnosis, clinical management, treatment and control. *Swiss Med Wkly* 142:w13727

World Health Organization: www.who.int

Ophthalmology

Allergic eye disease affects ~20% of the population and incidence is increasing. Peak age of onset is 20 years.[122] Acute allergic conjunctivitis is caused by an IgE-mediated type 1 hypersensitivity, triggering release of inflammatory mediators by mast cells. Most have a history or family history of atopy.

Chronic allergic disorders are characterized by an increase in the number of the local conjunctival T-cell population with a mixed cellular infiltrate of mast cells, eosinophils, neutrophils, and macrophages.

Seasonal allergic conjunctivitis (SAC) Up to 50% of allergic eye disease. Symptoms are seasonal and mild—but may continue long after allergen exposure. Examination shows small papillae on the tarsal conjunctiva. It is self-limiting and not sight-threatening. ℞: Antihistamine drops, eg **ketotifen**, azelastine, epinastine, emedastine, or **olopatadine**. 2nd line: diclofenac 0.1% drops. Mast cell stabilizers (eg nedocromil) may be used prophylactically.[123]

Perennial allergic conjunctivitis (PAC) Symptoms are mild and may persist all year with seasonal exacerbations. Small papillae are found on the tarsal conjunctiva. *Management: Prescription drops:* **olopatadine** (antihistamine and mast cell stabilizer), **lodoxamide**, or **nedocromil** (mast cell stabilizer). *Over-the-counter drops:* sodium cromoglicate 2% (/6h).

Vernal keratoconjunctivitis (VKC)[36] comprises only 0.5% of allergic eye disease. The typical patient is an atopic boy living in a warm, dry climate with severe bilateral symptoms in spring (itchy eyes, foreign body sensation, photophobia) and giant cobble-stone papillae under the upper eye lid (fig **5.28** on p434). Lid skin is spared, unlike AKC (see below). ℞: Start with drops, eg **olopatadine** or **lodoxamide** (BOX). If uncontrolled or if corneal disease develops, steroid drops are needed (eg 1% prednisolone acetate/2h; taper rapidly). Ciclosporin drops (1-2%) also help.[124] Corneal involvement needs careful eye clinic review and coverage with steroids, antibiotic drops, and lid hygiene to limit staphylococcal colonization. If severe blepharitis, oral **erythromycin** or **doxycycline** (in adults) can help. Topical lubricants also help soothe eyes and washout allergens.[125]

Atopic keratoconjunctivitis (AKC) affects 1.5% of the population. Symptoms are severe with pain, redness, and reduced vision. Associated with atopic dermatitis. Signs include conjunctival papillae and eventual conjunctival scarring which can lead to corneal opacification and neovascularization.

Giant papillary conjunctivitis (fig **5.28** on p434) Giant papillae on the tarsal conjunctiva is an iatrogenic condition related to foreign bodies, eg contact lenses, ocular prosthesis and sutures. *Management:* Involves removal of the foreign body and treatment with topical mast cell stabilizers or steroids.

Differential diagnoses Dry eyes, blepharitis, any causes of red eye (p430).

3 principles for successfully managing allergic eye disorders

1 Remove the allergen responsible where possible ('don't travel to places which make your symptoms worse').[126]
2 General measures: •Cold compresses •Artificial tears to wash out allergens and ↓itch •Oral antihistamines for symptom relief, eg **loratadine** 10mg/d PO •Nasal steroid sprays may help even if no nasal symptoms.[127]
3 Eye-drop specifics (rapid action + fewer SEs , being topical)—eg antihistamines (eg **azelastine**), drugs inhibiting mast cell degranulation (**cromoglicate**; **lodoxamide**), and accessory drugs, eg steroids (eg **dexamethasone**; beware inducing glaucoma), ± NSAIDs (eg diclofenac), immunosuppressants (**ciclosporin**, specialist use only), and vasoconstrictors (eg **xylometazoline**—not very effective, may cause rebound hyperaemia).

36 AKC and VKC are severe forms of bilateral allergic inflammation. Both affect the ocular surface and are potentially sight-threatening if not treated appropriately. Although both are chronic, VKC tends to be seasonal at first.

Leonardo da Vinci first outlined the principle behind contact lenses in his 1508 'Codex of the eye' where he explained a method of directly altering corneal power by either submerging the head in a bowl of water, or wearing a water-filled glass hemisphere over the eye.[128] However it was not until 1888 that Adolf G. Fick fitted the first successful contact lens.

Functions of a contact lens (See p459 for hygiene and wear tips)

- *Corrective vision*: More commonly used to correct refractive error (spherical lens), they also have a role in correction of astigmatism.
- *Correcting colour vision*: Some studies have been carried out on colour-blind patients using a red tinted lense. Whilst it doesn't completely correct their colour perception, it does slighty improve it.[129]
- *Purely cosmetic:* 80% of contact lenses are worn for cosmetic reasons. Only 20% are worn because lenses are better for the eye condition than spectacles. Among this 20% a minority wear the lenses to hide disfiguring inoperable eye conditions, a greater proportion have them for very high refractive errors.
- *Orthokeratology:* An old technique which appears to be making a come back. It uses gas-permeable contact lenses at night which reshape the cornea so that when the patient wakes up, they don't have to correct their refractive error during the day as the corneal surface has been remoulded. This occurs because the cornea is involved in 60% of the refractive process. Its effects are short lived, averaging 72 hours, therefore they would have to be worn every couple of nights.
- *Therapeutic:* Contact lenses are often used as bandages post cataract surgery or increasingly being considered as vehicles to deliver directed ocular treatment, eg stem cell thereapy. Contact lenses are commonly used in the early stages in the treatment of keratoconus.

Indications Myopia above −12 dioptres and hypermetropia above +10 dioptres because equivalent spectacles produce quite distorted visual fields.

Types of lens Hard lenses are 8.5–9mm in diameter and are made of polymethylmethacrylate (PMMA). Gas-permeable hard lenses are larger and allow gas to permeate through to the underlying cornea. They can only cope with a limited degree of astigmatism and do not wet as well as standard hard lenses, so may mist up in the day. Soft disposable lenses can be worn during the day for up to 4 weeks. Disposable contact lenses are now more common due to the lower risk of ocular infections.

Complications *CLARE:* Contact Lens-Induced Red Eye reaction typically presents as an acute inflammatory response of the anterior segment of the eye defined by severe conjunctival and circumlimbal hyperaemia. It is very common to see both diffuse and focal subepithelial infiltrates.[130] *Keratoconjunctivitis* or *giant papillary* change in the upper tarsal conjunctiva, possibly due to sensitization to the cleansing materials used, or to the mucus which forms on the lens. *Sensitivities:* Cleaning solutions made by different manufacturers should not be mixed. The storage solution should be washed off before the lens is inserted. Soft contact lenses, being permeable, tend to absorb chemicals, so weaker cleaning agents are used. Sensitivity to cleaning agents usually presents as redness, stinging, ↑lens movement, ↑mucus production, and thickened lids. It may be necessary to stop wearing lenses for several months. *Infection*: It is always imperative that when taking an eye history, you ascertain if the patient wears contact lenses as infective organisms such as *Pseudomonas aeruginosa* must be investigated for and treated with ofloxacin when suspected.

Further reading

Miraldi Utz V *et al.* (2014). Allergic eye disease. *Pediatr Clin North Am* 61(3):607-20.

Saban DR *et al.* (2013). New twists to an old story: novel concepts in the pathogenesis of allergic eye disease. *Curr Eye Res* 38(3):317-30.

Ophthalmology

Refractive procedures are increasingly undertaken as an alternative to wearing spectacles; mostly for cosmetic reasons. Occasionally they are undertaken for anisometropia (imbalance of prescriptions); for astigmatism after surgery; or for intolerance of spectacles or contact lenses. A variation of PRK (photorefractive keratotomy) may be undertaken for some corneal diseases. LASIK (see below) is now the most common procedure. It is well researched and in terms of surgical procedures is extremely safe but there are possible complications. It should be noted that most ophthalmologists wear spectacles!

Photorefractive keratotomy (PRK) This is an entirely laser treatment where the curved front of the cornea is altered by laser ablation. It is only done for low degrees of myopia and is less predictable than LASIK with some people having under-correction and others over-correction. Corneal haze with reduced vision, glare, and haloes are occasional problems. In most low myopes it gives good outcome but it is very painful for a few days.

LASIK (laser-assisted *in situ* keratomileusis) This is a combination of minor surgery where the cornea is incised and an extremely thin trapdoor-shaped flap hinged away and then excimer laser is applied to the bare corneal stroma underneath. Thereafter the flap is pushed back into position and adheres naturally. It is, surprisingly, virtually painless, settles very quickly, and is fairly predictable in its outcome. Corneal sensitivity recovers after ~6 months. A thin flap with a nasally placed hinge is associated with the most rapid recovery of corneal sensitivity.[131] It is possible to undertake surgery on much greater degrees of refractive error; with up to 5 dioptres of hypermetropia; 5 dioptres of astigmatism; and 15 dioptres of myopia (if >15, risk ↑↑).[132] Serious complications are rare but trauma to or infection of the flap may result in permanent corneal scarring. In one series of 779 eyes, no serious, vision-threatening, irreversible complication such as keratectasia or progressive endothelial cell loss was observed (follow-up: 5yrs). Warn that improved acuity tends to wane over time,[133] and also that the operation will not affect stiffening of the lens which occurs with age and that glasses will likely be required for the resulting presbyopia. Intraocular pressure often falls (eg by 4mmHg). Note that LASIK tourism to find cheap surgery abroad is associated with problems such as corneal ectasia, flap problems, keratitis, and under- and over-correction.[134]

LASEK (laser epithelial keratomileusis) This is different from LASIK in that the corneal epithelium is softened with an alcohol solution and lifted off. Laser is then used to reshape the cornea and the epithelium is carefully replaced.

Lens surgery Altering refraction by clear lens extraction with intraocular lens implantation with the appropriate corrective power is another option. Accommodation is lost, so reading needs correction. Another option is an intraocular lens implanted in front of the human lens (phakic implant).

Other procedures Uncommon. They include insertion of perspex rings into the cornea; other laser techniques to alter corneal curvature; and surgery to the sclera to attempt to correct presbyopia. They are much less certain in outcome and are best regarded as experimental.

Further reading

The bionic eye: A Review. Clinical & Experimental Ophthalmology. 2011.

NICE Guidelines. Photorefractive (laser) surgery for the correction of refractive errors. 2006

Google smart lens Google and Novartis are currently working together on developing a contact lens which can accurately measure glucose levels at all times from the tear film, potentially changing how we treat certain chronic disease in the future.[135]

The bionic eye The bionic eye has historically been considered a futuristic accessory restricted to the realms of science fiction; however, over the past years significant advances have been made towards making the restoration of vision a clinical reality. These devices target various components of the visual pathway (see p429); specifically the cortex, subcortex, optic nerve, and retina. The earliest studies looked at cortical stimulation but to date it is stimulation of the retina which has become the most advanced with multiple ongoing trials. Retinal devices are especially beneficial for degenerative retinal diseases such as retinitis pigmentosa (p448), for which there is no current cure. It does nothing for those lacking optic nerve function such as glaucoma (a major cause of international blindness, see p442). The *Argus II®* is currently the most advanced prosthesis (fig 5.54). It is approved for adults with profound retinitis pigmentosa who have previously had some useful vision but currently have bare light or no light perception in both eyes. The device consists of a small video camera which is mounted on a pair of glasses worn by the patient. A small computer (often attached to the patient's belt) then processes these images and sends the information back to the glasses via a cable. The information is then transmitted wirelessly from the glasses to a pre-inserted retinal implant which stimulate the retina's remaining cells to create perceptions of light. Watch the videos of the experimental outcomes here: www.2-sight.com and www.youtube.com/watch?v=Bi_HpbFKnSw. Learning to interpret the patterns of light with the retinal implant takes time and currently technology enables patients to simply gain an appreciation of light flashes to detect motion. The visual outcomes so far are basic but we are taking exciting steps forward.[136,137]

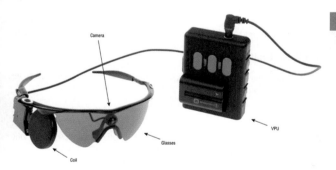

Fig 5.54 The Argus II® system.

Relevant pages elsewhere ►*Every page in all chapters and OHCM.* This is why the above contents list is oddly starved of nice meaty clinical topics.

We would like to thank Dr Chantal Simon, our Specialist Reader and author of the Oxford Handbook of General Practice *for her invaluable advice on developing this chapter. We are grateful for permission to use of some of the content (as acknowledged) from the* OHGP. *Thanks also to Cadamban Shanmugasundram, our Junior Reader.*

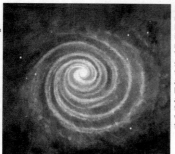

Fig 6.1 GPs may feel the weight of the universe as they navigate the seemingly infinite workload and resist collapsing into a black hole. However, the spiral shape of our own galaxy, the Milky Way, and the spiral symbol used at the start of each chapter is a reminder to think about opportunities for holistic and integrative care on an individual level; to pick up cues as to what is really important to our patients, and to try and make a real difference to their well-being, mental health, and social functioning.

An introduction to general practice

General practice is often the first point of access to healthcare services and in the UK it forms the cornerstone of primary care. Over 90% of the UK population are registered with a GP. A GP is defined by the Royal College of General Practitioners (RCGP) as *'personal doctors, primarily responsible for the provision of comprehensive and continuing generalist care to every individual seeking medical care irrespective of age, sex and state of health.'*[1] GPs are generalists who diagnose and treat illness within the community, promote better health, prevent disease, certify disease, monitor and treat chronic disease, and refer patients requiring specialist services.

Medical generalism *'Generalism describes a philosophy of practice which is person, not disease, centred; continuous, not episodic; integrates biotechnical and biographical perspectives; and views health as a resource for living and not an end in itself.'*[2] It is an approach to the delivery of healthcare that applies a broad and holistic perspective to the patient's problems and involves:
• Seeing the person as a whole and in the context of their family and wider social environment.
• Using this perspective as part of the clinical method and therapeutic approach to all clinical encounters.
• Being able to deal with undifferentiated illness and the widest range of patients and conditions.
• In the context of general practice, taking continuity of responsibility for people's care across many disease episodes and over many years.
• Coordinating care across organizations both within and between health and social care.

Scope of general practice Patients have an average 8.2 consultations with their GP every year in the UK, yet only 1 in 20 consultations results in a referral to secondary care. Everything else is dealt with within the primary care setting. To do this, GPs must:
• Have a working knowledge of the whole breadth of medicine.
• Maintain on-going relationships with their patients—they are the only doctors to remain with their patients through sickness and health.
• Focus on patients' response to illness, rather than the illness itself—taking into account personality, family patterns, and the effect of these on the presentation of symptoms.
• Be interested in ecology of health and illness within communities and in the cultural determinants of health beliefs.
• Be able to draw on a far wider range of resources than are taught in medical school, including intuition, knowledge of medicine, communication skills, business skills, and humanity.

General practice is the most efficient and cost-effective way of providing patient care. Over 90% of patient contacts in the NHS are dealt with in general practice, which operates on 8.39% of the total NHS budget. The main roles performed by GPs (outlined in a King's Fund report) include: [3]

- *Consultations:* To manage pre-existing conditions or make an effective diagnosis of a new problem. Consultations may lead to a combination of advice, a prescription, treatment, or referral to a specialist. The cost of a GP consultation in the UK is ~£13. The average cost of an ED attendance is £108. [4]
- *Prescriptions:* The NHS spends >£10 billion on prescription drugs each year. The vast majority of these are prescribed by GPs.
- *Treatments:* GPs provide advice and treatment for many illnesses and may also perform minor surgery, soft-tissue and joint injections.
- *Referrals:* GPs are seen as gatekeepers to other NHS services. Patients are usually referred to specialists only after seeing a GP, which helps ensure cost-effective care.
- *Screening and immunization:* Most practices run screening programmes (eg to detect cervical cancer) and undertake immunization for both adults and children.
- *Management of long-term conditions:* GPs manage patients with long-term chronic illnesses such as asthma or diabetes.
- *Health promotion:* GPs provide information to promote health and allow patients to understand their illness and enable self-care.

In addition to the day-to-day medical care of their patients, GPs have a number of additional roles.

- *Navigating:* GPs work with patients and carers to guide them effectively and safely through the health care system.
- *Service redesign and improvement:* GPs manage service provision within their own practices, and are involved in commissioning services for their community.
- *Research:* GPs need critical appraisal skills to understand and apply relevant evidence to inform clinical decision-making, and must collaborate effectively in primary-care based research.
- *Education:* GPs can be effective teachers in a wide range of contexts—educating patients, practice staff, medical students and junior doctors, fellow GPs, and the general public.
- *Leadership:* The majority of GPs have leadership roles.

Differences between GPs and specialists

The increasing sophistication, complexity and sub-specialization of hospital-based medicine also highlights the need for high-quality generalists, who deal with undifferentiated problems and 'illness'. Research by Marinker (see TABLE) encapsulates neatly the contrast in roles between GPs and specialists.

GPs	Specialists
Exclude the presence of serious disease	Confirm the presence of serious disease
Tolerate uncertainty—managing patients with undifferentiated symptoms	Reduce uncertainty—investigating until a diagnosis is reached
Explore probability of seeing patients from a population with a relatively low incidence of serious disease	Explore possibility seeing a pre-selected population of patients with a relatively high incidence of serious disease
Marginalize danger—recognizing and acting on danger signs even when a diagnosis is not certain	Marginalize error—ensuring accurate diagnosis and treatment

The material on this page has been adapted from the *Oxford Handbook of General Practice* 4th edition by Simon *et al*, and has been reproduced by permission of Oxford University Press.

Primary care

The term *primary care* is used (in the UK and North America) to describe primary medical care to individuals (eg family/general practice). *Primary health care* is a broader term which describes an approach to health policy and services.

The World Health Organization's (WHO) *Alma Ata* declaration[5] (below) describes an ideal model of primary health care and was adopted at the International Conference on Primary Health Care held in Alma Ata, Kazakhstan in 1978.

Primary health care should '*be made universally accessible to individuals and families in the community, by means acceptable to them, through their full participation, and at the cost that the community and country can afford to maintain in the spirit of self-reliance...[and] addresses the main health problems in the community, providing promotive, preventative, curative and rehabilitative services accordingly*'.

There is huge inequality in access to, and provision of health care services between and within countries, as well as vast differences in the health status of individuals. How can these issues be addressed? Is it possible to provide primary health care for all?

The ultimate goal of primary health care is better health for all. Outlined below are some of the basic principles identified in the Alma Ata Declaration, which should be incorporated into national policies in order to help develop and sustain primary health care as part of a comprehensive health system:[6]

- *Accessibility (equitable distribution of health care):* Health services must be provided equally to all people irrespective of economic status, race, or location. This concept helps shift accessibility of services from cities to rural areas.
- *Community participation:* Meaningful involvement of the community in planning and maintaining their health services. This grass-roots approach allows sustainability due to local ownership.
- *Health promotion:* Developing skills and understanding of health education, immunization, nutrition, sanitation, maternal and child health, and prevention/control of endemic diseases.
- *Use of appropriate technology:* Use of technology that is cost-effective and feasible, eg refrigerators for vaccine cold storage.
- *A 'multi-sectional approach':* Recognition that health cannot be improved by intervention within just the health sector and that other sectors are equally important, including: agriculture (eg food security); education; communication; housing; access to safe water and basic sanitation.

Critics argue that the declaration is too broad, does not have clear targets, and is generally not attainable, yet the approach has seen significant health gains in some of the world's poorest and politically unstable communities.

Targeted, selective, and cost-effective approaches have also been shown to save lives, such as UNICEF's GOBI–FFF program: Growth monitoring; Oral rehydration therapy for diarrhoea; Breast-feeding; Immunizations; Family planning; Female education; and Food Supplementation.

Primary health care strategy Analysis of the health care systems of 11 Westernized countries by The Commonwealth Fund[7] found the UK ranks first overall and scores highest in 9 of the 12 areas measured, including quality, access, and efficiency. The UK also spends the second lowest per head on health care—half the amount of the USA, which as the most expensive in the world consistently under-performs relative to other countries (most notably in its absence of universal health insurance coverage).

Research by Starfield shows that a good primary care system underpins a good health care system. Health systems that are orientated towards primary care are associated with better health for the population, lower costs of care, higher satisfaction of the population with its health services, and lower medication use. Specific features of the health care system that help to achieve this are universal access to services, equitable distribution of resources across a population, a high percentage of physicians who are primary care physicians (and who have earnings equitable to specialists) and a system that attempts to achieve a higher level of performance (through first-contact, comprehensive, co-ordinated, family-centred care).[8]

First contact Primary care is the 1st contact with health services. This is not just a routine appointment with a GP, but encompasses a wide spectrum of services: 1 *General practice* 2 *Out-of-hours GP* 3 *Phone advice* (NHS 111) 4 *Walk-in centres* 5 *ED* 6 *Pharmacies*.

The cornerstone of primary care is the responsibility that individuals and families have for their own physical and mental well-being. ►*75% of health problems are taken care of outside formal health systems*. Only 25% of patients who experience symptoms cross the threshold to consult a GP and of those, only 5% are subsequently referred to hospital. Unless individuals and families act on their own initiative to promote their health, no amount of medical care is going to make them healthy. In assessing how good a community is at primary health care, one needs to look not just at medical care, but also at social, political, and cultural aspects.

GPs with extended roles (GPwER) *(previously GPs with special interests—GPwSI)* GPs can develop special interests to enhance their skills and improve management of workload between primary and secondary care (by reducing and enhancing referrals to consultants). The GPwSI framework was originally designed to run outside GP practices but newer models allow GPs to offer extended roles within their day job (hence the change of name). Typical roles are in diabetes, dermatology, cardiology, women's health, and palliative medicine. They deliver a service beyond that of the GP, eg in requesting specialist investigations, starting treatment, or undertaking advanced procedures. Although GPwERs reduce waiting times, the chief issue for patients is not the wait to see a specialist but the thoroughness of the consultation and the expertise of the clinician.

Intermediate care This type of care lies between traditional primary care and secondary care. It integrates facilities from many areas to address complex health needs which do not require use of hospital services. There is a trend for more secondary care services to transfer to the community. Examples include pre-admission assessment units; early and supported discharge schemes; community (cottage) hospitals; domiciliary stroke units; hospital-at-home schemes (eg providing dialysis or parenteral nutrition); rehabilitation units. It is one of the mechanisms by which health and social services mesh to allow patients to receive the most appropriate care. Its main advantages are: 1 Care close to home 2 Best use of new technology, eg near-patient testing; phone-activated devices to summon help 3 Cost-effective use of resources 4 Less rigidly demarcated professional roles 5 Creative integration of working practices.

Simple self-care constitutes the health activities which we do on our own and within a family, eg brushing our teeth, or taking paracetamol for a headache or fever. Empowered self-care is what can happen when health care professionals work together with the patient and other services. Empowered self-care is a key strategy for primary care, both for disease prevention and chronic disease management.

Chronic disease management Most patients with diabetes will spend at most a few hours face-to-face with a health care professional over the course of a year. For the rest of the time they must manage the disease themselves and need to be given the resources and education to do this. Self-management plans are commonplace in primary care. They encourage an interactive partnership between the clinician and the patient to support self-management of chronic conditions. An example is the provision of standby 'rescue' medication to those with COPD, along with instructions on when to start these for an exacerbation. Self-management plans are commonly used in diabetes, asthma, and COPD.

Disease prevention A 'stages of change'[9] approach can be used to help patients change their behaviour and address addictions, lifestyle modification, and disease prevention. This model shows that a change in behaviour usually occurs gradually through identifiable stages:
- *Precontemplation:* Patients are uninterested, unaware, or unwilling to make a change (eg a patient may feel 'immune' to the problems caused by smoking or high cholesterol).
- *Contemplation:* Patients may assess barriers as well as benefits to change. Giving up an enjoyed activity may cause a sense of loss despite the perceived gain.
- *Preparation:* Patients prepare to make a specific change, eg trying a low-fat diet or decreasing their alcohol intake.
- *Action:* This demonstrates a desire for lifestyle change; however, glossing over the previous stages may show that action itself is not enough.
- *Maintenance and relapse prevention* involves incorporating the new behaviour in the long term.

Motivational interviewing[10] In all scenarios, motivational interviewing techniques can be helpful in empowering patients. It encourages both the doctor and the patient to discuss the gains and losses of changing behaviour in a non-judgemental manner (as opposed to the doctor telling the patient what to do). Compare *'You need to stop smoking, it's bad for you.'* with *'Have you ever thought about giving up? What do you think is stopping you?'*

Barriers to self-care
- *Patient factors:* Patient's may be blinkered ('It will never happen to me'); We like to rebel ('I know it's bad, but I like it'); there may be a lack of motivation ('I can't be bothered to change'—the path of least resistance). All of these can be influenced by those who are rendered helpless and hopeless by unemployment, poverty, and family strife. Others may have difficulty accessing care, eg the homeless, refugees, drug abusers, ethnic minority groups, and patients living in rural areas without public transport.
- *Health care professional factors: Time:* It takes time to educate people regarding self-care (eg why antibiotics aren't required for a viral illness). *Motivation:* Health education may be seen as repetitive and boring. *Money:* Health promotion requires personnel and resources.
- *Society factors: Responsibility lies with the GP:* Pharmacists, schools, and the media suggest GP appointments for minor ailments in order to 'cover their backs'; *pressure from business* (eg tobacco advertising); there are also those who want to monopolize and medicalize health.

The primary health care team incorporates a broad range of professionals who undertake a wide variety of activities. Each team member should understand and acknowledge the skills, knowledge, and role of others within the team, and should also recognize and include the patient, carer, or their representative as an essential member of the team.

General practitioner *GP principals/partners* are independent contractors, usually within a partnership who provide primary health care services (± additional services). These GPs are self-employed and run the practice as a business, with responsibility for staff, premises, and equipment. Pay depends on income and expenditure. *Salaried GPs* are employed by a practice or other organization under an agreed contract and salary. They may not want the commitment or managerial tasks associated with being a partner. *Locum GPs* are self-employed GPs providing medical cover to different practices on a regular or intermittent arrangement. *FY2 doctors* and *GP registrars* are qualified doctors in training programmes undertaking a rotation within a GP surgery.

Practice nurses are nurses caring for patients within a GP practice. Activities include: •*Tests:* Audiometry; ECGs; spirometry. •*Advice:* Contraception; diet; lifestyle; travel. •*Treatment:* Dressings; injections. •*Prevention:* Vaccinations; BP; cervical smears. •*Chronic disease management:* Diabetes, asthma, COPD, etc.

Nurse practitioners are registered nurses who have acquired expert knowledge and clinical competencies for expanded practice, and who work autonomously in carefully delegated roles. Within general practice they triage patients, diagnose, and initiate treatment. Patient satisfaction is high and no increase in adverse outcomes has been found.

District nurses provide nursing care to those who are housebound (eg frail elderly patients, or those who are terminally ill or disabled). Activities include dressing leg ulcers, changing urinary catheters, administering drugs and injections; providing emotional support to patients and their families; caring for those who wish to die at home; identifying social care issues and liaising with other services. *Community matrons* have case-loads of vulnerable patients, eg who have >1 chronic disease. They provide home care (*active case management*) with the aim of reducing emergency admissions to hospital.

Community midwives Provide advice, care, and support for pregnant women and their babies in the antenatal and postnatal period (including home deliveries). They provide parenting support and care for the newborn in the early postnatal period.

Health visitors have nursing and midwifery backgrounds, plus health visiting qualifications. Most of their work is focussed on families with children <5yrs old. They promote good health and prevent illness by offering practical help and advice (eg on breast-feeding; minor illness; prevention of accidents; and safeguarding).

Practice managers lead on finance; employment law; tax; risk assessment/reduction; health & safety; CQC requirements.

There are many pressures unique to general practice. Dealing effectively with these pressures is important in order to improve job satisfaction and prevent adverse effects on clinical work and home life.

Time The standard GP appointment is just 10 minutes long in the UK. How can you deal with everything that needs to be done for a patient in that time? GPs are often interrupted during surgeries and have a myriad of business management tasks and clinical administrative tasks to do, in addition to their face-to-face clinical work. Time management is a key skill and stressor.

Isolation GPs spend a lot of time working alone seeing patients. In smaller practices they may be the only doctor working in the practice.

Dealing with uncertainty Few GPs work in settings where investigations can be accessed immediately. GPs must therefore manage uncertainty regarding symptoms or diagnosis and use time (eg follow-up appointments) to guide further management.

Managing long-term relationships with patients Marriages fail but GPs have to see patients on an ongoing basis, often for years or decades—whether they get on with them personally or not. Relationship management (including setting boundaries) is very important for GPs and can cause considerable stress; it is a skill that is not taught at medical school.

Switching emotions GPs see 15–30 patients in a single surgery. Each appointment is just 10 minutes long and anybody can come with any problem. It is not uncommon to deal with a patient who has acute chest pain and immediately follow that with a patient who is suicidal. Switching emotions and maintaining empathy over such diverse and often conflicting situations so quickly can be very stressful.

Managing patient demand vs budget restraint As gatekeepers GPs have a constant conflict between being criticized for not referring or prescribing appropriately, but being criticized and financially penalized if arbitrary targets are exceeded.

Constant reorganization The pace of change in primary care has been immense. Keeping up with those changes and ticking every box required to maintain practice income is a major stressor.

Interventions and solutions These apply to us all, not just GPs!
- *Improve your working conditions:* eg develop a specialist clinical or academic interest within or outside the practice. Learn to decline extra commitments. GPs with higher stress levels do not necessarily have low morale, but there is a close correlation between levels of job satisfaction and morale—job satisfaction seems to protect against stress.
- *Look at your own behaviour and attitudes:* Stop being a perfectionist; resist the desire to control everything; don't judge your mistakes too harshly.
- *Look after your own health and fitness:* Set aside time for rest and relaxation; make time for regular meals and exercise.
- *Allow time for yourself and your family:* Do not allow work to invade family time. Consider changes in working arrangements if it does.
- *Don't be too proud to ask for help:* As well as formal channels for seeking help, there are several informal doctor self-help organizations and counselling services for those in need.

Primary care

The consultation is the central act of general practice. It is something that has been studied extensively and various models exist (see p476). The key to a good consultation is the successful exchange of information. There is no 'correct' way to perform a consultation and approaches vary depending on individual preference and style, and according to the patient and situation.

Potential barriers to effective communication There are many! Lack of time, language problems, differing age, gender, ethnic or social background of doctor and patient, 'sensitive' issues to address, 'hidden' or differing agendas, lack of trust between patient and doctor.

Patient centredness is an approach where the doctor focuses on what the patient thinks and feels is important to the problems they bring. The patient's views are considered and integrated into the diagnosis and decision-making process. This is a shift in value from the traditional doctor-centred consultation where the patient is passive and the doctor decides on what to discuss and do. It is easy for the patient's own needs to get crowded out of a busy surgery. Depressed patients, for example, frequently hold back information they would like to discuss, as the doctor seems too busy. This concern about 'not worrying the doctor' can be counterproductive. So, every so often try saying 'Take your time—I'm not in any hurry. Let's try to get to the bottom of what's going on ... [pause]'.

Consulting in a patient-centred way seems to improve patient satisfaction and may improve health outcomes. It consists of 6 interactive components:[11]

1 *Exploring both the disease and the illness experience:* Integrating the history, physical examination, and investigations with understanding of the unique experience of the patient's illness (their feelings, ideas, effect on day-to-day life and expectations). See fig **6.2**.

2 *Understanding the whole person:* Awareness of the multiple aspects of a person's life, family, employment, social support, and the context in which they live (eg cultural issues, community).

3 *Finding common ground regarding management:* Identifying the problem and priorities and establishing the goals of treatment.

4 *Incorporating prevention and health promotion.*

5 *Enhancing the doctor–patient relationship:* At each consultation try to build on the relationship. Include compassion, trust, and a sharing of power and healing.

6 *Being realistic:* About time and the wise use of resources.

Primary care

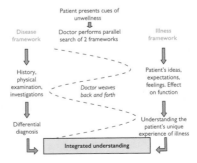

Fig 6.2 The patient-centred process.
Reproduced from Simon et al, *Oxford Handbook of General Practice* 4th edition (2014) with permission from Oxford University Press.

Consultation times have risen by 40% in the last 20 years (now on average ~12min). Short consultations are riskier than longer ones (eg less time to look things up and less time for safety netting ('If x, y, or z develops, you need to come back...'). ►Does heavy demand produce short consultations, or do short consultations produce heavy demand by failing to meet patients' needs?

The consultation time influences the degree of patient satisfaction, and may influence the consultation rate, with lower return visit rates for longer consultations (not shown in all studies), lower rates of prescription issue (esp. antibiotics), and more preventive activities. Running late is stressful for doctors (and patients). Factors which increase (↑) or decrease (↓) consultation rates (apart from season, distance to the GP, and sex—women consult more than men):

- Social deprivation (↑) and morbidity (↑).
- Increasing requirements to monitor almost all diseases and drugs, eg DMARDs for rheumatoid arthritis, diabetes reviews, etc (↑).
- Low frequency of contact associates with ↑educational status, paid employment in the health sector, and expectations of GP to care for minor illness (↑).
- The cheaper the housing (council tax band^{UK}) the higher the consultation rate.
- List size, and having personal lists (consultation rate ↓ by 7%—ie patients are encouraged to consult with only one doctor decreases overall attendance).
- Not prescribing for minor ailments—see p488 (?↓).
- New patients (for their 1st yr with a new GP), and patients over 65yrs (↑).
- If the GP is extrovert (↑) he or she recalls more, and his/her rate is higher than others (eg 6/yr vs 2/yr). GP age and sex also influence rates.
- High latitudes—within the UK (↑). The South-East has lowest rates.
- Preventive activities (↑; but this can reduce need to invite people to clinics).

There is some evidence for the Howie hypothesis that consultation duration is a valid and measurable marker of quality (effectiveness, safety, equity, and holistic patient experience, p488). It is certainly not true that extending consultation times will *automatically* increase health and satisfaction.[12]

Primary care

Consultation models can provide a useful framework for consulting in a structured or organized way, and can help develop consultation skills. As we learn to consult, they can give orientation to a consultation and a 'checklist' of things to do. Consultation models don't need to be followed from start to finish, pick areas from different models that work well for you. There are many different consultation models and the following list outlines just a few.

(Bio)Medical model *Traditional/hospital model* History-taking→examination →investigations→diagnosis→treatment→review. Whilst being thorough, it is time-consuming, doctor centred, and disease focussed.

Balint *The Doctor, His Patient and the Illness (1957)*[13]
A philosophy rather than a consultation model. Balint was a psychoanalyst who aimed to help GPs better understand the psychological aspect of practice.
• Psychological problems are often manifested physically.
• Doctors have feelings. Those feelings have a role in the consultation.
• Doctors need to be trained to be more sensitive to what is going on in a patient's mind during a consultation.

Byrne & Long *Doctors talking to patients (1976)*[14] Analysis of taped consultations led to a compilation of 6 areas covered in a consultation:
1 The doctor establishes a relationship with the patient.
2 The doctor attempts to/actually discovers the reason for attendance.
3 The doctor conducts a verbal or physical examination, or both.
4 The doctor, or the doctor and the patient, or the patient (in that order of probability) consider the condition.
5 The doctor (and occasionally the patient) detail treatment or further investigation.
6 The consultation is terminated—usually by the doctor.
This model was the first to include the tasks of introduction and finishing. It also involves the patient and introduces the notion of 'illness'.

The Stott & Davis model *Exceptional potential of the consultation (1979)*[15]
4 tasks that can take place in any consultation:
1 Management of presenting problems.
2 Management of continuing problems.
3 Modification of health-seeking behaviour eg advise self-treating minor illness.
4 Opportunistic health promotion.
Like Byrne & Long it does not actually tell us *how* to carry out the consultation.

Pendleton et al. *The doctor's tasks (1984)*[16]
This model involves exploring the patient's detailed thoughts, including their ideas, anxieties, and expectation, and identifying the effects of the illness.
1 Define the reason for attending: the nature and history; aetiology; the patient's ideas, concerns, and expectations; the effects of the problem.
2 Consider other problems: eg continuing problems and at-risk factors.
3 The doctor and patient choose an appropriate action for each problem (negotiation between doctor and patient).
4 The doctor and patient achieve a shared understanding of the problem.
5 The patient is involved in management of the problem and encouraged to accept appropriate responsibility.
6 The doctor aims to establish and maintain a relationship with the patient.
This model is the essence of patient centredness (see p474).

Neighbour *The Inner Consultation (1987)*[17]

The doctor works in 2 different ways throughout the consultation, as *The Organizer* and *The Responder*. Each consultation comprises 5 activities:

1 *Connecting* is the process of establishing rapport.
2 *Summarizing* marks the point at which the patient's reasons for attending, hopes, feelings, concerns, and expectations have been well enough explored, acknowledged, and summarized for the consultation to progress.
3 *Handing over* follows the doctor's assessment and diagnosis of the presenting problems and entails an explained, negotiated, and agreed management plan.
4 *Safety netting* allows the doctor the security of knowing that she has prepared, or could prepare for, contingency plans to deal with an unexpected event and some departures from the intended management plan (see p480).
5 *Housekeeping* allows the GP to deal with any internal stresses and strains.

This model thoughtfully re-defines the tasks of a consultation, but it is fairly complex.

Kurtz & Silverman *The Calgary–Cambridge Model (1996, update 2003)*[18] (fig 6.3).
A comprehensive (and daunting) list of 55 consultation skills contained within a framework that emphasizes patient-centred communication.

• *Initiating the session:* Establishing initial rapport and identifying the reason for the consultation.
• *Gathering information:* Exploring problems; understanding the patient's perspective; providing structure to the consultation.
• *Building the relationship:* Developing rapport; involving the patient.
• *Explanation and planning:* Providing the correct amount and type of information; aiding recall and understanding; achieving a shared understanding (by incorporating the patient's perspective); shared decision-making.
• *Closing the session.*

It is a useful teaching tool and allows structured analysis of a consultation, but possibly too much to remember!

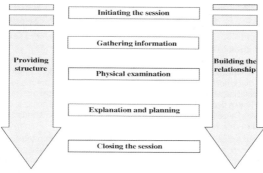

Fig 6.3 The Calgary–Cambridge model.
Reproduced with permission from Kurtz SM, Silverman JD, Benson J and Draper J (2003) Marrying Content and Process in Clinical Method Teaching: Enhancing the Calgary–Cambridge Guides *Academic Medicine* 78(8):802–809.

Further reading
Bevington, B (2013). *Talking with Patients: A Consultation Handbook* (6th ed) London: KSS Deanery.

When decision-analysts started observing consultations they were amazed at the number of decisions per minute, and the wide range of possible outcomes, such as 'no action; review next week' or 'ambulance direct to hospital' or 'refer' or 'prescribe x, y, and z, and stop q in a week...'. The average decision-analyst is disorientated by the sheer pace and apparent effortlessness of these decisions—so much so that doctors were often suspected of choosing plans almost randomly, until the idea of a 'perceptual filter' was developed.

Perceptual filters[19] This is the internal architecture of our mind—unique to each doctor—into which we receive the patient's history. It comprises our:
- Unconscious mental set: *tired/uninterested* to *alert, engaged, responsive*.
- Entire education, from school, to the last lecture we attended.
- Sum of all our encounters with patients. Ignore the fact that we can recall very few of these: this does not stop them influencing us strongly: does the rock recall each of those many, many waves which have sculpted it into extraordinary shapes, or which have entirely worn it away?
- Past specific, personal experience with this particular patient.
- Past specific, personal experience with the disease(s) in question.
- Non-personal subjective (eg 'endocarditis the most dangerous and stealthy disease...') or objective ideas (eg evidence-based medicine).

The mind's working space The perceptual filter achieves nothing on its own. What is needed is interpretation, rearrangement, comparison, and planning of executive action. The abilities of our mental working space are determined by the number of items of data that can be integrated into a decision. There is evidence that this vital number is 3-8.

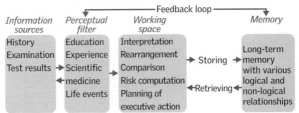

Fig 6.4 Consultation flowchart. After Sullivan.[19]

Thinking about thinking[1][20-22] The rapid decision-making often required by doctors can be aided by *heuristics*—strategies that provide cognitive 'short-cuts' to quick decisions (conscious or unconscious) which are made without full information or analysis. Understanding how we use heuristics (ie by considering how a decision is made) can help us make effective choices, but there are pitfalls. Failed heuristics (biases) interfere with judgement and can lead to diagnostic error. Important examples include:

Anchoring: A significant feature in the history is 'anchored' onto too early in the diagnostic process and is not adjusted for in light of later information. Adjusting probability by incorporating new information can help you become an intuitive thinker. Anchoring can be compunded by *confirmation bias*—the tendency to look for, notice, and remember information that fits with pre-existing expecations.

Availability: Explains our tendency to judge something more likely if it readily comes to mind. A recent experience with a disease increases the likelihood of it being diagnosed—problematic if the disease is rare, or has not been seen for a while.

Representativeness: A diagnosis is driven by the extent to which a patient resembles a classic case of a disease. When diagnosis is limited in this way, atypical variants can be missed.

Primary care

General practice is the art of managing uncertainty. Many patients present with problems or symptoms that are undifferentiated and unorganized and do not have an obvious diagnosis at presentation. Many symptoms are also medically unexplained (see p489). Almost any symptom can be made to seem fatal (is this lethargy due to cancer?), even seemingly trivial problems ('this pain in my toe...' —could it be due to an emboli or osteomyelitis?). Medicine is for gamblers (see below) and in order to survive we must learn to manage uncertainty and avoid lying awake at night worrying about the meaning of our patients' symptoms. (See also p521.)

Tips for dealing with uncertainty

Consider the differential diagnosis: A careful history and examination will allow you to consider the differential diagnosis. Making decisions when there is uncertainty and risk is difficult. Decisions are based not just on risk but also on possible outcome. High-risk problems should have a lower threshold for action (eg for possible MI or appendicitis).

Time as a tool: The skillful use of time (by reviewing a patient over a number of consultations across a period of time) can obviate the need for extensive investigation, or allow for incremental investigations as symptoms develop, or the results of initial investigations emerge.

Evidence-based medicine: When deciding on an investigation or treatment, consider what evidence exists for its use, how valid the evidence is, and if it is applicible to the patient you are seeing. No treatment is completely safe, entirely effective, or without side effects.

Sharing uncertainty: Sharing uncertainty with patients may increase trust and avoids deception. We can also share uncertainty with colleagues (eg discussing symptoms with another GP or referring to a specialist—this is also useful if you think the source of your uncertainty might be a gap in your own knowledge).

Safety netting: Discuss a contingency plan with the patient by informing them what to do if things don't go to plan (eg seeking urgent review if red flags develop with back pain, or educating a parent about the signs to look for that should prompt review of a febrile child).

Gamble safely: Making decisions under conditions of uncertainty is a form of gambling. We cannot refer and investigate every problem, yet we still need to make decisions. Some of these decisions will be scientific and rational. Some will be based on subtle clues or feelings. Make sure you assemble sufficient evidence to maximize your chances of being lucky.

Clinical governance: Defined as a systematic approach to maintaining and improving the quality of patient care. No matter how carefully we practise, adverse events will occur. It is important to discuss, reflect and learn from any errors and improve systems to try and prevent similar events.

1 This material was originally published in the *Oxford Handbook of Clinical Medicine* 9th edition by Longmore et al, and has been reproduced by permission of Oxford University Press.

Doctors are called on to make decisions about every patient they meet: few are curable at once, so making a plan for what to do for the best is the secret of success at the bedside. The aim here is to explain this secret, to enable you to flourish in the clinical world, and to keep you out of lawyers' offices.

Let us look at the steps of the history, physical, or mental examination, and investigations.

By the end of taking the **history**, you need to have acquired 3 things:

1 Rapport with the patient.
2 A diagnosis or differential diagnosis.
3 The placement of the diagnosis in the context of the patient's life.

Rapport: Consultations are shorter when rapport is good. The patient is confident that he or she is getting the full attention of the doctor, and these patients are more understanding, and more forgiving when things go wrong. Doctors are far from infallible, so we need to have confidence that the patient will feel able to come back if things are not right, tell us what has happened, agree on an adjustment of the treatment, and, by giving feedback, improve our clinical acumen.

Diagnosis: Studies have shown that skilled physicians have made a provisional diagnosis soon after the consultation starts, and they spend the rest of the history in confirming or excluding it. What happens if you are not skilled, and you have no hint as to the diagnosis? You need to get more information.

• Pursue the main symptom: 'tell me more about the headache...'
• Elicit other symptoms—eg change of weight or appetite, fevers, fatigue, unexplained lumps, itching, jaundice, or anything else odd?
• Get help from a colleague or even a diagnostic support system.
• Check you still have rapport with the patient. Are you searching for a physical diagnosis when a psychological diagnosis would be more appropriate? Here you might ask questions such as 'How is your mood?' 'What would your wife or partner say is wrong?' 'Would they say you are depressed?' 'What would have to change for you to feel better?'

▶Do not proceed to the physical examination until you have a working diagnosis: the answer is rarely found there (<10%).

Placing the diagnosis in the context of the patient's life: If you do not do this, you will not know what will count as a cure, and, more specifically, different patients need different treatments (see BOX on p241). Some factors to focus on might be: the motivation of the patient to get better ('I've got to get my knee better so that I stay strong enough to lift my wife onto the commode'); their general health; social situation; drugs (not forgetting nicotine and alcohol); is help available at home; work (yes/no; type)?

At the end of the history, occasionally there is enough information to start treatment. Usually you may be only, say, 70% sure of the diagnosis, and more information is needed before treatment is commenced (fig 6.5).

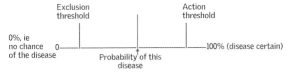

Fig 6.5 Probability of the disease after taking a history.

It is time for the physical **examination**. This aims to gain evidence to confirm or exclude the hypothesis, to define the extent of some process, or to assess the progress of known disease. At each step, ask 'What do I need to know?' Following the examination the diagram may look like this (fig 6.6):

Primary care

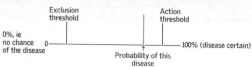

Fig 6.6 Probability of the disease after physical examination.

Investigations If the action threshold has not been crossed, further information is needed. Action thresholds vary from doctor to doctor, and from disease to disease. When the treatment is dangerous, the action threshold will be high (eg leukaemia). In self-limiting illnesses, eg pharyngitis, the action threshold will be lower. Note that 'action' may be that, in agreement with such a patient, only symptomatic treatment is needed, and future episodes could be managed without medical input. Similarly, it may be important to move the probability of a serious but unlikely disease beyond the exclusion threshold.

Once the probability of a disease passes the action threshold, treatment can commence, if the patient wishes (fig 6.7).

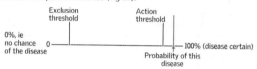

Fig 6.7 Passing the action threshold.

Supposing neither the action threshold nor the exclusion threshold is exceeded, then more information is needed, eg from pathology, imaging, or the passage of time. Time itself is an investigation: it may reveal sinister causes or the benign nature of the disease. To use time this way, you need to be reasonably sure that immediate treatment is not required.

If there is still not enough certainty to initiate management, get further information, eg from books, the internet, colleagues, further tests—or you may feel it appropriate to refer the patient. Or go round the process again, starting with the history—from a different viewpoint.

Once above the action threshold, it is time to decide what to do for the best. This is a decision shared by the doctor and the patient. It entails informed consent and consideration of:[23]
• The probability of the diagnosis.
• The likelihood of the different possible outcomes.
• The costs and side effects of treatment.
• The hope and values of those affected, particularly the patient.
• What is possible, considering the skills, resources, and time available.

Finally, tell your patient how they will know if they are on the path to improvement or relapse, and if so, at what point to seek help (safety netting or critical action threshold (fig 6.8; record this in the notes)—eg 'If your peak flow falls by 40%, start this prescription for prednisolone, and come and see me'.

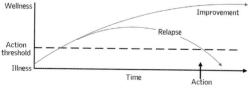

Fig 6.8 Pathway to improvement or relapse.

Here is a list of some of the things pundits tell us we should be doing when we meet patients:[24]

1 *Listen*—no interrupting or taking control of the agenda (how often are we guilty of implying: 'Don't talk to me when I am interrupting you')?

2 Examine the patient thoroughly (to establish the likelihood of competing diagnoses).

3 Arrange cost-effective incremental investigation.

4 Formulate a differential diagnosis in social, psychological, and physical terms.

5 Explain the diagnosis to the patient in simple terms (then re-explain it to relatives, and then try re-explaining it to the computer in terms *it* understands—ie 5-digit Read codes, see BOX, p531).

6 Consider additional problems and risk factors for promoting health.

7 List all the treatment options, and seek out relevant guidelines etc. (evidence-based bedside medicine).

8 Incorporate the patient's view on the balance of risks and benefits, harmonizing their view of priorities, with your own assessment of urgency.

9 Arrange follow-up and communicate with all of the health care team.

10 Arrange for purchase of all necessary care, weighing up cost implications for your other patients and the community, welcoming accountability for all acts and omissions, and for the efficient use of resources—with justifications based on explicit criteria, transparency, and principles of autonomy, non-maleficence, beneficence, and distributive justice.

The alternative Do your best.

The synthesis The alternative looks promising—even attractive, when compared with the 10 (im)possibilities just listed. But note that the alternative only looks attractive because it is vague. 'Do your best' is not very helpful advice—and once we start unpacking this 'best' we start to get a list like the 10 earlier points. *'Professionalism'* sums up *part* of what being a good doctor entails—ie: • Self-regulation • Self-actuating and self-monitoring of standards of care • Altruism • Commitment to service • Specialist knowledge and technical skills reflecting but not determined by society's values • Consistently working to high standards of probity and quality (no bribes, no favouritism, but a dynamic concern for distributive justice) • Self-determination—in relation to the range and pattern of the kinds of problems it is right to attempt to solve. For a further discussion, see *On Being a Doctor: Redefining Medical Professionalism for Better Patient Care* (King's Fund 2004).

Authenticity Trying to achieve authenticity is a meta-goal, and may be a better mast to nail your colours to than the 10 points listed earlier. Not because it is easier, but because paying attention to authenticity may make you a better doctor, whereas striving for all 10 of the points may make you perform less well (too many conflicting ideals). With *inauthentic consultations* you may be chasing remunerative activities, quality points, protocols, or simply be trying to clear the waiting room, at any cost, while the patient is trying to twist your arm into giving antibiotics or a medical certificate. *Authentic consultations* are those where there are no barriers; just 2 humans without status exploring and sharing hypotheses and beliefs and deciding what to do for the best (along the lines described in detail on p480)—with no ulterior motives and no conflicts of interest. Authentic consultations know and tell the truth where possible, and where this is not possible, the truth is worked towards—diligently and fearlessly.

Primary care

Continuity of care concerns the quality of care over time. It may be viewed from the perspective of the patient, in which the patient ideally experiences a continuous caring relationship with a clinician ('seeing the GP you know and trust' = *relationship continuity*). From the perspective of health care workers, continuity of care also relates to the co-ordination and sharing of information between different health professionals eg timely access to notes; case management or multidisciplinary team working (= *management continuity*).

Should we actively encourage patients to see the same GP? Do certain patients, eg those with chronic or multiple health problems, have a greater need for continuity? A 2010 Kings Fund report[25] found relationship continuity highly valued by patients and clinicians. The balance of evidence suggests it leads to more satisfied patients and staff, reduces costs, and improves health outcomes.

The importance of continuity of care Continuity of care has been identified as an assumed strength of general practice around the world. The patient and doctor build a relationship of trust and the GP accepts overall responsibility for co-ordinating care. However, recent developments in primary care, eg changing work patterns (more GPs working part time) and a focus on rapid access, suggest that relationship management is becoming more difficult to achieve. Good relationship continuity can also contribute substantially to good management continuity. A GP's clinical responsibility as co-ordinator of care can include helping patients understand their treatment, navigate unfamiliar services, and remain engaged with their care. Practice nurses and community matrons are also increasingly co-ordinating care, which is highly valued by their patients.

Patients' experiences of continuity Continuity becomes increasingly important for patients as they develop multiple health or complex problems, or become more socially or psychologically vulnerable; however, relationship continuity is also valued in other circumstances. Patients actually play a large part in securing continuity and this requires good negotiating skills, especially when access is difficult. Patients are often faced with making a choice between seeing the clinician of their choice or the need for an urgent appointment with anyone who is available. Those less confident or with poor language skills may need support in securing continuity.

Clinicians' perspectives on continuity GPs advocate the importance of continuity of care and consider access arrangements (particularly what happens at the front desk) as crucial to securing this. Quality of consultations (including sufficient time) helps cement 'committed' relationships. Management continuity is also important but GPs attempts to co-ordinate care with professionals outside the practice can be a source of frustration.

Despite professional recognition for continuity of care there is little practical guidance on how to achieve it.

Tips for good practice For relationship continuity: Encourage patients to establish a relationship with a particular professional; support patients to maintain these relationships by • providing patients with information on availability • That staff know who a preferred GP is • That sufficient capacity exists for same-day and advance appointments • That results, documents, and medication requests/reviews to go to the usual GP.

For management continuity: • Make full use of IT systems and electronic communications • Ensure timely availability of relevant clinical communication—particularly from hospitals • Arrange personal contact with other professionals, including meetings and informal discussions • Ensure pro-active follow-up after significant events.

Further reading
Freeman G et al. (2004). *Continuity of Care and the Patient Experience*. London: The King's Fund.

Primary care

Glory or drudge? We may dread home visits as requests filter in through a busy morning surgery, whilst patients are waiting to be seen, results are waiting to be filed, phone calls and referrals are waiting to be made and letters are waiting to be read and actioned. But when we are *doing* home visits, we might rather like them. We are less interrupted, and the possibilities of practising holistically are much enhanced. We see the family in their own context, and new diagnoses and treatment options may tumble out of cupboards, bathrooms, and larders. Home visits are greatly valued by patients, and are a good way to avoid unnecessary 999 calls.

Who should be visited? Home visits provide the best way to assess those who are acutely or chronically housebound. This includes those who are terminally ill or who are truly housebound and for whom travel to a GP surgery would cause unacceptable discomfort or deterioration. Home visits are not usually required to assess those who are able to travel by car to a doctor's surgery. This includes the elderly with poor mobility or general malaise; adults with common problems such as most cases of back pain or abdominal pain; and children with common symptoms such as fever, diarrhoea, and vomiting. It is not the doctor's job to arrange transport for these patients, which is usually readily available from family, friends, or taxi firms. Clinical effectiveness and efficiency of care must take precedence over patient convenience.

It is the doctor's decision whether a patient can be expected to attend the surgery. GPs are only obliged to visit if they feel it would be inappropriate for the patient to attend surgery. General practice is not an emergency service—there is not the infrastructure or workforce to try and attend patients who may be suffering from a serious medical emergency in the middle of a pre-booked surgery. In such circumstances it is unlikely that a GP could contribute beyond the care of a paramedic and an ambulance should be called.[26]

The doctor's bag

In order to undertake home visits you will need your own doctor's bag. Consider including the following:

Equipment Stethoscope; auroscope; ophthalmoscope; patella hammer; BP monitor; thermometer; pulse oximeter; peak flow monitor; urine dipstix; capillary glucose machine; needles; syringes; gloves/lubricating jelly; specimen bottles; sharps box.

Drugs Keep in date (check regularly) and consider carrying the following (exact contents will vary according to your location and circumstances): adrenaline; analgesia (opiate and NSAID); antibiotics (including benzylpenicillin + water for injection); antiemetic; antihistamine; aspirin; diuretic; GlucoGel®; glycerin suppositories; GTN spray; lorazepam/diazepam; naloxone; prednisolone; salbutamol inhaler. NB: if you carry controlled drugs your bag must be lockable and a record of drug use kept.

Other items BNF; headed notepaper; quick reference text; prescription pad; mobile phone + list of useful numbers eg chemists, ambulance, local hospitals; map/SatNav.

Primary care

Telephone consultations are increasingly used to try and manage workload and reduce unnecessary face-to-face consultations. Around 12% of GP consultations are now undertaken over the phone (a 4-fold increase over the last 20 years).

Routine calls Most GP surgeries offer telephone consultations to discuss conditions that do not require an examination, such as self-limiting minor illness; to answer patient queries, eg concerning prescriptions or management advice; and to follow-up chronic disease, eg hypertension or diabetes control. Phone consultations can also be used to discuss results of investigations.

The main drawback of telephone consultations is the inability to examine a patient and a lack of visual cues to aid communication. Be alert to verbal cues such as distress or hesitation and ask the patient about their ideas and concerns. Invite them to ask questions and only give advice once you have sufficient information on which to base your judgement. ►If examination is needed, see the patient.

Emergency calls Nearly all calls for emergency care are made by telephone. In some instances (eg trauma, suspected MI, burns, GI bleeds, or overdose) an emergency ambulance is more appropriate and should be called. In other instances you will need to collect enough information to assess whether a visit or urgent surgery appointment is indicated. If giving advice, make it simple and use language the patient can understand and ask them to repeat what you've told them. Give specific safety netting advice should symptoms change and inform the patient how to access further help if needed. Appear helpful, keep calm and friendly—worried callers often appear abrupt or demanding. If you feel the call is inappropriate, consider educating the patient as to why. ►If in any doubt about the problem or how to manage it, arrange to see the patient.

Phone consultations and triage seem a tempting way to reduce the need for precious appointments, but what is the evidence that they work? Research into the effectiveness of telephone consultations has found that phone services actually increase workload. Patients who had phone consultations with either a GP or nurse were 75% or 88% more likely to need a second consultation, compared to 50% if the first contact was face-to-face.[27] Interestingly the study found no difference in quality of care with telephone consultations.

Email consulting

Email has been used relatively little to consult with patients, however its use is likely to develop further. Successful use depends on a clear understanding of its role:

- Establish turnaround time for messages (do not use for urgent matters)
- Warn that email is not secure and confidentiality cannot be assumed
- Retain copies of email communication with patients in their notes
- Request patients to put their name and DOB in the email for identification
- Ask patients to be concise and to put the category of request in the subject line for appropriate filtering (eg prescription; appointment; advice)
- Append messages with standardized text containing the GP's full name, contact information, and reminders about security and alternative forms of communication for emergencies

Further reading

Campbell JL *et al.* (2014) Telephone triage for management of same-day consultation requests in general practice (the ESTEEM trial): a cluster-randomised controlled trial and cost-consequence analysis. *Lancet* 384:1859–68.

The predominant disease pattern in the developed world is one of chronic or long-term illness. In the UK, over 40% of adults (43% ♀; 41% ♂) report a long-term illness. Chronic disease is more prevalent in older people and in poorer social classes. People with chronic disease are intensive users of health services accounting for over half of all GP appointments; 65% of out-patient appointments; and 77% of hospital bed days.

Although details of chronic illness management depend on the type of illness, people with chronic diseases of all types have much in common with each other. They all have similar concerns and problems, and must deal not only with their disease(s) but also its impact on their lives and emotions.

Common patient concerns

- Finding and using health services and other community resources
- Knowing how to recognize and respond to changes in a chronic disease
- Dealing with problems and emergencies
- Making decisions about when to seek help
- Using medicines and treatments effectively
- Knowing how to manage stress or depression that go with chronic illness
- Coping with fatigue, pain, and sleep problems
- Getting enough exercise
- Maintaining good nutrition
- Working with their doctor(s) and other health care providers
- Talking about their illness with family and friends
- Managing work, family, and social activities.

Examples of chronic disease
• Coronary heart disease
• Diabetes
• COPD
• Cancer
• Heart failure
• Stroke
• Rheumatoid arthritis
• Chronic pain
• Renal disease
• Mental health problems
• Dementia

Effective chronic disease management Common elements include:

Involvement of the whole family: Chronic diseases do not only affect the patient but everyone in a family.

Collaboration: Between service providers, patients, and carers.

Personalized written care plan: Taking into account the patient and carers' views and using current evidence for disease management.

Tailored education in self-management: A patient with diabetes spends only 3h/year with a health professional—the other 8757h they manage their own condition. Helping patients with chronic disease understand and take responsibility for their condition is vital.

Planned follow-up: Planned follow-up according to the patient's care plan, disease registers and recall systems is important.

Monitoring of outcome and adherence to treatment: Use of disease/treatment markers (eg HbA1c in diabetes or CRP/ESR in rheumatoid arthritis); monitoring of concordance, eg checking repeat prescription use.

Tools and protocols for stepped care: Provide a framework for using limited resources to greatest effect; step professional care in intensity—start with limited professional input and systematic monitoring; and select subsequent treatment according to guidelines and the patient's progress.

Targeted use of specialist services: For those patients who cannot be managed in primary care alone.

Monitoring of process: Continually monitor management through clinical governance mechanisms.

Primary care

Depression and chronic disease

Depression is 2–3 times more common in patients with a chronic physical health problem than in people who have good physical health. A chronic physical health problem can both cause and exacerbate depression and treating depression in these patients has the potential to increase their quality of life and life expectancy. Depression is associated with:
• ↑ mortality, ↑ morbidity, ↑ disability, and poorer quality of life
• ↑ presence of smoking and a sedentary lifestyle
• Poorer chronic disease outcome measures (eg HbA1c)
• ↑ use of services and health care costs
• Poor concordance with medication and management plans.

The presence of a physical illness can complicate the recognition and assessment of depression, because some symptoms are common to both mental and physical disorders.

Detection of depression *Use* NICE *depression screening questions:*

During the last month, have you often been bothered by feeling down, depressed, or hopeless?

During the last month, have you often been bothered by having little interest or pleasure in doing things?

A positive response to either of these questions should prompt further assessment with the following 3 questions:

During the last month have you often been bothered by:
• Feelings of worthlessness?
• Poor concentration?
• Thoughts of death?

Further assessment and management p342.

Primary care

Further reading

NICE (2009). *Depression in Adults with a Chronic Physical Health Problem* (CG91). London: NICE. https://www.nice.org.uk/guidance/cg91

GPs may not want to spend much time on minor (minor for whom...?) conditions, but this may become unavoidable if a prescription is issued for each consultation on minor illness (rather pointless if all the patient wanted was reassurance). This reinforces attendance, as a proportion of patients will come to assume that a prescription is necessary. GPs rate a fifth of their consultations as being for minor illness (mild gastroenteritis, upper respiratory problems, presumed viral infections, flu, and childhood rashes). In some studies, 80% are likely to receive a prescription (but this number may be falling), and >10% are asked to return for a further consultation. Why does this great investment of time and money occur? Desire to please, genuine concern, defensive medicine, prescribing as a way to end a consultation, and therapeutic uncertainty all play a part.

Positive correlations with low prescribing rates include a young doctor, practising in affluent areas, and long consultation times. Patients in higher social classes are more likely to get a home visit for minor ailments than those in other social classes. Not everyone wants to reduce prescribing, but advice is available for those who do.

- Encourage *belief in one's own health* and innate powers of recuperation. '*The art of medicine is amusing the patient while nature cures the disease*' (Voltaire).
- Using a *self-care manual* explaining about minor illness.
- Using *self-medication* (eg paracetamol for fever).
- Using the *larder* (eg lemon and honey for sore throats).
- Using *time* (eg pink ear drums—follow-up if symptoms worsen).
- *Using deferred prescribing*: 'He'll get over it in a few days; but here is a prescription if I am wrong: it's good for him to learn to deal with these infections himself, but if this doesn't happen, this is plan B.'
- Using *pharmacists*, or *granny* (a more experienced member of the family).
- *Pre-empting requests* for antibiotics (eg for sore throat): 'I'll need to examine your throat to see if you need an antibiotic, but first let me ask you some questions ... From what you say, it sounds as if you are going to get over this on your own, but let me have a look to see.' [GP inspects to exclude a peri-tonsillar abscess.] 'Yes, I think you'll get over this on your own. Is that all right?'

Empowering patients Any illness, minor or otherwise, is an opportunity to empower patients. Use the time to enable patients to improve their ability to:
- Cope with life and to understand their illness.
- Cope with specific illnesses.
- Feel able to keep themselves healthy.
- Feel confident on handling health issues.
- Be confident about the ability to help themselves.

We know that time spent this way improves patient satisfaction and clinical outcome (although simply extending consultation times in the hope that this will happen is not enough).

Primary care

MUS are physical symptoms for which no organic cause can be demonstrated. GPs deal with MUS in 25% of consultations (costing the NHS £3.1billion/yr). MUS cause disability as severe as that originating from pathology. A third of patients will have a concurrent psychiatric diagnosis—usually anxiety or depression.

Risk factors for developing MUS • ♀>♂ • Physical illness/trauma • Stressful life events (history of child abuse) • Media campaigns that highlight specific diseases.

Classification 3 types of complaint (there are common overlaps):
• Pain of a specific location eg back pain, headache, fibromyalgia
• Functional disturbance in a particular organ eg IBS, palpitations
• Fatigue/exhaustion eg chronic fatigue syndrome

Underlying mechanism 2 mechanisms seem to underpin MUS:
• *Enhanced sense of bodily awareness:* A tendency to notice and amplify normal physical sensations such as heartbeat. Over-awareness ↑ anxiety and in turn makes the sensation more likely.
• *Mis-attribution of symptoms:* Rather than normalizing symptoms, patients attribute somatic explanations (eg a headache is due to a brain tumour rather than stress).

Assessment Consider in any patient with physical symptoms for >3 months that affects functioning but cannot be readily explained. Perform your assessment without prejudice—patients have the same chance as developing serious new illness. *Ask:*
• What are the symptoms? Are there signs on examination (rule out red flags)?
• What type of impairment do they cause?
• What are the patient's concerns and what would they like you to do?
• Does the patient have low mood or anxiety?
• Are there any other social/psychological factors triggering symptoms?

Investigation Review the notes carefully before requesting investigations (which usually clarify the diagnosis and reassure the patient and GP). In patients with MUS, 50% are not reassured following negative investigations. False positive results lead to ↑ anxiety and further investigation. Colluding with the patient ↑ illness behaviour. ▶Try to find a balance between appropriate investigation and risk of harm through over-investigation.

Management 4 key areas:
1 *Connecting:* Go back to the beginning, listen to the patient, acknowledge suffering, use existing knowledge of the patient.
2 *Summarizing:* Allow the patient to summarize problems, recap your understanding of the problem to the patient, and show an interest.
3 *Hand over:* Develop a shared action plan with realistic goals to improve functioning and provide reassurance about long-term outcome.
4 *Safety-netting:* Share uncertainty. Inform patients about red flags indicating serious disease; offer access should symptoms change.

Regular appointments (eg once a fortnight) might be helpful, as might a brief examination at each visit to check for signs of disease. Suggest increasing physical activity levels or voluntary work. Avoid referral unless a clear indication.

Treatment Amitriptyline 10mg ON (unlicensed) may help. Start with a low dose as response is not dose-dependent. Explain it is not being used for depression. CBT allows patients to change their thinking and cope more effectively.

4–10% of patients will have an alternative organic explanation.

Further reading

RCGP/Royal College of Psychiatrists/Trailblazers/National Mental Health Development Unit (2011) *Guidance for Health Professionals on MUS.* www.rcgp.org.uk

131 million working days were lost to sickness in the UK in 2011 costing >£100 billion. The most common reasons for sickness absence were:
• Musculoskeletal problems (35 million days lost)
• Minor illness (27.4 million days lost)
• Stress, depression, and/or anxiety (13.3 million days lost).

Sickness absence ↑ with age; ♀ have higher rates than ♂ The longer someone is not working, the less likely they are to return to work. ►Someone who has been off work for >6 months has an 80% chance of being off work for 5 years.

Returning to work can help recovery, improves physical/mental health and well-being, and decreases social exclusion/poverty. In contrast, long periods out of work can contribute to:
• Higher consultation rates, medication use, and hospital admissions.
• ×2-3 increased risk of poor general health, mental health problems and excess mortality.

The role of the GP When someone of working age presents with a problem that affects their ability to work, record a brief occupational history:
• Address the underlying health problem and any personal, psychological, organizational, or social factors preventing a return to work.
• Where possible, suggest adjustments to enable a return to work (eg amended duties or hours, or a phased return via the option of 'may be fit to work' on the Med 3 form—see BOX, p491).
• Involve occupational health professionals.

Time off work for emergencies In many cases, patients have the legal right to take time off work to deal with an emergency involving someone who depends on them, but they may only be absent for as long as it takes to deal with the immediate emergency. Employers do not have to pay for time taken off.

Dependants include spouse or partner, children, parents, or anyone living with the patient as part of their family, or others who rely wholly on the patient for help.

Emergencies include situations in which a dependant is ill and needs help; goes into labour; is involved in an accident or assaulted; needs the patient to arrange their longer-term care; needs the patient to deal with an unexpected disruption or breakdown in care (such as childminder or carer failing to turn up); needs to make funeral arrangements/attend the funeral.

Postoperative time off work The TABLE lists expected time off work for uncomplicated procedures. These are not hard and fast rules—alter them to fit individual circumstances (eg someone performing manual labour may need longer).

Operation	Minimum expected (wks)	Maximum expected if no complications (wks)
Angiography/angioplasty	<1	4
Appendicectomy	1	3
Arthroscopy (knee)	1	4
Cataract surgery	<1	2
Cholecystectomy	2	12
Colposcopy/cystoscopy/laparoscopy	<1	<1
CABG or valve surgery	6	12
ERPC or TOP	<1	<1
Femoral–popliteal grafts	4	12
Haemorrhoidectomy	2	4
Hysterectomy	2	8
Inguinal or femoral hernia	1	6
Laparotomy	6	12
Mastectomy	2	12
THR/TKR	6	26
TURP	2	8

Individuals must self-certify for the first 7 days of incapacity, then sickness certification from a GP is needed until Work Capability Assessment is carried out (below).

Own occupation test Applies to those claiming Statutory Sick Pay (SSP) for the first 28 weeks of illness. The GP assesses if the patient is fit to do his/her *own* job.

Work Capability Assessment (WCA) is carried out by employment advisors contracted to work for the Department for Work and Pensions (DWP). It is not diagnosis dependent and assesses a variety of different mental/physical health dimensions for ability to work. It is performed within the first 13 weeks of any claim for Employment Support Allowance (ESA) or Universal Credit and applies to:
• Everyone after 28 weeks incapacity.
• Those who do not qualify for SSP from the start of their incapacity.

Forms for certifying incapacity to work

SC1 Self-certification form for people not eligible to claim SSP who wish to claim ESA/Universal Credit. It certifies the first 7 days of illness.

SC2 As SC1 but for people who can claim SSP.

Med 3: Statement of Fitness for Work Completed by a GP or hospital doctor who knows the patient. It certifies periods of incapacity likely to be ≥7 days. Most are now computer issued.

During the first 6 months of incapacity a Med 3 can only be issued for a maximum period of 3 months. On the form there are 2 options:
• The patient is unfit for work.
• The patient may be fit for work—this allows the GP to recommend circumstances under which the patient may be able to return to work, eg with amended duties or reduced hours.

The form gives space for the GP to record the patient's functional limitations. This is designed to allow the employer to make adjustments to facilitate the employee's return to work.

The statement of Fitness for Work may be issued:
• On the day of your assessment of the patient (telephone consultations are acceptable).
• On a date after your assessment if you think it would have been reasonable to issue a Statement on the day of your assessment.
• After consideration of a report about the patient from another doctor or registered health care professional.

Only one Statement can be issued per patient per period of sickness. If mislaid, reissue and mark 'duplicate'.

Mat B1 Signed by a doctor or midwife. It is provided once to pregnant women within 20 weeks of EDD and enables her to claim statutory maternity pay and other benefits.

Further reading

Department for Work and Pensions (2013, updated 2015). *Getting the Most Out of the Fit Note: GP Guidance*. https://www.gov.uk/government/publications/fit-note-guidance-for-gps

Primary care

For UK drivers, the DVLA provides detailed condition-specific guidance about fitness to drive, which is regularly updated.[28] It is the responsibility of the driver to inform the DVLA. It is the responsibility of doctors to advise patients about medical conditions (and drugs/alcohol) which may affect their ability to drive. Drivers should also inform their insurance company. ►If in doubt, ask your defence union. The following guidance applies to group 1 (car and motorcycle) drivers.

Vascular disease

- *Acute coronary syndromes:* Don't drive for 4wks unless successful angioplasty.
- *Angioplasty or pacemaker:* Don't drive for 1wk post procedure.
- *Angina:* If symptoms at the wheel, at rest, or with emotion, don't drive until symptoms controlled; DVLA need not be informed.
- *CABG:* Don't drive for 1 month.
- *Arrhythmias:* May continue driving unless has caused/is likely to cause incapacity (inform DVLA; licence restored when attacks controlled for ≥4wks).
- *TIA/stroke:* Stop driving for 1 month; no need to inform DVLA unless there is residual deficit for >1 month.
- *Hypertension:* Continue driving unless symptomatic.
- *Abdominal aortic aneurysm >6.5cm:* Disqualification. (If 6-6.4cm: inform DVLA; needs annual review).

Diabetes

- *Insulin controlled:* Must inform DVLA. If meets medical standard a 1, 2 or 3yr licence is issued. Drivers must have adequate awareness of hypoglycaemia, must not have had >1 episode of hypoglycaemia requiring the assistance of another person in the last 12 months, and must monitor blood glucose levels 'appropriately'. Vision must conform to the required standard.
- *Tablets causing hypoglycaemia:* (eg sulphonylurea); OK to drive if regular review of DM and has not had >1 episode of hypoglycaemia requiring the assistance of another person in the last 12 months. No need to inform DVLA (otherwise inform DVLA and stop driving).

CNS disorders

- *Epilepsy:* Inform DVLA. Licence revoked until 1 year after last attack (special rules apply if fits only occur in sleep). If withdrawing medication, stop driving during period of withdrawal and 6 months afterwards.
- *Likely first fit/isolated seizure:* Don't drive for 6 months. If clinical factors/ investigations suggest seizure risk ≥20%/yr, = 12 months off driving.
- *Loss of consciousness:*
  - *Reflex vasovagal syncope:* No driving restrictions.
  - *Likely cardiovascular cause:* If abnormal ECG; clinical evidence of structural heart disease; >1 episode in 6 months; or syncope causing injury when sitting/lying inform DVLA and stop driving. If no cause found = 6 months off driving. If cause found and treated = 4wks off driving.
- *Chronic neurological disease:* eg Parkinson's disease, MS, dementia, MND. Inform DVLA. Licensing depends on clinical condition.
- *Sleep apnoea:* Don't drive. Restart if symptoms adequately controlled.
- *Significant head injury:* Inform DVLA. Usually 6-12 months off driving.
- *Sudden disabling giddiness:* Stop driving until symptoms controlled.

Psychosis

- Inform DVLA. Licence revoked. Restored if well and stable for ≥3 months, compliant with treatment, and free from adverse drug effects which would impair driving. Specialist report required.

Drug or alcohol misuse or dependency

- DVLA arranges assessment prior to licence restoration: 6 months—1yr off driving after detoxification for alcohol, opioid, cocaine or benzodiazepine dependence; or alcohol/drug related seizure.

Vision Acuity (±corrected with glasses) must allow reading a 79.4mm-high number plate at 20.5 metres (~6/10 on Snellen chart). Monocular vision is allowed if visual field is full. Binocular field of vision must be >120°. Diplopia isn't allowed unless *mild* and *eye-patch correctable*. *Diabetic retinopathy* matters, but applicants/licence holders may not need DVLA visual field tests on a regular basis if vision meets required acuity and visual field standards, and a consultant confirms that it is stable, eg: • Visual field shows no deterioration during the last yr • No further laser use in the last year or since their last licence renewal • No change in retinal signs in the last year or since renewal.

Drugs Many drugs affect alertness and driving ability (check *Data-sheets*), and many are potentiated by alcohol, so warn patients not to drive until they are sure of side effects, not to drink and drive, not to drive if feeling unwell, and never to drive within 48h of a general anaesthetic.

Prescription medication: It is illegal in England and Wales to drive with certain legal prescribed drugs if it impairs driving. These include benzodiazepines, methadone, morphine, and other opiate-based drugs (eg codeine and tramadol). Patients may drive if taking these medications so long as it does not cause them to feel impaired, and if medicines are taken as prescribed.

Recreational drugs: It is illegal to drive with certain abused drugs above a specified blood level including cannabis (THC), cocaine, MDMA (Ecstacy), LSD, methylamphetamine, and heroin/diamorphine.

Old age DVLA says: 'progressive loss of memory, impairment in concentration and reaction time with possible loss of confidence, suggest consideration be given to cease driving.' This is vague, as when reapplying for a licence (every 3yrs after 70) a driver simply signs to say 'no medical disability is present'.

Further reading

Department for Transport (July 2014). *Drug Driving and Medicine: Advice for Healthcare Professionals*. https://www.gov.uk/government/publications/drug-driving-and-medicine-advice-for-healthcare-professionals

DVLA (Aug 2015). *At a Glance Guide to the Current Medical Standards of Fitness to Drive for Medical Practitioners*. https://www.gov.uk/government/uploads/system/uploads/attachment_data/file/457961/aagv1.pdf

Each year >1 billion people travel by air. Air travel is increasingly accessible to all and health professionals may be asked to assess a patient's fitness to fly.[29] Most patients are able to fly safely and the following guidelines (from the UK Civil Aviation Authority) address the most common issues that may affect fitness to fly. Most in-flight medical emergencies occur when a passenger's individual medical condition is unknown to the airline and it is therefore essential that the airline is given adequate details in advance. Key information required: • The nature of the condition and its severity/stability • Medication being taken • Mobility issues. Patients should carry any medication in their hand luggage.

Physiology of flight The 'cabin altitude' in commercial aircraft should not exceed 8000ft and is typically between 5000–7500ft. This results in a decrease in the partial pressure of alveolar oxygen, but due to the shape of the oxy-haemoglobin dissociation curve, this only results in a fall of arterial oxygen to ~90% and is well tolerated by healthy travellers. Those with medical conditions associated with hypoxia or reduced oxygen carrying capacity (eg anaemia, respiratory/cardiac conditions) may not tolerate the reduction in barometric pressure without support.

Cardiovascular disease The majority of patients with cardiac conditions can travel safely. For contraindications and indications for oxygen see BOXES. *Angina* can fly if stable; *MI* may travel after 7–10 days if no complications; *CABG* (+other chest/thoracic surgery) may travel 10–14 days after surgery; *angioplasty/stent* may be fit after 3 days (individual assessment essential). *Symptomatic valvular heart disease* relative contraindication (individual assessment required). *Treated hypertension* OK to fly; *pacemaker/ICD* may travel once stable; *CVA* advised to wait 10 days (within 3 days if stable).

Diabetes Air travel should not pose significant problems if diabetes is well controlled. *Insulin treated diabetes* patients must carry adequate equipment and all insulin in hand baggage. Temperatures in the hold may degrade insulin (+ there is the potential for lost luggage). Insulin can be satisfactorily carried in a cool bag for long sectors. Individual regimens should be discussed. *General guidelines:* If travelling east (shorter day): fewer units of intermediate or long-acting insulin may be required. If travelling west (and day extended by >2 hours): supplemental short-acting or intermediate-acting insulin may be required. Those controlled with medication should not have a problem.

Haematological *Anaemia:* Hb ≥80g/L may travel without problems, assuming there is no co-existing cardiovascular/respiratory disease. If Hb <75g/L, special assessment is required (flying may be restricted). *Sickle cell anaemia* patients may need supplemental O_2 (+ delay travel for ~10 days following a sickling crisis). *Sickle cell trait* should not pose a problem. For air travel and DVT see *OHCM* p581.

Pregnancy Delivery in flight, or flight diversion is undesirable. For this reason, most airlines do not allow travel after 36 weeks for a single pregnancy and 32 weeks for multiple pregnancy. Most airlines require a certificate >28 weeks confirming EDD and that the pregnancy is progressing normally. Babies <2d old should not fly (preferably wait until >7d).

Respiratory If able to walk 50 metres at a normal pace or climb one flight of stairs without severe dyspnoea, it is likely they will tolerate flying. Those with significant disease may require O_2. *Asthma:* Ensure all medication is carried in hand baggage. Consider giving a rescue course of oral steroids. *COPD:* Supplemental O_2 may be required (some airlines charge for this; some allow passengers to carry their own O_2). *Bronchiectasis /cystic fibrosis:* Appropriate antibiotic therapy, adequate hydration, and O_2 may be required. ►*Pneumothorax:* Contraindicated until 2 weeks after successful drainage with full expansion of the lung. *Respiratory infection:* Postpone travel until infection has resolved and exercise tolerance is satisfactory.

Psychiatric illness Patients should not travel if they have disturbed or unpredictable behaviour that could disrupt the flight.

Ear problems Flying with otitis media or sinusitis may result in pain and perforation of the tympanic membrane. Patients are advised not to fly until symptoms resolve.

Surgery Patients should not travel <10d after surgery to the chest, abdomen or middle ear. *Laparoscopy* or *colonoscopy* patients may travel >24hrs; *Neurosurgery* patients may travel >7d.

Fractures Flying should be delayed 24h (if flight <2h) or 48h (for flights >2h) after application of a plaster cast. If needing to fly sooner, the airline will usually require the cast to be split along its full length.

Cardiovascular indications for medical oxygen
• Use of oxygen at baseline altitude
• CHF NHYA class III–IV or baseline PaO_2 <70mmHg
• Angina Canadian cardiovascular society class III-IV
• Cyanotic congenital heart disease
• Primary pulmonary hypertension
• Other CVD associated with known baseline hypoxemia.

Cardiovascular contraindications to commercial airline flight
• Uncomplicated MI within 7 days
• Complicated MI within 4–6 weeks
• Unstable angina
• Decompensated congestive heart failure
• Uncontrolled hypertension
• CABG within 10 days
• CVA within 3 days
• Uncontrolled cardiac arrhythmia
• Severe symptomatic valvular heart disease
• Respiratory contraindication = pneumothorax (see p494).

Further reading
UK Civil Aviation Authority (May 2012). *Assessing Fitness to Fly. Guidelines for Health Professionals from the Aviation Health Unit.* www.caa.co.uk

Primary care

Universal Credit Introduced in 2013 to replace •Income Support •Child Tax Credit •Working Tax Credit •Income-based Jobseeker's Allowance •Housing Benefit •Budgeting Loans/Advances •Income-related Employment and Support Allowance •Social Fund—Sure Start Maternity Grants, Funeral Payment, and Cold Weather Payments.

Low-income benefits not replaced by Universal Credit

• *Contributions-based Jobseeker's Allowance:* A non-income assessed benefit paid for ≤26wks to people ≥19yrs and under state pension age who are unemployed or working <16h/wk, capable and available for work, and have paid sufficient National Insurance in one of the two complete tax years before the start of the year the claim is made.

• *Local authority payments:* Council Tax Benefit, Community Care Grants, and Crisis Loans for general living expenses have been replaced with payments from local authorities.

• *Short-term advances:* Provided by the Department for Work and Pensions if financial hardship because of issues with benefit payments.

• *Automatic health benefits:* People claiming low-income benefits can claim free NHS prescriptions, dentistry, eye tests/glasses, etc.

Who can claim Universal Credit? Adults resident in the UK: •Adults >18yrs and under state pension age •Not in full-time education •Who have accepted a Claimant Commitment. NB: *Capital rules:* People with savings/capital £16,000 cannot claim. Payments are reduced for those with savings/capital £6000–£16,000.

Amount paid: Payments are paid monthly. Amount depends on:
• *Age:* Whether >25yrs and is single/has a partner
• *Children:* One rate for first child; lower rate for additional children
• *Childcare costs:* Up to 70% of childcare costs (criteria apply)
• *Inability to work:* Higher rates for those in the support group
• *Carer status:* If caring for a severely disabled person for >35h/wk
• *Housing:* If paying rent or a mortgage.

Benefits cap: Amount of benefit usually cannot exceed £500/wk if a lone parent or part of a couple, or £350/wk if single. Certain benefits are excluded when calculating the cap (eg Cold weather payments, Free school meals). The cap does not apply in certain circumstances (eg if anyone in the household is claiming Attendance Allowance, Disability Living Allowance, Personal Independence Payments, or either partner is unfit for work after Work Capability Assessment).

Both unemployed and working people can claim Universal Credit to supplement low income.

Claimant commitment: Claimants may be placed into one of four groups:
• *No work-related requirements:* No need to seek work if earning over individual threshold (national minimum wage if working 35h/wk); responsible for a child <1yr; over state pension age; carer; pregnant and <11wks prior to EDD; <15wks post-natal; aged 16–21yrs with no parental support and in full-time non-advanced education.
• *Work-focussed interview requirement:* (But no obligation to seek work.) If responsible for a child aged 1–5yrs or lone/nominated foster carer for a foster child aged <16yrs.
• *Work preparation requirement:* If assessed by the work capability assessment as having limited capability for work.
• *All work-related requirements:* Apply to everyone else—individuals must seek and be available to work.

Volunteering: People claiming Universal Credit can do voluntary work for a maximum of half the hours they are expected to seek work for.

Employment and Support Allowance

Eligibility
- Age ≥16yrs and under state pension age
- Not entitled to Statutory Sick Pay (p491)
- Unable to work due to sickness or disability—sc1 certification for the first 7d then Med3 certification until work capability assessment (p491)
- Sufficient NI contributions
- Unable to work and claiming ESA for <1yr.

Disability Living Allowance (DLA)

Eligibility
- Disability >3mo and expected to last >6mo more
- <16yrs at time of application
- *Mobility component:* Help needed to get about outdoors. Two levels; age restrictions apply
- *Care component:* Help needed with personal care. Three levels. If terminal illness, highest rate is automatically awarded.

Personal Independence Payment

Eligibility
- Age 16yrs–65yrs
- Disability requiring assistance present >3mo and expected to last >9mo more. Two payment components:
- *Daily Living Component:* Paid at the standard or enhanced rate depending on criteria scored (enhanced rate automatically paid if terminal illness).
- *Mobility component:* Paid at standard or enhanced rate.

Attendance Allowance (AA)

Eligibility
- Disability >3mo and expected to last >6mo more
- ≥65yrs and not permanently in hospital/local authority accommodation
- Needs attention/supervision
- Lower and higher rates—higher rate if 24h care required or terminal illness.

Carer's Allowance

Eligibility
- Aged ≥16yrs
- Spends >35h/wk caring for a person with a disability who is getting AA *or* Constant Attendance Allowance *or* enhanced rate of Personal Independence Payment *or* middle or higher rate of care component of DLA.
- Earning <£100/wk after allowable expenses
- Not in full-time education
- Other benefits (eg state pension) may affect eligibility.

How to apply Use the relevant form on www.gov.uk

English law does *not* require a doctor:
- To confirm death has occurred or that 'life is extinct'. A doctor is only required to certify what, in their opinion, was the cause of death.
- To view the body of a deceased person. There is no obligation to see/examine a body before issuing a medical certificate of cause of death (NB: cremation regulations *do* require the body to be examined after death if it is to be cremated).
- To report the fact that death has occurred.

English law *does* require the doctor who attended the deceased during the last illness to issue a certificate detailing the cause of death. ▶The death certification process in England and Wales is currently under review and likely to change in the near future.

Death in the community 1 in 4 deaths occur at home.

Expected deaths: You may need to visit and verify death. Advise the family to contact the undertakers and ensure the patient's own GP is notified. For deaths occuring in residential or nursing homes, the 'on-call' GP is often requested to visit. There is no statutory duty to do this but it is often reassuring for the staff at the home and often necessary before staff are allowed to ask for the body to be removed.

Unexpected and/or 'sudden' death: If called, advise the attendant to call the emergency services. If visiting, take a rapid history from any attendants. Then:
- *Resuscitate if appropriate.* Drowning and hypothermia can protect against hypoxic neurological damage; brains of children <5yrs old are more resistant to damage.
- *Report the death to the coroner.* If any suspicious circumstances, or circumstances of death are unknown/unclear—call the police. Alternatively if police or ambulance service are already in attendance and death has been confirmed, suggest the police surgeon is contacted.

Cremation Cremation Regulations (2008) require two doctors to complete a certificate to establish identity and that the cause of death is not suspicious before a person can be cremated. The person arranging the funeral may see the forms and pays a fee to each doctor. Two parts:
- *Cremation 4:* Completed by the patient's usual medical attendant—usually his/her GP if death occurs in the community.
- *Cremation 5:* Completed by another doctor who must have held full GMC registration for 5yrs and is not connected with the patient in any way nor directly connected with the doctor who issued cremation form 4. This is usually a GP from another practice.

▶Pacemakers and radioactive implants must be removed prior to cremation.

Notification of death to the coroner The coroner can be contacted via the local police. Reporting to the coroner does not automatically entail a postmortem. The coroner, once circumstances of the death are clear, may advise the GP to tick and initial box A on the back of the certificate, which advises the registrar that no inquest is necessary. See BOX (p499) for deaths that must be reported to the coroner.

Primary care

Deaths that must be reported to the coroner

The registrar of births, deaths, and marriages is obliged to refer a death to the coroner in any of the following circumstances. In reality, the coroner receives notification from a number of sources, including doctors and the police:[30]

• If it appears that the deceased was not attended during their last illness by a registered medical practitioner
• If the registrar has been unable to obtain a duly completed certificate of cause of death
• If it appears from the certificate that the deceased was not seen by the certifying medical practitioner either after death or within 14 days before death
• If it appears that the cause of death is unknown
• If the death appears to have been unnatural, violent, or suspicious
• If the death occurred during an operation or before recovery from anaesthesia
• If the death appears to have been due to industrial disease or poisoning.

Types of cases to refer

• Deaths which may be due to an accident, suicide, violence, or neglect
• Deaths which may be due to an industrial disease
• Deaths in or shortly after release from prison or police custody
• Deaths during or shortly after an operation or anaesthetic
• Drug abuse
• Non-therapeutic abortion
• Still births where there is a possibility that the child may have been born alive, or there is cause for suspicion
• Cases where the cause of death is unknown or uncertain
• Some coroners require notification of all deaths which occurred within 24 hours of admission to hospital.

When to consider making a Do Not Attempt CPR (DNACPR) decision

GMC guidance[31] If cardiac or respiratory arrest is an expected part of the dying process and CPR will not be successful, making and recording an advance decision not to attempt CPR will help to ensure that the patient dies in a dignified and peaceful manner. In cases in which CPR might be successful, it might still not be seen as clinically appropriate. When considering whether to attempt CPR, you should consider the benefits, burdens, and risks of treatment if CPR is successful. If such treatment is unlikely to be clinically appropriate, you may conclude that CPR should not be attempted. Some patients with capacity to make their own decisions may wish to refuse CPR; or in the case of patients who lack capacity it may be judged that attempting CPR would not be of overall benefit to them.

General principles[32] •The circumstances of cardiopulmonary arrest must be anticipated • When CPR would fail it should not be offered as a treatment option • Appropriate and sensitive communication and the provision of information are an essential part of good patient care • Quality of life judgements should not be part of the decision-making process for health care professionals • Where no advance decision about CPR has been made there should be an initial presumption in favour of providing CPR.

Responsibility for making a decision rests with the senior clinician who has clinical responsibility for the patient (eg consultant if in hospital; GP in Care Homes or the patient's home). DNACPR decisions should be made in consultation with other members of the care team. Junior doctors without full GMC license to practise (FY1) should not make this decision.

A DNACPR form should be completed and used to communicate this information to those involved in the patient's care. It is important that all relevant health care and social care professionals are aware that a DNACPR decision has been made.

The WHO definition of health as *'a state of complete physical, mental and social well-being and not merely the absence of disease or infirmity'* was formulated in 1948 and has never been adapted. At the time it was groundbreaking in its breadth and ambition. It overcame the negative definition of health as 'absence of disease' and included physical, mental, and social domains.

However, the requirement for 'complete' health would leave most of us unhealthy most of the time. Some argue that this contributes to the medicalization of society and lowers thresholds for intervention for conditions that were not previously defined as health problems. Disease patterns have changed: chronic disease previously led to early death, but is now burgeoning worldwide. People live with chronic disease for decades and ageing with chronic disease has become the norm. Are all these people definitively ill?

Redefining health is an ambitious and complex goal. There is support for moving towards a dynamic concept of health based on restoring integrity, equilibrium, & well-being through self-management—the ability to 'adapt and to self-manage.'[33]

▶ *If you haven't had a dialogue with a patient about what counts as health for them, and where they are in their lives, you haven't started to do medicine yet.*

Why does health matter?

Health is one of the few unqualified, self-evident goods (although it is rather pointless if it brings no pleasure). One person's health cannot be achieved at the expense of another's: if it seems to be, we end up substituting one problem for many others (eg global insecurity, through creation of an underclass). This is why health achieves a confluence of foreign and domestic policies of all enlightened government ministers, who at least in the UK state unequivocally that health improves *global security*, enhances *development*, *trade*, and *human rights*. Health creates a *standard* against which any action can be judged. If you are in a quandary, ask yourself: 'Which of my competing actions will promote health among those who have least access to health?'

What are the determinants of health?

Factors affecting access to health include finance, ideology, education, and *wealth*. With wealth comes more stable political systems, and these are what are necessary for literacy and education to flourish, which in turn lead to easy access to clean water (the key issue, as more than 1 billion people have no such access) and the possibility of developing equitable health delivery systems. After clean water, the next steps focus on better nutrition, smaller families, more self-help, and anti-HIV strategies.

▶ *How do you move a Western post-industrial population from a low level of health to a higher level of health?*

Future determinants of health are thought to rest on:

• Controlling climate change and reducing health inequalities.
• Decline in tobacco consumption in all age groups.
• Better health services with more effective, more acceptable treatments.
• Fewer under-doctored areas (currently defined as populations where there are fewer than 52.695 GPs per 100,000—ie a list size of >1898 per whole-time GP)—and more GPs in deprived areas. Funding more GPs has been calculated as one of the most efficient ways of reducing mortality.
• Education capable of influencing behaviour to ↓exposure to risk factors.
• Better protection of the environment and better housing.
• More patient-centred health care, so that patients are not passive recipients of care, but well-educated partners in the struggle against disease.

Primary care

The inverse care law and distributive justice

'Availability of good medical care varies inversely with the need for it in the population served. This operates more completely where medical care is exposed to market forces... The market distribution of medical care exaggerates maldistribution of medical resources.'

There is much evidence in support of this famous thesis formulated by Tudor Hart.[34] Premature death and long-term limiting illness are both strongly associated with deprivation. It is not just availability of care but access to services that matters: Those who need health care the least use services more, and more effectively, than those with the greatest need. Distributive justice is the fair distribution of health resources, based on the premise that all are equal in terms of health care provision. Ideally, sufficient health care would be provided to all, but the health budget doesn't allow for this. So, resources should preferably be distributed in relation to need, within a society that has equal access. In the UK, medical care does exist in deprived areas, but this does not ensure that services are accessed, or that they are of good quality.[2]

Social class and inequalities in health

With the introduction of the British NHS and its ideal of each according to need and equal access, we assumed that differences in the health of different social classes would be abolished. The reverse has happened![35] *The Black Report: Inequalities in Health*

Do health inequalities matter as long as overall health is improving? Yes, because justice matters too. It is the lack of justice which led to the NHS—which would have been the best invention of the 20th century, if only it had removed inequalities.

Mortality rates are higher in social class V (unskilled manual) vs class I (professional). This is true for stillbirths, perinatal deaths, infant deaths, deaths in men aged 15-64 and women aged 20-59, and for deaths due to lung cancer, heart disease, and stroke. Poor people living in North London live ~17yrs less than rich people in Chelsea.

Within occupations the effect of social class is seen in a 'purer' way than when groups of many occupations are compared: in a study of >17,000 Whitehall civil servants there was a >3-fold difference in mortality from all causes of death (except genitourinary disease) comparing those in high grades with those in low grades. Similarly in the army, there is a 5-fold difference in mortality from heart disease between highest and lowest ranks.

Illness makes us descend the social scale, but this effect is probably not big enough to account for the observed differences between classes. Cognitive ability can partly explain socio-economic inequalities in health ('intelligent people look after themselves'—has some truth). However, it is more likely that differences are due to *smoking, education, diet, poverty, stress,* and *overcrowding.*

Social, psychological, and physical factors are inter-related components which interact and play a significant role in the context of health, disease, and illness. Health is not purely a biological process but a combination of biological, psychological, and social factors.

The traditional biomedical model assumes that all illness can be traced back to a single disorder of a *part* of the body and that all symptoms are due to disease within the body.

Problems with the biomedical model:
- Symptoms are common—something we all experience on a daily basis and most of the time recognize as being within the limits of normal experience.
- All disease does not cause symptoms—much disease or pathology is asymptomatic (hence the need for screening programmes).
- Another problem is that patients are seen as 'passive victims' of disease, yet some diseases are closely related to behaviour (eg smoking and obesity), and so a proportion of diseases are caused in part by the patient. Similarly patients are not 'passive recipients' of treatment. For treatment to succeed, the patient needs to be an 'active partner' eg at its most extreme, medication will not work if it is not taken.
- The biomedical model also assumes people have two parts to their existence—the 'physical' and 'mental'—and that these aspects are separate and unrelated (this is reflected in the separation between 'physical' and 'mental' health services).
- The biomedical model cannot explain functional (non-organic) illness, which affects up to 20% of our patients. This group of disorders includes medically unexplained symptoms (p489), fibromyalgia, irritable bowel syndrome, and chronic fatigue syndrome.

Does illness arise from a disease which affects only a part of the whole body, or from a problem at the level of the whole person within their situation? In relation to illness, the reductionist biomedical model assumes there must always be a disorder of a part of the whole, and does not consider that the whole person may be ill without any specific part of the person being abnormal.

The biopsychosocial model first recognized the complex nature of illness, specifically the importance of biological, psychological, and social factors that contribute to illness—acknowledging the importance of factors other than disease.

A holistic approach to illness acknowledges objective scientific explanations of physiology, but also admits that people have inner experiences that are subjective, mystical (and, for some, religious), which may affect their health and health beliefs. It can help in understanding the problems faced by patients and emphasizes that in most illnesses there are many factors that may contribute to a person's experience. It predicts that in some people illness may arise without any disorder within the person (functional illnesses).

▶ The key for us is to try and understand our patients as a biopsychosocial 'whole' and develop skills to transform holistic understanding into practical measures. We must show tolerance and understanding of our patients' experiences, beliefs, values, and expectations. Empower your patient to value themselves by listening to their concerns, consider their mind–body connection, and take account of their emotional state. The whole-person approach strives to create health as well as treat illness.

Further reading

Wade DT (2009). *Holistic Health Care: What is it, and how can we achieve it?* http://www.ouh.nhs.uk/oce/research-education/documents/HolisticHealthCare09-11-15.pdf

Primary care

In order to act as advocates for our patients, an RCGP report 'The 2022 GP: A vision for general practice in the future NHS' states that a GP will:

- Act as 'gatekeeper' and 'navigator' to specialist services. This ensures effective resource utilization (eg referring appropriately, and referring to the most appropriate specialty), and coordination of care between different specialties or serivces.
- Retain his ability to be an independent advocate for patients and to meet professional obligations as a doctor first, irrespective of contractual arrangements or commissioning responsibilities, eg pressure not to refer x or prescribe y.

And herein lies the complexity and value of general practice: GPs must balance being gatekeeper and steward (of finite resources), whilst being able to advocate freely for patients and enable them to access services they need.

What does in mean to be a patient's advocate and navigator? GPs must support and represent a patient's best interests to ensure they receive the best and most appropriate health and social care. It means helping patients make choices concerning their own care, and co-ordinating this across an increasingly complicated health and social care system. In order to do this, GPs need to know the make-up of their practice population and understand the context of their patients and families. This includes socio-economic factors, ethnic and religious groupings, types of housing, and unemployment rates.

Primary care

Primary prevention is taking action to reduce the incidence of disease or health problems within the population either through universal measures that reduce lifestyle risks and their causes or by targeting high-risk groups.[36]

Why is it important? Primary prevention aims to reduce the overall burden of disease and improve health outcomes (and reduce the costs of treating disease). Prevention in childhood provides the greatest benefits, but it is valuable at any point in life. 80% of cases of heart disease, stroke and T2DM and 40% of cancers could be avoided if common lifestyle risk factors were eliminated. Lifestyle risk factors are known to cluster in the population, which has a dramatic effect on life expectancy. Addressing this clustering (and its socio-economic determinants) is likely to reduce inequalities and improve overall population health.

> **Current UK prevention programmes for health that involve GPs**
> - Over 40s health checks (which aim to prevent cardiovascular disease and diabetes)
> - Cancer screening: >90% of cervical cancer screening is done within primary care
> - Chlamydia screening for those aged 16–24yrs
> - Antenatal screening and care
> - Healthy child programme
> - Newborn bloodspot screening
> - Newborn hearing screening
> - Diabetic retinopathy screening
> - Renal, hypertension, and cholesterol screening for those with diabetes
> - Abdominal aortic aneurysm screening
> - PSA informed choice programme
> - Alcohol screening
> - Smoking screening/cessation
> - HIV screening on patient registration in high-risk areas
> - Dementia screening

How to do it: Supporting individuals to change behaviour, eg through brief advice during a consultation (*Have you ever thought about giving up smoking? What do you think is stopping you?*—see 'Motivational interviewing' p471); or through systematic community interventions such as reducing childhood obesity or 'no smoking days'.

Secondary prevention Secondary prevention is systematically detecting the early stages of disease and intervening before symptoms develop—eg treating hypertension and prescribing statins to reduce cardiovascular disease. Successful secondary prevention improves life expectancy and reduces complications of disease.

Why is it important? Secondary prevention interventions are highly cost-effective. In areas where the 'inverse care law' applies (p501), those in greatest need are likely to receive benefit. Identifying those at risk and intervening is one of the most effective ways in which GPs can reduce the widening gaps in life expectancy and health outcomes. However, there is substantial variation between practices in the implementation of secondary prevention—only a minority of patients receive all recommended interventions.

How to do it Secondary prevention largely involves the systematic application of standard, low-technology interventions and includes use of disease registers, systematic screening, and control of eg hypertension and diabetes. Try to engage with and provide services to patients who are not reached by mainstream services.

Tertiary prevention aims to reduce the impact of the disease by preventing disease-related complications eg retinal photography in diabetes. Where the condition is not reversible, tertiary prevention promotes quality of life through active rehabilitation.

Further reading

The Kings Fund (2015). *Transforming our Health Care System: Ten Priorities for Commissioners.* http://www.kingsfund.org.uk/sites/files/kf/field/field_publication_file/10PrioritiesFinal2.pdf

Barriers to prevention

Genetic barriers Not everyone responds to preventive measures. Some of us, because of our genes, are 'immune' to the benefits of exercise, for example. As genetic advances occur, our habitual blanket advice of 'take more exercise' looks increasingly old fashioned. What we should really do is get to know our patients psychologically and genetically, and tailor advice such as 'for you, diet advice is more important than exercise'.

Cognitive barriers When, if ever, we contemplate cataclysmic but preventable ill health in ourselves, we may either believe that *'It won't happen to me'* or we deliberately dare fate to *make* it happen to us. Some people are proud to announce that '... I eat everything, as much butter and fried foods as I can get ... I smoke 40-60 cigarettes a day ... To eat cornflakes, you've got to have sugar on them, otherwise there is no point in eating them ... As long as you keep smoking cigarettes, and drink plenty of whisky, you'll go on for ever'.

Psychological barriers All of us at times are prone to promote our own destruction as keenly as we promote our own survival. Knowing that alcohol may bring about our own destruction gives the substance a certain appeal, when we are in certain frames of mind—particularly if we do not know the sordid details of what death by alcohol entails. It provides an alluring means of escape without entailing too headlong a rush into the seductive arms of death. Gambling and taking risks are all part of this ethos.

Logistic barriers A general practice needs to be highly organized to be in a state of perpetual readiness to answer questions like 'Who has not had their BP checked for 3 years?' or 'Who has not turned up to attend for screening?' or 'Who has stopped sending in for their repeat prescriptions for antihypertensives?' UK IT systems have advanced a lot in the last years, enabling patient alerts to pop-up, allowing for opportunistic preventive activities. The price of this is that patient-centred activities are crowded out, and that, with many preventive activities offered, no guidance on prioritizing individual intervention is forthcoming.

Another example of logistical barriers is providing a sequence of working fridges in the distribution of vaccines to rural tropical areas.

Political barriers It is not unknown for governments to back out of preventive obligations as if influenced by groups who would lose if prevention were successful. Some countries are keener to buy tanks than vaccines.

Ethical barriers If child benefits were available only to those children who had had MMR vaccine, more mumps would be prevented (an unpopular approach!).

Financial barriers Practices must pay for extra staff to do effective screening. Angioplasty (for example) prevents some consequences of heart disease, but is too expensive to use on everybody whom it might benefit.

Motivation barriers Changing from a crisis-led work pattern to strategic prevention is one way that practice nurses can lead the way. They are particularly successful at the meticulous tasks on which all good prevention depends.

Primary care

This entails systematic testing of a population or a sub-group for signs of illness—which may be of established disease (pre-symptomatic, eg breast cancers), or symptomatic (eg unreported hearing loss in the elderly).

Wilson and Junger were the first to define criteria (in 1968) to guide the selection of conditions that would be suitable for screening. These help ensure a screening programme is viable, effective and appropriate:

Modified Wilson criteria for screening (1-10 spells IATROGENIC)[3]
1 The condition screened for should be an important one.
2 There should be an acceptable treatment for the disease.
3 Diagnostic and treatment facilities should be available.
4 A recognizable latent or early symptomatic stage is required.
5 Opinions on who to treat as patients must be agreed.
6 The test must be of *high discriminatory power* (below), *valid* (measuring what it purports to measure, not surrogate markers which might not correlate with reality) and be *reproducible*—with safety guaranteed (see BOX).
7 The examination must be acceptable to the patient.
8 The untreated natural history of the disease must be known.
9 A simple inexpensive test should be all that is required.
10 Screening must be continuous (ie not a 'one-off' affair).

Informed consent: Rees' rule Before offering screening, we have a duty to quantify for patients the chance of being disadvantaged by it as well as the chances of benefit eg anxiety while waiting for a false +ve result to be sorted out may be devastating; or there may be complications of subsequent tests (eg bleeding after biopsy after an abnormal cervical smear). We are all guilty of exaggerating benefits and avoiding discussion of controversial areas with patients. All tests have false-positive and false-negative rates, as summarized in the TABLE:

		Patients with condition	Patients without condition
TEST RESULT	Subjects appear to have the condition	True +ve (A)	False +ve (B)
	Subjects appear not to have the condition	False −ve (C)	True −ve (D)

Sensitivity: How reliably is the test +ve in the disease? A/A+C.
Specificity: How reliably is the test -ve in health? D/D+B.

Partly effective screening
Cervical smears (if >25yrs, p270)
Mammography (after menopause)
Finding smokers (+quitting advice)
Faecal occult bloods (colorectal ca)
Abdominal aortic aneurysm
Chlamydia screening for <25s.

Unproven/ineffective screening[4]
Mental test score (dementia, p366)
Urine dip (diabetes; kidney disease)
Antenatal procedures (p10)
PSA screening for prostate ca (detects too many harmless cancers?)
Elderly visiting to detect disease.[5]

Why screen in primary care? If screening is to be done at all, it makes economic sense to do it in primary care. In the UK, ≥1 million people see GPs each weekday, providing great facilities for opportunistic 'case-finding' (90% of patients consult over a 5yr period). Provided the GP's records are adequate, the last 10% are then asked to attend for special screening sessions. Private clinics do limited work, but there is no evidence that their multiphasic biochemical analyses are effective procedures, and NHS resources are wasted chasing false positive results.

---

3 ▶For an excellent critique of the Wilson criteria, see Gray J (2004) *Br J Gen Pract* 501:292-8.
4 There is evidence that some screening causes morbidity (mortality-awareness and hypochondriasis†)—so why is screening promoted? Because it is easier for governments to be optimistic than to be rigorous!
5 In one study (N=43,000 patients >75yrs old) neither in-depth assessment nor a targeted approach focused on those with ≥3 problems offered gains in survival or quality of life.[37]

Problems with screening

Take a healthy person, screen them, turn them into a patient, and then kill them. From a report on cervical screening: 'By offering screening to 250,000 we have helped a few, harmed thousands, disappointed many, used £1.5m each year, and kept a few lawyers in work.' Typical problems are:

• Those most at risk do not present for screening, thus increasing the gap between the healthy and the unhealthy—the *inverse care law* (p501).
• The 'worried well' overload services by seeking repeat screening.
• Services for investigating those testing positive are inadequate.
• Those who are false positives suffer stress while awaiting investigation, and remain anxious about their health despite reassurance.
• A negative result may be regarded as a licence to take risks and signs of interval disease (arising between screenings) may be ignored by patients who assume they are in the all clear.
• True positives, though treated, may begin to see themselves as of lower worth than hitherto.

▶Remember: with some screening programmes of dubious value, *it may be* healthier not to know.

Health education presumes that people are rational and want to promote their own survival. It begs the question: what should we live for? Unless an individual has an optimistic answer, health education will fail. For 60% of UK people, death is an attractive option compared with doing more exercise.[38] Alcohol and drugs—anything that achieves oblivion as soon as possible—is an ever more popular approach to life, despite years of health education. So society needs to ask itself 2 questions:

1 *Are we making it easy for people to make wise health choices?*
—and, more importantly,
2 *Are we making it easy for people to find something worth living for?*

In city after city, country after country, the answer is *No* and *No*. Britain is the worst place to live in the developed world, based on UNICEF measures of childhood well-being, so there is a long way to go before we get to the starting line where most people are amenable to health education.

Health education messages These must be *specific* and *direct*, eg in getting people to accept help for alcohol misuse, it is of little use saying:
- 'If you don't stop drinking you'll get these diseases …' (~25% may respond).
- Saying 'Accepting help is good for you because of these benefits …' (~50% will respond).
- 'If you don't accept help, you've had it' brings the biggest response.

Optimum messages must be specific about dates, times, and places of help. Well-chosen images and a degree of 'fear' in the message helps: in enlisting patients for tetanus vaccine a 'low fear' message gets a 30% response, while more fear can double this. Graphic images depicting the effects of smoking are mandatory on UK cigarette packets (evidence is rather flimsy) and it is possible that too high a level of fear is counter-productive. A gruesome film about the worst effects of dental caries produces petrified immobility, not self-help or trips to dentists. A better approach is **professional teaching**. Compared with parents, teacher-based oral health education has a better effect on oral health (at least in middle-school Chinese students).[39]

Changing attitudes The following paradigm holds sway: *knowledge → attitudes → intentions → behaviour*. As Chinese thought reformers knew so well, attitude changes depend on a high level of emotional involvement. In questions of belief, as in so many other questions, emotion trumps reason '*people don't demand that a thing be reasonable if their emotions are touched. Lovers aren't reasonable, are they?*'[Graham Green p115 The End of the Affair] Only resort to applying reason to attitudes if emotions are too hot to handle. NB: the arrows in the model above may be reversed: if our behaviour is inconsistent with our ideas (cognitive dissonance), it is often our ideas, not our behaviour which change.

Objective feedback Giving standard written advice about physical activity helps promote exercise. But to make big strides, it helps to give quantifiable feedback—ie a pedometer. This sort of feedback also improves quality of life.

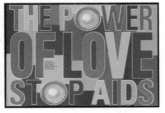

Fig 6.9 HIV/AIDS posters promoting safer sex through the use of condoms advanced beyond the simple messages of who is at risk and how HIV is transmitted by explaining how to prevent infection.
©Wellcome Library, London. Copyrighted work available under Creative Commons Attribution only licence CC BY 4.0 creativecommons.org/licenses/by/4.0/.

Primary care

Traditional approaches Leaflets and multimedia programmes can increase knowledge and change behaviour eg using graphic artists to provide emotionally charged, slick messages. See fig **6.10**.

Peer-to-peer methods Leaflets are authoritative, but this authority is itself a problem. Risk-takers are unlikely to listen to the prim and proper. So peer-education has been developed as a tool to reach certain groups, and evidence suggests that this is promising. Peers may be better than authority figures

Online education and training Online education and training for patients in the form of 'self-help' is increasing in provision and popularity. These include online cognitive behavioural therapy websites such as *MoodGym*, which provides free information and skills training to help cope with depression, and *Living Life to the Full,* a life skills course for people feeling distressed. Other examples include self-help modules for the management of symptoms of irritable bowel syndrome.

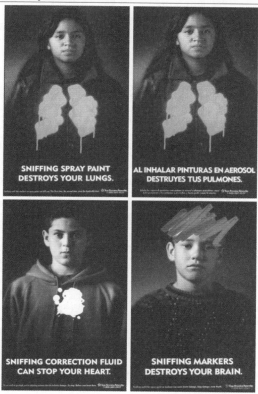

Fig **6.10** These bilingual posters, produced by the Texas Prevention Partnership, contributed to a campaign against inhalant misuse, which ran from 1990 to 1994. Use of inhalants fell by more than 32% in elementary schools and by ~20% in high schools.[59]

With permission from SYNERGIES, dba National Inhalant Prevention Coalition, www.
inhalants.org.

Cardiovascular disease (CVD) is a significant cause of mortality and morbidity and accounts for ~⅓ of all UK deaths. However, deaths from CVD have fallen in the UK since the late 1970s—due to better intervention and treatment, and greater preventative measures.

Goals of CVD risk assessment and management
- To reduce the risk of developing cardiovascular disease, which includes coronary heart disease (angina and MI), stroke and TIA, and peripheral arterial disease (ie all diseases caused by atherosclerosis)
- To improve quality of life and life expectancy.

Risk factors for developing CVD
Non-modifiable: ↑age; ♂>♀; family history; ethnicity (eg South Asian>European).

Modifiable: Smoking; low HDL-cholesterol/high non-HDL-c; sedentary lifestyle; unhealthy diet; excess alcohol; obesity.

Comorbidities (↑ risk): Hypertension; diabetes; CKD; dyslipidaemia; AF; RA/SLE; severe mental health problems.

Other factors: CVD risk is strongly associated with low income and social deprivation.

▶ *Targeting and modifying risk factors, and optimizing treatment of co-morbidities reduces risk of developing CVD.*

Strategies for preventing CVD
Primary prevention: eg NHS *Health Check Programme*—those aged 40-74 without CVD are invited every 5 years for a free health check, including CVD risk assessment (although evidence suggests general health checks do not have an effect on overall total mortality or mortality due to CVD).[40]

Secondary prevention: People who already have CVD can benefit from risk factor modification and cardiac rehabilitation (if appropriate).

Population-based strategies to prevent CVD: eg promoting walking and cycling as a means of transport or for recreation.

Assessing risk

CVD risk assessment tools assess the risk of developing cardiovascular disease (eg QRISK®2). This computer-based program uses details of age, sex, ethnicity, postcode, smoking status, selected medical and family history, blood pressure, BMI, and HDL-cholesterol ratio to determine a percentage risk of developing CVD over the next 10 years. NB: The following groups are excluded: those with T1DM; CKD; familial hypercholesterolaemia; or >85yrs.

The QRISK®2 score is expressed as a percentage (eg 14% risk of developing CVD within the next 10 years). Remember the risk score is an estimate. Everyone is at risk—low risk does not mean no risk.

Management of risk

CVD risk <10%: Although risk is low, advice can be given on reducing risk within relevant lifestyle factors or optimizing relevant co-morbidities.

CVD risk >10%: As well as advising on lifestyle factors and optimizing treatment of relevant co-morbidities, NICE recommend offering lipid-modifying therapy (eg *atorvastatin* 20mg OD; if no CI) to reduce risk. This can be delayed if lifestyle interventions are likely to reduce risk to <10%. Discuss the benefits and risks of starting a statin.

Lifestyle advice: Stop smoking; weight loss if overweight; eat a healthy diet; keep alcohol within recommended limits; encourage physical activity.

Further reading
NICE (2014). *Clinical Knowledge Summaries: CVD Risk Assessment and Management*. http://cks.nice.org.uk/lipid-modification-cvd-prevention

NICE (2014). *Lipid Modification: Cardiovascular Risk Assessment and the Modification of Blood Lipids for the Primary and Secondary Prevention of Cardiovascular Disease* (CG181). London: NICE.

NHS targets aim to decrease smoking from current levels (21%) to <15% by 2018. The smoking in public places ban in England in 2007 is estimated to have helped ≥400,000 people quit.[41][NICE]

Epidemiologists say that ~50% of smokers will die of smoking if they don't quit, losing ~25 years. Stopping smoking diminishes excess risk from tobacco, so that after 10-15yrs the risk of lung cancer approaches that of lifelong non-smokers. A similar but quicker decrease of excess risk (halved in 1st year) is found for deaths from coronary disease and, to a lesser extent, risk of stroke.[42]
►*60% of smokers want to give up*, and help with this achieves better outcomes.

Advantages of stopping smoking
• Less cancer—smoking accounts for ~29% of all cancer deaths
• Less chronic lung disease (COPD, recurrent chest infection, asthma exacerbation)
• Less cardiovascular disease (CHD, CVA, and peripheral arterial disease)
• Fewer problems in pregnancy—less pre-eclampsia, IUGR, preterm delivery, neonatal and late fetal death
• Less risk from passive smoking (cot deaths, lung disease, lung cancers)
• Return of the sense of taste and smell—and relative wealth.

To quit
1 Ask about smoking in all consultations (not just where relevant; be subtle; patients won't listen if agendas clash). Greet *any* success with enthusiasm!
2 Advise according to need. Ensure that advice is congruent with beliefs.
3 Motivate patients by getting *them* to list the advantages of quitting.
4 Assist in practical ways, eg negotiate a commitment to a 'quit date' when there will be few stresses; agree on jettisoning all smoking junk (cigarettes, ash trays, lighters, matches) in advance. Inform friends of new change.
5 Arrange follow-up—until that date consider texting patients (get consent) to send messages of encouragement (can ↑quitting from 13% to 28%).[43]

Pharmaceutical aids to smoking cessation (BNF 4.10)

Nicotine replacement therapy (NRT) Increases the chance of quitting by ×1.5. All preparations are equally effective. Start with higher doses for heavy smokers. Continue treatment for 3 months and tail off gradually over 2 weeks before stopping (except gum which can be stopped abruptly). *Contraindications:* Immediately post-MI, stroke or TIA; and if arrhythmia.

Nicotine withdrawal symptoms:
• Urges to smoke (70%)
• ↑ appetite mean (70%) 3–4kg weight ↑
• Depression (60%)
• Restlessness (60%)
• Poor concentration (60%)
• Irritability/aggression (50%)
• Night-time awakening (25%)
• Light headedness (10%)

Varenicline (eg Champix®) Smokers (>18yrs) start taking the tablets 1wk before the intended quit day (0.5mg OD for 3d; then 0.5mg BD for 4d; then 1mg BD for 11wks; 1mg OD if renal impairment/elderly). Cessation rate increased ×2. If the patient has stopped smoking after 12wks consider a further 12wk course to ↓risk of relapse. *Caution* in psychiatric disease. Advise to stop if agitated, depressed or suicidal.

Bupropion (eg Zyban®) Smokers (>18yrs old) start taking the tablets 1–2wks before an intended quit date (150mg for 3d then 150mg BD for 7–9wks). Cessation rate increased ×2. *Contraindications:* Epilepsy, or ↑risk of seizures, eating disorders, bipolar disorder.

► Prescribe *only* for smokers who commit to a target stop date. Initially prescribe enough to last 2wks after stop date. Only offer a further prescription if the patient demonstrates a continuing commitment to stop smoking. If unsuccessful the NHS will not fund another attempt for ≥6 months.

The problem isn't alcohol, it's life—lives in which sobriety poses insuperable problems: consciousness of futility, debt, responsibility, and social inhibitions. Alcohol obliterates all these, and will continue to do so, until other methods are more attractive. Cheap alcohol and peer pressure matter too. UK alcohol deaths: >20,000/yr.[44]

With the toll that excess alcohol takes in terms of personal misery and cost to the NHS (>£1.7 billion/yr[UK]), the need to reduce alcohol use and its root causes should be almost top of the government's social policy goals. But a powerful industry ensures that alcohol is cheaper (relatively) and more readily available than ever before—so that its use on an individually moderate scale arouses no comment. It is assumed to be safe, provided one is not actually an alcoholic. It is more helpful to view alcohol risks and benefits as a spectrum.

Prevalence of excess alcohol and recommended limits
- One unit is 8g ethanol, ie 1 measure of spirits, 1 glass of wine, or half a pint of ordinary-strength beer.
- Recommended limits: <21u/week ♂; <14u/week ♀ (NB: risk is a continuum).
- Binge drinking = >8u for ♂, or >6u for ♀ in 1d (affects 21% ♂; 9% ♀).
- Hazardous/harmful/problem drinking is excess intake causing potential or actual harm, but without dependence (affects 32% ♂; 15% ♀).
- Alcohol dependence results in withdrawal symptoms if alcohol consumption is decreased. It affects 6% ♂; 2% ♀.

▶A strategy to reduce bad effects of alcohol in your patients might comprise:
- If a symptom could be alcohol related, ask *in detail* about consumption.
- Question any patient with 'alerting factors'—accidents, driving offences, child neglect, assault, attempted suicide, depression, obesity. Question others as they register, consult, or attend for any health check.
- Use screening interventions (eg WHO *Alcohol Use Disorders Identification Test* AUDIT-C & AUDIT) to identify risk and offer education/advice.
- Screen for and manage any related health problems (see p376).

Helping people to cut down For specific treatment see p376 ▶Time interventions for when motivation is maximal, eg as (or before) pregnancy starts.
- Take more non-alcoholic drinks; reduce the sip frequency of alcoholic drinks.
- Limit opening hours; don't drink alone or with habitual drinkers; sip, don't gulp.
- Don't buy yourself a drink when it is your turn to buy a round of drinks.
- Go out to the pub later (but some pubs now open all night).
- Take 'days of rest' when no alcohol is used.

Agree goals to maintaining ↓drinking An alcohol diary helps get facts right.
- Teach how to estimate alcohol intake (u/week).
- Give feedback—eg if GGT (γ-glutamyl transpeptidase) falls are discussed, there is much lower mortality, morbidity, and hospitalization.
- Enlist family support; suggest a system of 'rewards' for sobriety.
- Community alcohol teams and treatment units may be required for alcohol dependency (see p376).

▶*Primary care is a good setting for prevention*: intervention leads to less alcohol consumption by ~15%, reducing the proportion of heavy drinkers by 20%—at one-twentieth the cost of specialist services. There is no evidence that GP intervention has to include more time-consuming advice such as compressed cognitive/behavioural strategies. Simple advice works fine as judged by falling GGT levels, at least for men. After interventions, women may report drinking less, but this is not reflected in a falling GTT.[45]

Further reading
NICE (2011) *Alcohol use disorders: diagnosis, assessment and management of harmful drinking and alcohol dependence* (CG115). London: NICE.

NICE (2010) *Alcohol use disorders: preventing the development of hazardous and harmful drinking* (PH24). London: NICE.

Primary care

Assessing and managing drug misuse

Assessment of drug misuse The most frequently abused drugs are cannabis, amphetamine, ecstasy, and cocaine. 14% of ♂ and 8% of ♀ aged 16–59 report taking illicit drugs in the last year. 3 factors appear important: availability; vulnerable personality; social pressures—particularly from peers. (See also p374.)

Detection: Suspicious requests for drugs of abuse eg opiate analgesia with no clear medical indication, or prescription requests which are too frequent. *Signs and symptoms:* • Inappropriate behaviour • Lack of self-care • Unusually constricted/dilated pupils • Evidence of injecting • Hepatitis or HIV infection. *Social factors:* Family disruption; criminal record.

Take a history of drug use/behaviour: Reason for consulting now; willingness to change; current and past usage; knowledge of risks; unsafe sex?

Take a medical and psychiatric history: Complications of drug abuse; alcohol use; overdose (accidental/deliberate). Consider urine toxicology to confirm drug misuse; consider blood for FBC, LFT, hepatitis, and HIV screening (with consent).

Management of drug misuse Aims to reduce drug-related morbidity and mortality; decrease risk of infectious diseases, and decrease criminal activity used to finance drug habits. The GP and primary care team have a vital role in:
• Identifying drug misusers
• Assessing health/willingness to modify drug behaviour (see stages of change model in the BOX on p471).

Education •Advise on safer routes of administration (eg smoking/rectal administration for heroin abusers); discourage IM/SC administration.
• Specific risks of drugs (eg psychosis with amphetamines; possible contamination)
• Safe injecting, overdose prevention, and basic first-aid training
• Safe sexual practices/condom use
• Discuss driving and drug misuse (see p492)
• Consider testing for/treating blood-bourne disease and offer hepatitis B immunization using the accelerated regimen (immunization at 0, 7, and 21d, and a booster after 12m) + offer immunization to close contacts of those already infected.

Treatment of dependence (See also p374)
• Set realistic goals—aim to help the patient remain healthy, until, with appropriate care and support, he/she can achieve a drug-free life. The aims of treatment are often best met by specialist services and substitute maintenance prescribing eg with methadone for heroin abuse.
• Set conditions for acceptable behaviour and treatment withdrawal. Agree on the pharmacy to be used and involve the pharmacist.
• Review regularly.
• Report patients who start treatment for drug abuse to the relevant authorities (see BOX). All types of problem drug misuse should be reported. NB: Databases cannot be used as a check on multiple prescribing as data are anonymized.
• Refer to community substance misuse team as needed.

National drug misuse databases/centres

England National Drug Treatment Monitoring System (NDTMS).

Scotland Substance Misuse Programme (SMP).

Wales Welsh National Database for Substance Misuse.

Northern Ireland Northern Ireland Drug Misuse Database (NIDMD).

Primary care

The prevalence of obesity (BMI >30kg/m²): USA 27%, UK 24%, Italy 10%. Obesity is the commonest disorder of childhood and adolescence (see *BMI charts*, p226–7 and *preventing adult diseases in childhood*, p156).

Body mass index (BMI)	
BMI = weight in kg / (height in m)²	
18.5–24.9	Healthy weight
25–29.9	Overweight
30–34.9	Obesity I (>27.5 if Asian)
35–39.9	Obesity II
>40	Obesity III (morbid obesity)

BMI (see MINIBOX) is the best measure of obesity. Waist circumference (measured midway between lower ribs and iliac crest) is an alternative measure of body fat correlated with CHD risk, DM, ↑BP, and ↑lipids. (See also 'Healthy diets', OHCM p236.)

Health risks of obesity
- *Greatly increased risk* (RR >3): Mortality (BMI >30); T2DM; gallbladder disease; dyslipidaemia; insulin resistance; breathlessness; sleep apnoea.
- *Moderately increased risk* (RR 2–3): CHD (5–6% of deaths are due to obesity); ↑BP; OA (knees); hyperuricaemia/gout.
- *Slightly increased risk* (RR 1–2): Cancer (breast, endometrial, oesophageal, colon); reproductive hormonal abnormalities; impaired fertility; PCOS; low back pain; stress incontinence; anaesthetic/surgical risks; suicide; bullying.

Causes • Physical inactivity • Cultural factors • Low education • Polygenic genetic predisposition • Smoking cessation • Childbirth (especially if not breastfeeding) • Drugs eg steroids, antipsychotics (olanzapine), contraceptives (especially depot-injections), insulin • Endocrine causes (rare; eg hypothyroidism, Cushing's, PCOS).

Typical needs Women: 2079kcal/d (♂ ≈2605); most eat ≥10% more than needed. Once weight goes up, physical activity lessens, and weight increases further.

Management Prevention begins in childhood with healthy patterns of exercise/diet. In obese adults, the main problem is maintaining lost weight.

Initial assessment: Assess willingness to change (see stages of change model in the BOX, p417), eating behaviour and diet, physical activity, psychological distress, and social and family factors affecting diet. Measure BMI and waist circumference. Check BP, blood glucose (for undiagnosed diabetes), and lipid profile.

Advice: Whether willing to change or not, provide advice on risks of obesity and benefits of healthy eating (OHCM p236) and physical exercise. Tailor your advice to the individual and if unwilling to change reinforce at each encounter.

Diet: Advise a weight loss diet for any patient who is overweight or obese and is willing to change:
- *Low-calorie diets:* All obese people lose weight on low-energy intake. Aim for weight loss of 0.5–1kg/week using a reduction of ~600kcal/d with a target BMI of 25, in steps of 5–10% of original weight. There is no health benefit of weight loss below this. If simple diet sheets are not effective, refer to a dietician. 500kcal/day reduction without any change of activity leads to ~0.45kg of weight loss/wk. Easy!

Drug therapy: Orlistat (120mg TDS with food) is the only drug licensed for treatment of obesity in the UK. It acts by ↓ fat absorption. Consider a 3-month trial if supervised diet/exercise has failed and BMI >30 (or >27 if co-morbidity). Continue after 3 months only weight ↓ is ≥5% initial body weight.

Group and behavioural therapy: Group activities (eg Weight Watchers®) have a higher success rate in producing and maintaining weight loss. Behavioural therapy together with low-calorie diets is also effective.

Surgery: Consider if BMI >40 and non-surgical measures have failed. Laparoscopic adjustable gastric banding is most commonly used (OHCM p628).

Further reading
SIGN (2010). *Management of obesity.* Edinburgh: SIGN.

Primary care

Insomnia describes a perception of disturbed or inadequate sleep. ~1:4 of the UK population (♀>♂) are thought to suffer in varying degrees. *Prevalence:* Increases with age (1:2 if >65yrs old). It can adversely affect quality of life, concentration and memory, performance of daytime tasks and cause relationship problems. 10% of traffic accidents are thought to be related to tiredness. Causes are numerous—common examples include:

• *Minor, self-limiting:* Travel, stress, shift work, small children, arousal.
• *Psychological:* ~½ have mental health problems: depression, anxiety, mania, grief, alcoholism.
• *Physical:* Drugs (eg steroids), pain, pruritus, tinnitus, sweats (eg menopause), nocturia, obstructive sleep apnoea.

What counts as 'a good night's sleep'? • <30min to fall asleep • Maintenance of sleep for 6–8h • <3 brief awakenings/night • Feeling well and refreshed on waking.

Management Careful evaluation. Many do not have a sleep problem themselves, but a relative feels there is a problem (eg the retired milkman who continues to wake at 4am). Others have unrealistic expectations: 'I need 12h sleep a night'. Reassurance may be all that is required. For genuine problems:

• *Eliminate physical problems preventing sleep:* eg treat asthma/eczema; give long-acting painkillers to last the night.
• *Treat psychiatric problems:* eg depression, anxiety.
• *Sleep hygiene:* see BOX.
• *Relaxation techniques:* eg self-help CDs.
• *Consider drug treatment:* Last resort 'only when insomnia is severe, disabling, or subjecting the individual to extreme distress'.

Drug treatment Zolpidem (5–10mg nocte), zopiclone (3.75–7.5mg nocte), benzodiazepines (eg temazepam 10mg nocte), and low-dose amitriptyline (10–30mg nocte) are all commonly prescribed for patients with insomnia. *Side effects:* Amnesia and daytime sleepiness. Most hypnotics affect daytime performance and may cause falls in the elderly. Warn about the effect on driving/operating machinery. Up to 40% of people with insomnia are thought to self-medicate with over-the-counter hypnotics that are available without prescription (eg sedative antihistamines).

▶Concerns about the use of benzodiazepines/z-drugs is that many people develop tolerance to their effects, gain little therapeutic benefit from long-term use, become dependent on them (both physically and psychologically), and suffer a withdrawal syndrome when they stop taking them. The Committee on Safety of Medicines recommend that the use of benzodiazepines for the treatment of insomnia should be restricted to severe insomnia and that treatment should be at the lowest dose possible and not be continued beyond 4 weeks.

▶▶Beware the temporary resident who has 'forgotten' his/her night sedation.

Primary care

Principles of 'sleep hygiene'	
• Don't go to bed until you feel sleepy	• Don't stay in bed if you're not asleep
• Avoid daytime naps	• Establish a regular bedtime routine
• Reserve a room for sleep only (if possible), do not eat, read, work or watch TV in it	• Make sure the bed is comfortable and avoid extremes of noise or temperature
• Avoid caffeine, alcohol, and nicotine	• Have a warm bath at bedtime
• Take regular exercise, but avoid late night hard exercise (sex is ok)	• Monitor your sleep with a sleep diary (length and quality of sleep)
• Rise at the same time every morning regardless of how long you've slept	

The material on these pages has been adapted from the *Oxford Handbook of General Practice* 4th edition by Simon *et al*, and has been reproduced by permission of Oxford University Press.

Recommended amounts of activity Adults: ≥30min/d of moderate intensity exercise ≥5d/wk; children ≥1h/d moderate intensity exercise every day. In the UK, 60% of adults are not active enough to benefit their health.

Health benefits of exercise *There is decreased risk of:* DM—through ↑insulin sensitivity; CVD—physically inactive people have ×2 ↑risk of CHD and ×3 ↑risk of stroke; osteoporosis—exercise ↓risk of hip fractures by ½; cancer— ↓risk of colon cancer; obesity (p514).

Exercise is a useful treatment for BP—can delay onset of hypertension and ↓BP by 10mmHg; MI; COPD; DM; hypercholesterolaemia— ↑HDL and ↓LDL; arthritis and back pain; mental health problems— ↓depression and anxiety. *In the elderly:* Exercise maintains functional capacity; ↓levels of disability and risk of falls/hip fracture; and improves quality of sleep.

Effective interventions
• *Practical advice* Enquire about activity levels and remind of the benefits of exercise; reinforce with leaflets/posters around the surgery. Assess willingness to change and suggest moderate exercise eg walking/cycling that can be incorporated into daily life (eg to work/school). Congratulate any success!
• *Health care* Counselling is as effective as more structured exercise sessions. Specialist rehabilitation schemes are available for specific conditions (eg post MI; COPD). Exercise schemes operate in some areas offering low-cost supervised gym exercise accessed via 'GP prescription'. Many sports facilities offer special sessions for pregnant women, the over 50s, and people with disability.

Healthy eating

The ideal diet should include a variety of foods. Advise patients to avoid snacking between meals.
• *Use starchy food* (eg bread,pasta, rice, potatoes) as the main energy source.
• *Eat plenty of fruit and vegetables* (>5 portions of fruit and/vegetables /d).
• *Eat plenty of fibre:* Good sources are high-fibre breakfast cereals, beans, pulses, wholemeal bread, potatoes (with skins), pasta, rice, oats, fruit/veg.
• *Eat fish:* At least ×2/wk, including one portion (max. ×2 if pregnant) of oily fish (eg mackerel, herring, salmon).
• *Choose lean meat:* Remove excess fat/poultry skin and pour off fat after cooking; use unsaturated oil to cook; boil/steam/bake in preference to frying. Use less cooked or processed red meat—consider substituting meat with vegetable protein (eg pulses; soya). Avoid fatty meats (eg sausages; salami).
• *Use skimmed milks:* And low fat yoghurts/spreads/cheese.
• *Avoid adding salt:* Aim for <6g of salt/d. Avoid processed foods, crisps, and salted nuts.
• *Avoid adding sugar:* And cut down on sweets, biscuits, and desserts.
• *Drink at least 2–3L of fluid daily:* Preferably not tea, coffee, or alcohol. Drinking a large glass of water with meals can reduce the urge to overeat.

Malnutrition 50% ♂; 25% ♀ >85y are unable to cook a meal alone. ▶ Malnutrition is common amongst the elderly. *Risk factors:* Low income; living alone; mental health problems; dementia; recent bereavement; gastric surgery; malabsorption; ↑metabolism; difficulty eating/swallowing (eg MND; CVA); chronic disease (eg IBD; IBS; cancer; CCF; COPD).

Management of malnutrition: Encourage to eat more and consider using nutritional, vitamin, and mineral supplements on dietician advice. Consider referral to social services if an inability to prepare meals/shop, or OT referral if difficulty with utensils.

We need to know about alternative medicine to understand our patients' undeclared distress, which use of these treatments is so often a sign of. We can also advise on the safety of various therapies. We must also learn from therapists about patient-centred care, and the sustainability of health care. This entails systems of interacting methods to restore and optimize health that have an ecological foundation, that are environmentally, economically and socially viable indefinitely, and that function harmoniously both with the human body and our wider environment, and that do not result in unfair or disproportionate impact on any ecosystem. *Alliance for Natural Health www.anh-europe.org*

Some alternative therapies are the orthodoxies of a different time (eg *herbalism*) or place (the *Ayurvedic medicine* of India), some are mainly diagnostic (*iridology*), some therapeutic (*aromatherapy*). Some doctors are suspicious of unorthodox medicine, and feel that its practitioners should not be 'let loose' on patients. But in many places the law is that, however unorthodox a practitioner may be, he or she cannot be convicted of unethical practice in the absence of clear harm. Many people (~5 million/yr in the UK) consult alternative practitioners, often as a supplement to orthodox treatment. Some will feel unable to tell their doctor about trips to alternative therapists, unless asked.

Modern medicine is criticized for sacrificing humanity to technology, and with little benefit for many people. In contrast to the orthodox doctor, alternative therapists are seen as taking time to listen, laying on hands rather than instruments, and giving medicines free (not always!) from side-effects.

Acupuncture Can treat many ailments; increasingly used in orthodox practice for pain relief (recommended by NICE in treatment of non-specific low back pain), control of nausea and treatment of addiction. Two predominant theories as to how it works are: **1** by causing muscle relaxation through trigger point stimulation and **2** through endorphin release. In some circumstances a combination of the 2 mechanisms are likely to make it effective (eg back pain). For migraines, endoprhin release is the likely predominant mechanism.

Homeopathy is based on the idea that 'like cures like', and that remedies are improved ('potentiated') by increasing dilution. Randomized trials show no greater efficacy than placebo, or suggest real (small) benefits, eg in asthma.

Manipulative therapies (osteopathy; chiropracty) are widely used and may help musculoskeletal and other problems, eg asthma.

Yoga This is an ancient Indian discipline with physical, mental, and spiritual components which aims to achieve a state of spiritual insight and tranquility. Randomized trials show that yoga can produce worthwhile benefit.

Holism Holism entails a broad view: of the patient as a person, of the role of the therapist, of the therapies used. The patient's autonomy is encouraged through involvement in decisions, and nurturing of self-reliance. ►*Specialism doesn't exclude holism:* nephrologists can be as holistic as naturopaths. As shown on p476, most models of the GP consultation are based on a patient-centred holistic approach. Compare the sequence 'bronchitis→antibiotic' with 'bronchitis→smoker→stressed→redundancy-counselling→?antibiotic'.

'Doctor, can I use alternative therapy for HRT?' One answer might be: 'Extracts from red clover (*Trifolium pratense*), soybean (*Glycine max*), and black cohosh (*Cimicifuga racemosa*; eg 8mg of standardized extract PO/24h) are often used. Some trials support their use,[46,47] but these are active agents that might have the same SEs as HRT. You could try them, and you might well be lucky. ►Beware advertising influences.'

Integrative medicine This is a patient-centred, interdisciplinary, non-hierarchical mix of conventional and complementary solutions to case management of patients with complex problems, eg chronic low back or neck pain.[48]

Domestic violence: the GP's role

Domestic violence is defined as any incident or pattern of incidents of controlling, coercive, or threatening behaviour, violence or abuse between those aged ≥16y who are/have been intimate partners, or family members regardless of gender or sexuality. This can encompass, but is not limited to, the following types of abuse: • Psychological • Sexual • Financial • Physical • Emotional.

Controlling behaviour: Acts designed to make people subordinate/dependent by isolating them from sources of support, exploiting their resources/capacity for personal gain, depriving them of means needed for independence, resistance ± escape, and regulating their everyday behaviour.

Coercive behaviour: Act/pattern of acts of assault, threats, humiliation, and intimidation or other abuse used to harm, punish, or frighten victims.

Prevalence Although men may be the victims of domestic violence, ~80% of reported domestic violence is against women by male partners. Domestic violence affects 1 in 4 women and is the most common form of inter-personal crime: 60%—current partner; 21%—former partner; half suffer >1 attack; 1 in 3 have been attacked repeatedly.

Effects High incidence of psychiatric disorders, particularly depression and self-damaging behaviours, eg drug/alcohol abuse, suicide/parasuicide.

Factors preventing the victim leaving the abusive situation
• Loss of self-esteem makes the victim think they are to blame
• Disruption of the family and children's relationship with partner
• Loss of intimate relationship with the partner
• Fear of partner
• Fall in income
• Risk of homelessness
• Fear of the unknown.

Presentation General practice is often the first place in which victims seek formal help, but only 1 in 4 actually reveals the true nature of the problem. Without appropriate intervention, violence continues and often increases in severity and frequency. By the time injuries are visible, violence may be a long-established pattern. On average, victims will be assaulted 35 times before reporting it to police.

Guidelines for care
• Consider the possibility of domestic violence—ask directly ►30% of domestic violence starts in pregnancy.
• Emphasize confidentiality.
• Document—accurate, clear documentation, over time, at successive consultations may provide cumulative evidence of abuse and is essential for use as evidence in court, should the need arise.
• Assess the present situation—gather as much information as possible.
• Provide information; offer help to make contact with other agencies.[6]
• Devise a safety plan, eg give the phone number of a local refuge; advise to keep some money and important financial and legal documents hidden in a safe place in case of emergency; help plan an escape route in case of emergency.

►Do not pressurize the victim into any course of action. If the patient decides to return to the violent situation, she or he will not forget information and support given. In time this might give them the confidence and back-up needed to break out of the situation.

►►If children are likely to be at risk you have a duty to inform social services or the police, preferably with the patient's consent.

6 Women's Aid 0808 2000 247 www.womensaid.org.uk; Police domestic violence units.

Primary care

This is a single or repeated act or lack of appropriate action, occurring within any relationship where there is an expectation of trust, which causes harm or distress to an older person. Prevalence is 4% (↑ with age; ♀:♂≈2:1). Older people often do not report abuse. Forms of abuse:

- *Physical:* eg cuts, bruises, unexplained fractures, burns
- *Psychological:* eg unusual behaviour, unexplained fear, appears helpless or withdrawn
- *Financial:* eg removal of funds by carers, new will in favour of carer
- *Sexual:* eg vaginal or anal bleeding, genital infections
- *Neglect:* eg malnourished, dehydrated, poor personal hygiene, late requests for medical attention.

Signs Inconsistent story from patient and carer; inconsistences on examination; fear in presence of carer; frequent attendance at ED; frequent requests for GP visits; carer avoiding GP.

Management Talk through the situation with the patient, carer, and other services involved in care. Assess the level of risk. Consider admission to a place of safety—contact social services and/or police as necessary; seek advice from Action on Elder Abuse.[7]

Adult safeguarding An adult (>18y) at risk of harm:
- May be in receipt of community care services by reason of mental/other disability, age, or illness, and
- May be unable to take care of him/herself, or
- Is unable to protect him/herself from serious harm/exploitation.

If suspected, contact local social services adult safeguarding lead (with consent if the patient is able to give consent).

The material on these pages has been adapted from the *Oxford Handbook of General Practice* 4th edition by Simon *et al*, and has been reproduced by permission of Oxford University Press.

7 Action on Elder Abuse 0808 808 8141 www.elderabuse.org.uk

GPs as managers GP partners have dual roles as both clinicians and managers of small businesses. There are 5 managerial functions:

1 *Planning:* Involves selecting missions and objectives, and the actions to achieve them—this requires decision-making

2 *Organizing:* Defining roles—ensuring all tasks necessary to accomplish goals are assigned to those people who can do them best

3 *Staffing:* Ensuring all positions in the organizational structure are filled with people able to fulfil those roles

4 *Leading:* Influencing people so that they will contribute to organization and group goals

5 *Controlling:* Measuring and correcting individual and organizational performance to ensure events conform to plans.

Management and teamwork Key features which contribute to successful teamwork are:

• *Communication:* Information sharing, feedback, and grievance airing
• *Clear team roles:* Especially with regard to responsibility and accountability
• *Sympathetic leadership:* A weak leader may allow the team to drift but an autocratic leader may be too directive and diminish the status of others, thus reducing the effectiveness of the team
• *Clear decision-making process:* Especially if there are differences of opinion
• *Pooling:* Knowledge, experience, skills, resources, and responsibility for outcome
• *Specialization of function:* Team members must understand and respect the role and importance of other team members
• *Delegation:* Work of the team is split between members and each member leaves the others to carry out functions delegated to them
• *Group work:* Team members share and are committed to a common, agreed purpose or goal which directs their actions.

Commissioning

The *Health and Social Care Bill* (2011) laid the foundations for groups of GPs and other clinical professionals to group together in *Clinical Commissioning Groups* to take on formal responsibility for commissioning the majority of NHS services in England, working in partnership with other health professionals, local communities, and local authorities.

Aims of commissioning: • To design improved patient pathways • To enable more efficient use of funds so that savings can be used to provide better patient services • To enable improved community and hospital services that better meet the needs of patients.

Clinical Commissioning Groups (CCGs): Every GP practice in England must be part of a CCG. The CCG governing body has decision-making powers, which meets in public and publishes minutes of meetings. The board is comprised of: • ≥2 lay members (one championing public and patient involvement and one overseeing governance) • One registered nurse, and • One secondary care doctor (neither employed by a local provider).

Principles of commissioning are the same whichever organization is undertaking it: *Planning*—assessing needs of the local population and resources available; *Contracting*—commissioning services for local patients; *Monitoring*—monitoring delivery of the service and ensuring the service is kept on track; *Revision*—revising the needs of the CCG and arrangements with providers.

Primary care

Primary care is about risk and uncertainty, but sometimes unnecessary risks cause ourselves and our patients unnecessary harm. Defence organization records suggest that ~½ of all successful negligence claims reflect poor clinical judgement on the doctor's part; the other ½ represent avoidable mishaps which would be susceptible to risk management approaches—often failures in simple administrative systems, communication failures, inadequate records, or lack of training.

Risk management means taking steps to minimize risk and keep ourselves and others as safe as possible. There are 4 stages:

1 Identify the risk—through analysis of complaints and comments from GPs, other practice staff, or patients; through significant event analysis/audit (p534) or by using defence organization material to identify common pitfalls.
2 Assess frequency and severity of the risk.
3 Take steps to reduce or eliminate the risk.
4 Check the risk has been eliminated.

Categories of risk relevant to general practice
• Clinical care, eg prescribing errors • Non-clinical risks to patient safety, eg security and fire hazards • Organizational risks, eg failure to safeguard confidential information or unlicensed use of computer software • Financial risks, eg employment of a new staff member.

Key safety issues for primary care
• *Diagnosis:* 28% of reported errors.
• *Prescribing:* 1 in 5 prescriptions contains a prescribing error; 1 in 530 prescriptions contain a serious error; 9% of hospital admissions are due to potentially avoidable problems with prescribed drugs. 4% of drugs are incorrectly dispensed each year.
• *Communication:* Poor communication is a major cause of complaints; 28% of patients have discrepancies between the drugs prescribed at hospital discharge and those they receive in the community.
• *Organizational change:* In industry, better teamwork, communication, and leadership decreases adverse incidents.

In each case, consider:
• *Organizational and management factors:* Financial resources/constraints; practice policies; organization
• *Work environment factors:* Staffing levels; skill mix; work load; equipment
• *Team factors:* Team structure; communication; supervision
• *Individual (staff) factors:* Knowledge; skills; competence; health
• *Task factors:* Availability/use of protocols/guidelines; availability of results
• *Patients factors:* Condition (complexity and seriousness); language and communication; personality and social factors.

Is this the right patient? Changing processes to reduce risk

Time and again at our significant events meeting a case would be discussed of the 'wrong' patient being booked into an appointment simply because they had the same name as the patient who should have been booked. As a result, consultations were written up in the wrong record, referrals made for the wrong patient, and prescriptions issued to the wrong person. At first we agreed that it was everyone's responsibility (reception and clinical staff) to check 3 identifiers when booking or seeing a patient (eg name, DOB, and address). However, mistakes kept happening. We then introduced a pop-up alert which appears for any patient who has the same name as someone else in the practice to highlight that extra care is required in checking and selecting the correct record.

Primary care

As we move away from providing care in expensive high-technology hospitals, more is expected of primary care, with implications for capital expenditure, acquiring new skills, and local access to procedures needing expensive equipment, eg endoscopy or us. Whole specialisms such as dermatology and day-case surgery may move out of the secondary sphere, as the distinction between primary and secondary care becomes redundant. Anticoagulant clinics are another example of a hospital service which 'might as well be done in the community'. How are these developments to be structured (taking the NHS as an example)? What are the dangers and opportunities?

Market-led models Well-capitalized companies take over running general practices, after winning provider contracts from Clinical Commissioning Groups. Such companies create free-standing polyclinics, or run a chain of GP surgeries. Alternatively, large supermarkets/pharmacies create in-store health centres. In both, GPs become salaried employees of the company providing services. However, there are clear problems with corporate health care: the United States differs from other industrialized countries with its absence of universal health insurance coverage. It is the most expensive health care system in the world yet it consistently underperforms relative to other countries (eg on access, efficiency and equity), and fails to achieve better health outcomes.[7]

Federated GP-led models General practices club together to purchase equipment and consolidate services. This is the model favoured by the Royal College of General Practitioners—as providing the most flexible model which can rapidly adapt to local priorities,[49] cause the least disruption to existing services—and maintain continuity of care. Under this model GPs develop special interests and 'portfolio careers' playing to their strengths in both the clinical and administrative spheres in an increasingly complex health environment—in which they both commission and provide care.

Various kinds of federated GP models exist, from informal alliances to limited companies owned and run by GPs, who hold shares in the company. One thing held in common is that they are part of the NHS family, and share core NHS values of inclusivity, fairness, and distributive justice. The primary motive for their creation is to maintain general practice-based primary care—and the system whereby patients can see the doctor of their choice near where they live.

Polyclinics The RCGP cautions against developing polyclinics that focus on diseases and technical care—but commends the value of co-location of services to reduce fragmentation. Champions of polyclinics say they are: •Cheap •More integrated (easy to refer across the corridor) •Better equipped •Available out-of-hours (24/7). But continuity of care suffers; this is highly valued by patients, and gives much job satisfaction to GPs. Whatever models are adopted, the cardinal values of general practice such as interpersonal care and continuity of care based on defined populations must be given full weight.

Quality control[8] If a service such as INR testing is taken out of the lab and fragmented to a number of smaller community-based clinics, quality control becomes problematic. Ditto for the validation of GPs with special interests.

Conflicts of interest If a GP federation is a for-profit organization (with funds flowing from the NHS) and if the doctors are sitting on boards deciding on which services are to be commissioned, there is a conflict of interest. The NHS is establishing procedures to minimize risk from this possibility—but nevertheless, probity is a vital issue, for doctors as well as other NHS staff.

---

8 If a batch of reagents is faulty, the lab will be onto this at once, but who would know in the community if a batch of INR test strips was faulty? Perhaps only after a series of bloody deaths was investigated.

►There is nothing better (for the doctor and the patient) than doing a job for the love of it—and not many people love targets set by other people—so the target has to entail great benefits to outweigh its unintended consequences.

►Beware accepting a protocol without knowing if it will affect your sympathy and time to communicate (a good example of this is the now redundant, but previously compulsive 'biopsychosocial' assessment of depression for QOF, which 'hijacked' the initial assessment of patients presenting with depression).

►Is the protocol independently validated? What is its *hidden objective*, eg cost-containment, conformity, self-advertisement, empire-building, or care?

►Reject protocols that don't specify conflicts of interest: most protocols (87%) are written by people with financial links to drug companies or public bodies wishing to curtail expense.[50]

Sympathy is a flower which has often withered before the end of morning surgery. If a protocol says that you must do 9 things to Mrs James who has diabetes, both of you may be irritated by the time you reach item 5: the doctor is running out of time, and the patient is running out of goodwill. She is worrying about her husband's dementia, having long since stopped worrying about her own illnesses.

Guidelines are seen as friendly, if flexible, allowing for the frailties of clinical science as it meets bedside reality; they can also be interactive, if computer programming is skilful. Protocols, particularly if they have been handed down from some supposedly higher authority, have a reputation for being strict, sinister, and stultifying instruments for thought control. How well do these stereotypes stand up in practice? It is known that doctors working in highly regulated environments with strict protocols perform suboptimally.[51] It is also worth noting that very few laws define their own exceptions. You could say that patients have a right to be asked if they want to participate in a protocol, and if so, that it should be done properly. Herein lies the paradox of protocols. They are designed to remove the many indefensible inconsistencies found in clinical medicine, yet protocols depend on the individual doctor's own flair and instinctive judgement so that they are applied in the best way.

The best approach is to welcome good protocols, and develop meta-protocols to be answered whenever (or almost whenever) such protocols are not adhered to. Why did you not adhere to the protocol? Please tick the appropriate box:
• My own convenience, eg too many other more important tasks to do.
• My patient's preference (well informed or otherwise).
• Evidence is shaky and may not apply to my practice population.
• Inefficient use of resources, eg scarce consultations are used up in follow-up.
• My instinct warned me not to apply the protocol in this case.[9]

To get round the problems of non-implementation of guidelines, some NHS primary care trusts sent in visitors from *pharmaceutical advisers* who had trained in outreach visiting (it is unfair to call them *thought-police*). But when this has been evaluated in randomized trials, no impact could be detected.[52]

Can we square guidelines & targets with patient-centred care? (p474)
Answer: *No*; discussing this issue with purveyors of guidelines is a good way to reveal the hidden agendas described above.

---

9 Understandably, many GPs don't follow protocols despite high awareness of them: other reasons include the fact that precise targets (eg for BP control) are always arbitrary, and should allow for some variation. Be prepared to defend your deviation from a guideline should it ever be questioned.

Clinical governance is the *'framework through which NHS organizations are accountable for continuously improving the quality of their services and safe-guarding high standards of care, by creating an environment in which clinical excellence will flourish.'* It links continuing professional development, multidis-ciplinary learning, audit, risk management, and significant event reporting/analysis. It is about defining quality (eg standards set by NICE, CQC, QOF), assur-ing accountability, and improving quality (by monitoring standards).

Essential elements
- *Risk avoidance:* Risk management; clear protocols; safe environment
- *Infrastructure:* Access to evidence; time; training strategies; IT support
- *Clinical effectiveness:* Sharing good practice; significant event audit (see 'Audit', p524); evidence-based medicine
- *Audit:* Regular review of practice against quality standards (p524)
- *Education/training:* Effective appraisal; performance feedback; targeted education
- *Staff:* Training; leadership; communication; common goals/teamwork.

What does clinical governance entail? Within practices, individual doc-tors must consider their own professional development and educational needs. There must also be continuous review and appraisal of procedures and standards. Deficiencies in knowledge, skills, or experience must be acted upon through appropriate education and professional development. Resources should be provided to help develop clinical governance (eg protected time for audit, funding for courses and educational activities).

Significant event analysis All practices should analyse and discuss episodes where there has been a significant occurrence (either beneficial or deleteri-ous). This should be done in a systematic and detailed way to asertain what can be learnt about the overall quality of care and to indicate changes that might lead to future improvements. One method of reporting is to record: •*De-scription of the event* •*Learning outcomes* and •*Action plan* (eg of changes implemented).

Audit is the systematic critical analysis of quality of heath care. Its purpose is to appraise current practice (*What is happening?*) by measuring it against pre-selected standards (*What should be happening?*) to identify and implement areas for change (*What changes are needed?*) and thus improve performance. Audit is a continual process and an integral part of clinical governance.

Aims of audit	
Improved care of patients	Aid to administration
Enhanced professionalism of staff	Efficient use of resources
Aid to continuing education	Accountability to those outside medicine

Criterion based audit—the audit cycle The process of identifying areas of care to be audited, implementing necessary changes and periodically review-ing the same issues is known as the audit cycle.

1 *Identify the issue:* This can be any practice matter—clinical or adminis-trative. Make sure the topic is important, manageable, clearly defined, and data are available to assess the criteria chosen. Good starting points are significant events, QOF targets, complaints, clinical guidelines, or personal observations.

2 *Agree criteria:* These are specific statements of what should be happening. They might be laid down for quality payments, 'gold standard' care, or gen-erated within the practice.

3 *Setting standards:* These are the minimum levels of acceptable performance for a criterion (100% achievement is unusual). Set realistic standards. These can be based on previous audit, comparison with other practices, or guidelines (eg '90% of patients with iron deficiency anaemia should be screened for coeliac disease; British Society of Gastroenterologists 2005)'.

4 *Planning and preparation:* What data will you use?; How will you search for it?; What Read codes (see BOX, p531) will you use? What literature has been consulted?

5 *First data collection:* What is current practice (compared to standards set)?; What changes are needed?

6 *Implement changes.*

7 *Second data collection:* Monitor the effects of change and compare data with the first round of data collection and against standards set.

8 *Summary of findings.*

Care Quality Commission (CQC)

The Health and Social Care Act 2008 required any individual, partnership, or organization providing health care services in the UK to register with the CQC as a service provider. The CQC inspects practices to ensure they meet essential standards.

Regulated activities Practices must register for any of the 'regulated activities' they perform. Of the 15 listed, those that apply to primary care include:
• Treatment of disease, disorder or injury • Diagnostic and screening procedures • Surgical procedures (if minor surgery performed) • Family planning procedures.

Essential standards eg 'Respecting and involving patients'; 'Consent to care and treatment'. Practices must provide evidence that they meet 16 standards and if non-compliant, must take steps to ensure compliance is met.

Complaints

Complaints are a fact of life for most GPs. The most constructive and least stressful approach is to view them as a learning experience and a chance to improve practice risk management. Always contact your local medical committee (LMC) ± defence organization if you are directly implicated in a complaint. Patients who complain generally want:
• Their complaint to be heard and investigated promptly; and handled efficiently and sympathetically.
• To receive a genuine apology if mistakes have occurred; and to be assured that steps will be taken to prevent a recurrence.

Time limit for complaints NHS complaints can only be accepted <1y after the incident which is the subject of complaint, or <1y after the date at which the complainant became aware of the matter. There is a 3y time limit placed on civil negligence cases.

Process Once a complaint is received in general practice, the complaints manager (usually the practice manager) should acknowledge the complaint within 48h and advise the complainant of the right to use the *Independent Complaints Advocacy Service*. The complaints manager investigates the complaint, consulting all involved, and makes a written summary of the nature of the complaint, investigation findings, ± apology, ± actions to remedy the situation/prevent further occurrences. This must be completed <25d after the original date of the complaint. If the complaint is not resolved at this point, the complainant can refer the matter to the NHS ombudsman.

Appraisal All uk doctors practising medicine undergo a yearly appraisal. It has moved from being an informal chat with a peer to a formal structured review on which revalidation (see later in topic) is based. The supporting information that doctors use at their appraisal falls into 4 broad categories:

1 *General information:* Gives context about what you do in all aspects of work
2 *Keeping up to date:* How you maintain and enhance the quality of your work
3 *Review of your practice:* Evaluating the quality of your professional work
4 *Feedback on your practice:* How others perceive the quality of your work.

There are six types of supporting information that you need to provide and discuss at your appraisal.

1 *Continuing professional development (cpd):* cpd is the process of tracking and documenting knowledge and experience gained both formally and informally as you work + how you apply this to your work. cpd should be relevant to the current and emerging knowledge and skills required for your work. You also need to reflect and evaluate on what you have learnt and how this improves your performance. 50 hours of cpd are required each year.
2 *Quality improvement activity:* Eg completion of an audit cycle or a case review. Curently this is only required once every 5-year revalidation cycle.
3 *Significant events:* Record any incidents or events ± any investigation or analysis of these, lessons learnt, and action taken/changes implemented.
4 *Feedback from colleagues:* and 5 *Feedback from patients:* These are collected once every 5-year cycle using standardized questionnaires.
5 *Review of complaints and compliments.*

Appraisal is a supportive developmental process, to reflect on our work, to consider developmental needs, to assess our career, and to consider how we might gain more job satisfaction. 'By giving feedback on performance it provides the opportunity to identify any factors that adversely affect performance, and to consider how to minimize or eliminate their effects. It is an important building block in a clinical governance culture that *ensures* high standards and the best possible patient care.'Chief Medical 53 Officer

There is a big question-mark over 'ensures', above. The effect of appraisal on patient care is unknown—but appraisal, it is hoped, can offer opportunities for interdependent support, self-education, self-motivation, and career development in the wider medical world. It may also be a catalyst for change and even a tonic against complacency.

Appraisal assumes gps aim to be professional, life-long learners (the 'move-&-grow' aspect of challenging appraisals). If this is not the case, the less cosy revalidation, performance management, assessment, and mediation will bite.

Licence to practise To practise medicine in the uk, all doctors are required to be registered with the gmc and hold a licence to practise. This gives a doctor the legal authority to undertake certain activities in the uk, eg prescribing, signing death or cremation certificates, and working as a doctor in the nhs. Re-licensing occurs every 5 years by the process of revalidation.

Revalidation aims to guarantee public safety. It is the process by which licensed doctors are required to demonstrate they are up to date and fit to practise. Licensed doctors have to revalidate every 5 years, and revalidation is acheived by having annual appraisals and by providing the required 'supporting information' listed earlier. Revalidation may be deferred if insufficient evidence is provided or there are unresolved concerns about a doctors performance.

Further reading
gmc (2012). *Supporting Information for Revalidation and Appraisal.* http://www.gmc-uk.org/doctors/revalidation/revalidation_information.asp
gmc (2015). *The Licence to Practise.* http://www.gmc-uk.org/doctors/licensing.asp

It would be nice for the public and the 'leaders' of our profession if there were a small number of under-performing doctors who could be retrained or struck off. Things are rarely so simple, and we may have to accept that, for many reasons, including chance, training, and resilience, the performance of *all doctors* will, at times, be, or appear to be, suboptimal.

Could differences in data comparing doctors (even if that data were accurate, validated, and stratified for risk) occur by chance? Imagine a thought-experiment in which 4 equal doctors use different strategies for predicting whether a tossed coin will land heads or tails. One always chooses heads, one always chooses tails, and the other two alternate their choices out of synchrony with each other. When I did this experiment for a pre-decided 14 throws each (56 throws in total), the best doctor only had 2 'errors', whereas the worst had 7 errors—over 3 times the rate. The public would demand that this doctor be retrained or struck off. So, must we all be prepared to be sacrificial lambs? The answer is Yes, but there are certain steps that can be taken to mitigate our own and our patients' risk exposure.

- When we encounter doctors who are clearly underperforming (eg due to addictions) we must speak out. This will encourage belief in the system.
- GMC guidance says *'All doctors have a duty to raise concerns where they believe that patient safety or care is being compromised by the practice of colleagues, or the systems, policies and procedures in the organisations in which they work. They must also encourage and support a culture in which staff can raise concerns openly and safely'.*[10]
- We should encourage an atmosphere of mutual support and trust—the sort of environment in which doctors feel safe to say 'All my cases of X seem to be going wrong—can anyone think why?' To stop this trust turning into cronyism we must be prepared to engage in, or be subjected to, audit (p524).

10 GMC (2012). *Raising and Acting on Concerns about Patient Safety*, p5. London: GMC.

On any day ~60% of people take medication, only half of which are prescribed. The others are sold over the counter (OTC). The commonest OTCs are analgesics, cough medicines, and vitamins; for prescribed drugs, the common groups are anti-depressants, cardiovascular drugs, and antibiotics. On average, 6-7 NHS prescriptions are issued/person/year (21 in Italy and 11 in France).

GPs account for 75% of NHS annual prescribing costs (~10% of the total cost of the NHS), although many of these 'GP drugs' will have been initiated in hospital. The cost of these prescriptions has risen faster than inflation and is ~£300,000/GP/year. Positive correlations with low prescribing include a young doctor, practising in an affluent area, and longer consultation times (extra time spent explaining about minor illness (p488) replaces expectation for a prescription by belief in one's own health).

Dispensing doctors Where there is no chemist's shop (eg rural areas) UK GPs are paid to dispense to their patients. Their annual prescribing rate can be as low as 70% of their non-dispensing fellow GPs.

Compliance (Does the patient take the medicine?) ►*There is no point in being a brilliant diagnostician if nobody can be persuaded to take your treatments.* Even in life-threatening conditions, compliance is a major problem occurring in up to 56% of patients (eg adolescents with acute lymphatic leukaemia). The following are associated with increased compliance:
• Being able to identify with a personal doctor
• Patient's overall satisfaction with the doctor
• Simple therapeutic regimens
• Written information
• Longer consultation times or prescribing on home visits
• Prescribing in association with giving health education
• Continuity of care, coupled with belief in efficacy of the treatment
• Short waiting time for appointments
• The encouragement of self-monitoring by the patient.

Monitoring compliance: Monitoring plasma drug levels is the most reliable way of doing this, but it is cheaper to ask patients to return with their tablets, so that you can count them (or to count during a phone contact)—or, better still, establish a basis of trust so that the patient can check for him- or herself.

✷Compliance or concordance? *Compliance* suggests that you know best and patients who lapse are foolish. But it is known that adapting GP advice to their needs leads to fewer side effects, eg GI bleeding: your prescription may read 'ibuprofen 400mg/8h', but the patient may, sensibly, only take the drug when his joints are bad. Don't think of this as the patient failing to do something. It is you who have failed to reach a shared understanding of the pros and cons of drug-taking. *Concordance* denotes more than this: think of it as a liberating concept, promoting egalitarianism in medicine. ►*There is no healthier ideal.* Are you nodding in the direction of concordance while still covertly believing in compliance? Then let us put the boot on the other foot and await the time *you* are monitored for compliance with some marvellous guidelines: we predict that concordance will now seem more rational and desirable!

Primary care

Formularies Aim is to make prescribing more cost-effective, by compiling an agreed list of favoured drugs. This voluntary restriction can work in tandem with compulsory NHS restricted lists, and lead to substantial savings.

ScriptSwitch is a computer program that uses software to flag up more cost-effective prescribing solutions, which can be swapped with one click, if the GP so desires (eg valaciclovir→aciclovir).

Generic prescribing Using generic names when prescribing is one of the simplest ways to reduce cost (eg prescribing ***desogestrel*** 75mcg/d, instead of using the brand name Cerazette®). All drugs have a chemical name, a generic name, and a proprietary or brand name. When a new drug is brought to market, the company that developed the drug will derive income from prescriptions—whether the generic or brand name is prescribed—whilst the patent is still valid. Once the patent expires, any company can manufacture and market the drug. At this point, if drugs are prescribed generically, the pharmacist can decide which brand to supply and market forces drive the price down.

Advantages of generic prescribing:
• *Cost:* Generic prescribing is cheaper.
• *Clarity:* There can be several brand names for the same drug. Using generic names allows everyone to be clear which drug is being used.
• *Convenience:* Pharmacists do not stock all brand names and may have to order a supply whereas generic preparations of all commonly used drugs are available.

NB: Reasons not to prescribe generic drugs include • Drugs with a low therapeutic index (where small differences in plasma concentration may be significant (eg lithium, phenytoin) • Modified-release formulations, where pharmacokinetic properties are not standardized eg diltiazem, sulfasalazine, nifedipine, aminophylline • Formulations containing ≥2 drugs.

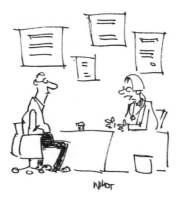

"I'd prescribe the drug, but considering the side effects, you're better off with the disease."

Fig 6.11 There is some truth in this humour: Consider the elderly gentleman with clinically insignificant prostate cancer and the side effects of hormone therapy—one of many possible examples.

With permission from CartoonStock.com.

There is great variability in individual GPs' referral statistics, which leads purveyors of government strategy to the error of saying 'Why is there a 4-fold difference in referral rates between GPs? Such variation is insupportable; some doctors must be referring too much ...' An advance is made when this issue is reframed as: '*There is information contained in this variability*'. This information can guide service development.

Referral rates Understanding the intricacies of purchasing health care depends on understanding referral patterns. If high-referring GPs refer needlessly, then the proportion of their referrals resulting in further action will be smaller than that of practices with low-referring GPs. Usually, this is not the case. Those with high referral rates have high rates of intervention. If I refer an ever-increasing number of my patients to an elderly-care clinic, must a time come when admissions level off? The idea of a 'levelling-off effect' is important. If the consultant is 'correct', and the GP's expectation as to the outcome of referral are uniform (probably never true) then when a levelling-off effect is observed, it may be true that the *average* referral rate is optimal, and that low-referrers are under-treating, and high-referrers are wasting money. In fact, levelling-off effects are rarely seen, except in general surgery. If the consultant is over-enthusiastic, and overstates treatment benefits, then the lower referrers are to be applauded for limiting the excesses of the consultant.

Appropriateness of referrals ▶ *In general, only agree that a referral is inappropriate if the patient, the GP, and the consultant concur on its lack of utility*. Each of these parties has different motivations—eg reassurance/explanation, medicolegal, as well as providing therapy. Despite the rhetoric, secondary care can be preoccupied by its own agendas and may have little interest in the unique needs of referred patients. Overall, referral rates are no more variable than admission rates, even in populations with similar morbidity. The reason may be that there is still a great deal of uncertainty underlying very many clinical decisions. We don't know who *exactly* should have knee replacements, cholecystectomy, etc.

▶ There is no known relationship between high or low referral rates and quality of care. Here are 3 cautions in interpreting referrals:

1 Don't accept GP list size as a denominator (takes no account of differing workloads in a practice). Consultations/yr is a better denominator.
2 If a GP has a special interest, this will influence referral patterns. More knowledge may lead to more referrals as partial knowledge leads to greater, not less, uncertainty. For example after a while all GPs with a special interest (GPSI) in dermatology will have been tricked by melanomas masquerading as seborrhoeic warts—so their referrals for histology will be higher than GPs who have less experience and have never been so tricked.
3 Years of data are needed to compare referrals to rarely used units.

Referral incentive schemes Are a complex and uncertain way to influence referrals. Local educational interventions with secondary care specialists and structured referral sheets can impact on referral rates. 'In-house' 2nd opinions and other primary care based alternatives to outpatient referral are promising. In 2013–14 >100 million out-patient appointments were scheduled by hospitals in England, an increase of 8.2% on the previous year.

Read codes are a hierarchical set of clinical terms that are used in patient electronic notes in UK general practice. They allow detailed coding of many areas, including symptoms, signs, investigations, diagnoses, treatments, and pathology results, as well as social information, eg occupation and ethnicity.

You do not need to learn the actual code to enter it, but simply choose a relevant term which has an associated code. The higher up the hierarchy, the less specific a code is. All codes contain 5 characters (with full stops used as 'padding' characters). The top level of the hierarchy is the chapter, or 'parent' code, and below that are associated 'daughter' codes. Eg:[54]

- G.... 'Circulatory system diseases'
- G3... 'Ischaemic heart disease'
- G30.. 'Acute myocardial infarction'
- G30y. 'Other acute myocardial infarction'
- G30y2 'Acute septal infarction'.

Using a coding system to record patient information allows for easy recording and retrieval of data; accurate reporting; income generation; research and data analysis. However, coding is only as good as the knowledge of coding by that doctor. Problems may arise when a 'diagnosis' code is entered for a symptom when the diagnosis is uncertain. Busy doctors have also learnt shortcuts by entering general codes such as 'Had a chat to patient' or 'Unwell generally'. Some codes are well known for being ridiculous (eg 'Accident caused by soap, stew or curries').[55]

Read codes have been in use in the NHS since 1985 and are continually updated. They were developed by a GP, Dr John Read and were purchased by the government in 1990 (owned by Crown Copyright). Read codes will eventually be replaced by a new coding system 'SNOMED Clinical Terms'—the aim being that all health care systems in the UK will use the same codes to allow for a unified patient record.

Patient participation groups (PPGs) ►Working *with* your patients is as important as working *for* them. The health care team meets with patients' representatives to discuss some of the following:

• Dealing with complaints (less adversarial than with formal methods—and independent of the NHS and doctors—hence reasonably credible).
• Harmonizing the 'consumer's' and the 'provider's' aims.
• Feedback to aid planning, implementation, and evaluation of services.
• Identifying unmet needs (eg among the isolated elderly).
• Improving links between the practice and other services.
• Health promotion in the light of local beliefs (p472).
• Pressurizing government institutions over inadequate services.

Owing to lack of interest, or to there being no clear leader or task, up to 25% of groups close over time. The complaint that participation mechanisms lead to tokenism (ie the democratic ideal has been exercised, but what has been created is just a platform for validating the *status quo*) does not turn out to be true if a group has power over funds which it has raised. Here, our experience is that analysis may be penetrating and decision swift, in a way that makes even the best-run health authorities/Trusts look pedestrian.

Another role for PPGs is to have dialogues with primary care organizations (PCOs) on proposed changes to services—eg whether practices are to be amalgamated or services withdrawn or replaced by provision via non-NHS private companies. PCOs have a statutory responsibility to consult, and patient participation groups have a valid role in bringing PCOs to account.[56]

The Patients' Association This group represents and furthers the interests of patients by giving assistance, advice, and information. It aims to promote understanding between patients and the medical world. Publications: *Patient Voice* and a directory of self-help organizations. See also the *Contact-a-Family* Directory: cafamily.org.uk

Self-help organizations Many thousands of these groups have been set up worldwide for sufferers of specific rare or common diseases. They offer information, companionship, comfort, and a lifeline to patients and their families, eg for sharing techniques and self-remedies. A danger is that they share nightmares as well, eg unnecessarily graphic descriptions of their children dying of cystic fibrosis may be spread, causing unneeded despondency. They raise funds for research, providing a 'welcome alternative to the expensive services of professionals'.

Groups as a way out of passive dependency If people learn in groups they take more control of their lives and they are more optimistic about being able to change things in their lives (such as their weight); self-esteem improves—and also objective measures of health (such as HbA_{1c}).

The term expert patient was coined to denote a well-informed patient in full possession of the facts about his or her case, and contributing to decisions in a valid way. Doctors often fear the expert patient, as so much time has to be spent investigating whether their viewpoints really are valid. This may lead to lack of harmony in the consulting room.

The inherent contradictions and strengths in the idea of expert patients are revealed through *reductio ad absurdum* (a logical technique beloved of Socrates).[57] Imagine a urologist consulting his GP about whether to have a radical prostatectomy or radiotherapy for his newly diagnosed prostate cancer. The GP might say to himself: 'Why on earth is he consulting me? He knows far more about the options than I do.' But let us imagine that his GP is, in fact, Socrates, who proceeds to ask various questions to reveal his inner fears (incontinence, erectile problems), and what he hopes to achieve by the various treatments on offer (to live long enough to see his disabled son through school). Socrates-the-GP is not adding any new facts. He is twisting the kaleidoscope, so that new patterns come into view. When a coherent pattern emerges he shows the urologist the door—saying 'Let me know what you decide'. The urologist sincerely thanks him. The man who leaves such a consultation is not the same as the one who entered. ▸*The expert patient has met a different sort of expert.*

Greater patient involvement in health issues and in the decisions relating to patients' own illnesses may lead to greater satisfaction, and better health. The more the patient knows about his or her own set of diseases, the better he or she will be able to decide what treatments to opt for. This is the rationale behind the expert patient programmes (MINIBOX). These are congruent with Bandura's social-cognitive theory of behaviour, which says that the main predictors of successful behaviour change are confidence (*self-efficacy*) in the ability to execute an action and expectation that a specific goal will be achieved (*outcome expectancy*). Expert patients (who are confident and assertive) are said to live longer, be healthier, and have a better quality of life,[58] and are exemplars of what health is all about (in chronic disease, health is not the absence of decay but an optimum, dynamic adaptation to it).

Nonetheless, there is a group of expert patients who tend to be middle-class know-alls who consult at great length about various maladies, arriving with sheaves of Internet printouts about treatments you have never heard of. Don't reject these patients out of hand. And don't assume any sort of superiority or inferiority. Just give your advice as best you can. You may get better results than Socrates—whose last attempt at *reductio ad absurdum* (during his famous trial) ended fatally when he was forced to drink hemlock. He was right—but it didn't do him much good. And so with you: you don't always have to be right. And by not insisting on this you may live to consult another day.

A 6-week course in self-management, eg in arthritis self-care
1 Course overview; acute and chronic conditions compared; cognitive symptom management; better breathing; introduction to action plans
2 Dealing with anger, fear & frustration; introduction to exercise; making an action plan
3 Distraction; muscle relaxation; fatigue management; monitoring exercise; action plans
4 Action plans; healthy eating; communication; problem-solving
5 Making an action plan; use of drugs; depression management; self-talk; treatment decisions; guided imagery
6 Informing the health care team; working with your health care professional; looking forward

7 Ear, nose, and throat

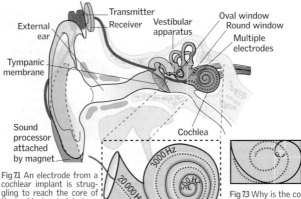

Fig 7.1 An electrode from a cochlear implant is struggling to reach the core of the cochlea's spiral, but unless it negotiates the ever tightening bends, lower tones (encoded near its core) are unheard. The shape of the cochlea was for decades thought simply to be efficient packaging—a way to conserve space within the skull, and that it had no effect on the function of hearing. However new theories propose the spiral shape acts to enhance low-frequency sounds. See fig 7.3 for more.

Cochlea (fig 7.2) is Latin for snail.

Fig 7.2 Our cochlea is a tapering spiral tube with 2.5 turns. Sometimes after an accident in the 7th embryonic week a child is born with only 1.5 turns (Mondini deformity; Incomplete partition type II). What is the result? Variable low-tone hearing loss. How is it diagnosed? Spiral CT.[1]

Fig 7.3 Why is the cochlea's spiral (blue) different to simple spirals based on Fibonacci sequences (black)? Low-tone hearing ranges in step with the pitch of the spiral; the tighter it is, the more sound energy in low-frequency waves is forced against the cochlea's outer wall. This 'whispering chamber effect' (where whispers cling to large curved walls and remain loud enough to be heard) augments low-frequency sound by ~20dB.[2]

We thank Mr Chris Potter FRCS, our ENT Specialist Reader and Cal Robinson our Junior Reader.
We would also like to acknowledge Mr Rogan Corbridge and Mr Nicholas Steventon, authors of the Ox-
ford Handbook of ENT and Head and Neck Surgery, which has been of great help in writing this chapter.

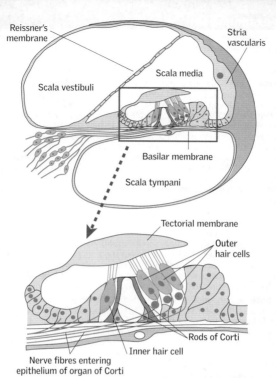

Fig 7.4 A cross-section of the cochlea. The basilar membrane is stiffer at the broad, outer end, so different frequencies peak at different positions along it.

Inside the spiral: the organ of Corti. Hearing and balance rely on the ability of hair cells to sense tiny mechanical stimuli. Outer hair cells are actively motile structures that feed energy into the vibration of the inner ear and enhance sensitivity to sound and movement. The sounds they produce are called otoacoustic emissions (OAE). Detecting OAE is a good test of a healthy inner ear and is used in neonatal screening tests. OAE and other hair cell functions are impaired by various types of hereditary deafness, syndromic hearing loss, and inner ear disease (eg Ménière's disease).

From the index...ENT emergencies

Examination in ENT differs from some other specialties in that its regions are rather inaccessible. An ENT department will have portable headlights and flexible fibre-optic scopes for nasendoscopy and laryngoscopy. However, if you are working in another speciality you are likely to have basic equipment only.

The ear Inspect the pinna (p538); any deformity? Look for *scars*—postauricular scars suggest mastoid surgery; endaural scars suggest middle ear surgery. Tragal tenderness points to otitis externa (p542).

Examine the auditory meatus: Pull the pinna up and back to straighten the cartilaginous bend. In infants, this has yet to fully develop so pull the pinna backwards. Swab any discharge and clean any debris carefully. Insert the largest comfortable aural speculum (don't probe too far—it's sensitive). Examine the external auditory canal. Any infection/inflammation? wax? foreign bodies? or exostoses? (p538). NB: There may be complete occlusion of the canal in severe otitis externa (p542).

Examine the tympanic membrane: Practice is the key (figs **7.8-7.14**, p539). Examine the quadrants in turn. Identify the pars tensa, pars flaccida, the handle of the malleus, and the cone of light (light reflex) that points to the toes. Note the colour, translucency, and any bulging or retraction. Any *perforations*? (Note size; position; site: marginal or central?). Perforation/retraction of the pars flaccida is potentially serious (p544). Assess drum mobility using a pneumatic attachment. Lack of movement suggests perforation or middle ear effusion (on squeezing the balloon, the drum should move). Drum movement on a Valsalva manoeuvre means a functional Eustachian tube. Also perform: free field voice testing; tuning forks (see BOX p537), + check facial nerve function.

The nose (Testing smell is often omitted, but often fascinating.[1]) Sit face-to-face. Inspect the external nose: skin, size, shape, scars? deviations? deformity? Lift the nose to inspect the vestibule (the skin-lined cavity of the anterior nose). Check patency of each nostril by occluding each nostril in turn with the flat of your thumb and asking the patient to breath in. Don't press on the side of the nose (it distorts the other nostril).

Inspect the nose internally: This can be done using a *Thudicum's speculum* or an otoscope with a large speculum (= *anterior rhinoscopy*). Insert gently; assess mucosa and septum (is it straight?; any bleeding points, crusting, or perforations?). Assess the size of the inferior and middle turbinates (are they hypertrophied?). Any polyps (see BOX p557)?

Examination of the posterior nose: Requires an endoscope (after spraying with **xylometazoline** & **lidocaine**). The middle meatus is a key nasal area as most of the sinuses ventilate via this cleft (between the middle and inferior turbinates (conchae). The postnasal space (nasopharynx) contains the Eustachian tube orifices & the pharyngeal recess, and may contain adenoids or naso-pharyngeal cancer. A postnasal mirror can be used to examine the nasopharynx via the oral cavity. Examine the palate, it is the floor of the nose.

The throat (fig 7.5) •Position yourself as for nasal examination; remove any dentures •Inspect lips and perioral region. Ask the patient to open their mouth without protruding the tongue. Use a tongue depressor to retract each cheek: inspect the buccal mucosa, the parotid duct opening (opposite the upper 2nd molar), gums, teeth, floor of the mouth, and the retromolar trigone (mucosa behind the 3rd molar over the ramus of the mandible—also known as 'coffin corner' due to its inaccesibility to casual examination and late presentation of tumours) •Depress the tongue; say 'ah then aye' (checks palate movement and exposes more mucosa) •Examine the tonsils (prominent tonsils aren't always enlarged; deep crypts with debris can be normal) •Put on a glove for bimanual examination of any oral lesion •Palpate the floor of the mouth (any submandibular gland stones or masses?) •Inspect the posterolateral borders of the tongue to ensure you do not miss any early tumours.

Cardinal ear symptoms	Cardinal nose symptoms	Cardinal throat symptoms
• Ear pain/discharge: p542	• Nasal congestion: p556	►► Stridor: p566
• Hearing loss: p551	• Epistaxis: p562	• Hoarseness: p568
• Tinnitus/vertigo: p554		• Dysphagia: p570
		• Neck lumps: p576

Prevalence of ENT symptoms

In one UK community study (n=>15,000), ~20% reported current hearing troubles, eg difficulty with speech in background noise (few wore a hearing aid regularly). 20% reported tinnitus lasting >5 minutes. ~15% reported hayfever [et al] in the last year, 7% sneezing or voice problems, and 31% had severe sore throat/tonsillitis. ~21% reported ever having had dizziness in which things seemed to spin around the individual, 29% unsteadiness/light-headedness, and 13% reported dizziness in which the person seemed to move.[3] Nasal polyp symptoms (p567): 2%.

Free field voice testing & tuning forks

Audiology phone apps Apps designed for measuring hearing have largely superseded traditional screening tests of hearing such as 'free field testing'. The listener is presented with a series of tones at different frequencies and is prompted to respond when the test signal is heard.

Modified Rinne's test Use a 512Hz activated tuning fork and place behind the ear against the mastoid process (tests bone conduction), then move to 2cm from the external auditory meatus (tests air conduction). Ask 'Which is louder?' *Positive test:* Air conduction is better than bone (=normal or sensorineural hearing loss; SNHL). ►If +ve in sudden SNHL refer the same day (p550). *Negative test:* Bone conduction is better than air conduction (=conductive deafness or a false −ve Rinne: in severe SNHL sound is actually being heard by the other ear).

Weber's test Place the activated tuning fork on the vertex or forehead. Sound localizes to the affected ear with conductive hearing loss, and to the contralateral ear in SNHL, and to the midline if both ears are normal (or there is bilateral SNHL). Rinne's and Weber's are performed together as a 'package' to help identify the type of hearing loss. These tests are popular in exams!

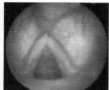
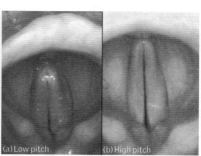

Fig 7.5 Vocal cords abducted for inspiration (above) and adducted for low- (a), and high-pitch phonation (b): NB elongation to raise pitch is done by the cricothyroid muscle.

(a) Low pitch   (b) High pitch

Courtesy of James Thomas.

---

1 *Sweat, darkness, dirt, and lust.* Smells are as hard to name as emotions: when we are told by a novelist or a chef, we say 'Yes: that's it!' Smells and emotions go hand in hand with memory. When we re-smell the smells of youth, or re-smell a perfume from a distant *affaire de coeur*, we are transported back to that moment. This expanding of the sense of smell to encompass all things struck Kipling on revisiting Lahore: '*the heat and smell of oil and spices, and puffs of temple incense, and sweat and darkness, and dirt and lust and cruelty.*'[4]

The external ear (fig 7.7). The pinna is fibroelastic cartilage, covered by skin. The ear drum (figs 7.6 & 7.8) is set obliquely, the external auditory canal is ~3cm anteriorly and ~2.5cm posteriorly. The canal's outer ⅓ is cartilage, having hairs and ceruminous (wax) glands in the skin; its inner ⅔ is bony and lined with sensitive skin.

Congenital anomalies The pinna develops from 6 hillocks derived from the 1st and 2nd branchial arches that appear at 4–6wks, with the intervening 1st branchial groove forming the external auditory canal. Any malfusion may give rise to accessory tags/auricles or a preauricular pit, sinus, or fistula. An infected sinus may be mistaken for an infected sebaceous cyst, but there is often a deep tract that lies close to the facial nerve. It must be removed to avoid further infection. ▶Auricular anomalies are frequently associated with middle ear anomalies.

Chondrodermatitis nodularis helicis This Latin describes an exquisitely tender, cartilaginous, inflamed nodule dwelling on the upper helix or antihelix (fig 7.7). It is commoner in men working outdoors and (legendarily) wimple-wearing nuns. *Cause:* Unknown. ?poor blood flow (avascular chondritis) from prolonged pressure; or vasoconstriction from cold. The affected side is usually the one on which the patient lies. ℞: Relieve pressure. If not helpful, excise skin and underlying cartilage (eg 'wide excision' or 'deep shave').[5]

Pinna haematoma Blunt trauma may cause bleeding in the subperichondrial plane elevating the perichondrium to form a haematoma. ℞: Arrange incision of the haematoma with primary closure (+ packing, to prevent reaccumulation). Aspiration is rarely adequate due to the thickness of the clot. Poor treatment leads to ischaemic necrosis, then fibrosis (cauliflower ear, p740). Secondary infection may cause major loss of cartilage; cover with antibiotics (eg ciprofloxacin).

Auditory exostosis (surfer's ear) These are smooth, multiple, bilateral swellings of the bony canals that represent local bone hypertrophy from cold exposure. *Symptoms:* None, so long as the lumen is sufficient for sound conduction (they are often picked up incidentally). If they hinder migration of wax or debris, occlude the canal to cause conductive deafness, or there is recurrent infection, surgical removal is indicated. Osteomas (p699) are usually solitary.

Wax (cerumen) Cerumen is the natural protective wax produced and secreted in the outer ⅓ of the canal. The amount of wax produced varies greatly from person-to-person. Excess wax may become impacted causing dulled hearing and a feeling of fullness in the ear ± tinnitus. Due to epithelial migration, the ear is self-cleaning; cotton buds are unnecessary. ℞: Optimal treatment for wax removal is suction under direct vision using a microscope. Irrigation (syringing) usually works too, eg after softening with olive oil or bicarbonate drops. Warn of post-procedure dizziness. Ear drops alone will often clear the wax. Instil the drops whilst lying with the affected ear uppermost. Pour in a few drops 2-3 times each day for 3-7 days. ▶Avoid irrigation if the drum is perforated; if grommets (or within 1½yrs); cleft palate; or after mastoid surgery. *Complications:* Pain; otitis externa; vertigo (0.2%); perforated drum (≤0.2%).

Ear FBs Foreign bodies are most common in children. There are many possible methods of removal. Soft FBs, eg cotton wool, may be grasped with crocodile forceps. Solid FBs are best removed by passing a wax hook or Jobson–Horne probe beyond the object and pulling back towards you. ▶*Always use instrumentation under direct vision.* Blind probing will cause damage. Avoid pushing objects deeper into the canal. *Irrigation* can be successful if you are sure there is no trauma to the ear canal or drum. Insects can be drowned and floated out with oil. The first attempt at FB removal will usually be the best tolerated. Difficult patients (eg children; the anxious) are best referred to ENT directly, without inexpert attempts at removal. This will increase the chance of successful removal with few complications.[6]

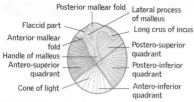

Fig 7.6 Left drum. The 4 arbitrary quadrants are indicated by solid lines and by the handle of the malleus. The light reflex points to the feet.

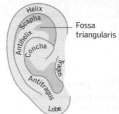

Fig 7.7 The pinna.

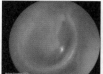

Fig 7.8 Normal right drum. If only patients could see how beautiful and delicate the drum is, amateur instrumentation of the ear would be far less common!

Courtesy of Michael Saunders FRCS.

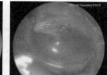

Fig 7.9 The left drum has *retracted*, as has the handle of the malleus (appears short). The lateral process will also become more prominent than normal.

Courtesy of Michael Saunders FRCS.

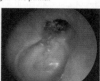

Fig 7.10 (Right drum) This crust in the attic represents a large underlying *cholesteatoma*.

Courtesy of Michael Saunders FRCS.

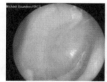

Fig 7.11 The (right) drum is opaque. There is prominence of blood vessels suggesting a *middle ear effusion*. This is one of several appearances of glue ear.

Courtesy of Michael Saunders FRCS.

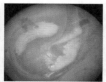

Fig 7.12 (Right drum) White patches are usually *tympanosclerosis* (calcium deposits), eg after infection or trauma. They are often of no significance; if severe can cause mild conductive hearing loss.

Courtesy of Michael Saunders FRCS.

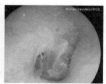

Fig 7.13 (Right drum) *Posterior perforation*. Posterior perforations may signify serious underlying disease, but this one is dry, and its posterior margin is defined. Traumatic perforations (eg barotrauma) are often posterior and linear, like a tear rather than a hole.

Courtesy of Michael Saunders FRCS.

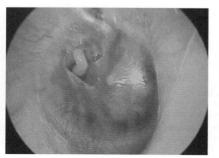

Fig 7.14 *Posterior perforation* exposing incudostapedial joint. The irregular perforation shape suggests the cause is trauma. These images may look surprisingly clear: this is because they were taken through a Hopkins rod, rather than an otoscope.

Courtesy of Rory Herdman FRCS.

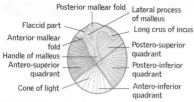
(labels: Posterior mallear fold; Lateral process of malleus; Flaccid part; Anterior mallear fold; Long crus of incus; Postero-superior quadrant; Handle of malleus; Postero-inferior quadrant; Antero-superior quadrant; Antero-inferior quadrant; Cone of light)

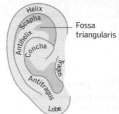
(labels: Helix; Scapha; Antihelix; Fossa triangularis; Concha; Tragus; Antitragus; Lobe)

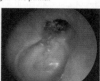

ENT

539

When assessing suspected hearing loss, determine its nature (conductive or sensorineural), its severity, and its cause: is it treatable, and is it part of some other disease process—eg unilateral sensorineural hearing loss (SNHL) in acoustic neuroma? Remember also to assess the degree of disability. ►If sudden sensori neural deafness refer urgently (same day) to ENT (see p551).

Tuning fork test See p537.

Pure tone audiometry is the most common method used to assess hearing. It quantifies hearing loss and determines its nature. Headphones deliver electronically generated tones at different sound pressure levels over frequencies of 250–8000Hz in a sound-proofed room. Air-conducted sound is initially played above the hearing threshold and then decreased in 10dB increments until it is no longer heard. The sound intensity is then increased in 5dB increments until a 50% response rate is obtained. A bone conduction threshold is also obtained by using a transducer over the mastoid process. NB: Masking (=narrowband noise to the untested ear) prevents cross-stimulation of the non-test ear. The results are recorded on a chart, with frequency (in Hz) on the x axis and decibels hearing level (dBHL;=deviation from normal) on the y axis—see figs 7.16.–7.22. See also 'normal hearing' BOX, p551.

Tympanometry (acoustic impedance audiometry) is an objective way of measuring pressure in the middle ear and establishing the cause of conductive deafness. *Principles:* In normal ears, compliance of the drum (the amount of displacement in mL for a given sound)—hence transmission of sound—peaks when middle ear pressure equals ear canal pressure. So the peak of the tympanometry curve reflects middle ear pressure. *Procedure:* A probe with an airtight seal is introduced into the meatus; it measures the proportion of an acoustic signal reflected back at varying pressures and generates a graph of compliance (fig 7.15). *Results:* A normal ear (middle ear space filled with air; ossicles intact) will show a normal peak with normal compliance (TYPE A, PURPLE). If there is disruption of the ossicles, or if part of the drum is flaccid, a large amount of energy will be absorbed into the drum which is free to move a lot—and it will move most when canal pressure=middle ear pressure (high compliance; TYPE AD, RED). Fluid in the middle ear makes the drum stiff, so most of the sound is reflected back to the probe—hence a low, flat result (low compliance, TYPE B, GREEN). This finding must be related to ear canal volume (also measured): if normal ≈ otitis media; if low ≈ wax occlusion; if high ≈ grommets or perforation. TYPE C (BLUE): Shift in peak of the curve to the left found with negative middle ear pressure, eg as in developing or resolving otitis media.[7]

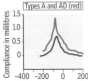
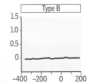
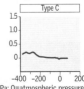

Ear canal air pressure—as set by the tympanometer in decaPascals (daPa; 0=atmospheric pressure)
Fig 7.15 Acoustic impedance audiometry (tympanometry).
Courtesy of Jane Jones, Oxford Radcliffe Hospitals NHS Trust.

Otoacoustic emissions (OAE) is used to assess function of the cochlea by recording sound vibration produced by the outer hair cells in the cochlea. It is most commonly used in neonatal screening (see p548).

Audiological brainstem responses (ABR) record electrical activity along the auditory pathway in response to a sound stimulus (see p548).

►Childhood deafness, see p548.

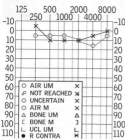

Fig 7.16 Normal hearing. © C Potter.

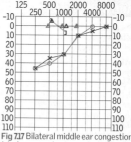

Fig 7.17 Bilateral middle ear congestion (air–bone gap due to conductive loss).
© C Potter.

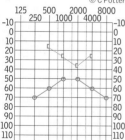

Fig 7.18 Right-sided Ménières (p554).
© C Potter.

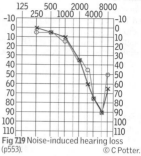

Fig 7.19 Noise-induced hearing loss (p553). © C Potter.

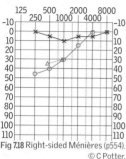

Fig 7.20 Right-sided otosclerosis, with Carhart's notch at 2kHz on masked bone conduction. © C Potter.

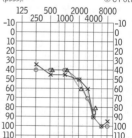

Fig 7.21 Typical presbyacusis—bilateral, symmetrical, high-frequency SNHL.
© C Potter.

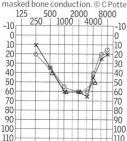

Fig 7.22 (left) Cookie-bite loss: as if someone took a bite out of the top of the audiogram (isolated mid-range hearing loss). It is likely to be hereditary. Test siblings. Referral to a geneticist may be indicated. © C Potter.

Abbreviations:
Right ear (red)
Left ear (blue)
m = masked
um = unmasked

►See also p551 'normal hearing'.

Legend (Fig 7.16):
O	AIR UM		✕
⌐	NOT REACHED		✕
O	UNCERTAIN		✕
△	AIR M		✕
⌐	BONE UM		⌐
⌐	BONE M		⌐
L	UCL UM		L
●	R CONTRA		✕

The cause is often non-otological (in 50%); look for sources of referred pain ('Referred otalgia' BOX, p543), eg throat and teeth: *does grinding/tapping hurt?*—see p580.

Otitis externa (OE)[8] Discharge, itch, pain, and tragal tenderness due to acute inflammation of the skin of the meatus, usually caused by excess canal moisture. Other causes: trauma eg fingernails (from itchy conditions, eg eczema/psoriasis); high humidity; absence of wax (from self-cleaning); a narrow ear canal; and hearing aids. *Pseudomonas* is the chief organism, though *Staphylococcus aureus* is another common offender. ΔΔ: Contact eczema.

• *Mild OE:* Scaly skin with some erythema. Normal diameter of external auditory canal (EAC). R: For all OE, cleaning the EAC is key (see 'Cleaning the external auditory canal' BOX, p543). Ears should be kept water free during treatment. In mild OE, use hydrocortisone cream to the pinna and EarCalm® Spray (2% acetic acid; acts as antifungal/bacterial).

• *Moderate OE:* (fig 7.23) Painful ear, narrowed EAC with malodorous creamy discharge. R: Swab for microscopy. Clean the canal. Prescribe topical antibiotic/± steroid drops (eg **Otosporin®**; **Sofradex®**; **Gentisone HC®**) NB: due to theoretical risk of ototoxicity, topical aminoglycosides are contraindicated in patients with a perforated TM or patent grommet. Topical *ciprofloxacin* drops are not licensed for treating OE but there is less potential for ototoxicity in those with grommets or perforation. Use drops for ≤7 days, as troublesome fungal infections can arise if used for longer (treat with **clotrimazole** 1% solution). If there is pinna cellulitis start antibiotics and refer.

• *Severe OE:* (fig 7.24) The EAC is occluded. A thin ear wick can be inserted with eg **aluminium acetate** (may require ENT referral). After a few days, the meatus will open up enough for either microsuction or careful cleansing.

▶Beware persistent unilateral otitis externa in diabetics/immunosuppressed/ the elderly: the risk is malignant/necrotizing otitis externa (below).

▶OE resistant to treatment can be a sign of malignancy eg SCC. Do biopsy.

Furunculosis This is a very painful staphylococcal abscess arising in a hair follicle within the canal. Consider lancing. If there is pinna cellulitis start oral antibiotics (eg flucloxacillin). Diabetes is an important predisposing factor.

Malignant/necrotizing otitis externa This is aggressive, life-threatening infection of the external ear that can lead to temporal bone destruction and base-of-skull osteomyelitis. 90% have diabetes. The cause is usually *Pseudomonas aeruginosa* (also *Proteus* and *Klebsiella*). Treatment is by surgical debridement, systemic antibiotics and specific immunoglobulins.

Barotrauma If the Eustachian tube is occluded, middle ear pressure cannot be equalized during descent in an aircraft or diving, so causing damage. *Symptoms:* Severe pain as the drum becomes indrawn initially then a secondary effusion may occur as a transudate or haemotympanum. *Prevention:* Not flying with an URTI; decongestants into the nose (eg **xylometazoline**); repeated yawns/ swallows/jaw movements. R: Supportive if simple; effusions usually clear spontaneously, and most perforations heal.

Temporomandibular joint (TMJ) dysfunction *Symptoms:* Earache, facial pain, and joint clicking/popping related to teeth-grinding or joint derangement, and, importantly, stress, making this a biopsychosocial disorder which may become a chronic pain syndrome (p636). *Signs:* Joint tenderness exacerbated by lateral movement of the open jaw, or trigger points in the pterygoids. R: Most patients improve without treatment. Reassure and explain. Simple analgesia. *Specialist treatment:* Dental occlusion therapy (eg oral splinting); physiotherapy; cognitive behavioural therapy (p374); surgery (rarely needed).[9]

Cleaning the external auditory canal[10]

Cleaning the ear canal facilitates application and effectiveness of topical treatment. Options include:

- *Gentle syringing or irrigation* to remove debris (provided the TM is intact).
- *Dry mopping:* Under direct vision using a Jobson Horne probe with a small piece of cotton wool on its serrated end, clean the auditory meatus with a gentle rotary action; don't touch the drum. Replace the cotton wool and continue until the wool is returned clean. Attend to the anterior-inferior recess, which often harbours debris. NB: Patients who have mastoid cavities (a surgical widened canal done to treat infection) should be followed up by ENT for irrigation and drying.
- *Microsuction* is very effective but not readily available in primary care, so may need referral to ENT. ▶Patients who have mastoid cavities are treated by microsuction, not irrigation.

Referred otalgia: when the cause is not in the ear

Referred (secondary) pain can arise from disease processes in the territories of the sensory nerves supplying the ear:

- *v:* The auriculotemporal nerve (a branch of the trigeminal nerve which supplies lateral upper half of pinna) may refer pain from dental disease and TMJ dysfunction (p542).
- *vii:* A sensory branch of the facial nerve (supplies lateral surface of ear drum) refers pain in geniculate herpes (Ramsay Hunt syndrome, p652).
- *ix:* Primary glossopharyngeal neuralgia is a rare cause of pain often induced by talking or swallowing.
- *ix & x:* The tympanic branch of the glossopharyngeal nerve and the auricular branch of the vagus (supplies medial surface of drum) refer pain from the posterior ⅓ of the tongue, pyriform fossa, or larynx, eg from cancer, or from the throat to the ear, eg in tonsillitis or quinsy. Otalgia is common post-tonsillectomy (esp. in adults), so it is worth warning all patients.
- *c2,3:* The great auricular nerve (c2,3, supplying lower ½ of pinna) refers pain from soft tissue injury in the neck and from cervical spondylosis/arthritis.

ENT

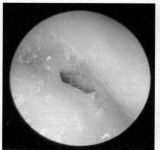

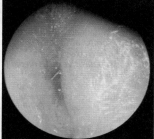

Fig 7.23 Moderate otitis externa.
Courtesy of Michael Hawke, MD, University of Toronto, hawkelibrary.com.

Fig 7.24 Severe otitis externa: the EAC is completely occluded.
Courtesy of Michael Hawke, MD, University of Toronto, hawkelibrary.com.

Further reading

NICE (2015). *Clinical Knowledge Summaries: Otitis Externa.* http://cks.nice.uk/otitis-externa

The character of the discharge provides clues:

Causes of discharge to consider
• Otitis externa/media • Cholesteatoma (rare but important). NB: crust in the attic/postero-superior quadrant often hides pathology, so remove it

• *External ear:* Inflammation, ie otitis externa (OE) produces a scanty discharge, as there are no mucinous glands—see p542. Blood can result from trauma to the canal. Liquid wax can sometimes 'leak' out.

• *Middle ear:* Mucous discharges are almost always due to middle ear disease. Serosanguinous discharge suggests a granular mucosa of chronic otitis media. An offensive discharge suggests cholesteatoma.

• *CSF otorrhoea:* CSF leaks may follow trauma: suspect if you see a halo sign on filter paper, or glucose is ↑, or β₂ (tau) transferrin is present.

Acute otitis media (OM) entails middle ear inflammation; it presents with rapid onset of pain, fever±irritability, anorexia, or vomiting often after a viral upper respiratory infection. Common organisms: *Pneumococcus, Haemophilus, Moraxella,* other streps and staphs. In acute OM, bulging of the tympanic membrane causes pain (fig 7.25), which eases if the drum perforates (there is associated purulent discharge). ℞: Optimize analgesia. Acute OM resolves in 60% within 24h without antibiotics. Consider immediate antibiotics if systemically unwell; immunocompromised; or no improvement in symptoms >4 days. Consider immediate or 2-day 'delayed' antibiotics if <3 months old; perforation/discharge; <2 yrs with bilateral OM. If required, give amoxicillin (40mg/kg/day in 3 divided doses) for 5 days (erythromycin if penicillin allergic).

Continuing discharge may indicate complications: mastoiditis which is rare (see below), and even rarer are petrositis; labyrinthitis; facial palsy; meningitis; intracranial abscesses. Mucopus may continue to drain when there is no mastoiditis, especially if grommets are in place. Treat with appropriate oral or topical antibiotics according to swab results. Clean the EAC to remove infected material from the meatus. ▶*If discharge continues, get expert help.*

Otitis media with effusion (glue ear) This occurs when an effusion is present after regression of the symptoms of acute OM, see p546.

Chronic otitis media (COM)[11] A variety of terms are used to categorize chronic infectious or inflammatory conditions of the middle ear. COM is defined as an ear with a tympanic membrane perforation in the setting of recurrent or chronic infections. Associated symptoms include hearing loss, otorrhoea, fullness, and otalgia.

• *Benign (or inactive) COM* is characterized by a dry tympanic membrane perforation without active infection.

• *Chronic serous otitis media* is characterized by continuous serous drainage (typically straw coloured).

• *Chronic suppurative otitis media (CSOM)* is diagnosed when there is persistent purulent drainage through a perforated tympanic membrane.

℞: Topical/systemic antibiotics (based on swab results); aural cleaning; water precautions; careful follow-up. Surgery may be required (myringoplasty; mastoidectomy—see box). *Complications:* Prolonged low middle ear pressure allows for the development of a retraction pocket of the *pars tensa* or *flaccida* (fig 7.9, p539), as this enlarges, squamous epithelium builds up and can no longer escape from the neck of the sac, resulting in a cholesteatoma.

Cholesteatoma (fig 7.26) has serious rare complications (meningitis; cerebral abscess; hearing loss; mastoiditis; facial nerve dysfunction). *Incidence:* 1:10,000. Peak age: 5–15yrs. It is a misnomer as it is neither cholesterol nor a tumour (it *is* locally destructive around and beyond the *pars flaccida*—from the release of lytic enzymes). Δ: Foul discharge ± deafness; headache, pain, facial paralysis, and vertigo indicate impending CNS complications. ℞: Mastoid surgery (see box) is needed to make a safe dry ear by removing the disease (preserving hearing is secondary).

ENT

Mastoiditis Middle ear inflammation leads to destruction of air cells in the mastoid bone ± abscess formation. Beware intracranial extension. Giving antibiotics for otitis media can prevent mastoiditis (NNT >4000). *Signs:* Fever; tenderness, swelling and redness behind the pinna (mastoid) + protruding auricle. *Imaging:* CT. *R:* Admit for IV antibiotics, myringotomy ± definitive mastoidectomy.

Surgery for chronic suppurative otitis media (CSOM)[12]

In patients with CSOM, surgery may be considered if aural cleaning and antibiotic treatment fail, and there is persistent perforation/discharge, conductive hearing loss, chronic mastoiditis, or cholesteatoma formation.

Myringoplasty (=repair of the tympanic membrane alone) A perforation in the tympanic membrane is patched using a graft (often using temporalis fascia or tragal perichondrium), and applied (usually) underneath the tympanic membrane. It acts as a scaffold for the tympanic membrane to grow across and has a ~90% success rate.

Mastoidectomy For patients with mastoiditis or advanced cholesteatoma, mastoid surgery and *tympanoplasty* (=surgical repair of the tympanic membrane and ossicles) is used to eradicate the source of chronic infection, excise the cholesteatoma and reconstruct the hearing mechanism. 'Canal wall up' mastoidectomy removes mastoid air cells whilst retaining the posterior canal wall. It leaves normal ear anatomy intact and prevents problems associated with a mastoid cavity (eg ongoing requirement for microscopic cleaning).

Risk factors for otitis media

- URTI (and autumn/winter)
- Bottle-feeding
- Passive smoking
- Dummy/pacifier
- Presence of adenoids (see p546)
- Asthma
- Malformations (eg cleft palate)
- Gastro-oesophageal reflux/BMI↑ in *adults.*

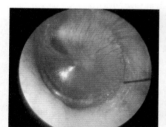

Fig 7.25 Acute otitis media. There is erythema and bulging of the pars flaccida and dilated circumferential vessels.
Courtesy of Michael Hawke, MD, University of Toronto, hawkelibrary.com.

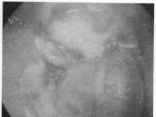

Fig 7.26 Attic cholesteatoma.
Courtesy of Rory Herdman FRCS.

Further reading

NICE (2015). *Clinical Knowledge Summaries: Otitis Media.* http://cks.nice.org.uk/otitis-media-acute

This is detected by otoscopy (fluid level or bubbles behind the drum) or indirectly, by tympanometry (p540). 50% of 3-yr-olds have ≥1 ear effusion/yr. *In adults, exclude a postnasal space tumour as the cause of middle ear fluid.*

Otitis media with effusion (OME)/Glue ear ►*Hearing impairment noticed by parents is the mode of presentation in 80%.* The fundamental problem lies with dysfunction of the Eustachian tubes. The exact cause is unclear, but there are associations with upper respiratory tract infections, oversized adenoids, narrow nasopharyngeal dimensions and presence of bacterial biofilms on the adenoids. OME is more common in boys; Down's syndrome; cleft palate; winter season; atopy; children of smokers and primary ciliary dyskinesia.[2] OME is the chief cause of hearing loss in young children, and can result in significant learning and behavioural problems. OME may cause no pain, so its presence may not be suspected.

History: Focus on poor listening, poor speech, language delay, inattention, poor behaviour, hearing fluctuation, ear infections/URTIs, balance problems and poor progress at school.

Examination: There is a variable appearance of the tympanic membrane on otoscopy (fig 7.27), eg retracted or bulging drum. It can look dull, grey, or yellow. There may be bubbles or a fluid level, or superficial radial vessels and ↓drum mobility when tested with a pneumatic attachment.

Tests: Refer for formal assessment of hearing, which should be appropriate for the child's developmental stage. *Audiograms:* Look for conductive defects. *Tympanometry:* Look for flat tympanogram (fig 7.15, p540). This helps distinguish OME from other causes eg otosclerosis. Also consider co-existing causes of hearing loss (p548).

Treatment:[13] OME is usually mild, transient, and resolves spontaneously: 50% of children with bilateral hearing loss of 20dB are likely to resolve in 3 months.

• *Active observation for 3 months:* If bilateral OME is confirmed, there should be a 3-month period of active observation. Give advice on strategies to minimize impact of hearing loss (eg reducing background noise (turn off the TV); sit at the child's level, and give short, simple instructions). Reassess with repeat hearing tests at 3 months.

• *Autoinflation* of the Eustachian tube may help during this period (eg using an Otovent® device—which involves inflating a special balloon via the nose).

• *Topical and systemic methods:* NICE doesn't recommend antibiotics, changes to diet, antihistamines, decongestants, steroids, or acupuncture.[etc]

• *Surgery:* If persistent bilateral OME + hearing level in better ear of 25–30dBHL (=decibel hearing level) or worse is confirmed over 3 months, consider insertion of ventilation tubes (*AKA* tympanostomy tube or grommets; fig 7.28). Surgery is also an option if hearing loss is less severe but there is a significant impact on development or education. The main complications of grommets are infections and tympanosclerosis (p539). Treat infections with aural cleaning and topical antibiotic/steroid ear drops; grommet removal may be needed. Adjuvant adenoidectomy at the time of grommet insertion should not be performed routinely.

• *Adults* with longstanding OME can be treated with tympanostomy tubes.

• *Hearing aids:* Should be reserved for persistent bilateral OME and hearing loss if surgery is not accepted.

Post-op: It is OK to swim with grommets, but avoid forcing water into the middle ear by diving. Some form of ear plug is wise. Grommets extrude after ~3–12 months; recheck the hearing at this point; ~25% need re-insertion. Rarely, a small perforation may persist after the grommet has come out, which may require surgery.

2 PCD/Kartagener's syndrome (p646) often causes otitis media and OEM throughout childhood (owing to loss of ciliary function in the Eustachian tube and middle ear), despite fairly continuous antibiotics. After 18yrs of age, the ear improves somewhat. Grommet placement does not improve middle ear function.

Grommets and hearing gain

Use of grommets to ventilate the middle ear is common but how much do they improve hearing? Cochrane review[14] on the effect of grommets on hearing in children with OME, as measured by standard tests, was found to be small (~12dB) and diminished after 6 months (4dB)—by which time natural resolution had led to improved hearing in non-surgically treated children. The raw numbers may look unimpressive, but due to the logarithmic decibel scale, even a 3dB increase in sound equates to a doubling of intensity and hearing sensitivity. For reference, a 16 to 25dB hearing loss may be mimicked by plugging the ears with the index fingers. In the classroom setting, this level of hearing loss presents an appreciable educational difficulty (see also 'normal hearing' box on p551).[15]

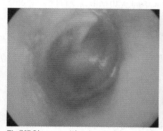

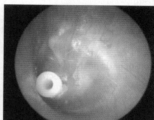

Fig 7.27 Glue ear with retracted drum & dull drumhead.
Courtesy of Rory Herdman FRCS.

Fig 7.28 A grommet.
Courtesy of Rory Herdman FRCS.

Further reading

NICE (2008). *Surgical Management of Children with Otitis Media with Effusion* (CG60). London: NICE. https://www.nice.org.uk/guidance/cg60

1 in every 500 newborns has bilateral permanent sensorineural hearing loss ≥40dB. Half of all prelingual deafness is genetic, 25% non-genetic, and 25% idiopathic.[16] ►*If you or a parent are worried, refer to audiology.*

Genetic hearing loss (50%)

Conductive hearing loss—CHL: Congenital anomalies of pinna, external ear canal, drum, or ossicles; Treacher–Collins (p655); Pierre Robin (p650); Goldenhar syndrome (oculoauricularvertebral [OAV] syndrome)—causes CHL and SNHL.

Sensorineural hearing loss—SNHL:

- *Autosomal dominant:* Waardenburg syndrome (SNHL, heterochromia + wide nasal bridge p425); Klippel–Feil syndrome (p648); Alport syndrome (p638); Branchio-oto-renal (BOR) syndrome (outer, middle, & inner ear + kidney malformations).
- *Autosomal recessive:* Pendred syndrome (SNHL with goitre); Usher's syndrome (SNHL+ retinitis pigmentosa); Jervell and Lange-Nielsen syndrome (SNHL +↑ QTc).
- *Non-syndromic SNHL:* Accounts for 70% of genetic hearing loss. Many genes are implicated and there are different patterns of inheritance (most are autosomal recessive). The degree of hearing loss and age of onset varies with type.
- *X-linked:* Alport syndrome (p638); Turner's syndrome (p655).

Non-genetic hearing loss (25%)

- *Intrauterine TORCH infection* eg CMV; rubella; toxoplasmosis; HSV; syphilis.
- *Perinatal causes:* Prematurity; hypoxia; IVH; kernicterus; infection (below).
- *Infections:* eg meningitis, encephalitis, measles, mumps.
- *Other causes:* Ototoxic drugs; acoustic or cranial trauma.

Universal newborn hearing screening (UNHS)

Screening within weeks of birth is the best way to ensure deafness is diagnosed and managed. Tests:

- *Otoacoustic emissions (OAE):* A microphone placed in the external meatus detects tiny cochlear sounds produced by movement of the outer hair cells, which occur spontaneously or in response to an auditory stimulus. OAE evaluates function of the peripheral auditory system, the area most often involved in SNHL (ie the sensory part of the cochlea and not the neural pathway, which is tested using ABR). OAE is abnormal or equivocal in 3–8%. Most of these 'failures' (84%) have external ear canal obstruction (collapsed ear canal or debris). For these patients arrange a repeat test or measure ABR (below).
- *Audiological brainstem responses (ABR):* The ears are covered with earphones that emit a series of soft clicks. Electrodes on the infant's forehead and neck measure brain wave activity in response to the clicks. ABR tests the auditory neural pathway from CNVIII to the lower brainstem.

Prevalence of deafness found at UNHS: 0.9–3.24:1000 for permanent bilateral hearing loss of >35dB; 5.95:1000 when unilateral and moderate hearing loss infants.[17]

Subjective hearing tests in older children

- *Distraction testing:* (6–18 months; not very accurate) An assistant in front of the child attracts their attention while a tester attempts to distract them by making noises behind and beside the child eg with a rattle, or voice.
- *Visually reinforced audiometry:* (6 mths to 2½yrs) The child turns their head to a sound stimulus and a toy lights-up to reward the listening behaviour.
- *Speech discrimination:* (at 24–60 months) The child touches selected objects cued by acoustically similar phrases, eg *key/tree.*

Management

Give support, advice, and information to the patient and family. Maximize the hearing a deaf child may have by use of hearing aids or cochlear implant (see BOX). Provide support to develop spoken or signed communication.

Further reading

NHS newborn hearing screening programme (NHSP): www.gov.uk/topic/population-screening-programmes/newborn-hearing

Smith RJH *et al.* (2014). Deafness and hereditary hearing loss overview. *GeneReviews®.* ncbi.nlm. nih.gov/books/NBK1434/

Cochlear implants

NICE recommends cochlear implants for children and adults with profound sensorineural deafness who do not benefit from a conventional hearing aid. Normal cochlear structure is essential, as is pre-op multi-disciplinary assessment.

Cochlear implants comprise a multichannel electrode inserted surgically into the cochlea that directly stimulates the auditory nerve when electrical signals are applied (see fig 7.1, p534). The electrode is attached to an external auditory processor through the skin via a magnetic coupler. The signal is not normal sound and intensive therapy is needed to understand the new sounds. Implants allow better lip-reading; provision and recognition of environmental sounds and relief of isolation. Quality is now sufficient for previously deaf people to have excellent hearing and, for example, use the phone.

BAHA: the bone-anchored hearing aid

BAHA Sound is transmitted to the cochlea via bone conduction (fig 7.29). *Indications:* Intolerance of conventional hearing aids (eg persistent draining ear; mastoid cavity; topical sensitivity); congenital malformations (eg microtia; atresia); single-sided deafness. BAHAs are becoming more widely used have a special benefit in some children with complex disorders because the children do not physically feel the presence of the hearing aid. On quality of life measures BAHAs do very well. *Complications:* include skin regrowth around the titanium screw and non-osseointegration. *Contraindications:* Average bone threshold worse than 45dB; non-compliance; poor hygiene; lack of bone volume.

ENT

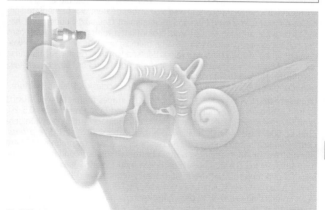

Fig 7.29 A bone-anchored hearing aid allows sound to be transmitted to the cochlea via bone conduction. A titanium screw implanted into bone allows attachment of the hearing aid.
© Cochlear Limited 2012.

I t is not the actual sound itself that matters, but the reverberations that it makes as it travels through our mind. These are often to be found far away, strangely transformed; but it is only by gathering up and putting together these echoes and fragments that we arrive at the true nature of our experience.
Virginia Woolf, 1926.

Deepening the emotional content of music, for example, by associating melody with concrete events in our lives, depends on dealings in ancient sub-neocortical limbic regions such as the hippocampus, amygdala, and anterior cingulate cortex, which form the hub of all our emotions, passions, and delights.

Many cope well with mild hearing loss if given comprehensive rehabilitation.

Classification Classify the type and possible cause of hearing loss:

- *Conductive hearing loss (CHL):* There is impaired sound transmission via the external canal and middle ear ossicles to the foot of the stapes through a variety of causes: external canal obstruction (wax, pus, debris, foreign body, developmental anomalies); drum perforation (trauma, barotrauma, infection); problems with the ossicular chain (otosclerosis, infection, trauma); and inadequate Eustachian tube ventilation of the middle ear (eg with effusion secondary to nasopharyngeal carcinoma). All result in conductive deafness.
- *Sensorineural hearing loss (SNHL):* Results from defects central to the oval window in the cochlea (sensory), cochlear nerve (neural) or, rarely, more central pathways. Ototoxic drugs (eg streptomycin, vancomycin, gentamicin, chloroquine and hydroxychloroquine, vinca alkaloids), postinfective (meningitis, measles, mumps, flu, herpes, syphilis), cochlear vascular disease, Ménière's (p554), trauma, and presbyacusis are all sensorineural. *Rare causes:* Acoustic neuroma (p553), B_{12} deficiency, multiple sclerosis, brain metastases.

▶ If unilateral SNHL exclude the dangerous: acoustic neuroma (MRI); cholesteatoma; effusion from nasopharyngeal cancer.

Sudden hearing loss • *If sensorineural: Definition:* Loss of ≥30dB in 3 contiguous pure tone frequencies over 3 days. Hearing loss may be sudden and abrupt, or rapidly progressive. Incidence: 5–20 per 100,000/yr. It is usually unilateral and the prognosis for some recovery is good (partial or complete spontaneous recovery occurs in 30–65%). *Management:* ▶▶Immediate specialist referral for investigation and management (see BOX). Sudden SNHL has many possible aetiologies. Detailed evaluation reveals underlying diseases (eg noise exposure; gentamicin toxicity; mumps; acoustic neuroma; MS; vasculopathy; TB) in 10%. Diagnose idiopathic sudden SNHL (ISSNHL) if no cause is found. Negative prognostic factors include: age <15yrs or >65yrs, ↑ESR, vertigo, hearing loss in the opposite ear, severe hearing loss.
- *Conductive:* A cause is 'always' found: infection, occlusion, trauma, fracture.

Otosclerosis New bone is formed around the stapes footplate, which leads to its fixation and consequent conductive hearing loss. *Prevalence:* 0.5–2% clinically, 10% subclinically. *Cause:* Autosomal dominant with incomplete penetrance; 50% have a family history. 85% are bilateral; ♀:♂ ≈ 2:1. *Symptoms:* Usually appear in early adult life and can be accelerated by pregnancy. There is conductive deafness (hearing is often better with background noise), ~75% have tinnitus; mild, transient vertigo is common too. 10% have Schwartze's sign—a pink tinge to the drum; audiometry with masked bone conduction shows a dip at 2kHz (Cahart's notch—see fig 7.20, p535). *Treatment: Hearing aid* (including BAHA) or *surgery*. Surgical options include stapedectomy or stapedotomy, to replace the adherent stapes. 90% enjoy an improvement in hearing. Microdrill and CO_2 laser stapedotomy give similar results. Many prefer surgery to wearing a hearing aid but careful selection is required as one complication of surgery is complete SNHL (1–4%). Surgery is only performed on the worse hearing ear; contralateral SNHL is a contraindication. **Cochlear implant** is another option (if severe).

Presbyacusis is age-related, bilateral, high-frequency SNHL. The exact mechanism is unclear but loss of high-frequency sounds starts before 30yrs and the rate of loss is progressive thereafter. Deafness (loss of hair cells: see fig 7.4, p535) is gradual and we do not usually notice it until hearing of speech is affected with loss of high-frequency sounds (consonants at ~3–4kHz are needed for speech discrimination). Hearing is most affected in the presence of background noise (try where possible to decrease this). Hearing aids are the usual treatment. See pure tone audiogram on p541 (fig 7.21), and BOX on p551.

▶▶Managing sudden sensorineural deafness[18]

▶▶ Take a full history, including drug history.

▶▶ Examine the EAC and TM to exclude wax/effusion. Perform tuning fork tests (p537; Weber goes to the other ear; Rinne AC>BC in affected ear).

▶▶ Get expert ENT help.

▶▶ Look for causes: FBC; ESR/CRP; U&E; LFT; TSH; autoimmune profile; clotting studies; fasting glucose; cholesterol.

▶▶ Arrange audiology: audiometry ± audiological brainstem responses.

▶▶ Treatment depends on the cause (if found). There are varied treatment regimens for ISSHL—no single treatment has been shown to be effective.

▶▶ High-dose steroids are commonly used (presumed inflammatory cause). One starting regimen is **prednisolone** 80mg/24h PO for 4 days tapered over 8 days. Intratympanic dexamethasone has a salvage role in treatment failure.

▶▶ There may be a response to hyperbaric O_2 therapy, if given promptly.

▶▶ Routine prescribing of antivirals, thrombolytics, vasodilators, vasoactive substances, or antioxidants to patients with ISSNHL is not recommended.[19]

The bounds of 'normal' hearing

Both frequency (Hz) and sound pressure (decibels, dB) are important for the detection of sound by the human ear, though the relationship between the two is also important. A person with normal hearing will hear sound frequencies between 20 and 20000Hz. Sound frequencies between 250

Is your hearing reduced?
• Do people 'mumble'?
• Do you keep saying 'What?'
• Do you misunderstand names?
• Is your TV volume 'too loud'?
• Are noisy rooms a problem?

and 8000Hz are the most important for speech interpretation. Vowel sounds have low frequencies (250–1000Hz) and are easier to hear. Consonants, at higher frequencies (1500–6000Hz) convey most of the meaning of what we say, which is why those with higher frequency loss (eg presbyacusis) have such difficulty.

The normal range of hearing is 0–140dB. Hearing is measured in decibels of hearing level (dBHL)—decibels relative to the quietest sounds heard with normal hearing. Normal hearing level =-10 to 25dBHL ('0' is average, hence minus scores are better than average). Hearing loss is categorized into mild (26–40dBHL); moderate (41–70dBHL); severe (71–90dBHL); and profound, which is defined as >90dBHL. Remember that decibels are a logarithmic scale, and that the range from 0 to 120dBs actually represents a million times relative increase in sound pressure. At high intensity (≥130dB), sound can also be a *painful* stimulus, showing an interesting (and variable) threshold relationship between useful information from special senses and painful stimuli (also present in the eye).

ENT

a *ou *ea* *e?

If you only hear vowels, understanding speech is difficult

Can you hear me?

Further reading

Mathur NN (2015). Sudden Hearing Loss. Medscape. http://emedicine.medscape.com/article/856313

Tinnitus (Latin *tinnire*, meaning to ring) is a perception of sound, typically in the absence of auditory stimulation. Tinnitus is often a symptom of an underlying abnormality. **Prevalence** 15% (0.5% severe). Two-thirds of patients have associated sensorineural hearing loss (SNHL). One-third have no identifiable cause.

Tinnitus character may help identify aetiology. It may be unilateral or bilateral, pulsatile or non-pulsatile. Ringing, hissing, or buzzing suggests an inner ear or central cause. Popping or clicking suggests problems in the external or middle ear, or the palate. Pulsatile tinnitus is often objective (below) but can also simply reflect an increased awareness of blood flow in the ear.

Classification[20] Tinnitus may be objective or subjective.
- *Objective tinnitus* (which is audible to the examiner) is rare and occurs due to • *Vascular disorders:* pulsatile vibratory sounds from eg AV malformations; carotid pathology; glomus tumours (fig 7.30). • *High-output cardiac states:* Paget's; hyperthyroidism; anaemia, causing pulsatile tinnitus. • *Myoclonus* of palatal or stapedius/tensor tympani muscles, resulting in an audible click. • *Patulous Eustachian tube:* prolonged opening, causing abnormal sound transmission to the ear.
- *Subjective tinnitus* is audible only to the patient. *Associations:* • Most commonly associated with disorders causing SNHL, eg presbyacusis; noise induced hearing loss; Ménière's (unilateral). • *Conductive deafness* is less commonly associated eg from impacted wax; otosclerosis. • *Ototoxic drugs:* cause bilateral tinnitus with associated hearing loss. Cisplatin and aminoglycosides can cause permanent hearing loss. Aspirin, NSAIDs, quinine, macrolides and loop diuretics are associated with tinnitus and reversible hearing loss. • *Otitis media* ± effusion. • *Other associations:* Hyper/hypothyroidism; diabetes; MS; ►acoustic neuroma (unilateral); trauma to the head or neck. Anxiety and depression is frequently associated with and may exacerbate tinnitus.

Pathophysiology Poorly understood. Possible mechanisms include spontaneous otoacoustic emissions; altered or increased spontaneous activity in the auditory nerve or central structures; plastic reorganization of central pathways; inappropriate feedback via descending pathways, and auditory–limbic interactions (BOX). Usually we are able to habituate tinnitus. If not, it becomes problematic.[21]

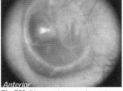

Anterior

Fig 7.30 Glomus tympanicum tumour: note red anterior mass and a small fluid meniscus around it.
Courtesy of Rory Herdman FRCS.

Tests Audiometry; tympanogram. ► Investigate unilateral tinnitus (MRI) to exclude acoustic neuroma (p553; 10% present this way).

R Treat any underlying cause. Take time to explain tinnitus—it is common and usually improves with time (via habituation). Ask their beliefs about tinnitus and address any underlying concerns. Manage depression, anxiety, or insomnia. Positive attitudes help. Treat the whole person, not just a malfunctioning ear. Treatment is aimed at reducing the impact of symptoms:
- *Hearing aids:* If hearing loss >35dB, a hearing aid that improves perception of background noise makes tinnitus less apparent.
- *Psychological support:* Psychoeducational counselling together with *sound therapy* (the use of background sound to reduce the impact of tinnitus by partially masking it, eg from a radio or fan) are the mainstay of rehabilitation.
- *Cognitive behavioural therapy:* (p390) To identify and modify unhelpful thoughts and behaviours.

Further reading

McKenna L (2011). *Tinnitus Explained.* http://www.tinnitus.org.uk/tinnitus-explained-1
NICE (2010). *Clinical Knowledge Summaries: Tinnitus.* http://cks.nice.org.uk/tinnitus

Acoustic neuroma

These are typically indolent, histologically benign subarachnoid tumours that cause problems by local pressure, and then behave as space-occupying lesions. They are misnomers as they usually arise from the superior vestibular nerve schwann cell layer, hence the name *vestibular schwannoma*. **Symptoms** Progressive ipsilateral tinnitus ± sensorineural deafness (cochlear nerve compression). Large tumours may give ipsilateral cerebellar or ↑ICP signs. Giddiness is common; vertigo rare. Trigeminal compression above the tumour may give a numb face. Nearby cranial nerves at risk: (v, vi, vii). **Tests** ▶Request MRI for all those with unilateral tinnitus/deafness. ∆∆ Meningioma. **Surgery** (difficult, and often not needed, eg if elderly); there are many methods with various ways of preserving hearing and the facial nerve. Sterotactic radiosurgery is increasingly popular.

Noise-induced hearing loss (NIHL)[22]

Exposure to loud noise will cause damage to the inner ear resulting in hearing loss. This can be a one-time exposure to an intense sound (=acoustic trauma, eg from an explosion) or, more commonly in occupational NIHL, continuous exposure to loud sounds that causes hearing loss over time. There is a relationship between volume of sound and its duration: 8 hours' exposure to a sound level of 85dB usually causes damage. Acoustic trauma is caused by sounds >180dB. Rupture of the drum and ossicular fracture may occur.

Symptoms There is bilateral symmetrical sensori-neural hearing loss ± tinnitus. There may be noise-induced temporary threshold shift, which occurs when hearing improves away from the source of exposure.

Audiometry Typically shows a 'notch' at 3, 4, or 6kHz with recovery at 8kHz (see fig 7.19, p541).

Management Reduce risk of occupational exposure: Abide by health and safety law; provide ear defenders; and screen occupations at risk. In established hearing loss use hearing aids.

The Jastreboff model of tinnitus[23]

The Jastreboff neurophysiological model proposes that the limbic and autonomic nervous systems are the primary systems for the development of tinnitus annoyance, with the auditory system playing a secondary role in tinnitus manifestation.

Tinnitus retraining therapy is based on this model and is aimed at habituating tinnitus-evoked reactions and perception. The two main components are educational counselling (to reclassify and neutralize tinnitus), and sound therapy (via constant low level broad band sound). Successful treatment results in patients who are not bothered by their tinnitus, even though they are aware of it.

ENT

Vertigo is a symptom—the sensation that you, or the world around you, is moving or spinning.

Vestibular (peripheral) vertigo is often severe, and may be accompanied by loss of balance, nausea, vomiting, ↓hearing, tinnitus, nystagmus (usually horizontal) and diaphoresis. Hearing loss and tinnitus are less common in *central vertigo* (usually less severe), nystagmus may be horizontal or vertical.

Is the symptom vestibular? 'I'm dizzy' is ambiguous. Elicit the illusion! Ask 'Did you or the world seem to spin (like getting off a playground roundabout?)' or 'Which *way* are things going?' Those with vertigo often know without hesitation; if not, this is a cue to pursue other causes (lightheadedness ± a 'sense of collapse' can be vascular, ocular, musculoskeletal, metabolic, or claustrophobic). ►Ask about duration of vertigo: seconds to minutes≈BPPV; 30min to 30h≈Ménière's or migraine; 30h to a week≈acute vestibular failure.

Causes (often multifactorial)
Peripheral:
• Ménière's disease
• Benign paroxysmal positional vertigo (BPPV)
• Vestibular failure
• Labyrinthitis
• Superior semi-circular canal dehiscence
Central:
• Acoustic neuroma
• Multiple sclerosis
• Head injury
• Migraine associated dizziness
• Vertebrobasilar insufficiency
Other:
• Multifactorial disequilibrium (causing falls in elderly)

Examination/tests Assess CNs & ears. Test cerebellar function & reflexes. Assess: nystagmus, gait, Romberg's test (+ve if balance is worse when eyes are shut, implying defective joint position sense or vestibular input). *Do provocation tests (Head thrust test; Hallpike test,* see BOX). If clinical doubt request audiometry ± electronystagmography; MRI.

Benign paroxysmal positional vertigo (BPPV) The commonest cause of peripheral vertigo. Attacks of sudden rotational vertigo lasting >30sec are provoked by head-turning. Other otological symptoms are rare. *Pathogenesis:* Displacement of otoconia (=otoliths) stimulate the semicircular canals. *Causes:* Idiopathic; head injury. *Diagnosis:* Establish important negatives: ►No *persistent* vertigo ►No speech, visual, motor, or sensory problems ►No tinnitus, headache, ataxia, facial numbness, or dysphagia ►No vertical nystagmus. *Hallpike test* is +ve (BOX). *R:* Usually self-limiting; if persistent, try: • Epley manoeuvre (fig 7.31) is 70–80% effective. • Home repositioning manoeuvres/vestibular habituation exercises (BOX). • *Drugs:* vestibular suppressant medication does not stop the vertigo • *Last resort:* Surgery eg vestibular nerve section (rare).

Ménière's disease Dilatation of the endolymphatic spaces[3] of the membranous labyrinth causes sudden attacks of vertigo lasting ~2-4h (nystagmus is always present); or there may be increasing fullness in the ears ± tinnitus followed by vertigo. Symptoms often become bilateral. Fluctuating SNHL is common (may become permanent). *Cause:* A mystery! *Δ:* Electrocochleography; posterior fossa MRI. *R:* *Acute:* Prochlorperazine (Buccastem® 3mg/8h bucally; short–term as vestibular sedative) *Prophylaxis:* betahistine 16mg/8h PO. Surgical approaches for persistent symptoms: Instillation of gentamicin via a grommet; Labyrinthectomy is 95% effective in controlling vertigo but causes total ipsilateral deafness; vestibular neurectomy (5% risk of hearing loss; 90% effective).

Acute vestibular failure *(AKA vestibular neuronitis/labyrinthitis)* (NB: the cochlea and semicircular canals =the labyrinth). Sudden attacks of unilateral vertigo and vomiting in a previously well person, often following a recent URTI. It lasts 1-2 days, improving over a week. *Signs:* Nystagmus away from the affected side. Audiogram if hearing loss. *R:* Vestibular suppressants eg Buccastem® 3mg/8h PO or cyclizine 50mg/8h PO. It is impossible to distinguish from 'viral labyrinthitis' and so this term is best avoided.

3 Also called *endolymphatic hydrops. Endolymph* is the fluid in the scala media (fig 7.4, p535) that is of a similar make-up to intracellular fluid. *Perilymph* is similar to CSF in composition, and is the fluid in the scala tympani and the scala vestibuli of the cochlea, that communicate at its apex via the helicotrema.

How to perform the (Dix-) Hallpike Test

- Ask the patient to keep their eyes open and look straight ahead at all times.
- Place the patient sitting on the couch in such a way that when they lie back, their head will be over the edge of the couch.
- With the patient sitting on the couch and positioned to allow them to lie backwards, turn their head 45° towards the test ear (this leads to maximal stimulation of the posterior circular canal on lying).
- Continue to hold the patient's head between your hands. Ask them to lie backwards and then quickly lower their head 30° below the level of the couch. Ask the patient if they feel dizzy and look for nystagmus.
- If +ve, there is vertigo and rotary nystagmus towards the undermost ear, after a latent period of 5–10sec. This lasts <30sec and is fatiguable. On sitting, there is more vertigo (± nystagmus). If any of these features are absent (no latency, no symptoms, and persisting nystagmus), seek a central cause.
- Watching online videos are an excellent way of learning how to do this + other tests such as the head thrust test and Epley or Semont manoeuvre.

Home treatment of BPPV

- A *modified Epley manoeuvre* can be taught to patients to perform at home. It is helpful in those who have frequent recurrence of vertigo or who do not respond quickly to therapist-led manoeuvres.
- *Brandt–Daroff exercises* were developed as a series of home exercises to reduce symptoms of BPPV. They are thought to work by repositioning, dispersing or dissolving inner ear debris, and through habituation from repeated exposure. They are usually used when other repositioning manoeuvres have been unsuccessful and are effective in 25–50% of patients.
- Cochrane review suggests repositioning manoeuvres are more effective than exercise based vestibular rehabilitation eg *Cawthorne Cooksey exercises*, although a combination of the two is effective for longer term recovery.[24]

ENT

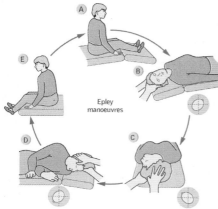

Fig 7.31 The Epley manoeuvre. The therapist moves the patients head through 4 sequential positions, resting for ~30sec between each movement. The aim is to reposition otoconia away from the sensitive posterior canals. This works in ~80% (a 2nd go may help). Some evidence supports postural restrictions post procedure (upright head posture for 48hrs, avoid lying on affected side for 7 days).

Epley manoeuvres

Rhinosinusitis in adults is defined as inflammation in the nose and paranasal sinuses with ≥2 symptoms, one of which must be nasal blockage/obstruction/congestion, or nasal discharge, ±facial pain or pressure, reduction or loss of smell, and either endoscopic or cⲧ signs. Rhinosinusitis symptoms are classified as mild, moderate or severe—and as acute (ARS) or chronic (CRS, if lasting >12wks).

Acute rhinosinusitis (common cold) Many episodes are self limiting. If symptoms persist >5 days, consider non-systemically bioavailable *intranasal corticosteroids* (eg mometasone; fluticasone; advise on correct technique, see fig 7.32). Avoid antibiotics unless severe or worsening symptoms (80% resolve in 14 days without antibiotics).[25] **Acute post-viral sinusitis** is defined as increase in symptoms after 5 days or persistant symptoms >10 days.

Chronic rhinosinusitis with nasal polyps see BOX, p557.

Chronic rhinosinusitis without nasal polyps *Intranasal corticosteroids* and *nasal saline irrigation* (p561) are central. If there is no improvement after 4 weeks and mucosal disease at subsequent endoscopy is moderate or severe consider microbiological cultures + add long-term (>12 weeks) antibiotics (if IgE is not elevated). Perform cⲧ scan and if poor response to treatment consider surgery.

Allergic rhinosinusitis may be seasonal (hay fever, prevalence ≈20%, common in childhood) or perennial (more common in adults). *Cause:* IgE-mediatied inflammation from allergen exposure to nasal mucosa causing inflammatory mediator release from mast cells, eg from house dust mite (perennial); pollens or animal dander. *Symptoms:* Sneezing; pruritus; nasal discharge (bilateral & variable); bilateral itchy red eyes. Check for asthma. *Signs:* Turbinates may be swollen and mucosae pale or mauve; nasal polyps. *R:*[26] •*Allergen/irritant avoidance* •*Nasal saline irrigation* (p561) •*Antihistamines* (non–sedating eg loratadine 10mg OD). If moderate/persistent symptoms: •*Intranasal corticosteroid sprays*—use non-systemically bioavailable corticosteroids (eg mometasone; fluticasone).

A short course of *prednisolone* can help rapid resolution of severe symptoms eg during exams (eg adults 10–20mg/24h; children 10mg/24h for 5–10 days). •*Immunotherapy:* Can induce long-term tolerance to allergens eg once-daily *sublingual immunotherapy* (SLIT) for grass-pollen-induced rhinosinusitis. The future for some patients may lie in same-season ultra-short course allergy vaccine (eg 4 injections of Pollinex Quattro®).[27]

Other causes of chronic rhinorrhoea/rhinitis Foreign body (see below), cSF (eg after head injury), bacteria (eg TB), HIV, CF, age (old man's drip[4]), pregnancy, decongestant overuse, antibody deficiency (p198), non-allergic rhinitis with eosinophilia (NARES), ASA triad.

Other causes of nasal congestion *Child:* Large adenoids; choanal atresia (congenital blockage of one or both nasal passages by bone or tissue); postnasal space tumour (eg angiofibroma); foreign body (►refer same day if *unilateral* obstruction ± foul/bloody discharge). *Adult:* Deflected nasal septum; granuloma (TB, syphilis, granulomatosis with polyangiitis, leprosy); topical vasoconstrictors; tricyclics. ►*Refer urgently if:* • Numbness • Tooth loss • Bleeding • Unilateral obstructing mass. *Ask:* do symptoms vary? Is it both sides? Any effects on eating, speech, smell, or sleep (snoring)? Assess nasal deflection. Is either nostril completely blocked (occlude each nostril)? Examine the postnasal space (nasal endoscope or mirror).

Further reading

British Society for Allergy & Clinical Immunology (BSACI) *Rhinitis Management Guidelines.* http://www.guidelines.co.uk/eye_ear_nose_throat_bsaci_rhinitis#.VjN8rX7hCM8

Fokkens WJ *et al.* (2012). EPOS 2012: European position paper on rhinosinusitis and nasal polyps 2012. A summary for otorhinolaryngologists. *Rhinology* 50(1):1–12.

4 Old man's drip often occurs on eating, and ipratropium nasal spray (Rinatec®) may help.

Chronic rhinosinusitis with nasal polyps

Simple nasal polyps are swellings of the nasal or sinus mucosa prolapsing into the nasal cavity. Prevalence is 2%. They are part of the spectrum of rhinosinusitis. **Cause** Unknown. **Typical patient** Male >40yrs old. **Sites** Usually bilateral. Middle meatus (most commonly). Single, benign maxillary polyps may arise in the maxillary antrum, and prolapse to fill the nasopharynx (antrochoanal polyps).

Symptoms Watery anterior rhinorrhoea, sneezing, purulent postnasal drip, nasal obstruction, sinusitis, mouth-breathing, snoring, headaches. **Investigations** Anterior rhinoscopy or nasal endoscopy. It can be hard to distinguish hypertrophied inferior turbinates from polyps. Polyps are pale, mobile, and insensitive to gentle palpation

Associations
• Allergic rhinitis
• Non-allergic rhinitis
• Chronic ethmoid
sinusitis
• Cystic fibrosis
• Aspirin hypersensitivity
• Asthma (eg non-atopic)

(fig 7.33). Turbinates are pink, mobile, and sensate. Consider allergy testing.

►NB: A single unilateral polyp requires urgent referral for biopsy as it may turn out to be a rare intranasal pathology (eg nasopharyngeal cancer, lymphoma).

Treatment

• *Medical:* Topical steroid drops shrink polyps eg **betamethasone 0.1%, 2 drops/12h** (both nostrils) for 2 weeks, followed by **fluticasone 100mcg (2 sprays)/24h** (both nostrils) for 3 months. Consider adding long–term antibiotics eg **doxycycline**. ►*Advise on correct posture* (fig 7.32): *simply tilting the head back doesn't work!*

• *Surgery: Endoscopic sinus surgery (ESS):* Consider if maximal medical treatment fails and ongoing severe symptoms. If more than simple polypectomy is planned, do CT to show anatomical variations. Complications of endoscopic surgery are rare, but can include damage to the optic nerve and CSF leak. *Post-op:* •'Don't blow your nose until you are better' • Watch for bleeding • Abide by epistaxis advice (p562).

Children ►Nasal polyps are rare if <10yrs old; rule out neoplasms, cystic fibrosis, and meningocele/encephalocele (esp. if unilateral and <2yrs old).

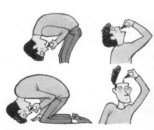

Fig 7.32 The left two images show how we should use nose drops; both the methods on the right are *equally* useless.

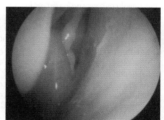

Fig 7.33 A polyp arising from right middle meatus. NB: the lower part of septum deviates to this side.

Courtesy of Rory Herdman FRCS.

ENT

These are air-filled cavities in the bones around the nose, in continuity with the nasal cavity (fig 7.34). They are lined by ciliated mucosa, which sweep debris and mucus towards and through the osteomeatal complex into the nostrils (fig 7.35). Obstruction impairs drainage and is due to anatomical problems (eg septal deviation/polyps), or mucosal problems (viruses cause mucosal oedema and ↓cilia action). Recognizing and correcting drainage problems is important.

Acute bacterial rhinosinusitis Is part of the rhinosinusitis spectrum (p536) and is suggested by the presence of at least 3 symptoms/signs of:
- Discoloured discharge (with unilateral predominance) and purulent secretion in the nasal cavity
- Severe local pain (with unilateral predominance)
- Fever (>38°C)
- Elevated ESR/CRP
- 'Double sickening' (ie a deterioration after an initial milder phase of illness).
▶*Swelling is uncommon: exclude carcinoma or dental root infections.*

Differential diagnosis of sinusitis (non-sinus pain): migraine, TMJ dysfunction (p542); dental pain; neuropathic pain; temporal arteritis; herpes zoster. Pain in the absence of symptoms described above is unlikely to be sinusitis.

Causes of bacterial sinusitis ▶Most follow viral infection. Other causes:
1 Direct spread (dental root infection or diving/swimming in infected water).
2 Odd anatomy: septal deviation, large ethmoidal bulla, polyps, large uncinate process (the part of ethmoid bone forming the maxillary sinus medial wall).
3 ITU causes: mechanical ventilation; recumbency; use of nasogastric tubes.
4 Systemic causes: Kartagener's; immunodeficiency; or general debility.
5 Biofilms[5]: type of infection which destroy mucosal cells of cilia and goblet cells.
Common organisms: S. pneumoniae, H. influenzae; and S. aureus, Moraxella catarrhalis, fungi.[6]

Investigations Diagnosis of acute bacterial sinusitis is usually clinical. Examine the nose and look for mucosal inflammation, oedema, nasal discharge ± polyps, and septal deviation. In recurrent acute or chronic sinusitis, CT of the paranasal sinuses and nasal endoscopy helps confirm the diagnosis and plan any surgery + identify any underlying anatomical problems (eg low cribiform plates). Normal x-rays cannot exclude sinus disease. NB: In recurrent acute sinusitis, CT may be normal in the absence of acute infection.

Treatment *Acute/single episode:* 98% of cases are viral, self-limiting and take ~2½ weeks to resolve. Simple analgesia, nasal saline irrigation (p561) and intranasal decongestants (eg **ephedrine** 0.5%, max. 1 week). Antihistamines are not routinely used as they may thicken secretions and complicate drainage. Give antibiotics if bacterial infection is suspected (eg **amoxicillin** or **doxycycline**). *Recurrent episodes:* Treat as above and refer for imaging/surgery (NB: results of surgery in patients with no evidence of sinus disease on CT or endoscopy are poor). If medical therapy fails, refer for ESS (endoscopic sinus surgery) tailored to the particular sinus affected. Smoking cessation helps as tobacco irritates nasal mucosa and ↓cilia function. Dental infection can be associated.

Complications ▶*Orbital cellulitis/abscess:* This is an emergency, p420. ▶*Intracranial involvement:* Meningitis, encephalitis, cerebral abscess, cavernous sinus thrombosis. *Mucocoeles* (esp. frontal sinus) may become infected pyocoeles (pus filled cavity). *Osteomyelitis:* Classically staph, eg frontal bone. *Pott's puffy tumour:* A subperiosteal abscess arising from frontal osteomyelitis.

---

5 Free-floating organisms become anchored to a living or inert surface (eg sinus mucosa; urinary catheter) and form a biofilm. This progressive organization facilitates further attachment and hinders removal.
6 Fungi can be isolated from the sinuses of almost every patient, so its causality is questionable.

Cancer of the paranasal sinuses

Suspect when chronic sinusitis presents for the first time in later life. *Early signs:* Blood-stained nasal discharge and nasal obstruction; cheek swelling. *Images:* MRI/CT ± endoscopy (with biopsy). *Differential histology:* Squamous cell (50%), lymphoma (10%), adenocarcinoma, adenoid cystic carcinoma, olfactory neuroblastoma, or chondrosarcoma, benign tumours. *R:* Radiotherapy ± radical surgery.

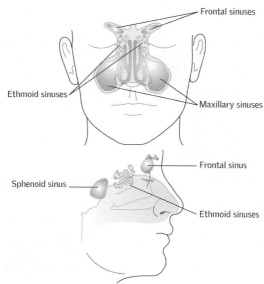

Fig 7.34 Sinus anatomy.

Redrawn with permission from Medtronic.

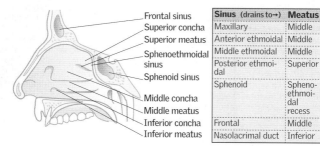

Sinus (drains to→)	Meatus
Maxillary	Middle
Anterior ethmoidal	Middle
Middle ethmoidal	Middle
Posterior ethmoidal	Superior
Sphenoid	Sphenoethmoidal recess
Frontal	Middle
Nasolacrimal duct	Inferior

Fig 7.35 The nasal turbinates (conchae) and meati. The TABLE shows the patterns of drainage of the sinuses & nasolacrimal duct.

Nasal fractures ►Always exclude significant head or c-spine injury. The most common cause is direct trauma from a punch, clash of heads, or a fall, often with brief but short-lived epistaxis. *Diagnosis*: New nasal deformity, often with associated facial swelling and black eyes. Examine the patient from behind and above, looking along the nose. x-rays are not required, but may help exclude other facial fracture. Look for a septal haematoma (a boggy swelling of the septum causing near-total nasal obstruction). ►If present it requires urgent incision and drainage. *R*: Treat epistaxis (p562); Advise on analgesia/using ice; close any skin injury. Reassess 5–7d post-injury (once swelling has resolved). If MUA is required, it can be performed 10–14d after the injury (before the nasal bones set).[28]

CSF rhinorrhoea Ethmoid fractures disrupting dura and arachnoid can result in CSF leaks. ►If not associated with trauma, ask: is it a tumour? Nasal CSF discharge tests +ve for glucose (dipstick unreliable; confirm with a lab glucose). CSF uniquely contains β_2 (tau) transferrin (needs >0.5mL; the gold standard). *R*: If traumatic, conservative management has high spontaneous resolution: 7–10d bedrest (head elevated 15–30°) ± lumbar drain. Avoid coughing, sneezing, nose-blowing. Surgery is often not needed. Cover with antibiotics and pneumococcal vaccine.

Foreign bodies Most are self-inserted by children. Organic material presents early with purulent unilateral discharge; inorganic bodies may remain inert for ages. Use an auroscope to examine the child's nose. *R*: Ask the child to blow their nose (if able) or ask a parent to try a 'parental kiss' by blowing into the mouth whilst occluding the other nostril (success rate >70%). If a child is co-operative it may be possible to grasp the object with crocodile forceps (avoid pushing deeper into the nose). Batteries need urgent removal. Refer to ENT if failed attempt or uncooperative patient.

Septal perforation Septal surgery is the most common cause (below). *Others: Trauma* (nose picking; foreign body; laceration; septal haematoma); *Inhalants* (nasal steroid/decongestant sprays; cocaine abuse); *Infection* (TB; syphilis; HIV); *Inflammation/malignancies* (SCC; Churg–Strauss, granulomatosis with polyangiitis). Perforations irritate, whistle, crust, and bleed. *R*: Symptomatic. Saline nasal irrigation (p562); petroleum jelly applied to the edge of the perforation. Progressive enlargement is a risk. Surgical closure may be via placement of a septal prosthesis ('button'). Only half of patients find this tolerable and continue use long term. Surgical repair has variable results (even in experienced hands). See fig 7.36 for nasal septal anatomy.

Septoplasty and septorhinoplasty

Septoplasty corrects a deviated nasal septum. It is most often performed where there is nasal obstruction with no other identifiable cause (eg polyps, hypertrophied turbinate) and where conservative treatment has failed.
Septorhinoplasty aims to straighten and/or refashion the shape of the nose—for cosmesis and to help breathing by improving the airway. *Post-operative care:* Avoid nose blowing for 1 week. Saline nasal irrigation (p561) with saline sniffs ×4/day for 2 weeks (prevents crusting).

Complications: Bleeding; CSF leakage; altered sensation of lips, gums and incisors. If a septal haematoma develops, incise and drain + give antibiotics to prevent a septal abscess (formal drainage may be needed, and may not prevent septal perforation). Adhesions between the septum and the lateral nasal wall may develop and may require division.

Naspharyngeal cancer (NPC)

Rare in the UK. **NPC** differs significantly from other cancers of the head and neck (HNSCC, p570). *Signs/symptoms:* Neck lump (cervical lymphadenopathy in 90%); Nasal symptoms (bleeding/obstruction/discharge). Hearing loss (usually unilateral due to conductive deafness from Eustachian tube blockage); Cranial nerve palsies (not I, VII, VIII) due to base of skull extension. Δ· Endoscopy/biopsy. NB: submucosal spread may mean the area *looks* normal. Stage by MRI. ℞: Radiotherapy is mainstay ± chemotherapy ± surgery (radical neck dissection). *Prognosis:* 5-yr survival >80% for stage I; <30% for advanced tumours.

Nasal saline irrigation (AKA nasal douching; 'saline sniffs')

Nasal irrigation A simple procedure that requires patients to 'sniff' a saline solution into the nostril. It helps keep the nose clean and removes any debris. It also prevents crusts from forming after surgery or epistaxis and is used in the management of rhinitis (p556), clearing away irritant allergens.

To make the saline solution: Place 1 flat teaspoon of salt and 1 flat teaspoon of bicarbonate of soda into a bowl and add ~1 pint of cooled boiled water. Stir until the salts have dissolved.

To use the solution: Pour some cooled solution into a *neti pot* or squeezy bottle with a nozzle (more effective than sniffing from the 'cup' of your hand). Close one nostril using your hand and pour or squeeze the solution up into your nose and let it run out. Repeat this action ~4 times up each nostril.[29]

ENT

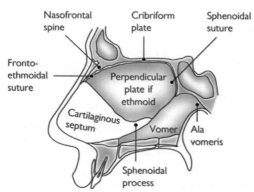

Fig 7.36 Nasal septal anatomy.
Reproduced from Warner et al, *Oxford Specialist Handbook of Otolaryngology and Head and Neck Surgery* (2009) with permission from Oxford University Press.

Respect all nosebleeds. Whilst they are common, they can be life-threatening. Epistaxis is *anterior* or *posterior*; anterior bleeds that can be easily seen with rhinoscopy are simpler to treat and are usually less severe. Proceed as follows: G-up (gown, goggles, gloves), then:

▸▸ Resuscitate as needed, eg if BP↓ or dizzy on sitting. ABCs; IVI, SaO₂, etc. Monitor vital signs.

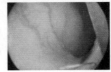

Fig 7.37 Vessels in Little's area (left side of septum). These are the main cause of epistaxis in children.

Courtesy of Rory Herdman FRCS.

▸▸ History: Which side? Trauma? How much loss? On warfarin/aspirin? Note past medical history.

▸▸ Ask the patient to apply pressure by pinching the *lower* part of nose for 20min. Breathe through the mouth; sit forward and spit blood into a bowl.

▸▸ Place an ice pack on the dorsum of the nose (ice may also be sucked). If this doesn't work...

▸▸ Prepare to cauterize the nose with silver nitrate:

▸▸ Encourage the patient to blow out nasal clots.

▸ Look inside; remove clots (gentle suction);

▸▸ Apply a cotton ball soaked in 1:200,000 adrenaline for 2 minutes (causes vasoconstriction); or use local anaesthetic spray (eg lidocaine).

▸▸ Find bleeding points (often on the anterior septum. Apply cautery for 2sec at a time, starting from the edge of the bleeding point moving in on a circle (this treats any feeding vessel).

▸▸ Remember: 'silver nitrate cauterizes everything it touches'. Avoid using if actively bleeding as this will wash the chemical away and may cause unwanted burns to the lips or throat.

▸▸ Never cauterize both sides of the septum, as this risks perforation.

Causes/associations
• Local trauma (eg nosepicking)
• Facial trauma
• Dry/cold weather
• Dyscrasia/haemophilia*et al*
• Septal perforation

After the bleed...
• Don't pick or blow!
• If you sneeze, send it through your open mouth
• Avoid bending, lifting, or straining.
• No hot food or drink[7]
• If it restarts, apply ice to the bridge of the nose, and hold the soft lower part *continuously* for 20 min; get help if this fails.

▸▸ If you cannot see the bleeding point, refer to ENT.

▸▸ If bleeding continues, try an *anterior nasal pack* (eg Rapid Rhino®; Merocel®). Lubricate/soak the pack as instructed; advance it into the nose horizontally and parallel to the hard palate (*not* up). Inflate if required, and tape securely to the face. If all is well, remove after 24h. If bleeding continues, try a *postnasal pack:* A variety are available, however a Foley urinary catheter (16–18G) is effective. Pass via the nostril into the nasopharynx. Inflate the balloon with >10mL water and pull anteriorly to occlude the posterior choana. Clamp (with padding over the skin) at the nasal vestibule, to prevent it falling backwards into the airway.

Anterior epistaxis is almost invariably septal; Little's area (Kiesselbach's plexus) is used to describe the area where anterior ethmoidal, sphenopalatine, and facial arteries anastomose to form an anterior anastomotic arcade (figs 7.37 & 7.38).

Serious posterior epistaxis More invasive procedures may be required:

1 *Examination under anaesthesia:* If a discrete bleeding point is found it can be treated directly, eg with diathermy, otherwise repacking may be needed. Correction of septal deviation may improve access.

2 *Arterial ligation:* Endoscopic ligation of eg the sphenopalatine artery is the cornerstone of serious epistaxis management in specialist units.

3 *Embolization* of eg the internal maxillary or facial artery can be lifesaving—but this can cause a stroke.

---

7 Clearly no-one will follow this advice, so suggest each mouthful is washed down with ice cold water to help keep the mouth cold and prevent vasodilatation.

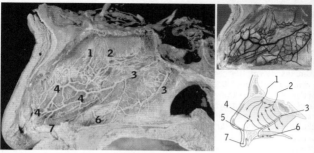

Fig 7.38 Blood supply to the nasal septum.
1 Anterior ethmoidal artery 2 Posterior ethmoidal artery 3 Sphenopalatine artery (≥2 branches, as on the dissection) 4 Little's area (anterior ethmoidal, sphenopalatine, and facial arteries anastomose to form this anterior anastomotic arcade) 5 Septal branch 6 Greater palatine artery 7 Superior labial artery and branches (from facial artery).

Courtesy of Prof Tor Chiu who performed the dissection.

ENT

An acute sore throat can be due to **acute pharyngitis** (inflammation of the oropharynx), or **tonsillitis** (fig 7.39).[30] It is commonly caused by a viral or bacterial infection and is generally self-limiting. Symptoms resolve in 40% within 3 days and within 1 week in 85%.

Causes: • *Viral:* 'The common cold' eg rhinovirus, coronovirus and parainfluenza virus account for ~25% of all sore throats; influenza type A and B (4%); adenovirus (4%); herpes simplex virus (2%); Epstein–Barr virus (glandular fever; 1%). • *Bacterial:* Group A β-haemolytic *Streptococcus* (GABHS) may cause pharyngitis, tonsillitis, or scarlet fever (below). It cannot be diagnosed on clinical features alone but the *Centor criteria* (below) can be used to assist the decision on whether antibiotics should be prescribed. GABHS accounts for ~15–30% of sore throats in children and ~10% in adults. • *Rarer infectious causes: Haemophilus influenzae* type B (▶epiglottitis, p566).

Tests: Throat swabs should not be taken routinely. Antistreptococcal antibody tests have no role in diagnosis, but can help confirm a history of GABHS in patients with suspected poststeptococcal glomerulonephritis or rheumatic fever.

Treatment Reassure. *Symptomatic relief:* Regular ibuprofen ± paracetamol to relieve pain and fever. Consider mouthwashes or spray (benzydamine eg **Difflam®**). *Antibiotics:* Do not routinely prescribe antibiotics (see BOX). Most cases are viral. Antibiotics won't provide symptomatic relief and should not be given to prevent complications. If *Centor criteria* are 3 or 4 (below), consider **penicillin V** for 10 days (lower relapse). Or **clarithromycin** or **erythromycin** for 5 days if penicillin allergic. Avoid amoxicillin, which causes a pathognomonic rash in almost all whose pharyngitis is from EBV. If immunosuppressed (eg leukaemia, aplastic anaemia, asplenia or HIV/AIDS), seek urgent specialist advice. If on DMARDS or carbimazole, check FBC urgently.

Centor criteria: • Presence of tonsillar exudate • Presence of tender anterior cervical lymphadenopathy • History of fever • Absence of cough. The presence of 3 or 4 of these criteria suggest infection due to *Streptococcus* (positive predictive value ~50%) and patients may benefit from antibiotics. If all 4 are absent, the negative predictive value is 80%.

Complications of tonsillitis • *Otitis media* (p544) • *Sinusitis* (p558).
• *Peritonsillar abscess (quinsy)* presents with sore throat, dysphagia, peritonsillar bulge, uvular deviation, trismus, and muffled voice. Antibiotics and aspiration (preferred to surgical drainage) are needed.
• *Parapharyngeal abscess:* A serious but rare complication, presenting with diffuse swelling in the neck. ℞: US to identify site; incise and drain under GA.
• *Lemierre syndrome:* Acute septicaemia and jugular vein thrombosis secondary to infection with *Fusobacterium* species + septic emboli (to lungs, bone, muscle, kidney, liver). Rare.

Differential diagnosis of unilateral tonsillar enlargement
• Apparent enlargement may be due to tonsillar shift because of peritonsillar abscess/parapharyngeal mass.
• If true asymmetry, perform excision biopsy to exclude malignancy (squamous cancer in 70%).

Scarlet fever[ND] is caused by exotoxins released from *Strep pyogenes* (a GABHS). If a rash develops on the chest, axillae or behind the ears, 12–48h after initial sore throat and fever, you are probably observing scarlet fever. *Signs:* Red 'pin-prick' blanching rash; facial flushing with circumoral pallor; a 'strawberry tongue'. ℞: Penicillin V (clarithromycin if allergic) for 10 days. *Complications:* Sydenham's chorea (p654) or even a post-infectious demyelinating disorder, eg acute disseminated encephalomyelitis. Scarlet fever used to be a major cause of infant mortality, but is now generally self-limiting in developed countries.

⁘ A holistic approach to the person with a sore throat

Don't focus on the throat, the swab, or the microbiology: home in on people's health beliefs and work to harmonize these beliefs with your own.

We often think patients expect antibiotics, and will be disappointed if they are not given. Often this is not the case. Do they attend with *every* sore throat? If not, why now? Symptoms may be worse than usual and ibuprofen may help. But what may *really* help is dialogue. Rich dialogue reduces symptoms rather than merely making them more acceptable.

But improving symptoms is not the only aim: dialogue may promote patients' trust in their own body and may be a stepping stone to active health rather than passive disease.

Don't do tonsillectomy unless you are sure that... ▸ 31

• Recurrent sore throat is in fact due to tonsillitis.
• The episodes of sore throat are disabling and prevent normal functioning.
• ≥7 well documented, clinically significant adequately treated sore throats in the preceding year; ≥5 episodes in each of the last 2 years or ≥3 in the last 3 years.

NB: there is now a risk that too few tonsillectomies are being done as more adults and children are being hospitalized for throat infections.

Other indications: children with OSA; suspicion of malignancy.

▸▸ Complications of tonsillectomy

• Primary haemorrhage (<24h) often requires a return to theatre.
• Secondary haemorrhage (>24h, but typically after 5–10 days) due to infection of the tonsillar fossa. As with primary haemorrhage, this is an ENT emergency and a common ED presentation: Use the ABC approach; gain IV/IO access; cross-match and give fluid boluses (see p234); summons an experienced anaesthetist and ENT surgeon. Major haemorrhage protocols vary. Surgery may be required. If bleeding stops, admit for hydrogen peroxide gargles, IV antibiotics and observation.

ENT

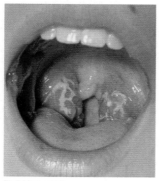

Fig 7.39 Tonsillitis.
James Heilman, MD, Wikipedia.

Further reading

NICE (2015). *Clinical Knowledge Summaries: Sore Throat – Acute.* http://cks.nice.org.uk/sore-throat-acute

SIGN (2010). *Management of Sore Throat and Indications for Tonsillectomy* (Guideline No. 117). Edinburgh: SIGN. www.sign.ac.uk/guidelines/fulltext/117/

Stridor is a high-pitched noise heard in inspiration from partial obstruction at the larynx or large airways. **Stertor** is an inspiratory snoring noise, coming from obstruction of the pharynx.

▶*Children's airways are narrower than adults, so obstruction happens faster and more dramatically. Poisseuille's law:* Resistance varies inversely with the 4th power of the radius, so 1mm oedema in a neonate's 4mm airway increases resistance 16–fold.

▶**Look for** swallowing difficulty/drooling, pallor/cyanosis, use of accessory muscles of respiration; downward plunging of the trachea with respiration (tracheal tug): all are grave signs and mean impending obstruction.

Causes • *Congenital:* Laryngomalacia, web/stenosis, vascular rings.
• *Inflammation:* Laryngitis, epiglottitis, croup, anaphylaxis.
• *Tumours:* Haemangiomas or papillomas (usually disappear without treatment).
• *Trauma:* Thermal/chemical—from intubation.

Laryngotracheobronchitis/croup
is the leading cause of stridor (predominantly inspiratory) with a barking cough ± respiratory distress due to upper airway obstruction. It is often worse at night. 95% are viral, eg

Severity grading of croup	
Mild	Occasional cough; no stridor at rest
Moderate	Frequent cough; stridor at rest
Severe	As moderate + respiratory distress

parainfluenza. ℞: Give all children with mild, moderate or severe croup a single dose of **dexamethasone** 0.15mg/kg (**prednisolone** 1–2mg/kg is an alternative). Advise parents it is usually self-limiting and resolves within 48hrs. Warn to seek help if severe signs. Humidified air (steam inhalations) are not recommended. Admit if moderate (and not settling), or severe croup. See also p158.

▶▶**Acute epiglottitis** is rapidly progressive inflammation of the epiglottis and adjacent tissues. It's an emergency as respiratory arrest can occur abruptly due to airway obstruction. Children (2-4 years old) present with a short history of fever, irritability, sore throat, pooling and drooling of saliva, and a muffled voice or cry. They prefer to lean forward and breathe tentatively. Cough is absent. It is now rare in children in the UK (*Haemophilus influenzae* type b vaccination has reduced prevalence). The typical patient now presenting is an adult, with severe sore throat and painful swallowing. See also p158.

Managing epiglottitis
▶▶ Keep the patient upright
▶▶ Do not examine the throat or cause distress
▶▶ Summon an anaesthetist and ENT surgeon
▶ Diagnosis is made by laryngoscopy and the patient intubated and treated with dexamethasone and antibiotics
▶▶ A surgical airway may be required if oral intubation is not possible

Laryngomalacia This is the main congenital anomaly of the larynx and is often noticeable within hours of birth (or up to a few months old). There is excessive collapse and indrawing of the supraglottic airways during inspiration leading to stridor, and breathing and feeding difficulties. Stridor may be most noticeable in certain positions, during sleep, or if excited/upset. In 85%, no treatment is needed and symptoms usually improve by 2 yrs old. Problems may occur with concurrent laryngeal infections or with feeding. Surgery can help in severe cases (aryepiglottoplasty).

Vocal cord palsy (laryngeal paralysis) accounts for 15-20% of all those with congenital laryngeal anomalies. *Cause:* Often unknown, but might be from vagal stretching at birth. *Unilateral:* May manifest during the first few weeks of life with a hoarse, breathy cry that is aggravated by agitation, feeding difficulties ± aspiration. ℞: Supportive; most recover by 2-3 years. *Bilateral:* Inspiratory stridor at rest that worsens upon agitation ± significant respiratory distress. ℞: Urgent airway intervention may be needed (intubation, tracheotomy) ± surgery.

▸▸Acute airway obstruction: management in adults

▸▸Give O_2 or Heliox® (a mixture of helium and O_2 that is less dense than air and *may* reduce work of breathing/respiratory distress).

▸▸Nebulized adrenaline (1mL of 1:1000 with 1mL saline).

▸▸Note O_2 saturation, respiratory rate, pulse, and blood pressure.

▸▸Call the on-call ENT registrar and anaesthetist for help.

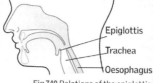

Fig 7.40 Relations of the epiglottis.

Epiglottis
Trachea
Oesophagus

▸▸Take a brief history from relatives, keeping in view the common causes of stridor.

Endotracheal intubation should be the first line of intervention where possible. Move on quickly if it proves difficult.

Emergency needle cricothyroidotomy and cricothyroidotomy kits eg Mini-Trach II® are temporary measures pending formal tracheostomy. A wide-bore cannula is inserted through the cricothyroid membrane. This will sustain life for 30–45min as jet insufflation oxygenates rather than ventilates and CO_2 builds up.

Surgical cricothyroidotomy is quicker and easier to perform than emergency tracheostomy but is not usually performed in children <12 years.

ENT

Why is this child drooling?

Drooling is often normal if <3yrs old (eg associated with teething). So don't assume that drooling + stridor must mean epiglottitis if drooling predated the stridor. Is drooling due to reduced cerebral control of oral function, hypersalivation, or an obstruction to swallowing?

• ▸▸Angioedema/anaphylaxis (p237) ▸▸Rabies (*OHCM* p432) ▸▸Epiglottitis
• Neurodisability, eg cerebral palsy, bulbar palsy (↓ oro-motor control)
• Muscle problems (oesophageal dysmotility; cricopharyngeal achalasia)
• Ingestion of a foreign body or chemical toxin
• Head and neck trauma
• Enlarged tonsils or adenoids
• Congenital lesions/nasal masses (eg an encephalocele or glioma).

Hoarseness entails difficulty producing sound, with change in voice pitch or quality ('breathy', 'scratchy', 'husky'). The majority of voice problems are due to viral upper respiratory tract infection and settle with little treatment. ▶Investigate hoarseness (esp. in smokers) lasting >3wks, as it is the chief (and often the only) presentation of laryngeal carcinoma (p571). *Ask about:* Gastro–oesophageal reflux (GORD), dysphagia, smoking, stress, singing & shouting. Voice overuse is a common cause.

Tests Laryngoscopy to assess cord mobility, inspect the mucosa and exclude local causes.

Differential diagnosis of a hoarse voice

Laryngeal cancer: Progressive and persistent gruff voice (see p571).

Vocal cord palsy: A weak 'breathy' voice. Often due cancer (see BOX).

Laryngitis: This is often viral and self-limiting, but there may be secondary infection with streps or staphs. It can also be secondary to GORD (see below) or autoimmune disease, eg rheumatoid arthritis. *Symptoms:* Pain (hypopharyngeal, dysphagia; pain on phonation); hoarseness; fever. ℞: Supportive. If necessary, give **phenoxymethylpenicillin** 500mg/6h PO for 1 week.

Reflux laryngitis (laryngo-pharyngeal reflux; LPR): There are chronic laryngeal signs and symptoms associated with GORD. ~15% of all visits to ENT clinics are because of LPR. ℞: PPI; diet/lifestyle modification; weight loss ± surgical fundoplication.

Reinke's oedema: Chronic cord irritation from smoking ± chronic voice abuse may cause a gelatinous fusiform enlargement of the cords, resulting in a deep gruff voice. Women often say they sound like a man. Seen almost exclusively in hypothyroid, elderly, female smokers. ℞: If conservative treatment fails (stop smoking, SALT), laser therapy may help.

Vocal cord nodules (fig 7.41) are caused by vocal abuse (eg poor singing technique, shouting or voice abuse) and result in a variable husky voice. Fibrous nodules (often bilateral) form at the junction of the anterior ⅓ and posterior ⅔ of the cords. This is the middle of the membranous vocal folds (the posterior portion of the vocal fold is cartilage), and it may receive most contact injury during speech. ℞: Speech therapy (if used early), or surgical excision.

Before saying 'no cause can be found', consider generalized infiltrating entities of the larynx, such as hyperkeratosis (as a result of smoking, alcohol abuse, pollution), leukoplakia, granulomata, papillomata (arising from HPV infection), polyps, and cysts.

Disorders of speech articulation causing a hoarse voice

- *Spasmodic dysphonia* is a focal laryngeal dystonia of unknown cause (a similar focal dystonia is blepharospasm =involuntary blinking of the eye). Involuntary spasms of the vocal cords produce strained strangled breaks in connected speech. Symptoms vary from day to day and can be worse with anxiety. ℞: Botox® injections into laryngeal muscles; no treatment is proven.
- *Muscle tension dysphonia* is a functional disorder due to abnormal laryngeal muscle tension. Patients complain of a husky hoarse voice that tires easily. It is associated with voice misuse and psychological stress. Globus-type symptoms are common (a feeling of a lump in the throat; frequent clearing of the throat). ℞: Reassurance and explanation ± speech therapy.
- *Children with functional speech disorders* have difficulty with specific speech sounds (eg /r/ /s/ /z/ /l/ and/or 'th'). Try to distinguish articulation disorders from phonological disorders and speech dyspraxia.

ENT

Laryngeal nerve palsy

The recurrent laryngeal nerve supplies the intrinsic muscles of the larynx (apart from cricothyroideus) and is responsible for both abduction and adduction of the vocal fold. It originates from the vagus nerve and has a complex course making it susceptible to damage. Symptoms of vocal cord paralysis are:
• A weak 'breathy' voice with a weak cough.
• Repeated coughing/aspiration.
• Exertional dyspnoea (a narrow glottis reduces air flow). NB: while at rest the contralateral cord can compensate by increased abduction.

Causes 30% are due to cancers (larynx; thyroid; oesophagus; hypopharynx; bronchus). 25% are iatrogenic, ie after parathyroidectomy, oesophageal, or pharyngeal pouch surgery. *Other causes:* CNS disease (polio; syringomyelia); TB; aortic aneurysm; 15% are idiopathic (postviral neuropathy).

Investigations If there is no history of recent surgery request a CXR. If this is normal, proceed to: CT (skull base to hilum); ± US thyroid; ± OGD.

Treating non-malignant causes Unilateral palsies can be compensated for by movement of the contralateral cord, but may need formal medialization via injections, or thyroplasty. *Reinnervation techniques* are also possible eg ansa cervicalis-to-recurrent laryngeal nerve (eg after damage during thyroidectomy).

Vocal hygiene...Don't whisper! Don't shout!

• Drink plenty (eg 2L of fluid each day prevents dehydration of the cords).
• Get plenty of sleep: tiredness kills the voice.
• Take adequate deep breaths whilst speaking.
• Steam inhalations help keep the vocal cords hydrated.
• Avoid shouting or whispering. If your voice feels tired or strained, rest it!
• Avoid excessive throat clearing (it bashes the vocal cords together).
• Avoid irritants (spicy foods, tobacco, smoke, dust, alcohol).
• Avoid eating late at night, as indigestion may affect the voice.
• Avoid throat lozenges; these numb the throat, and menthol is drying.

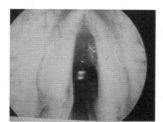

Fig 7.41 Vocal cord nodule (AKA Singer's nodule (right).
Courtesy of Rory Herdman FRCS.

Dysphagia is difficulty in swallowing: unless it is associated with a transitory sore throat, it is a serious symptom: ►*Endoscopy is essential.* *Painful swallowing* is termed 'odynophagia'.

The patient As examination is typically normal (unless anaemic), the history is key. Dyspepsia? Weight loss? Lumps? Progressive dysphagia?

1 Can fluid be drunk as fast as usual, except if food is stuck?
 Yes: Suspect a stricture (benign/malignant).
 No: Think of motility disorders (achalasia, neurological causes).

2 Is it difficult to make the swallowing movement?
 Yes: Suspect bulbar palsy, especially if cough on swallowing.

3 Is the dysphagia constant and painful?
 Yes (either feature): Suspect a malignant stricture.

4 Does the neck bulge or gurgle on drinking?
 Yes: Suspect a pharyngeal pouch (food may be regurgitated).

Malignant causes
• Oesophageal cancer
• Pharyngeal cancer
• Gastric cancer
• Extrinsic pressure, eg from lung cancer or node enlargement

Neurological causes
• Bulbar palsy (*OHCM* p510)
• Lateral medullary syn.
• Myasthenia gravis
• Syringomyelia (*OHCM* p520)

Other causes
• Benign strictures
• Pharyngeal pouch
• Achalasia*et al* (*OHCM* p240)
• Systemic sclerosis
• Oesophagitis
• Iron-deficient anaemia

Tests FBC; ESR; CXR; barium swallow; endoscopy with biopsy; oesophageal motility studies (requires swallowing a catheter containing a pressure transducer).

Nutrition Dysphagia can cause malnutrition. Nutritional support may be needed pre- and post-treatment, eg via a percutaneous endoscopic gastrostomy (PEG). Get expert dietician help; see *OHCM* p586.

Oesophageal carcinoma This is associated with achalasia, alcohol, smoking, Barrett's oesophagus (*OHCM* p709), tylosis (a hereditary condition causing hyperkeratosis of the palms), Patterson–Brown–Kelly (Plummer–Vinson) syndrome. *Symptoms:* Dysphagia, weight loss, hoarseness, cough. ℞: Surgery ± chemo/radiotherapy. Post-resection 5-yr survival is poor (*OHCM* p620).

Benign oesophageal stricture *Causes:* Oesophageal reflux; swallowing corrosives; foreign body; trauma. *Treatment:* Dilatation (endoscopic or with bougies eg under GA). **Barrett's oesophagus** *OHCM* p686. **Achalasia** *OHCM* p240.

Pharyngeal pouch The pharyngeal mucosa herniates through an area of weakness known as 'Killian's dehiscence', possibly due to incoordination of swallowing and increased pressure above the closed upper oesophageal sphincter. *Signs:* Dysphagia with gurgling, and regurgitation of undigested food; halitosis; a lump in the neck; aspiration/pneumonia. Often seen in elderly men. *Imaging:* Barium swallow (fig 7.42). Endoscopy must also be performed to exclude malignancy within the pouch. *Treatment:* (if symptomatic), endoscopic stapling of the wall that divides the pouch from the oesophagus.

Globus pharyngeus (AKA **globus hystericus**) is a sensation of a lump in the throat that is most noticed when swallowing saliva (rather than swallowing food or liquid). Patients may also complain of mucous in the throat which they are unable to clear. There is no primary swallowing difficulty and symptoms tend to come and go (worse when stressed or tired). *Cause:* Unclear. Possibly due to excess muscle tension in the pharynx, or ↑acid exposure at the laryngopharyngeal junction. *Treatment:* Reassure. It is worsened by anxiety, and stress can form a vicious circle, but don't dismiss these patients as '*globus hystericus*'. Endoscopy may be required to exclude malignancy (eg if unilateral symptoms, otalgia, neck lump or progressive swallowing difficulty).

ENT

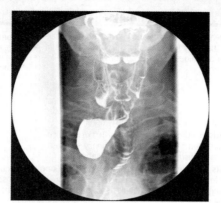

Fig 7.42 A pharyngeal pouch (called Zenker's diverticulum in the usa) 'I've got this cough…seems to get worse watching the news on tv'. When we hear this sort of absurdity, ask 'What are you doing *before* the News comes on?'. 'Eating my dinner…' At this point ask about dysphagia, choking, chronic cough, regurgitation of undigested food, halitosis, weight loss, and aspiration. Listen to the neck after eating: any gurgles? Any lateral fullness/swelling?

Oesophageal mucosa is herniating backwards between cricopharyngeus and inferior pharyngeal constrictors. *Typical patient:* A man over 60. *Incidence:* 2/100,000/yr. *Treatment:* Surgery, eg day-case endoscopic stapling; note that flexible endoscopy can cause perforation when a pouch is unsuspected; hence the need for barium imaging.

Reproduced from McGrath *et al*, *qjm* (2008) 101 (9): 747–748, with permission from Oxford University Press.

90% of head and neck cancers are squamous cell carcinomas (HNSCC).[32] HNSCC develops from the linings of the upper aerodigestive tract, comprising the:
• Oral cavity
• Oropharynx
• Hypopharynx, larynx, and trachea (see fig 7.44).

>80% arise in those >50 yrs old, but incidence amongst young people is increasing. Disease typically invades adjacent structures and spreads via lymphatics.

Associations • Cigarette smoking =×10↑ risk. • ↑ alcohol consumption • Vitamin A & C deficiency • Nitrosamines in salted fish • HPV • GORD • Deprivation.

Symptoms of HNSCC
• Neck pain/lump
• Hoarse voice >6wks
• Sore throat >6wks
• Mouth bleeding
• Mouth numbness
• Sore tongue
• Painless ulcers
• Patches in the mouth
• Earache/effusion
• Lumps (lip, mouth, gum)
• Speech change
• Dysphagia

Diagnosis Patients with suspicious symptoms (MINIBOX) should be referred urgently for ENT review. Investigations include fibre-optic endoscopy of the upper aerodigestive tract; fine-needle aspiration or biopsy of any masses and CT or MRI of the primary tumour site to stage the neck for nodal metastatic disease. Treatment and surgery is discussed and planned by a multi-disciplinary team.

Staging uses the 'TNM' system:
• *Tumour* (extent of primary tumour): T1 =<2cm; T4 =extension to bone, muscle, skin, antrum, neck.
• *Node* (involvement of regional lymph nodes): N0 =no involvement; N3 =any lymph node >6cm. For the purposes of surgical neck dissection, the lymph nodes of the neck are divided into 6 areas (levels) (see fig 7.43).
• *Metastases* (presence of metastases): M0 =no metastases; M1 =distant mets.

Oral cavity and tongue Uncommon in the UK. *Signs/symptoms:* Persistent, painful ulcers; white or red patches on the tongue, gums or mucosa; otalgia; odonophagia; lymphadenopathy. ℞: Surgery/radiotherapy. >80% 5-yr survival in early disease.

Oropharyngeal carcinoma is often advanced at presentation. ♂:♀≈5:1. *Typical older patient:* Smoker with sore throat, sensation of a lump, referred otalgia. *Risk factors:* Pipe smoking or chewing tobacco. 20% are node +ve at presentation. *Imaging:* MRI. ℞: Surgery and radiotherapy. Radiotherapy may be 1st line if the tumour is T1 (<2cm) or T2 (>2cm but <4cm). *Prognosis:* 5-yr survival ~50% for stage I. Tonsillar cancer has a better prognosis. *High risk HPV* (esp. type 16) has been linked to cancer of the tongue, tonsil and pharynx. HPV16 is most commonly transmitted during oral sex and cancer risk relates (partly) to number of partners. Cancers associated with HPV occur in younger people, and carry a better prognosis than those associated with smoking. Vaccination may ↓risk.

Hypopharyngeal tumours are rare. They can present as a lump in throat, dysphagia, odonophagia, pain referred to the ear, and a hoarse voice. The anatomic limits of the hypopharynx are the hyoid bone to the lower edge of the cricoid cartilage. *Premalignant conditions:* Leukoplakia (hyperparakeratosis ± underlying epithelial hyperplasia); Patterson–Kelly–Brown syndrome (Plummer–Vinson)—pharyngeal web associated with iron deficiency: 2% have postcricoid cancer. ℞: Radiotherapy and surgery. *Prognosis:* is poor (60% mortality at 1yr).

Laryngeal cancer (fig 7.45) *Incidence:* 2300/yr (UK). *Typical older patient:* Male smoker with progressive hoarseness, then stridor, difficulty or pain on swallowing ± haemoptysis ± ear pain (if pharynx involved). *Typical younger patient:* HPV +ve. *Sites:* Supraglottic, glottic, or subglottic. Glottic tumours have the best prognosis as they cause hoarseness earlier (spread to nodes is late). *Diagnosis:* Laryngoscopy + biopsy; HPV status; MRI staging. ℞: Radical *radiotherapy* for small tumours. Larger tumours are treated with partial/total *laryngectomy* ± block dissection of neck glands. See BOX for voice restoration after laryngectomy. 5-yr survival rate is 66%.

ENT

Voice restoration after laryngectomy[33]

Patients may fear not only losing 'their' voice, but that they will be unable to communicate after laryngectomy. Whilst surgery for small tumours may conserve a patient's voice, if the larynx is removed and the trachea brought to the skin as an end-stoma in the neck, a patient will require voice restoration.

Trans-oesophageal puncture (TEP) A one–way valve (voice prosthesis) is inserted between the trachea and the pharynx/oesophagus, which vibrates the pharyngeal-oesophageal (PE) segment. The valve is activated when the patient occludes their stoma and breathes out. Exhaled air is modified and shaped with the lips and teeth into speech.

Artificial larynx (Servox) If the above forms of speech are not achieved, an artificial vibrating larynx can be held firmly against the patient's neck, which causes the tissues (and as a result the air within the pharynx) to vibrate, producing a distinct electronic voice sound.

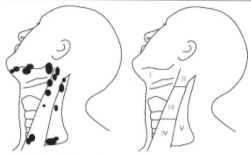

Fig 7.43 Lymph node levels in the neck.
The lymph nodes of the neck are described in six levels: level 1 (submandibular and submental), levels 2, 3, and 4 (high, mid, and low jugular chain), level 5 (posterior triangle) and level 6 (central neck).

Reproduced from Corbridge and Steventon, *Oxford Handbook of ENT and Head and Neck Surgery* 2nd edition (2010) with permission from Oxford University Press.

Neck dissection techniques include *radical neck dissection:* all neck lymph nodes removed (level I–V) + spinal accessory nerve, internal jugular vein and sternocleidomastoid muscle; *modified radical neck dissection:* as radical but with preservation of one or more non-lymphatic structures; *selective neck dissection:* one or more of the lymphatic groups is preserved, based on the patterns of metastases which are predictable for each site of disease; *extended neck dissection:* additional lymph node groups or non-lymphatic structures are removed.[34]

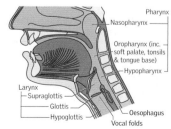

Fig 7.44 Anatomy of the head and neck.

Labels: Pharynx; Nasopharynx; Oropharynx (inc. soft palate, tonsils & tongue base); Hypopharynx; Oesophagus; Vocal folds; Larynx — Supraglottis — Glottis — Hypoglottis

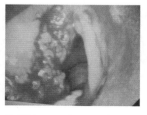

Fig 7.45 Laryngeal cancer along one vocal cord; it's just been biopsied, hence the bleeding.

Courtesy of Rory Herdman FRCS.

Arising in the medulla, and emerging between the pons and medulla, the facial nerve passes through the posterior fossa and runs through the middle ear before emerging from the stylomastoid foramen to pass into the parotid. Lesions may be at any part of its course.

Intracranial branches 1 The greater superficial petrosal nerve (lacrimation) 2 Branch to stapedius (lesions above these cause hyperacusis) 3 The chorda tympani (supply taste to anterior ⅔ of the tongue).

Extracranial branches (All are motor fibres that branch after emerging from the stylomastoid foramen.) •Posterior auricular nerve •Branch to posterior belly of digastric muscle and stylohyoid muscle. There are 5 major branches within the parotid: •Temporal •Zygomatic •Buccal •Marginal mandibular •Cervical.

Causes of facial palsy *Intracranial:* Brainstem tumours; strokes; polio; multiple sclerosis; cerebellopontine angle lesions (acoustic neuroma, meningitis). *Intratemporal:* Otitis media; Ramsay Hunt syndrome; cholesteatoma. *Infratemporal:* Parotid tumours; trauma leading to a complete palsy is an indication for urgent CT—if the nerve canal is disrupted, surgical exploration is advised. *Others:* Lyme disease; sarcoid; diabetes; Bell's palsy.

Signs Lower motor neuron lesions can paralyse all of one side of the face; but in upper motor neuron lesions (eg CVA), the forehead muscles and closing the eyes may still work (they are bilaterally represented).

Tests ESR; glucose; Lyme disease serology. Examine the parotid for lumps and the ears to exclude cholesteatoma and Ramsay Hunt syndrome (p652). Any head trauma? *MRI:* Space-occupying lesions; CVA; MS; temporal bone fracture.

Bell's palsy (AKA idiopathic facial palsy) (figs 7.46 & 7.47) is the cause of 70% of facial palsies and is a unilateral LMN facial palsy. It is partly a diagnosis of exclusion. *Incidence:* 15–40/100,000/yr. Risk increased in pregnancy (×3) and diabetes (×5). *Features:* The cause is unclear but is thought to be due to inflammatory oedema from entrapment of the facial nerve in the narrow bony facial canal. Onset is abrupt (eg overnight or after a nap), with complete weakness at 24–72h. The mouth sags and there is dribbling and watering (or dry) eyes + impaired brow-wrinkling, blowing, whistling, lid closure, cheek-pouting, taste and speech; ± hyperacusis from stapedius palsy.

Treatment:[35–37] There is good evidence that **prednisolone** results in improved rate of recovery and shorter time to recovery for people presenting within 72h of symptom onset. There is no consensus on the optimum dosing regimen. Options include 25mg/12h for 10 days, or 60mg/24h for 5 days reduced by 10mg each day thereafter. There is no role for antiviral treatment either alone or in combination with prednisolone—it has shown no effect on either rate of recovery or time to recovery. *Protect the eye* by keeping it well lubricated (drops during the day; ointment at night). If the cornea is exposed on trying to close the eye seek urgent ophthalmology advice.

Referral: Refer urgently to ENT or neurology if there is any doubt about the diagnosis; if recurrent Bell's palsy (~7%); in bilateral facial palsy (common causes: Lyme disease, Guillain–Barre syndrome, leukaemia, sarcoidosis, EBV, trauma, myasthenia gravis); and if paralysis shows no sign of improvement after 1 month.

Prognosis: ~80% will recover completely within 3 months. ~15% have axonal degeneration with delayed and possibly incomplete recovery, which can be complicated by aberrant reconnections. ~5% have permanent weakness that is cosmetically and clinically apparent (refer to a plastic surgeon >6 months).

Further reading

Lockhart P *et al.* (2009). Antiviral treatment for Bell's palsy (idiopathic facial paralysis). *Cochrane Database Syst Rev* 4:CD001869.

Salinas RA *et al.* (2010). Corticosteroids for Bell's palsy (idiopathic facial paralysis). *Cochrane Database Syst Rev* 3:CD001942.

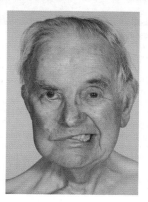

Fig 7.46 Right-sided Bell's palsy: the patient is trying to smile, but his right lower lid is drooping, the naso-labial fold is slack, and the lips do not move.

©OUP data bank.

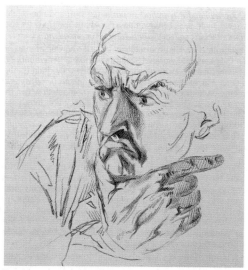

Fig 7.47 'Peevish melancholy' by Scottish surgeon, anatomist and neurologist, Sir Charles Bell (1774–1842) from his work 'Essays on the Anatomy of Expression in Painting' (1806). '...*In discontent the brow is clouded, the nose peculiarly arched, and the angle of the mouth drawn down very remarkably.*'

Bell is best known for describing the facial palsy that bears his name, but also first described the trajectory of the facial nerve. He combined neuroanatomy with practice and studied in detail the emotions of facial expression. A talented artist, he undertook numerous anatomical drawings, including many of injuries seen whilst operating on the wounded at the battle of Waterloo in 1815.

➤Refer urgently any possibly malignant neck lump to ENT.

Diagnosis First, ask 'How long has the lump been present?' If <3 weeks, reactive lymphadenopathy from a self-limiting infection is likely, and extensive investigation is unwise. Next ask: 'Which tissue layer is the lump in?'. Is it intradermal? (eg from sebaceous cyst with a central punctum, or a lipoma).

If the lump is not intradermal, and not of recent onset, you are about to start a diagnostic hunt over complex terrain. But remember—you are vastly outnumbered by a pack of diseases and possible pathology. Fig 7.50 shows an infected cyst.

Tests US shows lump architecture and vascularity and allows guidance of FNAC. CT defines masses in relation to their anatomical neighbours. Do virology and Mantoux test. CXR may show malignancy, or in sarcoid reveal bilateral hilar lymphadenopathy. Fine-needle aspiration cytology has a pivotal role in investigating suspicious lymph nodes (fig 7.52) in the neck (FNAC, figs 7.54 & 7.55).

Midline lumps •In patients <20yrs old, the likely diagnosis is a *dermoid cyst*. •If it moves *up* on protruding the tongue and is below the hyoid, it is likely to be a *thyroglossal cyst* (a fluid filled sac resulting from incomplete closure of the thyroid's migration path; treated by surgery). •If >20yrs old, it could be a thyroid mass (fig 7.49). •If it is bony hard it may be a *chondroma* (a benign cartilaginous tumour).

Submandibular triangle (Bordered above by the mandible and below by digastric.) •If <20yrs, self-limiting *reactive lymphadenopathy* is likely •If >20yrs, exclude *malignant lymphadenopathy* (eg firm and non-tender; any B symptoms: fever, night sweats, weight loss?) •➤Is TB likely? •If it's not a node, think of *submandibular salivary stone, tumour,* or *sialadenitis* (see fig 7.53).

Anterior triangle (Between the midline, anterior border of sternomastoid and the line between the two angles of the mandible.) •*Lymphadenopathy* is common: remember to examine the areas which they drain (is the spleen enlarged?—this ± B symptoms may indicate lymphoma). •*Branchial cysts* (fig 7.48) emerge under the anterior border of sternomastoid where the upper ⅓ meets the middle ⅓. The popular theory is that they are due to non-disappearance of the cervical sinus (where the 2nd branchial arch grows down over 3rd and 4th) but this is not universally accepted. Lined by squamous epithelium, their fluid contains cholesterol crystals. Treat by excision. •If the lump is in the superoposterior area of the anterior triangle, is it a *parotid tumour* (more likely if >40yrs)? •*Laryngoceles* are an uncommon cause of lumps in the anterior triangle: They are painless, more common in males, and are made worse by blowing. If the lump is pulsatile it may be a: •*Carotid artery aneurysm* •*Tortuous carotid artery* or •*Carotid body tumour* (chemodectoma). These are very rare, move from side-to-side, but not up and down, and splay out the carotid bifurcation. They are firm and pulsatile, and do not usually cause bruits. They may be bilateral, familial, and malignant (5%). Suspect in any mass just anterior to the upper third of sternomastoid. Diagnose by US/MRA. Treatment: extirpation by a vascular surgeon.

Posterior triangle (Behind sternomastoid, in front of trapezius, and above the clavicle.) •*Cervical ribs* may intrude into this area. These are enlarged costal elements from C7 vertebra. The majority are asymptomatic but can cause neurological symptoms from pressure on the brachial plexus or Raynaud's syndrome by compressing the subclavian artery. •*Pharyngeal pouches* can protrude into the posterior triangle on swallowing (usually left sided). •*Cystic hygromas* are macrocystic lymphatic malformations that transilluminate brightly. Treat by surgery or hypertonic saline sclerosant. •If there are many small lumps, think of *Lymphadenopathy*—TB or viruses, eg HIV or EBV or, if >20yrs, consider lymphoma (any B symptoms?) or metastases (fig 7.51).

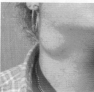

Fig 7.48 Branchial cyst.
© Bechara Ghorayeb.

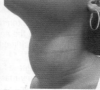

Fig 7.49 Goitre.
© Bechara Ghorayeb.

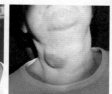

Fig 7.50 Infected cyst.
© Bechara Ghorayeb.

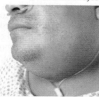

Fig 7.51 Deep cervical abscess.
© Bechara Ghorayeb.

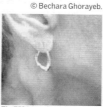

Fig 7.52 Lymph node metastases.
© Bechara Ghorayeb.

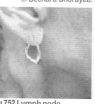

Fig 7.53 Submandibular abscess.
© Bechara Ghorayeb.

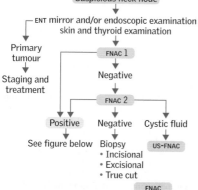

Fig 7.54 Fine-needle aspiration cytology (FNAC) in the investigation of a neck node.
Balm et al, 'Diagnosis and Treatment of a Neck Node Swelling', *International Journal of Surgical Oncology*, 2010.

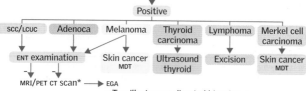

Fig 7.55 Procedure for suspicious node if pharynx is positive.
EGA: examination under GA; LCUC: large cell undifferentiated cancer; MDT: multidisciplinary team; SCC: squamous cell cancer; US: ultrasound.
Balm et al, 'Diagnosis and Treatment of a Neck Node Swelling', *International Journal of Surgical Oncology*, 2010.

The 3 major pairs of salivary glands are: *parotid* (on the side of the face in front of the ear), *submandibular* (below the jaw in the angle of the mandible), and *sublingual* (in the floor of the mouth). Many additional smaller glands are distributed throughout the mouth and throat.

Examination Look for external swellings, palpate for stones, test facial nerve function. Note size, mobility, and extent of any mass, as well as fixity to surroundings. Any tenderness? Assess surrounding skin as regional metastases from skin or mucosal malignancies may present as salivary gland masses.

Sialadenitis This is acute infection of the submandibular or parotid glands. It usually occurs in elderly or debilitated patients, who may be dehydrated and have poor oral hygeine. *Symptoms:* Painful diffuse swelling of the gland + fever. Pressure applied over the gland may lead to pus leaking out of the duct. *R:*Antibiotics + good oral hygiene. Sialogogues are helpful (eg lemon drops, which stimulate salivation). Surgical drainage may be required. Chronic inflammation or recurrent attacks may occur due to strictures (from previous infection) or salivary gland stones. Pain and swelling on eating are common.

Salivary stones (sialolithiasis) Usually affect the submandibular gland where secretions are richer in calcium and thicker. *Signs and symptoms:* Pain and tense swelling of the gland during/after meals. A stone may be palpable in the floor of the mouth. *Imaging:* Plain x-ray or sialogram if diagnostic doubt. *R:*Small stones may pass spontaneously (sialogogues may help). Larger stones may need surgical removal.

Other inflammatory conditions • *Sjögren's syndrome* (онсм p724) may cause diffuse enlargement of the parotid • *Viral infections* eg mumps and нιν may cause inflammation of the parotid or submandibular glands • *Granulomatous disease* eg тв and sarcoidosis.

Salivary gland tumours '80% of all salivary gland tumours occur in the parotid gland; 80% of these are benign pleomorphic adenomas; 80% of these are in the superficial lobe.' 50% of submandibular gland tumours are malignant. *Risk factors for malignancy:* Radiation to the neck; smoking. *Symptoms suggestive of malignancy:* Hard, fixed mass ± pain. There may be overlying skin ulceration and local lymph node enlargement • Tumours do not vary in size (eg when eating), as seen in inflammation or salivary stones. An associated facial nerve palsy suggests malignancy. ►Refer all patients with unexplained persistent salivary gland swelling, or any unexplained neck lump (or any previously undiagnosed neck lump that has changed over a period of 3–6 weeks). *Investigations:* us/мri, fnac/ст-guided biopsy. *R:*Surgery, radiotherapy.

Benign tumours	Low grade malignant	High grade malignant
Pleomorphic adenoma	Mucoepidermoid (grade I or II)	Mucoepidermoid (grade III)
Adenolymphoma (Warthin's tumour)	Acinic cell tumours	Adenocarcinoma
		Squamous cell cancer
Rarer: oncocytomas		Adenoidcystic

Pleomorphic adenoma: A slow-growing benign tumour occurring in middle-age that may turn malignant if present for many years. Usually diagnosed by fnac. *Treatment:* Surgical removal.

Warthin's tumour (adenolymphoma): Usually occur in elderly men, most commonly in the parotid gland. *Treatment:* Partial parotidectomy.

Mucoepidermoid carcinoma: Aggressive high-grade tumours require excision + radiotherapy. Low-grade tumours usually only need surgery.

Adenoidcystic tumours: Painful slow-growing tumours that tend to spread along the nerves ('perineural infiltration') + distant metastases and late recurrence. *Treatment:* Surgical excision + postoperative radiotherapy.

ENT

The dry mouth (xerostomia)

Signs • Dry, atrophic, fissured oral mucosa; also:
• Discomfort, causing difficulty eating, speaking, and wearing dentures.
• No saliva pooling in floor of mouth.
• Difficulty in expressing saliva from major ducts.

Complications Dental caries; candida infection.

Management • †oral fluids; take frequent sips.
• Good dental hygiene; no acidic drinks or foods that demineralize teeth.
• Try saliva substitutes/dry mouth products (eg biotene® products).

Typical causes
• Hypnotics & tricyclics
• Antipsychotics
• β-blockers; diuretics
• Mouth breathing
• Dehydration
• ENT radiotherapy
• Sjögren's syndrome
• SLE and scleroderma
• Sarcoidosis
• HIV/AIDS
• Parotid stones

ENT

Łucja Frey and her misconnection syndrome

'Doctor...when I eat, or even just *think* of food, a sweaty rash crops up on my cheek.' (fig 7.56).

Duphenix first described gustatory sweating in 1757, but its cause was mysterious until 1923, when a soldier presented to Łucja Frey, a pioneering Polish neurologist.[8] Her soldier had a bullet in his parotid, and with it, gustatory sweating. Frey's brilliant dissections showed how the auriculo-temporal branch of the trigeminal nerve sends parasympathetic fibres to the parotid and sympathetic fibres to facial sweat glands. During resprouting after injury, fibres switch course to cause gustatory sweating.

You don't have to be shot to get Frey's syndrome. Other causes: birth trauma; parotid surgery (in 23%, so pre-op counselling is vital but only understood fully by neuroanatomists). Management is difficult, but not always needed. Botulinum toxin has been tried.

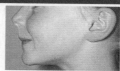
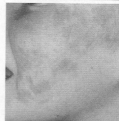

Fig 7.56 Frey's syndrome before and after eating.

Reproduced from *Postgraduate Medical Journal*, Nahin Hussain, Muthu Dhanarass, William Whitehouse, Frey's syndrome: a masquerader of food allergy, volume 86, pp. 1011, 2010 with permission from BMJ Publishing Group Ltd.

►Any oral ulcer which has not healed in 3 weeks should receive specialist assessment for biopsy to exclude malignancy (*онсм* p238).

Causes of facial pain Tooth pathology, sinusitis, temporomandibular joint (TMJ) dysfunction, salivary gland pathology, migraine, trigeminal neuralgia, atypical facial pain (no clear cause), trauma, cluster headache (*онсм* p461), angina, frontal bone osteomyelitis (post sinusitis), ENT tumours.

When helping a patient with a dental infection pay attention to the features below, before consulting a dentist, or a maxillofacial surgeon:

1 *Is it the teeth?* History: *Is the pain...*
- Worse with sugar and heat?⎫ Tooth is alive
- Worse or better with cold? ⎬► (pulpitis)
- Intermittent?   ⎭

  Is the pain...
- Worse with percussion?   ⎫► Tooth dead
- Constant/uninterrupted?   ⎬ (osteitis/abscess)
  Is the pain...
- Exacerbated by movement   ⎫► Abscess
  between finger and thumb   ⎭

X-ray (usually helpful): Orthopantogram (OPT) is useful for imaging molars and pre-molars. If incisors are suspected, request periapical x-rays of the tooth in question. Interpretation of x-ray (fig 7.57):

• *Abscess:*   • *Periodontal disease:*

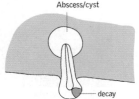

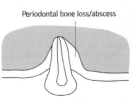

Fig 7.57 Distinguishing between (left) abscess of the tooth and (right) periodontal disease.

(Tooth tender to percussion)   (Tooth mobile)

2 *Trismus:* (Opening mouth is difficult because of spasm or pain.) This is a sign of severe infection. Ask the patient to open mouth wide and measure how many fingers breadth between the incisor teeth. Trismus always requires maxillofacial advice. Other causes: tetanus; neoplasia.

3 *Facial swellings due to dental infection:* Usually subside with oral antibiotics. ►If swelling is related to the lower jaw, assess for airways obstruction; if spreading to the eye, assess the second cranial nerve. If in any doubt, refer to a maxillofacial surgeon.

4 *Vital signs:* Check temperature, pulse, and blood pressure. Patients who are systemically unwell require maxillofacial advice/admission.

5 *Systemic disease complicating dental infection:* Any immunocompromise (eg HIV, leukaemia, diabetes, patients on steroids); patients at risk of endocarditis; coagulopathy (eg haemophilia or warfarin). Seek specialist advice.

Dental caries Declining in the West due primarily to fluoride, this condition i̶ increasing exponentially in developing countries. Causes: bacteria (esp. *S. mu̶ tans*), substrate (sugars), and susceptible tooth surface. In otherwise healthy individuals it is an entirely preventable disease.

Radiation caries (eg post head & neck radiotherapy, eg with jaw osteoradionecrosis). *Treatment and complications:* Pain ± infection. Toothache pain responds best to NSAIDs, eg **ibuprofen** 200–400mg/8h PO after food, and dental infection to **penicillin** and **metronidazole**, but drug treatment is never definitive, and a dental referral is required.

Periodontal disease Virtually all dentate adults have gingivitis, caused by bacterial and polysaccharide complexes at the tooth–gingival interface (=plaque). Toothbrushing is the only answer. Pathogens: herpes; streps.[etc...]

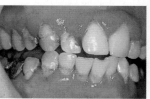

Fig 7.58 Periodontitis with damage to supporting tissue including bone.

Reproduced from *The BMJ*, Periodontal disease, Coventry et al., volume 321, 2000, with permission from BMJ Publishing Group Ltd.

Vincent's angina (necrotizing ulcerative gingivitis) is a smoking or HIV-associated, painful, foul-smelling gingivitis, caused by anaerobes (*Fusobacteria*) ± spirochetes (*Borellia vincentii*). ℞: **amoxicillin** 500mg/8h PO + **metronidazole** 400mg/8h PO + dental referral.

Causes of gingival swelling: Fibrous hyperplasia (congenital; or from phenytoin, ciclosporin, nifedipine); pregnancy, HIV, scurvy, leukaemic deposits.

Periodontitis (pyorrhoea) (fig 7.58) is a progression of localized inflammation from the gums into the ligament supporting a tooth. *Associations:* anaerobes; calcified bacterial deposits (calculi, tartar); poor oral hygiene. It needs a dentist.

HIV and periodontal disease: HIV causes candida, ulcers, linear gingival erythema, necrotizing ulcerative gingivitis, and necrotizing ulcerative periodontitis.

Causes of juvenile periodontitis: Poor nutrition; immunosuppression; wcc↓; neutrophil dysfunction (leucocyte adhesion deficiency, Chediak–Higashi or Papillon–Lefevre syndrome, with palmar keratosis), granulomatous disease.

Malocclusion Inappropriate positioning of the teeth in the jaws or between the jaws themselves is common. Those with prominent upper teeth are particularly prone to trauma, and those at risk (eg in epilepsy or involved in contact sports) should see an orthodontist. Those with severe facial or jaw disharmony who may be unable to chew or have psychological difficulty with their appearance may be amenable to surgical correction.

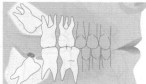

Fig 7.59 Impacting wisdom teeth.

Wisdom teeth These declare themselves in early adult life. Like the appendix, they are something of a vestigial organ. Impaction can cause pain (fig 7.59). If asymptomatic and not exposed to contamination by the mouth, they don't usually need removal. Complications are pain and infection and they may be involved in fractures of the mandible. Post-op recovery is often complicated by pain and swelling; pain responds well to NSAIDs and poorly to opiates. Infection complicates up to 30% not receiving antibiotics. Amoxicillin and metronidazole (as above) are standbys.

Teething An acute sore mouth during tooth eruption is often caused by viral infections. The onset of eruption of first deciduous teeth (p221) correlates with the fall-off in transferred maternal antibody.

8 Dermatology

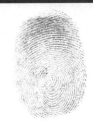

Fig 8.1 The spiral-like 'whorl' is one of a number of fingerprint patterns that offer an infallible means of personal identification, which unlike other visible characteristics are unique, and do not change over the course of a lifetime.

The epidermal ridges that make up a fingerprint help amplify vibrations detected by mechanoreceptors known as Pacinian corpuscles that respond to *changes* in pressure. Filippo Pacini, the Italian anatomist, saw the corpuscles in a hand he was dissecting as a medical student in 1831, when he was 19.

No one took his observations seriously, and Pacini heads our list of brilliant medical students ignored by their narrow-minded professors. He also discovered the cause of cholera in 1854, 30 years before Koch's 'first' description.

Pacini was the first medical student to understand what it is to feel pressure, without buckling. In his case, his chief pressure was the need to look after his two sick sisters—duties that eventually bankrupted him, and he died in a poorhouse in Florence in 1883.[1]

We dedicate this chapter to him, and everyone else feeling the strain.

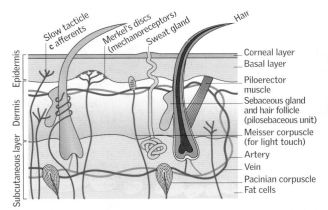

Fig 8.2 The anatomy of pleasure. All pleasure is sensory, and within our skin, this is thanks to unmyelinated tactile c afferents, which send impulses to our insular cortex—an area well suited to processing slow, gentle and pleasant touch (unlike our mundane somatosensory areas).[2]

⚙ Holistic approaches to dermatology

Because our skin is our most superficial organ, dermatology is never given due weight; but the skin is also our heaviest organ, and although its wounds may only seem skin deep, their effects can cast long shadows: people judge our health and beauty by the condition of our skin.

Our skin displays a more varied range of signs and reaction patterns than any other organ, but dermatologists do not confine themselves to the skin. Skin disorders such as psoriasis and eczema may be worsened by emotional stress (psychophysiologic disorders) and skin symptoms are features of many systemic diseases (p588). Primary psychiatric disorders may manifest as skin complaints, such as dermatitis artefacta and delusions of parasitosis (BOX, p611).

Common skin conditions such as eczema (p596) and psoriasis (p594) are not only the domain of dermatologists but are likely to be encountered by us all, regardless of our speciality. A practical knowledge and clinical confidence in diagnosing skin disease is a most valuable asset—and we *all* need to know how the dermatological aspects of our patients' lives interact with complex biological, social, and psychological events.

Latin^L & Greek^G for dermatology

Alba^L=white (as in albino).

Alopecia^G='fox-mange' (which causes patches of hair loss).

Atopy/Atopic^G=out of place/unusual (a predisposition to allergic responses).

Atrophy^G='without–food' (thinning and loss of skin substance).

Cutis^L=skin (sub^L=under, eg subcutaneous).

Derma^G=skin (intra^L=within).

Eczema^G, from *ekzein*, to break out, boil over.

Erythema^G=redness (eg of the skin).

Filiform^L=thread (long, irregular projections, seen in warts).

Impetere^L=to attack (as in impetigo).

Indurare^L=to harden (as in induration).

Lichen^L=tree moss (thick, bark-like skin caused by scratching, fig **8.4**).

Livedo^L=furious,red/blue; *reticulum*^{L}=net.

Lupus^L=wolf. The cutaneous manifestations of SLE appear similar to a wolf-bite.

Macula^L=stain/spot.

Papilla^L=nipple or teat (papule; papilloma).

Pilus/pili^L=hair.

Pityriasis^G=grain husk, flaky scales.

Psoriasis^G=psora=itch; NB: psoriasis often does not itch.

Purpura^L=purple (imperial) colour.

Rosea^L=pink.

Seborrhoeic=making *sebum*^{L} (suet, grease).

Telangiectasia^G...*telos*=end; *angeion*= vessel; *ekstasis*=extension (fig **8.3**).

Topicos^G=surface (hence creams are *top*ical).

Vesica^L=purse, bladder (fluid-filled blister).

Vitellus^L=spotted calf (as in vitiligo).

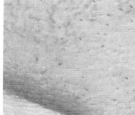

Fig 8.3 Telangiectasia.

Reproduced from Longmore et al, *Oxford Handbook of Clinical Medicine* 9e (2014) with permission from Oxford University Press.

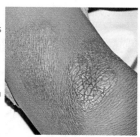

Fig 8.4 Lichenification.

We thank our Specialist Reader Dr Antonia Lloyd-Lavery and Bernard Ho our Junior Reader for their contribution to this chapter. We also thank and acknowledge Dr Susan Burge for her kind permission to use images from the Oxford Handbook of Medical Dermatology, a book which proved an invaluable resource in the writing of this chapter.

History *Ask about:* Duration of rash/lesions. Site of onset, spread, evolution, distribution of lesions. Symptoms (itch, pain). Aggravating or relieving factors (sunlight, heat). Any trauma? Previous treatments. Medical conditions and medications (any new medication?). Family history (psoriasis, atopy/eczema). Occupation (eg chemicals/detergents causing contact dermatitis). Change in shower gel/soap, cosmetics, or jewellery? Family and personal history of allergy/atopy, pets (eg allergy to animal danders). Sexual history (this may be important eg if considering herpes or syphilis). What is the impact of the condition on day-to-day life? Does it affect their mood or self-esteem? If itchy, is it interfering with sleep or concentration?

Examination Examine all the skin, scalp/hair, nails, and mucous membranes. Try to be as accurate as possible in describing lesions (see fig 8.5 on p585 for terminology). Is the problem epidermal or dermal?

* *Shape:* What shape are the lesions? Monomorphic (one form or shape) or polymorphic? Ring-like (annular) eg in fungal infections—active edge with healing centre, p598? Linear, eg from excoriations? Discoid (coin-like)?
* *Pattern:* Are lesions grouped, scattered, or generalized? Are there crops of lesions? (eg varicella) Target-like? (in erythema multiforme). Does it demonstrate a Köbner phenomenon (a predilection for areas of skin injury)?
* *Border:* Is the border distinct and well demarcated or indistinct?
* *Surface:* Is the surface scaly (suggesting epidermal pathology, eg in psoriasis) or smooth (dermal)? Are there excoriations or erosions from scratching? Lichenified skin looks thickened (from chronic rubbing). Any scarring?
* *Elevation:* Are the lesions raised or flat? If raised, is it due to a solid mass or fluid? Are blisters tense (subepidermal), or do they rupture easily (intraepidermal)?
* *Colour:* What colour is the rash? If red, does it blanch on pressure (suggesting erythema from increased blood in small vessels)? Non-blanching indicates purpura (from leakage of blood in the dermis).
* *Temperature:* Does the affected skin feel hotter or cooler than normal?
* *Evolution:* Ask the patient to show you lesions at different stages (if relevant).

Distribution • Symmetrical (suggesting an endogenous/systemic cause), or asymmetrical (suggesting an external cause eg insect bites, infection, trauma, or contact dermatitis)? • Is there a predilection for certain areas? eg flexural in atopic eczema (fig 8.29 on p597), or extensor in psoriasis (p594) • Areas in contact with jewellery or cosmetics (allergic contact dermatitis) • Areas exposed to sun, eg backs of hands, face, neck (photosensitivity; solar keratosis).

Ointments, creams, lotions: 3 ends of a spectrum

Creams are emulsions of oil and water and are well absorbed into the skin. They are generally more acceptable to patients than ointments because they are less greasy and easier to apply.

Ointments are greasy preparations that have no added water and are more occlusive than creams. They consist of varying amounts or combinations of soft, hard, or liquid paraffin, and are suitable for chronic, dry lesions. They often have a mild anti-inflammatory effect.

Lotions are used less commonly and have a cooling effect eg calamine lotion.

Emollients are ointments, lotions, creams, or sprays that soothe, smooth, and hydrate the skin. They are used in all dry, eczematous, and scaling disorders. The best emollient is the one the patient likes most, and choice depends in part on the severity of the condition. They should be applied frequently and liberally (in the direction of hair growth), and can also be used as soap substitutes or bath additives. If a large area of skin is involved, a large volume of emollient is needed, eg 500g/week. Most come as pump dispensers, which avoids bacterial contamination. If using tubs, remove cream with a clean spoon.

Flat, non-palpable changes in skin colour

Macule
Flat, non-palpable change in skin colour <0.5cm diameter. 'Freckles' are pigmented macules

Patch
Flat, non-palpable change in skin colour >0.5cm diameter

Elevation due to fluid in a cavity

Vesicle
Fluid within the upper layers of the skin <0.5cm diameter

Bulla
Large, fluid-filled lesion below the epidermis >10cm diameter

Blister
Fluid within the upper layers of the skin >0.5cm diameter

Pustule
Visible collection of pus in the subcutis

Elevation due to solid masses

Papule
A raised area <0.5cm diameter

Plaque
A raised area >2cm diameter

Nodule
A mass or lump >0.5cm diameter

Wheal
Dermal oedema

Callus
Hyperplastic epidermis, often found on the soles, palms or other areas of excessive friction/use

Loss of skin

Erosion
Partial epidermal loss Heals without scarring

Ulcer
Full thickness skin loss

Fissure
A linear crack

Atrophy
Thinning of the epidermis

Loss of tissue (epidermis/dermis +/or subcutis)

Surface changes

Scale
A small thin piece of horny epithelium resembling that of a fish

Crust (scab)
Dried exudate of blood/plasma or tissue fluid

Excoriation
A scratch mark

Lichenification
Thickening of the epidermis with exaggerated skin markings (bark-like) usually due to repeated scratching

Vascular changes

Telangiectasia
Easily visible superficial blood vessels

Spider naevus
A single telangiectatic arteriole in the skin

Purpura
A rash caused by blood in the skin—often multiple petechiae

Petechia
Micro-haemorrahge 1–2mm diameter

Ecchymosis
A 'bruise'. Technically a form of purpura

Erythema
A reddening of the skin due to local vasodilatation

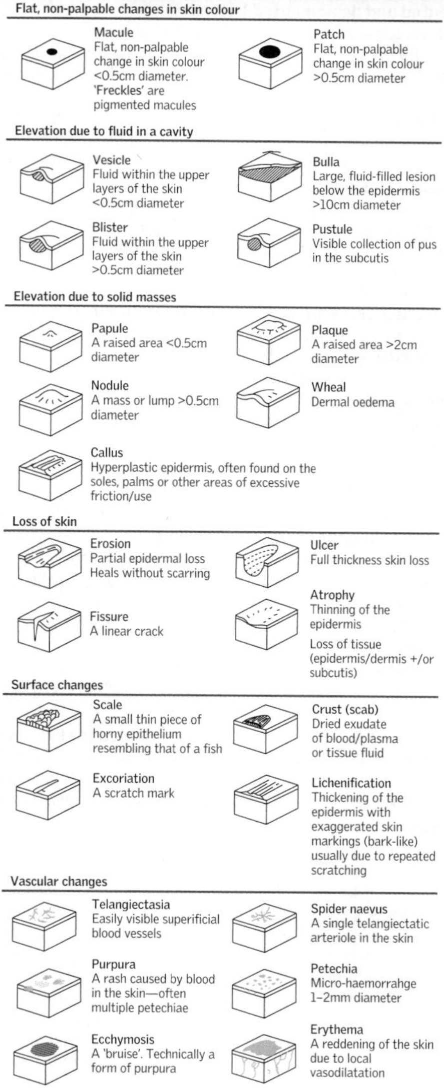

Fig 8.5 To communicate with a dermatologist, it is customary to translate your findings into the descriptive terms shown in the figure.

Adapted from Burge S, *Oxford Handbook of Medical Dermatology*, 2011, with permission from Oxford University Press.

Dermatology

Hypopigmented and depigmented lesions

- *Pityriasis versicolor:* Superficial slightly scaly infection with the yeast *Malassezia furfur.* Appears hypopigmented on darker skin. ℞: p598.
- *Pityriasis alba:* Post-eczema hypopigmentation, often on children's faces.
- *Vitiligo:* (fig 8.8) Smooth white depigmented patches or macules. *Associations:* Autoimmunity—particularly thyroid disease. ℞: Sun protection, cosmetic camouflage. Management is difficult: potent topical steroids may induce some repigmentation if recent onset; UVB phototherapy/PUVA (p595).

Hyperpigmented lesions

- *Lentigos:* Persistent brown macules, often larger than freckles, see BOX & fig 8.6.
- *Café-au-lait spots:* Faint brown macules; if >5, consider neurofibromatosis.
- *Melasma* (AKA chloasma): Smooth brown patches especially on the face, related to pregnancy or oral contraceptive use.
- *Melanocytic naevi:* 'moles' (p593).
- *Seborrhoeic warts/keratoses:* Benign greasy-brown warty lesions usually on the back, chest, and face; very common in the elderly, fig 8.7.
- *Systemic diseases*: Addison's (palmar creases, oral mucosa, scars); haemochromatosis; porphyria cutanea tarda (+ skin fragility and blisters).

Ring-shaped lesions

- *Basal cell carcinoma:* (p590) Pearly papule + central ulcer.
- *Tinea:* (p598) Ringworm lesions are round scaly & itchy with central healing.
- *Granuloma annulare:* (fig 8.11) Chronic non-infectious inflammatory ~1cm ring-shaped lesion, often on the back of hands. Cause unknown.
- *Erythema multiforme:* (p588) Target-like lesions, often on extensor surfaces.

Round, oval, or coin-shaped (discoid) lesions

- *Bowen's disease:* (p590; fig 8.17, p591) Slow-growing red, scaly plaque.
- *Discoid eczema:* Itchy, crusted/scaly eczema, worsened by heat.
- *Psoriasis:* Well-defined scaly red/pink plaques (p594). Distribution on extensor surfaces, scalp and natal cleft distinguishes it from discoid eczema.
- *Pityriasis rosea:* (p602) Herald patch; oval red lesions with scaly edge.
- *Erythema migrans:* (p588) is pathognomonic of Lyme disease, fig 8.9.
- *Impetigo:* Well-defined red patches, with honey-coloured crust, fig 8.10.

Linear lesions

- *Köbner phenomenon:* Lesions (eg psoriasis) related to skin injury, fig 8.12.
- *Dermatitis artefacta:* (p610) Bizarre-shaped lesions induced by the patient.
- *Herpes zoster:* (p599) vesicles/pustules in a dermatomal distribution.
- *Scabies burrows* (p608). • *Cutaneous larval migrans:* OHCM p442.

Itch (pruritus)

▶*Itch can be very distressing*. Skin will usually be scratched or rubbed and a number of secondary skin signs are seen: excoriations (scratch marks); lichenification (skin thickening, fig 8.4 on p583); papules or nodules (local skin thickening). *Causes:* Dry (and older) skin tends to itch. Determine if there is a primary skin disease or if itch is due to systemic disease (see also BOX p605).

- Itchy lesions: *scabies* (burrows in finger-webs, wrists, groin, buttock; p608); *urticaria* (transient wheals, dermatographism); *atopic eczema* (flexural eruption, lichenification, fig 8.29 on p597); *dermatitis herpetiformis* (very itchy blisters on elbows, shoulders); *lichen planus* (flat violet papules often on wrists).
- In ~22%, itch is caused by a systemic disease:[3] *iron deficiency* (koilonychia, pallor); *lymphoma* (nodes, hepatosplenomegaly); *hypo/hyperthyroidism; liver disease* (jaundice, spider naevi); *chronic renal failure* (dry sallow skin); *malignancy* (clubbing, masses); *drugs* (statins, ACE inhibitors, opiates, antidepressants). *Workup:* FBC, ESR, ferritin, LFT, U&E, glucose, TSH, CXR.

Treatment: Treat any primary disease; emollients (eg Diprobase®) to soothe dry skin; sedating antihistamines at night may be helpful.

Dermatology

Lentigos are brown macules/patches that persist in winter (unlike freckles). *Solar lentigos* are found on sun-damaged skin in older patients (fig 8.6). *Lentigo maligna* is a subtype of **melanoma** *in situ* and in ~5% may progress (over months or years) to *lentigo maligna melanoma* (a type of invasive melanoma; p592). Typical patient: Caucasian >40yrs with sun-damaged skin due to occupational exposure. The lesion is irregular, and variably pigmented (darker areas may be invasive). Not all show ABCDE signs of malignancy (p592). Use dermoscopes[1] ± full-thickness biopsy in equivocal lesions. Excision is best (>5mm margins).

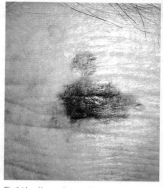

Fig 8.6 Lentigo maligna.　© Dr Suzannah Baron.

Dermatology

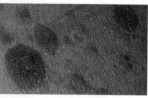

Fig 8.7 Seborrhoeic warts.
Reproduced from Warrell et al, *Oxford Textbook of Medicine*, 5th ed, 2012, with permission OUP.

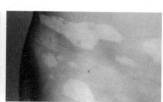

Fig 8.8 Vitiligo.
From Burge S, *Oxford Handbook of Medical Dermatology*, 2011, with permission OUP.

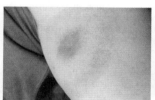

Fig 8.9 Erythema migrans (p588).
Courtesy of CDC/James Gathany.

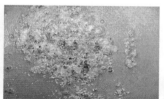

Fig 8.10 Impetigo (honey-coloured crusts).
Courtesy of Dr Samuel Da Silva.

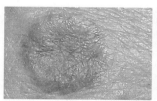

Fig 8.11 Granuloma annulare.
Courtesy of Dr Jonathan Bowling.

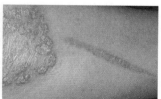

Fig 8.12 Köbner—psoriasis in a scratch.
From Burge S, *Oxford Handbook of Medical Dermatology*, 2011, with permission OUP.

1 The dermoscope is a handheld microscope using epiluminescence for evaluating pigmented skin lesions. It allows vision through the stratum corneum.

Diabetes *Flexural candidiasis; necrobiosis lipoidica* (waxy, shiny yellowish area on shins); *acanthosis nigricans* (pigmented, rough thickening of axillary, neck or groin skin); *granuloma annulare* (fig 8.11, p587); *folliculitis*.

Coeliac disease *Dermatitis herpetiformis* (very itchy/'burning' blisters on elbows, scalp, shoulders, ankles). *Treatment:* long-term gluten-free diet. It responds quickly to **dapsone** (50-200mg/day PO).

Inflammatory bowel disease •*Erythema nodosum* (tender ill-defined subcutaneous nodules, eg on shins; other causes: sarcoidosis, drugs, TB, streps). •*Pyoderma gangrenosum:* rapidly growing, very painful recurring nodulo-pustular ulcers, with tender red/blue overhanging necrotic edge. Often preceded by a tender pustule. Site: leg; abdomen; face. Other causes: Rheumatoid arthritis; myeloproliferative disorders (50% have no underlying disease).

Systemic lupus erythematosus (SLE) *OHCM* p556. *Facial butterfly rash; photosensitivity* (face, dorsum of hands, V of neck); *diffuse alopecia*. Patients may have cutaneous lupus erythematosus (see BOX).

Erythema multiforme (EM) (fig 8.13) A type of hypersensitivity reaction triggered most often by herpes simplex. *Minor form:* Erythematous well-defined round lesions appear on extensor surfaces of peripheries, palms, and soles and evolve at different stages (multiform) into pathognomonic target lesions. There is minimal mucosal involvement. *Major form:* (regarded as distinct from Stevens-Johnson syndrome/toxic epidermal necrolysis, p601). There is associated systemic upset, fever, and severe mucosal involvement. *Causes:* Herpes simplex (70%); mycoplasma; cytomegalovirus; orf; drugs. ℞: No treatment is required in the majority of cases. Potent topical steroid may

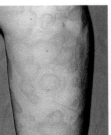
Fig 8.13 Erythema multiforme.

relieve any rash discomfort (but does not speed resolution). If needed, treat the cause eg aciclovir for HSV; antibiotics for mycoplasma; oral steroids if severe (controversial); supportive care. EM resolves spontaneously without scarring within 4 weeks. In recurrent disease consider aciclovir prophylaxis.

Erythema migrans (fig 8.7 p587) This is the best way to diagnose Lyme disease, as serology is difficult. ► <50% give history of a tick bite. The lesion is seen in 80% of cases and develops 7-10 days after the tick bite. A papule becomes a spreading red ring, lasting weeks to months. ℞: Get advice from someone experienced in managing Lyme disease. Antibiotics of choice are **doxycycline, amoxicillin** (unlicensed), or **cefuroxime** for 2-4 weeks.

Cutaneous vasculitis *Signs:* Variable, eg palpable purpura, eg on legs; nodules; painful ulcers; *livedo reticularis* (below). *Causes:* Idiopathic (often); systemic vasculitis, eg polyarteritis nodosa (PAN), Henoch-Schönlein purpura (vasculitic rash on legs/buttocks); granulomatosis with polyangiitis.

Livedo reticularis (fig 8.14) Non-blanching vague pink-blue mottling caused by capillary dilatation and stasis in skin venules, like diamond-shaped holes in a net, most often on the legs. *Causes:* A continuous network is physiological & disappears when the skin is warmed. Persistent and discontinuous is seen in connective tissue disease, vasculitis, cholesterol emboli, & hyperviscosity states. ℞: Treat the cause.

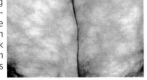
Fig 8.14 Livedo reticularis.
Reproduced from Longmore et al, *Oxford Handbook of Clinical Medicine* 9e (2014) with permission from Oxford University Press.

Dermatology

Connective tissue diseases and the skin

Lupus erythematosus (LE): An uncommon group of skin disorders:

1 *Chilblain LE:* Cold–induced plaques on fingers and toes.
2 *Chronic cutaneous (discoid) LE:* Inflamed scaly plaques+scarring±atrophy often localized to the head & neck. Most do not have significant systemic disease.
3 *Subacute cutaneous LE:* Widespread, non-scarring round or psoriasis-like plaques in photodistribution. 50% fulfil criteria for SLE.
4 *Acute SLE:* Seen in active SLE. Specific malar butterfly rash or widespread indurated erythema on upper trunk.
5 *Non-specific cutaneous LE phenomenon:* Vasculitis, alopecia, oral ulcers, palmar erythema, periungual erythema, Raynaud's phenomenon.

Systemic sclerosis features scleroderma (skin fibrosis) and vascular disease:

• *Limited cutaneous systemic sclerosis:* (formerly CREST syndrome) **C**alcinosis (subcutaneous tissues), **R**aynaud's, o**e**sophageal and gut dysmotility, **S**clerodactyly (swollen tight digits), and **T**elangiectasia. Skin involvement is 'limited' to the face, hands, and feet.

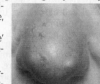

• *Diffuse cutaneous systemic sclerosis:* 'Diffuse' skin involvement (affecting the whole body if severe) and early organ fibrosis.

Sarcoidosis A multisystem granulomatous disorder. Skin is affected in 25% and lesions include • Hypopigmented patches • Yellow-brown firm (periorbital) papules • Scarring alopecia • Sarcoid in scars • Firm subcutaneous nodules (*Darier–Roussy sarcoid*) • *Lupus pernio* (fig 8.15) is diagnostic of sarcoidosis: chronic sarcoid plaques on nose, ears, lips, and cheeks ± permanent scarring.

Fig 8.15 Lupus pernio of the nose.

Reproduced from Warrell et al, *Oxford Textbook of Medicine*, 5th ed, 2012, with permission from Oxford University Press.

Paraneoplastic skin phenomena

If a tumour makes transforming growth factor (similar to epidermal growth factor and binds the same receptors), it is proposed that distant keratinocytes can flourish and a range of proliferative paraneoplastic signs erupt. Most are uncommon and are seen also in non-malignant conditions.[4]

Leser–Trélat sign: Sudden eruption of multiple *seborrheic keratoses* seen rarely in association with GI adenocarcinomas & genitourinary cancers.

Acanthosis nigricans: Darkened velvety skin, most commonly due to diabetes/obesity but can be associated with gastric cancer and lymphoma.

Dermatomyositis: Heliotrope (red/purple) eyelids (see fig 8 in *OHCM* p565); Gottron's papules (flat violet knuckle papules). 10–30% have an associated malignancy eg breast & ovary (♀), lung & prostate (♂), and colorectal.

Paraneoplastic pemphigus (rare): Severe mucosal and cutaneous erosions associated with lymphoreticular malignancy.

Acquired ichthyosis: Dry scaly skin seen in lymphoproliferative disorders.

Hypertrichosis lanuginosa: An increase in downy lanugo hair, most often associated with GI adenocarcinomas and lung cancer.

Tripe palms: Ridged velvety lesions on the palms, often in association with acanthosis nigricans & associated with GI adenocarcinoma and lung cancer.

Actinic (solar) keratoses (AK) (fig 8.16) Pre-malignant crumbly yellow-white scaly crusts on sun-exposed skin from dysplastic intra-epidermal proliferation of atypical keratinocytes. *UK prevalence:* 21% at 40yrs old; 52% if 70yrs old. *Natural history:* May regress/recur. Progression to scc <1 in 1000/yr. *ΔΔ:* Bowen's, psoriasis, BCC, seborrhoeic keratosis. If in doubt, biopsy. *Treatment:* See BOX p591. *Prevention:* Education; hats; sunscreens. Advise all patients to monitor their skin as AK is a marker for risk of developing skin cancer.

Bowen's disease (SCC *in situ*, fig 8.17) A well-defined slowly-enlarging red scaly plaque with a flat edge (asymptomatic). *Histology:* Full-thickness dysplasia/carcinoma *in situ.* 3–5% progress to squamous cell cancer (but the risk of metastases from the scc is high). *Cause:* UV exposure; radiation; immunosuppression; arsenic; HPV infection is associated with the development of anogenital disease. *℞:* Options include cryotherapy; topical **fluorouracil** or **miquimod** (unlicensed); photodynamic therapy; curettage; excision.[5]

Basal cell carcinoma (BCC, rodent ulcer) is the commonest skin cancer. *Nodular:* Typically, a pearly nodule with rolled telangiectatic edge on the face or a sun exposed site ± central ulcer (fig 8.18). Metastases are very rare. It slowly causes local destruction if left untreated. *Superficial:* Lesions appear as red scaly plaques with raised smooth edge, often on the trunk or shoulders. *Cause:* UV exposure; immunosuppression. *℞:* Depends on type, site, and whether primary or recurrent. Excision is often the treatment of choice. Other options: cryotherapy, curettage, radiotherapy, photodynamic therapy. Topical **imiquimod** or **fluorouracil** is reasonable for superficial lesions at low-risk sites.[6]

Squamous cell cancer (fig 8.19; the commonest skin cancer after BCC) A persistently ulcerated or crusted firm irregular lesion often on sun-exposed sites. It is locally invasive and may metastasize (↑ risk if lip, ear or non-sun exposed site; >2cm diameter; poor histological differentiation or host immunosuppression). Also related to chronic inflammation, eg leg ulcers, and HPV (eg genital area or periungual). *℞:* Local complete excision in primary scc.

Other malignancies & skin

Metastatic cancer Skin metastases (from direct tumour invasion or lymphatic/haematogenous spread) are uncommon but well recognized. The most commonly associated cancers causing cutaneous metastases are: • Breast (fig 8.21; skin of chest & scalp) • Stomach and colon (skin of abdominal wall–esp. periumbilical) • Lung (skin of chest & scalp) • Genitourinary system (uterus, ovary, kidney, bladder: skin of scalp, lower abdomen & external genitalia). Non-Hodgkin's lymphoma and leukaemia can also metastasize to the skin. Metastases are usually firm, intradermal, or subcutaneous nodules of varying colour.

Mycosis fungoides The commonest cutaneous T-cell lymphoma, which progresses from well defined itchy red scaly patches and plaques to red-brown infiltrated plaques and ulcerating tumours. *Δ:* Biopsy. *℞: Early stage:* Potent topical steroids, PUVA. *Late stage:* Radiotherapy. Sezary syndrome is a leukaemic form of cutaneous T-cell lymphoma characterized by erythroderma, lymphadenopathy, and malignant circulating CD4 positive T-cells (Sezary cells).

Paget's disease of the nipple (fig 8.20) An itchy, red, scaly, or crusted nipple, from direct extension of intraductal adenocarcinoma. *Δ:* Biopsy. *ΔΔ:* Eczema (but eczema is bilateral, non-deforming, and waxes and wanes, so... ►*always consider a biopsy in 'nipple eczema' + check for a breast lump. Surgery:* Mastectomy or lesser surgery ± radiotherapy.

Dermatology

Options in actinic keratoses (AK)

- *No treatment* or *emollient* is a reasonable option for mild AK.
- *Diclofenac gel* (3%) is moderately effective (mechanism unknown); used twice daily for 60–90 days it is well tolerated and cheap.
- *Fluorouracil* (5FU) 5% cream once or twice-daily for up to 6 weeks is effective for up to 12 months in clearing the majority of non-hypertrophic lesions. It works by causing erythema→vesiculation→erosion→ulcers→necrosis→healing epithelialization and leaves healthy skin unharmed.
- *Imiquimod* 5% 3×weekly for 4wks to lesions; assess after a 4wk treatment-free gap; repeat once if persisting; allow cream to stay on for 8h, then wash. It augments cell mediated immunity by inducing interferon-α and causes a similar inflammatory reaction to fluorouracil + occasionally 'flu–like symptoms.
- *Cryotherapy:* Effective for up to 75% of lesions.
- *Photodynamic therapy:* Effective in up to 91% but availability is limited. Useful if located at sites of poor healing eg lower leg.
- *Surgical excision and curettage:* Excise AKs if atypical, unresponsive to treatment or invasive scc is suspected.[7]

Dermatology

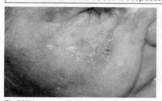

Fig 8.16 Actinic (solar) keratosis.
Courtesy of Dr Samuel da Silva:
www.atlasdermatologico.com.br.

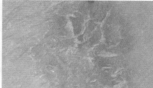

Fig 8.17 Bowen's disease.
Courtesy of Dr Jonathan Bowling.

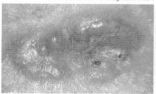

Fig 8.18 Basal cell carcinoma.
Courtesy of Dr Samuel da Silva:
www.atlasdermatologico.com.br.

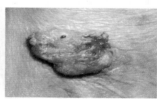

Fig 8.19 Squamous cell carcinoma.

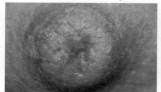

Fig 8.20 Paget's disease of nipple.
Courtesy of Dr Samuel da Silva:
www.atlasdermatologico.com.br.

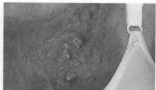

Fig 8.21 Breast cancer metastases.
Courtesy of Dr Samuel da Silva:
www.atlasdermatologico.com.br.

Further reading

de Berker D *et al.* (2007). Guidelines for the management of actinic keratoses. *Br J Dermatol* 56:222–30.

Morton CA *et al.* (2014). British Association of Dermatologists' guidelines for the management of squamous cell carcinoma in situ (Bowen's disease) 2014. *Br J Dermatol* 170:245–60.

Telfer NR *et al.* (2008). Guidelines for the management of basal cell carcinoma. *Br J Dermatol* 159:35–48.

Malignant melanoma (figs 8.22 & 8.23) The 5th commonest cancer in the UK. *UK incidence:* 20:100,000/yr (incidence has quadrupled since the 1970s). Nearly 1/3rd occur in those aged <50yrs and melanoma accounts for 75% of deaths associated with skin cancer. Most arise *de novo*, not in pre-exisiting melanocytic naevi.

Risk UV exposure†; sunburn, fair complexion, many (>50) melanocytic or dysplastic naevi, +ve family history, previous melanoma, old age (the highest incidence is in those >80yrs old). *Early diagnosis* ▶Everyone should know what early melanomas look like, and know how to get help.

Signs Use the ABCDEF criteria to identify suspicious pigmented lesions:
• Asymmetry in the outline of the lesion
• Border irregularity or blurring
• Colour variation with shades of black, brown, blue, or pink
• Diameter >6mm (cannot be covered by the end of a pencil)
• Evolution (all changing moles—in size, elevation and/or colour, are suspect)
• Funny looking mole—a mole that stands out or is different from others is better than ABCDE criteria for identifying nodular melanoma, which can be symmetrical, have regular borders, and be uniform in colour. Nodular melanomas are Elevated, Firm, and Growing.
▶▶Refer urgently (under the 2-week rule in the UK) any pigmented lesion you are concerned about. Prognosis is determined primarily by Breslow thickness and mortality is significantly improved if the tumour is removed when it is thin.

ΔΔ: Benign melanocytic lesions (see BOX); non-melanocytic pigmented lesions, eg *seborrhoeic keratoses* (p586), common if >50yrs.

Types of melanoma
• *Superficial spreading melanoma* (70%): Presents as a slowly enlarging pigmented lesion with colour variation and an irregular border. Initially growth is in the radial plane, where the lesion remains thin, but this may be followed by vertical invasion. Common on the trunks of men or legs of women.
• *Nodular melanoma* (15%): The most aggressive type of melanoma. There is no radial growth phase and lesions grow rapidly, invade deeply, and metastasize early. It is often darkly pigmented but may be amelanotic in 5%.
• *Acral lentiginous melanoma* (10%): Occur on the palms, soles, and subungual areas. It is the most common type of melanoma in black and asian skin. Refer urgently any new pigmented line in a nail, or growing under a nail (especially if it extends from the nailbed to the nailfold = *Hutchinson's nail sign*).
• *Lentigo maligna melanoma* (5%): Arises within a lentigo maligna (p587).

Treatment:[8] Surgery is the only curative treatment. For *any* unusual, growing, or changing pigmented lesion, excision biopsy of the whole lesion must be considered (with a 2mm *margin of normal skin* around the lesion + a cuff of subcutaneous fat). This allows for histological diagnosis and measurement of tumour depth (Breslow thickness). If malignant melanoma is confirmed, a wider excision margin is taken (up to 3cm) to ensure complete removal.

Prognosis: Depends on excision completeness and Breslow thickness. If <0.75mm thick, 5-yr survival is >95%; if >4mm it is 45%. Metastatic disease has a 5-yr survival of <10%. *Metastatic melanoma:* Adjuvant therapy eg **interferon alfa** (IFN-α) is used to minimize the risk of relapse in patients with resected node positive (stage III) disease. There is no curative treatment for stage IV disease. Treatment (aimed at palliating symptoms and maximizing quality of life) includes chemotherapy, biological therapy (IFN-α; IL-2) and novel therapies targeting specific molecular abnormalities eg **vemurafenib/dabrafenib** for those with BRAF mutations. Immunotherapy with **ipilimumab** (anti-CTLA-4) can result in prolonged survival in the minority of patients who respond. Melanoma is not responsive to radiotherapy.

Prevention: ▶Don't just diagnose today's melanoma: prevent tomorrow's.

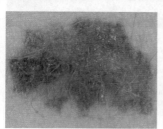

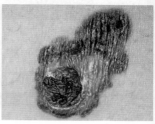

Fig 8.22. Superficial spreading melanoma.
© Dr Suzannah Baron.

Fig 8.23 Nodular melanoma.
© Dr Suzannah Baron.

Common benign melanocytic naevi (navus = mole)[9]

Congenital melanocytic naevi (usually >1cm) present at birth or in the early neonatal period. If >20cm there is increased risk for malignant change.[9]

Acquired melanocytic naevi present in childhood or in young adults and have a characteristic evolution (fig 8.24). They start as flat evenly pigmented naevi, in which 'nests' of melanocytes collect along the basal layer of the epidermis (= junctional naevi). As melanocytes migrate from the epidermis to the dermis, moles evolve into raised evenly pigmented dome-shaped naevi (= compound naevi). Finally the epidermal component is lost and moles change into pale brown papules (= intradermal naevi), before disappearing in old age.[9]

Halo naevi are common in adolescence. A 'white' halo develops around a benign melanocytic naevi. It is not sinister and results from loss of melanocytes by lymphocyte action. Halo naevi in adults (age 40–50yrs) may indicate melanoma elsewhere—check skin, eyes, and mucosal surfaces.[9]

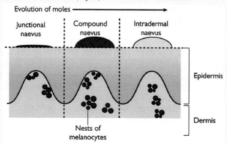

Fig 8.24 The life of a mole: evolution of melanocytic naevi.
Reproduced from Burge S, *Oxford Handbook of Medical Dermatology*, 2011, with permission from Oxford University Press.

Further reading

Marsden JR *et al.* (2010). Revised UK guidelines for the management of cutaneous melanoma 2010. *Br J Dermatol* 163:238–56.

Dermatology

Psoriasis is a chronic inflammatory skin condition characterized by scaly erythematous plaques, which typically follows a relapsing remitting course. *Pathogenesis:* The epidermis in psoriatic plaques is hyperproliferative. There is proliferation and dilatation of blood vessels in the dermis + infiltration of inflammatory cells (T-cells ± neutrophils). Plaque psoriasis is the commonest form (~90%). *Prevalence:* 1–3% (varying among ethnic groups eg 0.3% in China). 75% are affected before 46yrs old (uncommon in children). ♂:♀≈1:1. Susceptibility is inherited—if both parents have psoriasis, risk to offspring is ~50%. *Triggers:* Stress, infections (esp. streps), skin trauma (Köbner phenomenon), drugs (lithium, NSAIDs, β-blockers, antimalarials), alcohol, obesity, smoking, and climate.

۞Psychological and social effects of psoriasis are common and can be profound. 60% are depressed. Consider the impact on body image, mood, relationships, work/school, and any problems caused by treatment.

Types of psoriasis • *Chronic plaque psoriasis:* (fig 8.25) Symmetrical well-defined red plaques with silvery scale on extensor aspects of the elbows, knees, scalp, and sacrum. • *Flexural psoriasis:* Plaques in moist flexural areas (axillae, groins, submammary areas and umbilicus) are less scaly and often misdiagnosed as fungal infection (symmetry suggests psoriasis). • *Guttate psoriasis:* (fig 8.26) Large numbers of small plaques <1cm over the trunk and limbs are seen in the young (especially after acute streptococcal infection), usually lasting 3–4 months. • *Pustular psoriasis:* (palmoplantar psoriasis) yellow-brown pustules within plaques affecting the palms & soles; ♀:♂≈9:1. • *Generalized (erythrodermic) psoriasis:* (and generalized pustular psoriasis) may cause severe systemic upset (fever, ↑wcc, dehydration)—both are a medical emergency requiring urgent hospital referral. NB: Also triggered by rapid withdrawal of steroids. • *Nail changes* (in 50%): pitting, onycholysis (separation from nail-bed, fig 8.27), thickening and subungual hyperkeratosis (fig 8.28).

Psoriatic arthropathy 7% develop a seronegative arthropathy—5 types: **1** Monoarthritis or oligomonoarthritis **2** Psoriatic spondylitis **3** Asymmetrical polyarthritis **4** Arthritis mutilans (destructive) **5** Rheumatoid-like polyarthritis.

ΔΔ: Eczema; tinea (solitary or few lesions; asymmetrical; expanding); mycosis fungoides (asymmetric, less scaling, do biopsy); seborrhoeic dermatitis.

Management *Education* is vital; control, not cure, is realistic. Assess severity and proportion of skin affected. Find out what he/she finds most distressing. Consider phototherapy or systemic therapy if >10% body area affected. *Emollients* reduce scale and help relieve irritation. For all topical treatment select a base the patient prefers (ointment, cream, lotion, gel, or foam).

Topical treatment[10] *Plaque psoriasis:* Use a topical corticosteroid (eg Betnovate®) once a day (eg morning; <50g/wk) *plus* a topical vitamin D preparation (which affects cell division; eg Dovonex®) applied once a day (eg at night; max 100g/wk). NB: Dovobet® is a combined once-daily ointment or gel. Review at 4 weeks (advise patient to stop steroid before this if skin is clear). If response is good continue until the skin is clear or nearly clear. Potent corticosteroids should not be used for more than 8 weeks + there should be a treatment break of 4 weeks before being restarted (during which vitamin D analoagues can be continued). Tars: eg 1% coal tar lotion (eg Exorex®) is easier if widespread disease (not limited to the affected skin). Dithranol is an option in treatment resistance.

Scalp psoriasis: Potent topical steroid lotion (OD for max 8wks) or vitamin D analogue scalp preparation. Coal tar shampoos may help.

Flexural psoriasis: Use a mild–moderate potent topical steroid for up to 2 weeks (± antifungal/antibiotic combination). Break for 4 weeks between courses.

Localized pustular psoriasis & nail psoriasis is best managed by a dermatologist.

Psoriatic arthropathy: NSAIDs, DMARDs (eg methotrexate), and anti-TNF agents.

Phototherapy *Narrowband UVB phototherapy:* is most suitable for guttate or plaque psoriasis that cannot be controlled with topical treatments or when disease is widespread (± topical adjunctive or systemic treatment).

PUVA: psoralen + UVA is suitable for extensive large plaque psoriasis (oral psoralen) or localized pustular psoriasis (topical psoralen). There is increased risk of skin cancer (esp. squamous cell carcinoma).

Non-biologic oral drugs Severe psoriasis often needs oral drugs (get help).

Methotrexate 10-20mg/week PO; most useful in elderly patients; or if psoriatic arthropathy. Avoid if young in view of long-term risk of hepatic fibrosis. Monitor FBC & LFT.

Ciclosporin: 2.5-5mg/kg/day PO; good, but SE bad (BP↑; renal dysfunction).

Acitretin: Oral retinoid; useful for moderate/severe disease; SE: teratogenic; dry skin and mucosae; ↑lipids; glucose↑; ↑LFT (reversible). Check lipids, glucose, LFT at start, then every 2wks for 8wks, then every 12wks. In the UK, use is limited to hospitals. Starting at 25-30mg/24h PO. Exclude pregnancy, avoid donating blood for >1yr and pregnancy until >2yrs after the last dose.

Biological drugs[11] inhibit T-cell activation and function, or neutralize cytokines. They have revolutionized treatment of severe psorasis that hasn't improved with systemic treatments or light therapy (or where these are contraindicated/have caused side effects). Consider **infliximab**, **adalimumab**, and **etanercept** (TNF antagonists), or if these have failed, **ustekinumab** (an interleukin inhibitor). All are specialist use only.

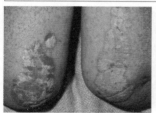

Fig 8.25 Plaque psoriasis on extensor surfaces.
Reproduced from Burge S, *Oxford Handbook of Medical Dermatology*, 2011, with permission from OUP.

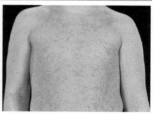

Fig 8.26 Guttate psoriasis.
Reproduced from Lewis-Jones, *Oxford Specialist Handbook of Paediatric Dermatology*, 2010, with permission from OUP.

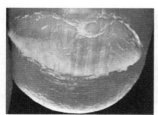

Fig 8.27 Onycholysis. Nail pitting may also be present.   © Dr Suzannah Baron.

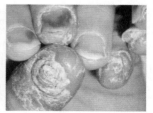

Fig 8.28 Psoriasis affecting the nails.
                    © Dr Suzannah Baron.

Dermatology

Further reading

NICE (2012). *Psoriasis: The Assessment and Management of Psoriasis* (CG153). London: NICE.
Smith CH *et al.* (2009). British Association of Dermatologists' guidelines for biologic interventions for psoriasis 2009. *Br J Dermatol* 161:987–1019.

Acute eczema causes a rash with inflamed red skin that is poorly demarcated and less scaly than psoriasis. The barrier function of the epidermis is abnormal and skin is easily irritated. Eczema is itchy and there is often associated excoriations. The pathophysiology is poorly understood and there are a number of patterns: Eczema may be *endogenous*, eg *atopic*, *seborrhoeic*, *varicose* (from venous stasis), or *discoid*; or *exogenous* eg *allergic contact* (type IV), or *irritant contact*. Different types may co-exist. Ask about impact on quality of life, school/work and sleep.

Atopic eczema[12,13] (fig 8.29) *Causes:* Multifactorial: •*Genetic:* A family history of atopy is common (70%). •*Infection:* staphs colonize lesions, suggested by weeping, crusting or pustules. •*Allergens:* Avoidance of allergens eg house dust mite or animal dander is difficult and of limited benefit. Food allergy is rarely the cause of eczema. Consider if there is a clear trigger with immediate symptoms (eg confirm a dairy allergy with specific IgE test; if +ve, get a dietician's help); or, in poorly controlled eczema associated with GI symptoms or failure to thrive. *Diagnosis:*[14] A child must have itchy skin (or parents report scratching) + ≥3 of: 1 Onset before 2yrs. 2 Past flexural involvement. 3 History of generally dry skin. 3 Personal history of other atopy (or history of atopy in 1st-degree relative if <4yrs). 5 Visible flexural dermatitis (or on cheeks/forehead and outer side of limbs if <4yrs). There may be lichenification (fig 8.4, p583, from chronic rubbing) or post-inflammatory hypo- or hyperpigmentation. Atopic eczema typically spares the nappy area. *Severity:* Mild, moderate, or severe, based on signs and symptoms, and quantity/strength of treatment required. Most children grow out of atopic eczema before 13yrs old. *Management:*
• *Explain:* Management involves control, not cure. Discuss the cause (multifactorial, causing a breakdown of the skin barrier). Eczema fluctuates and can be frustrating to treat. Say to report any severe weeping rash eg around the mouth: this may be ▸▸*eczema herpeticum* a primary herpes infection which may be fatal (get urgent help). Discourage elimination diets.
• *Emollients & soap substitutes:* Dry skin itches and is susceptible to irritants. Use emollients liberally (at least ×3–4/d), even when eczema is less active. They treat dryness and act as a barrier. The best emollient is the one the patient likes the most. Prescribe in large quantities (>500g/wk). Use emollient soap substitutes and bath oils. Intensive use ↓need for topical steroids.
• *Topical corticosteroids:* Use for exacerbations and only on active eczematous skin. Apply once each day 30min after emollient. Steroid-phobia and under-use are common. Explain treatment is safe if used as prescribed. Most infantile atopic eczema can be managed with mild to moderate corticosteroids (use only mild on the face and flexures). Potent corticosteroids may be needed—step up or down using the weakest steroid which is fully effective. As a guide, use should be limited to ≤1week for an acute flare (or 4-6 weeks to gain control in chronic disease). Haelan tape® (**fluordxycortide**) is good at healing fissured digits. Treat secondary bacterial infection (fig 8.30) with oral antibiotics. Topical **pimecrolimus** or **tacrolimus** can be used if eczema is not controlled with topical steroids. Systemic treatments such as **azathioprine**, **ciclosporin**, or **methotrexate** may be indicated in severe disease.
• *Itch:* Sedating antihistamines eg **hydroxyzine** used intermittently at night can reduce the itch/scratch cycle. Keep fingernails short and advise pressing the skin rather than scratching or rubbing.

Adult seborrhoeic dermatitis This common red, scaly rash affects scalp (dandruff), eyebrows, nasolabial folds, cheeks, and flexures. *Cause:* eg overgrowth of skin yeasts (*Malassezia*). It can be severe if HIV+ve. ℞: Mild topical steroid/antifungal preparations, eg **Daktacort**® or ketoconazole 2% cream or shampoo (or **metronidazole** 0.75% gel). Treat intermittently, as needed.

Dermatology

Irritant and allergic contact dermatitis

Irritant dermatitis We are all susceptible to irritants. Hands are often affected; redness ± weeping precedes dry fissuring. *Common irritants:* detergents, soaps, oils, solvents, alkalis; water (if repeated). It often affects bar staff and cleaners. ℞: Avoid all irritants; hand care (soap substitutes; regular emollients; careful drying; cotton or cotton-lined rubber gloves for dry and wet work respectively); as-needed use of topical steroids for acute flare-ups.

Allergic contact dermatitis (fig 8.31) (Type IV reaction) *Common allergens:* nickel (jewellery, watches, coins, keys); chromates (cements, leather); lanolin (creams, cosmetics); rubber (foam in furniture); plants (primulas); topical neomycin, framycetin, antihistamines, or anaesthetics (haemorrhoid creams). The pattern of contact gives clues to the allergen. There is often a sharp cut-off where contact ends. Secondary spread elsewhere is frequent (auto-sensitization). ℞: Consider patch testing and avoidance of implicated allergens; use a topical steroid appropriate for severity (↓ strength and stop as it settles).

Potency & side effects of topical corticosteroids

Mild hydrocortisone 0.5%, 1%; *with antimicrobials:* eg Canesten HC®, Daktacort®.
Moderate eg Betnovate–RD®, Eumovate®; *with antimicrobials:* eg Trimovate®.
Potent eg Betnovate®, Elocon®; *with antimicrobials:* eg Fucibet®, Betnovate-N®.
Very potent eg Dermovate®, Etrivex®.

Side effects Mild/moderate are associated with few. SEs depend on potency (caution in potent/very potent) and duration of use. *Local:* skin thinning, irreversible striae, telangectasia, worsening of untreated infection, contact dermatitis. *Systemic:* Adrenal suppression (rare).

The amount of topical steroid required can be estimated using the **fingertip unit** (FTU=the amount of cream squeezed from a standard 5mm nozzle along the palmar surface of the distal phalanx of an adult finger). 1FTU will cover an area equivalent to the palmar surface of 2 adult hands (including fingers).

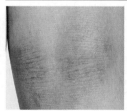

Fig 8.29 Atopic eczema. ©Dr S Baron.

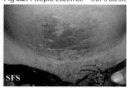

Fig 8.31 Contact dermatitis.
Courtesy Dr Samuel da Silva:
www.atlasdermatologico.com.br.

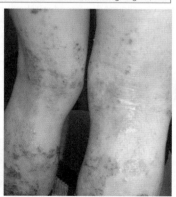

Fig 8.30 Atopic eczema with secondary bacterial infection causing crusting and weeping.
Reproduced from Burge S, *Oxford Handbook of Medical Dermatology*, 2011, with permission OUP.

Further reading

British Association of Dermatologists & Primary Care Dermatology Society (2015). *Management of Atopic Eczema.* http://www.pcds.org.uk/clinical-guidance/atopic-eczema
NICE (2007). *Atopic Eczema in Under 12s: Diagnosis and Management* (CG57). London: NICE.

Dermatology

Dermatology

Dermatophyte infections *(Ringworm; 'tinea'):* Fungal infections that invade and grow in dead keratin. Spread is most often transmitted indirectly from man to man. Species that infect only humans (=anthropophilic, eg *Trichophyton rubrum*, fig 8.32) are the most common. Fungi that infect animals (=zoophilic, eg *Microsporum canis*) cause a more inflamed rash in humans. Geophilic (soil) species rarely infect humans (eg *Microsporum gypseum*). A ringworm infection is a round, scaly, itchy lesion whose edge is more inflamed than its centre. It is called *tinea* followed, in Latin, by the part affected, eg tinea pedis (foot); cruris (groins); capitis (scalp); unguium (nail); corporis (body, fig 8.33). *Δ:* Send skin scrapings (from the active edge of a lesion), scalp brushings or nail clippings for microscopy (rapid result) and culture (4–6wks). *R:* *Skin:* Topical antifungal eg **terbinafine** or **imidazole** creams (eg clotrimazole) twice daily for 2wks. *Scalp:* Treat empirically with oral **griseofulvin** or **terbinafine** (unlicensed) + **ketoconazole** shampoo until culture results are known (*M. canis* responds to griseofulvin; *T. tonsurans* responds better to terbinafine). *Nails:* Nail infection is difficult to treat. Confirm diagnosis (microscopy/culture) before starting treatment. **Amorolfine** paint may be effective if mild (use for 6 months for fingernails; 9–12 months for toenails). **Terbinafine** PO for 6wks–3 mths (fingernail); or 3–6 months (toenails) if deemed essential. Explain about SEs and interactions.

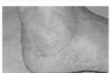

Fig 8.32 *Trichophyton rubrum*. Courtesy of Dr Jonathan Bowling.

Fig 8.33 Tinea corporis. Courtesy of Dr Susannah Baron.

Yeast *Candida albicans:* A commensal in the mouth and GI tract, it commonly infects skin, mainly affecting the mouth, vagina, glans of penis, skin folds/toe web, & nail areas. They are often pink and moist ± satellite lesions. Oral candida wipes off with a spatula (unlike lichen planus, p602) *R:* *Skin:* **imidazole** creams. *Mouth:* **nystatin** (eg oral suspension, 1mL/6h for 1 week) or **miconazole** oral gel. *Vagina:* **imidazole** cream ± pessary (eg Canesten Combi®).

Pityriasis versicolor: Malassezia species (eg *M. furfur*) cause multiple hypopigmented scaly macules on the upper trunk and back. The commensals produce azelaic acid which inhibits melanogenesis and prevents affected skin from tanning. *R:* **Imidazole** creams BD for localized disease; 2% **ketoconazole** shampoo daily for 5 days (wash off after 5min). Relapses are frequent.

Bacteria *Impetigo:* Contagious superficial infection caused by *Staph aureus* (±*Strep pyogenes*). Peak: 2-5yrs. Lesions (often well defined) usually start around the nose & face with honey-coloured crusts on erythematous base (±superficial flaccid blisters; fig 8.10, p587). *R:* Try topical **fusidic acid** for localized infection. Give oral antibiotics (eg **flucloxacillin** QDS for 7 days) if severe. Hygeine advice.

Erysipelas: Sharply defined superficial infection caused by *Strep pyogenes*. Often affects the face (unilateral) with fever and ↑wcc. *R:* See cellulitis (below).

Cellulitis: Acute infection of skin and soft tissues (eg legs). *Cause:* β-haemolytic streps ± staphs. It is deeper and less well-defined than erysipelas. *Signs:* pain, swelling, erythema, warmth, systemic upset and lymphadenopathy. *R:* ►Elevate the affected part. **Benzylpenicillin** 600mg/6h IV (or **phenoxymethylpenicillin** 500mg/4-6h PO) + **flucloxacillin** 500mg/6h PO. If penicillin-allergic, try **erythromycin** 500mg/12h PO.

Skin TB: Lupus vulgaris (a red-brown scarring plaque); *scrofuloderma* (suppurating nodules from direct extension of TB in lymph nodes); *TB verrucosa cutis* (indolent warty plaques); *TB gumma* (extension of TB from underlying foci); *tuberculids* (generalized exanthems eg erythema induratum/lichen scrofulosorum).

Warts (fig 8.34) Caused by human papillomavirus (HPV) in keratinocytes.
•*Common warts and plantar warts (verrucae):* Papules or nodules with a hyperkeratotic or filiform surface, most commonly seen at sites of trauma (fingers, elbows, knees; and pressure points on soles) in children. Warts may coalesce into confluent lesions (mosaic warts). Warts are contagious but risk of transmission is low. They rarely cause symptoms and will disappear spontaneously (within months–2yrs) without treatment and without scarring. *R:* Consider if painful, unsightly, or persisting. Any treatment should not cause more problems than the wart itself. •Topical salicylic acid (keratolytic), eg **Salatac**® gel daily for 12wks •Cryotherapy (not in younger children as it is painful) once every 3–4wks for up to 4 cycles •Duct tape occlusion—leave in place for 6d at a time for up to 8wks (probably a placebo).[15]
•*Plane warts:* Flat skin-coloured or brown lesions; tend to Köbnerize (p584) in scratch marks; they often resist treatment.
•*Genital warts (condylomata acuminata):* Sexually transmitted. *R:* NB There is significant treatment failure and relapse rate. •No treatment (⅓ resolve within 6m) •Self applied **podophyllin** or **imiquimod** cream (not if pregnant or in children) •Cryotherapy. Screen for other STIs. If a child, suspect abuse.[16]

Molluscum contagiosum *(pox virus)* These pink papules have an umbilicated (depressed) central punctum. Common in children. They resolve spontaneously (may take months). Treatment is often not recommended. Gentle cryo or squeezing/piercing may be tried.

Herpes simplex Recurrent genital or perioral infection, often preceded by symptoms of burning/itching. *Signs:* Grouped painful vesicles on erythematous base which heal without scarring (fig **8.35**). *Treatment: Oral:* Often none required. The benefits of topical **aciclovir** are small. *Genital:* Oral **aciclovir** (200mg 5×/day PO for 1wk, within 5 days of lesion onset). Hygiene measures + abstain from sex until lesions have cleared. Consider prophylaxis if >6 attacks/yr. Get expert advice if immunosuppressed or pregnant.

Herpes zoster Varicella-zoster virus becomes dormant in dorsal root ganglia after chickenpox infection has subsided. Recurrent infection affects one or more dermatomes (fig **12.36**, p762, esp. if immunosuppressed). Pain and malaise may precede the rash. *Signs:* Polymorphic red papules, vesicles, pustules (fig **8.36**). *R:* If mild, none. If >50yrs, ophthalmic involvement, severe, or immunosuppressed use an antiviral (eg **aciclovir** 800mg 5×/day PO for 1wk) starting within 72h of rash onset, to reduce pain and severity. Seek specialist advice if pregnant, immunocompromised or ophthalmic involvement. **Varicella-zoster vaccine** (eg Zostavax®) helps protect against herpes zoster and is given to those aged 70 and 79 (UK). **Immune globulin** can be used postexposure. *Complications:* Post-herpetic neuralgia; meningitis; encephalitis.

Fig 8.34 Common wart.
OUP.

Fig 8.35 Herpes simplex.
From Soames and Southam, *Oral Pathology*, 4th ed, 2005, with permission from OUP.

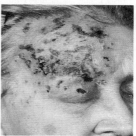

Fig 8.36 Ophthalmic zoster (shingles).

Dermatology

The 5 pillars of acne 1 Basal keratinocyte proliferation in pilosebaceous follicles (androgen- and corticotropin-releasing hormone driven), 2 ↑sebum production, 3 *Propionibacterium acnes* colonization, 4 inflammation, 5 comedones (white- & black-head) blocking secretions, hence papules, nodules, cysts, and scars (face, neck, upper torso). It is almost universal in teenagers: it causes much angst (nature picks the fairest skin at its vainest moment for her fiercest pustules). Most with acne don't have ↑androgens but their sebaceous glands are more sensitive to androgens.

℞ Be holistic; subtle doctors use acne consultations to promote mental health by giving patients a vocabulary to describe their misery, and so to control it. Dispel myths: it is NOT due to dirt, lack of washing, etc. & not infectious/contagious. Diet has little or no effect on acne. Ask about mood, effect on body-image/self-esteem & fears of social rejection. Suicidal ideation is a red flag.

Mild acne Mainly facial comedones. ℞: Topical **benzoyl peroxide** eg 2.5%, 5%, or 10% (start with a low strength), or **topical retinoid** (avoid in pregnancy) eg isotretinoin, or topical antibiotic alone (eg Dalacin T®). If poorly tolerated, try **azelaic acid** (15% gel). Treatment takes up to 8 weeks to be effective. If response is poor, consider a topical antibiotic combined with benzoyl peroxide or topical retinoid (eg Duac®; Isotrexin®).

Moderate acne Inflammatory lesions (papules and pustules) dominate, affecting face ± torso. ℞:• Topical antibiotic combined with benzoyl peroxide or topical retinoid (reduces bacterial resistance; for max 12wks). • Oral antibiotic—**tetracycline, oxytetracycline, doxycycline,** or **lymecycline** are first-line (**erythromycin** if pregnant or <12yrs old). Use for ≥4-6 months *with* topical **benzoyl peroxide** (start at 2.5% to avoid irritation). Do not use topical antibiotics at the same time. • A topical retinoid with benzoyl peroxide (Epiduo® gel) is an alternative; or if treatment has failed, a COCP with antiandrogen activity eg co-cyprindiol (eg Dianette®).[17,18]

Severe acne There are nodules, cysts, scars, and inflammatory papules and pustules. Refer to a specialist. ℞: Isotretinoin may be the best option (↓sebum production & pituitary hormones; specialist prescribing in UK). Marked benefit occurs in virtually all patients (permanent ~65%). SE: teratogenic (contraception must be used during + for 1 month after); skin & mucosal dryness; depression.

Rosacea

Rosacea is a chronic relapsing/remitting disorder of blood vessels and pilosebaceous units in central facial areas typically in fair-skinned people. *Prevalence:* 10%. *Pre-rosacea features:* Flushing triggered by stress/blushing, alcohol & spices. *Signs:* A central facial rash (usually symmetrical) with erythema, teleangiectasia, papules & pustules (without comedones), inflammatory nodules ± facial lymphoedema; blepharitis/conjunctivitis (ocular rosacea). In men, rhinophyma (swelling + soft tissue overgrowth of the nose) may occur. *Cause:* Unknown. ℞:[19] Use soap substitutes. Avoid sun overexposure & use sun-block.

• *Mild disease:* Topical **metronidazole** gel (0.75%) or cream (1%) ×2/day for 3–4 months or topical 15% **azelaic acid** gel (may cause transient stinging).

• *Moderate or severe disease:* An oral tetracycline (or erythromycin if contraindicated) taken for 4 months help control extensive papules or pustules but has little effect on redness. Low-dose **doxycycline** (40mg ×1/day) is also licensed and effective. **Isotretinoin** (above) and **lasers** are rarely needed.

• *Ocular rosacea:* Eyelid hygeine, ocular lubricants ± ciclosporin 0.5%.

Further reading

American Academy of Dermatology (2007). Guidelines of care for acne vulgaris management. *J Am Acad Dermatol* 56:651-63.

NICE (2014). *Clinical Knowledge Summary: Acne Vulgaris.* http://cks.nice.org.uk/acne-vulgaris

Dermatology

Cutaneous drug reactions are common, so...know the main culprits & how to treat.

- *Morbilliform* (=measles-like) or *exanthematous:* (fig 8.37) The commonest drug reaction, presenting with generalized erythematous macules and papules eg on the trunk ± mild fever, within 1–3wks of drug exposure. No mucosal involvement. *Drugs:* Amoxicillin (especially if the patient has glandular fever); cephalosporins, anti-epileptics, sulphonamides, allopurinol, captopril, thiazides. *ΔΔ:* Measles, scarlet fever, viral exanthema.

- *Urticaria: Signs:* Itchy erythematous wheals that move around appear rapidly after drug exposure ± angio-oedema/anaphylaxis. IgE mediated. *Drugs:* Penicillins and cephalosporins, opiates, NSAIDs, ACEi, thiazides, phenytoin. *R:* antihistamine ± IV hydrocortisone/IM adrenaline if anaphylaxis. (see p603).

⇢ *Erythroderma (exfoliative dermatitis): Signs:* Widespread erythema and dermatitis affecting ≥90% body surface. *Causative drugs:* Sulfonamides, allopurinol, carbamazepine, gold. Discuss management with a dermatologist.

⇢ *Stevens-Johnson syndrome (SJS):* Vague upper respiratory tract symptoms occur 2–3 weeks after starting a drug and ~2 days before a rash that affects <10% body surface. *Signs:* Painful erythematous macules evolving to form target lesions. Severe mucosal ulceration of ≥2 surfaces eg conjunctivae, oral cavity, labia, urethra. *Drugs:* Sulfonamides, anti-epileptics, penicillins, NSAIDs. *R:* See TEN.

⇢ *Toxic epidermal necrolysis (TEN):* Flu-like symptoms may precede skin involvement which affects >30% body surface. *Signs:* Widespread painful dusky erythema, then necrosis of large sheets of epidermis. Mucosae severely affected (fig 8.38). Mortality: ~30%. *Drug causes:* Sulfonamides, anti-epileptics, penicillins and cephalosporins, allopurinol, NSAIDs. *R:* Essentially supportive. Manage in ICU, HDU or burns unit. IV Ig is recommended (unproven). Avoid systemic or topical steroids (↑ risk of infection). Relieve pain; protect skin (do not debride).

- *Lichenoid:* Similar to lichen planus. Itchy flat topped purple–red papules. *Drugs:* β-blockers, thiazides, gold, antimalarials. *R:* Potent topical steroids.

- *Fixed drug eruption:* Lesions recur in the same area each time a particular drug is taken. *Drugs:* Paracetamol, tetracyclines, sulfonamides, aspirin.

Management principles A clear history of the onset and duration of the rash is essential. Record *all* drugs taken. Stop the likely offender. Drug withdrawal is not diagnostic—urticarial reactions settle in a few days; morbilliform in 7–10 days; most others last >8 weeks. Document the signs and symptoms including mucosal/systemic involvement. Assess the likelihood of this being a serious reaction and consider if it is likely to evolve. Give regular emollients for dryness or itch. Potent topical steroids reduce itch in widespread morbilliform, eczematous or lichenoid reactions. More severe eruptions are best managed by specialists. Rechallenge with the suspected drug is generally inadvisable.

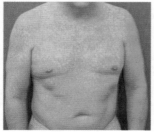

Fig 8.37 Morbilliform rash.
© DermNet NZ.

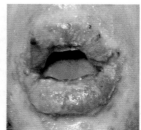

Fig 8.38 TEN/Stevens-Johnson syndrome.
© Dr Susannah Baron.

Dermatology

Lichen planus Lesions (eg on flexor aspects of wrists, forearms, ankles, and legs) are purple, pruritic, poly-angular, planar(flat-topped) papules, seen at any age + white lacy markings (known as Wickham's striae). Lesions elsewhere: scalp (scarring alopecia), nails (longitudinal ridges), tongue, mouth (lacy white areas on inner cheeks), and genitals. Lesions often arise at sites of trauma. Usually persists for 6-18 months. ℞: Topical steroids (± topical antifungals) are 1st-line (esp. in oral disease, eg fluticasone spray).

Strawberry naevae occur in neonates as a rapidly enlarging red spot. Most go by the age of 5-7yrs. No treatment is required unless a vital function is impaired, eg obscuring vision, impairing suck, or airway compromise.

Pyogenic granuloma (fig 8.39) is a vascular lesion thought to arise as a result of minor trauma, typically occurring on fingers. It appears as a fleshy moist red lesion which grows rapidly and often bleeds easily. ΔΔ: ▶Amelanotic malignant melanoma. *Treatment:* Curettage.

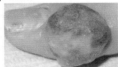

Fig 8.39 Pyogenic granuloma.
Courtesy of Dr Jonathan Bowling.

Pityriasis rosea A common, self-limiting rash which often may have a viral cause. The rash is preceded by a *herald patch* (oval red scaly patch, similar to, but larger than later lesions). It affects the neck, trunk (distributed in a 'christmas tree' pattern), and proximal limbs. There is no treatment. It will resolve in 2-12wks.

Alopecia Hair loss is *non-scarring* or *scarring*. Non-scarring causes may be reversible, but scarring alopecia implies irreversible loss.
• *Non-scarring alopecia: Alopecia areata:* Smooth well-defined round patches of hair loss on scalp; hairs like exclamation marks (short & tapering) are a typical feature; spontaneous regrowth occurs within 3 months in 80%. Total scalp hair loss = *alopecia totalis;* total body hair loss = *alopecia universalis.* ℞: Difficult. Consider topical or intralesional steroids. Psychological support. *Telogen effluvium* is shedding of telogen phase hairs after a period of stress, eg childbirth, surgery, severe illness. Other causes: nutritional (↓Fe or Zn); *androgeneic* (♀ & ♂ pattern) ℞: minoxidil.
• *Scarring alopecia:* Inflammatory disease damages follicular stem cells (eg lichen planus; discoid lupus); or follicles are damaged by trauma or tumour (BCC, SCC).

Blistering disorders *Causes:* Infection (eg herpes); insect bites; friction/trauma; eczema; drugs (ACEi; furosemide); immunobullous (dermatitis herpetiformis, pemphigoid, pemphigus). *Bullous pemphigoid:* The chief autoimmune blistering disorder in the elderly—due to IgG autoantibodies to basement membrane. *Signs:* Tense blisters (1-3cm in size) on inflamed or normal skin. *Skin biopsy:* +ve immunofluorescence (linear IgG and C3 along the basement membrane). ℞: Very potent topical steroids eg clobetasol (applied to lesions); prednisolone 0.3-1.0mg/kg/day PO (+bone & gastric protection; ↓dose gradually after 4 weeks if no new blisters). Blisters heal without scarring but the disease runs a relapsing-remitting course over 5-10yrs. *Pemphigus:* Affects younger people (<40yrs). It is due to IgG autoantibodies against desmosomal components (desmoglein 1 & 3), which leads to acantholysis (keratinocytes separate from each other). *Signs:* Flaccid superficial blisters which rupture easily to leave widespread erosions. The oral mucosa is often affected early. *Skin biopsy:* +ve immunofluorescence (intercellular IgG giving a crazy-paving effect). ℞: prednisolone (40-60mg/day PO, with gradual tapering). Rituximab and IV immunoglobulin in resistant cases.

Further reading

Harman KE *et al.* (2003). Guidelines for the management of pemphigus vulgaris. *Br J Dermatol* 149:926-37.

Venning VA et al. (2012). British Association of Dermatologists' guidelines for the management of bullous pemphigoid 2012. *Br J Dermatol* 167:1200-14.

Dermatology

Photosensitivity

Photosensitivity denotes conditions triggered by light. Rashes affect sun-exposed areas eg face, 'V' of neck, dorsum of hands and arms. They may be *primary* (rare, eg cutaneous porphyrias, xeroderma pigmentosum) or *acquired:*

Drug-induced photosensitivity Often due to phototoxicity (causing an exagerated sunburn response ± blisters), or photoallergy (delayed hypersensitivity reaction). Drugs may also cause pseudoporphyria or lichenoid reactions. Frequent offenders: thiazides; tetracyclines/sulfonamides; tricyclics; phenothiazines; NSAIDs; amiodarone.

Photoaggravated skin disease Cutaneous features of a disease are more severe on sun exposure eg rosacea, autoimmune blistering diseases, SLE.

Phytophotodermatitis Reactions from contact with light-sensitizing chemicals in plants (eg psolarens) cause linear erythema and blistering.

Polymorphic light eruption A common idiopathic disorder typically affecting young women in spring. After light exposure, itchy red papules, vesicles, and plaques develop on exposed sites, fading after 1–6 days. It often improves over the summer due to a phenomenon called 'hardening'. ℞: Sun-avoidance; sun-protection (high factor UVA + UVB sunscreen). Acute attack: potent topical steroids ± prednisolone 15–20mg/d for 3 days (eg to control if on holiday). Desensitization using UVB phototherapy or PUVA therapy (in severe cases).

Porphyria cutanea tarda (The commonest porphyria.) Reduced enzyme activity of uroporphyrinogen decarboxylase results in overproduction of photoactive porphyrins. Presentation is subacute and relationship to sun exposure is easily missed. *Causes:* Triggers eg HIV; hepatitis C; alcohol; OCP/HRT; ↑iron levels initiate disease in those genetically susceptible. *Signs:* Vesicles/bullae in sun-exposed sites, hypertrichosis, hyperpigmentation, skin fragility, and scarring (milia). *Tests:* faecal & urinary porphyrins; skin biopsy. ℞: Remove precipitants; sun-avoidance/protection; regular venesection; low-dose chloroquine.

Skin sensitivity to ultraviolet (UV) light (Fitzpatrick classification)		
Skin type	Do you burn or tan?	Those affected
I	Always burns, never tans	White/pale skin (freckles, blond/red hair)
II	Burns easily, tans poorly	Pale skin (blond hair, blue eyes)
III	May burn, tans lightly	Darker white skin (dark hair; brown eyes)
IV	Burns minimally, tans easily	Olive skin eg Mediterranean
V	Rarely burns, always tans	Asian, Middle Eastern, Latin American
VI	Never burns, tans darkly	Black African

Reproduced with permission from Fitzpatrick Thomas B, Ultraviolet-Induced Pigmentary Changes: Benefits and Hazards, in Hönigsmann H, Stingl G (eds): *Therapeutic Photomedicine*, Copyright © 1986 Karger Publishers, Basel, Switzerland.

Urticaria

Ordinary urticaria *Acute:* Smooth erythematous itchy hives and wheals are precipitated by eg infections and parasites (helminths); chemicals (insect bites, latex, drugs or food); or systemic disease. Skin prick or blood RAST tests (p596) may help. *Chronic:* Idiopathic in most, and lasts months–years (continuous or episodic). ~30% have histamine-releasing autoantibodies.

Physical urticaria is induced reproducibly by an external trigger, eg *dermographism* (a wheal develops on rubbing/stroking the skin); *cold contact* (occurs on exposure to cold air/water); *delayed pressure* (sustained pressue causes wheals after a delay of 30min–6h); *solar urticaria* (occurs on exposure of skin to UV). ℞: Antihistamine (several may need to be tried as response varies).

Urticarial vasculitis Cutaneous lesions resemble urticaria (tender wheals), and small-vessel cutaneous vasculitis (palpable purpura). If complement levels are low, it may be associated with SLE. ℞: Antihistamine, NSAIDs, but some patients may need immunosuppressive therapy.

Dermatology

Venous leg ulcers (fig 8.41) *Risk factors:* Varicose veins, DVT, venous insufficiency, poor calf muscle function, arterio-venous fistulae, obesity, leg fracture. Venous hypertension from damaged valves of the deep venous system causes superficial varicosities and skin changes (lipodermatosclerosis, fig 8.42). Minimal trauma, typically over the medial malleolus, causes ulcers.

Typical causes of ulcers
• Neuropathy
• Vascular: venous 75%; arterial 10%; mixed 15%
• Trauma

Rarer causes
• Pyoderma gangrenosum (eg with Crohn's; UC)
• Sickle-cell disease
• Vasculitis (eg SLE)
• Cryoglobulinaemia
• Malignancy
• Infection eg Leishmaniasis
• Drugs eg nicorandil

Management:[22] Graded compression bandaging promotes healing: Pressure reduces from the ankle (40mmHg) to the calf (15–20mmHg). This reduces superficial venous pressure. Do Dopplers first to exclude arterial disease (ensure the ankle-brachial pressure index is >0.8). Ulcers heal more quickly with occlusive dressings which absorb exudate and improve comfort. Infection should be treated with systemic antibiotics until definitive sensitivities are available (swab only if signs of infection). Avoid topical antibiotics as they ↑ the risk of resistance and contact dermatitis. Ensure adequate analgesia. **Pentoxifylline 400mg TDS PO** for up to 6 months should be considered to promote healing (unlicensed and not commonly used). Ulcers which don't heal on adequate treatment for 3 months must be investigated further (eg biopsy for malignancy). Once an ulcer is healed, patients should follow advice aimed at preventing recurrence: wearing compression stockings, skin care, leg elevation, calf exercises, and good nutrition.

Pressure ulcers

Pressure ulcers Result from uninterrupted pressure on the skin, leads to ulcers and extensive, painful, subcutaneous destruction, eg on the sacrum, heel, or greater trochanter[23,24] Shearing forces (from sliding down the bed); friction (when a patient is dragged across a bedsheet); and moisture (eg from incontinence) are implicating factors. *Risk factors:* Extremes of age, reduced mobility and sensation, vascular disease, and chronic or terminal illness make this more likely, particularly if nursing is poor. A full-thickness sacral sore causes much misery and extends hospital stay by *months*. ►This should make prevention a central preoccupation.

Staging	*Stage*	*I:* Non-blanching erythema over intact skin
	Stage	*II:* Partial thickness skin loss, eg shallow crater
	Stage	*III:* Full thickness skin loss, extending into fat
	Stage	*IV:* Destruction of muscle, bone, or tendons

Prevalence: ~3–14% of inpatients have pressure sores; most are over 70yrs. The prevalence in nursing homes is similar. 1/5th of pressure ulcers develop at home. Those with spinal injury are significantly at risk: 20–30% have a pressure ulcer within 1-5yrs of injury. *Complication:* Osteomyelitis.

Treatment: • Pressure-relieving mattresses and cusions • Frequent repositioning (turning charts help) • Optimize nutrition (get specialist help) • Treat systemic infection with antibiotics • Use modern dressings (eg hydrogels, hydrocolloids, films) to create an optimum environment to aid wound healing • Debride dead or necrotic tissue • Topical negative pressure treatment.

Prevention: Most pressure ulcers are avoidable. Initial and ongoing assessment of risk is vital, along with regular inspection of the skin + minimizing excess moisture. Proper positioning and regular turning (eg every 2h, alternating between supine, and right or left lateral position). Use pillows to separate the knees and ankles, and lifting devices to move patients.

Pruritus in the elderly

Pruritus is a common complaint in the elderly:
- *Skin causes:* Eczema (including *asteatotic eczema,* below); scabies (appearance can similar be in the elderly); *pemphigoid/pre-pemphigoid eruptions; asteatotic eczema; generalized xerosis.*
- *Medical causes:* Anaemia; polycythaemia; lymphoma; solid neoplasms; *hepatic* and *renal failure; hypo-* and *hyperthyroidism; diabetes (candidiasis).* Excluded by blood tests.

Asteatotic eczema (eczema craquelé)

Commoner in the elderly, this particularly affects the lower legs with a dry eczema that polygonally fissures into a crazy-paving pattern (fig 8.40). Emollients and soap substitutes help + moderately potent steroid (eg eumovate) for affected itchy inflamed areas. Rare (paraneoplastic) association is lymphoma (suspect if the eczema is difficult to treat).

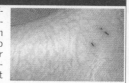

Fig 8.40 Eczema craquelé.
© Dr S Baron.

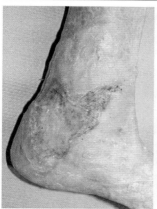

Fig 8.41 Venous leg ulcer (with eczema). Is there healthy granulation tissue on the ulcer floor? Remove all that over-ripe camembert pus to find out. Pain is frequent in these patients (who are often obese, so compounding immobility).

© Dr S Baron.

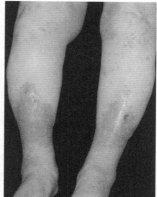

Fig 8.42 Varicose eczema with hyperpigmentation and lipodermatosclerosis (inflammation of layer of fat under the dermis and an ill-defined band resembling an inverted champagne bottle causing leg tapering down towards the ankle).

© Dr J Bowling.

Further reading

Grey GJ (2006). Pressure ulcers. *BMJ* 332:472.

NICE (2005). *Pressure Ulcers: The Management of Pressure Ulcers in Primary and Secondary Care* (cg29). London: NICE.

SIGN (2010). *Guideline 120: Management of Chronic Venous Leg Ulcers.* Edinburgh: SIGN.

Skin disease is a burdensome stigma for HIV patients.[25] Skin problems are markers of HIV progression, so understanding them is vital. Highly active antiretroviral therapy has helped HIV-related skin disease become less common, but it may trigger inflammatory reactions (immune reconstitution inflammatory syndrome; IRIS)—see below.

Acute seroconversion occurs 1-3 weeks after exposure; 70% experience symptoms. Features include an acute mononucleosis-type illness, usually accompanied by a non-specific maculopapular eruption affecting the upper trunk, associated with lymphadenopathy, malaise, headache, and fever. There may be oral or genital ulcers or candidiasis.

Infections There is increased risk from common pathogens and commensal organisms that don't normally cause disease. Signs may be florid and atypical.
- *Herpes virus:* See BOX.
- *Epstein–Barr virus:* Implicated in causing oral hairy leukoplakia (fig **8.43**).
- *Warts:* Widespread on oral mucosa, face, perianal region, + genital tract.
- *Molluscum contagiosum:* Widespread and atypical eg unusual sites; face, genitals. ℞: (difficult): cryotherapy, topical **retinoids**, cautery, or curettage.
- *Candidiasis:* May be severe, disseminated, and treatment-resistant, involving the oropharynx, vagina and skin. ℞: Topical **nystatin**; systemic **imidazoles**.
- *Tinea:* Generalized dermatophytosis/tinea capitis is common.
- *Syphilis:* Multiple ulcers (primary); rapid progression to tertiary disease.
- *Cryptococcosis:* Looks like facial molluscum contagiosum. ℞: **Fluconazole**.
- *Demodicosis:* Inflamed pruritic papular eruptions on face and upper trunk caused by *Demodex* (mite) folliculitis.
- *Scabies:* Severe variants, eg crusted are more common in advanced HIV disease. Paradoxically, patients may not complain of severe itch. A widespread scaly, crusted eruption occurs (highly infectious p608). ℞: **Permethrin** lotion.

Inflammatory disorders
- *Seborrhoeic dermatitis:* Widespread inflammatory red scaly patches on hairy areas and naso-labial folds & flexures. ℞: **Ketoconazole** cream.
- *Acquired ichthyosis:* (scaly skin) and *keratoderma* (thickened palm/soles).
- *Psoriasis:* HIV may lead to psoriasis, or cause pre-existing disease to worsen. Treating HIV will often improve response to standard therapy (p594).
- *Eosinophilic folliculitis:* The cause of this intensely itchy papulopustular eruption of sterile pustules is unknown Δ: Biopsy. ℞: 0.1% **tacrolimus**, topical **steroids**, UVB therapy, PUVA therapy.
- *Drug reactions* are common in HIV especially co-trimoxazole's maculopapular eruptions or erythema multiforme; toxic epidermal necrolysis, p601.
- *Pruritic papular eruption (PPE):* Common; small symmetrical red or skin-coloured itchy papules. Cause unknown. 80% have advanced immunosuppression.

HIV & nail changes Onychomycosis (eg *Trichophyton rubrum*; multiple fungi are often cultured in a single patient); nail pigmentation; Beau's lines. **HIV & hair** Diffuse alopecia or alopecia areata is associated with HIV.

HIV & skin neoplasia Kaposi's sarcoma (BOX), BCC, SCC, melanoma, skin lymphomas, Merkel cell cancer (a rare, aggressive neuroendocrine skin malignancy).

IRIS *(Immune reconstitution inflammatory syndrome):* With antiretrovirals, immunity begins to recover, but then responds to previously acquired opportunistic infection with a powerful inflammatory response, paradoxically worsening symptoms, often involving the skin. You may confuse this with serious HIV progression.

Lipodystrophy Subcutaneous fat is lost from the face and limbs (+ deposited on the trunk), as an effect of treatment with protease inhibitors.

Herpes simplex This can be increasingly troublesome as HIV progresses. Painful chronic ulcers and erosions develop, eg around mouth and genitals. *R:* High-dose **aciclovir** (oral or IV).

Varicella zoster This may occur with atypical signs (eg ≥1 dermatome; folliculitis; verrucous lesions). Ulceration and post-herpetic neuralgia may be more frequent and severe. In advanced disease, disseminated infection occurs. *R:* High-dose **aciclovir** (IV if systemic disease).

Kaposi's sarcoma (KS) An abnormally vascularized spindle cell tumour derived from capillary endothelial cells. Cause: HHV-8 (herpes hominis virus). It presents as purple papules or plaques on the skin and mucosa of any organ (fig 8.44). It metastasizes to nodes. 4 types: classic KS (typically on legs); endemic (African) KS; KS in immunosuppression (eg organ transplant recipients); and AIDS-related KS, often multi-organ (skin is not always involved). Incidence is falling thanks to HAART. *R: (if HIV +ve)* optimize HAART; **radiotherapy** can palliate symptomatic disease (esp. if unable to tolerate chemotherapy). Local treatment: intralesional chemotherapy, cryo, laser, photodynamic treatment, and excision. Systemic **interferon alfa** or chemotherapy (eg pegylated-liposomal **anthracyclines & paclitaxel**).

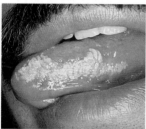

Fig 8.43 Oral hairy leukoplakia (adherent white plaques) is thought to be caused by Epstein-Barr virus. 'Corrugated' would be a better term than 'hairy' as there are no hairs. Associations: HIV (esp. if CD4 <200/mm³); immunosuppressives; lamotrigine.

© Prof D. Rosenstein

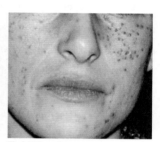

Fig 8.44 Kaposi's sarcoma.

© Dr S Baron.

Further reading

Schwartz RA *et al.* (2013). *Cutaneous Manifestations of HIV.* Medscape. http://emedicine.medscape.com/article/1133746-overview

Scabies (*Sarcoptes scabei*; fig **8.45**) A highly contagious, common disorder particularly affecting children and young adults. *Spread:* Direct person to person, eg by holding hands, sharing a bed. The ♀ mite digs a burrow (pathognomonic sign—a short, wavy, grey or red line on the skin surface) and lays eggs which hatch as larvae. The itch and subsequent red rash is probably due to allergic sensitivity to the mite or its products. *Signs:* It presents as very itchy papules, vesicles, pustules, and nodules affecting finger-webs (esp. first), wrist flexures, axillae, abdomen (esp. around umbilicus and waistband area), buttocks, and groins (itchy red penile or scrotal papules are virtually diagnostic). In young infants, palms and soles are characteristically involved. The eruption is usually excoriated and becomes eczematized. Mites can sometimes be extracted from burrows and visualized microscopically; eggs can be seen in skin scrapings. Crusted or Norwegian scabies is the same mite, but seen in the elderly or immunocompromised who harbour ~2 million mites, and are highly contagious.

Management: Treat all members of the household and all close contacts at the same time, even if asymptomatic. A good explanation (verbal + written) will aid concordance and promote the chances of successful cure. **Permethrin** 5% dermal cream is probably the most effective topical agent. It is also the drug of choice for pregnant women. **Malathion** is a good second choice (but not if pregnant or <6 months old). Oral **ivermectin** is recommended for severe scabies (200mcg/kg stat, repeated after 7–14 days). The rash and symptom of itch will take a few weeks to settle, occasionally longer. A suitable anti-pruritic such as **crotamiton** cream (eg Eurax®) (which also has anti-scabetic activity) can be useful during this period. *Example of advice to give for treating scabies:*
- Take a warm bath and soap the skin all over.
- Scrub the fingers and nails with a firm brush. Dry your body.
- Apply **permethrin** (or **malathion** 0.5% liquid) to *all* body parts from the neck down, including soles (+ scalp, face, and ears if <2yrs old, elderly, or immunosuppressed). Avoid the eyes! Save a small amount of cream and use this to reapply to any body part (eg hands) that is washed before the 24h is up.
- Wash off after 24h.
- Wash all sheets, towels, and clothing in a hot wash.
- Repeat treatment after 7 days.
- Treatment may worsen itch for 2 weeks—so use calamine lotion or crotamiton cream (eg Eurax®).

Headlice (*Pediculus capitis*; fig **8.46**) are common in children. Spread is only by head-to-head contact. Lice are 3mm long and have legs adapted to cling to hair shafts. Eggs (nits) are bound firmly to the scalp hairs and when empty appear white. *Signs:* Usually asymptomatic (presentation is upon seeing lice). Itch ± papular rash on the nape. *R̵:* All require 2 applications, 7 days apart. ●**Malathion 0.5%:** Apply to the hair from the roots to the tips. Leave lotion on overnight, then shampoo and rinse off. ●**Dimeticone 4%:** Leave lotion on overnight, then shampoo and rinse off. Resistance is a problem. ●**Isopropyl myristate and cyclomethicone:** Leave on hair for 10 minutes, then systematically comb using a fine-toothed comb to remove lice before washing with shampoo. (Not suitable if <2yrs old or in those with skin conditions.) *Combing* (see BOX). Only treat head-to-head contacts (over the past 5wks) if they have live lice (say to have a careful look).

Crab lice (*Phthiriasis pubis*) Often sexually transmitted and affect pubic hairs. Eyebrows, eyelashes, and axillae may also be involved. *Management:* Topical **malathion** 0.5% or **permethrin** to all affected areas. Wash off after 12h and repeat after 7 days. Screen for other sexually transmitted diseases.

Flea bites (*Pulicidae*) spread plague, typhus, and cat-scratch disease. The animal (eg cat or dog) which spreads the flea may not itch or scratch itself. Flea bites cause a papular urticaria in a sensitized individual. *Treatment:* De-flea pets; de-flea household carpets and soft-furnishings.

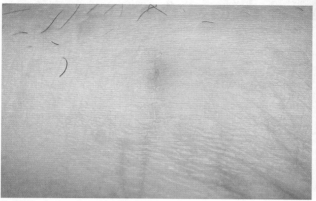

Fig 8.45 'Doctor, have I caught scabies?' 'Did you share bedding, clothing, or towels with anyone 4–6 weeks ago? Have you cuddled a pet? Or been to an institution? Is the itching worse at night?' Look for rows of irregular or s-shaped red furrows in web spaces, axillae, ventral skin on wrist or knee (also palms & soles in children). Here is a scabies burrow with a mite just visible (with the eye of faith) beyond the red area.

© Dr J Bowling.

Detection combing and combing treatment for head lice

Seeing lice[26] is hard; a special fine comb (prescribable, or bought at a chemist) can be used for detecting and treating lice. Here's what to do:

- Wash hair with ordinary shampoo, rinse, and apply lots of conditioner.
- Comb the hair with a normal comb to un-tangle it; then use the fine-toothed comb. Slot its teeth into the hair roots so they touch the scalp; draw it through to the hair tips.
- Ensure all hair is combed; check comb for lice after each stroke (use a magnifying glass). If lice are seen, clean comb by wiping it on a tissue, or rinse it before the next stroke. NB: nits (empty eggshells) don't mean live lice, as they can stick to hair even if lice have gone.
- After all hair is combed, rinse out conditioner.
- Treatment is only needed if ≥1 live lice are seen.
- *Wet combing treatment* involves the above steps with repeat combing at least 4 times every 4 days; only stop when no more lice have been seen for 12 days.
- For topical treatments—see p608.
- All affected people in the household need to be treated at the same time.

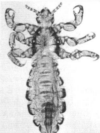

Fig 8.46 *Pediculus humanus.*
©Prof S. Upton, Kansas Univ.

Further reading

Knott L. (2013). *Head Lice*. Patient. http://patient.info/doctor/head-lice-pro

Dermatology

To construct a coherent identity, we must distinguish what belongs to the external, perceived world from what belongs to our inner world. The skin marks this boundary and can become the battle-field where different identities fight for dominance. A range of self-destructive skin phenomena exists, in which the primary problem is psychological:

Neurotic excoriations[27] Conscious compulsive picking, scratching, or gouging of the skin. It may be initiated by minor skin problems such as an insect bite or folliculitis, but it also occurs with previously normal skin. There is no known problem with the skin, so this is a physical manifestation of an emotional problem. Picking causes distress and there are often repeated attempts to stop. Lesions are usually similar in size and shape, and are grouped on easily accessible and exposed sites. Management is challenging.

Acne 'excoriée de la jeune fille' A form of neurotic excoriation, typically affecting young girls with mild acne who obsessionally pick at the skin causing scarred, infected lesions. The picking may continue long after the original acne has healed.

Trichotillomania Persistent and excessive hair-pulling resulting in noticeable hair loss, most frequently on the scalp, eyebrows, and eyelashes. It is common in children, who often deny hair-pulling. It is frequently precipitated or exacerbated by stress.

Dermatitis artefacta[28] is the deliberate and conscious production of self-inflicted skin lesions to satisfy an unconscious psychological or emotional need. Patients deny responsibility for the lesions and are resistant to the idea that they are important unconscious non-verbal messages (eg dealing with emotional deprivation), and as such are reluctant to accept psychiatric help.

Associations: Any chronic medical or skin condition, eg acne, alopecia, leg ulcer (which they may encourage); also psychosocial problems, eg emotionally unstable personality, see TABLE, p381; stress; unemployment; depression; anorexia nervosa (in 33%); chronic pain syndrome; sexual conflicts. There is overlap with Münchausen's and other pathomimicry, factious, or somatizing syndromes.

Epidemiology: ♀:♂≈6:1. In conscript armies, sex ratios may reverse (there is usually obvious secondary gain).

Signs: Variable (simply showing images can be very misleading). The morphology depends on how the lesions are induced but the outline is often different from the smooth outline of endogenous skin disease (eg irregular, jagged, linear geometric shapes). Look for unusual/inexplicable features. *Histology:* Non-specific, but may help establish a definite diagnosis.

ΔΔ: Always consider an alternative diagnosis eg pyoderma gangrenosum, contact dermatitis, photodermatitis, infection, or fixed drug eruption.

Treatment: Provide symptomatic care of skin lesions. Supportive care will only gain traction once issues surrounding emotional deprivation, isolation, insecurity, and other psychological states are addressed. Try to avoid confrontation—don't just prescribe antidepressants or antipsychotics and move on. Spend time with your patient and develop a therapeutic alliance. Include the family. Find a specialist (GP, dermatologist, or psychiatrist) who enjoys a holistic challenge of epic ectodermal proportions and who can roll skin and brain into a single unified management plan.

In this rare disorder,[29] patients have a fixed firm belief that they are infested with an insect or parasite which is causing pruritus. You will be shown excoriations and nodules, all caused by picking and scratching, that are produced by the 'insects'. Patients will often present pieces of skin, scale, or other debris (often contained in a matchbox) with the belief it is a carefully collected specimen of the parasite—and as proof of their affliction.

Primary skin lesions are not present and there is no true infestation or primary cause of pruritus. There is no obvious cognitive impairment. It typically occurs in white, middle-aged or older women.

Treatment is challenging. The patient believes there is a real and physical cause for a psychological problem. Try to encourage them to see a psychiatrist (this will be difficult). Olanzapine and risperidone are antipsychotics of choice. Do not use the delusion to encourage the patient to take medication 'in order to help kill the parasites'.

Morgellons disease is related to delusional parasitosis and affected individulas describe filaments or fibres growing from the skin that cause painful lesions (± biting or crawling sensations). Patients mistakenly believe they are infested with a parasite and present collected 'fibres' for examination and may pick at lesions with tweezers.

Dermatology

Further reading

Koo JYM (2013). *Dermatitis Artefacta*. Medscape. http://emedicine.medscape.com/article/1121933

Scheinfeld NS (2014). *Delusions of Parasitosis*. Medscape. http://emedicine.medscape.com/article/1121818

Scheinfeld NS (2015). *Excoriation Disorder*. Medscape. http://emedicine.medscape.com/article/112204

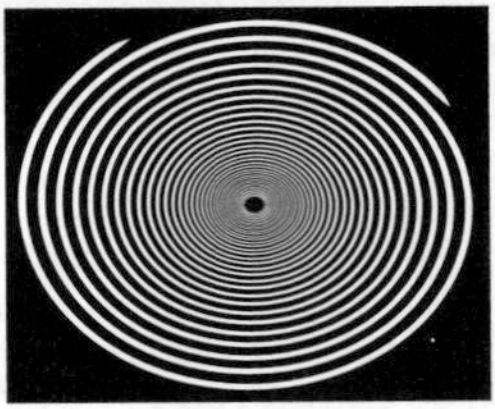

Fig 9.1 Reading this book the night before an exam, or staring at the centre of this spiral for long enough might just trick your mind into a hypnotic stupor, yet we suspect you would snap back to reality should a needle venture your way. The full triad of:
  Muscle relaxation
  Hypnosis and
  Analgesia
is required for effective anaesthesia to take place. Should one component be misplaced, situations such as awareness (p628), agitation and pain arise. Anaesthetists are masters at balancing and manipulating this triad to ensure the neccessary surgical procedure can take place; just attempting to understand the complex interactions can be hypnotic for any novice.

Other relevant pages Pain relief in labour (p66); resuscitation after delivery (p107); neonatal ITU (p108); ventilating neonates (p110); choosing the correct dose of lidocaine according to body weight (p773); **Online resources** www.frca.co.uk www.rcoa.ac.uk

Introduction

Anaesthesia evolved from humble origins in 1842 when CW Long gave ether, but he failed to report this landmark in pain relief. Then, in 1844, Horace Wells used nitrous oxide for tooth extraction, and in 1846 WTG Morton gave the first surgical anaesthetic with ether. It is now a highly sophisticated specialty in its own right. While the triad of anaesthesia (*hypnosis*, *analgesia*, and *muscle relaxation*) remains the fundamental principle behind general anaesthesia (GA) for surgery, the role of the anaesthetist has expanded to encompass not only the provision of ideal operating conditions for surgery, but also intensive care, resuscitation, alleviation of acute and chronic pain, obstetric anaesthesia, and anaesthesia for diagnostic procedures. A detailed knowledge of general medicine, physiology, pharmacology, the physical properties of gases, and the workings of the vast array of anaesthetic equipment are essential in order to practise well.

▶ We emphasize that this short chapter is no substitute for a specialist text or for experience on the ward and in theatre or clinic. The main aim is to enable understanding of the issues anaesthetists face, and to prepare one's mind for intelligent discussions on anaesthetic issues.

We thank Dr Melanie Osborne, our Specialist Reader, and Dillon Horth, our Junior Reader, for their help with this chapter.

►Ask about *allergy* to any drug, antiseptic, adhesive bandage, & latex. Remember to consider IV options for those patients nil by mouth. This is not an exhaustive list. Always check with local protocol.[1]

Which drugs can you take the morning of surgery?

• *ACE inhibitors:* No special action is required if BP & U&E are OK but many prefer to omit the morning dose due to the risk of perioperative hypotension. and kidney injury. ►Seek advice from the surgeon and anaesthetist.[2]

• *Antibiotics:* Aminoglycosides, colistin, and tetracycline prolong neuromuscular blockade, even *depolarizing* neuromuscular blockers.

• *Beta-blockers:* Continue; reduced risk of a labile cardiovascular response.

• *Digoxin:* Continue up to and *including* morning of surgery. Check for toxicity and check plasma K^+. Suxamethonium ↑serum K^+ by ~1mmol/L, and can lead to ventricular arrhythmias in the fully digitalized.

• *Statins:* Should be continued, especially in those at high risk of cardiovascular events but discontinue non-statin hypolipidaemic drugs.

• *Bronchodilators:* Continue and consider supplementing with nebulizers.

• *Proton pump inhibitors:* Should be continued.

• *Steroids:* If the patient is on or has recently taken steroids at an equivalent of >10mg prednisolone per day give extra cover for the perioperative period (p616). See *BNF* section 6.3.2 for steroid equivalence doses.

• *Anticonvulsants:* Give usual dose up to 1h before surgery. Give drugs IV (or by NGT) post-op, until able to take oral drugs.

• *Levodopa:* Possible arrhythmias when the patient is under GA.

Which drugs should you NOT take the morning of surgery?

• *Anticoagulants:* Know the indication. Check the INR, if needed switch warfarin to heparin preoperatively, leaving sufficient time for the INR to drop to <2 before surgery. Admit early, and discuss the plan of action so that all goes smoothly. Avoid epidural/spinal blocks. Beware of regional anaesthesia.

• *Aspirin* is controversial and dependent on indication and individual procedures, eg patients are given aspirin prior to percutaneous coronary intervention, but may be avoided in non-cardiac surgery due to bleeding risk.

• *Clopidogrel, prasugrel, & ticagrelor:* Stop 5–7 days before surgery.

• *Dual-antiplatelet therapy (DAPT) (often aspirin & clopidogrel/ticagrelor)* in patients already on DAPT for coronary stents, all elective non-cardiac surgery should be postponed until the minimal recommended duration of DAPT (typically 1 year) to minimize risk of stent thrombosis. ►It is a controversial area so involve the interventional cardiologist (needed if stent thrombosis occurs), surgeon, and anaesthetist if urgent non-cardiac surgery is needed. If possible, defer surgery for at least 6 weeks after bare metal stents and 6 months after drug-eluting stents.[1]

• *NSAIDs* should be discontinued due to renal and anti-platelet effects.

• *Diuretics:* Beware hypokalaemia and hypovolaemia. Check U&E.

• *Insulin:* Continue long-acting (basal) insulin, even when on a sliding scale. See *OHCM* p590 for diabetic patients undergoing surgery. Omit oral hypoglycaemics on the morning of surgery.

Which drugs should you consider ceasing earlier?

• *Contraceptive pill & HRT:* Stop 4 weeks before major surgery, restarting at 2wks post-op if mobile. Use heparin thromboprophylaxis + stockings.

• *SSRIs:* Stop 3 weeks prior to certain high-risk CNS procedures due to increased bleeding risk but in the majority of patients can be continued.

• *Ophthalmic drugs:* Anticholinesterases used to treat glaucoma may cause sensitivity to, and prolong duration of, drugs metabolized by cholinesterases, eg suxamethonium. Beta-blocker eye drops may cause systemic symptoms of bronchospasm/hypotension. Stop alpha-blockers as they can cause floppy iris syndrome making cataract surgery challenging.

Anaesthesia

Preoperative care aims to ensure that patients •Get the right surgery •Are happy and pain free •Are as fit as possible (see the ASA score on p615) •Have individualized decisions on type of anaesthesia/analgesia taking into account risks, benefits, and wishes. *It is the anaesthetist's duty to assess suitability for anaesthesia.* It requires an appreciation of the patient's wishes and desires, and pre-morbid state. It requires an understanding of the proposed surgery and the particular anaesthetic techniques to suit both the patient and surgeon. See p626 for attempting to predict a difficult airway. Assess neck movement and ability to open mouth. **The preoperative visit** Have the symptoms, signs, or patient's wishes changed? If so, inform the surgeon. Assess cardiovascular and respiratory systems, exercise tolerance, existing illnesses, drug therapy, & allergies. **Assess past history**—see MINIBOX.

Family history Ask about malignant hyperthermia (p628; dystrophia myotonica (*OHCM* p514); porphyria; previous problems with muscle relaxants; sickle-cell disease (test if needed). Does the patient have any specific worries?

Assess need for thromboprophylaxis—see p722 and also NICE guidelines.NICE

Past history screen
• MI or IHD
• Asthma/COPD
• Hypertension
• Rheumatic fever
• Epilepsy
• Liver/renal disease
• Dental problems
• Neck problems
• GI reflux or vomiting
• Past anaesthesia/ problems (eg intubation difficulty/PONV)
• Recent GA?

The *ward doctor* assists with a good history and examination, but should not be responsible for consent[1] (*OHCM* p570), though can discuss postoperative complications—both general (*OHCM* p578) and specific (*OHCM* p582). **Tests** Be guided by age, history, examination, proposed surgery, finding the safe balance between too many investigations and too few. Be guided by NICE, which grades the surgery, from grade 1 (eg abscess drainage) to grade 4 (complex+) and beyond: cardiovascular and neurosurgery.NICE NB: tests may not be needed for young fit adults having day surgery.

• *FBC* and *U&E*—see MINIBOX for when to check.
• *Group & save* for all major surgery; *crossmatch* according to local guidelines. Consider using autotransfusion devices.
• *LFTs* in jaundice, malignancy, or alcohol abuse.
• *Blood glucose* in diabetic patients (*OHCM* p576).
• *Clotting studies* in liver disease, DIC, massive blood loss, already on warfarin or heparin.

Check U&Es if:
• On diuretics
• Diabetes
• Burns victim
• Major trauma
• Hepatic/renal disease
• Intestinal obstruction/ ileus
• Parenteral nutrition

• *Virology:* HIV, HBsAg Hep C and Hep B.
• *Sickle-cell test* in those from Africa, West Indies, or Mediterranean area—and others whose origins are in malarial areas (including most of India). Take consent before performing the test, and offer genetic counselling.
• *Thyroid function tests* in those with thyroid disease.
• Pulmonary function tests ± arterial blood gas for ASA grades 3–4.
• *CXR & ECG:* If known cardiorespiratory disease, pathology or symptoms.
• *Lateral c-spine x-ray:* Consider in rheumatoid arthritis/anklyosing spondylitis/Down's syndrome to check for atlanto-axial instability.

►Be alert to risk factors (see BOX on p615). Communicate your concerns to the anaesthetist. Other issues:

• Perioperative antibiotics (*OHCM* p572)
• Frozen section (tell pathology)
• Bowel prep (*OHCM* p572)
• Post-op physio.

1 The consenting doctor must be capable of performing the procedure or have been specially trained in taking consent. Use only words the patient understands. Ensure he believes your facts and can retain pros and cons long enough to inform his decision. Make sure his choice is free from pressure from others. A patient may complain if: •He is unaware of what will happen •He has not been offered all options •He was sedated at the time of consent •He changed his mind •He was not told a treatment was experimental •A 2nd opinion has been denied •Details of prognosis were glossed over.

Risk factors associated with perioperative morbidity

- *Age:* The risk of dying doubles every 7 years from the age of 10. Such that the mortality risk at 90 is 5000× greater than the risk at age 10.
- *Sex:* Men are 1.7× more likely to die than women of the same age.
- *Socioeconomic status:* The impoverished are 2× as likely to die as the rich.
- *Functional status* is a reflection of the health of the patient at the time of surgery. NB: in most (but not all) studies ASA correlates with morbidity.[6]

ASA score	ASA = American Society of Anesthesiologists
1	Normally healthy
2	Mild systemic disease, but with no limitation of activity
3	Severe systemic disease that limits activity; not incapacitating
4	Incapacitating systemic disease which poses a threat to life
5	Moribund. Not expected to survive 24h even with operation
6	Brain-dead patient whose organs are being removed for donor purposes

- *Aerobic fitness:* A patient's functional capacity can be measured in metabolic equivalents (METs), where 1 MET equals the resting oxygen consumption of a 40-yr-old 70kg male. Ask the patient if they can walk indoors or 100m on level ground (2–3 METs), or climb 2 flights of stairs (4 METs) or participate in strenuous sport (eg singles tennis ~10 METs). When functional capacity is high, the prognosis is excellent, even in the presence of other risk factors. A functional capacity of < 4 METs has been associated with poorer outcomes in thoracic surgery, although it has less predictive power with non-cardiac surgery.[6] In the pre-assessment clinic aerobic fitness can be assessed by a shuttle walk, or cardio-pulmonary exercise testing (CPEX).
- *Diagnosed myocardial infarction (MI), heart failure, stroke, kidney failure* (creatinine >150μmol/L), *peripheral arterial disease:* Multiply long-term mortality risk by 1.5. Angina (without MI) and transient ischaemic attacks increase risk to a lesser degree.
- *Other:* Ask about COPD/asthma, diabetes, hypertension, and hypercholesterolaemia as these may contribute to perioperative risk. ▶Post-op chest infections are ×6 more likely in smokers. (see p719 for smoking risk).

Pre-op fasting Assoc. of Anaesthetists of Great Britain & Ireland 2010 [5]

Pulmonary aspiration of even 30mL of gastric contents is associated with significant mortality and morbidity; minimize this risk by aiming for an empty stomach. For elective surgery, if there is no GI co-morbidity, allow clear fluids (inc. black tea, coffee or pre-op drinks, see p630) ≥2h pre-op; all other intake (ie food/solids) up to 6h beforehand. In emergency surgery, restrict all oral intake to ≥6h pre-op. Involve the anaesthetist in any decisions if the situation is unclear. Children undergoing elective surgery are allowed formula/cows' milk/solids upto 6h pre-op; breast milk up to 4h pre-op; and clear fluids up to 2h pre-op. Chewing gum may be allowed up to 2h pre-op.

Patient safety: the WHO Surgical Safety Checklist

The WHO published their surgical checklist in 2008 and worldwide implementation has been associated with a reduction of postoperative complications and mortality.[7] It contains 19 questions which every team member is asked and must respond to: • Identity • Procedure • Consent • Equipment check • Site marked • Allergies? • Aspiration risk? • Anticipated blood loss >500mL (7mL/kg if a child)? • Have team members introduced themselves by name & role? (this includes students!) • Any patient-specific concerns? • Post-op: have equipment failures been addressed? • Have surgeon & anaesthetist liaised over recovery? *Full checklist:* www.who.int/patientsafety/safesurgery

Further reading

NICE (2003). *Routine Preoperative Tests for Elective Surgery* (CG3). London: NICE.

Historically most patients would have received some sort of preoperative anxiolytic to contribute to a smooth induction of anaesthesia by decreasing secretions (more important when ether was used), promoting amnesia and analgesia, and decreasing vagal reflexes (see MINIBOX). However, through increased use of day surgery, newer short-acting agents of induction, and enhanced recovery programmes (see p630) the use of routine premedication is no longer clinically advocated. It is really only those patients with special requirements (such as a patient with autism) or particular phobias that would require anxiolytics. These patients should be identified in the pre-op assessment. Careful planning can help to minimize concerns on the day.

Premedication: 7As
• Analgesia
• Anxiolysis
• Amnesia
• Antacid
• Anti-emesis (see BOX)
• Antibiotics
• Anti-autonomic

Anxiolysis The most common agents used are benzodiazepines. *Examples for the 70kg man:* Diazepam 5mg PO or temazepam 10–30mg PO. *Timing:* ~2h pre-op for oral drugs but this is difficult to plan on a busy surgical ward.

Children: will normally not require any anxiolytics. Topical anaesthetic creams are frequently used: Tetracaine 4% (Ametop®; apply 45min before inserting IVI) is more popular than EMLA®, as it does not vasoconstrict. *The presence of a parent and play therapist at induction is more powerful than any pre-medication*[8] and relaxing music may be as effective as anxiolytics in reducing anxiety.[9] If required though, use oral **midazolam syrup** (0.5mg/kg) in children as first choice, sometimes it is mixed with **ketamine**.[10]

Specific premedications *Analgesia:* Theoretically, pre-emptive analgesia in elective patients dampens the pain pathways *before* the signals start to arrive, thus modulating longer-term pain response. Large studies are lacking though.[11] **Gabapentin** can be given prior to knee/hip operations to reduce analgesic consumption after surgery (unlicensed use).[12] *Antacids:* For reflux either **ranitidine** 150mg PO or **omeprazole** 40mg PO/IV the night before and then 2h pre-op can be given—ranitidine reduces both gastric pH and volume. Emergency caesareans: see p78. *Antibiotic prophylaxis:* See OHCM p572. *Beta-blockers* can be used to reduce the risk of perioperative ischaemia. *Broncho-dilators:* eg salbutamol nebulizer. *Steroids: Minor operations:* eg 25–50mg **hydrocortisone** IV at induction. *Major operations:* 50mg hydrocortisone IV at induction, then repeat 3 times (8-hourly before restarting oral); ditto if adrenal insufficiency or adrenal surgery, or steroid therapy within last 3 months with over 10mg of prednisolone per day.

Day surgery is becoming more common, accounting for approximately 70% of all surgery performed in the UK.[13] The leading reason for surgery to be cancelled is lack of hospital bed availablity; delivering selected operations as day-cases is advantageous to both the hospital (see p764) but also to the patient who gets to sleep in their own bed, eat their own food, and mobilize freely. Avoidance of a stressful preoperative night has helped mitigate the need for preoperative anxiolytics in the majority of patients. The most common reasons for admission after day surgery include post operative nausea and vomiting (PONV; p631), uncontrolled pain, and lack of social care at home.

Common reasons for cancellation
• Insufficient ITU/ward beds, staff, theatre, time or other logistical problems.
• Current respiratory tract infection or exacerbation of other medical illness.
• Patient not in optimum condition, eg poor control of drug therapy (insulin for diabetic patients, digoxin, thyroxine, phenytoin).
• Recent myocardial infarction (eg within last 3 months).[14]
• U&E imbalance (particularly K⁺); anaemia.
• Inadequate preparation (results not available, not crossmatched/fasted).

Anaesthesia

Definition Sedation is a range of depressed conscious levels from relief of anxiety (minimal sedation) to general anaesthesia (see BOX).

Doctors in many specialties may be required to administer sedation. ►*The doctor giving moderate or deeper sedation must not also be responsible for performing any procedure* (such as manipulation of a dislocated joint). Her sole responsibility is to ensure that the sedation is adequate, and to monitor the patient's airway, breathing, and circulation. Sedation is not a shortcut to avoid formal anaesthesia, and it does not excuse the patient from an appropriate work-up or reasonable fasting (►risking aspiration of gastric contents, p624). Monitoring is mandatory, and must include at least pulse oximetry, HR, and BP.[15] It is easy for sedation to become general anaesthesia, with its attendant risks (see p628). The loss of the 'eyelash reflex' (gentle stroking of the upper eyelashes to produce blinking) is a good guide to the onset of general anaesthesia. ►Remember the need for oxygen and equipment to support ventilation as well as appropriate monitoring when undertaking any form of sedation.

Agents

• *Midazolam:* Initial adult dose 2mg IV over 1min (1mg if elderly). Further 0.5–1mg IV as needed after 2min. Usual range 3.5–7.5mg (elderly max 3.5mg). *SE:* psychomotor function↓.[16]

• *Propofol:* Widely used for sedation, see p620. Rapid acting anaesthetic—but may lead to hypotension and apnoea. In many circumstances (eg manipulation of large joint; painful dressing changes) a *narcotic analgesic* may be used too (eg morphine in 1–2mg aliquots IV, or shorter-acting opioids such as fentanyl) as propofol doesn't have analgesic properties.

• *Ketamine* may be used. This is a dissociative anaesthetic agent which can be used as an induction agent (p621), or for procedural sedation (p812). It produces deep analgesia with superficial sleep without loss of airway reflexes or hypotension.

Level of sedation

Minimal sedation (anxiolysis) is a drug-induced state where the patient is still able to respond to speech. Cognitive function and coordination are impaired but airway, breathing, and cardiovascular systems are unaffected.

Moderate sedation (conscious sedation) is drug-induced reduction of consciousness during which the patient is able to make a purposeful response to voice or *light touch*. Response to pain only indicates deeper sedation. At this level of sedation no airway adjuncts are required, breathing and cardiovascular function should be adequate.

Deep sedation is drug-induced reduction in consciousness to a point where the patient cannot be easily roused but does respond *purposefully* to painful stimuli (withdrawal is *not* purposeful). At this level airway intervention may be required (jaw thrust/ chin lift). Spontaneous ventilation may become inadequate.

General anaesthesia is drug-induced loss of consciousness during which patients are not able to be roused, even with repeated painful stimulation. Airway typically requires intervention, spontaneous ventilation is frequently inadequate and cardiovascular function may be impaired.

(Based on American Society of Anesthesiologists Guidelines, 2009)[15]

►*Typically procedural sedation of patients outside of the operating theatre or ICU for is confined to ASA 1 or 2 category patients (see p615).*

Further reading

British Association of Day Surgery: www.daysurgeryuk.net

Maurice-Szamburski A *et al.* (2015). Experience of sedative premedication on patient experience after general anaesthesia: a randomised clinical trial. *JAMA* 313(9):916–25.

Anaesthesia

Meticulously check all equipment before anaesthetic or sedative procedures.
• Check anaesthetic machine (*plugged in* and *on*).
• Tilting bed or trolley (in case of vomiting).
• High-volume suction with rigid Yankauer/long suction catheters.
• Reliable oxygen supply, capable of delivering 15L/min.
• Self-inflating bag with oxygen reservoir, non-rebreathing valve, and compatible mask (a 'bag-valve-mask' system).
• Oropharyngeal, nasopharyngeal, and laryngeal mask airways.
• A range of anatomical facemask sizes.
• Anaesthetic circuit: make sure that there are no obstructions to the flow. Check the vaporizers, flowmeters, and ventilator.
• Laryngoscope with range of blade sizes, spare bulbs, and batteries.
• Tracheal tubes (range) and catheter mount.
• Intravenous infusion cannulae and fluids (warmed if necessary).
• Anaesthetic drugs (& gasses) resuscitation drugs (& defibrillator).
• Monitoring equipment (eg pulse oximeter ± end-tidal CO_2 monitor, p628). See Association of Anaesthetists of Great Britain & Ireland.[16,17]

Inhalational anaesthetic agents

These are volatile liquids which readily vaporize, permitting administration by inhalation in O_2-enriched air or an O_2/N_2O mix. They help maintain anaesthesia and decrease awareness (by an unclear mechanism). Inhalational agents differ in their levels of respiratory irritation, taste (pungency), odour, and speed of onset-offset. Reflect on the properties of the ideal inhalational agent (BOX p619) before attempting to understand agent choice.

Halothane (fig 9.2) No longer used in the UK—it has been replaced by safer inhalational agents (below), due to the rare but serious complication of postoperative hepatitis. It is still commonly used in developing countries as it is cheap and widely available. It is a colourless, pleasant-smelling gas with little analgesic effect.

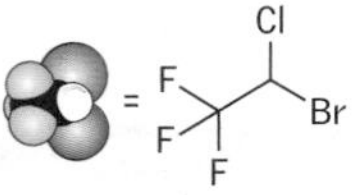

Fig 9.2 Halothane.

Sevoflurane (fig 9.3) is a halogenated ether which is well tolerated. It is the agent of choice for inhalation induction of general anaesthesia due to its combination of being low irritant, and having relatively fast onset–offset.

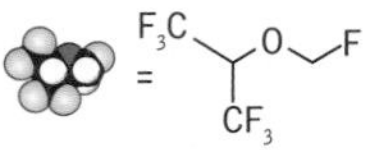

Fig 9.3 Sevoflurane.

Isoflurane (fig 9.4) A halogenated ether. Theoretically induction should be quick, but isoflurane is irritant, so coughing, laryngospasm, or breath-holding may complicate the onset of anaesthesia. Opioids can help reduce coughing.

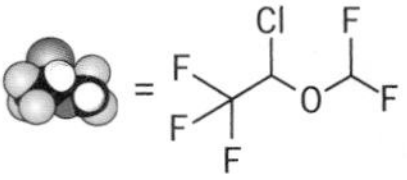

Fig 9.4 Isoflurane.

Desflurane (fig 9.5) is another halogenated ether with a rapid onset of anaesthesia, and quick recovery. It has a low absorption into fat so desflurane is often chosen for surgery in the morbidly obese as it provides for the quickest recovery post surgery.[16] However, it is more of a respiratory irritant than sevoflurane,

Fig 9.5 Desflurane.

so is sometimes only used for maintenance rather than induction of anaesthesia. It may also have greater depressant effects of the cardiovascular system than sevoflurane. All inhalational agents need to first be vapourized, desflurane has a much higher boiling point and thus needs a more specialized vapouriser.

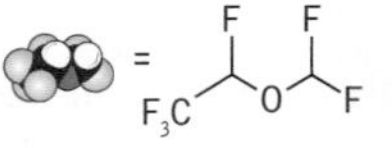

Stopping inhalation reverses all the above effects (except for hepatitis resulting from drug metabolism). ►►All can cause malignant hyperthermia (p628).

Commonly used iv anaesthetic agents

Propofol (2,6-diisopropylphenol; $t_{1/2}$=30–600min)[2] This lipophilic phenol derivative is in an emulsion in soybean oil and has become the most commonly used iv anaesthetic agent in the developed world. Its good recovery characteristics and anti-emetic effect make it popular, especially in day-case surgery.[17] It is fast-acting and its offset of action is due to rapid redistribution, and not metabolism.

- *Dose examples:* Induction = 2-3mg/kg ivi (at least) at 2–4mg/sec. Maintenance = 4–12mg/kg/h ivi. NB: ▶Rapid injection can cause cardiovascular depression (↓BP), and respiratory depression can occur when combined with iv narcotics. For procedural sedation: 0.5–1mg/kg ivi over 1–5min. Dose needs

  ▶*Contraindications:*
  - Extremes of age
  - <17yr for sedation
  - Egg or soy allergy[18]
  - Compromised airway[2]

  to be reduced in the elderly, debilitated, and shocked. Dose also depends partly on premed use: with midazolam induction dose requirements for propofol are reduced by 20–50%. This effect may be more pronounced in the elderly.[19,20]
- *Uses:* It is used in induction and maintenance of GA, and for sedation during regional anaesthesia, short procedures, and as a sedative in ITU (though contraindicated in children for this last use). Once opened, use ampoules or discard, because of the risk of bacterial growth. See p625 for total intravenous anesthesia (TIVA).
- *Problems: Pain on injection* occurs in up to 40% of patients. This can be minimized by either adding a small amount of lidocaine (eg 2mL of 1%) to the propofol, or by pre-injection of local anaesthetic.[21]

Thiopental sodium is the other common iv agent (see p620) and has in recent years been replaced by propofol as the most popular induction agent.

The ideal (but imaginary) *iv* anaesthetic agent

The ideal iv agent would be stable in solution and in the presence of light, be water-soluble and have a long shelf-life. It would be painless when given iv; non-irritant if injected extravascularly (with a low incidence of thrombosis) with some pain (as a warning) if given intra-arterially. Furthermore:
- It should act rapidly within one arm–brain circulation
- Recovery should be quick and complete with no hangover effect
- It should provoke no excitatory phenomena
- Analgesic properties are advantageous
- Respiratory and cardiovascular effects should be minimal
- It should not interact with other anaesthetic agents
- There should be no hypersensitivity reactions
- There should be no post-op phenomena, eg nausea or hallucinations.

The ideal (but imaginary) *inhaled* anaesthetic agent

Inhaled agents have advantages (eg no iv access required, more precise control) and disadvantages (eg claustrophobic) over iv agents.[22] The ideal inhaled agent should:
- Have low solubility in blood and tissues (to allow rapid recovery)
- Be resistant to any degradation
- Have no injurious effects on vital tissues
- Be administrable in a reliable and known concentration.

The ideal (but imaginary) *muscle relaxant*

Neuromuscular blockers are either depolarizing or non-depolarizing:[23]
- Non-depolarizing mode of action
- Rapid onset, short duration of action with high potency
- Spontaneous predictable reversal
- No cardiovascular effects
- Pharmacologically inactive metabolites
- Unaffected by renal or hepatic failure.

2 The pharmacokinetics are best modelled by a three-compartment model.

Anaesthesia

Thiopental sodium (t½=11h) a barbiturate that is typically mixed with water to give a 2.5% solution (ie 25mg/mL). It has a rapid onset of action (arm–brain circulation time about 30sec). Effects last 3–8min, and awakening is due largely to redistribution, not metabolism. Some 30% of the injected dose is still present in the body after 24h, giving rise to a hangover effect.

- *Dose examples:* 100–150mg (less if elderly/debilitated) IV over 10–15sec (longer if elderly/debilitated), followed by further quantity if needed according to response after 30–60sec (or up to 4mg/kg; max 500mg).

- *Uses:* Induction of GA; it is also a potent anticonvulsant—used in status epilepticus management when other measures have failed (p208).

- *Problems:* Anaphylaxis is rare (1 in 20,000). Is a negative inotrope so can drop cardiac output by 20%. May also lead to bronchoconstriction.

▶*Intra-arterial injection* produces pain and blanching of the hand/limb below the level of injection due to arterial spasm, followed by ischaemic damage and gangrene—following inadvertent brachial artery puncture in the antecubital fossa. This is less of a problem now that an indwelling cannula is obligatory (compared with the historical use of a needle). Extravascular injection causes severe pain and local necrosis. ▶Get expert help. Infiltrate with hyaluronidase 1500IU dissolved in 1mL water through the cannula.

> ▶*Contraindications:*
> - Airway obstruction
> - Barbiturate allergy
> - Fixed cardiac output states
> - Hypovolaemia/↓BP
> - Porphyria
> - Compromised airway[3]

Etomidate (t½=3.5h) This is a carboxylated imidazole. *Dose:* 0.15–0.3mg/kg. *Uses:* Histamine release is not a feature, but rapidity of recovery and cardiovascular stability are. Use is mostly restricted to induction for acutely unwell patients with trauma/head injuries for whom avoidance of even a brief episode of hypotension is important. *Problems:* Be aware it can induce involuntary muscle movements and nausea. Etomidate can lead to lethal adrenal suppression which is why prolonged use is avoided. Local thrombophlebitis can occur after injection.

Ketamine (a phencyclidine derivative, produced as a racemic mixture; *N*-methyl-D-aspartate receptor antagonist; t½=2.2h) *Dose example:* 2mg/kg usually gives 5–10min of surgical anaesthesia (for long procedures—see *BNF*).

Uses: Mainly for paediatric anaesthesia and procedural sedation; it is especially useful in facilitating the positioning of patients for spinal anaesthesia in the setting of painful limb fractures such as a fractured neck of femur. (see p812 for pre-hospital procedural sedation). It can also be used as a premedication with midazolam in patients requiring anxioysis (p616). Cardiac output is unchanged or increased, and so it is a good 'on site' or 'in the field' agent, as it can be given IM, producing profound analgesia without compounding shock. Ketamine has potent bronchodilatory properties, so can be considered during intubation in status asthmaticus.[24]

Problems: Hypertonus and salivation, but there is some maintenance of laryngeal reflexes (but do not rely on this). Recovery is slow. Emergence phenomena are troublesome (delirium, hallucinations, nightmares; all made worse if the patient is disturbed during recovery). ▶Avoid in the hypertensive patient, those with a history of stroke or raised intracranial pressure (↑ ICP further), patients with a recent penetrating eye injury (risk of ↑ intra-ocular pressure), and psychiatric patients. Avoid adrenaline infiltrations. In the UK, the Home Office classifies it as a class C drug as it is prone to misuse ('Special-K').

---

3 A compromised airway is a relative contraindication to any IV induction, regardless of the agent used.

Autonomic learning...

The autonomic nervous system (ANS, fig 9.6) is primitive, but not simple. It responds sensitively to intraoperative stress and many of the drugs used in anaesthesia (eg atropine, β-blockers) have a further effect on this system.

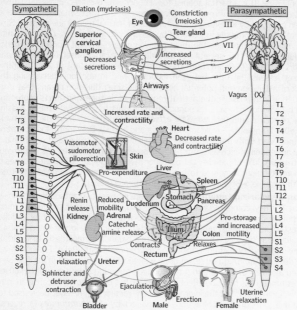

Fig 9.6 The autonomic nervous system.

Sympathetic

Site		Neurotransmitter	Receptor type
Pre-ganglionic	All	ACh	NAChR
	Adrenal gland[1]	ACh	NAChR
Post-ganglionic	Sweat glands	ACh[2]	MAChR[2]
	All other	NA	NAR

Parasympathetic

Site		Neurotransmitter	Receptor type
Pre-ganglionic	All	ACh	NAChR
Post-ganglionic	All	ACh	MAChR

Key: ACh = acetylcholine, NAChR = nicotinic acetylcholine receptor, MAChRs = muscarinic acetylcholine receptor; NA = noradrenaline; NAR = noradrenaline receptor
1 The sympathetic fibres that innervate the adrenal gland are pre-ganglionic
2 This is the main oddity: sweat glands have MAChRs in the sympathetic system
NB: there are a number of other (co-)transmitters in the autonomic system (such as ATP to adenosine receptors). The gut also has a large independent neuronal network.

Further reading

Pratt O et al. (2006). The Autonomic Nervous System: Basic Anatomy and Physiology. http://www.anaesthesiauk.com/article.aspx?articleid=100506# [Gives a detailed summary.]

Wood MJ et al. (2011). Drugs affecting the autonomic nervous system. Anaesth Intens Care Med 12:73–77.

These act on the post-synaptic receptors at the NMJ. There are two main types:

Depolarizing agents Suxamethonium (=succinylcholine) is the only one commonly used. It is a partial agonist for acetylcholine (ACh) receptors and causes initial fasciculation through depolarization of the post-synaptic membrane, then paralysis by inhibiting the restoration of normal membrane polarity. Suxamethonium is rapidly inactivated by plasma cholinesterases. *Dose:* 1–1.5mg/kg. *IV uses:* It has been the most popular paralytic agent in rapid sequence inductions (RSI) for several decades due to its rapid onset (30–60sec), and short duration (3–5min). Both these aspects are important in RSI. The rapid onset lessens the time between induction and intubation—decreasing the risk of aspiration and potential hypoxia. The short duration means that if intubation is impossible, the patient regains muscle tone, and starts protecting their own airway again. Its popularity may start to wane with the increasing use of rocuronium (below). *Side effects:* ↑K⁺ (enough to raise the plasma K⁺ by ~0.5–1.0mmol/L—avoid in paraplegia and burns!). Beware that K⁺ liberation is increased with multiple sclerosis, Guillain–Barré, stroke, and crush injury. Suxamethonium increases intra-ocular pressure (eg increases risk of vitreous extrusion). 30% of patients get postoperative muscle pains. Repeated doses of suxamethonium may lead to bradycardia—more common in children—treat with atropine. ▶Beware suxamethonium apnoea (p628).

Non-depolarizing agents These drugs are competitive antagonists of ACh—that is, they compete with ACh at the NMJ—but without producing initial depolarization (so no fasiculations). Their action can be reversed by anticholinesterases (eg neostigmine) which lead to an increase in the amount of ACh available at the NMJ. They are used during balanced anaesthesia to facilitate IPPV and surgery. Examples include: *Rocuronium:* Lasts 20min. Typically given at dose of 0.6mg/kg (ideal body weight p621)—although in RSI has been used at doses of 0.9–1.2mg/kg to produce intubating conditions within 60sec. Rocuronium has few side effects—although has been known to cause anaphylaxis. Excretion is via the liver. Historically, rocuronium has not been used for RSI due to its duration of action. The availability of *sugammadex* (a reversal agent for rocuronium) is allowing this to change. At doses of 16mg/kg (given 3–5min post rocuronium) sugammadex is able to reverse rocuronium faster than the time taken for suxamethonium to wear off.[25] Given its lower side effect profile, RSI with rocuronium could be considered an attractive alternative to RSI with suxamethonium. *Vecuronium:* Lasting 30–40min, it is used if cardiovascular stability is important. *Adult dose:* 0.1mg/kg IV then 20–30mcg/kg IV as needed. Sugammadex also reverses vecuronium. *Atracurium:* lasts ~25min. Metabolism is by *Hoffman elimination* (spontaneous molecular breakdown), so it is the drug of choice in renal and liver failure. *Dose:* 0.5mg/kg IBW IV then 100–200mcg/kg IBW IV as needed.

Other non-depolarizing agents include cisatracurium and mivacurium.

Note on neuromuscular blockers in those with myasthenia In general, these patients are resistant to suxamethonium and very sensitive to non-depolarizing relaxants (action may be prolonged: lower doses may be needed). Warn patients that mechanical ventilation may be needed post-op. Liaise closely with a senior anaesthetist. A small dose of atracurium is most commonly used. ▶ Any patient with neuromuscular disease should be considered at risk when neuromuscular blockers are used and post-op care should be delivered in a high dependency unit (HDU).

Further reading
Raghavendra T (2002). Neuromuscular blocking drugs: discovery and development. *J R Soc Med* 95(7):363–7.

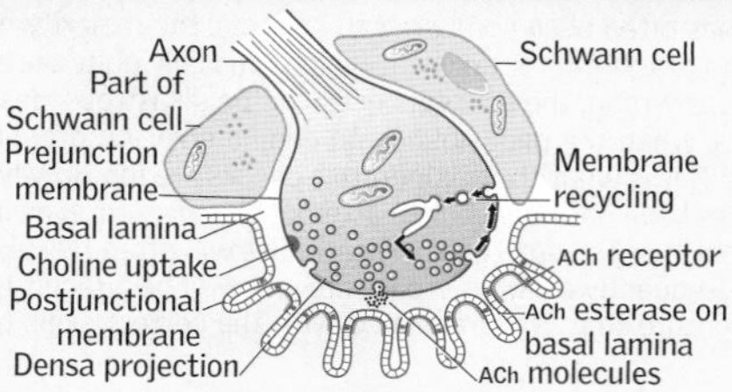

Fig 9.7 Procession at the synapse: with the arrival of an action potential at the nerve terminal comes the release of acetylcholine (ACh) by exocytosis of vesicles at the presynaptic membrane. ACh then diffuses across the synaptic cleft (~75nm wide)

Actions of ACh within the synaptic cleft (fig 9.7):
1 Hydrolysis by acetylcholinesterase (AChE) to choline and acetate.
2 Diffusion into circulation (then broken down by pseudocholinesterase).
3 Binding to post-synaptic nicotinic ACh receptors (NAChRs).
4 It is the last of these that continues the signal procession at the post-synaptic membrane by opening an ionophore channel linked to the receptor, allowing the influx of Na^+ cations. Membrane depolarization ensues, creating an endplate potential that results in muscle contraction. Hydrolysis of ACh whilst bound to the receptor causes termination of the endplate potential, bringing the trigger to contraction to an end.

Although there is a degree of receptor redundancy in the system for safety, the skeletal neuromuscular junction is nonetheless a site where lethal paralysis can take place. But agents that meddle here are not all bad.

Mayhem...
• *Curare:* Eg tubocurarine, reversible NAChR blocker; poison used in South America extracted from plants and used to tip darts for hunting.
• *α-Neurotoxins:* Eg α-bungarotoxin, irreversible NAChR blockers found in snake venom; multiple research uses; eg immunostaining techniques.
• *Organophosphates: Eg sarin* irreversibly inhibit AChE, causing prolonged binding of ACh at the post-synaptic membrane & depolarization. see p804.

...mischief...
• *Nicotine:* Mimics the effect of acetylcholine at the receptor.
• *Myasthenia gravis:* Autoimmune depletion of NAChRs on the post-synaptic membrane (*OHCM* p516).
• *Eaton–Lambert syndrome:* Defective ACh release at the pre-synaptic membrane; paraneoplastic or autoimmune syndrome, with antibodies vs the pre-synaptic voltage-gated Ca^{2+} channels—*OHCM* p516.

...or medication?
• *Suxamethonium:* Depolarizing NAChR blocker (see OPPOSITE).
• *Vecuronium:* Non-depolarizing NAChR blocker (see OPPOSITE).
• *Neostigmine:* Anticholinesterase that prevents breakdown of ACh in the synaptic cleft, increasing the efficacy of ACh.
• *Edrophonium:* Another anticholinesterase, which was used diagnostically in myasthenia gravis (Tensilon® test); also used to reverse effects of non-depolarizing blockers, but worsens effect of depolarizing blockers.
• *Botulinum toxin:* Neurotoxin produced by Clostridium botulinum which blocks ACh release causing flaccid paralysis and respiratory failure (see p421 *OHCM*) *causes* **Mayhem**. *But* commercial production has become widespread as controlled injections can weaken skeletal muscle to relieve focal spasticity and associated disability. First used clinically in strabismus (p422), it is now part of mainstay treatment of blepharospasm, spasmodic torticollis, dystonias, cerebral palsy, multiple sclerosis, and severe hyperhidrosis. Botulinum toxin A (more common) & B are the two serotypes in use. Cosmetic surgery relies on serotype A.

Practising anaesthetics has often been compared to aviation: the majority of time is spent planning and practising for an event which is usually quite unremarkable. Yet when it goes wrong, the consequences can be disastrous. Just like in commercial flights, when the pilot notices an engine error on ground then the flight is delayed. This is what the preoperative checks are for. However in conflict, the air forces have no choice but to attempt the mission; even in the face of identified problems. The emergency theatre list will often feel like this. An anaethesist will frequently encounter patients who will be difficult to anaesthesize; you must ensure that you are armed with the correct skills to face any consequence.

►*Check equipment before even the shortest anaesthetic procedure*, see p618. Ensure that the appropriate monitoring is on before induction. Assess for a difficult airway (p626) and be familiar with rescue plans (p628).

Induction May be IV *or* inhalational, usually IV. *A trained & dedicated assistant must be present.*[26] *Intravenous:* •Establish IV access •Pre-oxygenate, and give co-induction agents (eg fentanyl/midazolam) •Give a sleep-inducing dose of, eg propofol. ►*Beware:* Stimulation before adequate anaesthesia can have drastic consequences (coughing, breath-holding, laryngospasm). Noise is a stimulus too. *Gaseous:* •*Either* start with sevoflurane in oxygen according to age and clinical state •*Or* give nitrous oxide: oxygen 60%:40% mixture with a volatile agent, eg sevoflurane •Establish IV access as soon as asleep.

Indications for gaseous induction
• At the patient's request •Difficult IV access •Children •Some patients with partial airway obstruction (actual or potential, eg foreign body, tumour, or abscess), though awake fibre-optic intubation is often used (see p626).

Airway control It is essential to confirm that ventilation is possible before muscle relaxants are administered. Airway control is maintained by holding a mask onto the face held in jaw thrust, by inserting a laryngeal mask airway, or by intubation (p627). Ensure the patient is adequately anaesthetized (see box p625), as laryngoscopy and tracheal intubation can produce a harmful *adrenergic stress response* with adverse increases in pulse and BP (see p621). Concurrent short-acting opiates or esmolol IVI can attenuate this in a dose-dependent way.[27] Airway adjuncts (eg oropharyngeal or nasopharyngeal) *may produce vomiting or laryngospasm* at light levels of anaesthesia.

Intubation Passing an ET tube through the cords into the trachea protects the airway and facilitates reliable ventilation. (see p626 for the technique). Most commonly needed in:
• Risk of vomiting/aspiration (►►p629) of gastric contents: eg reflux oesophagitis, abdominal disease, major trauma, non-fasted, hiatus hernia, pregnant >15wks.
• Management of difficult airways. If difficulty is suspected, ensure senior help is available and consider fibre-optic or awake intubation.
• An inaccessible or shared airway (eg as in head and neck surgery).
• Conditions when paralysis facilitates surgery, eg abdominal surgery.

►*Paralysed patients cannot breathe—and so require ventilation.*

Muscle relaxation (paralysis with neuromuscular blocking agents) enables intubation—the norm is a short- or long-acting muscle relaxant, as appropriate: *Short-acting:* Suxamethonium, typically 1-1.5mg/kg IV. Use if risk of vomiting ↑ or when difficulty with intubation is anticipated. *Long-acting:* Many are available, eg rocuronium/vecuronium (see p622), but they take longer to provide suitable conditions for intubation. Rocuronium provides suitable intubating conditions in 60–90sec, but vecuronium may take >2min.

Further reading
Yuill G *et al.* (2002). An introduction to total intravenous anaesthesia. *BJA CEPD Rev* 2(1):24–6.

Options for maintaining anaesthesia

1 Volatile agent. Either spontaneously breathing or ventilation, with or without opiates. If the patient is ventilated, muscle relaxants are generally used.

2 IV infusion anaesthesia, eg propofol ± opiates. See following section on TIVA.

3 High-dose opiates with mechanical ventilation. ►NB: There is a considerable risk of awareness (p628) so it is only used in exceptional circumstances.

Total intravenous anaesthesia (TIVA) Historically, the maintenance of anaesthesia was provided by inhalational agents as perioperative monitoring of blood concentrations and adjusting to patient needs was easier. TIVA is a continuous infusion of (typically) propofol & remifentanil (an ultrashort-acting opioid) which is delivered through a pump which uses pharmacokinetic data to calculate an infusion rate to give a target concentration (blood or effect site) which is set by the anaethesist depending on surgery, stimulation, etc. It is especially useful for patients with a history of PONV (p631) or operations on the airway (eg tracheal stent) as there are no inhalational agents involved. TIVA is associated with a higher risk of awareness.[28]

Gauging depth of general anaesthesia

Whatever the technique, the dose and concentration of each drug is adjusted according to the level of anaesthesia achieved vs the desired level (determined by monitoring vital signs—eg HR, BP, signs of sympathetic stimulation). Lack of inappropriate levels of general anaesthesia in a patient should be suspected in the presence of:

• ↑HR[s] and/or ↑BP[s]
• Lacrimation[s]
• Dilated pupils[s]
• Movement or laryngospasm
• Note that many of these responses are mediated by autonomic sympathetic drive (=[s], see p621), and *all* should be picked up with appropriate and continual monitoring (p628).

Other measures Bispectral index (BIS) EEG monitoring can help assess the depth of GA—and can also reduce PONV and anaesthetic consumption, but not cost or time to discharge.[29] Evoked potentials (auditory and somatosensory) have also been used.[30]

►*No single method is reliably accurate, and these cannot replace the vigilance and clinical suspicion of the anaesthetist.*

Monitoring during anaesthesia [26] AAGBI

The continuous presence of the anaesthetist with a dedicated assistant is by far the most important monitor. Clinical monitoring supplemented by (not substituted by) a range of monitors of the patient and the anaesthetic delivery apparatus is mandatory. The process begins prior to induction of anaesthesia and continues throughout. ►*A warm, pink, and well-perfused patient is the aim.* Sweating and lacrimation invariably indicate something is wrong: *Respiration:* Rate, depth. *BP:* Intra-arterial in long/high-risk cases may be sighted after induction (also allows ABG analysis). *T°:* Particularly important in infants, as the large surface area to body mass may lead to hypothermia. A warm environment, warming blankets, and warm IV fluids, are important in long cases. *Pulse oximetry:* Computes HR and arterial O_2 saturation. *ECG:* Reveals rate, arrhythmias, and ischaemia. *CVP:* Helps differentiate hypovolaemia from ↓cardiac function. Insert when large blood loss is anticipated, or in unstable patients. *Capnography* is essential: a low end-tidal CO_2 warns of a displaced ET tube, emboli, and more. Inspired oxygen concentration and end-tidal volatile agent concentration should also be monitored. Also monitor urine output, neuromuscular status, and ventilator pressures. Alarms should be set to appropriate levels prior to the case.

Preparation is the key. Assess the neck pre-op.

Prediction of difficult intubation may be possible with assessment of the Mallampati classification (fig 9.8), thyromental and sternomental distances; these subjective predictive tests vary between users and should simply be employed as a guide.[31] Be prepared for a difficult airway even if the prediction has been for an easy intubation and vice versa.

Difficult intubation
• Obese
• Short neck
• Limited neck movement
• Receding chin/mandible
• Protruding teeth.
• Limited mouth opening

Anaesthesia

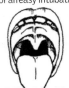   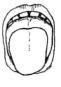

Fig 9.8 The Mallampati Test (with Samsoon and Young's modication). Examine the patient's oropharynx with the patient opening their mouth maximally and protruding their tongue without phonation. Class 1: Soft palate and uvula visible. Class 2: Uvula tip masked by base of tongue. Class 3: Only soft palate visible. Class 4: Soft palate not visible. When used alone it correctly predicts 50% of difficult laryngoscopies and has a false +ve rate of >90%.

Reproduced from Allman and Wilson, *Oxford Handbook of Anaesthesia*, 2011, with permission from OUP.

Technique Endotracheal tube (ETT) sizes: (mm internal diameter, ID):

> *Adult ID:* ♂ = 8.5mm, ♀ = 7.5mm *Children ID* = [age in years/4] + 4.0mm
> *Length for child: Oral* = [age /2] + 12.5cm. *Nasal* = [age/2] + 14.5cm

NB: Broselow tape-measures are said to be more accurate for children.
• Lubricate the tube, and check that its cuff and the laryngoscope work.
• Position the patient with neck flexed and head extended using a pillow.
• Hold the laryngoscope in the left hand; open the mouth with the right.
• Slide the blade down the right side of the tongue into the vallecula (area between tongue and epiglottis), guarding the lip and teeth with the fingers of your right hand. ▶*Do not lever on the teeth; you may damage them.*
• Lift the laryngoscope blade upwards and away from yourself.
• Lift the epiglottis from view: the cords should become visible. When they are, insert the tube with your right hand (anatomy—p567).
• Once the cuff of the ET tube is beyond the cords, remove the laryngoscope; ask the assistant to inflate the cuff to prevent air leak.
• Attach to the circuit. Gently inflate lungs. Watch the chest move. Do both sides move equally? Is the abdomen moving and not the chest?
• Auscultate both sides of the chest. Is air entry equal? Fix the tube with a tie.
• Confirm correct placement with capnography (detects CO_2, p628).

▶*Remember: if in doubt, take it out.* It is safer to re-intubate than to risk leaving a tube in the oesophagus. Tubes may slip down a main bronchus (usually right). If so, withdraw until both sides of the chest move equally and air entry is equal (so avoiding collapse in the unventilated lung, or pneumothorax on the overventilated side). If you are having problems intubating:

If difficult intubation is predicted use of video laryngoscope or awake fibre-optic laryngoscopy is recommended to guide ETT placement. Give mild sedation (see p616), an anti-cholinergic (to reduce secretions), and local anaesthesia to the nasal cavity & pharynx (not just for comfort, they will gag and cough too much without it; this distress could lead to loss of airway). Deep anaesthesia is only initiated once ET intubation confirmed (by vision and capnography).

If unable to intubate? see p628.

Indications Ventilators are used in anaesthesia when there is an operative need for muscle paralysis, or when muscle paralysis is part of a balanced GA for a long operation. (Ventilators are used in intensive care for ventilatory support in reversible acute respiratory failure—this is a different topic: see eg p110.) Familiarity with ventilators is best gained from direct observation of their use. If you are interested in finding out more, then pursue a placement in the intensive care unit. ►Mandatory alarms for ventilators include disconnect, high-pressure, and oxygen failure alarms.

Modes[4]

When the patient is paralysed and intubated, *intermittent positive pressure ventilation (IPPV)* is mostly used. These ventilators have controls to alter:

- Tidal volume—which provides precise control of volume and $PaCO_2$ (ie volume controlled)
- Pressure necessary to inflate the lungs (ie pressure controlled)—which reduces risk of barotrauma
- I:E ratio (I:E = the ratio of inspiratory to expiratory time)
- Respiratory rate
- Inspiratory time.

Other controls may be available to adjust:

- Inspiratory flow waveform
- End-tidal pause.

Overview of ventilator modes
• Pressure controlled
• Volume controlled

Controlled mandatory ventilation (CMV) is another form which controls the drive and rate of ventilation in the presence of paralysed spontaneous breathing, and is in practice the same as IPPV.

Some ventilators deliver *synchronized intermittent mandatory ventilation (SIMV)* which allows the patient to start breathing spontaneously when paralysis wears off, providing assistance if these breaths are inadequate. These are less common in theatre, and more often used in intensive care.

Whichever mode is used, *positive end-expiratory pressure (PEEP)* is often a useful adjunct. PEEP allows a pressure to be exerted at the end of expiration, which help splint open alveoli, increasing the surface area available for gas exchange, thereby reducing the amount of 'shunt'(areas of lung which are perfused but not ventilated). A typical PEEP value would be ~5cmH$_2$O. High levels of PEEP may lead to reduced venous return due to a rise in intrathoracic pressure.

Lung compliance
$$\text{Compliance} = \frac{\text{change in volume}}{\text{change in pressure}}$$
This is a useful concept in ventilation, as it relates to the behaviour of various parts of the respiratory tract. Poor compliance means only a small change in volume for a big change in pressure.

Laryngeal mask airway (LMA) is used in >50% of elective UK surgery, and in cardiac arrests where a skilled intubator is not present. It consists of a tube with a cuff; lubricate the cuff, and slide over the palate so the device sits over the larynx. A cuff takes ~30mL of air (depends on size, sizes range from 1.0 to 5.0). It is safe and effective. It is more efficient than masks. Advantages are that no laryngoscope is needed (no damage to teeth or cord stimulation), ease of insertion and it is safer for minor surgery as it does not require the same depth of paralysis and anaesthesia as endotracheal intubation. Specialized LMAs can assist with difficult intubation (eg an intubating laryngeal mask airway, ILMA), and may allow air/fluid to be aspirated from the stomach (eg Proseal®).

Further reading

Gupta S *et al.* (2005). Airway assessment: predictors of difficult airway. *Indian J Anaesth* 49(4):257–62.
Verma SP *et al.* (2013). Video laryngoscopy and fiberoptic assisted tracheal intubation. http://emedicine.medscape.com/article/110880-overview

4 High-frequency oscillatory ventilation (HFOV) is used in preterm infants and neonates (p110).

The most important cause of mortality and morbidity attributable to anaesthesia is associated inadequate airway management. Patients do not die from failure to intubate, they die from failure to ventilate. The majority of cases are due to unexpected difficulty or poor preparation for patients with predicted difficulty. ►Predicting barriers to rescue techniques (eg in obese patients it will be difficult to access the cricothyroid membrane) are just as important as planning for difficult intubation.[32] See p626 for difficult airways.

If unable to intubate? Prior to induction you must know the plan should intubation fail: PLAN A (eg tracheal tube); PLAN B (ILMA/LMA p627); PLAN C (bag-mask ventilation/wake patient if able); and PLAN D (needle/surgical crycothyroidectomy) before you start.[33] There are national failed intubation guidelines: www.das.uk.com Difficult Airway Society ►Adequate oxygenation is top priority: • Get senior help; *can't intubate, can't ventilate* is an emergency • Do not repeat the dose of suxamethonium: allow the relaxant to wear off whilst maintaining oxygenation. This scenario is vitally important and all junior anaesthesists must demonstrate that they can deal with this in a simulated setting before they are allowed to give anaesthetics without immediate senior supervision.

Atelectasis and pneumonia Atelectasis is best seen on CT (not CXR). Starts within minutes of induction, and is partly caused by using 100% O_2. ℞: Good pain relief aids coughing. Arrange physiotherapy + antibiotics (онсм p161).

Awareness This is most distressing for patients and can lead to post-traumatic stress disorder. The patient can become aware of events during the operation; ~½ recollect conversations between theatre staff, ~¼ feel the presence of the ETT, ~⅓ experience pain. *Incidence:* ~1:19,600 anaesthetics. It is more frequently reported in cardiac and obstetric surgery as they typically undergo lighter anaesthesia. Paralysis makes diagnosis difficult and relies on close monitoring (p625) for signs of physiological distress. Residual paralysis during emergence from anaesthesia can be perceived by patients are awareness.[34]

Bronchospasm If intubated, check tube position (carina stimulation may be the cause: withdraw tube slightly). Check for pneumothorax. Ventilate with 100% O_2. ↑ concentration of volatile agent if he is 'light'—most volatiles (esp. sevoflurane) are good bronchodilators. Salbutamol±aminophylline 250mg IV. $MgSO_4$ 2g IV may help. Give hydrocortisone 100mg IV. ►►**Anaphylaxis** See онсм p806.

►►**Laryngospasm** The cords are firmly shut. Treat with 100% oxygen. Deepen anaesthesia—attempt to ventilate. It may be necessary to paralyse and intubate.

►►**Malignant hyperthermia** Rare, autosomal dominant, life-threatening condition triggered by exposure to suxamethonium or volatile anaesthetics. Suspect when there is unexpected ↑oxygen consumption, hypercapnia, and tachycardia. Rapid temperature rise (>2°c/h) may be a late sign. *Treatment:* Hyperventilate with 100% O_2; maintain anaesthesia with IV agent; abandon surgery; muscle relaxant with *non-depolarizing muscle relaxant*. Give *dantrolene 2.5mg/kg IV* as initial bolus. Check for hyperkalaemia, arrhythmias; acidosis; myoglobinaemia; coagulopathy; raised creatinine kinase. Take to ICU.[35]

Damage to teeth occurs in around 1:4500 GA and is a risk even when the anaethesist uses the appropriate technique with care. Dental damage is the leading cause for litigation against anaethetists so ensure that your patient's dental hygiene is well documented in the preoperative assessment.[36] Give patient information leaflets: 'Damage to teeth, lips and tongue'. www.rcoa.ac.uk

Suxamethonium apnoea Rare. Abnormal cholinesterase leads to prolonged drug effect lasting 2–24h. Ventilate & sedate until relaxant effect wears off. Consider fresh frozen plasma (for plasma cholinesterase activity).[37]

Shivering Be aware that shivering increases O_2 consumption 5-fold. Not always due to hypothermia. Treatment options include tramadol, nefopam.[38]

Anaesthesia

Aspiration of foreign material into the respiratory tract can occur at any time around anaesthesia. It is unlikely to occur if a tracheal tube is *in situ*. It may occur with a LMA (p627). ►Aspiration is a much greater risk in emergency surgery, pregnancy, diabetes, and with a hiatus hernia, causing fatality in ~1 in 70,000 of all anaesthetics. It can be the result of passive regurgitation, or of active vomiting. If suspected (direct visualization at laryngoscopy, coughing, vomiting, laryngospasm, bronchospasm, $S_AO_2\downarrow$, tachypnoea, wheeze and crepitations on auscultation), then immediately do the following:

▸▸ Apply cricoid pressure (unless actively vomiting; risks oesophageal rupture).
▸▸ Use suction to clear the mouth of debris.
▸▸ Endotracheal intubatation, use soft catheters to suction the upper airway.
▸▸ Refrain from ventilating whilst undertaking these procedures, providing oxygenation levels are acceptable (to prevent dispersion of aspirate).
▸▸ Empty the stomach with an NGT at the first available opportunity.
▸▸ Put the patient head down and in the left lateral position.
▸▸ Cancel surgery, unless it is for an emergency.
▸▸ Consider ongoing ventilatory support to ensure adequate oxygenation.
▸▸ Arrange a CXR. Further investigation may be needed, eg bronchoscopy.

Rapid sequence induction (RSI) is the method of endotracheal intubation used in the emergency setting when the airway of an acutely unwell patient is threatened and the subsequent risk of aspiration is high. ►As patients are unlikely to be fasted it relies on prompt induction and paralysis in order to minimize risk of aspiration. If haemodynamically unstable, take the time to resuscitate your patient to optimize their ability to cope with anaesthesia.

• Pre-oxygenate with 100% O_2 for 3min to provide an O_2 reservoir in the lungs for use during the period of induced apnoea.

• *Apply cricoid pressure* (fig **9.9**) and give induction agent (eg propofol) then immediately give muscle relaxant (eg suxamethonium).[39] Wait 60sec for muscle relaxant to work (patients will often twitch before relaxing).

RSI: a quick overview
• NGT and IV access
• Pre-oxygenate
• IV induction
• Fast muscle relaxant
• Cricoid pressure
• ET intubation

• The trachea is then intubated and cuff inflated, cricoid pressure may be released, and a volatile agent added to maintain anaesthesia.

• Give a longer-acting muscle relaxant (ie non-depolarizing) when suxamethonium wears off.

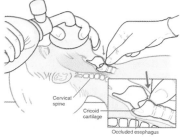

Fig 9.9 You may be asked to apply cricothyroid pressure during RSI. Apply firm backward pressure (aim for force of 10–30N) on the cricoid cartilage (used because it is a full ring of cartilage which can be pushed down) to occlude the oesophagus in an attempt to stop gastric reflux to the larynx. It is a skill to practise as poor placement of fingers will fail to occlude the oesophagus and pressure on the larynx may make intubation more difficult. Possible risks include disruption of cervical spine injuries and oesophageal injury. There is controversy over whether this pressure actually prevents aspiration.

Cervical spine
Cricoid cartilage
Occluded esophagus

Reproduced with permission of Goodman & Green Current Procedures Pediatrics ©McGraw Hill.

Further reading

Ellis DY *et al.* (2007). Cricoid pressure in emergency department rapid sequence tracheal intubations: a risk-benefit analysis. *Ann Emerg Med* 50(6):653–65.

Watch Keith Greenland's talk on 'Emergency Surgical Airway: Facts and Fiction': http://lifeinthefastlane.com/ccc/cant-intubate-cant-ventilate/

Anaesthesia

What to do at the end of anaesthesia

- Change inspired gasses to 100% O_2 then stop anaesthetic drug infusions.
- After ascertaining that some spontaneous reversal has occurred (use a peripheral nerve stimulator), reverse any residual muscle paralysis with neostigmine (~2.5mg in adults) + an anticholinergic to prevent muscarinic side effects (↓HR, salivation), eg atropine (1.2mg)/glycopyrronium (0.5mg).
- Once spontaneously breathing, inspect mouth and oropharynx under direct vision. Remove ET tube then administer oxygen by facemask for as much and for as long as necessary to counteract hypoxia due to diffusion hypoxia, respiratory depression, or ventilation/perfusion mismatch.[5]
- If no problems, transfer to recovery, but be ready to reassess at any time.

Recovery

- Look for hypoventilation (?inadequate reversal—check with nerve stimulator; narcosis—reverse opiates with naloxone—*cautiously* to minimize pain; check for airway obstruction). Ensure adequate analgesia.
- Monitor temperature, HR & BP; return the patient to the ward when you are satisfied with his cardiovascular and respiratory status and pain relief.
- Give clear instructions on postoperative fluid regimens, blood transfusions, oxygen therapy, pain relief, and physiotherapy.

Enhanced recovery programmes (ERPs) aim to improve the physiological disruption and psychological distress of surgery. Key principles include the preoperative optimization of medical co-morbidities, carbohydrate drinks 2h prior to surgery to avoid the metabolic state associated with fasting,[40] careful intraoperative fluid management with use of minimally invasive surgical techniques when appropriate. Postoperative care focuses on early mobilization and prompt return to normal nutrition; this includes vigorous treatment of pain. There should be clear discharge instructions with an aim to get the patient home early, if not on the same day. ERPs are effective in reducing length of hospital stays and complication rates in surgery.[41]

Patient-centred anaesthesia

♣ Anaesthetists must form brief but intimate relationship with their patients, often under difficult circumstances. As well as doing a good technical job, they need to be aware of subjective areas that are of particular importance to patients. In one study, ratings for information provision, involvement, and emotional support were rated significantly less important than physical comfort and respect. Ratings did not differ very much *vis à vis* inpatient vs day surgery, surgical service, type of anaesthetic, or anaesthetist.[42] NB: Comfort may centre around needle-less induction of anaesthesia and good perioperative care in non-frightening surroundings.[43] Avoiding nausea/vomiting (BOX, p631) is a top priority.[44] NB: information booklets can improve satisfaction.[45] Patient-centred anaesthesia cannot flourish in a vacuum: if the whole context of care is patient-centred the need for anaesthetic care itself may be less. Eg, in obstetrics where there is a one-to-one relationship between the midwife and the mother, the need for epidurals is ~50% less (and the 2nd stage of labour shorter) than with less personal methods.[46]

One way to improve patient-centred anaesthesia is to control distractions in the anaesthetic work place: time and motion studies show that it is relatively easy for anaesthetists to be distracted by extraneous interruptions.[47] Exactly how to limit this in busy NHS practice is a challenge.

Patients can be confused by an uncertain locus of responsibility. In some cultures (eg in Japan), chief responsibility for perioperative care lies with the surgeon. In other cultures, responsibility is shared—with confusing results unless the surgeon and the anaesthetist co-operate closely.[48]

---

5 For a short duration (<5min) while very soluble nitrous oxide is diffusing out of the circulation into the alveoli, the concentration of O_2 in alveolar gas will be falling (diffusion hypoxia).[49]

Postoperative nausea and vomiting (PONV)

PONV is one of the most unpleasant side effects imposed by anaesthesia. It is experienced by ~25% of patients (up to 80% if high-risk). [50] Control symptoms to optimize patient comfort and minimize post-op complications:

- PONV is the most common cause of delayed discharge after surgery
- Electrolyte imbalance and dehydration
- Pulmonary aspiration
- Wound dehiscence or bleeding
- Damage to site of surgery (direct, eg ENT, or indirect, eg neurosurgery)
- Inability to take oral medication.

The exact mechanisms of action for all the factors involved (see MINIBOX) are unknown, though the central mechanisms behind the vomiting reflex are somewhat better understood. It is initiated in the vomiting centre of the medulla (fig 9.10), which itself receives input from higher centres, the chemoreceptor trigger zone (CTZ), afferent somatic and visceral fibres, and the vestibular apparatus of the middle & inner ear. Of these, the CTZ in the *area postrema* (located in the floor of the 4th ventricle) is probably the most important.

PONV risk factors

- *Patient factors:*
  - Female (3× risk)
  - Previous history
  - Obesity
  - Motion sickness
  - Preoperative anxiety
- *Anaesthetic agents:*
  - Opioids
  - Nitrous oxide (N₂O)
  - Etomidate/ketamine
  - Volatile agents
- NB: total IV anaesthesia with propofol ↓PONV
- *Surgery type:*
  - GI/GU/Gynae
  - Neurosurgery
  - Middle ear
  - Ophthalmic
- *Post-op factors:*
  - Dehydration
  - Hypotension
  - Hypoxia
  - Early oral intake [51]

For specific anti-emetics see *OHCM* p241, and in this book on p617. Neurokinin 1 (NK₁) receptor antagonists, eg **aprepitant** (80mg PO, given 3h prior to anaesthesia), are a new class of antiemetics which appear more effective than 5-HT₃ antagonists (eg ondansetron). [52,53] Non-pharmacological approaches such as P6 acupuncture point stimulation are effective. [54]

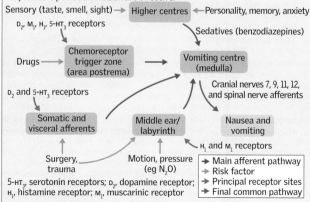

Fig 9.10 The neural pathways, receptor sites and triggers for PONV.

Reprinted from *Anaesthesia & Intensive Care Medicine*, Vol 7, issue 12 Barry Miller, Postoperative nausea and vomiting, 99, 453–55, ©(2006), with permission from Elsevier.

Further reading

Gan TJ *et al.* (2014). Consensus guidelines for the management of postoperative nausea and vomiting. Anesth Analg 118(1):85–113. (Erratum in *Anesth Analg* 2014; 118(3):689 and 2015; 120(2):494.)

PONV calculator: http://daysurgeryuk.net/en/resources/ponv-calculator/

Regional anaesthesia is broadly split into peripheral nerve blocks (PNBs) or neuraxial anaesthesia (see p634). The aim is to reduce nerve conduction of painful impulses to higher centres (via the thalamus), where the perception of pain occurs. It is used either alone or to supplement general anaesthesia (GA) by providing prolonged and effective postoperative analgesia. Regional anaesthesia is especially useful for operations on the lower limbs and abdomen where avoidance of a GA is desirable due to medical co-morbidities (notably cardiac & pulmonary). ►Regional techniques may still lead to loss of airway and so require the same resuscitation facilities as for a GA.

Continual regional anaesthesia involves placement of a catheter near the nerve to allow continuous delivery of LA, as compared to a *single dose* of LA.

Locating peripheral nerves requires sound knowledge of anatomical landmarks. Historically, nerves were located by direct nerve stimulation with the needle (invoking a sensory or motor response), but visualization with US or use of peripheral nerve stimulators is now common to minimize nerve trauma and maximize success rates. [55]

Types of local anaesthetic (LA) agents

1 **Lidocaine (lignocaine):** Max dose in healthy adult=3mg/kg IBW (see p733).
2 **Prilocaine** ($t_{1/2}$=2h): Moderate onset. Dose is 3–5mg/kg IBW. Max 400mg Low toxicity; the drug of choice for Bier's block (IV regional anaesthesia).
3 **Bupivacaine** ($t_{1/2}$=3h): Slow onset and prolonged duration. More cardiotoxic than others. Contraindicated in IV regional anaesthesia (Bier's block). Dose for local infiltration is 2mg/kg IBW to a max of 150mg.
4 **Levobupivacaine** (isomer of bupivacaine) is less cardiotoxic. Dose for local infiltration or peripheral nerve block: 2mg/kg (max 150mg). Use <150mg (use 5–7.5mg/mL solution) for epidural; <15mg for intrathecal.
5 **Ropivacaine** ($t_{1/2}$=1.8h): Dose: 3mg/kg IBW. Less cardiotoxic than bupivacaine. Less motor block when used epidurally. Contraindicated for IV regional anaesthesia and paracervical block in obstetrics.
6 **Tetracaine** ($t_{1/2}$=1h): Slow onset. High toxicity. Eye *drops* for topical anaesthesia, and now *topically* (AMETOP®) as an alternative to EMLA®. Also available as a gel (combined with adrenaline & lidocaine) for open wounds

NB: 0.5% solution=5mg/mL. 1% solution=10mg/mL. So for a 70kg man, the maximum dose of lidocaine is 20mL of 1% or 10mL of 2% solution.

Adrenaline slows systemic absorption of LA (thus increases duration of LA effect) and is useful in areas of increased vascularity (eg intercostal blocks) where risk of systemic absorption is higher. Systemic effects from adrenaline are esp. hazardous in CVS disease or ↑BP. ►*Adrenaline is contraindicated in digital or penile blocks, and around the nose/ears (risk of local ischaemia).*

Complications *Failure* is user and procedure dependent, always have a backup which is likely to be GA. *Nerve injury* is rare and tend to settle within weeks if it does occur. *Bleeding* ►Abnormal coagulation is a relative contraindication since even small haematomas can cause enough compression to cause long term nerve damage, especially for neuraxial techniques. *LA toxicity:* From excess dose, too rapid absorption, or direct IV injection. Inital features: Perioral tingling; numb tongue; anxiety; lightheadedness; tinnitus. Signs of severe toxicity: seizures; apnoea; direct myocardial depression; coma. ►►Stop injection of LA; ►Call for help and follow national protocol which guides the use of lipid emulsion (Intralipid®). [56] This may work by binding to the LA and thus reducing the amount of free LA in the circulation. If in circulatory arrest manage with standard ALS protocols plus Intralipid®. Recovery from LA-induced cardiac arrest may take >1h. *Seizures:* Benzodiazepines/propofol/thiopental in small incremental doses.

Specific peripheral blocks and their uses

Block type	Examples of use
Bier's block (p728) (IV regional anaesthesia)	Hand/forearm manipulation or surgery
Cervical plexus	Carotid endarterectomy
Interscalene (brachial plexus)	Shoulder surgery (good prolonged post-op analgesia)
Axillary block	Hand/forearm surgery
Lumbosacral plexus (psoas compartment block)	Hip surgery (combined with a sciatic nerve block)
Ilioinguinal–iliohypogastric nerve	Inguinal hernia repair
Femoral nerve (see 'Further reading')	Femoral fracture, knee surgery (when combined with a sciatic block)
Sciatic nerve	Surgery below the knee
Popliteal & saphenous nerves	Ankle or foot surgery

►Ensure that the anaesthetized area is positioned and protected sufficiently both intra- and postoperatively to avoid injury.

Anaesthesia

Transversus abdominal plane (TAP) nerve block

This block is frequently used as part of the analgesic regimen for any surgery on the lower abdomen involving the anterior abdominal wall. **Anatomy** The anterior abdominal wall comprises of three key muscle layers: external oblique (EO) (most superficial), internal oblique (IO) and transversus abdominis (TA) muscle (most internal). Sensory innervation is composed of the anterior rami of T7-L1. **Target** Aim to deliver the LA to lie in the plane between IO and TA since this is where the sensory nerves travel through to reach the abdominal wall. Place the US probe midway between the costal margin and iliac crest; the needle should pierce the skin just above the iliac crest through the triangle of Petit (figs 9.11 & 9.12). In this lateral position, the EO muscle is still present as fascia so you will feel two 'pops' as the needle passes through EO and IO to enable LA injection (30mL each side, volume is more important than concentration to encourage spread to as many nerves as possible) between IO and TA. A catheter is often left for continuous analgesia.[57]

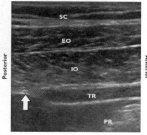

Fig 9.11 US is an essential piece of equipment for siting a TAP block.

Reproduced from Warman et al, *Regional Anaesthesia, Stimulation, and Ultrasound Techniques* (2014) with permission from OUP.

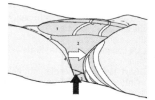

Fig 9.12 Diagram to indicate the markings of the lumbar triangle of Petit. 1 rectus abdominis muscle; 2 external oblique muscle; 3 latissimus dorsi muscle; 4 iliac crest; white arrow, inferior costal margin; black arrow, lumbar triangle of Petit.

Reproduced from Warman et al, *Regional Anaesthesia, Stimulation, and Ultrasound Techniques* (2014) with permission from OUP.

Further reading

Anaesthesia UK (2006). *Does Regional Anaesthesia Improve Outcome?* http://www.frca.co.uk/
Bogacz A et al. (2012). *Femoral Nerve Block – A Guide for Medical Students and Junior Doctors.* New York School of Regional Anaesthesia: www.nysora.com

Spinal anaesthesia Anaesthetic into the *subarachnoid space*. (fig 9.13). The aim is to anaesthetize the spinal roots passing through here.

- Insert IV cannula and start IV crystalloid.
- Check BP; position patient—sitting or left lateral.
- Surgical scrub & prepare back.
- Infiltrate skin with 1–2mL 1% lidocaine.
- Insert a 25G spinal needle at L3/4 space (ie below spinal cord). Small needles are used to reduce risk of postdural puncture headache. Free flow of CSF confirms correct placement. Rotate the needle through 180° to ensure that all the needle aperture is in (avoids patchy blocks).
- Inject 1–3mL 0.5% Marcain Heavy® (bupivacaine + glucose, a hyperbaric solution that falls by gravity). NB: much less LA is needed in pregnancy. Consider adding a small amount of opioid to prolong the analgesic effect.

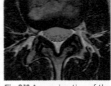

Fig 9.13 Approximation of the subarachnoid space in red on this T2-weighted MRI. Note spinal nerve roots.
Courtesy of Norwich Radiology Department.

- Achieving a low, high, or unilateral block is only possible if the patient is left in position for a protracted period prior to surgery (usually unrealistic).
- Monitor BP—may ↓; if so, give crystalloid ± vasopressors (eg **ephedrine** 3–6mg IV repeated as needed (p632), or **phenylephrine** 50–100mcg).

A small total drug concentration is required—producing sympathetic blockade (vasodilation, ↓BP), sensory blockade (numbness) and finally motor blockade (↓ or absence of lower limb power).

Complications of spinal anaesthesia: •Total spinal block (↓BP, ↓HR, anxiety, apnoea, LOC)—see below •Headache—see below •Urinary retention •Permanent neurological damage (very rare).

Extradural (epidural) anaesthesia[58]

This is anaesthetic into the *extradural space*. (fig 9.14). Insertion of indwelling catheter allows prolonged instillation of LA and/or opiates. Larger volumes of LA are required than with spinal anaesthesia. Opiods enhance sensory and not motor block. Lumbar most common site, but cervical/thoracic possible (needs great skill).

- Use aseptic technique, with patient sitting, or in the left lateral position.
- Check BP. Start IV crystalloid—eg 500mL.
- L3/4 commonest site. Infiltrate 1–2mL 0.5% lidocaine.
- Insert 16G Touhy needle until held firm in ligamentum flavum (~2–3cm).
- 'Loss of resistance' technique finds epidural space: 10mL 0.9% saline via Touhy needle is difficult to inject while in ligaments, but once in the epidural space, sudden loss of resistance enables easy injection.

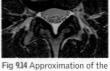

Fig 9.14 Approximation of the extradural space in yellow on this T2-weighted MRI.
Courtesy of Norwich Radiology Department.

- Fine-bore epidural catheter threaded, needle withdrawn, and catheter placed to needle depth plus 3–5cm. Check you can't aspirate fluid from catheter.
- Administer 2mL test dose of anaesthetic and wait 3min. If there has been inadvertent intrathecal placement this will result in spinal anaesthesia.
- Inject required dose, eg 10mL 0.25% plain bupivacaine in 5mL aliquots.
- Secure catheter in place.
- Monitor BP every 5min for 15min (slower onset than spinal; therefore hypotension takes longer to be revealed).

Complications of epidural anaesthesia *Dural puncture:* <1%. CSF leak may not be obvious; hence the importance of test dose. Push oral fluids, with caffeine. Nurse flat. Give analgesics for headache, laxatives to prevent constipation/straining. Blood patch[6] is usually necessary if headache lasts >24–48h, most patients benefit after the 1st blood patch, nearly all after the 2nd.[59] *Vessel puncture and inadvertent injection:* Treat with ABC remembering: O_2, IVI, pressor drugs, atropine if bradycardia (due to block of sympathetic outflow to heart T2–4). *Hypoventilation:* Motor block of intercostals; may need control of ventilation. *'Total spinal'*—ie injection of a large epidural dose into the CSF. Marked hypotension. Apnoea. Loss of consciousness. Treatment: ABC resuscitation and 100% O_2. Treat ↓BP. ►►*Death will occur from asphyxia if treatment is not prompt. Epidural haematoma or abscess:* Aim for early diagnosis to prevent permanent CNS damage. ►►Get emergency neurological review and MRI.[60] *Other:* Patchy or unilateral block. Nerve root damage.

Benefits of epidural anaesthesia In obstetric practice (p66) there is no excess risk of caesarean section,[61] though superior outcome with regional anaesthesia compared with GA has not been confirmed.[62] Epidural local anaesthetics cause less GI paralysis compared with systemic or epidural opioids, with comparable pain relief.[63] Epidurals may also ↓post-op risk of respiratory failure.[60]

Caudal (sacral epidural) Left lateral; prone or semi-prone positions; aseptic technique. Palpate sacral hiatus (4–5cm above coccyx tip). This is often not easy. Another method is to palpate the posterior superior iliac spines: the line joining them forms the base of an equilateral triangle with the sacral hiatus at the apex. Insert 21G block needle perpendicular to skin through the sacrococcygeal membrane into the sacral canal. A 23G needle may be useful for infants. Aspirate, and inject up to 20mL 0.5% bupivacaine in the adult. If injecting is difficult (there should be no resistance), or swelling occurs, the needle is in the wrong place—so *stop!* Withdraw the needle and start again. *Indications* Provides anaesthesia for the sacral region—commonly used in children. Useful, eg in scrotal surgery, low cavity forceps (needs experience because of risk of injecting into baby's head), hernias or haemorrhoids.

GA or regional anaesthesia? Abdominal, pelvic, and lower limb surgery are ideal for regional techniques (eg hernia repair, THR). However, in day-case surgery, neuraxial techniques may be associated with a prolonged stay.[64] For some operations, outcome may be better with neuraxial techniques—one study found marginal benefits of fewer deaths and DVTs in hip fracture surgery.[MET 65] They can also be used as an adjunct to GA, reducing the stress response and postoperative pain.[66]

Absolute contraindications to **all** *neuraxial anaesthesia:*
1 Anticoagulant states (the risk is pressure damage to cord from bleed—there is an extensive local vertebral venous plexus).
2 Local sepsis (risk of introducing infection to CSF).
3 Shock or hypovolaemic states (effective reduction in circulating volume due to vasodilatation).
4 Raised intracranial pressure (→coning).
5 Unwilling or uncooperative patient.
6 Fixed output states (eg mitral and aortic stenosis).

Relative contraindications to **all** *neuraxial anaesthesia:*
• Neurological disease—procedure may be blamed for change in state.
• Ischaemic heart disease.
• Spinal deformity or previous surgery.
• Bowel perforation (theoretical risk of ↑parasympathetic activity, peristalsis, and peritoneal soiling).

6 An epidural blood patch is a relatively straightforward procedure where the patient's own blood is injected into the epidural space at the site of the previous LP. The benefit is 2-fold; the volume replacement helps build up pressure again and the blood eventually seals the CSF leak.

Analgesia promotes well-being, sleep, and facilitates recovery or, in the case of palliative medicine (*OHCM* p522) the easeful passage into oblivion. Pain relief also aids physiotherapy (allowing coughing and mobility), preventing pneumonia. Pain also exacerbates hypo/hyperventilation, hypertension, and tachycardia, and can lead to urinary retention.

Methods of analgesia (See *OHCM* p576 and *OHCM* p534)[7]

1 *Oral:* Try paracetamol: 1g/6h—then:
  • *NSAIDs:* Diclofenac 250mg/8h (remember danger of GI bleed; cover with PPI; caution in asthma). Effects on renal function are minimal if pre-op U&E is normal[67] but be cautious if hypovolaemic.
  • *Tramadol* 50–100mg/4–6h PO/IV. Fewer SEs than morphine, but less potent.
  • *Opioids,* eg codeine, **morphine sulfate** solution. NB: most are poorly absorbed from the gut.
  • *Neuropathic agents:* eg **gabapentin** for neuropathic pain associated with chronic regional pain syndrome (CRPS, p723) or diabetic/vascular neuralgia. See *BNF* section 4.8.1.

2 *Sublingual:* **Buprenorphine** (an uncommonly used synthetic opiate; 'controlled' drug): 0.4mg/6h sublingually, or buccal fentanyl drops/lozenges.

3 *Inhalational:* **Nitrous oxide/oxygen** (Entonox®), useful for labour pains, changing dressings, and physiotherapy.

4 *Intramuscular:* Rarely used—eg morphine 10mg IM; pethidine 100mg IM.

5 *Subcutaneous:* Used in palliative care eg **diamorphine**.

6 *Intravenous:* Boluses or continuous infusion. Patient-controlled analgesia (PCA). The patient can give himself boluses, avoiding the risks of continuous infusion. Remember to program maximum dose limit.

7 *Regional anaesthesia (RA):* p634. Epidurals (opiates, or LA, boluses or continuous infusion). Many techniques used (intercostal nerve, brachial plexus, femoral nerve blocks).

8 *Transcutaneous fentanyl patches.*

9 *Transcutaneous electrical nerve stimulation* (TENS).

Chronic pain Some anaethesists dedicate significant amounts of their workload to the management of chronic pain, it is an extremely important topic which is only briefly touched upon here. No single treatment will be effective for every patient. Treatment may be broadly categorized into three categories—pharmacological, physical, and psychological. The British Pain Society recommends individualized pain management programmes based on the principles of cognitive behavioural therapy for those with chronic pain which cannot be remedied with drug and physical treatments alone. These consist of education on pain physiology, psychology, and self-management of pain problems.[68] Pharmacological treatments include simple analgesia, opioids, tricyclic antidepressants, neuropathic pain medicines (eg **gabapentin**), and epidurals for low back pain. Interventions which may help certain patients include acupuncture and hypnosis.

Pain in children See p196 for narcotic and other analgesia in painful conditions such as sickle-cell disease.

See p810 & 812 for analgesia in the pre-hospital environment.

Further reading

Pergolizzi Jr JV *et al.* (2014). The WHO pain ladder: Do we need another step? *Pract Pain Manage* 14. http://www.practicalpainmanagement.com/resources/who-pain-ladder-do-we-need-another-step
SIGN (2013). *Management of Chronic Pain* (SIGN 136). Edinburgh: SIGN.

7 Contexts such as barbiturate poisoning and Bickerstaff's brainstem encephalitis can give a brain-death picture—*but are reversible* (worryingly so—more for ethicists than the patient).

8 Patients who have 'confirmed' brain death and who are suitable for organ donation would be heart-beating donors. However, organ retrieval is never straightforward, and so the Maastricht criteria exist for the categorization of non-heart-beating organ donors: 1 Dead on arrival at hospital; 2 Unsuccessful resuscitation; 3 Awaiting cardiac arrest (eg after withdrawal of treatment); 4 Cardiac arrest after confirmation of brainstem death.[69]

Making the diagnosis Persistent vegetative states (vs) are rare, and liable to misdiagnosis by non-specialists—it requires careful repeated assessment and taking into account observations made by family and carers. ▸*The harder you look, the more likely you are to find signs of active cognition, thus negating the diagnosis of a vs.* The patient

Causes
• Trauma
• Anoxia
• Vascular causes
• Encephalitis

in a vs 'appears at times to be wakeful, with cycles of eye closure and eye opening resembling those of sleep and waking'. But they lack signs of awareness—there is no evidence that they can perceive the environment or their own body. Persistent vs is defined as > 4 weeks, and permanent vs is defined as 12 months following a traumatic brain injury, or 6 months following other causes of brain injury. Patients that show awareness are said to be in a minimally conscious state rather than a vs.

Investigations There are a number of methods that can be used to aid the decision as to whether there is cognitive brain function present: eg somatosensory evoked potentials (SSEPs) and electroencephalography (EEG). However, the problem is that these tests not only have to be 100% specific (an impossibility) but they also need to be able to predict *return* of cognitive function, and not just its presence. To make matters even more complicated, pharmacological and metabolic changes can also interfere with the accuracy of such tests. One review has quoted that with the absence of somatosensory evoked potentials in patients with hypoxic ischaemic encephalopathy, the chances of waking are less than 1%.[70]

Another method of showing awareness and cognition is by demonstrating communication, eg by following a simple request to look at a named object. Other ways of communicating include listener scanning: the therapist goes through A–Z slowly, and the patient buzzes when the required letter is reached. It may take months to establish that the patient can communicate.

Management While waiting for any recovery, aim to provide vigorous nursing care to maintain nutrition, and to prevent pressure sores, and tracheostomy and muscle contracture complications. No drugs are known to help, although there is anecdotal evidence that bromocriptine may do so. Multimodal stimulation (arousal programmes) may help; these programmes involve stimulation of all senses every 15min for up to 11h per day. Once it is agreed that there will be no recovery (the difficult issue), discussions on withdrawing active treatment and nutrition raise big ethical questions—which are only partly mitigated if the patient has an advance directive (an unlikely event). Ethicists, medical specialists, nurses, physiotherapists, judges, and the family must all be allowed to have their say. None is infallible. (See also Death *OHCM*, p6.)

Muddled over death, brain death, and persistent vegetative states?

When the Buddha was ailing, he was at first mispronounced dead by Ananda, his attendant for 25 years. Ananda was then 'corrected' by a top monk who stated that the Buddha had entered a deep yogic trance in which no vital signs could be discerned (as might occur in hypothermia).[71] How do you tell? First, recognize that death is a *process*. Next, accept that absent brainstem reflexes is a only a useful shorthand for death of the brainstem—which itself is only a shorthand for brain death (functions remain, such as thermoregulation and production of CNS hormones, etc). And death of the brain becomes a shorthand for death itself. According to Buddhist authorities, death occurs when the body is bereft of *vitality*, *heat*, and *sentiency*. In many ways the senior monk was right. First know your patient, and take into account past history[7] and the medical and moral context in which the diagnosis of brain death or permanent vs is being made. Then ask a colleague, and keep an open mind—esp. when organ donation is contemplated.[8]

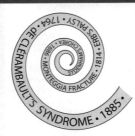

Fig 10.1 We like eponyms. What better way to achieve immortality and recognition than have your name live on—even if no one remembers anything about you other than what you discovered. That's if you *did* discover it in the first place (this is often contentious!). *Stigler's Law of Eponomy* states 'No scientific discovery is named after its original discoverer'—see *OHCM* p708.

Eponyms sound far more glamorous than histologically driven disease titles, the names of which often evolve as more becomes known. Whilst the golden age of eponyms may be behind us, we hope those that remain—like the spiral—will carry on forever.

Alphabetical list of eponymous syndromes

See also *OHCM* p708-31. Biographical details sourced from www.whonamedit.com.

Alport's syndrome A group of inherited, progressive, haematuric nephropathies which may also affect the cochlea (sensorineural deafness) and eye (lenticonus; dot-and-fleck retinopathy). It is associated with mutations in genes encoding the $\alpha 3,4,5$ chains of collagen IV, the major constituent of the basement membrane. *R:* No effective treatment is available. Those with end-stage renal disease usually undergo transplantation.[1,2]   *Arthur C Alport, 1880–1959 (South African physician)*

Asperger's syndrome An autistic spectrum disorder characterized by poor social skills and restricted interests, but with normal language and IQ. There is difficulty interpreting emotions, body language, and understanding non-literal use of language, such as sarcasm.   *Hans Asperger, 1906–1980 (Austrian paediatrician)*

Bardet–Biedl syndrome Autosomal recessive A rare multisystem disorder of underlying ciliary dysfunction and a key genetic cause of chronic renal failure in children.[3] *Features:* Renal failure (dysfunction of renal tubule cilia), GU tract malformations, obesity, cognitive impairment, poor visual acuity, and limb deformities. $\male : \female \approx 1.3:1$.   *Georges L Bardet 1885–1970 (French physician); Artur Biedl 1869–1933 (Hungarian pathologist)*

Batten disease (neuronal ceroid–lipofuscinoses) A group of severe neuro–degenerative diseases. Neuronal loss occurs due to increased apoptosis and altered autophagy from defects in the CLN genes (pathogenesis unknown). *Features:* Visual loss, seizures, loss of motor and cognitive function and early death. *Tests:* Molecular testing for CLN1-3 mutations.[4]   *Frederick E Batten 1865–1918 (British Neurologist)*

Becker's muscular dystrophy x-linked recessive There are mutations in the dystrophin gene (xp21), but unlike Duchenne (p642, where there is near-total loss of dystrophin) there is 'semifunctional' dystrophin, with later onset, milder symptoms, and slower progression. Cardiac involvement is the main factor influencing survival. *Tests:* ↑CK, MM biopsy, genetic tests/counselling (p154). *R:* Supportive (exercise programmes, physio; managing complications).   *Peter E Becker 1908–2000 (German physician)*

Beckwith–Wiedemann syndrome An overgrowth syndrome characterized by macrosomia, macroglossia, hemihyperplasia, and abdominal wall defects. There is predisposition to embryonal tumours (esp. Wilm's, p133) in ~10%.[5]

J Bruce Beckwith b1933 (American pathologist); Hans-Rudolf Wiedemann 1915–2006 (German paediatrician)

Bourneville's disease (tuberous sclerosis complex) (epiloia =EPIlepsy, LOW INtelligence + Adenoma sebaceum, see fig 10.2) Autosomal dominant A multi-organ disorder resulting in hamartomatous lesions that affect virtually every organ system. The main complication is epilepsy or developmental delay from 'tubers' within the brain. *Cause:* Mutation of tumour suppressor genes TSC1 (loci on 9q34, making *harmatin*) or TSC2 (16p13 makes *tuberin*; mutations here are worst). *Prognosis:* Highly variable. *Diagnosis:* See BOX.   *Désiré-Magloire Bourneville 1840–1909 (French neurologist)*

Johnnie Walker or Dandy–Walker?

We are surrounded by eponyms commemorating the Great and the Good, from the Nobel Prizes and the Ryder Cup, to Jack Daniels and Johnnie Walker. Medical eponyms are pickled in something almost as intoxicating: the hidden recesses of our own minds. We store away the bizarre, the fearsome, and the mundane—and then, years later, as if playing some game of snap, we match these features with the person sitting in front of us, and say: 'Dandy–Walker!' or 'Prader–Willi!'. But as the years go by we may wonder more and more about the people behind the eponyms. We might read about these quacks and geniuses—yet it is always rather unsatisfying. History shows us everything except the one thing we want to see: the spark that made these eponymous characters truly original.

Diagnosing tuberous sclerosis (Bourneville's disease)[6]

Clinical diagnostic criteria

Definite diagnosis: 2 major features, or 1 major and 2 minor features.
Possible diagnosis: Either 1 major, 1 major + 1 minor, or ≥2 minor features.

Major features		Minor features
1	Hypomelanotic (ashleaf) macules (≥3)	1 'Confetti' skin lesions
2	Angiofibromas (≥3) (fig 10.2)	2 Dental enamel pits (≥3)
3	Ungal fibromas (≥2) (fig 10.3)	3 Intraoral fibromas (≥2)
4	Shagreen patch (sacral plaque, like shark skin)	4 Retinal achromic patch
5	Multiple retinal hamartomas	5 Multiple renal cysts
6	Cortical dysplasias* (≥3)	6 Non-renal hamartomas
7	Subependymal nodules* (≥2)	
8	Subependymal giant cell astrocytomas*	
9	Cardiac rhabdomyoma	
10	Lymphangioleiomyomatosis	
11	Angiomyolipomas	

*=brain lesions.

Genetic criteria: Identification of a pathogenic mutation of TSC1 or TSC2 is sufficient to make a definite diagnosis. However, a negative result does not exclude diagnosis as ~15% have no mutation identified by conventional testing.

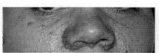

Fig 10.2 Angiofibromas (adenoma sebaceum).

Courtesy of Dr Samuel da Silva.

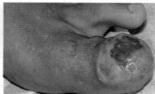

Fig 10.3 Ungual fibroma.

Courtesy of Dr Samuel da Silva.

Briquet's syndrome (somatization disorder) Chronic, multiple, medically unexplained, difficult to treat (but unfeigned) symptoms, affecting any body part. Psychological cause. Onset <30yrs (see BOX). *Paul Briquet 1796–1881 (French physician)*

Bruton agammaglobulinaemia See BOX, p199. *Ogden Carr Bruton 1908–2003 (US physician)*

Buchanan's syndrome A single artery arises from normally formed ventricles (the **truncus arteriosus** fails to divide into the pulmonary trunk and aorta). There is cyanosis from birth. *Ŗ:* Surgical correction. *A Buchanan; described 1864*

Capgras syndrome A delusional misidentification where the patient believes a person has been replaced by an exact clone, an impostor. *Cause:* Psychosis; head injury; B₁₂↓. See BOX. *Jean Marie Joseph Capgras 1873–1950 (French psychiatrist)*

Castleman's disease (angiofollicular lymph node hyperplasia) A lymphoproliferative disorder comprising 2 distinct diseases: *unicentric* with solitary mediastinal lymph node; *multicentric* systemic disease + associated immunosuppression. POEMS syndrome may be present (BOX).[7] *Benjamin Castleman 1906–1982 (US pathologist)*

Chediak–Higashi syndrome ^{Autosomal recessive} Hypopigmentation (skin, eyes, hair), prolonged bleeding, recurrent infection, abnormal NK cell function. Morbidity results from frequent infections or lymphoproliferation into organs.[8] *Cause:* 1q43 mutation (CHS1/LYST gene). Fatal in 90% by 10yrs of age without marrow transplant.[9] *Otokata Higashi 1902–1981 (Japanese paediatrician); Alexander M Chédiak 1903–1993 (Cuban physician)*

Conradi–Hünermann syndrome (chondrodysplasia punctata) A group of skeletal dysplasia disorders characterized by skeletal abnormalities (shortening of limbs, X-ray epiphyseal stippling), cataracts, and skin lesions (icthyosis, alopecia). *Cause:* Genetic (most are X-linked dominant; severity is variable); warfarin teratogenicity.[10] *Erich Conradi 1882–1968; Carl Hünermann 1904–1978 (German physicians)*

Cornelia de Lange syndrome A multi-system malformation syndrome causing characteristic facial dysmorphism in association with growth retardation, IQ↓, and upper limb anomalies. ~50% are due to NIPBL gene mutation. There is wide clinical variability.[11] *Cornelia Catharina de Lange 1871–1950 (Dutch paediatrician)*

Corrigan's syndrome Congenital aortic regurgitation (AR). Corrigan's pulse is the collapsing pulse of AR. *Sir Dominic John Corrigan 1802–1880 (Irish physician)*

Cotard's syndrome (nihilistic delusions) The patient may state he is already dead and demand burial, deny his existence, or believe his insides are rotting away. *Cause:* Psychotic depression (especially elderly patients), alcohol, syphilis, parietal lobe lesion, or just being born. *Jules Cotard 1840–1887 (French physician)*

Crigler–Najjar syndrome Two rare syndromes of inherited unconjugated hyperbilirubinaemia presenting in the 1st days of life with jaundice ± CNS signs. *Cause:* Mutation in UGT enzyme activity causing absent (type 1) or impaired (type 2; mild) ability to excrete bilirubin. *Ŗ:* T1: Liver transplant before irreversible kernicterus (p115). *John F Crigler b1919; Victor A Najjar b1914–2002 (US paediatricians)*

Dandy–Walker syndrome Congenital obstruction of the foramina of Luschka and Magendi leads to progressive head enlargement, congested scalp veins, bulging fontanelle, separation of cranial sutures, papilloedema, and bradycardia (fig 10.4). *Ŗ:* CSF shunt. *Walter E Dandy 1886–1946 (US neurosurgeon); Arthur E Walker 1907–1995 (US neurologist)*

De Clerambault's syndrome (erotomania) The patient (usually female) is persistently deluded that a person of higher social status is in love with them (eg a politician or celebrity). Stalking is one manifestation. There may be a persecutory delusional belief that individuals are conspiring to keep them apart. *Ian McEwan Enduring Love* *Gaëtan Gatian de Clérambault 1872–1934 (French psychiatrist)*

Diamond–Blackfan anaemia (erythrogenesis imperfecta) An inherited red cell aplasia. *Features:* ↓marrow erythroid production (→normochromic macrocytic anaemia); growth retardation; ~30–50% have craniofacial, upper limb, heart, and urinary system malformations. *Cause:* 25% due to mutations in RPS19 gene on 19q13.[12] *Ŗ:* Steroids ± bone marrow transplant; or stem-cell transplant from a donor embryo (pre-implantation genetic diagnosis confirms HLA matching).[13] *Louis K Diamond 1902–1999; Kenneth D Blackfan 1883–1941 (US paediatricians)*

Eponymous syndromes

Helping people with Briquet's syndrome

- Give time—don't dismiss these patients as just the 'worried well'.[14]
- Explore with the patient the factors perpetuating the illness (disordered physiology, misinformation, unfounded fears, misinterpretation of sensations, unhelpful 'coping' behaviour, social stressors).
- Agree a management plan which focuses on each issue and makes sense to the patient's holistic view of him- or herself.
- Treat any depression (p342); consider cognitive therapy; make the patient feel understood; broaden the agenda, negotiating a new understanding of symptoms including psychosocial factors.[15]

Castleman's lymph node hyperplasia with POEMS syndrome

POEMS syndrome entails: Peripheral neuropathy, Organomegaly/hyperplasia, Endocrinopathy, a Monoclonal paraprotein, and Skin lesions. Interleukin-6 excess is also a feature. Children with unexplained chronic inflammatory symptoms ± PUO ± failure to thrive may need detailed soft tissue tests to reveal associated vascular tumours.

☺ Cloning our wives

In idle moments, we might think that it would be useful to clone our wives. This is what men with Capgras syndrome have accomplished. But could we really cope with this? Men with Capgras syndrome get very destabilized by not knowing who they are talking to—the genuine, or the fake wife.[16] It is an example of a delusion called the 'clonal pluralization of identities'.[17] As such, it is the best example we have of a purely metaphysical disease. When a man with Capgras syndrome asks his wife with all solicitude: '*How are we today?*'—he means *every word* he utters. And he never knows the answer.

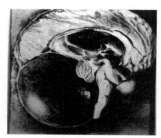

Fig 10.4 Dandy–Walker dilatation of the 4th ventricle. The large cyst is actually an enlarged 4th ventricle and not separate from it. The 3rd and lateral ventricles are much enlarged, secondarily.

Courtesy of Professor Ralph Józefowicz.

DiGeorge's syndrome A severe form of the chromosome 22q11.2 deletion syndromes. *Signs:* Congenital heart disease, abnormal facies, cleft palate, underactive parathyroids ($\therefore$Ca$^{2+}\downarrow$), thymus hypoplasia, $\downarrow$T-cell-immunity and cognitive/behavioural problems. *Angelo Mari DiGeorge 1921–2009 (US paediatrician)*

Di Guglielmo's disease A subtype of acute myeloid leukaemia (AML) characterized by invasion of pathological dysplastic RBCs into the liver, spleen, lymph nodes, kidneys, & heart. 3 stages: **erythromyelosis, erythroleukaemia, & AML.** *R̷:* chemotherapy ± bone marrow transplant.[18] *Giovanni Di Guglielmo 1886–1961 (Italian haematologist)*

Duchenne muscular dystrophy $_{\text{recessive}}^{\text{x-linked}}$ Mutations in dystrophin gene (xp21.2) result in near-total loss of dystrophin (muscles get replaced by fibrocalidue tissue). *Presentation:* Boys aged 1–6yrs, with a waddling, clumsy gait, and classic Gower's manoeuvre: on standing, he uses his hands to climb up his legs. No abnormality is noted at birth. Distal girdle muscles are affected late; selective wasting causes calf pseudohypertrophy. Wheelchairs are needed at 9–12yrs. There is respiratory impairment and infections; cardiomyopathy and orthopaedic complications (tendon contractures, scoliosis, osteoporosis). *Prevalence:* 1:3600—6000 male births. *Creatine kinase* is ↑; ►measure in all boys not walking by 1½yrs. *Muscle biopsy:* Abnormal fibres surrounded by fat and fibrous tissue. *R̷:* Interdisciplinary management and co-ordinated clinical care is crucial. Aim to maintain walking (eg using knee–ankle–foot orthoses). **Prednisolone** slows decline in muscle strength and function in the short term.[19] A disease-modifying agent (AVI-4658) is under development.[20] Gene therapy may be an option. *Prognosis:* Mechanical ventilation improves longevity (median age at death is now 31yrs). *Carrier ♀:* ~10% show some disease manifestation. *Prenatal screening* is available. *Guillaume Benjamin Amand Duchenne de Boulogne 1806–1875 (French neurologist)*

Ebstein's anomaly A congenital defect with downward displacement of the tricuspid valve (±deformed leaflets) atrializing the right ventricle causing right-sided heart failure. There may be no symptoms, or cyanosis, clubbing, arrhythmias, systolic, and diastolic murmurs. It can be associated with other cardiac malformations. *Tests:* Echo; ECG: tall P waves, ↑P–R interval; RBBB. *Prognosis:* varies according to severity. *Wilhem Ebstein 1836–1912 (German physician)*

Edwards syndrome (trisomy 18) The 2nd commonest trisomy (Down's is 1st p152) causing extensive and characteristic congenital malformations (see fig 10.5). There is severe psychomotor and growth retardation in the 5–10% who survive beyond the first year of life. *Prevalence:* 1:~7000 live births (80% ♀).[21] *John Hilton Edwards 1928–2007 (British physician)*

Ehlers-Danlos syndrome A clinically diverse condition with skin fragility (figs 10.6 & 10.7), ligament laxity, short stature, spinal deformity, vascular fragility, and (rarely) retinal detachment. *9 sub-types:* Hypermobility (type III) is the most common and probably synonymous with joint hypermobility syndrome. Vascular rupture is a major concern in type IV. *Δ:* Primarily clinical; genetic testing (via skin biopsy).[22] *Edvard L Ehlers 1863–1937 (Danish dermatologist); Henri-Alexandre Danlos 1844–1912 (French physician)*

Eisenmenger syndrome Refers to any congenital heart defect with a left-to-right shunt (eg large septal defects) in which the development of pulmonary hypertension leads to subsequent shunt reversal. *Victor Eisenmenger 1864–1932 (Austrian physician)*

Erb's palsy is caused by damage to the brachial plexus (usually C5/C6 nerves) from birth trauma. See p76, p750. *Wilhelm Heinrich Erb 1840–1921 (German neurologist)*

Fallot's tetrad (*OHCM* p151) **1** Ventricular septal defect (VSD) **2** Pulmonary stenosis **3** Right ventricular hypertrophy **4** The aorta overriding the VSD. It is the commonest cyanotic congenital heart disorder (10%; 3–6/10,000). *Signs:* Severity depends on degree of pulmonary stenosis. Cyanosis, dyspnoea, faints, clubbing, thrills, harsh systolic murmur at left sternal base. *Tests:* Echo shows anatomy & degree of stenosis. Cardiac CT/MRI helps plan surgery. *R̷:* 'Total repair' entails VSD closure and correcting pulmonary stenosis, eg before 1yr, and may result in normal life. *Prognosis:* Without surgery, mortality rate is ~95% by age 20. 20-yr survival is ~90–95% after repair. *Etienne-Louis Arthur Fallot, 1850–1911 (French physician)*

x-linked muscular dystrophies

1 Duchenne's muscular dystrophy (severe)
2 Becker muscular dystrophy (later presentation; much slower progression)
3 Emery–Dreifuss muscular dystrophy (benign; early contractures)
4 McLeod syndrome (benign with acanthocytes)
5 Scapuloperoneal (rare).

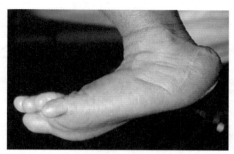

Fig 10.5 Rockerbottom feet, as seen in Edwards syndrome. Other signs: microcephaly, microphthalmia, micrognathia, microstomia, rigidity with limb flexion, odd low-set ears, receding chin, proptosis, cleft lip/palate ± umbilical/inguinal herniae; short sternum (makes nipples look widely separated). The fingers cannot be extended + 2nd and 5th fingers overlap 3rd and 4th.

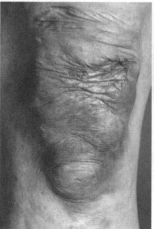

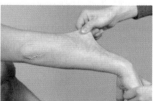

Fig 10.7 Elastic skin in Ehlers–Danlos (EDS). Bennett's paradox: the woman at a drag ball is the true impostor for, unlike everyone else, she is what she seems. So with EDS, which doesn't behave like a connective tissue disease *because it really is one* (a true disease of collagen). Other 'connective tissue diseases' are really diseases of something else.

Fig 10.6 In Ehlers–Danlos syndrome, skin is poor healing, fragile, and easily bruised or torn, with wide scars as thin as cigarette paper. Look for piezogenic papules (easily compressible outpouchings of fat through defects in the dermis on the sides of the feet).

Fanconi anaemia x-linked or auto-somal recessive Defective stem cell repair and chromosomal fragility leads to progressive marrow failure and aplastic anaemia. There is increased risk of acute myelogenous leukaemia and solid tumours. Congenital anomalies include absent radii, thumb hypoplasia, syndactyly, missing carpal bones, skin pigmentation, microsomy, microcephaly, strabismus, cryptorchidism, IQ↓, deafness and short stature. 15 causative genes have been identified. R: Stem cell transplant has increased survival (~90% with well-matched donors), and is the only proven cure for the haematopoietic manifestations of FA. Gene therapy trials are in progress.[23]
Guido Fanconi, 1892–1979 (Swiss paediatrician)

Galeazzi fracture Distal radial shaft fracture with associated dislocation of the distal radio–ulnar joint (fig **10.8**). *Ricardo Galeazzi, 1866–1952 (Italian orthopaedic surgeon)*

Ganser symptom A patient gives repeated wrong but 'approximate answers' to questions eg 'How many legs does a horse have?'—'3'; 'What colour is snow?'—'Black'. The nature of the answer reveals an understanding of the question posed. **Ganser syndrome** has varying definitions and includes approximate answering + clouding of consciousness, hallucinations and conversion symptoms. It may be organic, psychiatric or factitious (a form of malingering in those feigning mental illness).[24] *Sigbert Josef Maria Ganser, 1853–1931 (German psychiatrist)*

Gaucher disease Autosomal recessive The commonest lysosomal storage disease, caused by mutations in glucocerebrosidase gene on chromosome 1q21. Three subtypes are defined based on the presence or absence of CNS signs. 1 *Non-neuronopathic* presents with painless splenomegaly, anaemia, thrombocytopenia, & skeletal disease. 2 *Acute neuronopathic* (rare) characterized by rapid and progressive neurodegeneration, organomegaly, and death in infancy (usually by aspiration and respiratory compromise). 3 *Chronic neuronopathic* appears like type 1 *plus* with progressive slowing of oculomotor horizontal saccades ± learning disability, epilepsy, or dementia. 75% present before the age of 20 but severity varies widely for type 1 & 3. Δ: Measure acid β-glucosidase activity in peripheral WBCs. R: Enzyme replacement therapy eg **imiglucerase** helps haematology and organomegaly, but not bone indices, in type 1 & 3.[25] *Philippe Charles Ernest Gaucher, 1854–1918 (French dermatologist)*

Hand–Schüller–Christian syndrome (HSC; Langerhans' cell histiocytosis (LCH); histiocytosis X) The group of disorders now known as *LCH* were initially divided into a number of diseases (including *HSC*), depending on the site and severity. Monoclonal Langerhans-like cells are pathognomonic of this destructive, infiltrative disease in which bone, liver, skin, and spleen show lytic foci of eosinophils, plasma cells, and histiocytes. Lesions may show on a ⁹⁹technetium-labelled bone scan. It occurs in children and adults, eg starting with a polyp at the external auditory meatus. Other signs: see MINIBOX. R: Bone surgery, steroids, cytotoxics, and radiotherapy may induce remissions.

Signs of HSC
• Diabetes insipidus*
• Exophthalmos*
• Lytic bone lesions*
• Failure to thrive; dyspnoea
• Scalp lumps/skin erosions
• Eczema-like rash/pustules
• Cord compression± fits
• Ear discharge, stomatitis
• Honeycomb lung
• Hepatosplenomegaly
• Lymphadenopathy
• T°↑; anaemia; ↓platelets
*Classic triad; seen in 10%

Alfred Hand Jr, 1868–1949 (US paediatrician);
Artur Schüller, 1874–1957 (Austrian neurologist); Henry A Christian, 1876–1951 (US physician)

Hartnup's disease Autosomal recessive Increased GI & urinary loss of neutral amino acids causes pellagra-like photosensitive skin rash, cerebellar ataxia, and aminoaciduria. Causative gene: SLC6A19. R: High-protein diet; avoid sun exposure if symptomatic; **Nicotinamide** if niacin deficient.[26] *Baron et al (1956) described this disorder in the Hartnup family of London*

Hunter syndrome (mucopolysaccharidosis II) x-linked recessive (33% are new mutations). Iduronate sulfatase (IDS) deficiency results in glycosaminoglycan accumulation in the lysosomes of organs and tissues. *Signs:* Deafness, IQ↓, short stature, chronic diarrhoea, unusual face, hepatosplenomegaly, joint contractures, spinal stenosis. In the severe form (MPSIIA), life expectancy is 10–15 years. Δ: Enzyme analysis for IDS. R: None is curative. Enzyme replacement (**idursulfase**); bone marrow transplant.[27] *Charles A Hunter, 1873–1955 (Scottish–Canadian physician)*

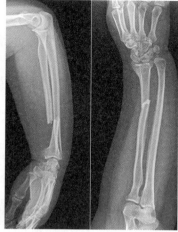

Fig 10.8 X–rays of a Galeazzi fracture show a short oblique fracture of the distal radius with distal ulnar dislocation from disruption of the distal radio–ulnar joint.

Emergency Radiology Cases edited by Hani H Abujudeh (2014): 2 x-rays on p. 139. By permission of Oxford University Press, USA.

Huntington's disease *Autosomal dominant* A progressive neurodegenerative disorder with spiny neuron loss in the neostriatum due to excessive CAG repeats in the huntingtin gene (chromosome 4). Normally, there are <28 repeats. 29-35 CAG repeats means no signs but they may pass Huntington's to their children. 36-39 CAG repeats means ↓penetrance. If >40 CAG repeats there is full penetrance (+ anticipation). Symptoms usually do not appear until adulthood (~30-50yrs). *Early findings*: ↓auditory & visual reaction times, then mild chorea (flitting, jerky movements), odd extraocular movements, ↑reflexes, ↓rapid alternating movements. Unpredictable motor impairment is found until chorea starts. *Late signs:* Personality change, self-neglect, apathy, clumsiness, fidgeting, fleeting grimaces, dementia and progression to death 10-30yrs from diagnosis. ℞: None prevents progression. Ethical dilemmas surround testing, as symptoms may only start after completing a family. *George Huntington, 1850–1916 (US physician)*

Hunt's syndrome (pyridoxine [vitamin B₆]–dependent seizure; PDS) Classic PDS: intractable neonatal seizures resistant to conventional anticonvulsants respond rapidly to parenteral **pyridoxine**. *James Ramsay Hunt, 1872–1937 (US neurologist)*

Hurler syndrome *Autosomal recessive* A severe form of mucopolysaccharidosis type 1, a lysosomal storage disorder caused by deficiency of α-L-iduronidase with resultant inability to breakdown dermatan sulfate & heparan sulfate (essential for normal growth). There is accumulation of mucopolysaccharides in urine, cartilage, periosteum, tendons, valves, meninges, & eye. After briefly normal growth, there is physical and mental decline, hydrocephalus, thick skin, hirsutism, and CCF. *Cause:* IDUA gene mutation (chromosome 4). *Tests:* Metachromatic Reilly bodies in lymphocytes; x–ray. ℞: Multidisciplinary approach; enzyme replacement with **laronidase**. Death is often ≤10yrs.[28] *Gertrud Hurler, 1889–1965 (German paediatrician)*

Hutchinson's triad (congenital syphilis) VIIIth nerve deafness + interstitial keratitis + notched, pointed incisors. *Sir Jonathan Hutchinson, 1828–1913 (British surgeon)*

Ivemark syndrome The association of asplenia with visceroatrial heterotaxia (abnormal organ position; AKA situs ambiguus). *Björn Ivemark, 1925–2005 (Swedish pathologist)*

Kartagener syndrome *Autosomal recessive* Primary ciliary dyskinesia (inflexible, poorly beating cilia) **associated with** situs inversus (dextrocardia). Clearance of mucus & bacteria is poor, hence chronic sinusitis and bronchiectasis. ♂ infertility, ♀ salpingitis and otitis media are common. ℞: Antibiotics, continuous or intermittent, for airway infections; immunization.[29] *Manes Kartagener, 1897–1975 (Swiss physician)*

Kawasaki disease A febrile vasculitic syndrome causing coronary aneurysms. *Cause:* Unknown. *Median age:* 18-24 months. 3 phases: 1 *Acute febrile:* Lasts 1-2wks; the child has fever ≥5 days + major signs (see BOX & fig 109). 2 *Subacute:* Lasts from remission of fever to weeks 4-6. Hallmarks of this phase include the development of coronary artery aneurysms (& the risk for MI and sudden death), desquamation of the digits, thrombocytosis, irritability, and conjunctival injection. 3 *Convalescent:* Resolution of clinical signs and normalization of inflammatory markers (weeks 6-12). *Tests:* ESR & CRP↑; bilirubin↑, AST↑, α₁-antitrypsin↑, platelets↑; serial echocardiogram; MRA accurately defines aneurysms. ℞: **Immunoglobulin** 2g/kg as a single IVI dose within 10d of symptom onset decreases new coronary aneurysms.[30] IVIG+prednisolone if non-responsive to initial dose;[31] **Aspirin**. *Prognosis:* Good with prompt treatment. Mortality ~1%. *Tomisaku Kawasaki, b1925 (Japanese paediatrician)*

Klinefelter syndrome (47, XXY karyotype) The chief genetic cause of male hypogonadism presenting with gynaecomastia and infertility. *Associations:* Psychosocial issues, mild learning disability, autoimmune disease, osteoporosis, ↓sexual maturation. ℞: Androgen therapy; mastectomy. Lifespan is normal, but arm span may exceed body length. *Harry Fitch Klinefelter Jr, 1912–1990 (US physician)*

Klippel-Feil syndrome *Autosomal recessive or dominant* Congenital fusion of cervical vertebrae ± neurological symptoms. The clinical triad seen in 50% is short neck, low posterior hairline, and limited neck movement *Mirror movements* (synkinesia) may occur (=*voluntary* movements in one limb cause the same *involuntarily* movement in the other). *Maurice Klippel, 1858–1942; Andre Feil, b1884 (French neurologists)*

Diagnostic criteria for Kawasaki disease[32]

Fever for ≥5 days + at least 4 of the following:*
1 Bilateral non-exudative conjunctivitis.
2 Cervical lymphadenopathy (often unilateral, firm, tender nodes).
3 Pharyngeal injection, dry fissured lips, strawberry tongue. No mouth ulcers.
4 Polymorphous rash (especially on the trunk).
5 Changes in extremities: arthralgia, palmar erythema or later, ►swelling of the hands/feet ± skin desquamation.

*Kawasaki disease may be diagnosed with <4 of these features if coronary artery aneurysms (CAAs) are present. Fever is often high (>40°C) and can persist for ≥2 weeks if untreated.

►Incomplete forms exist, so get expert help *today* while wrestling with this difficult, important diagnosis. There is paradoxical data that incomplete or atypical forms are *more* likely to have complications such as CAA.

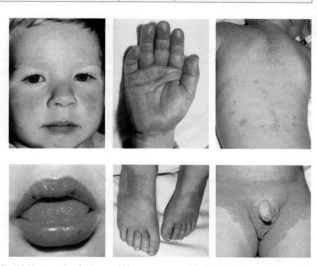

Fig 10.9 Photographs of a 4-year-old boy show some of the typical features of Kawasaki's disease including (from top left–right), bilateral nonexudative conjunctivitis; erythematous and oedematous hands and (below) feet; an erythematous truncal rash; dry, fissured, erythematous lips with a 'strawberry' tongue; and a desquamating perineal rash.

Kugelberg–Welander (spinal muscular atrophy type 3) $\frac{\text{Autosomal}}{\text{recessive}}$ Weakness and hypotonia from loss of LMN in the spinal cord & brainstem nuclei. Usually manifests >18 months old. *Erik KH Kugelberg, 1913–1983; Lisa Welander, 1909–2001 (Swedish neurologists)*

Landouzy–Dejerine (facioscapulohumeral) **muscular dystrophy** $\frac{\text{Autosomal}}{\text{dominant}}$ Distinct and slowly progressive (asymmetrical) regional weakness appears at 12–14yrs of age. There is shoulder weakness, winged scapulae, difficulty in closing the eyes, sucking, blowing, and whistling. Extraocular and pharyngeal muscles are spared. *Associations:* Foot drop (anterior tibialis weakness); high-frequency hearing loss. *Joseph J Dejerine, 1849–1917 (French neurologist); Louis TJ Landouzy, 1845–1917 (French physician)*

Laurence–Moon syndrome $\frac{\text{Autosomal}}{\text{recessive}}$ Retinitis pigmentosa, obesity, polydactyly, hypogenitalism, ↓IQ, ↓body hair, azoospermia (♂), learning disability, speech delay, and renal abnormalities (calyceal clubbing, cysts, or diverticula; end-stage renal failure in 15%). It is distinct from Bardet–Biedl syndrome, p638 (no polydactyly). *John Z Laurence, 1829–1870; Robert C Moon, 1844–1914 (British ophthalmologists)*

Leber's hereditary optic atrophy Bilateral, painless, irreversible blindness occurring in young adults (♂:♀=4:1), caused by mutations in mitochondrial DNA (transmitted by maternal inheritance). **Idebenone** may help.[33]
Theodor Karl Gustav von Leber, 1840–1917 (German ophthalmologist)

Lesch–Nyhan syndrome $\frac{\text{X-linked}}{\text{recessive}}$ Deficiency of hypoxanthine-guanine phosphoribosyl transferase (HPRT) causes 3 problems: **1** *Uric acid overproduction:* Hyperuricaemia (orange crystals in the nappy) causing renal stones ± renal failure, and gout. **2** *CNS:* Motor delay, IQ↓ (eg <65), severe generalized dystonia ± choreoathetosis and fits. **3** *Behavioural problems:* Cognitive impairment, persistent and severe self-injurious behaviour (lip/foot biting, head banging, face scratching). Smiling aggression to others may occur. *Δ:* Measurement of HPRT enzyme activity. Diagnosis is confirmed by identifying a mutation in the HPRT gene. Nearly all cases are in males. *Prognosis:* Death is usually before 40yrs, from renal failure or infection. Sudden death may occur. *R̠:* Good hydration (urine flow↑); **allopurinol** prevents urate stones, but not CNS signs. Protective devices to prevent self–injury. Deep brain stimulation can stop self-injurious behaviour.[34] Milder variants exist. *Michael Lesch, 1939–2008; William L Nyhan, b1926 (US physicians)*

Lewy body dementia Dementia with intracytoplasmic neuronal inclusion bodies (fig **10.10**) in brainstem/cortex + fluctuating cognitive impairment, parkinsonism, hallucinations, & visuoperceptual deficits. *R̠:* Cholinesterase inhibitors (eg **rivastigmine**). Overlap with Alzheimer's and Parkinson's disease makes treatment hard as antiparkinsonian agents can precipitate delusions, and antipsychotics worsen parkinsonism.[35] *Friedrich H Lewy, 1885–1950 (German neurologist)*

Li-Fraumeni syndrome $\frac{\text{Autosomal}}{\text{dominant}}$ A familial cancer predisposition syndrome in which patients are at risk for a wide variety of malignancies. It devastates families, but fascinates geneticists due to germ-line mutations of the tumour suppressor gene TP53; see BOX. *Frederick P Li, b1940; Joseph F Fraumeni, Jr, b1933 (US physicians)*

Martin-Bell (fragile X) **syndrome** $\frac{\text{X-linked semi}}{\text{dominant}}$ The leading monogenic cause of cognitive impairment (♂1:4000; ♀1:8000). *Cause:* The FMR1 gene (fragile X mental retardation-1) on xq27 includes a CGG-repeat that lengthens as it is passed from generation to generation. Once the repeat exceeds a threshold length (>200), no fragile X protein is made, and disease results. *Signs:* Delayed speech & language; delayed motor milestones (secondary to hypotonia). ↓IQ, hyperactivity, emotional and behavioural problems, anxiety, mood swings, autism, and tactile defensiveness (little eye contact; no hugging). 15% have seizure disorders. *Physical features:* A long narrow face, large ears, prominent jaw, big testes (♂). *Tests:* Molecular genetic testing of FMR1 gene. Prenatal screening is possible. *R̠:* Improvement in general behaviour has been shown with **minocycline**.[36] *James P Martin, 1893–1984 (British physician); Julia Bell 1879–1979 (British geneticist)*

Fig 10.10 Lewy body (arrow). NB: there are no generally accepted biomarkers to distinguish dementia with Lewy bodies (DLB) from other dementias. Think of DLB whenever there is progressive anxiety, depression, apathy, agitation, sleep disorder with psychosis and memory disorders.

The best imaging candidate may be striatal dopamine transporter system scintigraphy using FP-CIT SPECT.[37]

Courtesy of Kondi Wong and the National Human Genome Research Institute.

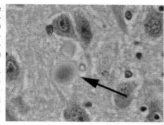

Li–Fraumeni syndrome, p53, and the guardian of the genome

TP53 is a tumour-suppressor gene that codes for p53, a protein that regulates the cell cycle (chromosome 17p13.1; encoding nuclear phosphoprotein, a transcription factor allowing passage through the cell cycle). In Li–Fraumeni syndrome, as only one allele is affected, development is normal until a spontaneous mutation affects the other allele. Somatic mutation of p53 occurs at both alleles in 50–80% of spontaneous human cancers. Cells with a p53 mutation do not pause in G1 (a phase in which DNA repair takes place, and faulty DNA purged), but proceed straight to S1 (DNA replication), which is why p53 protein is known as the 'guardian of the genome'. Examples of cancers caused this way include early-onset breast cancer, brain tumours, sarcomas, leukaemia, lymphoma, melanoma, & adrenal cortex carcinoma.[38]

Note that tumours are associated with more than one syndrome, eg adrenal cortex tumours are associated with familial cancer syndromes such as the Beckwith–Wiedemann and Li–Fraumeni syndromes, the Carney complex, multiple endocrine neoplasia type 1, congenital adrenal hyperplasia, and the McCune–Albright syndrome (p650).[39]

In a retrospective study of 200 cancer-affected carriers of TP53 germline mutations, 15% developed a 2nd cancer, 4% a 3rd cancer, and 2% a 4th cancer. In some populations (eg in South Brazil) there is a high prevalence of otherwise rare mutations in p53, partly explaining high rates of colon and other cancers (eg fatal stomach cancers in children as young as 12).[40]

McCune–Albright syndrome ≥2 of: **1** Polyosteotic fibrous dysplasia of bone, **2** Irregular areas of skin pigmentation, **3** Autonomous endocrine hyperfunction (eg precocious puberty). See fig 10.11 and BOX.

Donovan J McCune, 1902–1976; Fuller Albright, 1900–1969 (US physicians)

Monteggia fracture Fracture of the proximal ⅓ of ulna, with dislocation of the radial head (IV types). *Giovanni Battista Monteggia, 1762–1815 (Italian surgeon)*

Morquio's syndrome (mucopolysaccharidosis IV) $\frac{Autosomal}{recessive}$ Lysosomal storage disease caused by GALNS gene mutation (type A) or β-galactosidase gene mutation (type B). Overlapping clinical features of short stature and skeletal dysplasia, with no CNS involvement & normal IQ. *Luis Morquio, 1867–1935 (Uruguayan paediatrician)*

Niemann–Pick disease (sphingomyelinase deficiency) $\frac{Autosomal}{recessive}$ A neurovisceral lysosomal lipid storage disorder. *Type A:* Early-onset, rapidly progressive neurodegenerative course, systemic disease, and death in early childhood. *Type B:* Traditionally non-neuronopathic, milder, with later onset and variable severity (often detected by hepatosplenomegaly or lung symptoms). Δ: Sphingomyelinase activity in peripheral blood white cells; targeted gene mutation analysis.[41]

Albert Niemann, 1880–1921 (German paediatrician); Ludwick Pick, 1868–1944 (German pathologist)

Noonan syndrome $\frac{Autosomal}{dominant}$ A multisystem disorder characterized by short stature, characteristic facial features (ptosis, down-slanting eyes, low-set ears), congenital heart defects (in 50%, most commonly hypertrophic cardiomyopathy and pulmonary stenosis), ± chest and spine deformities, webbed neck, clotting disorders, and learning disability. *Cause:* 4 disease-causing mutations in the RAS-MAPK signalling pathway (a regulator of cell growth) have been identified.[42] *Prevalence:* 1:2500. *Jacqueline Anne Noonan, b1928 (US paediatric cardiologist)*

Ondine's curse (congenital central hypoventilation syndrome) Autonomic dysfunction causes central alveolar hypoventilation and apnoea (especially during sleep). There is variable requirement for ventilatory support. *Cause:* PHOX2B gene mutation. Ondine was a nymph who sacrificed her immortality by falling in love with a prince who promised to honour her with every waking breath. When the prince lost interest, Ondine uttered her curse: 'for as long as you are awake, you shall breathe. But should you ever fall asleep, that breath will desert you'.

Othello syndrome (delusional jealousy) A lover has a fixed belief that their partner is being sexually unfaithful. They may go to great lengths to provide delusional 'evidence' to back up this belief (engaging a spy; examining underwear). *Associations:* Alcohol, schizophrenia, depression, frontal lobe dysfunction, dementia. ►Get psychiatric help: jealousy is the most deadly of all the passions and there is a significant association with violence. In Shakespeare's play, Othello murdered his wife as a result of a false belief that she had been unfaithful (but he was deceived rather than deluded—so did Othello actually have the Othello syndrome?).[43] *Othello, 1603–∞ (Described in 1955 by John Todd, British psychiatrist)*

Patau's syndrome (trisomy 13) Cleft lip & palate (± other midline facial defects), microcephaly, neural tube defects, omphalocele, hernias, cardiac defects (seen in 80%, eg patent ductus arteriosus, VSD ± dextrocardia). Hands show flexion contractures ± polydactyly. *Typical survival:* A few days; 5% survive >6 months. *Prevalence:* 1 in 7500 births.[44] *Klaus Patau, 1908–1975 (German born US geneticist)*

Pick's dementia Early-onset progressive frontotemporal dementia. 15:100,000 aged 45–64yrs. *Signs:* Before cognitive loss, look for: personality change, social disinhibition, emotional blunting, impaired insight, dietary changes, perseverative behaviours (eg drinking from an empty cup). *Tests:* MRI. ℞: AChEIs unlikely to be beneficial. *Arnold Pick, 1851–1924 (Czech neurologist & psychiatrist)*

Pierre Robin syndrome (AKA PR sequence) A *sequence* of events due to a small mandible (± cleft palate), causing posterior tongue displacement and airway obstruction + poor neonatal feeding. ℞: Prevent the tongue slipping back by prone positioning; surgery if severe airway compromise. *Pierre Robin, 1867–1950 (French dentist)*

In the McCune–Albright syndrome (MAS), precocious puberty is not the only endocrinopathy: hyperthyroidism and Cushing's also occur. In the case of the 'Taiwanese giant' (an unfortunate name for a 14-year-old), excess growth hormone production has also been found.[45] Deformities, fractures, and pain further complicate the picture (pain can be relieved by bisphosphonates). The craniofacial fibrous dysplasia may encroach on the optic nerve, causing visual problems.

Precocious puberty in MAS is gonadotropin-independent and does not respond to GNRH agonists (but they may be used as adjuncts to treatment). The largely experimental treatment for precocious puberty includes aromatase inhibitors for females (which block the effects of oestrogen), and anti-androgen (eg spironolactone) + aromatase inhibitors for males.

The cause may be a mutation of the GNAS1 gene coding the α subunit of the stimulatory guanine-nucleotide binding protein, G-protein, which activates adenylate cyclase ($\therefore$ ↑intracellular cyclic AMP).[46]

Eponymous syndromes

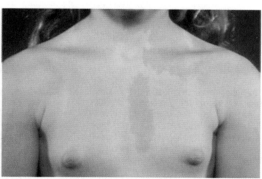

Fig 10.11 Hyperpigmented café-au-lait macules (which frequently predominate on one side of the body without crossing the midline) and gonadotropin-independent precocious puberty in a young female with McCune–Albright syndrome.

Reproduced with permission from Mehta A, Hindmarch P. Precocious Puberty. BMJ *Best Practice* Copyright © 2014 BMJ. http://bestpractice.bmj.com/best-practice/monograph/1127.html

Pompe disease (glycogen storage disease–II; acid maltase deficiency) _{Autosomal recessive}
Glycogen accumulation in lysosomes due to ↓lysosomal $α_{1,4}$-glucosidase activity causes myopathy and systemic disease. 3 forms. 1 *Infantile:* Progressive and rapidly fatal if untreated. There is hypotonia, cardiomyopathy, respiratory distress, & failure to thrive. 2 *Juvenile:* Delayed motor milestones, weakness, & hypotonia. 3 *Adult:* Proximal weakness ± respiratory symptoms. Glycogen accumulates in heart, muscle, liver, CNS, & kidneys. *R:* Alglucosidase alfa prolongs life and can reverse cardiomyopathy. *Joannes Cassianus Pompe, 1901–1945 (Dutch pathologist)*

Prader–Willi syndrome (PWS) *Cause:* Loss of paternal contribution of the proximal part of the long arm of chromosome 15. *Prevalence:* 1:25,000. *Signs: Infancy:* Hypotonia, poor feeding, genital hypoplasia, delayed motor milestones. *Childhood:* Hyperphagia with progressive obesity; food seeking behaviour (eg shop-lifting food, eating spoiled foods); short stature; behavioural problems, eg obsessive–compulsive traits; psychosis in 5–10%; ↓IQ. *Δ:* Chromosomal analysis. *Andrea Prader, 1919–2001; Heinrich Willi, 1900–1971 (Swiss paediatricians)*

Ramsay Hunt syndrome (herpes zoster oticus) This is herpes zoster infection of the facial nerve. Often in the elderly, severe otalgia precedes VII cranial nerve palsy (± VII, IX, V, VI in order of frequency). Zoster vesicles appear around the ear, in the deep meatus (± soft palate & tongue, fig 10.12). There may be vertigo, tinnitus, or deafness. *R:* Aciclovir + prednisolone. *James Ramsay Hunt, 1872–1937 (US neurologist)*

Rett syndrome A neurodegenerative disorder occurring almost exclusively in females. After initially normal perinatal development there is neurological regression. 4 stages: 1 *Developmental arrest* (6–18 months): Developmental delay, hand wringing, ↓head growth. 2 *Rapid regression* (1–4yrs): Loss of acquired skills, hand sterotypies, autistic behaviour, seizures, breathing irregularities. 3 *Pseudostationary* (2–10yrs): Some improvement in behaviour/communication. 4 *Late motor deterioration* (>10yrs): Slow motor regression. *Cause:* Monogenic x-linked dominant disorder due to mutations in MECP2 gene.[47] *Andreas Rett, 1924–1997 (Austrian paediatrician)*

Reye's syndrome Acute encephalopathy and liver failure occurs days after a febrile viral illness (eg URTI, varicella, influenza). Aspirin intake is a risk factor and there was a dramatic decline in incidence of the disease following its association. *Tests:* Transaminases↑; blood ammonia↑ (correlates with survival); INR↑; glucose↓ (none are specific). Liver biopsy: swollen, pleomorphic mitochondria (ATP↓, gluconeogenesis & ureagenesis↓). *CT:* Cerebral oedema; but may be normal. *ΔΔ:* Inborn errors of metabolism. *Prognosis:* Mortality <20%; full recovery in >60%.[48] *Ralph Douglas Kenneth Reye, 1912–1977 (Australian pathologist)*

Russell–Silver syndrome A clinical and genetically heterogeneous congenital disorder, characterized by severe intrauterine and postnatal growth retardation, dysmorphic facial features, small stature and relative macrocephaly. *Cause:* Genetic and epigenetic alteration can be detected in around half of all cases, including hypomethylation in the chromosome 11p15 imprinting centre, and maternal uniparental disomy (inheritance of both alleles from the mother) of chromosome 7. *Prognosis:* Relatively good. Growth hormone improves linear growth. *Alexander Russell, 1914–2003 (British paediatrician); Henry K. Silver, 1918–1991 (US paediatrician)*

Shakhonovich's syndrome (hypokalaemic periodic paralysis) _{Autosomal dominant} Recurrent attacks of flaccid paralysis triggered by emotional stress, carbohydrate loads, & rest after exercise. Duration and frequency of attacks varies greatly. Speech, eye movements, & swallowing are not affected. *Onset:* ~7–21yrs. *Signs:* During attacks, muscles feel firmer than usual. Reflexes: diminished. *Genes:* Mis-sense mutations of CACNA1S (type 1) & SCN4A genes (type 2) affecting the voltage sensor of the transmembrane segment of Ca^{2+} channels (type 1) and Na^+ channels (type 2). *Tests during attacks:* $^{s+}K^+$↓; PO_4^{3-}↓; urate↑; WCC↑; glycosuria. *R:* IVI/oral K^+ can help; acetazolamide prevents some attacks, depending on genetic diagnosis. *Genetic counselling.* *ΔΔ:* Hypokalaemic thyrotoxic periodic paralysis.[49] *Who was Shakhonovich?*

Prader-Willi syndrome (pws), imprinting, and epigenetics

Chromosome 15q11–q13 is a critical region for pws, which results from loss of expression of paternally expressed genes at this site. Angelman syndrome, a rare disorder characterized by severe physical and intellectual disability, seizures, and frequent laughter, occurs from loss of maternally expressed genes at the same locus. But how do our genes know where they come from?

pws was the first human disorder attributed to genomic imprinting, where certain genes can be expressed in a parent-specific manner. Normally, we inherit 2 copies of a gene, one from each parent, and both copies shape how we develop. In genomic imprinting, one copy of a gene is inactivated. If the remaining functional gene is defective, this may cause disease. The processes whereby genes can be activated or deactivated is referred to as epigenetic. In general, methylation of the DNA in a gene will cause that gene to be inactivated whereas acetylation of histones (simple proteins around which DNA is coiled) can activate inactive genes. Such changes, known as imprints, appear prior to germ cell (sperm or oocyte) maturation, and hence in the embryo.[50] Russell Silver syndrome and Beckwith–Wiedemann syndrome are other examples of imprinting disorders.[1]

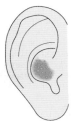 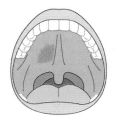 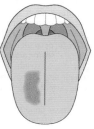

Fig 10.12 Shingles is generally a disease of sensory nerves, however Ramsay Hunt syndrome is distinctive in that there is a motor component causing facial paralysis. The rash of herpetic blisters is in the distribution of the *nervus intermedius* (part of the facial nerve) and may include the anterior two-thirds of the tongue, the soft palate, the external auditory canal, and auricle.

1 Our thanks to Dr Guy Bradley-Smith for his advice on this section.

Still's disease (systemic-onset juvenile idiopathic arthritis/sJIA) Accounts for ~10% of all JIA and presents with systemic upset and spiking fevers that typically occur around the same time once or twice each day. There is arthralgia and generalized myalgia. Fever spikes are usually accompanied by a salmon–pink macular (often linear) rash on the trunk and limbs. There may be hepatosplenomegaly & lymphadenopathy (esp. axillary). Serositis causes chest pain or shortness of breath (± pleural and pericardial effusions).[51] *Other subgroups:* Juvenile ankylosing spondylitis; psoriatic arthritis; ulcerative colitis-associated arthritis; juvenile-onset rheumatoid arthritis—here Rh factor is +ve, and systemic upset is rarer. There is also *adult-onset Still's disease.* *Tests:* WCC↑; ESR↑; CRP↑ (≈poor response); Hb↓; ferritin↑; LFT↑; albumin↓; echo. ℞: The goal is to prevent joint damage & loss of function and control pain. A multi-disciplinary approach is used and includes physiotherapists, OTs, dieticians, & counsellors. Medication is aimed at inducing remission. NSAIDs may be adequate for patients with low disease activity. Systemic corticosteroids (eg **prednisolone**) have a short-term role. **Methotrexate** is used in those with ongoing active disease. **Tocilizumab** (IL-6 receptor blocker that results in decreased inflammatory cytokine production) is the 1st-line biologic therapy for those intolerant of or not responding to methotrexate._{NICE} The IL-1 receptor antagonist **anakinra** is also effective. *Sir George Frederick Still, 1868–1941 (British paediatrician)*

Sydenham's chorea (St Vitus dance) A neurological manifestation of acute rheumatic fever (p166) and the chief cause of chorea in children. It may be the *only* feature, appearing up to 6 months after clinical signs of strep infection have abated. *Pathogenesis:* Thought to involve molecular mimicry with *Streptococcus*-induced antibodies cross-reacting with antigens of the basal ganglia. *Motor signs:* Involuntary purposeless movement, worsened by stress and disappearing on sleep, with clumsiness, grimacing, a darting lizard's tongue and unclear speech. *Non-motor features:* Include obsessions, compulsions, attention deficit, ↓verbal fluency, ↓executive function.[53] The term PANDAS (Paediatric Autoimmune Neuropsychiatric Disorder Associated with *streptococcus*) denotes a putative subset of obsessive–compulsive disorder and Tourette's syndrome (OHCM p714) that bears some resemblance to Sydenham's chorea. ΔΔ: Wilson's disease, juvenile Huntington's, thyrotoxicosis, SLE, polycythaemia, Na⁺↓, hypoparathyroidism, kernicterus, phenytoin, neuroleptics, hereditary chorea. ℞: Spontaneous remission occurs in the majority. **Sodium valproate** can help control chorea. Despite treating active and recurrent strep infections vigorously, chorea may persist. *Thomas Sydenham, 1624–1689 (British physician)*

Syme's amputation Amputation of the foot through the articulation of the ankle with removal of the malleoli. *James Syme, 1799–1870 (Scottish surgeon)*

Tay–Sachs disease _{recessive}^{Autosomal} Type I GM2 gangliosidosis affecting ~1:4000 Ashkenazi Jewish births (1:320,000 in the general population). Decreased lysosomal hexosaminidase A enzyme activity results in accumulation of gangliosides in neurons and progressive neurodegeneration. Low levels of enzyme are detectable in carriers. Children are normal until ~6 months old, when developmental delay, photophobia, hyperacusis, and irritability occur. There is progression to uncontrolled seizures, spasticity, blindness, and dementia. Death occurs at ~3–5yrs, typically from pneumonia. Δ: HEX A enzyme activity; DNA analysis. *Ophthalmoscopy:* Cherry-red spot at macula. The condition is now rare due to genetic screening, prenatal diagnosis (made by amniocentesis), & pre-implantation genetic diagnosis. *Warren Tay 1843–1927 (British ophthalmologist); Bernard Sachs, 1858–1944 (US neurologist)*

Tolosa–Hunt syndrome Painful ophthalmoplegia and ipsilateral ocular motor nerve palsies, from non-specific granulomatous inflammation in the cavernous sinus or superior orbital fissure. The cause is unknown. MRI may show inflammatory changes. Corticosteroids are the treatment of choice, but may not resolve ophthalmoparesis. *Eduardo Tolosa 1900–1981 (Spanish neurosurgeon); William E Hunt, 1921–1999 (US neurosurgeon)*

Treacher Collins syndrome (mandibulofacial dysostosis) ^{Autosomal dominant} Craniofacial deformities with characteristic flattening of malar bones, hypoplastic zygoma, micrognathia, cleft palate, oblique palpebral fissures, external ear anomalies and conductive hearing loss. *Cause:* TCOF1 gene mutations. *Reconstructive surgery* is an option. *Edward Treacher Collins, 1862–1932 (British ophthalmologist)*

Turner's syndrome 45 X0 monosomy in 40–60% or mosaic pattern in remaining karyotypes, eg 45,X/46,XX or 45,X/47,XXX. *Prevalence:* 1:2000 girls. *Signs: Newborn:* lymphoedema of the hands & feet; cardiac and renal abnormalities (coarctation of aorta; absent kidney). *Infancy:* short stature, webbed neck, behavioural difficulties, recurrent otitis media, and hearing loss. *Adolescence:* Gonadal dysgenesis (streak ovary) results in absent or incomplete puberty, amenorrhoea and impaired growth. Δ: Chromosomal analysis. *Association:* Autoimmune disease (screen for thyroid disorders, diabetes, & coeliac disease). ℞: Recombinant human growth hormone is used to treat short stature. Supplemental oestrogen (started ~12yrs) initiates pubertal development and prevents osteoporosis. Treatment is progressed to maintenance with larger oestrogen doses cycled with progesterone (eg as COCP). Surveillance and screening of cardiac, renal, ENT, & autoimmune problems. Psychological support. Almost all affected women are infertile but pregnancy with donor embryos is possible.[54] *Henry Turner, 1892–1970 (US endocrinologist)*

Ulysses syndrome After the Trojan war, Ulysses decided to come home, but it took him 10 years and many perilous and perhaps pointless adventures before he returned to his starting place. Similarly, our patients with Ulysses syndrome find themselves caught in a web of further investigations, referrals, and sometimes treatment before finally being recognized as healthy, which they were in the first place. It is a side effect of unnecessary and inappropriate investigations or wrong interpretation of results. Patients start out with a problem, and end with the same problem, after many risky and futile tests have advanced their case not one bit, as we have not had the courage to say: 'Let's not *do* anything'. *Described by Mercer Rang, 1933–2003 (British paediatric orthopaedic surgeon)*

Von Gierke's syndrome (type 1a glycogen storage disease; GSD 1a) ^{Autosomal recessive} Glucose-6-phosphatase deficiency blocks the final steps of glycogenolysis and gluconeogenesis causing clinically significant end-organ disease. Δ: Mutation analysis of G6PC gene. *Signs:* Hepatomegaly (glycogen & fat accumulation), renomegaly, growth retardation, hypoglycaemia, hyperuricaemia, failure to thrive, dyslipidaemia, xanthomata over joints and buttocks, and platelet dysfunction. ℞: Diet therapy to prevent hypoglycaemia. *Complications:* Hepatic adenoma; hepatocellular cancer; kidney disease.[55] *Edgar Otto Conrad von Gierke, 1877–1945 (German pathologist)*

Werner syndrome (WS; progeria) ^{Autosomal recessive} The commonest premature ageing syndrome. *Signs:* Lack of pubertal growth spurt & scleroderma; prematurely aged appearance (20–30yrs old) + typical associated problems: loss or greying of hair, cataracts, dyslipidaemia, diabetes, atherosclerosis, and ↑malignancy. The complex molecular and cellular phenotypes of WS involve features of genomic instability and accelerated replicative senescence. The gene involved (WRN) has been cloned, and its gene product (WRNP) is a helicase. Helicases play important roles in a variety of DNA transactions, including DNA replication, transcription, repair, and recombination, and in WS unwinding of DNA pairs is disordered.[56] ℞: None specific; treat related problems. *C. W. Otto Werner, 1879–1936 (German physician)*

Wiskott–Aldrich syndrome (WAS) ^{X-linked recessive} A severe primary immunodeficiency (p198) with eczema, recurrent infections, thrombocytopenia, autoimmune disorders, IgA nephropathy ± haematopoietic neoplasia. Platelets are too few and too small. Without marrow transplant, most die before adulthood. Prenatal diagnosis is possible. ℞: *Antibiotics* ± IV immunoglobulin for infections. Haematopoietic stem cell transplant is 1st-choice therapy. Gene therapy is awaited. *Alfred Wiskott, 1898–1978 (German paediatrician); Robert A Aldrich, 1917–1998 (US paediatrician)*

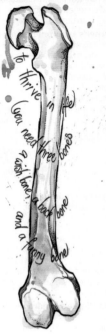

Fig 11.1 Quote from Reba Mcentire: 'To thrive in life you need three bones; A Wish bone, a Back bone and a Funny bone.'

© Gillian Turner.

Orthopaedics offers a vast range of fascinating applications which can capture every medical interest. Attention to detail and addressing the individual needs of each patient is critical to any orthopaedic intervention as we strive to restore and preserve normal function of the musculoskeletal system. It is easy to look at a single joint in isolation, yet the masters of this speciality are able to take a step back and optimize the entire body structure. Orthopaedic surgery embraces the entire patient journey from diagnostic assessment, operative interventions, and rehabilitation. Knowledge of anatomy is therefore key; you won't be able to identify the abnormal if you don't know what normal is!

Further reading and other relevant pages

www.orthoworld.com
www.anatomy.tv
Metabolic bone disease: OHCM p698;

www.wheelessonline.com
www.e-anatomy.org
Rheumatology: OHCM p540–65;
Trauma management: Chapters 12 and 13

We thank our Specialist Reader Mr Chris Peach for reviewing this chapter. We also thank Mr Jamie A'Court, and Mr Yousaf Khan for their invaluable contributions. The work of our junior readers Mayooreshan Anandarajah and Raj Dattani is also much appreciated.

For the reflexes (p744):
1,2 Buckle my shoe *S1/S2* Ankle
3,4 Kick the door *L3/L4* Knee
5,6 Pick up sticks *C5/C6* Biceps & Brachioradialis
7,8 Shut the gate *C7/C8* Triceps
Serratus anterior is supplied by the long thoracic nerve.
C5, 6, & 7 Raise your arms up to heaven (Nerve root for Long Thoracic Nerve)

Musculocutaneous nerve supplies the 'BBC' (p744):
Biceps, **B**rachialis, & **C**oracobrachialis

Superficial forearm flexors: **P**layers **F**ollow **P**imps **F**or **F**un:
Pronator teres, **F**lexor Carpi Radialis **P**almaris longus, **F**lexor carpi ulnaris, **F**lexor digitorum superficialis

Radial nerve supplies the 'BREAST':
Brachio**R**adialis, **E**xtensors, **A**nconeus, **S**upinator, **T**riceps

Median nerve in the hand supplies 'LOAF' (p749):
Lateral 2 lumbricals, **O**pponens pollicis, **A**bductor pollicis brevis, **F**lexor pollicis brevis

The hand interossei: 'PAD/DAB': **P**almar **AD**duct, **D**orsal **A**bduct

Hand deformities: 'DR CUMA' (p744):
Drop wrist **R**adial nerve, **C**law hand **U**lnar nerve, **M**edian nerve **A**pe hand

Femoral sheath: 'NAVeL': **N**erve, **A**rtery, **V**ein, (empty space), **L**ymph nodes

Femoral triangle: **S**o **I** **M**ay **A**lways **L**ove **S**urgery:
Superior (**I**nguinal), **M**edial (**A**dductor longus), **L**ateral (**S**artorius)

External hip rotators: **P**retty **G**irls **O**ften **G**row **O**ld **Q**uickly:
Piriformis, **G**emellus **S**uperior, **O**bturator internus, **G**emellus inferior, **O**bturator externus, **Q**uadratus femoris

Foot evertors: E: p**E**rineus longus/br**E**vis/t**E**rtius

Foot invertors: I: t**I**bialis posterior/anterior

Structures behind medial malleolus: **T**om, **D**ick and **A** **V**ery **N**ervous **H**arry
Tibialis posterior, **F**lexor **D**igitorum longus, **A**rtery (posterior tibial), **V**ein (posterior tibial), **N**erve (posterior tibial), **F**lexor hallucis longus (fig 11.61, p711)

Paediatric bone fractures—Star Wars 'GO C3PO' (p727):
Greenstick, **O**pen, **C**omplete, **C**losed, **C**omminuted, **P**athological, **O**thers (epiphysis)

Salter–Harris fractures: I–V—SALTR *(in relation to epiphysis)* (p719):
Separation, **A**bove, **L**ower, **T**hrough, **R**ammed (Compression)

CRITOL: *age of ossification in paediatric elbow* (p719):
Capitellum: 1 year
Radial head: 3 years
Internal (medial) epicondyle: 5 years
Trochlea: 7 years
Outer (lateral) epicondyle: 9 years
OLecranon: 11 years

x-ray features of OA: LOSS (p683):
Loss of joint space, **O**steophytes, **S**ubchondral sclerosis and **S**ubchondral cysts.

Orthopaedics

Typical presenting features of musculoskeletal disease

- Trauma
- Sequalae from previous trauma
- Pain (traumatic or atraumatic)[1]
- Deformity
- Swelling
- Weakness
- Loss of function
- Stiffness
- Neurological.

A patient's report of pain, stiffness, swelling, and weakness/loss of function are key components of any orthopaedic story. Careful dissection of details within these sections is required.

Questions to ask Any recent or past trauma to site? Hand dominance? Assessment of the patient's baseline function and expectations is also essential, is she expecting to regain the ability to perform fine needlework? Occupation and hand dominance plays a major role, is he a professional piano player reliant on fine finger movements or a builder dependent on physical strength?[2] General health ok? If aches and pains all over, is it fibromyalgia or polymyalgia?

Medical conditions affecting orthopaedic function (See Chapter 12, OHCM.)

Mnemonic: RPT—MSK—DHS [3]

- **R**heumatic fever (or childhood arthritis)
- **P**soriasis (think of psoriatic arthritis)
- **T**B (affects joints as well)
- **M**usculo**s**keletal disorders (such as SLE, hypermobility, bone malignancy, osteoarthritis)
- **D**iabetes
- **H**ypo/**H**yperthyroidism and other metabolic bone disease
- **S**exually transmitted diseases such as reactive arthritis (Reiter's syndrome).

Also consider:

- Medications (eg steroids aggravating osteoporosis and subsequent bisphosphonate treatment)
- Smoking (reduced healing time)
- Neuromuscular disease.

'Look, Feel, Move' and special tests

Going through clinical examination with an expert is the best way to learn, but this experience can be reinforced by taking principles and background reading with you into the arena. Most orthopaedic examinations can be developed by following the 'LOOK, FEEL, MOVE' structure.

- **LOOK** for deformity and resting joint position, skin changes (scars/erythema/bruising) and soft tissues (muscle wasting/swelling/contractures)
- **FEEL** for anatomical landmarks, warmth, swelling, and tenderness. Allow patient to actively
- **MOVE** joint first before you assess passive range of movement and power (see MRC scale). With respect to movement limitation: *active loss* = neuromuscular deficit; *passive loss* = bony/soft tissue is blocking movement.

Special tests Finally assess joint function and include any special tests (eg knee meniscal tests, hip fixed flexion deformities). Establish neurovascular status by cappillary refill time (CRT) and sensation/power of local nerves.

Key points • Always examine *the joint above* and *below* the joint being examined, ie for the hip, examine the knee and lumbar spine. This will uncover any referring pathology. • Always compare with the same joint on the other side • Assess the neurovascular status (especially in trauma) • Exposure should be appropriate but remember to respect patient dignity.

---

1 Use SOCRATES to help take a history of pain. Site, Onset (Sudden, gradual), Character (Ache? Stabbing? Burning?) Radiation, Associated symptoms, Time (when did it start), Excerbating/Releiving factors, Severity (use a scale out of 10).
2 Be aware of patient expectations. *Patient:* Will I be able to play the piano after these bandages come off? *Doctor:* Yes, you can expect full recovery *Patient:* Great! I've never been able to play the piano....
3 See p734 for why the acronym DHS will stick in your mind!

Quantifying strength: The UK MRC scale objectives strength (reasonably well):	
Grade 0 No muscle contraction	**Grade 3** Active movement against gravity but not against resistance
Grade 1 Flicker of contraction	**Grade 4** Active movement against resistance but not achieving full power.
Grade 2 Active movement with gravity eliminated	**Grade 5** Normal power

Grades 4−, 4, and 4+ describe movement against slight, moderate, and strong resistance. To test proximal muscle power: ask patient to sit from lying and to rise from squatting. ►Observe gait (easy to forget, even if the complaint is of walking difficulty!). See p682 and *OHCM* p471 for gait disorders.

When you examine, it's useful to have a picture in your mind's eye of the pathology you are looking for and which investigations could help. Here are the *Ottawa ankle rules* (Fig 11.2); a decision aid for excluding fractures of the ankle and mid-foot. They have a sensitivity of almost 100%, which allow you to confidently rule out fractures in ankle sprains without the need for an x-ray. As a consequence though, the specificity is somewhat lower. In this case, specificity is an indicator of the number of unnecessary x-rays which could be avoided if following these rules.

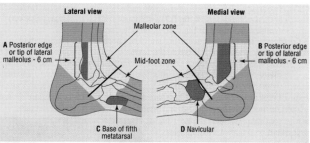

Fig 11.2 Use the Ottawa ankle rules to guide the need for an x-ray. Ankle x-rays are required only if there is pain in the malleolar zone and tenderness at either point *A*, point *B*, or inability to weightbear both immediately and in the ED. Foot x-rays are required if there is pain in the midfoot zone and tenderness at either point *C*, point *D*, or inability to weightbear both immediately and in the ED. Reproduced from *The BMJ*, Bachmann et al., volume 326, issue 7386, p.417, copyright notice 2003 with permission from BMJ Publishing Group Ltd.

Three wise men

Reaching the correct diagnosis can be difficult and this paper² gives a very thought provoking overview in the diagnostic challenges faced in clinical medicine. Diagnostic errors are the leading cause of litigation in the USA. Is this new lesion a metastases from the existing lung cancer or is it a new primary? The answer dictates your treatment. The authors draw inspiration from three wise men. *Occam's razor* states that a single unifying diagnosis is likely the cause of all the symptoms. In contrast, *Hickam's dictum* quotes that 'patients can have as many diseases as they damn well please'. *Crabtree's bludgeon* puts the latter two into perspective and reminds us of the risk of ignoring key facts as we insist on finding evidence to support our ideal diagnosis instead. How many times have you diagnosed a rarity and then enthusiastically searched the case notes to find further evidence to back your claim, whilst ignoring features supportive of another theory? As patients live longer and chronic diseases are more prevalent, Hickam's dictum may be more appropriate and Occam's razor better applied to the younger, healthier population. Reflect on those approaches as embark on your own diagnostic journey (see p478).

Orthopaedics

▶▶If you suspect a cervical spine injury, immobilize the neck with 3-point immo-bilization: hard collar, sandbags, and tape. NB: if very restless, use hard collar only, as otherwise the neck is vulnerable when the body moves on an immobilized head (see p753 for advice on when to image the c-spine; p716 for x-ray requests).

Imaging Supervise all movements closely during transport to radiology. If there is a spinal cord injury, and the patient is stable, CT is the first line of imaging. Image the whole spine as there may be more than one injury. MRI shows fractures, subluxations, disc disruption and protrusion, and cord contusion—and helps es-tablish prognosis. ▶NB: it is hard to arrange in emergency settings, and takes a lot longer than CT (eg 20min vs 20s). Consider CT myelography if MRI is contraindicated.
When examining the image, follow 4 simple steps (ABCS):
1 *Alignment:* Check alignment of the following: •Anterior vertebral bodies
•Posterior vertebral bodies •Posterior spinal canal •Spinous processes (fig 11.4).
    • A step >3mm is abnormal (<25%=unifacet; >50%=bifacet dislocation).
    • Atlas–dens interval (ADI)—normal if <3mm (adults) or <5mm (children).
    • 40% of <7-yr-olds have anterior displacement C2 on C3 (in this pseu-do-subluxation the posterior spinal line is maintained).
2 *Bone contour:* Trace around each vertebra individually.
    • Anterior/posterior height difference of >3mm (implies *wedge fracture*). In general <25% difference is stable and >25% difference is unstable.
    • Pedicles (*hangman's #*, fig 11.7) & spinous processes (*clayshoveller's #*).
    • Avulsion fractures of the vertebral body (*teardrop #*).
3 *Cartilages:* The disc space margins should be parallel (>11° is abnormal).
4 *Soft tissues:* Check the soft tissue shadows:
    • Retropharyngeal—C1–C3 <7mm; C4–C7 <22mm/1 vertebral body (fig 11.5).
    • Spinous process separation (interspinous ligament rupture). CT can help diagnose fractures here.

▶All 7 cervical vertebrae must be seen, along with the C7–T1 junction: do not accept an incomplete image—a 'swimmers' view of C7–T1 may be needed.

▶A cross-table lateral in the best hands will still miss at least 15% of injuries.

Other views and investigations
• Open mouth 'peg' view (OMV, fig 11.6) for suspected odontoid peg fractures and C1 fractures (*total* lateral mass over-hang of C1 on C2 should be <8mm).
• CT is used to image areas not adequate-ly assessed on plain films (p779).
• MRI is vital for assessing ligamentous disruption, disc prolapse, and the neu-ral elements (spinal cord and nerve roots), all of which can only be inferred from CT and plain x-ray. Whole spine as-sessment is best.

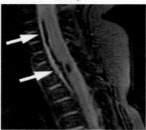

Fig 11.3 An 11-month-old with a normal CT neck on admission, developed paraplegia 6 hours after his stroller was hit by a car. An urgent MRI was performed; T1 weight-ed image showing anterior subdural haemorrhage from C2 to C7 (arrows).

Reproduced with permission from Silman, Langdorf, Rudkin, Lotfipour, Pediatric Spinal Cord Injury without Radiographic Abnormality, *Western Journal of Emergency Medicine,* © 2008.

Spinal cord injury without radiological abnormality (SCIWORA) is becoming less common as pathology may be visible on MRI (fig 11.3). It is a condition in which there is a neurological deficit in the absence of a lesion on plain x-rays. It typically occurs in paediatric cervical spine injuries and is treated in the same manner as a spinal fracture with appropriate immobilization and referral. Clinical evidence of the injury in children may be delayed in up to 50%, so always consider spinal cord injury if the mechanism is appropriate.[3]

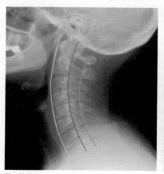
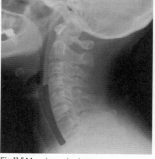

Fig 11.4 The lines to check for discontinuity on a lateral c-spine x-ray:
Yellow = anterior spinal line
Red = posterior spinal line
Green = spinolaminar line
Blue = tips of spinous processes.
Note that we can see all the way to C7–T1.
Courtesy of The Norfolk and Norwich University Hospitals (NNUH) Radiology Dept.

Fig 11.5 More important areas
Yellow = ADI should be <3mm in adults
Red = before C1–C3 should be <7mm
Blue = before C4–C7 should be <22m.
ADI is the distance between the anterior aspect of the odontoid peg and the posterior of the anterior arch of C1.

▶ *Do a detailed neurological examination in all fractures of the c-spine and seek advice from the on-call neurosurgical or spinal team.*

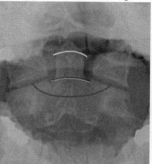
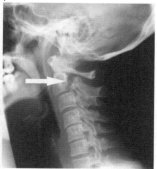

Fig 11.6 Odontoid peg fractures are best seen on the OMV. There are 3 types:
Type I = through the tip (stable)
Type II = through the base (unstable)
Type III = into the body of C2. (?stability)
Remember to check for the overhang of C1 on C2 (<8mm in total). Courtesy of The Norfolk and Norwich University Hospitals (NNUH) Radiology Dept.

Fig 11.7 Lateral x-ray of the c-spine showing a fracture through the pedicles of the C2 vertebra—the hangman's fracture, which is traumatic spondylolisthesis of C2.
Courtesy of Professor Peter Scally.

The paediatric cervical spine

Below the age of ~9yrs, the cervical spine needs to be assessed as an entirely different entity, as it creates very different patterns of normality and abnormality. The most important point to make here is it is best to ask a specialist's opinion—ie ask a Paediatric Radiologist. Nonetheless, remember:
▸▸ Injury is commonest in the upper spine.
▸▸ SCIWORA (see p660).
▸▸ Growth plates (physes) and synchondroses can be mistaken for fractures.
▸▸ C2-3 and C3-4 can demonstrate pseudosubluxation.
▸▸ C7–T1 does not need to be visualized unless ≥9yrs old.

Cervical spondylosis (See *онсм* p512.) Degenerative changes of the cervical spine (eg featuring degeneration of the annulus fibrosus and bony spurs) tend to narrow the spinal canal and intervertebral foramina. Very common: ~90% of men >60yrs and women >50yrs. Usually asymptomatic, but can cause neck and arm pain with paraesthesiae. 5–10% of symptomatic patients develop *cervical myelopathy* (progressive cord compression with spastic weakness). Acute myelopathy requires urgent neurosurgical refferal). See *онсм* p512.

Cervical spondylolisthesis Displacement of one vertebra upon the one below. *Causes:* 1 Congenital failure of fusion of the odontoid process with the axis, or fracture of the odontoid process (skull, atlas, & odontoid process slip forward on axis). 2 Inflammation softens the transverse ligament (fig 11.9) of the atlas (eg rheumatoid or complicating throat infections), so the atlas slips forward on the axis. 3 Instability after injuries. The most important consequence of spondylolisthesis is the possibility of spinal cord compression. Treatments used include traction, immobilization in plaster jackets, and spinal fusion.

Prolapsed cervical disc (See p676, back pain.) Central protrusions (typically C5/6 & C6/7) may give symptoms of spinal cord compression (p756). Posterolateral protrusions may cause a stiff neck, pain radiating to the arm, weakness of muscles affected by the nerve root, and depressed reflexes. *Tests:* MRI is preferred (fig 11.10). *Treatment* is with NSAIDs, and sometimes a collar. As pain subsides, physiotherapy may help to restore mobility. Surgery is occasionally indicated, in the light of CT/MRI findings.

Cervical rib Congenital development of the costal process of the C7 vertebra is often asymptomatic but may cause thoracic outlet compression (figs 11.8 & 11.11). Similar symptoms with no radiological abnormality is called a scalenus or 1st rib syndrome. Thoracic outlet[3] compression involves the lowest trunk of the brachial plexus (fig 12.37, p751) ± the subclavian artery. Pain or numbness may be felt in hand or forearm (often on the ulnar side); there may be hand weakness and muscle wasting (thenar or hypothenar). *Diagnosis:* Weak radial pulse ± forearm cyanosis. Specific manoeuvres (eg Adson's test) are not reliable. x-rays may not reveal cervical ribs, as symptoms may be caused by fibrous bands. Arteriography may show subclavian compression. *Treatment:* Physiotherapy to strengthen the shoulder elevators may improve symptoms, but rib removal or band division may be needed.

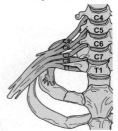

Fig 11.8 Cervical rib causing compression of the inferior trunk of the brachial plexus (p751). The distal part of the rib can also cause stenosis in the subclavian artery, with post-stenotic dilatation (visible on arteriography).

Spasmodic torticollis (cervical dystonia) The commonest adult focal dystonia. Episodes of a sudden stiff painful neck with torticollis are due to trapezius and sternocleidomastoid spasm. Social withdrawal can be a problem. *Causes:* Idiopathic; genetic; trauma. *Treatment:* Is notoriously challenging. 20% experience spontaneous recovery within 5 years of symptoms but generally it is a life-long disorder. Heat, manipulation, relaxants, and analgesia offer limited benefit. Try anticholinergics, benzodiazepines and baclofen. Botulinum toxin (p417) is a safe and effective option.[4] Surgical intervention is becoming more successful and includes selective ramisectomy for cervical musculature, deep brain stimulation from electrodes[5] and selective peripheral denervation of the cervical musculature which participates in the abnormal neck postures.[6] ■ **Infantile torticollis** May result from birth damage to sternocleidomastoid. *Typical age:* 1–36 months. *Treatment:* Self-limiting in 97%. If persistent, physio helps by lengthening the muscle; surgical division is more drastic.[7]

3 The thoracic outlet is the space between the 1st rib and clavicle.

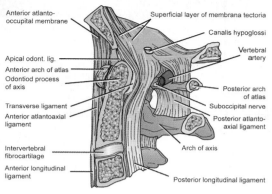

Fig 11.9 Cut-away sagittal view of the atlas and the axis cervical vertebrae, showing the ligaments around the odontoid peg.

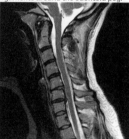

Fig 11.10 T2-weighted sagittal MRI of the cervical spine showing intervertebral disc protrusion at the C5/6 level.

Courtesy of The Norfolk and Norwich University Hospitals (NNUH) Radiology Dept.

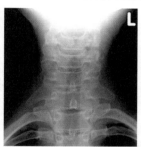

Fig 11.11 AP x-ray of the cervical spine showing bilateral rudimentary cervical ribs in the form of prominent transverse processes (the condition is a spectrum). They are usually a unilateral x-ray finding, though the contralateral side may still have a ligamentous band present. The presence of a cervical rib increases the likelihood of the brachial plexus being *prefixed*—ie arise from C4–C8 rather than C5–T1.

Courtesy of The Norfolk and Norwich University Hospitals (NNUH) Radiology Dept.

Whiplash injury

'Whiplash' injury is cervical strain caused by sudden neck extension with rebound flexion. It is common, often in rear-end crashes. Hyperextension causes damage to the anterior musculoligamentous structures. Subsequent protective muscle spasm causes pain and stiffness, which may be severe. *Treatment:* Reassure physical injury is rare. Emphasize positive attitudes to prognosis and recovery are important. Encourage prompt return to usual activity and occupation. Suggest active mobilization (if tolerated). Aim to prevent chronicity and 'disuse syndrome' through advocating self-management with analgesia. Collars, rest, and negative attitudes can contribute to delayed recovery and chronicity. If symptoms last for >1yr, they are likely to be permanent.[8] Always give a patient information leaflet.

Further reading

Jinnah HA *et al.* (2013). The focal dystonias. *Mov Disord* 28(7):926–43.

National Spasmodic Torticollis Association: www.torticollis.org

ST Dystonia: www.spasmodictorticollis.org/index.cfm

History Where is the pain: shoulder or neck? Past dislocations? Does shoulder movement make it worse? If all movements worsen pain, suspect arthritis or capsulitis; if only some movements, suspect impingement.

Examination Strip to waist. **LOOK** Wasting of rotator cuff muscles, deltoid, pectorals, hands. Posterior glenohumeral dislocation causes internal rotation, anteromedial mass seen on anterior dislocation. **FEEL** Anatomically, the glenohumeral joint is lax and depends far more on surrounding rotator-cuff muscles than bony structures for stability. (figs 11.13 & 11.14). **MOVE** To assess glenohumeral movement, feel the lower half of the scapula to estimate degrees of scapular rotation over the thorax. Half the range of normal abduction is by scapula movement (fig 11.12).

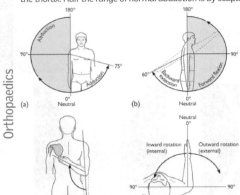

Fig 11.12 Internal rotation of shoulder 'imagine you are doing up a bra'. This is the last movement to recover after shoulder soft-tissue surgery.

Reproduced from Bulstrode et al., *Oxford Textbook of Trauma and Orthopaedics*, with permission from OUP.

The muscles used for movement at the shoulder joint
- *Flexion:* (Forward movement) Pectoralis major, deltoid (ant. ⅓), coracobrachialis.
- *Extension:* Deltoid (posterior ⅓); latissimus dorsi, pectoralis major, and teres major begin the extension if the shoulder starts out flexed.
- *Abduction:* Supraspinatus for first 15°, then deltoid.
- *Adduction:* Pectoralis major, latissimus dorsi, teres major, subscapularis.
- *Medial rotation:* Pectoralis major, deltoid (middle ⅓), latissimus dorsi, teres major, subscapularis.
- *Lateral rotation:* Teres minor, infraspinatus.

Scapula movement on the chest wall NB: serratus anterior prevents 'winging' of the scapula as pressure is placed on the outstretched hand.
- *Elevation:* (Shrug shoulders) Levator scapulae, trapezius.
- *Depression:* Serratus anterior, pectoralis minor.
- *Forward action:* (=protraction, eg punch) Serratus anterior; pectoralis major.
- *Retraction:* (Brace shoulders) Trapezius, rhomboid.

The importance of shoulders
We shrug our shoulders to show we don't know, or don't care. We give the cold shoulder to someone we dislike yet we offer our shoulder for a friend to cry on and we help shoulder their burden. We stand shoulder-to-shoulder, united, in a common cause. We pull onto the hard shoulder of the motorway when our car breaks down. Take any shoulder pathology seriously as loss of upper limb function can have a large impact on many aspects of life.

Further reading
www.shoulderdoc.co.uk

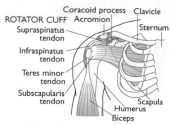

Fig 11.13 Shoulder anatomy (without deltoid: anterior view). Rotator cuff muscles: Supraspinatus (abduction), Subscapularis (internal rotation), Infraspinatus (external rotation), Teres Minor (external rotation + extension). (Mnemonic: SITS (supraspinatus, infraspinatus, Teres Minor, subscapularis). Biceps' long head traverses the cuff attaching to top of the glenoid cavity.

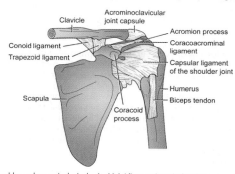

Fig 11.14 Shoulder and acromioclavicular (AC) joint ligaments: anterior view.

Some specific specialist shoulder examination tests

There are over 100 shoulder tests, many of which are not performed as they were first described. Here is a useful quotient for the budding orthopod.

Tests for impingement A painful arc between 60° and 120° abduction; exacerbated by thumb pointing down (empty can) and better with thumb pointing up (full can). *Neer's test:* Passive flexion of shoulder with a pronated arm, whilst scapula is stabilized. *Hawkin's test:* Shoulder and elbow both flexed to 90°, pain on passive internal rotation as the rotator cuff rubs on the undersurface of the acromion.

Tests for rotator cuff tears *Jobe test (supraspinatus weakness or injury):* Patient internally rotates arm whilst in 45°abduction and 30° forward flexion with an extended elbow. Attempt to further abduct against resistance on the elbow results in pain. *Belly-press test* (subscapularis) patient presses on their abdomen (+ve if elbow drops posteriorly as there is pain on internal rotation of shoulder). *Infraspinatus and teres minor:* Flex elbow to 90° and externally rotate against resistance. *Drop arm sign:* Patient lowers arm slowly from 160° abduction. If patient can't control the arm, and it drops quickly to the side = rotator cuff tear.

Test for AC joint disease *Scarf test:* Forced adduction of arm across the neck.

Biceps tendonitis *Speed's test:* Patient starts with arm flexed forward 60°, elbow extended and forearm in supination, and attempts to flex shoulder forward against resistance. Pain on palpation of long head of biceps tendon during this manoeuvre.

Orthopaedics

More prevalent in occupations such as builders and hairdressers due to repetitive awkward upper limb movements.

Rotator cuff tears Tears in supraspinatus tendon (fig 11.15), or adjacent sub-scapularis and infraspinatus, may present insidiously from degeneration in the elderly or, more rarely, after trauma in younger patients. Patients complain of shoulder *weakness* and pain. Night pain may affect sleep as patient is unable to keep the arm in a comfortable position. Typical age: >40yrs. *Imaging:* US and MRI are useful; US is quicker and cheaper to perform and gives information about tear or no tear, but MRI can quantify muscle wasting which can be a useful prognostic indicator.[9] *Treatment:* Incomplete: surgery if symptoms persist. Complete: prompt referral for assessment for open or arthroscopic repair.

Impingement syndrome (on abducting 45°–160°) Only a proportion will have a painful arc (others have increasing pain up to full abduction), which is why the term *impingement syndrome* (as the tendon catches under the acromion during abduction between, eg 70° and 140°) is preferred (rather than painful arc syndrome).

Causes of pain on abduction:

1 *Supraspinatus tendinopathy* or partial rupture of supraspinatus tendon gives pain reproduced by adducting pressure on the partially abducted arm. Typical age: 35–60. *Treatment:* Active shoulder movement with physiotherapy and pain relief; subacromial bursa injection of corticosteroid with local anaesthetic may help.[10] Refer patients with refractory symptoms lasting 6 months for consideration of arthroscopic subacromial decompression.[11] Patients with the following features are most likely to respond well to surgery; temporary benefit following steroid injection, mid-arc pain on abduction, consistently positive Hawkins test.[12] The 'sourcil sign' (sclerosis under the acromion) on xray does not aid diagnosis.[13]

2 *Calcifying tendinopathy:* One of the acute calcific arthropathies. Typical age about 40yrs. There is acute inflammation of supraspinatus. Pain is maximal during the phase of resorption. *Treatment:* Physiotherapy; NSAIDs; steroid injection; rarely, excision of calcium. See fig 11.16.

3 *Acromioclavicular joint osteoarthritis:* This is particularly common in young weightlifters. *Treatment:* Rest; NSAIDs; steroid injections. Excision of the ACJ only if resistant to non-operative measures.

Long head of biceps tendinopathy Pain is in the anterior shoulder and characteristically ↑ on forced contraction of biceps. *Treatment:* Pain relief; corticosteroid injection to the tendon may help, but risks tendon rupture. *Technique:* p710.

Rupture of long head of biceps Discomfort occurs after 'something has gone' when lifting or pulling. A 'ball' appears in the muscle on elbow flexion, like a 'Popeye' muscle. *Treatment:* Repair is rarely indicated as function remains.[4]

Frozen shoulder (adhesive capsulitis) normally has no obvious triggers for shoulder pain. Pain may be severe and worse at night (eg unable to lie on one side). The natural history is divided into: **1** The painful phase (up to 1 year). Active and passive movement range is reduced. Abduction↓ (<90°) ± external rotation↓ (<30°) **2** Frozen phase where pain usually settles but the shoulder remains stiff (6–12 months) **3** Thawing phase as the shoulder slowly regains range of movement (1–3 years). It may be associated with cervical spondylosis (more global restriction of movement), diabetes, and thyroid disease (always check fasting glucose and TFTs). *Treatment:* Early physiotherapy and NSAIDs if tolerated. Corticosteroid joint injections may reduce pain in early phases.[14] Oral steroids provide short-term improvement but benefits are not maintained beyond 6 weeks and therefore not use in clinical practice.[15] Surgical release with either manipulation under anaesthesia or arthroscopic arthrolysis is currently the most effective treatment. Resolution may take years.

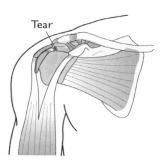

Tear

Fig 11.15 Rotator cuff tear in the supraspinatus tendon. See fig 11.13, p665 for muscle names. Distinguishing between tendinopathy and partial tears can be difficult as both cause a painful arc syndrome as the tendon catches in the subacromial space during abduction. Partial tears cause a painful arc (below); complete tears limit shoulder abduction to the 45–60° given by scapular rotation. NB: tendon rupture can also be asymptomatic.[20] If the arm is passively abducted beyond 90° deltoid's contribution to abduction comes into play, which is then possible from this point. Full-range passive movement is present.

Courtesy of The Norfolk and Norwich University Hospitals (NNUH) Radiology Dept.

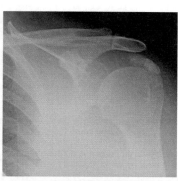

Fig 11.16 AP X-ray of the left shoulder showing calcifying tendinopathy in the left supraspinatus. The glenohumeral joint also appears subluxed, though this is most likely 'deltoid inhibition' caused by pain. Supraspinatus involvement is common since the tendon is susceptible to minor trauma due to poor vascularity at the insertion point.

Courtesy of The Norfolk and Norwich University Hospitals (NNUH) Radiology Dept.

Shoulder osteoarthritis

▶Remember that the neck may refer pain via C5 to the deltoid region and via C6, C7, and C8 to the superior border of the scapula. If aches & pains all over; think about polymyalgia or fibromyalgia. If shoulder tip pain is present examine for diaphragmatic irritiation. Shoulder OA (fig 11.17) is not so common as hip or knee OA. Good success rates (especially for pain relief) are being achieved by joint replacement. Timing of surgery is important, so that the rotator cuff and glenoid are not too worn for good stability.[18] See OHCM p543 for features of OA on x-ray.

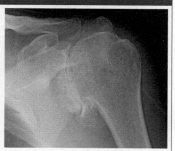

Fig 11.17 AP X-ray of the left shoulder showing osteoarthritis: loss of joint space, subchondral sclerosis, osteophytes, glenoid erosion and humeral head deformity are all present.

Courtesy of The Norfolk and Norwich University Hospitals (NNUH) Radiology Dept.

Further reading

Favejee MM *et al.* (2011). Frozen shoulder: The effectiveness of conservative and surgical interventions – systematic review. *Br J Sports Med* 45(1):49-56.

4 Conversely, if it is the biceps *insertion* that is avulsed, surgical repair will be required.

Lateral epicondylitis (tennis elbow) Inflammation where the common extensor tendon arises from the lateral epicondyle of the humerus. (see fig 11.19). *Presentation:* Often a clear history of repetitive strain. Pain is felt at the front of the lateral condyle, and is exacerbated when the tendon is most stretched (wrist and finger flexion with hand pronated). Ask the patient to extend the wrist, and then to resist extension of the middle finger: is pain elicited? *Treatment:* Most cases will naturally resolve through restriction of activities which overload the tendons. Cases typically last 6–24 months and 90% recover within 1 year. Physiotherapy in motivated patients is the most effective non-surgical treatment, using eccentric loading exercises, acupuncture, and deep friction manual therapy. Epicondylitis braces have no proven efficacy but are helpful in some patients. Corticosteroid joint injections (see p788) are no longer recommended; although giving excellent short-term results (6wks) they are disruptive in the long term (>3 months). One study showed that success rates at 1yr for physiotherapy and 'wait and see' policies was superior to injections.[17] Novel therapies such as platelet-rich plasma injections (expensive, invasive, and not currently recommended by NICE).[18] Only severe cases unresponsive to conservative management should be considered for surgical tendon release.

Medial epicondylitis (golfer's elbow) Inflammation of the forearm flexor muscles at their origin on the medial epicondyle. Most common cause of medial elbow pain, but $1/5$ as common as tennis elbow. Pain is exacerbated by pronation and forearm flexion. Occasionally associated with ulnar neuropathy as the ulnar nerve runs behind the epicondyle. Treatment and prognosis is similar to tennis elbow.

Olecranon bursitis (student's elbow) This is a traumatic bursitis following pressure on the elbows, eg while engrossed in a long book. There is pain and swelling behind the olecranon. If there is overlying skin cellulitis then consider antiobiotics. A rare complication of olecranon bursitis is abscess formation; septic bursitis should be formally drained by the orthopaedic team and will need IV antibiotics. Send aspirate fluid for Gram stain and microscopy for crystals. Other causes include gouty bursitis (look for tophi).

Osteoarthritis of the elbow (fig 11.18) Osteochondritis dissecans[5] and fractures involving the joint are risk factors. *Tests:* Flexion, extension, and forearm rotation may be impaired. Loose bodies may cause restriction of movement, eg loss of full extension. *Treatment:* Surgery is indicated for pain or stiffness not responding to conservative measures or if there are signs of locking. Whilst total elbow replacement in rheumatoid arthritis is very effective, it is less so in the treatment of OA.

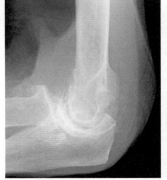

Fig 11.18 Lateral x-ray of the elbow showing degenerative changes of osteo-arthritis. There is loss of joint space, osteophyte formation, bony deformity, and subchondral sclerosis. Movement is painful and severely restricted.

Courtesy of The Norfolk and Norwich University Hospitals (NNUH) Radiology Dept.

5 *Osteochondritis dissecans:* subchondral bone becomes avascular, and may progress to fragments of bone and overlying cartilage (osteochondral fragments) breaking away from the bone to form loose bodies. *Cause:* Unknown. *Typical site:* Lateral side of the medial femoral condyle of 13–21-year-olds. *Symptoms:* Pain after exercise with intermittent knee swelling. *Treatment:* Stable lesions are treated conservatively, as spontaneous healing can occur. Unstable fragments may be pinned.

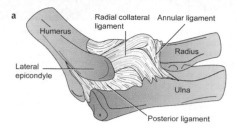

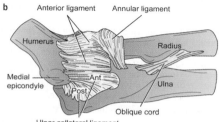

Fig 11.19 The ligaments around the elbow joint—posterolateral view of the right elbow (a) and anteromedial view of the left elbow (b). Stability of this joint is mainly from bony factors, though ligaments do play an important part—eg the annular ligament wraps around the head of the radius (which can pop out in a 'pulled elbow' and also allows smooth pronation/supination). Remember that the joint is made up from 3 articulations: radio-humeral, proximal radioulnar, and humeroulnar. The elbow joint is formed by an articulation of the distal humerus with the proximal radius and ulna. Flexion/extension occur at the ulnohumeral joint and is possible through a range of 0°–150°. With the elbow flexed, supination/pronation of 90° should be possible—this occurs at the radiohumeral and proximal radioulnar articulations. Pain at the elbow may radiate from the shoulder.

Ulnar neuritis (cubital tunnel syndrome) Osteoarthritic or rheumatoid narrowing of the ulnar groove and constriction of the ulnar nerve as it passes behind the medial epicondyle, or friction of the ulnar nerve due to cubitus valgus (a possible sequel to childhood supracondylar fractures) can cause fibrosis of the ulnar nerve and ulnar neuropathy. *Presentation:* Sensory symptoms usually occur first, eg ↓ sensation over little finger and medial half of ring finger. Patients may experience clumsiness of the hand and weakness of the four small muscles of the hand innervated by the ulnar nerve (see p744). *Tests:* Nerve conduction studies may confirm the site of the lesion. *Treatment:* Surgical decompression. See p749 for nerve compression syndromes.

Pulled elbow (subluxation of radial head) Typical patient: 1–4-yr-old who has been lifted by the arm in play, causing the radial head to slip out of the annular ligament. The arm is held slightly flexed and twisted inwards. Reduction can be achieved through the examiner cradling the elbow, with thumb/forefingers over the radial head and either hyperpronating or supinating (limited evidence to support that pronation may be less painful) and flexing the elbow and function is quickly restored. Imaging is not needed. Caution parents not to avoid future pulling of the arm, as this condition recurs in up to 25%.

Further reading

Orchard J et al. (2011). The management of tennis elbow. *BMJ* 342:d2687.

Dupuytren's contracture Progressive, painless fibrotic thickening of the palmar fascia with skin puckering and tethering. Ring and little fingers are chiefly affected. It is often bilateral and symmetrical. As thickening occurs there may be MCP joint flexion. If interphalangeal joints are affected the hand may be quite disabled. Early disease may benefit from less invasive treatments eg injectable *Clostridium histolyticum* or percutaneous needle fasciotomy. [19] Splinting and corticosteroid injections are no longer recommended. *Surgery* Fasciectomy aims to remove affected palmar fascia and release contractures. [20] As a guide, if the patient cannot place his palm flat on a flat surface (*Hueston's table-top test*), refer for surgery. There is a high tendency for recurrence.

Causes/associations
Often multifactorial:
• Genetic (AD)
• Smoking
• Diabetes
• Antiepileptics
• Peyronie's disease (OHCM p722)

Ganglia These smooth, multilocular swellings are cysts containing jelly-like fluid in communication with joint capsules or tendon sheaths. Treatment is not needed unless they cause pain or pressure (eg on median or ulnar nerve at the wrist). They may disappear spontaneously. Local pressure may disperse them (traditionally a blow from a Bible!). Aspiration may work, but surgical dissection gives less recurrence. [21] Problems include painful scars, neurovascular damage (esp. in palmar wrist ganglia), and recurrence.

Carpal tunnel syndrome (see p749) is the most frequent cause of hand pain at night and the most common nerve compression syndrome (fig 11.20).

De Quervain's disease This refers to stenosing tenosynovitis (thickening and tightening) of the 1st extensor compartment (there are 6 in total), abductor pollicis longus and extensor pollicis brevis tendons (at the anterior border of the anatomical snuff box) as they cross the distal radial styloid (fig 11.20). Pain is worst when these tendons are stretched (eg lifting a teapot), and is more proximal than that from osteoarthritis of the 1st carpometacarpal joint. *Finkelstein's sign* is pain elicited by gripping the thumb into the palm of the same hand with passive ulnar deviation. *Cause:* Unknown but symptoms can be exacerbated by overuse of the tendons (eg wringing clothes). *Treatment:* First try rest (thumb spica splint), ice, and NSAIDs. Corticosteroid injection (p706) at tendon site during the 1st 6 months of symptoms is effective in 90% of patients. If conservative measures fail, decompression of the tendons is provided by splitting the tendon sheaths. >80% do well post-op. [22]

Volkmann's ischaemic contracture Is fortunately now rare. It follows poorly managed compartment syndrome or interruption of the brachial artery near the elbow (eg after supracondylar fracture of humerus, p727). Muscle necrosis (esp. flexor pollicis longus and flexor digitorum profundus) results in contraction and fibrosis causing a flexion deformity at wrist and elbow. ►Suspect compartment syndrome if a damaged arm has no radial pulse, and passive finger extension is painful (a crucial sign, p727). *Treatment:* see p722 for compartment syndrome. *Treating contractures:* Prevention is key! To restore lost function, surgery to release compressed nerves ± tendons.

'You have strong, clever hands...' She looked up at me questioningly. 'What do you do for a living?' 'I play the lute' _{Patrick Rothfuss} _{The Wise Man's Fear} There are no minor injuries of the fingers or hand, especially for those who rely on dexterity for a living. This musician would not only be stripped of his ability to earn, but also of his coping mechanism. What is your coping mechanism to survive the turmoils medicine throws at you? In the UK, alcohol and tobacco use are common coping strategies and in Pakistan students reported music and sports. Stress amongst undergraduates is prevalent; ensure that you find and protect a *positive* coping mechanism.

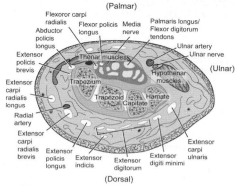

Fig 11.20 Cross-sectional view of the wrist showing the contents of the carpal tunnel and the extensor tendons of the hand. When trying to describe local anatomy of the hand, it is easier to use the terms *ulnar* and *radial (thumb side)*, rather than medial and lateral, which can cause confusion. *Dorsal* refers to the posterior surface, while *palmar (also known as volar)* refers to anterior surface.[6] See p749 for carpal tunnel syndrome.

Orthopaedics

Flexor tendons pulley mechanisms[6]

In order to stop the long flexor tendons of the hand bowing when the fingers are flexed, the fingers have a number of pulleys (well-placed thickenings in the flexor sheath) attached to the bones and palmar plates beneath. Named morphologically as either 'A' for annular, or 'c' for cruciate, there are 5 A-pulleys and 3 c-pulleys. The most important are A2 (which is at the proximal end of the proximal phalanx) and A4 (at the middle of the middle phalanx), both of which need to be preserved during any surgery to prevent bowing of the flexor tendons. Sometimes mountaineers, and others hanging on by their fingertips, partially damage the A2 pulley (typically). Apply ice and buddy-taping/splinting. Then do only light exercises (rubber doughnut squeezes; mild stretches) until 2wks after pain and swelling subside. Visible bowing of the tendon may indicate that surgery is needed. See fig 11.21.

Trigger finger (tendon nodules) Caused by a swelling of the flexor tendon or tightening of the sheath. Ring and middle fingers most commonly affected. Swelling of the tendon sheath, along with nodule formation on the A1 pulley (fig 11.21) prevents the tendon gliding smoothly and instead 'catches' causing the finger to lock in flexion. As extension occurs, the nodule moves with the flexor tendon, but then becomes jammed on the proximal side of the pulley, and has to be flicked straight, so producing triggering. Much more common in diabetes where recurrence is also higher ℞: Simple rest and sometimes splinting helps most patients. If severe, steroid injection into the region of the nodule may be tried. See p709 (fig 11.59). Risk of recurrence is high, so surgery may be needed.[23]

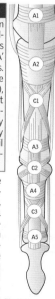

Fig 11.21 Pulley system.

Further reading

Black EM *et al.* (2011). Dupuytren disease: an evolving understanding of an age-old disease. *J Am Acad Orthop Surg* 19(12):746–57.

Pettitt DA *et al.* (2012). Clinical review: Volkmann's ischaemic contracture. *Eur J Trauma Emerg Surg* 38:129–37.

6 The International Federation for Societies for Surgery of the Hand recommends the term 'palmar'.

Orthopaedics

History Attention should be paid to the nature of the pain, exacerbating and relieving factors, and the history of onset. Review the sinister causes of back pain to help structure your history taking. ▶You must document the presence of red flags (p680 and MINIBOX). These signify cord or cauda equina compression and should set alarm bells ringing: refer at once (needs an MRI in <4h). Remember that motor deficits and bowel or bladder disturbances are more reliable than sensory signs.

Red flags of sinister pain
• ≤20 or ≥55 years old
• Violent trauma
• Minor trauma in osteoporosis
• Alternating or bilateral sciatica
• Weak legs
• Weight loss/fever
• Taking oral steroids
• Progressive, continuous, non-mechanical pain
• Systemically unwell
• Drug abuse or HIV +ve
• Pain unrelated to mechanical events
• Local bony tenderness
• CNS deficit at more than one root level
• Thoracic spine pain
• Worse pain whilst supine
• Previous neoplasia

Examination starts the moment your patient walks into the room. Observing gait and function can elicit any discrepancies in a patient's descriptions of reduced function. With the patient standing and wearing only underwear, inspect the back for abnormality or surgical spinal scars. Palpate bony landmarks (fig 11.22) for local tenderness and deformity. Localized sacro-iliac joint tenderness suggests spondyloarthropathy (sacroiliitis is suggested when there is pain on hip adduction as the hip and knee are flexed). Spinal movements assessed are *forward flexion* (stretch forward to touch toes with knees straight)—look to see how much movement is due to back flexion and how much by flexion at the hips—with back flexion the back has a gently rounded contour. On bending fully forwards, the distance between vertebral spines should increase. *Schobers test* determines any limitations to forward flexion. Locate where L5 lies, then place one finger 5cm vertically below and another finger 10cm above. Lumbar flexion is considered limited if the distance increase is <5cm as the patient leans forward to touch their toes. Look for a rib hump—a sign of scoliosis (p674); *extension* (arch spine backwards), *lateral flexion* (lean sideways so hand moves down corresponding thigh), and *rotation* (keep pelvis fixed but move shoulders round to each side in turn—mostly from the thoracic spine). Movement at the costovertebral joints is assessed by the difference in chest expansion between maximal inspiration and expiration (normal=5cm). Iliac crests are grasped by the examiner and compressed to move sacroiliac joints and see if this reproduces the pain. Compare leg length; quantify discrepancy and muscle wasting (measure thigh and calf circumference). If there are leg symptoms ensure *neurologic assessment* of L4 (knee reflex), L5 (weakness of ankle and great toe dorsiflexion, sensory loss in medial foot and 1st/2nd toe web space) and S1 (ankle reflex, weakness of plantar flexion) roots.

Testing for an underlying herniated disc 98% of which will be at the L4–S1 levels. You can try to incorporate these tests into the rest of your examination as they may prove pain free if the patient is not genuine. *Straight leg raising* aims to stretch the sciatic nerve and reproduce root pain (a characteristic lancinating pain distributed in the relevant dermatome, and made worse by coughing or sneezing). Keeping the knee extended, lift the patient's leg off the couch and note the angle to which the leg can be raised before eliciting pain. If 30–70°, Lasègue's sign is said to be positive. The crossed straight leg raise involves lifting the unaffected leg. If this reproduces pain in the affected side it is said to be positive. It is less sensitive but more specific for an underlying herniated disc. All these tests may still give false positives and negatives, hence the importance of a good history combined with the examination. Other causes of sciatica include spinal stenosis, cauda equina syndrome, and pregnancy.

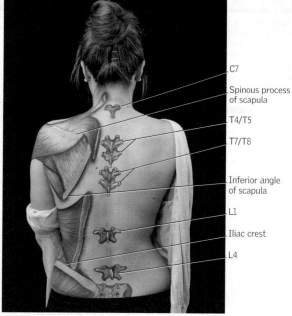

Fig 11.22 Surface anatomy of the back.

Reproduced courtesy of Art and Anatomy Edinburgh. Copyright © 2015 Art and Anatomy Edinburgh. Contributors Megan Anderson, Nichola Robertson, Kimmie Simpson, Philip Stewart, and Alex Haddon.

Other causes of back pain

The commonest musculoskeletal complaint is back pain, yet do not apply your orthopaedic blinkers until other causes of back pain have been ruled out:
- Retroperitoneal (duodenal ulcer, AAA; pain is often lumbo-dorsal and spine movements pain-free and full)
- Local infection or systemic TB causing osteomyelitis
- Renal colic or pyelonephritis
- Neoplasia (eg myeloma, pancreatic cancer)
- Bone metastases: The commonest tumours to metastasize to bone are: breast, bronchus, kidney, thyroid, and prostate so it may be relevant to examine these. Less than 1% of patients presenting to primary care have spinal malignancy as a cause for back pain. Historically, if the following features were absent then spinal malignancy was considered unlikely: >50 yrs old, PMH of cancer, pain >1 month, raised ESR and low Hb. However, a Cochrane review in 2013 questioned the diagnostic accuracy of these screening questions. Only a PMH of cancer increased the likelihood of spinal malignancy.

Other parts of the body to examine ▶Remember to examine gait and hip joints (p687) as hip flexion can reproduce nerve root pain. Other relevant areas are the iliac fossae (important in days when tuberculous psoas abscesses were common), abdomen, pelvis, rectum, and major arteries.

Further reading

Sandella BJ (2014). *Examination of Low Back Pain Technique*. Medscape. http://emedicine.medscape.com/article/2092651-technique

Kyphosis is an excessive curvature of spine in the sagittal plane (>40°), typically the thoracocervical spine, sometimes with a lordosis of the lumbar spine. Less common than scoliosis, but potentially more dangerous are dislocations of the spinal column into cord can cause cord compression and paraplegia which sometimes develops rapidly, eg during adolescence.

Causes of kyphosis
• Congenital
• Osteoporosis
• Spina bifida
• Calvé's vertebrae
• Cancer; wedge fractures
• Tuberculosis; polio
• Paget's disease
• Ankylosing spondylitis

Scheuermann's disease[7] One of the osteochondroses (p702). The commonest cause of kyphosis in 13–16-yr-olds. It typically presents when parents notice poor posture and kyphosis. Aetiology remains unknown. The normal ossification of ring epiphyses of several thoracic vertebrae are affected. Deforming forces are greatest at their anterior border, so vertebrae are narrower here, causing kyphosis. During the active phase, vertebrae may be tender. Patients appear round shouldered and 'hunched'—they tend to present for deformity rather than pain. *x-rays:* Irregular vertebral endplates, Schmorl's nodes, and ↓disc space ± anterior wedging causing thoracic kyphosis of more than 40°. Three adjacent vertebral bodies of at least 5° of wedging is pathognomonic. Schmorl's nodes are herniations of the intervertebral disc through the vertebral endplate. *Treatment* involves posture control and exercise (eg swimming). Physiotherapy ± spinal braces can help, though curvature may recur after discontinuation of bracing. Surgery may be tried for severe kyphosis (>75°) with curve progression, refractory pain, or neurological deficit.

Scoliosis This is lateral spinal curvature with secondary vertebral rotation. There is lateral curvature (Cobb angle) of the thoracic or lumbar spine of >10°. It is usually accompanied by a degree of rotation of the spinal column. The chief cause is idiopathic with no serious underlying pathology, and normally involves muscle spasm. The UK screening programme was discontinued in 2012 since clinically significant cases would have been detected anyway. *Classification:*
• Idiopathic (may be infantile, juvenile, adolescent, or adult onset)
• Neuromuscular (neuropathic or myopathic)
• Syndromic (eg Marfan's, *OHCM* p720, or neurofibromatosis, *OHCM* p518).
• Other (eg tumour, osteoporosis, infection etc.).

Adolescent idiopathic scoliosis is the most common spinal deformity, most frequently affecting girls. Complications in later life revolve around pain, cosmesis, and impaired lung function. Curvature increases while the affected person continues to grow, so usually the earlier the onset the worse the deformity. Risk of progression is also higher with greater Cobb angles at presentation (>25°), double curves progress more than single curves, and a scoliosis in girls is more likely to progress than one in boys. *Treatment:* All should be referred to specialist clinics for observation and measurements of Cobb angle. ~¹⁄₆ patients require treatment and only ¼ of those treated need surgery. When curvatures are progressing, attempts to halt it may be made using braces but benefit is limited by pyschosocial issues and adherance to wearing a brace for the optimal ≥20h/day. Bracing will not correct the deformity but has a role in slowing/preventing curve progression. Surgery in <7-yr-olds attempts to optimize further growth of spine and lungs, however surgery in older patients is only indicated if existing deformity is causing problems or progression is likely. Surgery involves deformity correction with spinal fusion and stabilization (fig 11.24). Intraoperative spinal cord monitoring reduces the most feared post-op complication—paralysis (it now occurs in 0.2%). ►When scoliosis in youth gives pain (especially at night), exclude osteoid osteoma (p699), osteoblastoma, spondylolisthesis (p676), and spinal tumours.

Orthopaedics

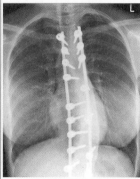

Atlas
Axis

7th cervical
1st thoracic

12th thoracic
1st lumbar

5th lumbar

Coccyx

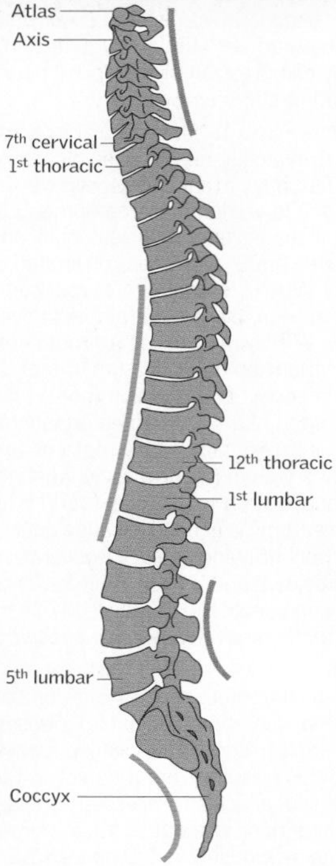

Fig 11.23 The spine.

During development, the vertebral column initially has a *primary curvature* (anteriorly concave, as for the thoracic and sacral curvatures in red), then goes on to develop *secondary curvatures* in the cervical and lumbar regions (in blue, fig 11.23). The normal vertebral body count is 7 cervical, 12 thoracic, 5 lumbar, 5 sacral, and then some coccygeal (3–5). There is some variation, eg L5 can be fused to the sacrum (sacralization) or S1 can be distinct from the sacrum (lumbarization), though total numbers remain constant (even across some mammalian species, especially in the cervical region—eg the giraffe also has 7 cervical vertebrae).

Remember that there are 8 cervical spinal nerve roots, with the C1 root arising from above the C1 vertebra, the C8 root from above the T1 vertebra, and from T1 onwards the root exiting below the corresponding vertebra. This occurs because during development the incipient spinal nerves develop through the embryonic sclerotomes, with the upper part of the C1 sclerotome joining with the last occipital sclerotome to form the base of the occipital bone, and the lower part of the C1 sclerotome forming the C1 vertebra with the upper C2 sclerotome—and so on. Failure of formation and segmentation during development can lead to *congenital scoliosis* (rare). Defective induction of vertebral body formation on one side of the body (=hemivertebra) may cause a severe *scoliosis*, and incorrect or absent induction of vertebral arch closure by the neural tube causes the degrees of *spina bifida* (p140).

Fig 11.24 Kyphoscoliosis.
This chest x-ray of a 21-year-old female demonstrates spinal stabilization sugery with pedicle screws and longitudinal rods performed aged 11. Thoracic problems tend to give more severe deformity than lumbar. Rib deformity causes a characteristic hump on the convex side of the curve which manifest on asking the patient to bend forwards, see www.SAUK.org.uk (Scoliosis Association UK) for examples.
© Nina Hjelde.

Further reading

Tribus C (2010). *Scheuermann Kyphosis.* Medscape. http://emedicine.medscape.com/article/1266349-overview

7 Scheuermann also described a seperate condition involving lumbar disc spaces (now called juvenile disc disorder to avoid confusion between disease processes).

Orthopaedics

Backache is often from low back strain or degenerative disease. *Local pain* is typically deep and aching (from soft tissue and vertebral body irritation). *Radicular pain* is stabbing, and is caused by compression of the dorsal nerve roots, and projects in a dermatomal distribution. *Other causes:*

Intervertebral disc disorders 1 *Disc prolapse:* (fig 11.25): Lumbar discs are those most likely to rupture (esp. L4/5 & L5/S1). Typically, one is seized by severe pain on coughing, sneezing, or twisting a few days after back strain (onset may be insidious). Pain may be confined to the lower lumbar area (lumbago), or may radiate to buttock or leg (sciatica) if the herniated nucleus pulposus compresses a nerve root. *Signs:* Forward flexion (p672) and extension limited, ± lateral flexion—unilaterally and inconstantly. With L5/S1 prolapse, S1 root compression causes calf pain, weak foot plantar flexion, ↓sensation (pinprick) over sole of foot and back of calf, and ↓ankle jerk. With L4/5 prolapse (L5 root compression), hallux extension is weak and sensation↓ on outer dorsum of foot. If lower lumbar discs prolapse centrally, cauda equina compression (p681) may occur. *Tests:* MRI (or CT) if intervention is contemplated—▶▶an emergency if cauda equina compression is suspected—or if rest fails and symptoms are severe, with CNS signs such as reflex or sensory changes, or muscle wasting. *Treating disc prolapse:* Brief rest and early mobilization + pain relief (p679) is all that is needed in 90% (±physiotherapy). Discectomy is needed in cauda equina syndrome, progressive muscular weakness, or continuing pain. 2 *Degenerative disc disease:* The exact aetiology remains unknown and is likely multifactorial and not only due to ageing as it occurs in young people too. It may lead to herniation. Surgical interventions include prosthetic disc replacement. 3 *Discitis:* (see p680).

Spondylolisthesis There is displacement (usually forward) of one lumbar vertebra upon the one below (usually L5 on S1, sometimes palpable). *Causes:* Spondylosis (age-related degeneration resulting from joint deformity, associated with osteophyte formation), spondylolysis (results from a defect in the pars interarticularis), congenital malformation of articular processes, osteoarthritis of posterior facet joints. Onset of pain with or without sciatica is often in adolescence ± hamstring tightness causing a waddling gait. *Diagnosis* is by x-rays and MRI to assess nerve compression. *Treatment:* Only temporary relief is achieved with conservative bracing and physio, curative treatment involves spinal fusion (essential for slips >50%).

Lumbar spinal stenosis (LSS) and lateral recess stenosis (figs 11.26 & 11.27) Generalized narrowing of the lumbar spinal canal or its lateral recesses causing nerve ischaemia. Typically caused by facet joint OA (the only synovial joints in the back) and osteophytes. Unlike the pain of lumbar disc prolapse, this can cause: • Pain worse on walking with aching and heaviness in one or both legs causing the person to stop walking (= 'spinal claudication') • Pain on extension • Negative straight leg raising test • Few CNS signs. Watch out for the patient who prefers to lean over shopping trollies, walk uphill rather than down, and cycle as these activities help flex the back and release tension on compressed nerves. *Tests:* MRI is preferred, but when insufficient or contraindicated, myelography (injection of contrast into subarachnoid space) is available. *Treatment:* Decompressive laminectomy gives good results if NSAIDs, epidural steroid injections, and corsets (to prevent exaggerating the lumbar lordosis of standing) fail to help.

Inflammatory back pain: spondyloarthropathies (p552 OHCM) (figs 11.28 & 11.29) Inflammatory diseases which affect axial and peripheral joints. The most common is ankylosing spondylitis. Key questions in history: insidious onset over months, early morning stiffness >45min, diffuse non-specific buttock pain, pain improves with activity and worsens on rest, other joint, bowel or eye involvement.

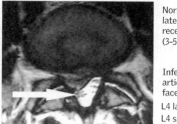

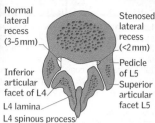

Fig 11.25 Axial MRI image at the L5/S1 level showing a right-sided paracentral disc prolapse. Observe the displaced nerve roots within the CSF-filled dural sac (arrow). Remember that CSF is white on T2-weighted MRI.

Courtesy of Mr Mark Brinsden, FRCS.

Fig 11.26 L5 cross-section showing lateral recess stenosis. This is usually caused by degenerative disease of the facet joint, but rarely can be from congenitally shortened pedicles.

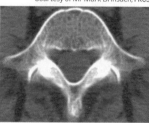

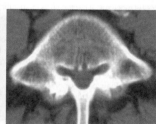

Fig 11.27 Cross-section CT images at L5, one with spinal stenosis (right). Observe the difference in spinal canal shape and dimensions caused by osteoarthritis of the facet joints posterolaterally. Factors contributing to spinal stenosis: disc prolapse, spondylolisthesis, hypertrophy of the ligamentum flavum. Identify the spinal canal contents at this level, including the thecal sac and the two L5 nerve root sheaths that occupy the lateral recesses.

Courtesy of Mr Mark Brinsden FRCS.

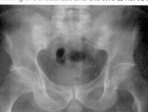

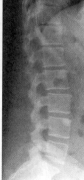

Fig 11.29 Lateral view of the lumbar spine demonstrating early changes of ankylosing spondylitis. There is squaring of the vertebral bodies with associated sclerosis of the corners (Romanus lesions).

Reproduced from Watts et al., *Oxford Textbook of Rheumatology* 4e (2013), with permission from OUP.

Fig 11.28 X-ray findings in a patient with established ankylosing spondylitis. Bilateral sacroiliitis with subchondral erosions and sclerosis. X-rays are used as a diagnostic criteria for ankylosing spondylitis. MRI is useful in cases with normal xrays but high clinical suspicion.

Reproduced with permission of the Cleveland Clinic Center for Continuing Education. Bunyard MP. Ankylosing Spondylitis. Disease management project ©2000–2015 The Cleveland Clinic Foundation. All rights reserved.

Further reading

Hughes SP *et al.* (2012). The pathogenesis of degeneration of the intervertebral disc and emerging therapies in the management of back pain. *J Bone Joint Surg Br* 94(10):1298–304.

Issack PS *et al.* (2012). Degenerative lumbar spinal stenosis: evaluation and management. *J Am Acad Orthop Surg* 20(8):527–35.

Orthopaedics

Lower back pain is extremely common; ~80% of people in the UK suffer at some stage in their lives. 50 per 1000 industrial workers have time off work because of it each year, with each employee taking an average of 19 days off work. In the UK it accounts for 4.9 million lost working days/yr.[24] A GP expects 20 people per 1000 on her list to consult with it each year (only ~10% are referred to hospital of which less than 10% need surgery). ~90% of backache can be attributed to non-specific lower back muscular strain or degenerative disease. Typically affects 30–50yr olds. The spine is a complex series of articulations (see p675), with spongy discs between vertebral bodies acting as shock absorbers, and a multitude of articulating facet joints. Problems in one part affect function of the whole. Spasm of vertebral muscles can cause significant pain. Upright posture provokes big forces on the spine, eg when lifting, and discs may rupture (if young), vertebrae fracture (elderly) or soft tissues tear (low back strain). NB: with low back strain the exact mechanism may be elusive. It is not uncommon for patients to develop sciatica p679 or other nerve root signs. *A variety of terms* can be used to describe mechanical back pain; non-specific, uncomplicated, or simple back pain. Be cautious of telling your patient you have diagnosed 'simple' back ache since, for them, the pain is everything but 'simple'! Carefully explain that these terms simply declare a lack of sinister features (p680). *Key questions to ask* The goal is to rule out serious pathology (p680). Were there any triggers to pain starting? Any previous back problems? Adequate analgesia taken? What are their expectations for recovery and current coping mechanisms? (See 'Yellow flags' in BOX.)

Imaging Plain x-rays correlate poorly with symptoms; only consider in the acute setting if suspecting malignancy or fractures (ie trauma, osteoporosis)[25] as a 2-view lumbar spinal x-ray irradiates gonads and can be the equivalent radiation dose of one CXR every day for a year. Reserve CT/MRI and bloods for when symptoms are chronic (>4 weeks) or in sinister causes.[8]

Why do some people get intractable back pain?

The worldwide prevalence of chronic back pain is 23%.[26] Much energy is expended on frequently fruitless searches for pathology. Imaging may be non-specific. The patient's attitude towards rehabilitation is pivotal and the following list demonstrates potential psychosocial issues which can prolong recovery and spiral into chronic back pain.[27]

Yellow flags
• Belief that pain and subsequent activity are harmful
• Pain behaviour (such as extended rest, avoidance of normal activities)
• Over-reliance on passive treatments (such as ice packs, analgesia, etc.)
• Depression, anxiety, personality disorders
• Unsupportive home environment or over-protective family
• Inappropriate expectations and failing to actively engage with treatment.

Other risk factors for chronicity Poor work conditions, low income/social class, and number of children (for women and men). Be cautious of blaming sedentary lifestyles, sitting at work, or occupational carrying as studies do not find in favour of this popular association.[28–30] Associations with smoking and co-existing cardiorespiratory disease may be due to vascular problems, and pain may be maintained by involvement of the sympathetic chain, which mediates hyperaesthesia, hyperpathia (excess pain from minor noxious stimuli), allodynia (pain from minor skin stimulation)—but surgical sympathectomy often only provides temporary relief. This implies central neuromodulation of stimuli producing a complex regional pain syndrome (p723). Dorsal horn receptor fields may expand and have their thresholds changed by peripheral injury, so pain is more intense, and appreciated over a wider area than simple anatomy would predict.

---

8 Only offer MRI for non-specific lower back pain if assessing patient for potential spinal fusion.

Management of lower back pain

Most simple back pain is self-limiting: of those attending GPs, 70% are better after 3 weeks, 90% by 6 weeks, irrespective of treatment. Lower back pain is especially challenging to manage as it disrupts patients physically, socially, and psychologically. Focus on:

- Pain relief
- Exercises to improve function
- Identifying yellow flags which impede recovery (see box on p678)
- Lifestyle changes to prevent recurrence

'*Get on with your life within the limits of the pain*' gives better results than physiotherapy with lateral bending exercises. Encourage patients to return to work. Avoid bed-rest after the 1st 48h (a board under the mattress helps). *Analgesia* breaks the pain–muscle spasm cycle (paracetamol ≤4g/24h PO, ± NSAID, eg **ibuprofen** 400mg/8h PO or **naproxen** 500mg/12h PO). Opioids may be needed early. *Warmth* helps, as does swimming in a warm pool. If acute spasm persists, try a *muscle relaxant* such as **diazepam** 2–4mg/8h PO for 3 days and warn about side effects (eg drowsiness). *Cognitive therapy in groups* (p400) helps tackle unhelpful beliefs about backache and fears about restarting activity. The role of *antidepressants* is disputed but may help refractory pain, but not level of functioning.[31] *Physiotherapy* in the acute phase can ↓pain and spasm. Many consult osteopaths or physiotherapists or chiropractors for *manipulation*, but studies show that it is unlikely to provide relief beyond that attained from other standard therapies. Referral for epidural anaesthesia. Corsets may help. Note that orthopaedic referral for spinal fusion is no better than intensive rehabilitation.

Referral criteria to specialist services (orthopaedics or spinal surgeons). The current guidelines advocate earlier referral than previously practised.

Red Flags present =	Immediate referral
Progressive/severe neurological deficit=	To be seen by specialist within 1 week
Disabling pain > 2 weeks =	Early referral to physio, consider corticosteroid injections.
Disabling pain > 6 weeks (despite physio & analgesia)	To be seen by specialist within 2 weeks

A large RCT compared early surgery (<12 weeks) versus conservative treatment for sciatica caused by lumbar disc herniation. Although early surgery generated faster pain relief (especially if sitting aggravated pain), at the end of 1 year both groups had similar rates of dissatisfaction.[32]

Laid flat by a wealth of evidence

Entering the search term 'back pain' in Pubmed for the previous edition of this book delivered 42,099 entries, with 392 meta-analyses. At the time of writing, the same search now yields 49,498 entries and 558 meta-analyses! Holding back throes of exasperation: where do you start, what do you look for, and how can you filter? (See also p636.) Does this wealth of evidence exist because back pain is such a common condition, because there are so many different treatment options, or because we are not yet able to offer definitive therapy to our patients?

As we stand up to the challenge laid down by evolution (and search engines alike), those without back pain can count themselves lucky, while those struck horizontal by our primitive postural problems try not to think of the irony that we are lying in the plane in which our vertebral column originally worked!

Further reading

Knott L (2013). *Lower Back Pain and Sciatica*. Patient. http://patient.info/doctor/low-back-pain-and-sciatica

NICE (2015). *Clinical Knowledge Summaries. Scenario: Management of Sciatica*. http://cks.nice.org.uk/sciatica-lumbar-radiculopathy#!scenario

Sahrakar K (2015). *Lumbar Disc Disease*. Medscape. http://emedicine.medscape.com/article/249113-overview

Age is important (see box on p681): only 3% of those aged between 20 and 55 have 'spinal pathology' (eg tumour, infection, inflammatory disease) compared with 11% of those <20yrs, and 19% >55yrs. ▶Pain brought on by activity and relieved by rest is rarely sinister. If cancer or infection is suspected, refer promptly.

Spinal tumours These may be of spinal cord, meninges, nerves, or bone. They may be primary, secondary, lymphoma, or myeloma. They may compress the cord, causing pain, lower motor neuron signs at the level of the lesion, upper motor neuron signs and sensory loss below—or bowel and bladder dysfunction. Peripheral nerve function may be impaired resulting in pain along the course of the nerve, weakness, hyporeflexia & ↓sensation (p746). With cauda equina involvement there is saddle anaesthesia ± urinary retention (see BOX, p681). When the deposit is in the spinal canal and there is no bone involvement, there may be no pain, just long tract signs. When bones of the back are involved there is progressive, constant pain and local destruction of bone. Metastases tend to affect cancellous bone, but focal lesions cannot be seen on x-rays until 50% of bone mass is lost. There may be muscle spasm and local tenderness to percussion. Bone collapse may result in deformity, or cause cord or nerve compression. *Tests:* ▶Do FBC, ESR, LFT, bone profile in presence of red flags or whenever pain lasts >4 weeks, whatever the age. Do a myeloma screen if >50 years. Plain x-rays; CT; MRI; isotope bone scans; bone biopsy. In those with past cancer and current back pain, it is best to do a bone scan first (fig 11.30), with plain x-rays of any hot spots suggesting metastases.

Pyogenic spine infections This is a notoriously difficult diagnosis as all signs of infection may be absent (eg no fever, tenderness, or WCC↑, but the ESR is often↑). It may be secondary to other septic foci. Pain occurs, and movement is restricted by spasm. It is usually an infection of the disc space (discitis). *Risk factors:* Diabetes mellitus, immunosuppression, urinary surgery, or catheterization. Half of infections are staphylococcal. *Streptococcus, Proteus, E. coli, Salmonella typhi,* and TB also occur. *Tests:* ESR↑; WCC↑; x-rays show bone rarefaction or erosion, joint space narrowing ± subligamentous new bone formation. Technetium bone scans and MRI (fig 11.31) are better. *Treatment:* As for osteomyelitis (p696), resting the back with bed rest, brace, or plaster jacket. Surgery may be needed if unresponsive to medical therapy.

Pott's disease (spinal TB) A frequent form of extra-pulmonary TB (represents 1–3% of all TB and incidence is rising), especially if co-infected with HIV. Tends to affect young adults who present with systemic symptoms, gradual onset localized back pain, and stiffness of all back movements. Most commonly affects T10-L1. Spinal deformity is common, especially kyphosis when thoracic vertebrae are affected. Abscesses (esp. of psoas muscle) and cord compression may occur (Pott's paraplegia). *Differential diagnoses:* Malignancy; other infections; gout; rheumatoid. *Tests:* ESR↑. x-rays tend to be normal until >50% bone mass, later images show narrow disc spaces, local osteoporosis, and bone destruction leading to wedging of vertebrae. MRI is more specific than CT in the diagnosis of spinal TB and is the ideal way to delineate cord compression. Bone scans can help differentiate from malignancy. One meta-analysis showed PET to be superior to all other forms of imaging, with a sensitivity of 96% and a specificity of 91%.[33] Consider the imaging resources available in each country though, naturally the majority of research into spinal TB is based on x-rays. Cultures of synovial tissue or bone from needle biopsy are often needed. Always do CXR to check for co-existing pulmonary TB. *Treatment* (see p696, 'Osteomyelitis'). There is insufficient evidence for the rouine use of surgery alongside medical treatment. [34]

Typical causes of back pain according to age	
15–30yrs	Prolapsed disc, trauma, fractures, ankylosing spondylitis (*OHCM*, p552), spondylolisthesis, pregnancy
>30yrs	Prolapsed disc, malignancy (lung, breast, prostate, thyroid, kidney)
>50yrs	Degenerative, osteoporosis, Paget's disease (*OHCM* p699), malignancy, myeloma (*OHCM* p362); lumbar artery atheroma (which may itself cause disc degeneration)

The *cauda equina* (=horse's tail)

The cord tapers to its end, the *conus medullaris*, at approximately (can be variable) L1 in adults. Lumbar and sacral nerve roots arising from the *conus medullaris* form the *cauda equina*. These spinal nerve roots separate in pairs, exiting laterally through the nerve root foramina, providing motor and sensory innervation of the legs and pelvic organs. Compression is most frequently from large prolapses or herniation of lumbar discs, but may be from extrinsic tumours, primary cord tumours, spondylosis, spinal stenosis. Compression to the cauda equina clinically produces a lower motor neuron lesion. Keep an eye out for the following danger signs: ▸▸Poor anal tone (do PR) ▸▸Severe back pain ▸▸Saddle-area (perineal) sensation↓ ▸▸Incontinence/retention of faeces or urine ▸▸Paralysis ± sensory loss. Diagnosis can be tricky. See p756 for the functional anatomy. Although most patients present with sudden onset back pain and neurological signs progressive over hours/days, the syndrome can be painless and develop over weeks. Although this syndrome is rare (affects 2% of herniated lumbar discs) it must always be considered because delay in diagnosis can lead to permanent neurological damage to sexual, bladder, and bowel function. Subsequently, for medico-legal purposes, it is critical that clinical documentation *must always* make comment on these signs whenever a patient presents with back pain. If suspected, refer to neurosurgery/spinal teams immediately who will expect an MRI within 4 hours. See *OHCM* p470 for metastatic spinal cord compression.

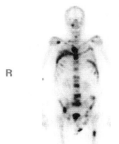

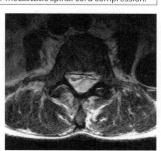

Fig 11.30 Bone scan showing multiple metastases from prostatic cancer, including infiltration of the pelvis, ribs, left femur, and spinal column. Bone scans in spinal TB are not as useful since infection typically causes a hotspot but avascular bony fragments from TB can be cold spots.

Fig 11.31 Axial T2-weighted MRI of the lumbar spine showing an epidural abscess in the posterior portion of the spinal canal causing mild stenosis.
Courtesy of The Norfolk and Norwich University Hospitals (NNUH) Radiology Dept.

Courtesy of The Norfolk and Norwich University Hospitals (NNUH) Radiology Dept.

Further reading

Gardner A *et al.* (2011). Cauda equina syndrome: a review of the current clinical and medico-legal position. *Eur Spine J* 20(5):690–7.

Garg RK *et al.* (2011). Spinal tuberculosis: a review. *J Spinal Cord Med* 34(5):440–54.

Jutte PC *et al.* (2006). Routine surgery in addition to chemotherapy for treating spinal tuberculosis. *Cochrane Database Syst Rev* 5:CD004532.

Problems with the hip joint usually remain clinically silent until patients present with secondary dysfunction, often of lower limb and back, arising from long-term compensatory movements. (For hip prostheses, see p706.) It can be difficult to differentiate between hip and back pathology. Pain in the knee may be referred from the hip (and vice versa). The movements examined at the hip are described in fig 11.33. Internal rotation is often the first movement to be restricted by hip disease. **Questions** Are activities of daily living affected?—walking distance, ability to climb stairs (only one at a time possible?), difficulty getting out of low chairs. **Examination** Follow the routine for joint examination (p658).

Also examine Spine, knee, sacroiliac joints/pelvis.

Measurements Apparent leg length disparity (with the lower limbs parallel and in line with the trunk) is called either 'apparent shortening' (eg due to pelvic tilt or fixed adduction deformity—which gives the apparent shortening on that side) or 'apparent lengthening' (eg due to fixed hip abduction). In these cases, there is no true disparity, as detected by measuring between the anterior superior iliac spine and medial malleolus on each side with the pelvis held square (fig 11.32) and the lower limbs held equally adducted or abducted or by comparing leg length by positioning the lower limbs perpendicular to a line joining the anterior superior iliac spines.

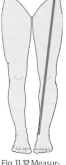

Fig 11.32 Measuring leg length: from the anterior superior iliac spine to the medial malleolus.

Fixed deformity Joint or muscle contractures prevent limbs from being put in the neutral position. With fixed adduction deformity, the angle between the limb and the transverse axis of the pelvis (line between both anterior superior iliac spines) is <90° but with fixed abduction deformity it is >90°. Fixed flexion deformity is detected by the ***Thomas test:*** With the patient supine on an examination couch, flex the good hip up towards the chest until the lumbar lordosis is obliterated (check by finding it impossible to pass a hand between the patient and the couch in the small of the back). If there is a fixed flexion deformity the thigh on the affected side will lift off the couch as the lumbar lordosis is obliterated. NB: to assess the full range of extension, have the patient prone on the table and then extend the hip.

The Trendelenburg test is a test of the function of hip abduction and the ability to support the pelvis when standing on one leg. In this state, it is normal for the pelvis to rise on the side of the lifted leg. Weakness of the abductors on the weight-bearing leg cause a 'positive' Trendelenburg test; the pelvis falls on the side of the lifted leg. A common mnemonic is 'sound side sags'. *Causes:* **1** Abductor muscle paralysis (gluteus medius and minimus are supplied by the superior gluteal nerve), ie nerve root lesions, pain, postoperative nerve damage, weakened muscles due to OA **2** Upward displacement of the greater trochanter (severe coxa vara, fig 11.34, or dislocated hip) **3** Absence of a stable fulcrum (eg un-united fractures of the neck of femur).

Gait If a hip is unstable or painful, a stick is used on the opposite side (the reverse is true for knees) so as to off-load the hip abductors on the affected side. *Antalgic gait:* Shortening of the stance phase[9] on the painful leg occurs, with quick and short steps. *Short-leg gait:* Discrepancy in length is compensated for by adduction of the long leg at the hip and abduction of the short leg creating pelvic drop, or an *equinus* deformity. *Trendelenburg gait:* A waddling gait caused by weak hip abductors, in which the trunk tilts over the weakened side (can be bilateral) in the stance phase. See *OHCM* p459.

9 The *stance phase* of gait starts when the forward foot foot makes contact with the ground. Then there is loading, mid- and terminal stance (+preswing)—before the shorter *swing phase* starts.

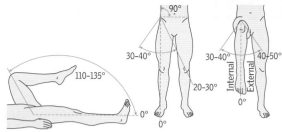

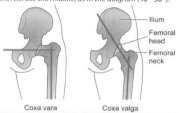

Fig 11.33 Ball and socket (eg the hip) joints have 3 axes of movement: flexion–extension (left); ab- & adduction (middle); and external & internal rotation. External rotation of the ball in the socket is achieved by movement of the shin across the midline, as in the diagram (40°–50°).

Fig 11.34 Coxa vara and coxa valga. Coxa vara is more common; the angle between the neck and the shaft of femur is less than the normal 125°; causes true shortening of limb and Trendelenburg 'dip' on walking with resultant limp. Causes: Congenital; SUFE, malunion # of neck of femur or trochanteric #; softening of bones (rickets, osteomalacia, Paget's disease).

Coxa vara   Coxa valga

Osteoarthritis of the hip

In addition to the secondary risk factors for OA mentioned on p692, hip OA can follow AVN (see p735) and paediatric hip disease (see p686). Note that BMI does not increase risk of hip OA as it does in knee OA. See also OHCM p546.

History Pain is poorly localized around groin, thigh, or buttocks. Pain can be referred to the knee. Worse on weightbearing with stiffness when attempting activities which flex the hip (eg tying shoe laces).

On examination there is an antalgic gait with a positive Trendelenburg sign. Expect reduced ROM (especially on internal rotation). Figs 11.35 & 11.36 show examples of hip arthoplasty. Most patients won't know what type of prosthesis they have, you must become familiar with the x-ray appearances. Re-surfacing of the hip is rarely performed now but there remains a cohort of patients with them *in situ*.

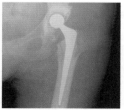

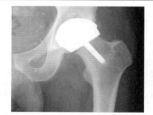

Fig 11.35 AP x-ray of a cemented total hip arthroplasty.

Courtesy of The Norfolk and Norwich University Hospitals (NNUH) Radiology Dept.

Fig 11.36 AP x-ray of the left hip after Birmingham hip resurfacing.

Courtesy of The Norfolk and Norwich University Hospitals (NNUH) Radiology Dept.

Further reading

Byrd JW (2007). Evaluation of the hip: history and physical examination. *N Am J Sports Phys Ther* 2(4):231–40.

Sabharwal S *et al.* (2008). Methods for assessing leg length discrepancy. *Clin Orthop Relat Res* 466(12):2910–22.

►When a child complains of pain in the knee, always examine the hip (fig 11.38). Localizing the source of pain can be difficult. Any limp warrants further investigation (see BOX, p685). A 4-yr-old presents with a pyrexia and a limp due to hip pain; differentiating between septic arthritis (an emergency) and transient synovitis (benign) can be difficult. There are 4 prognostic clinical signs: • Temp >38.5° • wcc> 12 • CRP > 20 • Non-weight bearing. If three or more are present, then there is >93% chance of septic arthritis.[35] If so, do urgent blood culture ± US-guided aspiration. The hip is a deep joint so local signs (eg warmth, erythema) will appear late in the disease process. The most common source of atraumatic pain is the hip, here are some important causes:

Differential diagnosis
You must rule out:
• Septic arthritis (p546 *OHCM*)
Then consider:
• Tubercular arthritis[2–5yr]
• Perthes' disease[4–7yr]
• SUFE[10–16yr]
• Inflammatory arthritis
• Osteomyelitis
And by exclusion:
• Transient synovitis

Transient synovitis of the hip (irritable hip) is the chief cause of hip pain in children aged 4–10 years but is a diagnosis of exclusion. Acute onset and self-limiting with rest ± analgesia. Aetiology considered to be viral illness preceded by recent viral URTI or autoimmune. On examination there is pain in the extremities of movement, bloods and radiology are normal. If other joints are involved, consider juvenile idiopathic arthritis (see 'Still's disease', p654).

Perthes' disease (fig 11.40) For no known reason, avascular necrosis of the femoral head occurs, although this ischaemia is self-healing, it is the subsequent bone remodelling that distorts the epiphysis and generates abnormal ossification. It affects those aged 3–11yrs (typically 4–7yrs). It is bilateral in 10–15%. ♂:♀≈4:1. It presents with pain in hip or knee and causes a limp. On examination all movements at the hip are limited, especially internal rotation and abduction. Early x-rays ± MRI show joint space widening. Later there is a decrease in size of the femoral head with patchy density. Later still, there may be collapse and deformity of the femoral head with new bone formation. Long-term prognosis is governed by the risk of OA in the deformed hip. Severe deformity of the femoral head risks early arthritis and likely need for joint replacement. The younger the patient (<6yrs) the better the prognosis (due to increased ability to remodel). For those with less severe disease (<½ the femoral head affected on lateral x-rays, and joint space depth well preserved) treatment is bed rest and NSAIDs until pain-free, followed by x-ray surveillance. If prognosis poorer (>½ femoral head affected, narrowing of total joint space) surgery may be indicated.

Slipped upper femoral epiphysis (SUFE)[10] Affects those aged 10–16yrs. 20% are bilateral. ♂:♀≈3:1. The exact cause is unknown, though it is likely to be a combination of hormonal & biomechanical factors. About 50% are obese. There is displacement through the growth plate (fig 11.39) with the epiphysis always slipping down and back. It usually presents after minor injury (or atraumatic) with limping and pain in the groin, anterior thigh, or knee. 90% are able to weightbear (stable) and 10% are not (unstable). Flexion, abduction, and medial rotation are limited (eg lying with foot externally rotated). Δ: anteroposterior (fig 11.37) + frog-leg lateral x-rays of both hips. Delayed diagnosis can lead to progression of slip with increased risk of early OA and stable lesions becoming unstable. Treatment is surgical with early internal fixation to stablize any slippage and encourage physeal closure. Prophylactic fixation remains controversial and assessed on individual basis. If untreated, consequences may be avascular necrosis of the femoral head (p735) or malunion predisposing to arthritis. ►Symptoms may be mild so have a high index of suspicion if in correct age group. If occurring in those <10 or >16yrs, then consider an endocrinopathy, eg hypothyroidism or growth hormone imbalance.

---

10 It may be that unrecognized SUFE can cause later osteoarthritis of the hip.

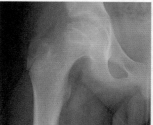

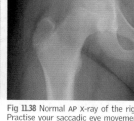

Fig 11.37 AP X-ray of the right hip showing a SUFE. The changes are subtle, but note that a line (the line of Klein) drawn along the upper edge of the femoral neck in fig 11.38 would intersect the femoral head, but would not in fig 11.37. More reliable, though even harder to appreciate, is the widening of the physis—most prominent at the lateral edge.

Courtesy of The Norfolk and Norwich University Hospitals (NNUH) Radiology Dept.

Fig 11.38 Normal AP X-ray of the right hip. Practise your saccadic eye movements between the two to appreciate the slip downwards and medially.

Courtesy of The Norfolk and Norwich University Hospitals (NNUH) Radiology Dept.

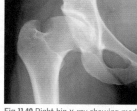

Fig 11.40 Right hip X-ray showing modelling deformity of the femoral head, consistent with prior Perthes' disease.

Courtesy of The Norfolk and Norwich University Hospitals (NNUH) Radiology Dept.

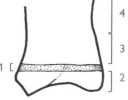

Fig 11.39 Bones such as the femur grow from a cartilaginous growth plate called a *physis* (1); the end of a bone beyond the growth plate is called the *epiphysis* (2); the shaft of a long bone is called the *diaphysis* (4); the ossified portion of bone in a transitional zone between the epiphysis and diaphysis is called the *metaphysis* (3) and it should always have a smooth cortex. The diaphysis continues (arrow) to the metaphysis at the other end of the bone. The stem, *-physis*, comes from the Greek for 'growth'. An *apophysis* is a bony outgrowth independent of a centre of ossification. Epiphyseal injuries: p719. © Tom Turmezei

The limping child

Pain in the hip is the main cause for a limp in children, a presentation which must be taken seriously. You must assume it is septic arthritis until proven otherwise (see MINIBOX). Examination can prove difficult since children will often inadvertently exaggerate their limp and are poor historians. Challenging a little one to race you down the hall or see who can jump the highest is an excellent motivator to make children forget their ailment and engage in activity with you. This trick was learned from an ED consultant who got the child I had been desperately trying to mobilize, leap out of the room. She simply suggested that the noise outside meant that the new toys had arrived. Other non-hip causes of limp in children: malignancy (leukaemia), infection (discitis), metabolic (rickets) and inflammatory (reactive arthritis, juvenile idiopathic arthritis).

Further reading

BMJ Best Practice (2015). *Assessment of Gait Disorders in Children.* http://bestpractice.BMJ.com/best-practice/monograph/709.html

Shah H (2014). Perthes disease. *Orthop Clin North Am* 45(1):87–97.

Walter KD (2015). *Slipped Capital Femoral Epiphysis.* Medscape. http://emedicine.medscape.com/article/91596-overview

DDH refers to a spectrum of pathology from stable acetabular dysplasia to established hip dislocation. It has replaced the term congenital dislocation of the hip (CDH) to reflect the progressive course of this condition. Affects 1-3% of newborns. ♀:♂≈6:1; left/right hip incidence≈4:1; bilateral in ⅕.

At-risk babies
• Breech birth
• Caesar for breech
• Other malformations
• Sibling with DDH
• Birth weight↑
• Oligohydramnios
• Primip/older mother
• Postmaturity

Diagnosis Early diagnosis is important since, if appropriately aligned in the first few months of life, a dysplastic hip may spontaneously resolve.[11] Delays in diagnoses (termed >7 weeks late) require more complex treatment and has less successful outcomes. A Norwegian study showed that DDH was responsible for 29% of hip replacements in patients aged <60 yrs.[36] All babies should have their hips examined in the 1st days of life and at 6 weeks (fig 11.41). If high risk (see MINIBOX), the infant should have a US at 2–4 weeks, with treatment instigated by 6 weeks if not spontaneously resolved. ►Be alert to DDH throughout child surveillance (p150) as a hip may be normal at birth, and become abnormal later.

Ultrasound is the imaging of choice, up to 4.5 months, as it is non-invasive and dynamic. Pelvic x-rays are better for older infants. Routine US screening for DDH remains controversial on account of the high rate of spontaneous resolution of dysplasia and due to insufficient evidence (based on a recent Cochrane review),[37] however targeting high-risk babies (BOX) is advised. Bear in mind though that in a large UK series, 40:1000 babies had evidence of instability on routine US screening; only 3:1000 required treatment.

Treatment If neonatal examination suggests instability arrange US. A recent Cochrane review confirmed that delaying treatment by 2-8 weeks allows time for spontaneous resolution, thus reducing need for treatment without increasing risk of later complications in infants who have clinically unstable hips (but not dislocated) or have mild dysplasia on US. Hips that remain unstable at 6 weeks require prompt treatment. Typically treatment involves long-term splinting in flexion-abduction in a Pavlik® harness (see fig 11.38). *From 6–18 months* examination-under-anaesthetic, arthrography and closed reduction are performed followed by a period of immobilization in a *spica* hip bandage (*spica* refers to the pattern of bandaging, from the Latin for an 'ear of corn'), as the harness is <50% successful beyond 6 months of age. Open reduction is sometimes required if closed techniques fail. *After 18 months* (delayed presentation) open reduction is required with corrective femoral/pelvic osteotomies to maintain joint stability.

Club foot (talipes equinovarus)

A common congenital deformity with unknown aetiology. Mostly an isolated idiopathic finding, but 20% are associated with genetic syndromes or other congenital conditions. ♂:♀ >1:1; bilateral in 50%. The foot deformity consists of: **1** Inversion **2** Adduction of forefoot relative to hindfoot (which is in varus) **3** Equinus (plantarflexion) deformity. The foot cannot be passively everted and dorsiflexed through the normal range. The preferred treatment, starting as early as possible, is the *Ponseti method*, in which the foot is manipulated and placed in a long leg plaster cast (which aims to correct the forefoot adduction and hindfoot varus deformity) on repeated occasions. It is important that deformity correction is *gradual*. If this does not work, soft tissue release between ages 6–12 months (with further surgery on bones if required in later childhood).[38]

11 The importance behind picking up DDH is that for a hip to develop normally the femoral head must articulate with the acetabulum. Failure to identify the problem early means that there is no development of the acetabulofemoral joint, posing real problems for any prospect of surgical correction.

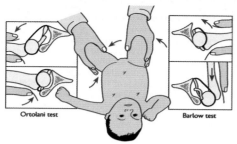

Fig 11.41 Hip tests: the Ortolani test and the Barlow manoeuvre. Beware repeated Ortolani and Barlow manoeuvres which may induce instability.

Hip tests for DDH

Clinical detection of DDH is user dependent, but improves with training and guidance.[39] The manoeuvres in fig 11.41 detect unstable hips, but will both be negative in an irreducible dislocated hip, so use other tests as well.

Ortolani manoeuvre This test relocates a subluxed or partially dislocated hip. With the child's hips flexed and abducted, place your fingers on the greater trochanter and try to lift up the femoral head and relocate it into the acetabulum. The test is positive when there is a palpable 'clunk' as the hip relocates. The test will be negative if there is an *irreducible* dislocation.

Barlow manoeuvre This test aims to sublux or dislocate an unstable hip. Start with hip flexed and adducted slightly. Gently apply axial load to the femur and try to dislocate the femoral head. The test is positive when the femoral head is felt to dislocate; may be accompanied by a 'clunk'.

Galeazzi test Looks for apparent shortening of femur caused by dislocation of femoral head. The child lies supine on an examination table with the hips flexed, the feet flat on the table, and the ankles touching the buttocks. The test is positive when the knees are at different heights. This test will be negative if both hips are dislocated as there will be no apparent discrepancy.

Other signs A widened perineum and buttock flattening on the affected side. Unequal leg length and asymmetrical groin creases may also suggest DDH (although not present in bilateral cases). If >3 months old, limited abduction (<60°) of hip whilst in flexion may be the most sensitive test for DDH. Signs in older children: delay in walking and waddling gait (affected leg is shorter). Bilateral involvement will increase the lumbar lordosis.

Pavlik® harness

A Pavlik® harness is adjusted during growth to help maintain hip reduction and stability (fig 11.42). Excess abduction (in splint) may cause *avascular necrosis* of the head of femur—the worst possible outcome of treatment. Monitor patient carefully to ensure that harness fits well and hips are adequately reduced; US is helpful here. Continue to wear harness until hip remains stable both clinically and on US. Contraindicated if >4.5 months old or hips are irreducible.

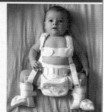

Fig 11.42 The Pavlik® harness. © Anna Williams 2012.

Further reading

Eastwood DM *et al.* (2010). Clinical examination for developmental dysplasia of the hip in neonates: how to stay out of trouble. *BMJ* 340:c1965.

Sewell MD *et al.* (2009). Developmental dysplasia of the hip. *BMJ* 339:b4454.

The knee is the largest human joint in terms of volume and surface area of cartilage and is most susceptible to injury, age-related wear, inflammatory arthritis, and septic arthritis. It consists of a hinge joint between the femur and tibia. The patella is the largest sesamoid bone and is embedded in the quadriceps tendon. It articulates with the trochlear groove of the femur and increases the mechanical advantage of the quadriceps. **History** Traumatic? (think ligament/meniscal damage) Atraumatic? (think overuse problem or degenerative changes). Did patient hear/feel a pop? (often occurs with anterior cruciate ligament (ACL) tears). How long did swelling take to develop? (immediate: # eg tibial plateau; within hours: ACL tear; over night: meniscal tear). Does the knee lock? Is squatting difficult? (both potentially present when mensical tears flip in/out of joint) Does the knee give way? (non-specific for muscle weakness, meniscal tears or ligament instability).

Examination Fully expose the leg. LOOK for alignment, quadriceps wasting, and for swelling. Even 5–10mL of fluid will 'fill in' the medial and lateral peripatellar dimples giving the knee a general fullness. FEEL Confirm by placing the palm of one hand above the patella over the suprapatellar pouch, and thumb and forefinger of the other hand below the patella. Fluid can be moved between the two by squeezing one hand, then the other. If >15mL fluid is present it may be possible to feel a *patellar tap* (milk fluid towards centre of knee then ballott patella against the anterior surface of the femur). Palpate the medial and lateral joint lines (for osteoarthritis/meniscal/plateau injuries), the patella, the popliteal fossa and femoral condyles. MOVE Flexion should be enough for the heel to touch the buttock. Check to see no evidence of crepitus or 'locking'. Ensure patella tendon is intact by examining active knee extension/straight leg raise.

Examine the *medial* and *lateral collateral ligaments* (fig 11.43) with the knee flexed 20°–30° (to relax the posterior capsule and the cruciate ligaments); one hand lifts the ankle, the other stabilizes the knee. Stress the knee by abducting the ankle while pushing the knee medially with the hand behind the knee (tests the *medial* ligament with a *valgus* stress force). Reverse the pressures to give adducting force to test *lateral* ligament (ie *varus* stress). If these ligaments are torn the knee joint opens more widely when the relevant ligament is tested (compare knees against each other, as general laxity may be present). Tenderness over lateral joint line could be iliotibial band tendinitis.

Test the *cruciate ligaments* (figs 11.44 & 11.45) with the knee 90° flexed (anterior/posterior drawer tests) and at 20° of flexion (Lachman's test); immobilize the patient's leg by sitting on his foot, and then with the knee in flexion, grip the upper tibia and try to draw it towards you, away from the femur. The ACL prevents *anterior* glide of the tibia on the femur; the posterior cruciate ligament (PCL) prevents *posterior* glide. Excessive glide in one direction suggests damage to the relevant ligament. The 'pivot shift test'[12]; a more sensitive test to determine if symptoms really are due to cruciate damage (can be asymptomatic).

McMurray's rotation test is an unreliable way of detecting pedunculated *meniscal tears*.[13] With the knee flexed, the tibia is laterally rotated, then the knee is extended. This is repeated with varying degrees of knee flexion, and then again with the tibia medially rotated on the femur. The test is designed to jam the free end of a torn meniscus in the joint—a click being felt and heard and it is postive if pain is experienced by the patient as the jammed tag is released as the knee straightens. NB: normal knees often produce patellar clicks. Apley's grinding test is more reliable and easier to perform; with the patient lying prone, flex the knee to 90° and rotate the tibia with axial pressure whilst distracting the femur.[40]

12 This is so-called because it was found to be positive in patients (eg American Football players) who reported to their surgeon that 'When I pivot (on my leg) something shifts'.
13 Meniscal tears are especially difficult to clinically diagnose because the menisci are avascular and only the outer ⅓ is innervated; there can be little pain or swelling after injury.

Orthopaedics

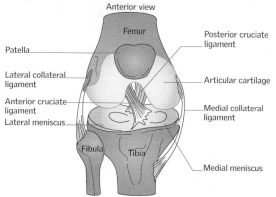

Anterior view

Femur

Patella

Lateral collateral
ligament

Anterior cruciate
ligament

Lateral meniscus

Fibula   Tibia

Posterior cruciate
ligament

Articular cartilage

Medial collateral
ligament

Medial meniscus

Fig 11.43 The anatomy of the right knee—as seen from in front. The medial collateral ligament is much broader than the lateral ligament, and its deep fibres are firmly attached to the medial meniscus. The lateral ligament and the lateral meniscus are interposed by the popliteal tendon (see fig 11.40), and hence are not connected. Four ligaments stabilize the knee: anterior and posterial cruciate ligaments, medial and lateral collateral ligaments. The secondary stabilizers include the menisci, iliotibial band, and biceps femoris.

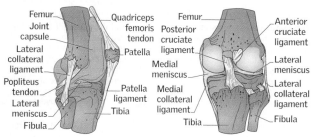

Femur

Joint
capsule

Lateral
collateral
ligament

Popliteus
tendon

Lateral
meniscus

Fibula

Quadriceps
femoris
tendon

Patella

Patella
ligament

Tibia

Femur

Posterior
cruciate
ligament

Medial
meniscus

Medial
collateral
ligament

Tibia

Anterior
cruciate
ligament

Lateral
meniscus

Lateral
collateral
ligament

Fibula

Fig 11.44 The synovium of the right knee joint: lateral (left) and posterior views. Note that the synovium extends up behind the patella (remember for joint aspiration, p706), and that both cruciate ligaments are extrasynovial (but are intracapsular). NB: the joint capsule is distended in these images by infusion of fluid.

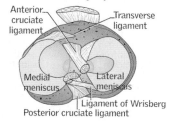

Anterior
cruciate
ligament

Medial
meniscus

Transverse
ligament

Lateral
meniscus

Ligament of Wrisberg

Posterior cruciate ligament

Fig 11.45 Tibial plateau and ligaments.

The ACL prevents anterior translation and rotation of the tibia on the femur.
The PCL prevents posterior subluxation of tibia on the femur.
The medial meniscus is securely attached to the joint capsule, and consequently more frequently torn compared to the lateral meniscus which is more mobile.

Arthroscopy enables internal structures of the knee to be seen and a definite diagnosis may be made. It also enables a wide range of operations to be done as day-case surgery. This is routinely preceded by MRI.

Further reading

Rossi R *et al.* (2011). Clinical examination of the knee: know your tools for diagnosis of knee injuries. *Sports Med Arthrosc Rehabil Ther Technol* 3:25.

The common symptoms are anterior knee pain and swelling. Anterior knee pain can be due to many causes:

Patellofemoral pain syndrome (PFPS) Is common in young athletes—esp. runners and may be associated with overuse as well as lower limb malalignment, muscle imbalance, and patella tracking abnormalities. Patella aching is felt after prolonged sitting or on climbing/descending stairs. There may have been a recent increase in sporting activity or trauma, ask about a history of patella subluxation/dislocation. Effusion is rare. Medial retropatellar tenderness and pain on patellofemoral compression occur: +ve Clarke's test = pain on patellofemoral compression with tensed quadriceps muscles. There may be either decreased or increased patella mobility. *Diagnosis* is clinical. *Treat* by relative rest—if due to increased training employ a structured rehabilitation. Quadriceps and hip strengthening exercises are the mainstay of treatment. NSAIDs may only reduce pain for a few months. Surgery is rarely indicated. [41]

Bipartite patella (fig 11.46) is a congenital fragmentation of the patella, found in ~1%. Usually an incidental x-ray finding (often falsely interpreted as a fracture pattern), but may give pain if the superolateral fragment is mobile with tenderness over the junction. Excision of fragment may relieve pain.

Patella tendinopathy (jumper's knee) is usually initiated by micro- or macro patella tendon tears, eg associated with sudden sporting loads. It can occur anywhere in the patellar tendon, and settles with rest ± NSAIDs. If unable to rest, steroid injection around (not into) the tendon may help. Eccentric contraction exercises (tension whilst lengthening the muscle) may also help. [42]

Hoffa's fat pad syndrome This is a very painful impingement of the infrapatella (Hoffa's) fat pad thought to be caused by maltracking of the patella. Typically caused by over-extension of knee (such as an awkward fall or lifting weights with locked knees). Extending a bent knee while putting pressure on the patellar tendon margins elicits pain and a defensive behaviour. [43] Think of it in those with meniscus or ligament-type symptoms when imaging shows they are intact. MRI may show a hypertrophic Hoffa pad impinging between articular surfaces (which causes pain under the patella). There may be hydrarthrosis or haemarthrosis (from arteriole rupture).

Chrondromalacia patellae Softening of the articular cartilage of the patella.

Osgood-Schlatter disease (p703) pain ± swelling over tibial tuberosity.

Bursitis (fig 11.47) The *prepatellar bursa* is the most commonly affected causing anterior knee pain following trauma or overuse (kneeling for prolonged periods of time) earning it the name 'house maid's knee'. May also occur with infection, crystalarthropathies, and rheumatoid arthritis. Typically presents with swelling and tenderness anterior to patella, and pain on kneeling. Prepatellar bursae may be aspirated, ± corticosteroid injected to decrease recurrence. If very persistent it may need excision. Pain may be relieved by topical NSAIDs. Aspiration distinguishes friction bursitis from suppurative bursitis, which needs drainage and antibiotics, eg **flucloxacillin 500mg/6h PO (adults).▶** Always consider septic arthritis of joint (p546 *OHCM*).

The *infrapatellar bursa* leads to 'clergyman's knee' as they kneel more upright. The *semimembranous bursa* lies in the popliteal fossa (a popliteal cyst which differs from the 'Baker's cyst' which is a herniation from the joint synovium) and causes popliteal discomfort.

You will notice the strong association of overuse injuries with occupation—housemaid's knee has also been referred to as nun's knee, miner's knee, etc. So remember to ask about occupation or repetitive sport movements such as tennis or golf in elbow injuries.

Further reading

LLopis E *et al.* (2007). Anterior knee pain. *Eur J Radiol* 62:27–43.

Orthopaedics

'All these hags'

Once, after a stay in hospital with a fracture, a patient who was not quite as deaf as she was supposed to be, told one of us (JML) how she had overheard a newly arrived orthopaedic surgeon say to the ward nurse 'What are we going to do with all these hags?'. As he progressed down the ward, turning first to the left and then to the beds on the right, his mood became morose, then black—as if he was getting angry that all these 'hags' were clogging up his beds, preventing his scientific endeavours. But what was really happening, my patient suspected, was that, as he turned to left and right, he was really nodding goodbye to his humanity, and, dimly aware of this, he was angry to see it go. On this view, these rows of hags were like buoys in the night, marking his passage out of our world. We all make this trip. Is there any way back? The process of becoming a doctor takes us away from the very people we first wanted to serve (Captain Pollard syndrome, p652). Must medicine take the brightest and the best and turn us into quasi-monsters?

The answer to these questions came unexpectedly in the months that followed: sheer pressure of work drove this patient's observations out of my mind. It was winter, and there was 'flu. In the unnatural twilight of a snowy day I drifted from bed to bed in a stupor of exhaustion with a deepening sense of a collapse that could not be put off...It was all I could do to climb into bed: but when I awoke, I found I had somehow climbed into a patient's bed, who had kindly moved over to make space for me, and was now looking at me with concern in her eyes. Herein lay the answer: the hag must make room for the doctor, and the doctor must make room for the hag: *we are all in the same bed.*

Orthopaedics

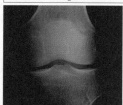

Fig 11.46 Bipartite patella at the usual position of the superolateral edge. This x-ray has been 'windowed' to make the lesion more obvious (the bean-sized fragment is between 1 and 2 o'clock). This has been one of the major advantages of digitized image viewing.

Courtesy of The Norfolk and Norwich University Hospitals (NNUH) Radiology Dept.

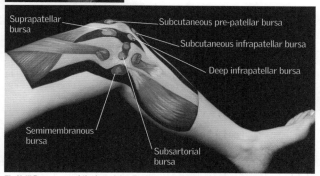

Suprapatellar bursa

Subcutaneous pre-patellar bursa

Subcutaneous infrapatellar bursa

Deep infrapatellar bursa

Semimembranous bursa

Subsartorial bursa

Fig 11.47 Bursa around the knee joint. Bursae are small fibrous sacs of fluid with a synovial lining, typically found around joints and between tendons and ligaments where they pass over bones. They function to reduce friction. Bursitis is inflammation of a bursa with consequent increases in synovial fluid production & swelling. There are ~16 bursae surrounding the knee, see p690 for those most commonly affected.

Reproduced courtesy of Art and Anatomy Edinburgh. Copyright © 2015 Art and Anatomy Edinburgh. Contributors Megan Anderson, Nichola Robertson, Kimmie Simpson, Philip Stewart, and Alex Haddon.

Osteoarthritis (OA) (also see p546 *OHCM*) Knee OA is the most common joint disease in Europe. Women (especially if >55yrs old) are at greater risk.[44] Knee swelling may occur with any arthritic process.

Primary osteoarthritis can be defined as degeneration of the articular cartilage and surfaces of a joint with no predisposing factors—in this sense, the disease is idiopathic, though current research

Secondary OA causes
• Post-traumatic
• Postoperative
• Post-infective
• Malposition
• Mechanical instability
• Osteochondritis dissecans (p668)

is suggesting many of these cases have subtle underlying congenital/developmental defects. In *secondary* OA there is an underlying precipitant to the degenerative process (see MINIBOX). OA is associated with ↑BMI, genetic factors, age, and occupation. Weight loss in women reduces risk of getting OA symptoms.[45][n=796] Patients complain of pain on initiating movement. Stiffness follows inactivity, but often resolves in <30min. In the knee, OA particularly affects the posterior patella and the medial compartment, so tending to varus deformity (osteotomy is an attractive alternative to total knee replacement (TKR) for early OA in young, active patients since a prosthesis will only last approx 15 years). Osteotomies can delay TKR for up to 10 years. On examination, an arthritic knee will have a limited range of motion with crepitus during both active and passive movements. There may be joint deformity and bony overgrowth from osteophytes. *Treatment:* NSAIDs (topical ibuprofen may be as good as oral in older patients, and has fewer SE), quadriceps strengthening exercises, weight loss, local steroid injections (gives some relief in the short term, but long-term benefit is unclear).

Knee replacement Consists of resection of articular surfaces of the knee, then resurfacing with metal and polyethylene components. Replacement may be total or partial (unicompartmental). Pain correlates poorly with radiological signs. Success rate: 95%. Consider referral for joint surgery in those patients with significant disabling pain (even at rest or disturbing sleep) which has a detrimental impact on QOL despite adequate conservative approaches. Postoperative knee swelling is relatively common; due to the close proximity of the joint to the external environment any suspicion of infection must be dealt with seriously. ▶▶Prosthetic joints must only be aspirated in an orthopaedic theatre; never in ED or clinic. *Joint survival:* 90% last 15yrs (better than hips). Revision rates are similar. Quality of life can be transformed, even if >80yrs old. TKR is highly cost-effective with respect to QALYs gained.[46]

Meniscal cysts *Typical patient:* A young man, with past trauma, then insidious development of cyst. *Pain:* Over the joint line. Lateral cysts are 5–10× more common than medial. Swelling may disappear with full flexion. The meniscus is often torn radially (an otherwise unusual direction) so there may be knee clicking and giving way. Δ: MRI. *Treatment:* Arthroscopic decompression.

Ligament tears, meniscus lesions, patellar dislocation See p737.

Baker's cyst is the most common swelling of the popliteal fossa. Primary cysts in young people tend to be asymptomatic. Secondary cysts are a misnomer, since they result from fluid building up within the semimembranosus bursa associated with chronic knee effusions from OA. Patients present with posterior knee swelling and aching. ▶▶Always consider DVT, especially if cyst has ruptured causing calf swelling. US helps determine nature of cystic lesions and presence of vascular flow. Treatment is mostly conservative with analgesia, spontaneous resolution can occur in young people. To date, there is no gold standard approach and treatment is aimed at the underlying articular disorders.

The acutely swollen hot joint

▶You must suspect septic arthritis (p546 *OHCM*) in any acutely painful and swollen joint as this is the most serious diagnosis.

Differential diagnosis	
Inflammatory disease	**Disorders in bone/cartilage**
Septic arthropathy	Trauma
Crystal arthropathy (gout and pseudo-gout(CPPD)) (p550 *OHCM*)	Haemarthrosis (associated with high bleeding tendency)
Rheumatoid arthritis	Fracture
Reactive arthritis	
Psoriatic arthropathy	

Osteoarthritis, many of the rheumatological conditions, and malignancy can also present with chronic swelling. Note that acute polyarthritis is associated with multiple systemic rheumatological and infective disease processes.
▶▶Always ask if other joints are affected and if patient is systemically unwell.

On **examination** feel the joint margins for bogginess (suggestive of chronic inflammatory arthritis) and palpate for effusions. Look for erythema and feel for warmth.

Investigations *Aspiration* of synovial fluid from the affected joint is the key investigation. Analysis (see TABLE on p707) helps to diagnose haemarthrosis, infectious and crystal arthropathies. Be mindful that one cannot rule out sepsis simply because crystals are present or initial Gram staining is negative—use your clinical judgement and treat if you suspect infection. ▶*Aspiration of a replaced joint must be done under sterile conditions in theatre.* See p708. *Bloods:* Do CRP, FBC, U+Es, LFTs, bone profile (for calcium and phosphate) and blood cultures. Also request a serum urate but note it may be normal in acute attacks of gout. Consider rheumatoid factor, anti-CCP, and antibody titres if rheumatological cause is suspected. Ask the rheumatology team for help if no obvious cause.

X-rays are usually normal in septic arthritis but may shows signs of chronic gout (well-defined 'punched out' erosions in juxta-articular bone see fig 3 on p543 in *OHCM*).

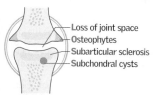

Loss of joint space
Osteophytes
Subarticular sclerosis
Subchondral cysts

Fig 11.48 Features of osteoarthritis.
Reproduced from Longmore et al., *Oxford Handbook of Clinical Medicine* (2014), with permission from OUP.

Further reading
Eid AS *et al.* (2012). As we managing knee effusion well? *BJMP* 5(1):a504. www.bjmp.org/files/2012-5-1/bjmp-2012-5-1-a504.pdf

Examination 25° of extension (dorsiflexion) and 30° of flexion (plantarflexion) are the norm at the tibiotalar joint. Inversion and eversion are from the sub-talar and midtarsal joints. Toes should have between 60° and 90° extension. Note callosities. Examine the arches (fig 11.46). Watch as the toes are lifted off the ground, and on standing on tiptoe. Examine gait and shoes (normal wear pattern: medially under ball of foot, posterolaterally at heel).

Hallux valgus (bunion) The big toe devi-ates laterally at the metatarsophalangeal joint (fig 11.49). Typically present bilaterally. Pressure of the metatarsophalangeal joint against the shoe leads to bunion formation; some have gross relatively painless deform-ity which only causes problems with shoe-fittings, others can report high levels of pain with minimal deformity. Risk factors in-clude female gender, age, type of footwear, a positive family history, conditions caus-ing joint hypermobility, and neuromuscular disease. Secondary OA in the joint is com-mon. Educate the patient on appropriate footwear (wide, low-heeled shoes) and foot exercises to strengthen musculature around the big toe. Bunion pads and plastic wedges between great and second toes may relieve pain, but this is a progressive condition and correction of deformity requires surgery. Painful bunions which inhibit lifestyle and footwear choices should be considered for surgery. Surgery is not indicated for

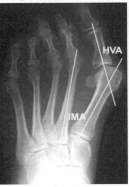

Fig 11.49 Weightbearing AP image showing a hallux valgus deformity and the hallux valgus angle (HVA) and intermetatarsal angle (IMA).

Courtesy of Professor Peter Scally.

cosmetic reasons. Many different operations are used with no accepted gold standard and each patient is considered individually. Surgery achieves toe alignment and alleviates pain in ~90%.[47] Complications include chronic pain, recurrence, and joint stiffness.

Lesser toe deformities may accompany a halux valgus as they have similar biomechanical risk factors. All present with painful calluses when walking and difficulties finding shoes that are comfortable. Typically affects >60-year-olds. Initially the deformity will be flexible, over time the joint stiffens and becomes fixed. ▶Always investigate for diabetic neuropathy. Examine the lower limb neurovascular status and musculature. Management is similar to halux valgus with orthotics and surgery reserved to correct painful, debilitating deformi-ties.

1 *Hammer toes:* These are extended at the MTP joint, hyperflexed at the PIP joint, and extended at the DIP joint. The toes look curled. Associated with contracture of flexor digitorum longus tendon. Second toes are most com-monly affected.

2 *Claw toes:* Extended at the MTP joint but flexed at PIP and DIP joints giving a clawed appearance where the toe digs into the sole of the foot. The operative treatment for both hammer and claw toes is metatarsal shortening (flexible deformity) or PIP joint arthrodesis (fixed deformity).

3 *Mallet toes:* Flexion deformity of the DIP joint in isolation treated with flexor tenotomy (flexible deformity) or DIP joint arthrodesis (fixed deformity).

Our feet have carried us through the history of mankind. Although many of our problems today arise from the strained biomechanics of walking on two feet, the foot remains a remarkable structure. Historically, pain in the foot has not captured much interest amongst the medical profession and research has moved slowly. Often dismissed as trivial, we now increasingly have started to recognize the importance of physical inactivity and how very limiting chronic foot pain can be.[48] So just like we tend to forget to nurture our souls, don't leave these soles out of your assessment.[14]

Ingrowing toenails (onychocryptosis) Typically the big toe in young adults. Incorrect nail cutting ± pressure of shoes predispose to the lateral nail digging into its fleshy bed, which reacts by becoming heaped up infection—'proudflesh'. *Conservative treatment* involves tucking cotton-wool soaked in surgical spirit under the proudflesh and awaiting nail growth (then cut it straight with edges protruding beyond flesh margins). However, a recent Cochrane review has shown that *surgical interventions* (whole-nail avulsion or wedge resection of affected side) are more effective in preventing recurrence, especially when combined with the application of phenol.[49]

Adult forefoot pain (metatarsalgia) Increased pressure on the metatarsal head causes pain in the ball of the foot. Associated with ↑BMI, high heels, toe deformities, high-impact sports and inflammatory arthritis. Occupational therapy can provide orthotic supports for shoes. Advise rest and gentle strengthening exercises. Surgery other than for rheumatoid arthritis is unpredictable.
Morton's neuroma: A common cause of metatarsalgia in women. Pain is from pressure from an interdigital neuroma[15] between the metatarsals (eg from tight-fitting shoes). Pain usually radiates to the lateral side of one toe, and the medial side of its neighbour (eg toes 3 & 4). Compressing the affected web space is quite specific. MRI helps diagnosis, as does us if by an experienced operator. Neuroma excision may be needed.[50]

March (stress) fractures occur in the shaft of 2nd or 3rd metatarsals. May follow excessive walking: the history should raise suspicion and prompt a scouring search of the metatarsi. x-rays may be normal, or have subtle periosteal changes. Radionuclide bone scans are more discriminating. Treatment is rest and analgesia, crutches for a few weeks may be useful. If pain is severe, try a plaster cast while awaiting healing.

Pain in the heel can be a diagnostic challenge, consider use of x-rays (to see calcaneal spurs), MRI (to highlight degenerative tendon changes), or bone scans (diffuse uptake in inflammatory arthritis or stress fractures). *Causes:*
- Diseases of the calcaneum
- Rupture of calcaneal tendon (p710)
- Postcalcaneal bursitis (back of heel)
- Post-traumatic (eg calcaneal #)
- Arthritis of the subtalar joint
- Systemic diseases
- Seronegative spondylarthopathy
- Infection.

Plantar fasciitis The plantar fascia supports the arch of the foot. The most common cause of plantar heel pain. Arises from degenerative changes from microtrauma; it is not inflammatory as the suffix 'itis' would suggest. Obesity, inactivity, and excessive walking are risk factors. Treatment should be instigated promptly (immobility is a risk factor for chronicity). No clear superiority between stretching of the achilles tendon, orthotics, and shockwave therapy. Injections have fallen out of favour due to risk of tendon rupture. Prognosis is usually good with minimal treatment, the trick is to encourage athletes to be patient and discourage immobility in inactive patients.

14 Corns: Focal friction-dependent hyperkeratotic intradermal nodules develop at bony pressure points. A bursa-like structure may form around these islands. Likelihood↑ if neuropathy eg diabetes. Unlike calluses (thickened areas of skin) they have a core of keratin, occur only on the foot, and cause pain.[51] Optimize footwear, chiropody, or excise the corn.[52]
15 It is not a true neuroma, but rather degenerative and inflammatory changes to the interdigital nerve resulting in entrapment neuropathy.[53]

Orthopaedics

This is an infection of bone. Incidence is reducing as living standards rise. It can be categorized as acute haematogenous, secondary to contiguous local infection (with or without the presence of vascular disease), or direct inoculation from trauma or surgery. All forms can progress to chronic osteomyelitis. Infection may spread from boils, abscesses, pneumonia, or genitourinary instrumentation, though often no primary site is found.

▶Always look for osteomyelitis in diabetic feet and deep pressure sores.

Common organisms
• Staphylococcus aureus
• Pseudomonas
• E. coli
• Streptococci
Other organisms
• Salmonella (esp. with sickle cell disease)[54]
• Mycobacteria
• Fungi

Clinical features See BOX, p697. **Tests** ESR/CRP↑, WCC↑. Blood culture (+ve in 60%) and most useful in haematogenous spread of infection. Bone biopsy and culture is gold standard for pathogen identification and if diagnosis remains uncertain—but rarely required for acute osteomyelitis. Swabs from discharging sinuses, or needle aspiration of material near bone, may give misleading results.[55] x-ray changes are not apparent for 10–14 days but then show haziness ± loss of density of affected bone, then subperiosteal reaction, and later, sequestrum and involucrum (see BOX & figs 11.51–11.53). NB: infected cancellous bone shows less change. MRI is sensitive and specific (88% and 93%, vs 61% and 33% for isotope scans)—and avoids ionizing radiation, but isotope scans are still sometimes required (eg in presence of prostheses causing imaging artefact).[56]

Treatment Before antibiotics, the treatment was amputation, now surgery aims to simply drain abscesses and remove sequestra (culture all sequestra). The key is 6 weeks of antibiotics: **vancomycin** 1g/12h and **cefotaxime** 1g/12h IVI until the organism

Complications
• Septic arthritis
• Fractures
• Deformity
• Chronic osteomyelitis

and its sensitivities are known. Alternative treatments for adults are **fusidic acid** or **clindamycin**. Ciprofloxacin 500mg/8–12h PO is suitable for *Pseudomonas* osteomyelitis, but be guided by sensitivities and a microbiologist. In children, prevalence of *Haemophilus influenzae* osteomyelitis is reducing due to the HIB vaccination.

Chronic osteomyelitis Poor treatment results in pain, fever, sequestra (infected dead bone) and sinus suppuration (presence of a sinus tract is pathognomonic) with long remissions. Always suspect chronic development in vascular insufficiency with non-healing tissue ulceration overlying bony prominences. Diabetic ulcers have a high risk of osteomyelitis, even before bone becomes exposed. If bone can be felt on probing the ulcer, then this is sufficient to diagnose chronic osteomyelitis.[57] x-rays show thick irregular bone. Treatment involves radical excision of sequestra, skeletal stabilization, 'dead-space' management (often needs plastic surgical input) and antibiotics (as above, modified according to sensitivities) for ≥12 weeks. *Complications:* Amyloid, squamous carcinoma development in sinus track.

Bone TB (eg vertebral body = Pott's disease[16]).This represents 1–3% of all TB; incidence is rising, but remains rare in UK. Spread is haematogenous or via nearby nodes. *Treatment:* Drain abscesses, immobilize affected large joints. Standard 6-month courses (OHCM p386) of eg **isoniazid** (300mg/day), **rifampicin** (600mg/day) and **pyrazinamide** (1.5g/day) may not be long enough and treatment is likely needed for 1 year. Bed rest and bracing is no longer recommended, and gentle exercise is encouraged. A Cochrane review has found no evidence to support routine surgical intervention; it is only neccessary in advanced cases with marked deformity, abscess formation or paraplegia.[34] Prognosis in patients with no neurological defecit tends to be good.

Patterns of infection Cancellous bone is typically affected in adults—commonly in vertebrae (IV drug use) and feet (diabetics). In children, vascular bone is most affected (eg in long-bone metaphyses—esp. distal femur, upper tibia). Infection leads to cortex erosion, with holes (*cloacae*). Exudation of pus lifts up the periosteum interrupting blood supply to underlying bone and necrotic fragments of bone may form

Risk factors
• Diabetes
• Vascular disease
• Impaired immunity
• Sickle cell disease
• Surgical prostheses
• Open fractures
• Impaired immunity

(*sequestrum*). The presence of sequestra is typical of chronic infection. New bone formation created by the elevated periosteum forms an *involucrum*. Pus may discharge into joint spaces or via sinuses to the skin.

The patient Pain of gradual onset and unwillingness to move over the course of a few days. Local findings include tenderness, warmth, erythema, and slight effusion in neighbouring joints. Look for signs of systemic infection. All signs are less marked in adults.

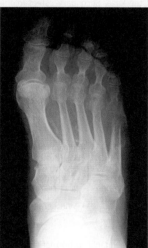

Fig 11.50 Osteomyelitis causing destruction of the 5th metatarsal head and the base of the 5th proximal phalanx. Note also the vascular calcification in this patient, who had diabetes.

Courtesy of The Norfolk and Norwich University Hospitals (NNUH) Radiology Dept.

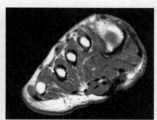

Fig 11.51 Axial T1-weighted MRI of the foot through the metatarsals, showing reduced signal within the first metatarsal (from replacement of the marrow fat with pus) consistent with osteomyelitis.

Courtesy of The Norfolk and Norwich University Hospitals (NNUH) Radiology Dept.

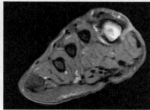

Fig 11.52 Axial T1-weighted MRI of the same patient as fig 11.51, this time with FAT SAT (fat saturation) and IV gadolinium contrast. The effect of this technique is to suppress the marrow fat and enhance the infection.

Courtesy of The Norfolk and Norwich University Hospitals (NNUH) Radiology Dept.

Orthopaedics

Further reading

Howell WR *et al.* (2011). Osteomyelitis: an update for hospitalists. *Hosp Pract* (1995) 39(1):153–60.

Termaat MF *et al.* (2005). The accuracy of diagnostic imaging for the assessment of chronic osteomyelitis: a systematic review and meta-analysis. *J Bone Joint Surg Am* 87(11):2464-71.

16 Mr Percivall Pott has an interesting story, he's not only famous for Pott's Disease of the spine. www.rsc.org/education/eic/issues/2006Mar/PercivalPott.asp

Orthopaedics

Bone is a common site for secondaries (prostate, thyroid, lung, kidney, breast)[17] whilst primary bone neoplasia is rare: incidence of 9 per million population/year. Delays in diagnosis are common. Metastases are blood-borne and usually arise in the lungs or other bones. Staging is done with MRI or combination techniques such as PET-CT.[58] Treatment of these rare and highly aggressive primary tumours is best carried out in multidisciplinary specialist treatment centres.

Bone sarcoma presentation
• Non-mechanial bone or joint pain
• Bone pain at night
• Bony swellings
• Pathological fractures

Multiple myeloma (*OHCM*, p362) is the most common primary malignant bone tumour and accounts for 45% of all malignant bone tumours. Bony manifestations include multiple punched-out osteolytic lesions.

Osteosarcoma[18] The second most common primary malignant bone tumour. Primary osteosarcoma typically affects adolescents and arises in the metaphyses of long bone, especially around the knee. Secondary osteosarcoma may arise in bone affected by Paget's disease or after irradiation. Classically presents between ages 10–20 with a peak in adolescent growth spurt. *Imaging:* Bone destruction and new bone formation (sunray spiculation), often with marked periosteal elevation (Codman's triangle). 50% of lesions are around the knee joint. Patients often present with pain before a mass develops. Staging MRI of the area will assess intramedullary spread. Do an HRCT chest to screen for pulmonary metastases, especially if ALP is raised. *Treatment:* Historically, the affected extremity was usually amputated but >80% of patients devloped recurrent disease (typically pulmonary metastases) which highlights that most patients probably have micrometastatic disease at diagnosis. Neoadjuvant (prior to surgery) chemotherapy is advised. A 5-year survival rate of ~60–70% is achievable.[58]

Ewing's sarcoma This malignant round-cell tumour of long bones (typically diaphysis) and limb girdles, usually presents in adolescents. See MINIBOX for x-ray features. MRI is helpful. Typically patients have a T11:22 chromosomal translocation. *Treatment:* Chemotherapy, surgery, and radiotherapy are required. The key adverse prognostic factor is metastases at diagnosis (5-year recurrence-free survival is 22%—vs 55% if no metastases).[59, n=975]

Radiological features
• Bone destruction
• New bone formation in concentric layers 'onion ring' sign
• Soft tissue swelling
• Periosteal elevation

Chondrosarcoma may arise *de novo* or from malignant transformation of chondromas. It is usually associated with pain, or a lump, and presents in the axial skeleton of the middle-aged. 'Popcorn calcification' is typical on x-ray. MRI/CT will better define tumour extent. *Treatment:* No response to chemotherapy or radiotherapy, so treatment is by excision. Inadequate surgery is accompanied by local recurrence, often of a higher grade of malignancy. The cure rate depends on the type and grade of chondrosarcoma at diagnosis.

Limb-sparing surgical reconstruction (after excising a bone tumour) may involve replacing affected bone with a metal and polyethylene endoprosthesis—as an alternative to amputation. Excellent and durable reconstruction is possible using massive endoprostheses or bone allografts. Amputation is reserved for exceptional cases. 85% of patients now have limb salvage following chemotherapy for primary bone tumours.

---

17 Mnemonic for tumours which commonly metastasize to bone: Particular Tumours Love Killing Bone.
18 There are many different subtypes, including intramedullary, periosteal, parosteal, & telangiectatic.

Bone tumours: benign

Osteochondroma[19] is the commonest benign bone tumour, usually occurring about the knee, proximal femur, or proximal humerus. Presents as a painful mass associated with trauma. Seen on x-ray as a bony spur arising from the cortex and usually pointing away from the joint. *Treatment:* Remove if causing symptoms, eg pressure on adjacent structures. Any osteochondroma continuing to grow after skeletal maturity must be removed because of risk of malignancy (arises rarely in solitary osteochondromas but in up to 10% of patients with ***hereditary multiple exostoses***—an autosomal dominant inherited condition causing short stature as well as forearm, knee, and ankle deformity see p700).

Osteoid osteoma is a painful benign bone lesion that occurs most commonly in long bones of males 10–25yrs old (and also often in the spine). It appears as local cortical sclerosis on x-rays with a central radiolucent nidus. Within the nidus there may be a small nucleus of calcification. The nidus produces prostaglandins leading to pain unrelated to activity, and relieved by Ibuprofen (and other prostaglandin inhibitors). *Treatment:* CT-guided biopsy and radiofrequency ablation.[60] Plain x-rays may miss these tumours. CT is the best imaging modality.[61]

Chondroma These benign cartilaginous tumours may arise from bone surfaces or within the medulla (=enchondromata). They may cause local swelling or #. *Treatment* is rarely needed, exclude malignancy (chondosarcoma).

Fibrous dysplasia of bone is a developmental abnormality where bone is not properly formed. May lead to pain and increased risk of fracture. Surgical stabilization is sometimes needed. In the polyostotic form bisphosphonates may help relieve symptoms.

Sarcoma versus carcinoma

A sarcoma is any malignant neoplasm arising from mesenchymal cells (which give rise to connective and non-epithelial tissue). There are three broad categories: **1** Soft tissue cancers **2** Primary bone cancers **3** Gastro-intestinal stromal tumours (GIST). Carcinomas affect epithelial cells and frequently cause breast, bowel, and lung cancers.

Soft tissue sarcomas (STS)

STS are uncommon (~1500/yr in UK) but can arise in any mesenchymal tissue, originating from fat, muscle, etc. presenting as a painless enlarging mass. Risk factors include neurofibromatosis type 1 (OHCM, p518) and previous radiotherapy.

Diagnosis Any lump that has any feature from the MINIBOX is to be considered malignant until proved otherwise. **Imaging** with MRI followed by needle biopsy. Pathological diagnoses include rhabdomyosarcoma (most common in children), liposarcoma, leiomyosarcoma, fibrosarcoma, etc. Gene

Consider STS malignant if
• Bigger than 5cm
• Increasing in size
• Deep to the deep fascia
• Painful

expression profiling is helping to improve diagnosis and indicate tumours which may respond to chemotherapy. **Treatment** is by excision with wide margins followed by radiotherapy for most. Adjuvant chemotherapy with doxorubicin may be appropriate, trabectedin has a role.[62] **Prognosis** is related to histological grade, size and depth of the tumour. High-grade, large, deep tumours have <50% 5yr survival. STS in children often respond well to chemotherapy; survival is better.

Further reading

Skinner HB *et al.* (2015). *Current Diagnosis & Treatment in Orthopaedics* (5th ed). New York: McGraw-Hill Medical.

19 Cartilage tumour classification: Is the lesion benign or malignant? Is the lesion a pure or impure cartilaginous tumour? Is the epicentre of the lesion intraosseous, juxtacortical, or in the soft tissues? The most common benign tumours are enchondroma, osteochondroma, chondroblastoma, and chondromyxoid fibroma. Chondrosarcoma is malignant.

Osteogenesis imperfecta (OI) 'brittle bone disease' is an inherited disorder of type I collagen that results in joint laxity and fragile, low-density bones which recurrently fracture. It affects 1 in 20,000. OI has historically been classified into four forms (although type IV has recently been expanded into IV–VII). Since patients initially present with inconsistent histories of injury frequency and severity, this condition can be mistaken for child abuse (p146).

I	The mildest and most common form. It is autosomal dominant (AD). Associated with blue sclerae (due to increased corneal translucency) and 50% have hearing loss. Fractures typically occur before puberty. Normal life expectancy.
II	Lethal perinatal form with many fractures, blue sclera, & dwarfism. Recessive.
III	Severe form—occurs in about 20%. Recessive. Fractures at birth + progressive spinal and limb deformity, with resultant short stature; blue or white sclera; dentinogenesis imperfecta common (enamel separates from defective dentine, leaving teeth transparent or discoloured); life expectancy is decreased.
IV	Moderate form. AD. Fragile bones, white sclerae after infancy.

x-rays: Many fractures, osteoporotic bones with thin cortex, and bowing deformity of long bones. *Histology:* Immature unorganized bone with abnormal cortex. *Treatment:* Prevent injury. Physio, rehab, and occupational therapy are key. Osteotomies may correct deformity. Intramedullary rods are sometimes used in long bones. Bisphosphonates may increase cortical thickness.[63] As OI is a genetic disease, gene therapy is being explored in hopes to alter the course of the collagen mutations. This is especially challenging due to genetic heterogeneity and that most OI mutations are dominant negative (the mutant allele product interferes with normal allele function).[64]

Achondroplasia (fig 11.53) The most common form of disproportionate short stature. It occurs due to reduced growth of cartilaginous bone. It is AD, but ~80% are from spontaneous mutation.[65] Gross motor skills develop later—only 50% sit unsupported at 9 months, and only 50% walk alone at 18 months. *x-rays:* Short proximal long bones & wide epiphyses. *Treatment:* Involves monitoring for potential complications. Growth hormone has been tried.[66]

Hereditary multiple exostoses An AD disorder in which certain proteins accumulate leading to cartilage-capped tumours (exostoses/osteochondromata) developing from affected cartilage at the end of long bones. These point away from the nearby joint. If severe, bones are badly modelled, causing short stature as well as forearm, knee, and ankle deformity. Beware of malignant transformation to chondrosarcomas or osteosarcomas (see p698). *Treatment:* Remove symptom-producing exostoses.

Osteopetrosis Lack of differentiation between cortex and medulla of bone (from underlying failure of osteoclastic bone resorption) results in very hard, dense 'marble' bones that are brittle. Anaemia and thrombocytopenia may result from decreased marrow space. Deafness and optic atrophy can result from compression of cranial nerves. Lack of remodelling preserves variations of ossific density causing the characteristic 'bone within a bone' appearance.

See Neurofibromatosis (OHCM p518), Marfan's (OHCM p720), Ehlers–Danlos & Morquio's, p143.

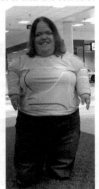

Fig 11.53 Adults with achondroplasia are short with ↑lumbar lordosis, bow legs, and short proximal arms & legs. Lifespan, mental, & sexual development are normal. Complications include tibial bowing, joint hypermobility, hydrocephalus, foramen magnum compression (5–10%), recurrent otitis media, and hearing loss, sleep apnoea (75%) and ↑BMI.   © Nina Hjelde.

Orthopaedics

Developmental bone biology

Because bone is ossified, we tend to think of it as the architectural rock around which our living tissues are constructed. But bone maintenance and development is a highly dynamic and regulated process sensitive to a wide variety of hormones, inflammatory mediators, growth factors, and genetic influences which become aberrant whenever there are deletions, insertions, and missense mutations. The concept of a *master gene* is useful to indicate how genes relate and interact. Master genes encode proteins that can control other genes by directly binding to their DNA, for example, the transcription factor OSF2 (osteoblast specific transcription factor 2) gene is thought to serve as a master gene regulating expression of other genes, allowing mesenchymal stem cells to differentiate into osteoblasts. NB: master genes make a mockery of genes vs environment questions. One gene is an environment for another, and the effects of each may be catastrophic in some environments or negligible in others.

Remain in light...the different types of bone

- *Cancellous (spongy bone):* Trabeculations form a network of parallel lamellae, the spaces being filled with connective tissue or bone. This type of bone does not make callus when healing (a type of lamellar bone).
- *Compact:* Non-cancellous bone that is formed from Haversian canals and concentric lamellae (a type of lamellar bone).
- *Cortical:* Superficial layer of compact bone.
- *Endochondral:* Develops in cartilage that has been destroyed by calcification and subsequent resorption.
- *Heterotopic:* Forms outside the normal skeleton either from a pathological process (eg in the heart) or as a reaction to local trauma/surgery.
- *Lamellar:* The overall normal type of adult bone (subdivided into cancellous and compact), characterized by repeating architectural patterns (fig 11.54).

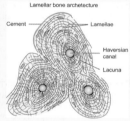
Lamellar bone archetecture.

Cement — Lamellae

Haversian canal

Lacuna

Fig 11.54 Lamellar bone architecture.

- *Membranous:* Formed from intramembranous ossification (eg clavicle).
- *Sesamoid:* Bone formed in a tendon where it passes over a joint (eg the pisiform bone in flexor carpi ulnaris, and the patella).
- *Cartilagenous:* Formed from growth plates (p683).

Remain in light...the different types of joint

- *Cartilagenous, primary:* Hyaline cartilage between the bone ends. Only types are the costochondral and sternochondral (1st rib) joints.
- *Cartilagenous, secondary:* As above, but with a layer of fibrocartilage between the layers of hyaline cartilage. Only types (that all lie in the midline) are the manubriosternal, intervertebral, pubic symphysis, xiphisternal, and sacrococcygeal joints.
- *Fibrous:* Fibrous tissue between bones; eg radio-ulnar interosseous membrane.
- *Synovial:* Joint cavity containing synovial fluid, with hyaline cartilage on the bone surface; eg acetabulofemoral, glenohumeral.
- *Synovial, atypical:* Joint cavity containing synovial fluid, with fibrocartilage on the bone surface ± a fibrocartilage disc; eg acromioclavicular and sternoclavicular joints (with discs). NB: fibrocartilage is found on the articulating surface of any bone that undergoes intramembranous ossification.

Further reading

Glorieux FH (2008). Osteogenesis imperfecta. *Best Pract Res Clin Rheumatol* 22(1):85–100.

Renaud A *et al.* (2013). Radiographic features of osteogenesis imperfecta. *Insights Imaging* 4(4):417–29.

Wright MJ *et al.* (2011). Clinical management of achondroplasia. *Arch Dis Child* 97(2):129–34.

The osteochondroses are a group of conditions characterized by the abnormal endochondral ossification of epiphyseal growth during childhood. Osteochondrosis (also called osteochondritis) occurs in the wrist, elbow, hip, knee, ankle, fingers, toes, and spine. The underlying cause of most osteochondroses is unknown, although inheritance, overuse/trauma, rapid growth, and anatomic configuration may be predisposing factors. All osteochondroses undergo an interruption of blood supply to the epiphysis, followed by bone and cartilage necrosis, revascularization, and regrowth of bone.

Kienböck's disease Avascular necrosis of the lunate carpal bone after single or repetitive injuries. Affects young adults 20–40 years; typically gymnasts. Pain is felt over the lunate (esp. during active wrist movement). Grip is impaired due to pain. Associated with negative ulnar variance. *x-rays:* (fig 11.5) Sclerotic lunate with a little depth reduction early; more marked flattening later, leading later to osteoarthritis. *Treatment:* Early disease is managed symptomatically with splinting and analgesia; if sufficiently symptomatic then surgery attempts to ease compression of the lunate by ulnar lengthening or radial shortening and fusion of the capitate. Late, symptomatic presentation: proximal row carpectomy, intercarpal arthrodesis, total wrist arthrodesis. Once arthritis is established, lunate excision does not help. Wrist arthrodesis is the last resort.

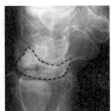

Fig 11.55 Kienböck's disease. Lunate sclerosis with central lucency.

Reproduced from Bulstrode et al., *Oxford Textbook of Trauma and Orthopaedics* 2e (2011), with permission from OUP.

Panner's disease/osteochondritis dissecans (OCD) of the elbow represent a continuum of disease of the capitellum. Panner's disease is the avascular necrosis of the ossific nucleus of the capitellum. Mostly presents in boys under 10yrs, causing lateral elbow pain and swelling. Conservative managment is usually all that is required. OCD of the elbow affects the surface below the cartilage of the anterior capitellum. A loose body is formed from a convex joint surface when a segment of subchondral bone and cartilage becomes avascular and separates from underlying bone. Adolescents experience early aching and effusions after use, and sudden painful locking of joints once pieces have separated to make loose bodies. *x-rays:* Look for lucent areas in a piece *about* to separate, the defect from which the piece *has* separated, and loose bodies *after* separation. *Treatment:* Stable lesions are managed conservatively with activity modification. Unstable lesions may need fixation ± removal of loose bodies. Closed wedge resection may lead to revascularization.

Köhler's disease Rare, affects the navicular bone.[20] Children affected are 3–5-yr-olds. Pain is felt in the mid-tarsal region and they limp. *x-rays:* Dense, deformed bone (fig 11.52). *Treatment:* Symptomatic: resting the foot or wearing a walking plaster. *Prognosis:* Excellent, with few long-term problems.

Freiberg's disease This may be classed as an OCD of the lesser metatarsal heads (commonly the 2nd). Presents as forefoot pain that worsens with pressure. Usually starts around the time of puberty. There may be microfractures at the junction of the metaphysis and the growth plate—precise aetiology is unknown. *x-rays:* Epiphysis of a metatarsal head becomes granular, fragmented, and flattened. *Treatment:* Good shoes ± metatarsal pad. Limit activity for 4–6 weeks. If severe, consider removal of affected bone with bone grafting or arthroplasty and use of a walking plaster.

20 The navicula is the bone at the top of the foot and is separated from the metatarsals by the 3 cuneiform bones with which it articulates. Moving proximally, it articulates with the talus. Navicula is Latin for a small ship. The term carpal navicular was formerly used for the scaphoid bone in the wrist.

Osgood–Schlatter disease is tibial tuberosity apophysitis that affects children 10–15yrs old. ♂:♀≈3:1. The 'accepted theory' suggests that repeated traction causes inflammation and chronic avulsion of the secondary ossification centre of the tibial tuberosity, leading to inflammation, hence its association with physical overuse. The pain below the knee is worse on strenuous activity and quadriceps contraction (lift straight leg against resistance). The tuberosity looks enlarged and is tender. Osgood–Schlatter disease is self-limiting in >90% of cases. *x-rays:* Tibial tuberosity enlargement (± fragmentation) (fig 11.57). Note the appearance of a normal immature tibial tuberosity, fig 11.56. MRI shows the tendonitis. NB: diagnosis is clinical, not simply radiological. *Treatment:* Standard treatment is limitation of activity, ice, oral anti-inflammatories, knee padding, and physiotherapy. Plaster cast immobilization is now uncommonly used as it leads to quadriceps wasting. Tibial tubercle excision once skeletally mature may be recommended if the above fail.[67]

Sinding–Larsen's disease (jumper's knee) has a similar pathophysiology and treatment to Osgood–Schlatter's disease (above) but the onset tends to be 1–2yrs earlier. Traction tendinopathy with calcification in the proximal attachment of the tendon, which may be partially avulsed.

Sever's disease This common calcaneal apophysitis is probably from strained attachment of the Achilles tendon. It is usually self-limiting. Typical age: 8–13yrs. There is pain behind the heel (bilateral in 60%) ± limping, and tenderness over the lower posterior calcaneal tuberosity. *x-rays:* Often normal. *Treatment:* Physiotherapy and heel raise. If needed, a below-knee walking plaster may give pain relief. Most are well after 5 weeks.[68]

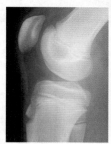

Fig 11.56 Normal x-ray. appearance of an immature tibial tuberosity. Courtesy of The Norfolk and Norwich University Hospitals (NNUH) Radiology Dept.

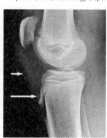

Fig 11.57 Osgood–Schlatter disease. Patellar tendon oedema (small arrow) and thin osseous density anterior to the apophysis of the tibial tuberosity (large arrow).

Reproduced from *BMJ Case Reports* 2013, Osgood–Schlatter disease, Patrick Joseph Maher, Jonathan S Ilgen, with permission from BMJ Publishing Group Ltd.

Eponyms of osteochondroses	
Eponym	**Site affected**
Blount disease	Proximal tibial epiphysis
Freiberg's disease (p702)	Head of 2nd or 3rd metatarsal
Friedrich disease	Clavicle
Köhler's disease (p702)	Navicular bone
Osgood–Schlatter disease (p703)	Tuberosity of the tibia
Panner's disease (p702)	Capitellum of humerus
Perthes' disease (p684)	Hip
Scheuermann's disease (p674)	Vertebral ring epiphyses
Sever's disease (p703)	Calcaneal apophysis
Sinding–Larsen disease (p703)	Secondary patellar centre

Further reading

Cooper G (2014). *Osteochondritis Dissecans*. Medscape. http://emedicine.medscape.com/article/1253074

Maher PJ *et al.* (2013). Osgood-Schlatter Disease. *BMJ* Case Reports. http://casereports.*bmj*.com/content/2013/bcr-2012-007614.full

It always starts with studying biomechanics and designing implant systems which closely mimic normal function. Joint replacement has been used for ~75yrs.[21] From 2003 to 2013, 620,400 primary hip and 676,082 knee replacements were implanted in England and Wales. That equates to an average of 170 hips and 185 knees per day over 10 years! The number of procedures has risen annually and is predicted to continue rising. 93% of hips and 96% of knees were done for OA with a median age of 63 (hips) and 70 (knees).[69]

Preoperative assessment (6wks prior to operation) of co-morbidities and ability to cope with rehabilitation must be thorough, it is likely to be complicated in this patient population. Give written information.[70]

Early complications
● VTE [4%]
● Dislocation [3%]
● Deep infection [2%]
● Fracture [1%]
● Nerve palsy [1%]
● Limb-length discrepancy [1%]
● Death [0.4-0.7%][71]

Hip replacement is carried out to relieve pain and disability caused by arthropathies of the hip. Other conditions which may result in replacement are: rheumatoid arthritis; avascular necrosis of head of femur; congenitally dislocated hip; fractured neck of femur. 60% are women but incidence in men is increasing. *Total hip replacement (THR)* both the articular surfaces of femur and acetabulum are replaced. This can either be conventional (replacing femoral head and neck) or simply resurfacing the femoral head (considered in younger patients with OA so that femoral neck is preserved). In *hemiarthroplasty* only the articular surface of femoral head is replaced (indicated in patients with #NOF who have no arthritis but are at high risk of femoral head avascular necrosis. Many prostheses are available; most consist of a metal femoral component with an intramedullary stem sometimes held in place by bone cement, and a plastic acetabular component—fig 11.35 on p683. 95% of UK hip replacements are cemented.[69] Younger patients typically receive uncemented prostheses as they are easier to revise once the prosthesis is worn. *Outcomes* can be determined by persistance of pain or proportion of patients who require revision. Early success of operation occurs in 90%. Later problems of loosening or infection are heralded by return of pain. If plain x-rays are inconclusive in the case of loosening, strontium or technetium scans may reveal increased bone activity. Suspected sepsis should be investigated by WCC, ESR, and US-guided aspiration. Revision arthroplasty is more successful for loosening than for infection.[72,73] *Joint survival:* By 9–10yrs post-op 11% of implants have been revised. Be cautious in recommending replacement to those less than 60 years old as they will have a high chance of revision in their lifetime. Revision operations are more demanding both for surgeon and patient than the primary operation. Earlier replacement is used for rheumatoid arthritis as joints tend to be grossly affected younger—and excessive delay may result in technically difficult surgery upon very rarefied osteoporotic bone.

Other joints Total joint arthroplasty is now used with success in most joints, including shoulder, elbow, wrist, finger, ankle, and toes. The national joint registry records data on every joint arthroplasty implanted in the UK. It is critical in evaluating which areas of the body and which prostheses are successful. Joint spacers are used in finger joints for rheumatoid.

Knee replacement (see p692) **Thromboembolic events** (see p722)

---

21 The first hip replacement was done by Philip Wiles at the Middlesex Hospital in 1938. The Charnley low friction arthroplasty was first used in the 1960s.
22 CRP returns to normal after 3 weeks and ESR returns <20mm/hr after 6 weeks.

Dislocation (mostly THR) occurs in 0–5% of primary THR but risk is higher with revision surgery due to existing weakening of surrounding tissues. Causes for recurrent dislocations are multifactorial and include neuromuscular disease, inappropriate choice, or incorrect placement of implants. Typically relocation takes place under GA and rarely needs open surgery, but recurrent dislocations may require surgical revision. Preventable by comprehensive patient education and rehabilitation programmes.

Prosthetic loosening is the most common contributor to failure of TKR in the long term. It can present with chronic pain or increased risk of fracture. Metal on metal hip replacement where both components are metal have a high incidence of loosening and pain. In addition they can cause aseptic lymphocyte dominated vasculitis associated lesion (ALVAL), pseudo tumours, and soft tissue reactions.

Periprosthetic fractures occur most commonly around hip arthroplasties (1% after primary but 4% after revision [74]) and incidence is likely to rise as the age of the population increases. Typically present after trauma which can be minor (especially if prosthesis has started to loosen). Factors predisposing to periprosthetic fractures are osteoporosis and loosening of the implant (both septic and aseptic). Recently bisphosphonates have also been implicated. [75]

Infection is a disastrous complication of joint replacement. Occurs in 1–2% of cases. It can be early (<3 months) or late. May present acutely with fever and suppuration or in a more indolent fashion with pain and loss of function due to loosening of components. Perioperative wound complications, obesity, increased age, diabetes mellitus, steroid use, and rheumatoid arthritis increase risk. Coagulase-negative staphylococci are the common infective organisms. *Investigations:* Although essential in diagnosis of chronic infection, CRP [22] is not helpful in early stages due to recent traumatic surgery, but joint aspiration with high WCC and clinical findings of acute joint swelling, erythema and warmth with a fever is indicative. [76] Take blood cultures. Plain x-rays may show periprosthetic loosening. CT/MRI may be of limited use due to artefact. Gallium/labelled leucocyte imaging may be useful in hard to diagnose cases. *Treatment:* Early on, debridement + antibiotics may be enough. Later, with loosening of components, radical debridement must include removal of all prosthetic material, as well as any involved bone and soft tissue. Antibiotics may be needed for months. The joint is usually washed out and a 2-stage revision is performed which involves removing the prosthesis and cement mantle to debride the debris from the inside of the bone followed by implantation of an antibiotic-loaded cement spacer. This is functionally debilitating for the patient. If the infection is cleared, then reimplantation after >2 months can occur.

Antibiotic prophylaxis against prosthesis infection [77]

• *Dentistry* Infection with oral bacteria is rare; prophylaxis is not needed.
• *Colonoscopy + polypectomy* may be more risky than dentistry; some recommend prophylaxis, if <6 months since replacement.
• *Antibiotic-impregnated cement?* The best prophylaxis might be achieved with a combination of gentamicin-impregnated cement, systemic antibiotics for >24h post-op, and surgery performed in ultra-clean environments (laminar air flow theatres/surgeons in 'space suits').

Further reading

Buckley R (2014). *General Principles of Fracture Care Treatment & Management*. Medscape. http://emedicine.medscape.com/article/1270717

NICE (2011). *The Management of Hip Fractures in Adults* (CG124). London: NICE.

Norris R *et al.* (2012). Occurrence of secondary fracture around intramedullary nails used for trochanteric hip fractures: a systematic review of 13,568 patients. *Injury* 43(6):706–11.

Orthopaedics

Joint aspirations *Diagnostic role:* Any blood, crystals, or pus? (see BOX on p707 for diagnostic analysis). *Therapeutic role:* For tense effusions, septic effusions, and haemarthroses. Approaches for specific joints are given below and on p708. ▶Remember that aspiration of a joint with a prosthesis should only be done under the strictest sterile conditions (ie in the operating theatre) to minimize risk of introducing infection. *Equipment:* Check you have swabs, needles, and sterile bottles. For aspiration of viscid fluid (eg haemarthrosis) use a 19G needle. For the larger joints use a 21G needle, and for fingers and toes a 23G needle. Locate joint margins carefully before cleaning; once the skin is clean use scrupulous aseptic no-touch technique but even then, the skin is clean but not sterile. Samples for microbiology should be sent in sterile containers (also for cytology) and blood culture bottle. Radiological guidance may be needed for certain joints (eg hip, spine).

Gauge	Colour of needle base
23G	Blue
21G	Green
20G	Yellow
19G	White

Steroid injections to inflamed joints, bursae, or tendon sheaths aim to ↓inflammation and relieve pain, perhaps by ↓prostaglandin synthesis, stabilizing mast cells, or ↓tissue calcification, or increasing vascularization and permeability of synovium. *Preparations* include **cortisone acetate** (cheapest, shortest acting), **methylprednisolone**, and **triamcinolone** (intermediate acting). They may be mixed with 1% lidocaine. When triamcinolone is used for injecting near short tendons, 10mg strength is preferred to 40mg as tendon rupture has been reported after the latter. Despite our best intentions 'joint' injections often fail to meet their target (50% in one study in which contrast material was also injected); those off-target are less likely to relieve symptoms.[78]

Conditions responding to steroid injection Localized subacromial bursitis; large and small joint arthritis eg hip, knee, acromioclavicular, and sternoclavicular joints; arthritis of elbow, radioulnar, acromioclavicular, and sternoclavicular joints; ganglia; trigger fingers; de Quervain's disease; strains of collateral and cruciate ligaments of knee; suprapatellar, infrapatellar, and Achilles tendinopathy; plantar fasciitis; traumatic arthritis of metatarsophalangeal joints; and sesamo-first-metatarsal joint, rheumatoid arthritis.

Be cautious in immunosuppressed patients, diabetics, blood clotting disorders, active infection, and nearby tumours. ▶ Never inject through cellulitis or into a prosthetic joint.

Side effects: Typically include pain at the injection site and skin atrophy/fading of skin pigment. Other side effects include: haemarthrosis, facial flushing, urticaria, post-injection flare syndrome (synovitis with fever), paresis, and septic arthritis (≤1 in 14,000 injections). ▶*It is essential that steroids are not used in septic conditions* and, if any doubt at all exists, results of synovial fluid culture should be awaited. Remember the possibility of tuberculous synovitis—especially in recent foreign travel. Repeated injections increases the risks of side effects: beware ligamentous laxity, joint instability, calcification, or tendon rupture.

Further reading

Courtney P *et al.* (2009). Joint aspiration and injection and synovial fluid analysis. *Best Pract Res Clin Rheumatol* 27(2):137–69.

Peterson C *et al.* (2011). Adverse events from diagnostic and therapeutic joint injections: a literature review. *Skeletal Radiol* 40(1):5–12.

Synovial fluid in health and disease

Blood, crystals, or pus? Aspiration of synovial fluid is used to diagnose haemarthroses, or infectious or crystal (gout and calcium pyrophosphate deposition CPPD—old name =pseudogout) arthropathies.

	Appearance	Viscosity	WBC/mm³	Neutrophils
Normal	Clear, colourless	High	<200	<25%
Non-inflammatory eg OA	Clear, straw	High	<5000	<25%
Haemorrhagic, eg tumour haemophilia, trauma	Bloody, xan-thochromic	Variable	<10,000	<50%
Acute inflammatory[23]	Turbid, yellow	Decreased		
• Acute gout			~14,000	~80%
• Rheumatic fever			~18,000	~50%
• Rheumatoid arthritis			~16,000	~65%
Septic	Turbid, yellow	Decreased		
• TB			~24,000	~70%
• Gonorrhoeal			~14,000	~60%
• Septic (non-gonococcal)[24]			~16,000	~95%

Orthopaedics

Managing carpal tunnel syndrome (CTS)

See p749 for clinical features.

Tests Nerve conduction studies can be helpful in complex or mixed symptoms as well as monitoring responses to surgery. Ultrasonography and MRI can help identify lesions. [79]

Management Treat any treatable association (see MINIBOX). Rest, weight reduction, and wrist splints are first line for both alleviation of symptoms and also reducing risk of recurrence. 20% of cases will spontaneously resolve. *Splinting* in a neutral position alone was sufficient to relieve symptoms and avoid surgery in 37% of patients.[80,n=176] *Corticosteroid injections* are widely used for short-term (10 weeks) pain relief in mild to moderate disease but when compared to placebo at 1 year there was no difference and 75% of patients still needed surgery within 1 year. [81] There are no adequate guidelines for repeated injections after the first successful injection wears off. Seek expert help before injecting patients with clinically severe or complex disease, diabetes or the elderly as outcome may be worse.

CTS associations
• Hypothyroidism
• Pregnancy; the Pill
• Gout & pseudogout
• Diabetes; obesity
• Cardiac failure
• Acromegaly
• Rheumatoid arthritis
• Premenstrual state
• Amyloidosis

Injection technique: Introduce the needle angled at ~45°just proximal to the distal wrist crease, to the ulnar side of palmaris longus. ►*Do not use local anaesthetic.* If the patient reports an 'electric shock' then you are probably touching the nerve. Redirect the needle towards the ulnar side and then inject 25mg hydrocortisone acetate. The intention is to deliver steroid around the flexor tendons and not into the carpal tunnel itself. A splint worn for the next few days may mitigate symptoms which can occur at the time of injection. *Carpal tunnel decompression:* Release of the flexor retinaculum has a well-documented success rate for more permanent results. [82] Endoscopic release is as effective as the standard open approach in terms of symptom relief and functional status, although the endoscopic approach may be associated with better grip strength and a faster return to work. [83] Complications are rare, but persistence of symptoms, reduced grip, and pillar pain (deep aching pain at the base of the thenar eminence and across wrist) can persist up to 2 years and must be explained to the patient.

23 Includes eg Reiter's syndrome, pseudogout, SLE etc.
24 Includes Staphs, Streps, Lyme, and *Pseudomonas* (eg post-op).

Shoulder injection As shoulder pain from soft tissue causes are common (lifetime incidence ~10%), and pain can be chronic (≤23% resolve within 4wks), this is one of the most commonly injected joints. A cochrane study based on moderate evidence showed no difference between intraarticular steroid injection and systemic IM injection; nor was there a significant advantage to US-guided approaches versus blind use of landmarks.[84] There is no difference between 40mg and 80mg of steroid, however use large volumes eg 5–10mL as small volumes are at risk of being injected into structures rather than around them.

Subacromial injection (impingement syndrome, calcific tendinitis, see p666): Whilst standing behind, seat the patient with arm resting on lap. Palpate 2cm medial and inferior to the end of the spine of the scapula (easily palpable). Aim tip of needle towards the anterolateral tip of the acromion. *Intra-articular injection* (arthritis, frozen shoulder): Whilst standing behind, seat the patient with arm resting on lap. Palpate 2cm medial and inferior to the end of the spine of scapula (easily palpable). Aim needle directly towards the coracoid process felt anteriorly. If the needle hits bone, then external rotation of the arm will help the needle drop into the joint. ▶Do not go medial to the coracoid process (neurovascular structures, p751 figs 12.38 & 12.39).

Lateral approach (subacromial bursitis, impingement syndrome): Inject 25–50mg hydrocortisone acetate with lidocaine just below the lateral tip of the acromion, pointing downwards and advancing medially. If the needle is withdrawn from touching the head of humerus with slight pressure on the plunger, a drop in pressure is felt as the bursa is entered.

Knee joint The patient lies with knee supported, slightly flexed and muscles relaxed. Palpate the joint space behind patella either medially or laterally—the lateral approach may be less reliable.[85] Insert a needle horizontally between the patella and femur. Slight resistance is felt on traversing the synovial membrane; it should be possible to aspirate fluid, and injection fluid should flow easily. Ultrasound guidance may result in less procedural pain, greater synovial fluid yield, and improved clinical outcomes.[86] *Usual doses:* 25–50mg **hydrocortisone acetate**, 40mg **methylprednisolone**, 20mg **triamcinolone**. Repeat injections should be longer than 3 months apart. If injection is used for prepatellar bursitis, give 25mg hydrocortisone acetate into the most tender spot.

The ankle Plantar flex foot slightly, palpate joint margin between tibialis anterior (the most medial) and extensor hallucis longus (lateral to tibialis anterior) tendons just above tip of medial malleolus. Inject 25mg **hydrocortisone** acetate into the joint. See fig 11.58a.

Biceps tendinopathy is no longer injected as the risk of biceps tendon rupture was high, US-guided injection lessens the risk.[87]

Wrist injection Inject 25mg hydrocortisone acetate 1–1.5cm deep between extensor tendons of ring and little fingers between ulnar head and lunate.

De Quervain's tenosynovitis Extensor pollicis brevis and abductor pollicis longus tendons—on traversing the extensor retinaculum on the dorsal wrist—may cause a tender swelling (p670). With needle almost parallel to skin pointing proximally, inject 25mg hydrocortisone acetate slowly just distal or proximal to the radial styloid, at the site of maximum tenderness. If needle in tendon, injection is difficult so withdraw until easy flow occurs. See fig 11.58b.

Trigger finger (fig 11.59) Insert needle at MCP skin crease parallel to flexor tendon, pointing to palm. Palpate tendon thickening in palm; proceed as for de Quervain's. See p671 for more information on trigger fingers.

First carpometacarpal joint of thumb Avoiding radial artery, inject 25mg hydrocortisone acetate at base of first metacarpal at 1cm depth in anatomical snuffbox (aim at base of little finger). ▶In all areas, learn from an expert.

Orthopaedics

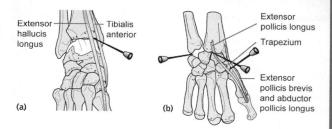

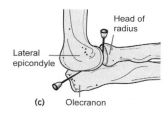

Fig 11.58
(a) Dorsal aspect of the right ankle indicating anatomical landmarks—shown here is the anterior ankle approach.
(b) Dorsal aspect of the right wrist indicating anatomical landmarks—shown here from left to right are the injection sites for the wrist joint, de Quervain's tenosynovitis, & the 1st carpometacarpal joint.
(c) The right elbow, flexed—shown from left to right the posterior and lateral approaches.[88]

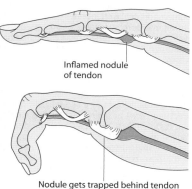

Inflamed nodule of tendon

Nodule gets trapped behind tendon sheath, and finger becomes stuck in flexed position

Fig 11.59 Trigger finger.

▶ When injecting a trigger finger, ask the patient to flex and extend the finger to ensure that the tip of the needle is not in the tendon.

Orthopaedics

Further reading

Vitale MA (2014). Doc, will this injection make my trigger finger go away? *Bone Joint Surg Am* 96(22):e191.

Orthopaedics

The main tendons to rupture are the extensor tendons of the fingers, the Achilles tendon (fig 11.61), the long head of biceps (p664), supraspinatus (p664), and the quadriceps expansion (fig 11.60). The cause may be sharp or blunt trauma (anything from sporting injuries to rubber bullets). Ultrasound aids diagnosis, but its usefulness is largely operator dependent.

Mallet finger Often caused by a sudden blow to an extended finger (eg hit by cricketball on outstretched finger) which leads to rupture of the extensor tendon at the distal phalanx. *Treatment:* Splint the affected digit for 6 weeks (in slight hyper-extension) using a Stack or moulded aluminium splint. If untreated, the mallet finger may develop into a swan-neck deformity. See p540 *OHCM*. If conservative treatment fails, or it is associated with a large avulsion # (>30%), refer to a hand surgeon for consideration of surgical fixation.[89] (see Mallet toes p694.)

Boutonnière deformity Rupture of the central slip of the extensor tendon (at the base of the middle phalanx) allows the lateral bands of the extensor mechanism to slip towards the palm, turning them into flexors of the PIP joint, giving the appearance of poking a finger through a button hole (=Boutonnière in French). The result is flexion at the PIP and hyperextension of the DIP joint. It can occur following injury (forced flexion of extended PIP joint or volar dislocation of distal finger at PIP joint) or secondary to rheumatoid arthritis. Acute injuries are typically treated by splinting PIP in complete & constant extension, allowing movement at DIP and MCP joints. Refer to hand therapy.

Achilles (calcaneal) tendon rupture Typified by sudden pain at the back of the ankle during running or jumping as the tendon ruptures. Pain may be perceived as a 'kick' rather than actual pain. It is possible to walk (with a limp), and some plantar flexion of the foot remains, but it is impossible to raise the heel from the floor when standing on the affected leg. A gap may be palpated in the tendon course (particularly within 24h of injury). *The squeeze test* (Simmonds' or Thompsons' test) is sensitive: ask the patient to kneel on a chair, while you squeeze both calves—if the Achilles is ruptured, there is less plantar flexion on the affected side. *Treatment:* Tendon repair (percutaneous or open) is often preferred by young, athletic patients. Conservative treatment may be most suitable for smokers, diabetics, and those >50yrs old. Conservative management usually requires initial casting in equinus position brought to neutral over 6–8 weeks. Typically there is no weight bearing for 6–8 weeks. Late-presenting ruptures usually need reconstructing. Open surgery significantly reduces the risk of rerupture compared with conservative cast immobilization or functional bracing; however wound breakdown from open intervention can be catastrophic as the tendon then becomes exposed.[90]

Quadriceps expansion rupture (fig 11.62) is quite rare and typically affects >40-yr-olds. Injury may be direct (eg blow) or indirect (stumbling causing sudden contraction of the apparatus). Jumper's knee (p690) may predispose. *Look for systemic causes of tendon weakening:* Steroid abuse (especially in spontaneous rupture in athletes); pseudogout (CPPD); Wilson's disease; renal failure with hyperparathyroidism.[91] *Treatment:* If the extensor mechanism is disrupted (no straight leg raising) then surgery is mandatory. After repair, the knee is immobilized for >4 weeks with immediate postoperative weightbearing; then intensive physiotherapy helps regain knee function. Many have persistent extensor mechanism weakness as compared to the other leg.

Distal biceps rupture Occurs in men typically involved in heavy lifting. Presents with a history of something 'tearing' or 'popping' and pain in the antecubital fossa with bruising over the medial forearm. Needs urgent surgical repair.

Further reading

Taylor DW *et al.* (2011). A systematic review of the use of platelet-rich plasma in sports medicine as a new treatment for tendon and ligament injuries. *Clin J Sport Med* 21(4):344-52.

Wilkins R *et al.* (2012). Operative versus nonoperative management of acute Achilles tendon ruptures. A quantitative systematic review of randomized controlled trials. *Am J Sports Med* 40(9):2154-60.

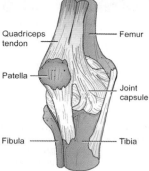

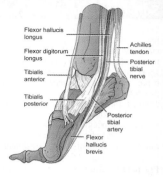

Quadriceps tendon

Femur

Patella

Joint capsule

Fibula

Tibia

Flexor hallucis longus

Flexor digitorum longus

Tibialis anterior

Tibialis posterior

Flexor hallucis brevis

Achilles tendon

Posterior tibial nerve

Posterior tibial artery

Fig 11.60 The quadriceps (extensor) expansion encloses the patella and inserts into the tibial tuberosity as the patellar tendon. Rupture can occur at the site of quadriceps insertion to the patella, through the patella by fracture, or by avulsion of the patellar tendon from the tibial tuberosity.

Fig 11.61 The medial aspect of the ankle, showing the extensor and flexor tendons of the foot. The Achilles tendon tends to rupture ~5cm proximal to its insertion into the calcaneus. Also note the ordering of the flexor tendons posterior to the medial malleolus, from anterior to posterior—this can be remembered with the mnemonic on p657: **T**om, **D**ick and **A V**ery **N**ervous **H**arry.

The foot arches

Pes planus (flat feet) The medial longitudinal arch (fig 11.62) collapses—leading to the whole sole nearly coming in contact with the ground. Flat feet are normal when a child is learning to walk. The medial arch develops over the next few years. In adults flat feet are associated with dysfunction of the posterior tibialis tendon (PTT) (a dynamic stabilizer of the medial arch). In most, it is asymptomatic and may not need intervention if the arch restores itself on standing on tiptoe (eg a 'mobile' flat foot). Pain may develop medially over the PTT

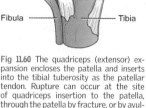

Fig 11.62 The medial (1) and lateral (2) longitudinal arches of the foot.

and there may be progressive forefoot abduction and hindfoot valgus deformity with loss of ability to heel rise, as the condition progresses. Weight loss, supportive shoes (with insoles), orthosis may help in mild cases. [92] Pain and limitations in sport tend to be post-op complications so don't advise surgery lightly.

Pes cavus Accentuated longitudinal foot arches which do not flatten with weight-bearing. May be idiopathic, or associated with an underlying neurological condition (see MINIBOX). Claw toes may occur, as weight is taken on metatarsal heads when walking (hence causing pain). *Other symptoms:* Difficulty with shoes; foot fatigue; mobility↓; ankle instability/sprains; callosities. *If foot used to be normal, refer to a neurologist.* If orthoses and custom footwear fail, surgical procedures include soft-tissue releases, tendon transfers, arthrodesis. [93]

Pes cavus associations
• Spina bifida
• Cerebral palsy
• Polio
• Muscular dystrophy
• Charcot–Marie–Tooth dis.
• Syringomyelia
• Friedreich's ataxia
• Spinal tumour

Sport and exercise medicine (SEM) is a relatively new and often poorly understood medical specialty. While the central theme is the diagnosis and management of injury arising from participation in sport, including but not exclusively elite athletes, it has an increasingly important public health role: promoting healthy living and chronic disease management through exercise. (see MINIBOX).

In the practice of SEM, special consideration must be given to specific population groups—eg females (± pregnancy), children, older people, and those with physical impairments/spinal cord injury—and their unique physiological demands.

Benefits of exercise[94]
Reduced risk of:
• Cardiovascular disease and stroke
• Diabetes
• Obesity
• Osteoporosis
• Dementia
• Certain cancers
Improved:
• Immune response
• Psychological well-being
• Sleeping patterns

Pre-participation Preparation and safety is paramount in minimizing risk of injury and improving performance outcomes both recreationally and at an elite level; avoiding adverse outcomes should always be regarded as preferential to their management. You should carefully consider the impact of known medical conditions but also those that are potentially undiagnosed, eg the need for cardiac screening in elite athletes.

The medical practitioner should encourage the patient to control factors that can be controlled and prepare for those that cannot. Initial measures to be taken include: appropriate training and technique prior to participation; comprehensive warming up and cooling down to protect the participant from soft tissue and joint injuries; the correct use of strapping for the provision of additional joint support and proprioceptive feedback; and extra care if over-reaching to avoid overtraining syndrome.

Potential factors influencing risk of injury and performance	
External factors	**Internal factors**
Environment (climate, altitude, playing surface)	Pre-existing health conditions
Sports type	Previous injury
Opponent	Current fitness level and correct technique
Equipment	Hydration and nutrition
Technology	Warm up and cool down

Injury assessment SEM spans primary to tertiary care and encompasses a large multidisciplinary team: medics, surgeons, radiologists, physiotherapists, nutritionists, psychologists, epidemiologists, orthotics and sports scientists, among others. Each sport and activity possesses a particular injury profile, whereby certain injuries are more likely due to the nature of the specific sport. For example, shoulder injuries are more frequent in contact sports such as rugby than they are in football, due to the physicality required in the tackle. As in other areas of medicine, a thorough history and understanding of the injury mechanism is paramount, and is complemented by appropriate clinical examination. Investigations are more readily available at the elite level, with near-patient US a desirable skill of the sports medicine doctor.[95]

When working 'pitch-side' for a sports team be aware of the variety of complaints and injuries that may emerge; you can find yourself as general practitioner, emergency doctor, and musculo-skeletal specialist. In one afternoon the sports medic may have to deal with earache, a traumatic eye injury, head injury with loss of consciousness, and knee pain, highlighting the importance of versatility and a broad knowledge base.

We thank Dr Gemma Phillips for help with this page.

Orthopaedics

Concussion and sport-specific protocols

Concussion is a minor traumatic brain injury. It has a variable presentation that includes (to name a few) nausea, dizziness, headache, unsteadiness, and visual disturbance. It is not always associated with loss of consciousness and when subtle can be very tricky to spot. Emerging evidence has suggested not only immediate concerns of subsequent increased injury risk and second impact syndrome, but a long term potential for chronic neurological impairment. Many sports have implemented specific guidance for the assessment and management for head injuries, including a graduated return to play- protecting players and empower medical teams. Please refer to the 2012 Zurich consensus statement on concussion in sport for more information. [96]

Injury management Overuse injuries are widely seen in all levels of SEM, where repetitive mechanical stress outweighs the body's mechanism for recovery. An example would be *iliotibial band syndrome*. The iliotibial band (ITB) passes over the lateral tibial tuberosity during knee flexion, friction here causes local inflammation producing lateral knee pain on movement and direct palpation. As with all soft tissue injuries, a protocol of 'RICE' (rest, ice, compression, and elevation) is recommended in the first instance (NB: Icing should be limited to maximum of 20-minute sessions, with a barrier between the cold surface and skin, to limit local cold injuries). Judicial use of NSAIDs in those without contraindications in the short term can be helpful for analgesia and treatment, followed by a suitable rehabilitation programme: stretching exercises of the ITB, gluteal strengthening, and a graduated return to the ITB-stressing activity. In severe cases, specialist review and steroid injection is an option but the risk of tendon rupture must be balanced. [97] For elite athletes, the threshold for specialist intervention and active management (including surgery) is lower for all injuries. In professional sport always be aware of antidoping regulations, it is highly recommended to become an accredited UK anti doping (UKAD) Advisor (www.ukad.org.uk).

Ethics in sports medicine

A fundamental aspect of medicine is to first do no harm, a principle that can be difficult to define, let alone follow, when the objective of the patient is personal and professional success in a career that is anything but health promoting. Ethics is a pertinent feature of SEM with the typical doctor–patient relationship mixed with potentially competing interests. You should consider the individual's understanding of, and capacity to make, each decision in a given situation bearing in mind the combined personal and external (coach/team/media/fans/timing) pressures. Remember careers are often short lived, athletes are competing for their livelihoods—a drive which must not be underestimated or ignored. Consider their perspective: 'If I come off the pitch injured today does it compromise my first team position? I have a family that needs to be supported, will this impact upon my future contract and income? How will I be perceived by my team mates and coaches?' You may find yourself deciding during the half time break of a cup final, whether you should permit the star-player carrying an injury to remain on the field despite the potential for longer-term adverse implications. As an SEM practitioner in a professional sporting environment it is inevitable that a fine line will exist between maintaining doctor–patient trust, prioritizing patient welfare and protecting your own professional integrity, all the while trying to balance good working relations with coaches and management. At times you may find yourself advocating for the athlete's longer-term interests, often these decisions are the most difficult.

Further reading

British Association of Sport and Exercise Medicine: www.basem.co.uk

Holm S *et al.* (2009). Ethics in sports medicine. *BMJ* 339:b3898.

McCrory P *et al.* (2012) Consensus statement on concussion in sport: the 4th International Conference on Concussion in Sport. *Br J Sports Med* 2013;47:250–58 doi:10.1136/bjsports-2013-092313.

Orthopaedics

Managing trauma patients involves having a systematic approach. These patients commonly have both internal and external injuries, usually in combination, which are potentially life-threatening. When assessing major trauma patients a focused history and A (+ c-spine) B C D E examination is mandatory (as per ATLS® principles, see p781). Appropriate imaging must be arranged urgently but this must not delay the treatment of life-threatening issues.

This chapter aims to guide you through orthopaedic trauma, look to the emergency medicine chapter to address major trauma (see p778).

The Koru is frequently used in M(a)ori art as a symbol of perpetual movement and creation. (fig 12.1). It is based on the unfurling fern frond which eventually points inward to indicate an eventual return to the beginning. Just like your career through medicine, life will flow through stages of change but to achieve harmony there will always remain an undercurrent of stability and adherence to your inner values. As the fern unfurls, the people of New Zealand view the Koru as a new beginning. Each of your patients is a new start, a new opportunity to do your best. Don't let the tough shifts pull you down, instead tuck them into your Koru so that your return to equilibrium is hastened. Those experiences will stay with you but it's your choice how you let them affect your next patient. Victims of trauma, no matter how trivial, have suddenly been ripped out of their comfort zone. It's our job to guide their Koru back to harmony and facilitate their new beginning.

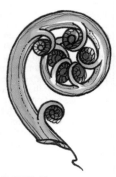

Fig 12.1 The Koru.
© Gillian Turner.

Sources/further reading The image bank at: www.trauma.org

www.radiologymasterclass.co.uk   Trauma management: Trauma, Chapter 12

We thank our Specialist Reader Mr Chris Peach for reviewing this chapter. We also thank Mr Jamie A'Court, and Mr Yousaf Khan for their invaluable contributions. The work of our junior readers Mayooreshan Anandarajah and Raj Dattani is also much appreciated.

Trauma

Describing an x-ray

Describing a fracture over the phone can be intimidating. Know your anatomy and the basic descriptive terms below before you start.

Seven key questions
• How many fractures?
• Can I see all the bone?
• What is broken?
• Are the bones normal?
• Any trapped air?
• Any foreign body?
• More plain films needed (IVU, CT, arteriogram)?

Description

• *Site:* Bone(s) fractured; part of bone (proximal, shaft, distal, etc.) see p685, fig 11.39.

• *Intra-articular involvement?*

• *Epiphyseal involvement?* (see TABLE on p719 for Salter Harris classification).

• *Obliquity:* Transverse; short oblique; spiral; multi-fragmentary.

• *Displacement:* Can be described in terms of rotation, angulation, shortening and translation. Compare placement (in degrees or %) of distal fragment with respect to proximal fragment so when giving a displacement description, this refers to the *distal* fragment. For angulated fractures, the terms 'apex dorsal' and 'apex palmar' can be used in the hand.

• *Impaction* can cause shortening, try and estimate the extent.

• *Fracture pattern* can be simple (spiral, oblique, or transverse), buckle, greenstick, wedge or comminuted (splintered fragments), segmental (multiple breaks in the bone creating at least 3 fragments). Avulsion of a fragment occurs when a tendon or ligament pulls a fragment of bone away.

• *Soft tissues* are typically assessed on examination. Neurovascular status? Always consider compartment syndrome (see BOX, p722). Open (formerly known as compound) or closed? The Gustilo classification is most commonly used for open fractures (TABLE, p718).

▸▸ Take a full history. Was the fall due to sudden dizziness that may need an ECG and a medical review? Is the fracture you are focusing on part of a larger trauma case (see p781 for ATLS® principles)? Look for more occult signs of injury.

A game of trauma?

We encourage you to think about the mechanism of injury when assessing a fracture (see p787, 'Read the wreckage'). Is it a little grandmother who FOOSH (fell on outstretched hand) (see p728 for Colles type fractures)? Or is it a young chap falling off a horse (see p752 for spinal cord injuries)? Each era has been associated with different accidents (fig 12.2). Consider the Hangman's fracture (forced hyperextension of the neck causing fracture of both C2 pedicles, fig 11.7 p661). This was historically named after judicial hangings, yet post-mortem studies showed that only a few hangings actually demonstrated this injury pattern.[1] The majority of eponyms arise from recent times, but the medieval era was a vicious and bloody one—yet there are no residual eponyms. This time was called the Dark Ages, not because there were so many (k)nights, but because there is a paucity of historical records kept as compared to the wealth of knowledge which is now documented. It is likely they did have eponymous fracture patterns amongst each community. Next time you watch any battles onscreen, pay attention to the mechanisms of injury. Archeological studies have demonstrated that fracture immobilization and reduction likely took place[2] and that farming injuries were very common.

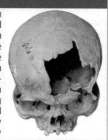

Fig 12.2 This adult skull was found amidst medieval remains in Norway. Just like modern medicine, the clues to aetiology lie in noting the surroundings. Was farming equipment used in defence against a Viking raid, or was this a more formal battle scene? Reproduced with permission from Brodholt and Holck, Skeletal trauma in the burials from the royal church of St. Mary in medieval Oslo.

International Journal of Osteoarchaeology © 2010 John Wiley & Sons.

The aim is to provide information that will alter management, without exposing patients to unnecessary radiation, think especially of the radiation exposure to thyroid in c-spine x-rays, gonads in pelvic views, and to the eyes in skull and facial x-rays (lens cataracts are the risk). It is impossible to protect the ovaries. For example, each lumbar spine x-ray=2.2mSv=40 CXRs. The Sievert (Sv) is the SI unit of radiation absorbed by biological tissues—see *OHCM* p733. This dose may be expected to cause 16 malignancies/yr in the UK at current rates of exposure. Guidelines which help clinicians make sensible radiology requests yield substantial savings in costs and in patients' waiting times, without compromising patient care. ▶Remember to treat and assess the patient, not just the radiological findings.

When an x-ray is indicated, consider the Rule of Twos:
• Two joints (above and below the fracture site of an extremity)
• Two times (pre- and post any intervention to the dislocation or fracture)
• Two views (often AP and lateral views, but some need joint-specific views such as the AP mortise view[1] for ankles and the odontoid peg for c-spine).

Twisting injury of foot/ankle Follow the Ottawa rules on p659 (see fig 11.2) but all rules have exceptions, and, on occasion, we've all seen patients walk on a fractured ankle.

Injury to the cervical spine The consequences of a missed c-spine injury are disastrous, and so imaging is always performed for major trauma. But in patients who have been subjected to less violent trauma, when should imaging be requested? Based on the *Nexus criteria*[3] for imaging of blunt injury, the following factors (mnemonic NSAID) are important, though may have the drawback of a low sensitivity if applied as the sole criteria for imaging:
• Neurological exam reveals a focal deficit.
• Spine exam reveals tenderness (posterior midline).
• Alteration in consciousness.
• Intoxication.
• Distracting injury—ie long bone #, clavicle #, chest trauma, etc.

The *Canadian C-spine*[4] rules are more specific but more complicated. High-risk factors (dangerous mechanism, age >65, focal neurology) mandate an x-ray. Absence of these allows consideration of low-risk factors (simple rear end RTA, sitting up in ED, ambulatory at any time, delayed onset of pain, absence of midline c-spine tenderness)—the presence of any one low risk factor allows clinical examination of the neck: if the patient can rotate their neck 45° left and right they do not need an x-ray. Don't rely on mobile equipment; if possible, take to the radiology department, supervising all movements closely. If there is a clear spinal cord injury, and the patient is stable, CT is the first line of imaging (see p717). Image the whole spine as there may be more than one injury. MRI shows fractures, subluxations, disc disruption and protrusion, and cord contusion—and helps establish prognosis. ▶NB: MRI is hard to arrange in emergency settings, and takes a lot longer than CT (eg 20min vs 20s). Consider CT myelography if MRI is contraindicated.

See p790 for head injury associated with neck injury.

Nose injury Imaging in ED is not indicated in simple nasal injury.

Rib injury A CXR is only indicated if you suspect a pneumothorax; rib views are not needed in uncomplicated blunt injury as presence of a rib fracture will not alter your management.

Lumbar spine pain Avoid x-rays in 1st 6 weeks if there are no factors suggesting serious disease, eg trauma, focal neurology, fever, malignancy. See p678.

Foreign bodies Always do x-ray if the presence of glass is possible (glass is usually radiopaque). Ultrasound can also be used in foreign body detection and to guide removal, especially for those that are not radio-opaque (eg splinters).

---

1 AP mortise view (foot is held in 15° internal rotation) to assess presence of talar shift.

Trauma

Quick, accurate, and available: good reasons to think of CT as 1st-line imaging for trauma patients. But there are caveats, as any radiologist who has seen images arriving at their workstation monitor, only to have to comment that the patient's heart has stopped, will tell you. The appropriateness of scanning in an acute trauma must be decided on the balance of risk and benefit to the patient. It is not that radiologists don't want sick patients in their department; radiology departments just aren't the best place to be if you are very sick. ▶*Ensure that the patient is haemodynamically stable before moving them to the relatively resource-poor radiology department.* Some centres have tried to overcome this problem by bringing CT to the emergency department, imaging patients as they come through the door, and while CT may well become the new stethoscope, this approach will also have its faults. Remember that *radiation can do harm:* It cannot be used limitlessly (*OHCM* p733). *Imaging is just a snapshot:* A 'normal' scan mustn't allow for complacency in patient observation. ▶*Always be on the lookout for clinical deterioration requiring prompt intervention. Imaging takes time:* Transfers and interpretation take the longest: CT itself may only take 20s. This is time that the patient is at risk and also time delaying definitive management. For this reason, you may be paradoxically encouraged to request *more* imaging (eg including c-spine), given that having to come back for a second scan doubles the risk.

CT of the cervical spine CT assessment of the cervical spine is quick and effective. Meta-analysis suggests that CT be used as the 1st-line investigation in those with a depressed mental status, though not as a matter of course for less severe injury, in which plain x-ray should still be used.[5] It also has cost–benefit implications. It is also indicated if an injury is seen on the plain film series and if there is inadequate visualization (C7/T1 can be difficult to image in full with plain x-ray.) A similar approach applies for other spinal injuries, but remember that MRI will be needed to assess the vital soft tissue structures.

CT guidelines for head injury (see p790)

CT of the chest Evidence of traumatic injury on CXR that warrants further imaging: • Haemothorax • Pneumothorax • Widened mediastinum (all difficult to spot on a supine film) • Pneumomediastinum • Posterior rib fractures • Fractures of ribs 1 or 2 • Pulmonary contusion.

CT of the abdomen and pelvis Usually done together. Indications may include: • Free fluid noted on FAST scan (p785) • Suspicion of retroperitoneal haemorrhage (if shock is present, but no cause found) • Renal trauma (macroscopic haematuria, microscopic haematuria + shock).

CT of the appendicular skeleton Part of preoperative planning for complex injury patterns. ▶*Remember to think of patterns of injury:* eg rib fractures with bilateral pulmonary contusions have a high coincidence of intra-abdominal injury.

MRI is esp. useful for bony lesions such as tumours, osteomyelitis, or osteonecrosis and soft-tissue pathology such as mensical or shoulder rotator cuff tears.

Further reading

Stiell JG *et al.* (2001).The Canadian C-spine rule for radiography in alert and stable trauma patients. *JAMA* 286:1841–8.

Vinson DR (2001). Nexus cervical spine criteria. *Ann Emerg Med* 37:237–8.

'Is it a fracture or just a break in the bone?' What would you reply? Consider their state of distress at being both in pain and a patient; the latter aruguably more painful. As they face the unknown they defend themselves in the best manner possible, arming themselves with familiar terminology. Doctors hide behind jargon, naturally patients would attempt the same. However, in gently educating the patient (that these two terms are one and the same) you transport them back to reality. Perhaps a break in the bone really is a better thing; something more tangible for them. Explore what they perceive the difference to be. In many cases, our patients consider a fracture as an injury neccessitating major operation. Or they may think a fracture is not 'as bad' as a break. Although jargon is to be approached with caution in this situation, always use appropriate terminoley when *describing x-rays* (p715).

Fracture healing (fig 12.3) x-ray changes showing hard callus formation around the fracture site can only be seen 8-12 weeks post-injury. A rule-of-thumb for fracture healing is given by the 'rule-of-3s'. A *closed, paediatric, metaphyseal, upper limb* fracture is the simplest and will heal in 3 weeks. Any 'complicating factor' *doubles* the healing time, ie adult; diaphyseal; lower limb; open injury. For example an *adult (6), diaphyseal (12) forearm* fracture may take 12 weeks to heal. Likewise an *open (6), adult (12), diaphyseal (24), tibia (48)* may be expected to take 48 weeks (almost a year!) to heal. Metaphysis and epiphysis are defined on p685 (fig 11.39). See also fig 12.4.

Fracture healing depends on the position and stability of the bone segments, but is also influenced by the patient's general health (MINIBOX) and difficulties with wound such as local infection and neurovascular compromise.

Use the **Gustilo classification** to describe the soft tissue damage incurred by open fractures. Note that grade 3 implies significant neurovascular compromise. It is the most commonly used, but other classification systems may offer enhanced evaluation (eg Tscherne and Hanover fracture scales).

Pathological fractures (see p761).

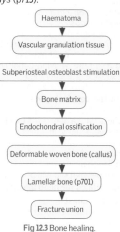

Fig 12.3 Bone healing.

Haematoma → Vascular granulation tissue → Subperiosteal osteoblast stimulation → Bone matrix → Endochondral ossification → Deformable woven bone (callus) → Lamellar bone (p701) → Fracture union

Risk factors for poor healing
• Older age
• Co-morbidities (esp. diabetes)
• Recent trauma
• Smoker (see p719)
• Osteoporosis
• Corticosteroids
• NSAIDs
• Local complications to fracture

Gustilo classification of open fractures	
Type I	*Low-energy* wounds <1cm long, eg caused by bone piercing skin
Type II	*Low-energy* wounds >1cm, causing moderate soft tissue damage
Type III	All *high-energy* injuries irrespective of wound size: • IIIA fractures have *adequate* local soft tissue coverage • IIIB fractures have *inadequate* local soft tissue coverage • IIIC implies arterial injury needing repair

Reproduced with permission from Gustilo, Prevention of infection in the treatment of one thousand and twenty-five open fractures of long bones: retrospective and prospective analyses, *Journal of Bone and Joint Surgery American*, Volume 58, Issue 4, pp.453–458, © 1976 Journal of Bone and Joint Surgery.

Smoking and tissue healing—the consequences of a cigarette break

Trauma patients need to knit back together well, and they face a number of complications without adding tobacco into the physiological equation. Smokers have increased risk of perioperative complications (VTE, respiratory tract infection, & cardiac ischaemia) and reduced fracture healing.

What damage are smokers doing? Nicotine increases the time it takes for a fracture to unite *and* reduces quality of bone healing. Tobacco smoking also reduces tissue oxygenation and wound healing. This is particularly pertinent for operations on the lower extremities—eg Achilles tendon repair (p710) or calcaneal fracture ORIF—because of the precarious local blood supply combined with a propensity for compartment syndrome, ▶p722.

Is it justifiable to withhold surgery from smokers?[2] Perhaps 'yes', if a given problem has a non-operative alternative with similar outcome yet potentially disastrous complications exacerbated by smoking: eg a calcaneal ORIF spiralling out of control into an amputation. Also perhaps 'yes', if resources must be distributed across a population in whom smokers are shown to fare much worse with a given operative management. The ethical counterpoise would be from a discriminatory angle, both in terms of costs and the concept of self-inflicted harm—eg in comparison to dangerous sporting activity.

How to approach the issue Careful informed consent will be vital, though whether scare tactics are allowed is another matter altogether. Abstaining for 6 to 8 weeks prior to elective surgery will reduce many of the side effects of smoking, but this is not a luxury afforded to trauma patients, and for some the stresses of what has happened may be too much to place on top of stopping smoking.[3] Do smokers mobilize more keenly in the post-op period in response to their craving to get off the ward for a cigarette? There appear to be no studies to answer this yet! For giving *advice on stopping smoking*, see p511.

Salter and Harris classification of epiphyseal injury

I	Seen in babies or pathological conditions (eg scurvy)
II	The commonest injury, with the fracture line *above* the growth plate
III	There is a displaced fragment, with the fracture line *through* the growth plate
IV	Union across the growth plate may interfere with bone growth
V	Compression of the epiphysis causes deformity and stunting

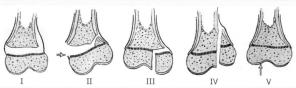

Fig 12.4 Salter and Harris classification of epiphyseal injury.
Salter R, Harris W, Injuries involving the epiphyseal plate, *The Journal of Bone and Joint Surgery*, Volume 45, Issue 3, pp. 587–622, 1963—a simple summary of the five stages of the classification.

Injuries to and around the growth plate can be difficult to distinguish from normal appearances, especially when they are viewed obliquely. Most physes are in a plane that makes it relatively easy to diagnose the injury (eg distal radius, and to a lesser extent proximal femur), whereas some cross the plane of the x-ray at multiple angles (eg proximal humerus). With these trickier physes, it is wise to liaise with someone with experience. Also consider comparison with the contralateral side.

2 With pressure to provide a cost-effective and fair service in the NHS, there are strong arguments from both parties. The debate certainly does not allow for smoke without fire...'
3 Though even stopping just one day before surgery has been shown to improve outcome.[8]

The following principles of fracture management aim to re-store the limb to its maximal biomechanical function:

1 Anatomic reduction (realignment) of fracture fragments
2 Stabilization of fragments to enable normal activity (eg surgical fixation or splinting in a cast)
3 Maintaining neurovascular (NV) supply
4 Encouraging early rehabilitation.

Conservative management uses splints (see p811), casts, and traction to realign and stabilize displaced fractures. This also allows freeing of any structures trapped between bone ends which aids revascularization (vital in subcapital fractures of the femur) and prevents later degeneration if fractures involve the joints. ▸▸Occasionally reduction will be required immediately to preserve NV status, ie in ED before an x-ray is even taken (eg for fracture-dislocation of the ankle or knee). Manipulation under anaesthesia (for analgesia and muscle relaxation) and x-ray screening. NB: if under GA, obtain consent for ± ORIF in case closed reduction is unsuccessful.

Methods of traction Internal and external fixation has removed the need for much traction in adults, but it is still used for children. Traction or fixation helps hold the reduced fracture in place for healing, which takes from 2 weeks (babies) to >12 weeks (p718).

- *Skin traction* uses adhesive strapping to attach the load to the limb. The problems are that the load cannot be very great, and that sensitivity to the adhesive may develop.
- *Skeletal traction:* Using a pin through bone, bigger forces can be employed such as fixed and balance traction:
  - *Fixed traction:* The Thomas' splint (fig 12.5). Weight can be added over a pulley (at the foot end) to relieve pressure on ischial tuberosity.

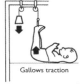

Fig 12.5 Thomas' splint.

  - *Balanced traction:* (fig 12.6) The weight of the limb balanced against the load. This can enable the patient to easily lift the leg off the bed, eg for a bed pan.
  - *Gallows traction* (fig 12.6) is suitable for children up to 2 yrs of age. The buttocks rise just above the bed.

The nurses on the specialists units will be experts at setting up and adjusting traction devices, so ask if you can watch and help.

Complications of casts:
- Avoid these by providing education on good cast care and rehabilitation courses
- Muscle atrophy
- Stiff joints
- Pressure ulcers
- NV disturbance
- Osteoporosis

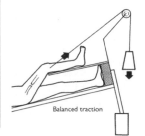

Balanced traction

Gallows traction

Fig 12.6 Traction: balanced traction, and gallows traction.

Trauma

1 *Give IV antibiotics* as soon as possible, ideally within 3 hours of injury: Co-amoxiclav (1.2g) 8-hourly and continue for 72 hours or definitive wound closure, which ever is sooner. Consider tetanus status.
2 Continuous assessment of *neurovascular status* of limb.
3 *Immediate surgery* in vascular impairment or compartment syndrome.
4 *Urgent surgery* if wound is heavily contaminated, eg sewage matter.
5 Plastic and orthopaedic surgical teams should work together; the primary surgical treatment of severe open tibial fractures only takes place in a non-specialist centre if the patient cannot be transferred safely.
6 *Debridement* is performed by plastic & orthopaedic surgeons working together within 24 hours of the injury (unless there is contamination).
7 *Cover wound* in saline-soaked gauze to prevent desiccation; only handle to remove gross contamination and allow photography.
8 *Splint the limb*, including the knee and ankle.
9 If definitive skeletal and soft tissue reconstruction is not to be undertaken in a single stage, then vacuum foam dressing or an antibiotic bead pouch is applied until definitive surgery.
10 *Definitive skeletal stabilization and wound cover* are achieved within 72 hours and should not exceed 7 days.

Open reduction internal fixation (ORIF)

If possible, fractures involving joint articulations should be treated by ORIF which allows open reduction and rigid fixation of the joint surfaces such that immediate movement can occur—see MINIBOX for the other indications for ORIF. The trick is then to achieve stable internal fixation in order to facilitate healing and also reduce serious complications (p722).

Indications for ORIF:
• Failed conservative R̖
• 2 #s in 1 limb
• Bilateral identical #s
• Intra-articular #s
• Open #
• Displaced unstable #

• *Plates* provide strength & stabilize # involving articular surfaces. Specifically designed types exist to counteract the various forces experienced in different joints (eg compression plates for long bones).
• *Screws* are often combined with other devices. Many different sizes exist.
• *Intramedullary nails* are placed in the medullary cavity (centre) of long bones, typically used in femoral and tibial shaft fixation.
• *Kirschner wires (K-wires):* Often used for closed reduction and percutaneous or internal fixation of fractures (rarely just for ORIF). K-wires are less rigid than plates and screws but can easily be removed after use.

External fixation is useful when there are burns, loss of skin and/or bone, or in case of open fractures since external fixation causes less disruption to the fracture site and associated soft tissue. It can be both definitive or tempory. Pins/wires are placed away from the zone of injury in various configurations giving varying degrees of stability. Pins are inserted into the bones directly; either just through the far bone cortex or directly through the opposite side of the limb. Pins are connected using a series of clamps and rods. Stability of fixation can be increased in a number of ways; use additional or larger dimeter pins, move rods closer to the bone, pins in different planes, etc.

Damage control orthopaedics (DCO) is a novel, and somewhat controversial, concept used in haemodynamically unstable polytrauma patients who receive temporary external fixation (eg pelvis) to facilitate haemorrhage control and resuscitation in order to optimize the patient for more permanant surgery later. Immediate invasive surgery provokes further inflammatory damage already induced by trauma so DCO aims to perform the minimal amount of orthopaedic surgery to achieve heamodynamic stability (p786).

Further reading
Taljanovi MS *et al.* (2003). Fracture fixation. *Radiographics* 23:1569–90.

See MINIBOX. **Fat embolism** Typically after pelvic or femur #. The mechanical theory—fat emboli are released from disrupted bone marrow. The biochemical theory—release of free fatty acids directly damage the penumocytes. Usually arises on day 2–3. *Signs:* altered mental state (few have fits), pyrexia (even low grade), SOB, hypoxia, tachycardia, petechial rash. ▶▶Consider ITU. Treatment is mainly supportive for respiratory failure. Mortality is 5–15%. Early immobilizszation has reduced incidence of femoral shaft #. ▶▶Major differential is PE.

Neurovascular injury is increasingly likely as deformity worsens, vascular injury is common in knee dislocations and supracondylar humeral #.

Infection The most common complication following # surgery is infection <1% in elective surgery to 20% in open fractures. Cellulitis, osteomyelitis, and sepsis can occur. See p705; prosthetic infections.

Delayed union is when the # has not healed within the expected time (see p708). *Causes:*
- # in a bone which has finished growing
- Poor blood supply (eg tibia) or avascular fragment (eg scaphoid)
- Comminuted/infected fracture
- Systemic disease (eg malignancy or infection)
- Distraction of bone ends by muscle; ORIF prevents this.

Complications
Immediate:
• Internal bleeding
• External bleeding
• Organ injury, eg brain
• Nerve or skin injury
• Vessel injury (limb ischaemia: *OHCM* p658)
Later—local:
• Skin necrosis/gangrene
• Pressure sores
• Infection
• Non- or delayed union
Later—general:
• Venous/fat embolism
• Pulmonary embolism
• Pneumonia
• Arthritis

Non-union This is said to have occurred when there is no evidence of progression towards healing, clinically or radiologically, by 6 months. Broadly, a non-union occurs from inadequate or abnormal biology or mechanics. Management is aimed at optimizing biology (infection, blood supply, bone graft) or the mechanics (skeletal stabilization). Avascular necrosis is also a cause, seen typically in femoral neck (p734) and scaphoid fractures (p731).

Malunion occurs when the fragments have not healed in anatomical positions causing loss of function, risk of secondary OA and contractures.

Thromboembilic events DVT occurs in ~⅔ of major orthopaedic events, but fatal PE in only 0.1–0.2%. Patients undergoing repair of hip # have the highest risk of fatal PE. Up to 70% have asymptomatic DVTs after TKR.[10] LMWH halves DVT rate and lowers risk of fatal PE by ~75%.[11] Compression stockings are less effective. Initiate enoxaparin 40mg 12-24 h post-op and a further 7-10 days (minimum) to reduce risk of VTE whilst minimizing risk of bleeding. Warfarin can also be used (INR 2-3) but had 33% higher risk of DVT and bleeding as compared to LMWH. Fondaparinux 2.5mg/day may be better than enoxaparin.[12] n=1049

Late complications include CRPS (p723):
- *Failure of fixation:* eg plates or nails break, or dislodge.
- *Psychological problems in mobilizing:* eg 'compensation neurosis'.

Compartment syndrome

▶▶Life- and limb-threatening. Occurs when swelling of tissues in an anatomic compartment (can occur anywhere, most commonly in the leg) occludes the vascular supply leading to hypoxia and eventually necrosis. Subsequent rhabdomyolysis can cause renal failure. Correct hypovolaemia vigorously. Watch out for ↓ urine output & ↑ plasma K. On examination there is swelling, redness, mottling, and pain on passive muscle stretching. Pain is often disproportionate to injury. Intracompartmental pressures can be measured (>30mmHg is defined as critical), this should not delay surgical review as the diagnosis is clinical and prompt fasciotomy is life/limb saving.[9]

CRPS type I is a deranged sequel to limb trauma *without* nerve injury (CRPS I ≈ algodystrophy ≈ reflex sympathetic dystrophy, RSD). *CRPS type II* has an identifiable nerve lesion. Here it is helpful to bear in mind that after a partial nerve lesion there is ↑activity in undamaged afferent c fibres with neuropeptide release (∴ vasodilatation within their innervation territory). But CNS phenomena are important too. Animal studies show ↑expression of the N-methyl-D-aspartate (NMDA) receptors in models of neuropathic pain (and NMDA receptor blockers such as memantine can improve symptoms).[13] Another proof of central effects is the finding of substantial reorganization of somatotopic CNS maps—leading to mislocalization of tactile stimuli.[14] Overall, however, this condition is poorly understood.

CRPS I is a 'complex disorder of pain, sensory abnormalities, abnormal blood flow, sweating, and trophic changes in superficial or deep tissues'. The central event may be loss of vascular tone or supersensitivity to sympathetic neurotransmitters. Pathogenesis is obscure, the idea of exaggerated regional inflammatory responses is supported by the fact that IgG labelled with indium (^{111}In) is concentrated in the affected extremity.[15]

Causes Injury esp. distal and esp. upper limb—eg fractures, carpal tunnel release, ops for Dupuytren's, tendon release procedures, mastectomy, transradial cardiac catheterization, knee surgery, crush injury, ankle arthrodesis, amputation, hip arthroplasty, rotator cuff injury, zoster, myocardial infarction, stroke, cancer, spontaneous/idiopathic.

Presentation Typically patients have initial trauma—commonly in a hand or foot—which may be trivial or severe. This is followed weeks or months later by pain, allodynia/hyperalgesia, vasomotor instability, and abnormal sweating. Pain is often burning in nature and may extend to the whole limb. The limb may be cold and cyanosed, or hot and sweating (locally). T° sensitivity may be heightened. The skin of the affected part may be oedematous, or, later, shiny and atrophic. Hyperreflexia, dystonic movements, and contractures may occur. Symptoms are often worse after exercise, and may include weakness, hyperalgesia, clumsiness, inability to initiate movements, spasms, dystonias, and allodynia (a stimulus not usually painful now hurts). There are no systemic signs (no fever, tachycardia, or lymphadenopathy).

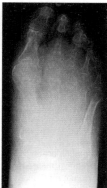

Fig 12.7 CRPS type I, with diffuse osteopenia and destruction of the 2nd and 3rd metatarsals.

Courtesy of The Norfolk and Norwich University Hospitals (NNUH) Radiology Dept.

Imaging *x-rays:* Patchy osteopenia greater than expected from disuse; joint space *not* narrowed (*no* thinned cartilage)—see fig **12.7**. *Bone scintigraphy:* Characteristic uniform uptake, with increased limb perfusion on the dynamic phase.

    Treatment ▶Refer to pain clinic/multidisciplinary team (physio + OT).

- Encourage optimism and pleasurable things. Ultimately, with appropriate care, CRPS is self-limiting.
- Avoid bad habits of trying to protect the affected limb by keeping it immobile, (leads to stiffness). Educate on using the limb in activities of daily living.
- Effective painkillers eg amitriptyline 25mg ON PO ± NSAIDs.

Further reading

Singh JA *et al.* (2011). Cardiac and thromboembolic complications and mortality in patients undergoing total hip and total knee arthroplasty. *Ann Rheum Dis* 70:2082–8.

Talbot M *et al.* (2006). Fat embolism syndrome: history, definition, epidemiology. *Injury* 37(Suppl 4):S3–7.

Fracture of the clavicle Historically thought to be caused by a fall onto an outstretched hand (FOOSH), most seem to occur after a direct blow to the clavicle and is common in cyclists. Fractures are most common in the middle third where proximal fragment is pulled superiorly by sternocleidomastoid. Management is typically a broad arm sling with follow up x-rays at 6 weeks to ensure union. ORIF of displaced # significantly reduces the risk of non-union; deformity may lead to functional problems in adulthood (figs 12.8, 12.9, & 12.10). ▶Remember the possibility of neurovascular injury (brachial plexus; subclavian vessels) + pneumothorax as complications.

Scapula and acromion fractures Rarely need fixation. These represent high-energy transfer injuries, so assess carefully to exclude other injuries.

Acromioclavicular (AC) joint dislocation is typically caused by a direct blow to top of the shoulder in young contact-sport athletes. The patient has a tender prominence over the AC joint and adduction of arm across the body will ↑ pain. Assess neurovascular status. *Imaging:* On x-ray check for congruity of the underside of the acromion with the distal clavicle. Radiography may be normal. *R:* Depends on displacement of the AC joint on x-rays. Minimal displacement can be rested in a broad arm sling, more severe disruption will likely require open reduction and ligament reconstruction.[16]

Anterior shoulder dislocation is most common (95%) (fig 12.11). Typically young males present following contact sports which have forced the arm into abduction, extension, and external rotation. Eldery patients can simply have a history of falling on an outstretched hand. *Signs:* Loss of shoulder contour (flattening of deltoid), an anterior bulge from the head of the humerus, which may also be palpated in the axilla. ▶Check pulses and nerves (including the axillary nerve supplying sensation over lower deltoid area) pre- and post-reduction. Before reduction, do x-ray (*is there a fracture?*). Relieve pain (eg intra-articular local anaesthetic, parenteral opioid, Entonox®) throughout the procedure. *Treatment: Simple reduction:* Apply longitudinal traction to the arm in abduction, and replace the head of the humerus by gentle pressure. *Kocher's method:* Flex the elbow to 90°, abduct the shoulder, externally rotate the shoulder/humerus and then abduct the upper arm back across the front of the body before internally rotating the shoulder. *Risk:* humeral #. Remember to obtain an x-ray post-reduction. Support the arm in internal rotation with a broad arm sling and refer to fracture clinic for follow-up. Surgery may be needed eg if young/athletic, or recurrent dislocation.

Posterior dislocation of the shoulder is rare and presents with a limitation of external rotation. May be associated with epileptic seizures or electrical shocks. It may be hard to diagnose from an anteroposterior x-ray ('light-bulb' appearance of humeral head); lateral x-ray views are essential.

Fracture of the proximal humerus Most are stable osteoporotic fractures in the elderly following a fall on an outstretched arm. Minimally displaced fractures may be managed conservatively. Open fractures, pathological fractures, 3 or 4 part fracture-dislocations or those with neurovascular injury (brachial plexus/axillary artery) will need operative management. Prognosis and complications (eg avascular necrosis) worsen with ↑ number of fragments.

Fracture of the humeral shaft Typically after a fall onto the arm, rarely onto the outstretched arm. Most do not need surgery; splinting with a humeral brace and gravity traction by means of 'collar and cuff' sling usually gives satisfactory reduction. Immobilize for 8–12 weeks. Surgical options include locking or compression plating. ▶Radial n. injury may cause wrist-drop, but damage can also be a complication of surgery, so *document function preoperatively.*

Fractures of the distal humerus See p726.

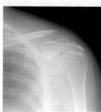

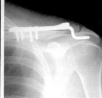

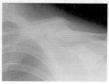

Fig 12.8 Comminuted distal clavicular fracture—an injury requiring ORIF.

Courtesy of The Norfolk and Norwich University Hospitals (NNUH) Radiology Dept.

Fig 12.9 Hook plate repair of fig 12.8-type injury. Remember nearby vessels!

Courtesy of The Norfolk and Norwich University Hospitals (NNUH) Radiology Dept.

Fig 12.10 Healed mid-clavicular # (different patient)—note deformity. Often, surgical repair is not needed for clavicle #, as healing and long-term function are good.

Courtesy of The Norfolk and Norwich University Hospitals (NNUH) Radiology Dept.

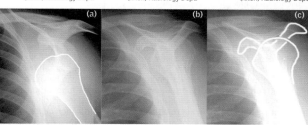

Fig 12.11 Due to the ligamentous laxity (see p664) the shoulder joint comprises 45% of all dislocated joints. Anterior dislocation of the shoulder (a)[4] and a post-reduction image (b)—copied and highlighted, (c). The dislocation can be painful, so positioning is difficult for the radiographer. These are attempted lateral views of the scapula. After reduction, the head of the humerus lies in the centre of the 'Y' with the coracoid process anterior and the acromion posterior.

Courtesy of Prof. Peter Scally.

Recurrent shoulder dislocation

Is there an underlying connective tissue disorder? 2 types: **Atraumatic** (5%) Often a teenager with no history of trauma, but having general joint laxity. Remember AMBRI: atraumatic (ie 'born loose'); multidirectional; bilateral; treat by: rehabilitation; inferior capsular shift surgery only if rehab fails. Beware of habitual dislocations; a patient who deliberately causes dislocations as their 'party trick' (less likely to respond to operative intervention). **Traumatic** Dislocation is anterior (sometimes inferior, rarely posterior) and secondary to trauma (may be mild); abduction + lateral rotation of the arm (eg donning a coat) may cause dislocation. Remember TUBS: traumatic (ie 'torn loose'); unilateral; Bankart lesion; surgical treatment. Recurrent dislocations cause further instability through the creation of damaged joint capsule components: *Bankart lesions* arise from avulsion of the glenoid labrum from the glenoid and *Hill–Sachs lesions*; an impaction # of the humeral head following anterior dislocations (seen on x-rays with arm medially rotated). Those <25 years have a higher risk of recurrent events compared to >40-year-olds, but this latter group requires imaging of rotator cuff as high risk of traumatic rupture rather than labral injury. **Treatment** depends on the cause and typically requires arthroscopic investigation. Both open and arthroscopic repair is possible, the latter however is gaining popularity, further supported by a recent study suggesting that the majority of patients have successful outcomes and relatively low risk of recurrence with arthroscopic fixation too.[17] Care of elderly patients focusses more on physio exercises to strengthen rotator cuff muscles.

4 The humeral head can sometimes lie low in the glenoid fossa with surgical neck fractures, from 'deltoid inhibition'—relaxation of the muscle from pain, causing subluxation; it is *not* a fracture-dislocation.

▶ Look for neurovascular compromise! The antecubital fossa contains (from lateral to medial) the radial nerve, biceps brachii tendon, brachial art. and median nerve (typically anterior interosseous branch). The ulnar nerve passes posteriorly at the medial epicondyle.

The elbow *Imaging:* Presence of an elbow fracture is suggested by an 'anterior sail sign' or 'posterior fat pad sign'.[5] *Management:* If no # obvious, but an effusion is present, treat initially with a broad arm sling. Re-x-ray after 10d (# more easily seen): if clear, start mobilization. For fractures, internal fixation may be needed. Physiotherapy & early mobilization are vital in preventing stiffness.

Fractures of the distal humerus • *Supracondylar fractures* (see p727).
• *Fracture of the medial epicondyle:* These may require surgery if a fragment is in the joint or if there are ulnar nerve compression symptoms.
• *Fracture of the lateral epicondyle:* Surgical fixation may be required. Complications include cubitus valgus and ulnar nerve palsy.
• *T-shaped intercondylar humerus fracture:* This is a supracondylar fracture with a break between the condyles. Notoriously difficult to surgically fix; requires rigid fixation to allow early mobilization.

Fractures of the radial head Most common elbow # in adults. The elbow is swollen and tender over the radial head; flexion/extension may be possible but pronation & supination hurt. Radiography often shows an effusion, but minor fractures are often missed. Undisplaced fractures can be treated in a collar and cuff, there remains dispute over whether early mobilzation actually improves function without increasing risk of complications. If displaced or fragment prevents supination/pronation then internal fixation or excision of the radial head may be needed. *Complications:* 3–14% are associated with the 'terrible triad' of radial head fracture, elbow dislocation, and coronoid process #; resulting in joint instability and post-traumatic complications.[18]

Elbow dislocations are commonly posterior (90%) and result from a fall on a not yet fully outstretched hand, with elbow flexed; this causes posterior ulna displacement on the humerus, and a swollen elbow, fixed in flexion. ▶ Associated fractures, brachial artery and nerve injury must be considered. *Closed reduction (±GA):* Stand behind the patient; flex the elbow to relax biceps brachii. With your fingers around the epicondyles, push forwards on the olecranon with your thumbs, and down on the forearm. Hearing a clunk heralds success. This may be aided by traction at the wrist. A post-reduction image is needed to exclude fractures. Immobilize in a backslab for 10 days. *Complications:* Stiffness, instability, radio-ulnar joint disruption, failure to identify neurovascular compromise leading to severe morbidity with limb ischaemia, compartment syndrome and neurological changes.[19]

Olecranon fractures either occur after a direct blow or as an avulsion injury when triceps (which inserts onto olecranon) contracts during a fall on the semiflexed supinated arm. Treat with ORIF, eg tension band wiring, if displaced fracture.

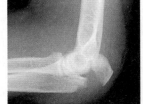

Fig 12.12 Displaced olecranon fracture needing fixation.

Courtesy of The Norfolk and Norwich University Hospitals (NNUH) Radiology Dept.

Elbow joint replacement is typically performed in patients with rheumatoid arthritis, but also increasingly in complex fractures, post-traumatic instability and OA.[20]

---

5 The *anterior fat pad* can be seen on lateral elbow x-ray as a radiolucent triangle in front of the distal humerus. It can be present in a normal elbow, and is only abnormal when raised off the bone by an effusion. A visible *posterior fat pad* is always abnormal. Absence of either of these signs makes a fracture very unlikely. Other things to check on the lateral x-ray: *anterior humeral line* (which should cross the anterior third of the capitellum) and *alignment of the radial shaft* with the capitellum (which it should bisect).

The Salter Harris classification of physeal injuries (see p719) helps predict the risk of growth disturbance. Paediatric elbow x-rays can be difficult to interpret because of the ossification centres (see mnemonic p657). Physeal # tend to heal quickly (~4 weeks) but monitor carefully to ensure normal growth has not been disrupted. Paediatric bone is softer and leads to unique # patterns not seen in adults eg: *greenstick #* (cortex fails in tension and develops a partial transverse crack), *torus #* (buckle of one cortex as it fails in compression), *plastic deformation* (the bone bends with no evidence of #). Typically these are treated with closed reduction (if needed) and cast immobilization.

Pulled elbow (subluxation of radial head) See p669.

Supracondylar fracture is the most common # of childhood (rare in adults).
Present with pain, swelling, and inability to move elbow. Most (95%) are due to hyperextension. The Gartland classification uses lateral x-rays to describe the severity of displacement from extension injuries.

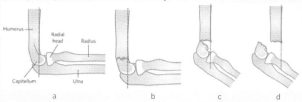

Fig 12.13 (a) In a normal elbow, a line drawn along the anterior surface of the humerus.
(b) Gartland type I: The anterior humeral line passes through the middle of the capitellum. Non-displaced. Difficult to see on x-ray so look for the fat pad signs. See footnote on p726.
(c) Gartland type II: The anterior humeral line passes anterior to the middle of the capitellum. The distal fragment is angulated with an intact posterior cortex.
(d) Gartland type III: Unstable posterior displacement.

> Republished, with permission, from resources at The Royal Children's Hospital, Melbourne, Australia http://www.rch.org.au/clinicalguide/guideline_index/fractures/Supracondylar_fracture_of_the_humerus_Emergency_Department/

Gartland type IIIa is *posteromedial* and threatens the radial n. IIIB is *posterolateral* and threatens the median n., esp. the anterior interosseous branch, which innervates deep flexors to the index finger and flexor pollicis longus (pincer grip); entirely a motor nerve, so injury is easily missed. *Management:* ▶ Check neurovascular status. Keeping the elbow in extension after injury prevents exacerbating brachial artery damage from the time of injury. Type I fractures can be managed with and above elbow back slab and sling. Type II fractures may require reduction under sedation/GA. Type III fractures generally require GA and fixation with K-wires.[22] *Complications:* A cubitus varus deformity of the elbow can result from malunion, but should pass through the middle ⅓ of the capitellum.

Further reading

Chen HW *et al.* (2014). Complications of treating terrible triad injury of the elbow: a systematic review. *PLoS One* 9(5):e97476.

Jie KE *et al.* (2014). Extension test and ossal point tenderness cannot accurately exclude significant injury in acute elbow trauma. *Ann Emerg Med* 64:74–8.

Trauma

Distal radial and ulnar fractures are very common, especially in osteoporotic post-menopausal women who fall on an outstretched hand. ▶ Compartment syndrome can occur in forearm injuries, as can damage to the ulnar, radial, and median nerves (especially the anterior osseous branch).

Treatment is guided by evidence of neurovascular compromise and patient criteria. Traditionally, the majority of wrist fractures were 'pulled' (closed reduction) in the ED using either a haematoma block or Bier's block (IV regional anaesthetic using an inflatable cuff around the upper arm). The general consensus in the literature is that Bier's blocks are more effective overall then haematoma blocks and are preferable.[23] Current practice, however, varies and there is an increasing number of wrist # undergoing surgical fixation; there remains dispute over whether ORIF or K-wires (not strictly ORIF) is best.[24] Closed reduction in the ED is being reserved more and more for those patients with neurovascular compromise or where manipulation in the department is likely to be the definitive treatment (eg frail patients with low functional demands). See p729 for procedure. If closed manipulation is performed, x-rays must be obtained.

Use your eponyms wisely (also see p708 in *OHCM*) It is so tempting to fire off 'Colles' fracture' or other names that spring to mind whenever faced with an x-ray suggestive of distal radial injury... Have a quick think before scrambling for eponyms; modern practice has shifted towards simply describing the anatomic fracture pattern that you see (see p715) as eponyms are frequently incorrectly applied. Here are a few in the forearm:

Colles' fracture: An extra-articular # of the distal radius with dorsal displacement of the distal radius. Note that Colles originally based his descriptions solely on clinical examination (since Rontgen only discovered x-rays in 1895) and described this injury as a wrist dislocation with 'dinner-fork' deformity (the fingers are the prongs). Avulsion of the ulna styloid process may also occur.

Smith's fracture: (Reverse Colles) Volar displacement and angulation of the distal radial fragment. Fixation is needed in these fractures more commonly than in Colles' fractures, as the fracture fragment tends to migrate palmarly.

Barton's fracture is an intra-articular fracture involving the dorsal aspect of the distal radius (fig 12.14 is a reverse Barton's, involving the palmar surface).

Chauffeur's fracture: Fracture of the radial styloid (historically seen in drivers who drove old cars which needed cranking to engage the engine).

Monteggia/Galeazzi fractures: See p650 & p644.

Night-stick fractures are isolated ulnar shaft #s, typically associated with a direct blow to a forearm held up in self defence against a truncheon (a 'night stick'). Look for other injuries as this fracture pattern requires a large force.

Wrist dislocation Although wrist injuries are very common, dislocations are in the minority. They most commonly involve the carpal bones, especially at the scapholunate or lunotriquetral junctions. May be anterior or posterior. Typically young athletes. x-rays help rule out fracture. Manipulation and often open reduction, and plaster immobilization eg for 6 weeks. Median nerve compression may occur.[25] See p731 for scaphoid fractures.

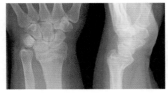

Fig 12.14 AP and lateral views of the left wrist. Does it matter what eponym denotes which type of wrist fracture this is? Colles', Smith's, or Barton's? Try describing it anatomically instead.

Courtesy of The Norfolk and Norwich University Hospitals (NNUH) Radiology Dept.

Reduction of a fracture of the distal radius (Colles' type)

- Ensure that there is adequate local or regional anaesthesia. Traction should be applied to the hand with an assistant to provide counter-traction at the elbow. The fracture can often be felt to disimpact with 'clunk'.

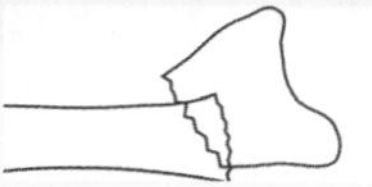

Dorsally angulated
Dorsally displaced
Loss of ulna tilt
+/- Impacted

Fig 12.15 View before reduction (radius shown alone in lateral view only).

- *Exaggerate* dorsal angulation while maintaining distal traction to stop the inelastic dorsal periosteum from preventing reduction by longitudinal traction.

- Correct dorsal and radial angulation, again maintaining distal traction. Aim for anatomical alignment:

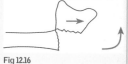

Fig 12.16

- Apply plaster backslab (p774), moulded to maintain reduction in ulnar deviation with some wrist flexion. Backslabs are more popular than full casts; an advantage is that you do not need to split the cast.

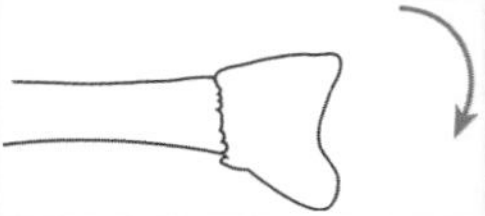

Fig 12.17

- Maintain traction while the POP is applied. This is most easily done by pulling on the thumb and 1st finger against counter-traction. This applies to both palmar and ulnar deviation.

- Support in a sling, once an x-ray has shown a good position (fig 12.18).

- Check x-ray in 5d, when swelling has reduced; the plaster is then completed.

▶ Inability to get a good position may indicate soft tissue interpositioning.

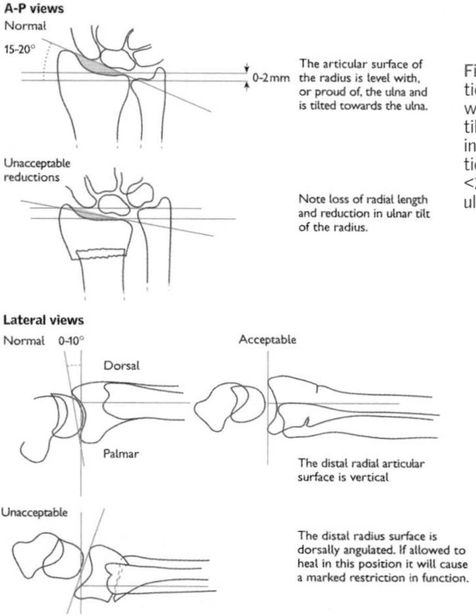

A-P views

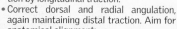

Normal

15–20°

0–2mm

The articular surface of the radius is level with, or proud of, the ulna and is tilted towards the ulna.

Unacceptable reductions

Note loss of radial length and reduction in ulnar tilt of the radius.

Fig 12.18 Acceptable positions post-reduction of wrist fractures (dorsal tilt <10°; radial shortening <2mm; radial inclination >15°; articular step <2mm; and distal radioulnar joint congruence).

Lateral views

Normal   0–10°

Dorsal

Palmar

Acceptable

The distal radial articular surface is vertical

Unacceptable

The distal radius surface is dorsally angulated. If allowed to heal in this position it will cause a marked restriction in function.

Further reading

Hoynack BC (2015). *Wrist Fracture in Emergency Medicine*. Medscape. http://emedicine.medscape.com/article/828746

Trauma

Metacarpal fractures The base of the 2nd and 3rd metacarpals (MCs) form the functional centre of the hand around which the movement of the hand is centred (fig 12.20). Thus, whilst malalignment and imperfect reduction may be tolerated in the 5th MC (<40° volar angulation), far less is permitted in the 2nd MC (<10°). The 5th MC is most commonly involved, often from a punch. Management may vary depending on whether the fracture is in the head/neck/shaft or base of the MC, however, stable closed fractures can be managed in a splint/cast for ~2 weeks, with the wrist in partial extension (20–30°), MCP joints in 70–90° flexion with fingers in extension. Unstable fractures may require K-wires/ORIF. Longer periods of splinting in plaster or a 'boxing glove' bandage can cause a stiff hand, eg from joint adhesions/contracture, flexor tendon fibrosis, and collateral ligament shortening. Rotational fractures disclose themselves by producing a rotation of the fingers—see BOX; they usually require operative fixation (plate & screws), as do fractures of ≥2 MCs.

▶Beware wounds overlying metacarpophalangeal joints (often contaminated from the punched victim's teeth, and may communicate with the joint). These almost always need washout and exploration in theatre.

Fractures of the proximal phalanx Spiral or oblique fractures occurring at this site are likely to be associated with a rotation deformity—and this must be corrected (see BOX). Often, the only way to do this accurately is by open reduction and fixation, eg with a single compression screw.

Middle phalanx fractures Manipulate these; splint in flexion over a malleable metal splint, strapping the finger to its neighbour ('neighbour strapping'). The aim is to control rotation, which interferes with later finger flexion.

Distal phalanx fractures may be caused by crush injuries and are often open. If closed, symptoms may be relieved by trephining the nail (see p733).

Mallet finger The tip of the finger droops because of avulsion of the extensor tendon's attachment to the terminal phalanx or rupture of the terminal part of the tendon. If the avulsed tendon includes a piece of bone, union is made easier—using a special splint, eg with 0° of extension. Use for 6 weeks. Surgical intervention may be indicated if the fracture fragment is >30% of the joint surface. Poorer outcome is associated with delay in splinting (see p710).

Gamekeeper's thumb This is so called because of the laxity of the ulnar collateral ligament of the metacarpophalangeal joint of the thumb during the forced thumb abduction that occurs when wringing a pheasant's neck. The same injury is described in dry ski slope participants who fall and catch their thumb in the matting ('skier's thumb'). Diagnosis can be difficult as the thumb is so painful to examine, but to miss this injury may condemn the patient to a weak pincer grip—inject 1–2mL 1% lidocaine around the ligament to facilitate examination. Differentiation of complete vs partial tears of the ligament is crucial because the treatment for complete tears is surgical. Radiological evaluation will detect a bony avulsion fragment. Partial tears (clinically stable), or those associated with undisplaced avulsion fractures of the proximal phalanx, can be adequately treated using simple short-arm thumb spica casting.

Finger tip amputation distal to the DIP joint can include damage to nail, bone and soft tissues. Although not as exciting as p809, this injury is very common and surrounded by false belief that the severed tip should be placed directly in ice—discourage this first-aid practice as it may worsen damage. Transport of tip should be made in a clear bag near ice for preservation. Look for associated fracture or foreign bodies. Minor soft tissue loss is treated conservatively with dressings as it will likely heal by secondary intention after 3–5 weeks.[6] More significant injury requires skin grafting, most likely from another part of the hand.

---

6 This link shows an excellent demonstration of finger tip healing post injury.[26]

Assessing rotational deformity

Refer any fractures with obvious rotational deformity (a clinical, not a radiological decision, fig 12.19), as this can be disabling. Assessing for rotational deformity in finger and metacarpal fractures is essential. It cannot be accurately assessed with the fingers extended, so ask the patient to flex their fingers: they should all point to the scaphoid. Alternatively, look at and assess the nails end on in this position. Refer to a specialist if rotation is detected, as manipulation may be required; function and perhaps livelihood are at stake.

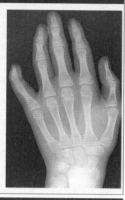

Fig 12.19 Salter Harris II fracture of base of 5th proximal phalanx. The finger can be appreciated to be angulated, but the degree of rotation must still be assessed clinically. See p719 Salter Harris fractures.

Image courtesy of The Norfolk and Norwich University Hospitals (NNUH) Radiology Dept.

Scaphoid fractures

Common and easily missed on x-ray; results from falls on the hand. *Signs* Tender in anatomical snuff box and over scaphoid tubercle, pain on axial compression of the thumb, and on ulnar deviation of the pronated wrist, or supination against resistance. *Imaging* Request a dedicated 'scaphoid' series. If −ve, and fracture is suspected MRI has been shown to be sensitive and cost-effective.[27] CT is an alternative. If neither is available, cast and re-x-ray in 2 weeks. Non-displaced fractures involving the waist may be immobilized in a neutral forearm cast for several weeks until union. Percutaneous cannulated screw fixation allows the patient to return to work earlier but does not affect the long-term outcome. *Complications* Avascular necrosis: the proximal pole relies on interosseous supply from the distal part.

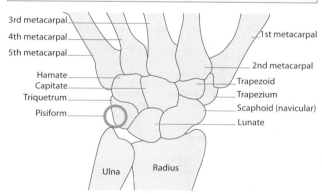

Fig 12.20 Naming the carpal bones doesn't have to be tedious, there are several mnemonics. Some less appropriate than others and we encourage you to seek them out! One more sensible option to describe the carpal bones in the proximal row, then distal row is: She Left The Party To Take Cathy Home. (Scaphoid, Lunate, Triquetrium, Pisiform, Trapezium, Trapezoid, Capitate, Hamate).

Further reading

Mallee WH *et al.* (2014). Clinical diagnostic evaluation for scaphoid fractures: a systematic review and meta-analysis. *J Hand Surg Am* 39(9):1683-91.

▶*There are no minor injuries to the hand*. Any breach of the integument may be the start of a chain of events that leads to loss of our most useful appendage. *Hands are very frequently injured simply because they are how we tend to explore our surroundings. The complexity of anatomy and biomechanics in our hand truly deserves its own chapter but here are a few things to consider.*

Infections *Staph aureus* is the most common bacteria associated with hand infection (80%). Others include Streps and Gram –ves. *Paronychia:* Infection causing painful cellulitis around the finger nail (see fig 12.21). In the early stages, antibiotics may cure this, but once a collection forms, drainage of the abscess is required. Chronic fungal infections typically develop in workers whose hands are repeatedly exposed to wet conditions. They describe a of history frequent bacterial infections with abscess formation and nail deformities. *Felon:* An abscess in the pulp of the distal finger. X-ray to look for a foreign body as the source of infection. Incise into area of maximal fluctuance; blunt antibiotics is needed to break up septae, and

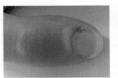

Fig 12.21 Acute paronychia
© DermNet NZ.

a drain left in place and treat with ıv antibiotics.[28]
Infective flexor tenosynovitis: Bacterial infection of flexor tendon sheath—which can spread via the carpal tunnel to the forearm; this potential for rapid spread makes it a surgical emergency. Look for 'Kanavel's 4 signs': **1** Symmetrical swollen fingers. **2** Tenderness over flexor sheath **3** Pain on passive extension of fingers so the patient preferentially chooses to **4** hold the finger in slight flexion. Treat urgently with ıv antibiotics and either repeated visits to theatre or post-operative in-dwelling catheter irrigation (see fig 12.22). Even previously healthy patients can expect residual digital stiffness despite optimal therapy.

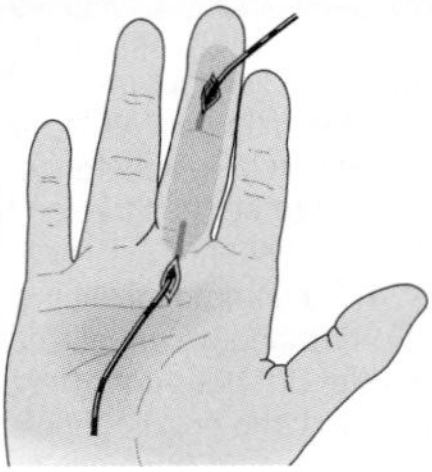

Fig 12.22 Drainage and closed irrigation for flexor sheath infection. The antibiotic solution drips in through the distal catheter and drains out the proximal one.

Reproduced with permission of Way LW ed. '*Current Surgical Diagnosis and Treatment*', 10th ed. Appleton & Lange 1994 © McGraw Hill.

Flexor tendon injuries Failure to flex the DIP joint against resistance ≈ flexor digitorum profundus division (fig 12.23). If this is intact but flexion of the PIP joint is affected, there is division of superficialis. Flexor pollicis longus section leads to inability to flex the interphalangeal joint of the thumb. In general, flexor tendon injuries are best treated by primary repair (most are open injuries). If there is loss of tendon substance or delayed presentation, a staged repair with a silastic implant to keep the tendon sheath open, followed by a tendon graft, may be needed. Intensive hand physiotherapy with supervision is essential.

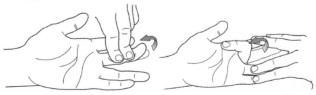

Fig 12.23 Examination of flexor digitorum profundus (FDP) and flexor digitorum superficialis (FDS).

Reproduced from Warwick et al., *Oxford Specialist Handbook of Hand Surgery* (2009), with permission from OUP.

Trauma

In the absence of fingernails, the ability to manipulate small objects is significantly reduced, the distal phalynx is rendered defenceless, and the cosmetic appearance is flawed. Yet injuries to the nail are still frequently ignored when multiple injuries affect the hand.[30] The anatomy of the nail is far more complex than people initially consider. The nail bed is adherent to the periosteum of the distal phalynx below and the nail plate above. This rich vascular layer enables nail plate growth; allowing the average nail to completely regrow within 9 months. Note that various systemic diseases can also affect the nail (eg psoriasis, liver disease, thyroid disease).

Injury to the nailbed is often associated with subungal haematomas and damage to the distal phalynx ►Always do an x-ray as 50% of nail bed injuries are associated with fractures of the distal phalynx. Crush injuries (such as door closures or hammers) are the most common cause.

Subungal haematoma is seen under the nail when the highly vascular nailbed is disrupted after trauma to the fingertip. The nail is often still intact. Small, pain-free haematomas tend to settle spontaneously and patients do not attend the doctor. It can become painful if the build up of blood increases the pressure under the nail. Trephination of the haematoma should be considered to release this pressure, approaches include electric cautery, 18-gauge needle and a heated paper clip. This can be performed without anaesthesia in the ED. The key question to ask before attempting this is: is there evidence of complex laceration to the nail bed? Lacerations may require suturing and exploration of the nail bed. Studies have suggested that when the haematoma covers >50% of the nail then further examination may be warranted.[31] Failure to address nailbed injuries appropriately can result in nail bed deformities and abnormal growth, and infections of both soft tissue and bone (osteomyelitis). ►Trephination performed in the presence of a fracture converts it into an open fracture. Do an x-ray if in doubt!

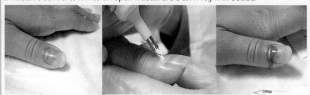

Fig 12.24 Trephination of a subungal haematoma. Clean the site well to minimize risk of infection. Once the trephination device reaches the collection of blood then you will see it ooze out, multiple trephination holes may be required. Watch this video for the technique.[32]

Image reprinted with permission from Medscape Drugs & Diseases (http://emedicine.medscape.com/), 2015, available at: http://emedicine.medscape.com/article/827104-overview

Nail bed repair is required when repairing avulsed nails, bed lacerations, and after injuries which have crushed the finger tip. Use a digital nerve block[7] and sterilize the area well. Elevate (avulse) the nail using a fine clamp at one nail edge which you turn on its long axis (like opening a sardine can); the nail will wrap around the clamp and peel off the nail bed. Use absorbable sutures and keep debridement to a minimum to reduce scarring. Replace the nail to serve as a splint and secure it with either sutures or tissue adhesives. Refer to hand surgeons in complex injuries.

Further reading

BMJ Best Practice (2015). *Paronychia.* http://bestpractice.bmj.com/best-practice/monograph/350.html

British Society for Surgery of the Hand: www.bssh.ac.uk

Haneke E (2006). Surgical anatomy of the nail apparatus. *Dermatol Clin* 24(3):291–6.

7 A ring block (digital block) which anaesthetizes the distal phalynx is required for treating most painful finger tip injuries. Inject 1% lidocaine on both medial and lateral midpoints of the middle phalynx. Do not mix the lidocaine with adrenaline which can cause end artery spasm and finger tip ischaemia.

Trauma

Fractures of the femoral shaft and distal femur (supracondylar femur) usually involve significant trauma in young adults whilst relatively minor trauma in the elderly can typically cause intracapsular neck of femur (NOF) fractures.

Intracapsular fractures occur just below the femoral head and include subcapital (most common), transcervical, and basicervical (see fig 12.25). These often cause *external rotation, adduction, & shortening of the affected leg*.[8] The injuring force can be trivial and the patient may be able to walk (but with difficulty). Intracapsular # have a higher incidence of AVN and non-union due to the femoral head blood supply (p735). If displacement is minimal, internal fixation *in situ* gives the best outcome (rate of displacement, risk of AVN, and non-union are all reduced). In displaced # the head is excised and a prosthesis inserted. NB traumatic hip # tend to receive a hemiarthroplasty, predominently due to patient comorbidity. The acetabulum is not replaced unlike elective THR.

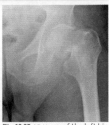

Fig 12.25 AP X-ray of the left hip showing a sub-capital fracture of the femoral neck. This may be easily appreciated on this view, but a lateral is vital for less obvious injuries.

Courtesy of The Norfolk and Norwich University Hospitals (NNUH) Radiology Dept.

Garden classification for intracapsular femoral neck fractures is based purely on the AP X-ray and correlates with prognosis, IV being the worst risk of AVN. The key is to differentiate between undisplaced (I&II) versus displaced (III&IV).

I	Incomplete undisplaced fracture with the inferior cortex intact
II	Complete undisplaced fracture through the neck
III	Complete neck fracture with partial displacement
IV	Fully displaced fracture

Reproduced with permission and © of the British Editorial Society of Bone and Joint Surgery, Garden RS. Low-angle fixation in fractures of the femoral neck. *J Bone Joint Surg [Br]* 1961;43-B:647–663 (the Garden classification).

Extracapsular fractures (between insertion of the hip joint capsule & 5cm below the lesser trochanter fig 12.26) are subclassified as trochanteric or subtrochanteric. Compared to intracapsular #s, the blood supply to the femoral head is not disrupted so AVN/# non-union is rarer. Fixation uses either intramedullary screws or sliding hip screws (for which the trade name Dynamic Hip Screw (DHS) is often used). A DHS will stabilize the # but allow compression at the site due to sliding of the screw in the femoral head, on weight bearing.

Types of proximal femoral fractures (fig 12.26)
• *Intra-[itn] and extra[ext]-capsular fractures:*[33]
  1 Subcapital [itn]
  2 Transcervical [itn]
  3 Basicervical [itn]
  4 Intertrochanteric/pertrochanteric [ext]
  5 Reverse oblique/transtrochanteric [ext]
  6 Subtrochanteric [ext]

Fracture type (eg displaced/undisplaced) and site determines management:
• Undisplaced intracapsular (1 or 2) → cannulated hip screw
• Displaced intracapsular (1 or 2) → (hemi)arthroplasty or THR if normally ambulant & medically fit
• Basicervical (3)/intertrochanteric (4) → DHS fixation
• Transtrochanteric (5)/subtrochanteric (6) → Intramedullary hip screw (but note that a DHS can be used in selected cases).

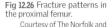

Fig 12.26 Fracture patterns in the proximal femur.

Courtesy of The Norfolk and Norwich University Hospitals (NNUH) Radiology Dept.

Blood supply to the femoral head

The primary blood supply to the femoral head are the retinacular arteries from the medial and lateral femoral circumflex arteries (arising from profunda femoris artery) (fig 12.27). This blood supply can be compromised by intracapsular fractures and SUFE (p684) and place the femoral head at risk of **Avascular necrosis (AVN)**. There is a small contribution from the foveal artery which runs in the ligament attached to head of femur, but this is frequently inadequate to prevent AVN. Risk of AVN is <10% if undisplaced, but can be >80% if displaced.[34] Subsequently NICE recommend that surgery should be performed on the day or day after admission.[33] *Sites at risk of AVN:* Hip (commonest), knee, scaphoid, shoulder.

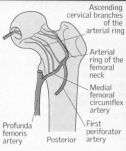

Fig 12.27 Blood supply to the femoral head.

Imaging: MRI is best. *Local causes:* Trauma; secondary to rheumatoid, severe OA, psoriatic arthropathy, or neuropathic joints. *Systemic:* Atraumatic AVN can initially be painless and incidentally discovered on x-rays, make sure you educate this patient group to report symptoms promptly. Thalassaemia, sickle-cell (+ any cause of microthrombi, eg platelets↑ in leukaemia), NSAIDs/steroids (eg post-transplant). *Treatment:* Immobilization; analgesia; for hips, arthroplasty. >50% will require operative intervention within 3 years. AVN will eventually cause necrosis with bone collapse and secondary OA.[35]

More femoral and hip injuries

Femoral shaft fracture ►Requires considerable force—look for injuries elsewhere. 500–1500mL of blood may be lost in a simple #; check distal pulses (possible femoral artery injury). Sciatic n. injury may also occur. The proximal bone fragment is flexed by iliopsoas, abducted by gluteus medius, and laterally rotated by gluteus maximus. The lower fragment is pulled up by the hamstrings and adducted (with external rotation) by the adductors. *Treatment:* Stabilize patient in ED and traction with a Thomas splint (fig 12.5 p720). Definitive treatment is typically with a locked intramedullary nail introduced proximally over a guide wire. This allows early mobilization. See also p794.

Distal femoral & proximal tibial fractures are divided into intra- or extra-articular (supracondylar). Intra-articular # needs internal fixation with anatomically contoured locking plate. Tibial plateau # are intra-articular and difficult to treat; non-operative treatment is appropriate in the elderly, however internal fixation is normally required to restore the articular surface and minimize later OA. Hinged cast braces locked in extension can reduce the risk of chronic flexure contacture following tibial plateau fractures.[36]

Posterior hip dislocation (eg to front-seat passengers if the knee strikes the dashboard). Feel for the femoral head in the buttock. The leg is *flexed*, **internally** *rotated, adducted,* and *shortened.* Frequently associated with # of femoral head, neck or shaft. ►The sciatic n. may be lacerated or stretched/compressed; early MRI diagnosis may prevent later equinus foot deformity. *Treatment:* Reduction under GA within 4 hours to reduce risk of AVN. Traction for 3 weeks promotes joint capsule healing.[37]

Further reading

Baker PN (2014). Evolution of the hip fracture population: time to consider the future? *BMJ Open* 4:e004405.

BMJ Best Practice (2014). *Hip Fractures.* http://bestpractice.bmj.com/best-practice/monograph/387/resources.html

8 This is opposed to the internal rotation found in hip dislocation. These positionings are explained by the changes in the fulcrum for the force applied by iliopsoas to the proximal femur in either condition.
►NB: *pathological fractures* are discussed in the BOX on p761.

Trauma

▶Around 80,000 people suffer a hip fracture annually in the UK. This number is set to rise to >100,000 by 2020 in line with the predicted 88% rise in people >65 years old over the next 25 years. Hip fractures are the most common reason for admission to the orthopaedic ward.[38]

Amidst your desperate attempts at identifying and describing the type of fracture that you think you might see,[9] take a peek past the computer screen towards your patient. This is most likely a life-changing injury. ~¼ of patients are admitted from institutional care and ~20% of those previously independant enough to live at home will eventually need to move into care homes. The mortality and morbidity is vast with hip fractures. 8% will die within 1 month of this fracture; 30% will die within 1 year. Be kind, and gently explain that we haven't offered a cup of tea because she needs to remain nil by mouth (NBM). Take a moment to explain the severity of this injury to the family also; in those patients who had significant morbidity and frailty prior to this injury it might be worth discussing issues surrounding resuscitation.

Management

Assess obs. Treat shock with crystalloid, but beware of incipient heart failure.
- Relieve pain (eg morphine 0.1mg/kg IV + femoral nerve block (or a fascia iliaca compartment block (see p633) + an antiemetic).
- Imaging: a good quality lateral is essential (see fig 12.25, p734). 2–10% of fractures can be missed on x-ray, consider CT/MRI.[39]
- Prepare for theatre: FBC, clotting, U&E, CXR, ECG, crossmatch 2u, consent.
- Sort out medical problems pre-op: ▶Get help from an ortho-geriatrician.

Preventing hip fractures

Preventing hip fractures is the best approach to reducing mortality, elective hip replacements have a 0.5% 30-day mortality risk whilst those following traumatic hip fractures have 8% risk.[41]
- Prevent falls: eg good lighting, less sedation, & keep-fit programmes.
- Teach exercise and balance training, eg with tai chi classes for the elderly. This lessens fear of falling, and can halve rates of multiple falls.
- Prevent osteoporosis: eg exercise, bisphosphonates.
- Ensure good vitamin D intake (plasma levels ≥30nmol/L; esp. in northern climes). A lack of vitamin D and calcium is associated with hip fractures whether or not patients are osteoporotic.
- Follow-up meta-analyses have cast doubt over whether hip protectors decrease risk of hip fracture in the elderly. Acceptability by users remains a problem, because of discomfort and practicality.[42]

The following may prevent complications after hip injury
- Early mobilization and post-procedure anticoagulation (p722).
- Co-ordinated multidisciplinary inpatient rehabilitation.
- Good nutrition—but meta-analyses do not provide much support for specific multi-nutritional commercial food supplements.

Further reading

Butler M *et al.* (2011). Evidence summary: systematic review of surgical treatments for geriatric hip fractures. *J Bone Joint Surg Am* 93:1104–15.

Hu F *et al.* (2012). Preoperative predictors for mortality following hip fracture surgery: a systematic review and metaanalysis. *Injury* 43:676–85.

Ongley D (2014). *Fractured NOF Patient: Killing me softly with my song...* http://www.aqua.ac.nz/upload/resource/NOF%20patient%20killing%20me%20softly.pdf

9 If you cannot see a fracture on the lateral and AP x-rays, but the patient still cannot weight bear then consider an MRI (or CT if MRI is contraindicated or not possible within 24h).[40]
10 (Also known as O'Donoghue's unhappy triad.)[47]

Trauma

The patella *Dislocation:* Is typically lateral—often as the result of twisting the lower leg, combined with contraction of the quadriceps. The knee is flexed with a lateral deformity. Reduction is achieved with firm medial pressure whilst extending the knee. Post reduction: do x-rays to check for patellar # and check the extensor mechanism of the knee. Ensure a period of immobilization in cast/posterior splint or brace. Rehabilitation will require quadriceps strengthening exercises. *Recurrent patella subluxation* may be related to developmental abnormalities around the knee. A tight lateral retinaculum causes the patella to sublux laterally, giving medial pain. The knee may give way. It is commoner in girls and with valgus knees. It may be familial, or associated with joint laxity, a high-riding patella (*patella alta*), or a hypotrophic lateral femoral condyle. *Signs:* Increased lateral patellar movement, accompanied by pain and the reflex contraction of quadriceps (ie a +ve patellar apprehension test). It may warrant surgery to strengthen the medial expansion.[43] *Patella fracture* usually results from a fall onto a flexed knee or due to dashboard injury in motor vehicle collision. Non-displaced fractures with an intact extensor mechanism may be managed conservatively. Displaced fractures are likely to require operative fixation.

The knee *Injury to a collateral ligament* is common in sport. *Mechanism:* The medial ligament is most commonly injured by a blow to the lateral aspect of the knee whilst the foot is fixed (putting valgus stress on the knee); vice versa for the lateral ligament. *Signs:* Effusion ± tenderness over affected ligaments. Rest is needed, then firm support. NB: surgery is rarely needed for isolated medial collateral ligament injury. Lateral injury is less common but tends to be more extensive and involve cruciates and common peroneal nerve injury; surgery is required if there is instability. *Anterior cruciate ligament (ACL) tear:* Typically follows a twisting injury to the knee with the foot fixed to the ground. Unable to continue playing. *Signs:* Effusion; haemarthrosis; +ve 'draw' sign (p688). Examination under GA may be needed. *Treatment:* This is problematic. 3 weeks' rest and physio may help. In the young, or ↑knee instability, consider ligament reconstruction (autograft).[44] Chronic ACL deficiency results in the knee giving way with laxity on examination and risk of OA. *Posterior cruciate ligament (PCL) tear* The PCL is twice as strong as ACL and less frequently damaged. Menisci are rarely involved. Occurs in car crashes as the knee strikes the dashboard. Often missed in the acute injury. Do a posterior draw test (p688). Most are treated conservatively, PCL reconstruction is more difficult and less predictable than ACL reconstruction.[45]

Meniscal (semilunar cartilage) tears are the most common reasons for knee arthroscopy. See p689 for anatomy. Medial meniscus tears (eg 'bucket-handle') follow twists to a flexed knee (eg in football). Adduction + internal rotation causes lateral meniscus tears. Extension is limited (knee locking) as the displaced segment lodges between femoral and tibial condyles. The patient must stop what he is doing, and can only walk on tiptoe, if at all. The joint line is tender, and McMurray's test is +ve (p688). If the 'handle' of the 'bucket' becomes free at one end (= 'parrot beak' tear), the knee suddenly gives way, rather than locking. MRI gives tear location, morphology, length, depth, and stability, and helps predict tears requiring repair. Look for avulsions on x-ray. Management is conservative when possible, small asymptomatic tears tend to heal spontaneously, though arthroscopy is usually needed for locked knees, cysts, or persisting symptoms after injury. Surgery aims to preserve the meniscus. Peripheral tears in young, stable knees can be considered for meniscal repair, but repairs do not do well with a combined ACL tear and the knee remains unstable; the meniscus must then be reconstructed.[46]

Typical injury triad: ACL + medial collateral ligament + medial meniscus following valgus stress with rotation of the knee.[10]

Trauma

The ankle is composed of two joints: the subtalar joint (consists of calcaneus and talus to facilitate eversion/inversion) and the 'true' ankle joint (consists of tibia, fibula, and talus to facilitate dorsi- and plantar flexion).

Ankle ligament strain is usually (85% of sprains) an inversion injury which injures the anterior talofibular part of the lateral ligament (ATFL). 5% are eversion sprains (damaging medial deltoid ligament) and 10% are syndesmotic injuries.[48] *Signs:* Stiffness, tenderness over the lateral ligament, pain on inversion. ▶Follow the Ottawa ankle rules to decide if an x-ray is needed to rule out # (see fig 11.2 on p659). *Treatment:* Consists of 'POLICE' (Protection from further injury, Optimal Loading, Ice, Compression, Elevation) for simple sprains, ensure good analgesia to enable patient to gently exercise ankle as early as pain allows. In contrast, severe sprains (ligament is completely ruptured with inability to weightbear) require below knee immobilization for at least 10 days. Rehabilitation is advised to reduce recurrent injury. Advise patient to return if there is evidence of neurovascular compromise or pain hinders any weight on injured limb by 24 hours and not full weightbearing by 4 days.

Ankle fractures In general, stable fractures only involve one side of the ankle (Weber A/B fractures—see fig 12.28). Stable or minimally displaced fractures may be treated non-operatively in a cast. Unstable or displaced fractures require surgery.

Maisonneuve's fracture: Proximal fibular fracture + syndesmosis rupture, and medial malleolus fracture or deltoid ligament rupture. If 2 bones dislocate where no true joint exists, the term *diastasis* ('standing apart') is used. ▶Always examine the proximal fibula with 'ankle sprains'. ℞ is surgical as fractures are unstable and require fixation to restore the ankle mortise and placement of 1-2 suprasyndesmotic screws.

Lisfranc fracture-dislocation at the 1st tarsometatarsal joint: ▶A commonly missed fracture in multitrauma patients, but it can also occur by stepping awkwardly off a kerb. It may cause compartment syndrome of the medial foot (± later arthritis and persistent pain) so must be treated promptly. *Imaging:* On x-ray look for widening of the gap between the medial cuneiform and the base of the 2nd metatarsal. Because of the overlapping bones, subluxations can be hard to see. MRI helps. ℞: Achieve precise anatomic reduction with screw fixation across the 2nd tarsometatarsal joint (Lisfranc joint).[49]

Fractured neck of talus can occur after forced dorsiflexion, and is a serious injury because interruption of vessels may lead to avascular necrosis of the body of the talus. ℞: Displaced fractures require ORIF.

Calcaneus (os calcis) fractures: Often bilateral, after serious falls in manual workers. The outcome is frequently poor and many patients are left disabled and unable to return to their previous work. ▶Always look for associated spinal fracture. *Signs:* Swelling; bruising; inability to weight bear. ℞: ▶*Does the fracture enter the subtalar joint?* For years there has been debate and insufficient evidence to distinguish between conservative and operative approaches; a recent RCT[n=151] report that operative treatment compared to non-operative care (POLICE—p738, splints, and early mobilization) showed no advantage after 2 years in patients with typical displaced intra-articular fractures of the calcaneus. This risk of complications was also higher post surgery.[50]

2nd metatarsal fracture: ▶Look for Lisfranc dislocations. Usually heal well with non-operative cast and weightbearing as pain allows.

5th metatarsal fracture has two main types: proximal avulsion # typically associated with ankle inversion (treat conservatively) and Jones # (transverse fracture near base) which tends to require surgical intervention due to risk of non-union. See p695 for march fractures.

▶▶Consider venous thromboprophylaxis in all immobilized lower limbs.

Trauma

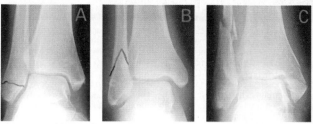

Fig 12.28 A simplification of the *AO Weber classification* of malleolar fractures.
A Below   B At the level of   C Above

Images courtesy of Professor Peter Scally.

The Danis–Weber classification defines ankle fractures by the level of fibula fracture relative to the tibiofibular syndesmosis. Involvement of the medial/lateral/posterior[11] malleoli are described as malleolar, bimalleolar, or trimalleolar. The Lauge–Hansen classification is more complicated (involves mechanism of injury, position of foot at time of injury in addition to x-ray findings).

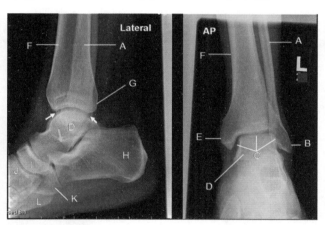

Fig 12.29 Identifying individual bones on x-ray (AP and lateral views of the ankle). Labelled are the fibula (A), lateral malleolus (B), mortise joint of ankle (C), talus (D), medial malleolus (E), tibia (F), posterior malleolus of talus (G), calcaneus (H), navicular (I), superimposed cuneiforms (J), cuboid (K), base of 5th metatarsal (L).

Reproduced with permission of Nicholas Joseph, CEO CE Essentials.

Further reading

Bleakley CM *et al.* (2012). PRICE needs updating, should we call the POLICE? *Br J Sports Med* 46:220–1.

Kaminski TW *et al.* (2013). National Athletic Trainers' Association position statement: conservative management and prevention of ankle sprains in athletes. *J Athl Train* 48:528–45.

11 The posterior malleoli refers to the posterior part of the distal tibia.

Assault is the commonest cause of facial trauma; young men are most affected.[51] Facial laceration and mandible fracture are the most frequent injuries. Always consider associated neck, eye, or head injury. Remove blood, loose/false teeth, and vomit from the mouth. Lie in the semi-prone position to prevent airway obstruction (fig 13.2, p762). See p660 for assessing neck injuries. Fibre-optic nasoendoscopy can be performed by the ENT team to look for pharyngeal/laryngeal trauma; try gentle intubation—if impossible, do cricothyrotomy (OHCM p786), then tracheostomy.▶ Airway compromise requires urgent expert help (anaesethtics & ENT).

Lacerations of the face Clean meticulously. Alignment of the tissues and antisepsis must be exact to produce a good cosmetic result.
- *Simple lacerations:* Consider glue or skin closure strip (eg Steri-Strip®) (p772).
- *Complex lacerations:* Ask for a plastic/ENT/maxillofacial surgeon.
- *Mammal bites:* See p772.
- *Ruptured ear drum:* NSAIDs for analgesia, and advise to keep ear dry.
- *Eye injury, nose fractures, and nose bleeds:* See p740-3.

Mandible injury *Signs:* Local tenderness and swelling; jaw malocclusion; a mobile fragment; bone may protrude into the mouth in open fractures; if comminuted, the tongue may make airway management extremely difficult, so get expert help. *Diagnosis:* Orthopantogram (OPG) x-rays. Enlist dental help. *Treating TMJ dislocations:* Place (gloved) thumbs over the back teeth and press downwards, while at the same time levering the chin upwards with your fingers (both hands). Consider midazolam sedation: see p617. Blows to the chin may cause fracture at the impact site, or indirect fractures near the temporomandibular joint. *Fractures:* Usually require ORIF with miniplates in theatre; conservative treatment involves wiring teeth together for 6 weeks. Complicated fractures may benefit from lag osteosynthesis. *Complications:* infection; non-union. *Avulsed teeth* may be replaced (p774). If inhaled, do expiratory CXR. *Bleeding socket:* ask patient to bite on adrenaline-soaked pads or suture.

A badge of honour? A common facial injury in wrestlers and rugby players is a direct blow to the pinna, the resultant shearing force causes separation of the auricular perichondrium from the underlying cartilage. The adherent network of perichondrial blood vessels tear and cause a haematoma to develop (see also p538). This vascular disruption leads to compromised cartilage viability giving rise to a 'cauliflower' ear deformity; players can be surprisingly proud of these (fig 12.30). If the patient presents within 7 days attempt to drain the haematoma, beyond this, formation of scar tissue complicates drainage. There is no perferred method of drainage, options include needle aspiration and incision & drainage. Review after 24 hours to check for recaccumulation and re-drain if needed. Apply a pressure bandage after drainage by stuffing saline-soaked gauze in the external auricular crevices and wrap bandages around the head. Specialist bandages also exist. Give broad-spectrum antibiotics to cover soft tissue infection.[53]

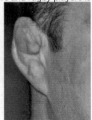

Fig 12.30 Cauliflower ear. See this excerpt from a UK newspaper which shows an interesting display of cauliflower ears.[52]

© Nils Jorgenson/REX Shutterstock

Further reading
Bell RB et al. (2004). Management of cerebrospinal fluid leak associated with craniomaxillofacial trauma. *J Oral Maxillofac Surg* 62:676–84.

Laski R et al. (2004). Facial trauma: a recurrent disease? The potential role of disease prevention. *J Oral Maxillofac Surg* 62:685–8.

Reuben AD et al. (2005). A comparative study of evaluation of radiographs, CT and 3D reformatted CT in facial trauma: what is the role of 3D? *Br Jr Rad* 78(927):198-201.

Trauma

The face forms a shock absorber which protects the brain from injury. The most common #s to the facial bones lie along 2 hoops, from ear to ear. One is formed by the zygomatic arch, body, infraorbital rim, and nose. The other is formed by the mandible (fig 12.31). Major blunt trauma can cause a # to the entire middle third of the face, which has been classified by Le Fort, but since the advent of seat belts these are less common.

Zygoma fractures *The arch:* Before swelling arrives, there is a depression in front of the ear, and lateral jaw excursions or jaw opening may be limited and painful. A suitable x-ray is the submentovertex view (smv). *The complex:* The zygoma's body has 4 extensions: **1** frontozygomatic **2** arch **3** maxillary buttress (in mouth) **4** infraorbital rim. Fractures may be palpated at these points, or disproportionately severe pain elicited on palpation. Occipitomental views are most suitable. *Orbital floor injuries:* Blunt trauma around the eye can cause # to the orbital floor. Imaging: ct is best, but om views may show trap door sign in the maxillary sinus (fig 12.32).

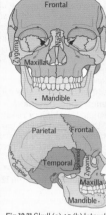

Fig 12.31 Skull (a) AP (b) lateral.

Clinical exam for periorbital trauma:
• Is there csf rhinorrhoea (yes in ≤25%)? See p560.[54]
• Check zygomatic arch by assessing range of mandibular lateral excursions and opening. Also palpate over the arch (just under the skin) and compare with the unaffected side.
• Patient sitting, doctor standing above and behind, place index fingers on the cheeks and look down from above for asymmetry.
• Check the orbit floor for: diplopia on upward gaze (≈trapped orbital contents); enophthalmos; numbness in the distribution of the infraorbital nerve (suggests fracture).
• Small risk of retrobulbar haemorrhage: catastrophic if missed: severe pain at back of eye; proptosis; loss of visual acuity. ►Prompt eye exam is essential.

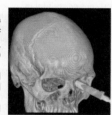

Fig 12.32 3D CT of a nasty injury to the eye. ►►On no account remove the knife.

Courtesy of Prof Peter Scally.

NB: if the eye is very swollen, application of a rubber glove filled with ice is invaluable, especially if you ask a specialist to travel to check patient; they can no more open a swollen eye than you. *Treatment:* Unless vision↓, or there is significant risk of infection, admission on presentation is not mandatory: seeing at the next fracture clinic is adequate. If in doubt, consult the relevant specialist. Explain about not blowing the nose in fractures in continuity with the maxillary sinus (risks periorbital emphysema and infection).

►**Medicolegal issues** Facial injuries commonly result from assault. Your notes may be used in criminal injuries claims or as evidence in court. Often the individual is drunk and abusive, it is late, and you are busy, but you must make accurate notes with diagrams. Other people will definitely take time to study and criticize what you have written. Don't forget photographs if assault is particularly serious or children are involved. Document that the patient has given, or refused, permission for statements to be made to the police or legal professionals (the medical notes are confidential).

▶Prevention is the key, eg wearing goggles, or plastic glasses when near small, moving objects or using tools (avoids splinters, fish-hooks, and squash-ball injuries). *Always record acuity* (both eyes; if the uninjured one is blind take all injuries *very* seriously). Take a detailed history of the event.

If unable to open the injured eye, instil a few drops of local anaesthetic (**tetracaine 1%**): after a few mins, comfortable opening may be possible. Examine lids, conjunctiva, cornea, sclera, anterior chamber, pupil, iris, lens, vitreous, fundus, and eye movement. An irregular pupil may mean globe rupture. Afferent pupil defects (p424) do not herald well for sight recovery. Note pain, discharge, or squint. CT may be very useful (foreign bodies may be magnetic, so avoid MRI).

Penetrating trauma Refer urgently: delays risk of ocular extrusion or infection. Uveal injury risks of sympathetic ophthalmia in the other eye. ▶A history of flying objects (eg work with hammers and chisels) prompts careful examination + x-ray to exclude intraocular foreign bodies (±skull x-ray or CT to exclude intracranial involvement). ▶*Don't* try to remove a large foreign body (knife; dart). Support the object with padding. Transport supine. Pad the *unaffected* eye to prevent damage from conjugate movement.

Foreign bodies (FBs) (fig 12.33) *Have a low threshold for getting help*; FBs often hide, so examine *all* the eye and evert the lid. FBs cause chemosis, subconjunctival bleeds, irregular pupils, iris prolapse, hyphaema, vitreous haemorrhage, and retinal tears. If you suspect a metal FB, x-ray the orbit. With high-velocity FBs, consider orbital US: pick-up rate is 90% vs 40% for x-rays; skill is needed (not always to hand in a busy ED!). Removal of superficial FBs may be possible with a triangle of clean card (**chloramphenicol 0.5%** drops after, to prevent infection).

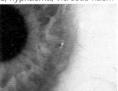

Fig 12.33 Corneal FB (centre).
© Bristol Eye Hospital.

Corneal abrasions (fig 12.34; often from small fast-moving objects, eg children's finger-nails; twigs.) They may cause intense pain. Apply a drop of local anaesthetic, eg 1% **tetracaine** before examination. They stain with **fluorescein** and should show sign of healing within 48h. Send the patient home with analgesics. Re-examine after 24h. If still having a foreign body sensation after removing the pad, stain again with fluorescein. If the cornea stains, repeat the procedure for another 24h. If it still stains after 48h, refer. NB: A Cochrane review of small corneal abrasions do not favour using pads.[55] See also p434.

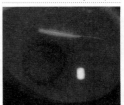

Fig 12.34 Corneal abrasion just above the pupil.
© Bristol Eye Hospital.

Burns Treat chemical burns promptly: instil anaesthetic drops (**tetracaine 1%**) every 2min till the patient is comfortable. Bathe the eyes in copious clean water while the specific antidote is sought. Often the lids close tight from severe pain. Late serious sequelae: eg corneal scarring, opacification, and lid damage. Alkali burns are more serious than acid. Refer promptly.

Photokeratitis 'Arc eye' Welders and sunbed users who don't use UV protection may damage the cornea (FB sensation, watering, blepharospasm). Intense pain (has been compared to child birth!) starts 6–12hrs after UV exposure. R: Generous oral analgesics, analgesic eye drops for home use are not advised due to ocular toxicity. Give antibiotic ointment and it will recover in 24h.[56]

Finally, remember **fat embolus** in trauma patients with visual problems.

Trauma

Contusions and intraocular haemorrhage

Our eyes are protected by bony orbital ridges; significant force is needed to fracture these so look for associated peripheral and head injuries. Severe contusions from large objects may damage the eye, but smaller objects such as squash balls and airgun pellets cause local contusion, eg resulting in lid bruises and subconjunctival haemorrhage which usually settles in 2 weeks.

Intraocular bleeds ►*Get expert help:* acuity may be affected. Blood is often found in the anterior chamber (hyphaema, fig **5.3**, p413): small amounts clear spontaneously but if filling the anterior chamber, evacuation may be needed. It is often recognizable by pen-torch examination. Even small hyphaemas must be carefully evaluated (so refer): it may signify serious injury. *Late complications:* Glaucoma; corneal staining; re-bleeding.

Secondary haemorrhage This may occur within 5 days and may produce sight-threatening secondary glaucoma. Sometimes the iris is paralysed and dilated due to injury (called traumatic mydriasis). This usually recovers in a few days but sometimes it is permanent. Vitreous haemorrhage will cause a dramatic fall in acuity. There will be no red reflex on ophthalmoscopy. Lens dislocation, tearing of the iris root, splitting of the choroid, detachment of the retina, and damage to the optic nerve may be other sequelae; they are more common if contusion is caused by smaller objects rather than large.

Blows to the orbit Blunt injury (eg from a football) can cause sudden ↑ in pressure within the orbit, and may cause blowout fractures with the orbital contents herniating into the maxillary sinus. Tethering of the inferior rectus and inferior oblique muscles causes diplopia. Test the sensation over the lower lid skin. Loss of sensation indicates infra-orbital nerve injury, confirming a blowout fracture. CT may show the depressed fracture of the posterior orbital floor. Fracture reduction and muscle release is necessary.[57]

Types of major injury, and prognosis

The ocular trauma score (OTS) gives prognostic information (the higher the better prognosis): to get the score, assign a point value for initial visual acuity from row 1 of the table. Then subtract the appropriate points for each diagnosis from subsequent rows. A patient with an initial visual acuity of <6/60, scleral rupture, and retinal detachment has a score of 80-23-11= 46.

Visual acuity (p414)	No light perception	60
	Light perception/hand movement only	70
	<6/60	80
	6/50-6/15	90
	>6/12	100
Globe rupture		-23
Endophthalmitis		-17
Perforating injury		-14
Retinal detachment		-11
Afferent pupillary defect (Marcus Gunn pupil)		-10

In one series, the chief injuries were corneal wounds (68%), lens injury (50%), retinal lesions (50%), vitreous haemorrhage (25%), and endophthalmitis (14%). Multiple foreign bodies causing perforating injury with retained posterior segment foreign body occurred in 7%. Outcome was worse if acuity was affected, presence of a large foreign body, or there was bacterial endophthalmitis or proliferative vitreo-retinopathy.[58]

Further reading

Magarakis M et al. (2012). Ocular injury, visual impairment, and blindness associated with facial fractures: a systematic literature review. *Plast Reconstr Surg* 129:227-33.

Roth FS et al. (2010). Pearls of orbital trauma management. *Semin Plast Surg* 24:398-410.

Wipperman JL et al. (2013). Evaluation and management of corneal abrasions. *Am Fam Physician* 87:114-20.

Trauma

Upper limb		
Nerve root	**Muscle**	**Test by asking the patient to:**
C3,4	Trapezius	Shrug shoulder (via accessory nerve).
C4,5	Rhomboids	Brace shoulder back.
C5,6,7	Serratus anterior	Push arm forward against resistance.
C5,6	Pectoralis major (clavicular head)	Adduct arm from above horizontal, and push it forward.
C6,7,8	Pectoralis major (sternocostal head)	Adduct arm below horizontal.
C5,6	Supraspinatus	Abduct arm the first 15°.
C5,6	Infraspinatus	Externally rotate arm, elbow at side.
C6,7,8	Latissimus dorsi	Adduct arm from horizontal position.
C5,6	Biceps	Flex supinated forearm.
C5,6	Deltoid	Abduct arm between 15° and 90°.
Radial nerve (C5–8)		
C6,7,8	Triceps	Extend elbow against resistance.
C5,6	Brachioradialis	Flex elbow with forearm half way between pronation and supination.
C5,6	Extensor carpi radialis longus	Extend wrist radially with fingers extended.
C6,7	Supinator	Arm by side, resist hand pronation.
C7,8	Extensor digitorum	Keep fingers extended at MCP joint.
C7,8	Extensor carpi ulnaris	Extend wrist to ulnar side.
C7,8	Abductor pollicis longus	Abduct thumb at 90° to palm.
C7,8	Extensor pollicis brevis	Extend thumb at MCP joint.
C7,8	Extensor pollicis longus	Resist thumb flexion at IP joint.
Median nerve (C6–T1)		
C6,7	Pronator teres	Keep arm pronated against resistance.
C6,7	Flexor carpi radialis	Flex wrist towards radial side.
C7,8,T1	Flexor digitorum superficialis	Resist extension at PIP joint (while you fix his proximal phalanx).
C8,T1	Flexor digitorum profundus I & II	Flex the DIP of the index finger, with the PIP held in extension.
C8,T1	Flexor pollicis longus	Resist thumb extension at interphalangeal joint (fix proximal phalanx).
C8,T1	Abductor pollicis brevis	Abduct thumb (nail at 90° to palm).
C8,T1	Opponens pollicis	Thumb touches base of 5th finger-tip (nail parallel to palm).
C8,T1	1st and 2nd lumbricals	Extend PIP joint against resistance with MCP joint held in flexion.
Ulnar nerve (C7–T1)		
C7,8,T1	Flexor carpi ulnaris	Flex wrist towards ulnar side.
C7,C8	Flexor digitorum profundus III & IV	Flex the DIP of the little finger, with the PIP held in extension.
C8,T1	Dorsal interossei	Abduct fingers (use index finger).
C8,T1	Palmar interossei	Adduct fingers (use index finger).
C8,T1	Adductor pollicis	Adduct thumb (nail at 90° to palm).
C8,T1	Abductor digiti minimi	Abduct little finger.
C8,T1	Flexor digiti minimi	Flex the little finger at MCP joint.
The musculocutaneous nerve (C5–6)		
C5,6	This may be injured at the brachial plexus, causing weakness of biceps, coracobrachialis, and brachialis. Forearm flexion is weak, ± some loss of sensation.	

Sources: MRC Handbook; www.rad.washington.edu/atlas; www.medmedia.com/05/324.htm

See p746–7 for dermatomes and peripheral nerve distributions.

NB: root numbers in **bold** indicate that root is more important than its neighbour. ►Sources vary in ascribing particular nerve roots to muscles—and there is some biological variation in individuals. The above is a reasonable compromise, and is based on the MRC guidelines.

Lower limb		
Nerve root	**Muscle**	**Test by asking the patient to:**
L**4,5**, S1	Gluteus medius & minimus	Internal rotation at hip, hip abduction.
L5, S1,2	Gluteus maximus	Extension at hip (lie prone).
L**2,3,4**	Adductors (obturator nerve)	Adduct leg against resistance.
Femoral nerve (L2–4, posterior division)		
L1,2,3	Iliopsoas	Flex hip with knee flexed and lower leg supported: patient lies on back.
L2,3	Sartorius	Flex knee with hip external rotated.
L2,3,4	Quadriceps femoris	Extend knee against resistance.
Obturator nerve (L2–4, anterior division)		
L2,3,4	Hip adductors	Adduct the leg.
Inferior gluteal nerve		
L5,S1,S2	Gluteus maximus	Hip extension.
Superior gluteal nerve		
L4,5,S1	Gluteus medius & minimus	Abduction and internal rotation of hip.
Sciatic nerve (including the common peroneal nerve^{cp} & tibial nerve)		
L4,5^{cp}	Tibialis anterior	Dorsiflex ankle.
L5,S1^{cp}	Extensor digitorum longus	Dorsiflex toes against resistance.
L5,S1^{cp}	Extensor hallucis longus	Dorsiflex hallux against resistance.
L5,S1^{cp}	Peroneus longus & brevis	Evert foot against resistance.
L5,S1^{cp}	Extensor digitorum brevis	Dorsiflex 2nd–4th toes (muscle of foot).
L5,S1,2^{T}	Hamstrings	Flex knee against resistance.
L4,5^{T}	Tibialis posterior	Invert plantarflexed foot.
S1,2^{T}	Gastrocnemius	Plantarflex ankle joint.
L5,S1,2^{T}	Flexor digitorum longus	Flex terminal joints of toes.
S1,2^{T}	Small muscles of foot	Make sole of foot into a cup.

Trauma

Quick screening test for muscle power					
Shoulder	Abduction	c5	Hip	Flexion	L1,2
	Adduction	c5, 7		Extension	L5,S1
Elbow	Flexion	c5, 6	Knee	Flexion	s1
	Extension	c7		Extension	L3,4
Wrist	Flexion	c7,8	Ankle	Dorsiflexion	L4
	Extension	c7		Plantarflexion	s1,2
Fingers	Flexion	c7–8			
	Extension	c7			
	Abduction	T1 (ulnar)			

See TABLE on p659 for MRC grading of muscle power.

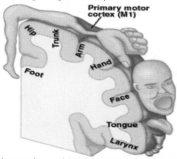

Fig 12.35 The motor homonculus—a pictorial representation of the anatomical divisions of the primary motor cortex. © BrainHQ from Posit Science.

Trauma

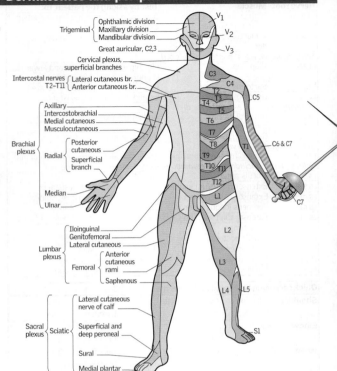

Fig 12.36 (a) These images reflect the 2011 evidence-based dermatomes, which have revealed much more individual variation than originally thought, so much so that some areas have been left blank (white) because no single best option can be given.

(b) Feet and hands.

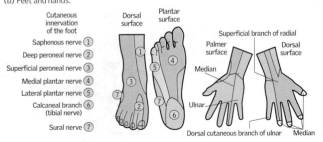

Cutaneous
innervation
of the foot

Saphenous nerve ①
Deep peroneal nerve ②
Superficial peroneal nerve ③
Medial plantar nerve ④
Lateral plantar nerve ⑤
Calcaneal branch ⑥
(tibial nerve)
Sural nerve ⑦

See p744-5 for testing peripheral motor nerves.

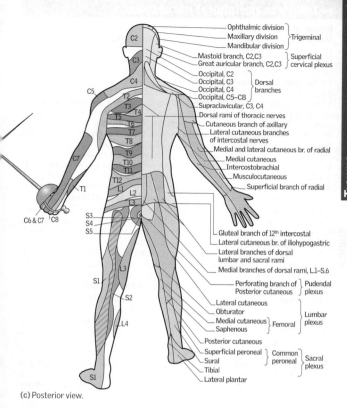

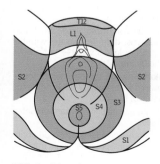

(c) Posterior view.

(d) Perineal dermatomes.

Aim to keep a few key dermato-mes up your sleeve	
C3–4	Clavicles
C6–7	Lateral arm/forearm
T1	Medial side of arm
C6	Thumb
C7	Middle finger
C8	Little finger
T4	Nipples
T10	Umbilicus
L2–L3	Anterior & inner leg
L5	Medial side of big toe
L5, S1–2	Posterior & outer leg
S1	Lateral margin of foot and little toe
S2–4	Perineum
The above is a rough approximation	

Trauma

Repair of nerve injuries (p744 & p746) Examine sensory and motor function. Repair of any peripheral nerve injury is challenging and requires a senior hand or plastics surgeon to be involved. *Neurapraxia* implies temporary loss of nerve conduction often via ischaemia following pressure (eg to the lateral popliteal nerve as it crosses the neck of the fibula, see below). In mixed nerves, the motor modality is the more vulnerable component. eg Saturday night palsy (compression of radial nerve at the spiral groove after falling asleep with the arm overhanging the chair). *Axonotmesis* entails damage to the nerve fibre but the epineural tube is intact, providing guidance to the regrowing nerve. Good recovery is the rule. Growth rate is 1-3mm/day. *Neurotmesis* means division of the whole nerve. As there is no guidance from the endoneural tube, regrowing fibrils cause a traumatic neuroma if they are unable to bridge the gap. The current surgical standard is epineural repair with nylon sutures. To span gaps that primary repair cannot bridge without excess tension, nerve-cable interfascicular autografts are used. Results of nerve repair are fair (at best), with ~50% regaining useful function. There is much current research regarding the pathophysiology of nerve regeneration and how to optimize repair.[60]

Median nerve (c5-T1) The nerve of *grasp*. Injury above the antecubital fossa causes: •Inability to flex index finger interphalangeal joints on clasping the hands (Ochner's test) •Inability to flex the terminal phalanx of the thumb (flexor pollicis longus) •Loss of sensation over the thenar half of the palm.

If the lesion is at the wrist, the only muscle reliably affected is abductor pollicis brevis. Test it by holding the hand palm up. Can the patient raise the thumb out of the plane of the hand? The area of sensory loss is smaller than that for more proximal lesions. See box, 'Median nerve anatomy'.

Ulnar nerve (c8-T1) This is the nerve of finger abduction and adduction (among other roles). One subtle sign of an ulnar nerve lesion is inability to cross the fingers in the 'good luck' sign. Injury level determines severity of the claw deformity. In a distal lesion of the ulnar nerve, there will be more clawing of the 4th and 5th fingers compared with a proximal, more complete lesion at the elbow. This is the *ulnar paradox* as you would expect a lesion higher up to produce more clawing and deformity, but a proximal lesion disrupts the ulnar part of flexor digitorum profundus leading to unopposed extension and therefoe less clawing; the closer the paw the worse the claw. *Froment's paper sign:* On holding a piece of paper between thumb & finger (both hands), there is flexion of the thumb's distal phalanx on trying to pull apart (flexor pollicis longus, is recruited to overcome adductor pollicis weakness). Sensory loss is over the little finger & a variable area of the ring finger.

Radial nerve (c5-T1) This is the nerve of extension of the elbow, wrist, and fingers. It opens the fist. Injury will produce wrist-drop. Test for this with the elbow flexed and the forearm pronated. Sensory loss is variable, but always includes the dorsal aspect of the root of the thumb.

Lateral popliteal (common peroneal) nerve (L4-s2) The commonest lower limb nerve injury. Lesions lead to equinovarus with inability to dorsiflex the foot and toes. Sensory loss is over the dorsum of the foot.

Tibial nerve (s1-3) Loss causes calcaneovalgus and inability to stand on tiptoe or invert the foot. Sensory loss is over the sole.

Common peroneal compression Nerve compression against the head of fibula (eg plaster casts, thin patients lying unconscious, proximal fibula fracture, squatting, obstructed labour) causes inability to dorsiflex the foot. Sensation may be ↓ over the dorsum of the foot. *Treatment:* Most recover spontaneously but surgical decompression may be needed (eg if >3 months without improvement). Physiotherapy and splint until foot-drop recovers.

Trauma

Carpal tunnel syndrome (CTS)[12] ► This is the commonest cause of hand pain at night. It is due to compression of the median nerve as it passes under the flexor retinaculum. ♀:♂>1:1. *Signs* are in the median nerve distribution:

• Tingling or pain is felt in the thumb, index, and middle fingers.
• When the pain is at its worse, the patient characteristically flicks or shakes the wrist to bring about relief. Pain is especially common at night and after repetitive actions. Affected persons may experience clumsiness.
• Wasted thenar eminence & ↓sensation over the lateral 3½ digits (*not* 5th).
• Lateral palmar sensation is spared as its supply (the palmar cutaneous branch of the median nerve) does not pass through the tunnel.
• *Phalen's test:* holding the wrist hyperflexed for 1min reproduces the symptoms. (This is more reliable than *Tinel's test*—tapping over the tunnel to produce paraesthesiae. Note: Phalen's flexing, Tinel's tapping.)

Investigations and management see p707 and fig **12.46**, p761.

Median nerve anatomy

The median nerve arises from C5, C6, C7, C8, & T1 as a condensation of lateral & medial cords of brachial plexus (fig **12.37**, p751). It crosses medial to the brachial artery in antecubital fossa. It has no branches above the elbow. ~5cm distal to elbow it gives off its anterior interosseous branch (motor to flexor policis longus (FPL), flexor digitorum profundus (FDP), index finger & pronator quadratus). The palmar cutaneous branch (sensory to thenar skin) arises ~5cm proximal to wrist and overlies the flexor retinaculum. The recurrent motor branch to the thenar muscles arises at the distal end of carpal tunnel. The median nerve is motor to PT (pronator teres), FCR (flexor carpi radialis), PL (palmaris longus), FDS (flexor digitorum superficialis), LOAF (see p657). Sensation: radial 3-and-a-half digits. See fig **11.20**, p671 for a cross-sectional diagram of the carpal tunnel.

Anterior interosseous nerve compression This median nerve branch may be compressed under the fibrous origin of flexor digitorum profundus, causing weakness of pinch and pain along the forearm's radial border. The patient will be unable to flex the DIP joint of the index finger and PIP joint of the thumb to make a rounded 'o' shape *Treatment:* Initial conservative managment with surgical decompression if required.

Posterior interosseous nerve (PIN) compression This branch of the radial nerve is compressed on passing through the proximal supinator muscle, eg after forearm fracture or excessive exercise. Patients experience weakness of thumb and finger extension. Electromyographic studies are typically positive. **Radial tunnel syndrome** involves compression of the same nerve, but presents with lateral forearm pain rather than weakness. Electrodiagnostic studies tend to be negative. *Examination* may show weakness of long finger extensors, and short and long thumb extensors, but no sensory loss. *Treatment:* Rest, splints, NSAIDs are first line. Steroid injections may help. In resistant cases surgical decompression of areas of potential compression of the PIN.

Ulnar nerve compression at the wrist Uncommon. See *OHCM*, p507.

Meralgia paraesthetica (lateral femoral cutaneous nerve) is a symptom complex of numbness, paraesthesiae, and pain (eg burning/shooting) in the anterolateral thigh. Most cases are idiopathic. *ΔΔ*: Lumbar disc hernia. *℞:* (often self-limiting but may recur). Lose weight if needed, rest, NSAID ± carbamazepine ± cortisone and local anaesthetic injection at the anterior superior iliac spine gives unpredictable results.[61]

Further reading

Heaton S *et al.* (2012). Entrapment syndromes. In Simpson DM *et al.* (eds) *Neuropathic Pain: Mechanisms, Diagnosis and Treatment*, pp281–305. New York: OUP.

Sawardeker P *et al.* (2015). Nerve compression: ulnar nerve of the elbow. In Trail IA *et al.* (eds) *Disorders of the Hand*, pp243–65. New York: Springer.

The brachial plexus extends from the intervertebral foramina to the axilla spanning a distance of ~15cm. Useful landmarks on its route from cord to arm worth remembering are:

- The roots leave the vertebral column between the scalenus medius and anterior muscles (see fig 12.38).
- The creation of divisions from trunks takes place under the clavicle, *medial* to the coracoid process.
- The plexus has an intimate relationship with the subclavian and then axillary arteries, with the median nerve forming from the medial and lateral cords anterior to the latter. Look for the characteristic 'M' formation: see fig 12.39.

Traumatic causes *Direct:* eg shoulder girdle fracture, penetrating or iatrogenic. *Indirect:* eg avulsion/traction injuries, due to excessive lateral flexion of the neck—as may occur in motorcycle injuries, or to the newborn during delivery.

Atraumatic causes Tumours (eg Pancoast, from lung), radiation, neuropathy.

Root injuries There are 4 types: high, middle, low, and complete. The position of the arm at time of injury determines the nerves involved.

- *High lesions: Erb's palsy* (c5, c6) Damage affects the suprascapular, musculocutaneous and axillary nerves. This leads to paralysis of supraspinatus (abduction), infraspinatus (external rotation), biceps (supination), brachialis (flexion of elbow), deltoid (abduction) and teres minor (external rotation). As a result the arm is held internally rotated, pronated, extended and adducted in the *'waiter's tip'* position. Sensation is impaired over deltoid, lateral forearm, and hand. Difficult deliveries (or any trauma in a downwards direction) can produce this sign in neonates.
- *Low lesions: Klumpke's paralysis* (c8, t1) Occurs when the arm is pulled superiorly (forced abduction)—eg trying to break a fall from height by grabbing onto something. Damage to the c8, t1 roots leads to a combination of median and ulnar nerve injury which may produce 'claw hand' (extension at MCP joints, with flexion at DIP/PIP joints) due to loss of lumbrical function. The arm is held in adduction. Horner's syndrome (p424) may also occur.

Injury to the cords

- *Injury to the lateral cord of the plexus*: Absent power in the biceps and brachioradialis (flexes the forearm at the elbow).
- *Posterior cord injury:* Teres major & deltoid inaction; radial nerve palsy.
- *Medial cord injury:* Affects the ulnar and median nerves. Sensation is absent over the medial arm and hand. See fig 12.37.

Recovery is difficult to determine as each lesion and patient must be assessed individually. Intensive rehabilitation with physiotherapy and occupational therapy is needed to encourage spontaneous healing if nerves are not completely disrupted. Minimize contracture development by using braces. With incomplete trunk lesions recovery may take >5 months. Prognosis is poor in lesions proximal to the dorsal root ganglion (DRG). Surgical intervention is complex. Early liaison with a regional centre is advised as early exploration improves the outcome of nerve repair. Surgical options include nerve grafting of viable roots, nerve transfer (from intercostal or phrenic nerves) free functioning muscle transfers and tendon transfers.[62]

Further reading

British Orthopaedic Association (2012). BOAST 5: *Peripheral Nerve Injury*. https://www.boa.ac.uk/wp-content/uploads/2014/12/BOAST-5.pdf

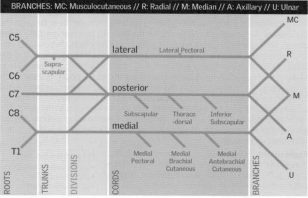

BRANCHES: MC: Musculocutaneous // R: Radial // M: Median // A: Axillary // U: Ulnar

Fig 12.37 The brachial plexus, the *bête noire* of medical students. This diagram should be just memorizable the night before an exam.   Image courtesy of Luke Famery.

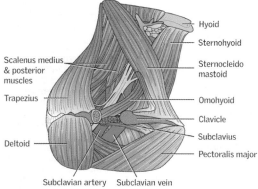

Fig 12.38 The proximal brachial plexus. The purpose of this figure and fig 12.39, is to show where the brachial plexus is, and not what the brachial plexus is.

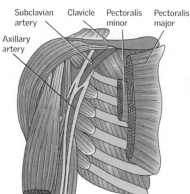

Fig 12.39 The distal brachial plexus: note the relationship with the axillary artery.

The spinal cord is a precious bundle of nerves which travels down through the 33 bones of the spinal column to enable the body to function normally. Even though <5% of spinal injuries result in spinal cord injury (SCI), the resulting motor, sensory, and autonomic dysfunction are too devastating to ignore. It is the lack of motor function that one immediately thinks of when considering life in a wheelchair. However, most patients with significant SCI prioritize their wishes for restoration of functions in this order: bowel and bladder control; sexual function; hand function; breathing. **Causes** Most commonly due to trauma; especially RTAs but as the population ages, falls are becoming more frequent. For this reason, pay particular attention to the need for examining and imaging the neck in head injuries (p790). Other causes include tumours, prolapsed discs, and inflammatory disease.

Assessment Follow the ATLS® principles (p781). Plan movements carefully and use the log-roll technique (p782) and c-spine immobilzation. Prevent and treat hypotension (aim for SBP >90). Look for, and exclude other injuries before assigning cause of hypotension to neurogenic shock. Restore intravascular volume (don't overload) then consider use of vasopressors (see below for fluid balance). Monitor and treat symptomatic bradycardia. Monitor and regulate temperature. ▶Perform serial neurological examinations to assess for deterioration; test for root lesions (see MINIBOX); test the reflexes: (biceps

For root lesions, test:
• C5: shoulder abduction
• C6: elbow flexion
• C7: elbow extension
• C8: finger flexion (grip)
• T1: finger abduction
• L2: hip flexion
• L3: knee extension
• L4 : ankle dorsiflexion
• L5: great toe extension
• S1: ankle plantarflexion

C5; brachioradialis C6; triceps C7). Motor nerve roots and dermatomes are given on p744-7. The main sites of injury are C6 & 7, followed by C2. ~10% of c-spine fractures will have another spinal fracture elsewhere, so always examine the whole spine. ▶▶NB: Remember that a spinal cord injury causing anaesthesia may be masking serious injury below the lesion (eg compartment syndrome, acute abdomen). **Imaging** See p660. Good knowledge of anatomical and developmental variation is also required when assessing x-rays—eg pseudosubluxation of C2 on C3 mimicking injury.

Consequences of injury Injury to the cervical spine causes tetraplegia, but injury above the segmental level of the phrenic nerve (C3, 4, 5 keeps the diaphragm alive) results in paralysis of the diaphragm. Intubate and ventilate patients with high tetraplegia early on. Thoracic spine damage causes paraplegia and lumbar spine lesions give rise to symptoms of cauda equina compromise. Lesions above T6 can be associated with autonomic dysreflexia (see p758). Incomplete spinal cord injuries display specific patterns (see p754). *Respiratory insufficiency:* arises both from neurological dysfunction and associated trauma to chest wall or head. Check vital capacity repeatedly. If <500–600mL, intubation and ventilation will be needed. Monitor arterial blood gases. Intubation may produce vagal bradycardia, so consider **atropine** 0.3–0.6mg IV before intubation and suction. If abdominal distinsion is causing respiratory compromise, pass an NGT as there is high risk of aspiration. *Fluid balance:* There is likely to be hypotension below the lesion (sympathetic interruption and resultant *neurogenic shock*—↓BP and pulse rate). This is not due to hypovolaemia, and it is dangerous to give large volumes of fluid. Use IV not oral fluids for 48h and while ileus persists. *The skin:* Turn every 2h between supine and right/left lateral positions. The Stoke Mandeville bed does this electronically. Use pillows to separate the legs and maintain a lumbar lordosis. *The bladder:* Pass a urinary catheter before the bladder volume exceeds 500mL (overstretching of detrusor can delay the return of automatic bladder function).

Treatment starts on-scene with controlled movement of the patient and optimizing conditions in head injury (p790) in order to minimize secondary insults.

▶Arrange early transfer to a spinal injuries unit. *Steroids:* ◆✲ IV Methylprednisolone use is still controversial and may only marginally improve motor strength if given within 8 hours.[63] Seek specialist advice. *Early surgical decompression and stabilization:*◆✲ Should be attempted when feasible but there may be no difference in neurologic or functional improvement with early vs late surgery.[64] *Traction:* Skeletal traction will be needed for cervical injuries. Spring-loaded Gardner–Wells skull tongs are preferable to Crutchfield calipers, which need incisions. *Anticoagulation:* Acute cord injury patients are at very high risk of developing VTE, with asymptomatic DVT demonstrable in 60-100% of patients. LMWH (eg enoxaparin 40mg/24h sc) is currently recommended over unfractionated heparin regimens for prevention of VTE.[65] Start warfarin later and continue for at least 3 months or until completion of inpatient rehabilitation.[66]

Immobilization of the cervical spine collar

Which patients should be immobilized? In trauma with a significant mechanism of injury (eg high-speed RTA), head injury with neck pain or patients found collapsed with suspected trauma then a c-spine injury should be assumed until otherwise proven. Patients who are GCS 15, sober with no neurology and no neck pain or midline tenderness do not need collars. **When can I remove the collar?** If your patient is painfree, GCS 15, cooperative, with no neurological signs then remove the collar for examination: Note the posture of the neck and any bone tenderness (midline and over the spinous processes). If safe to remove collar, check the range of movements: flexion & extension (mainly atlanto-occipital joint); rotation (mainly atlanto-axial joint); lateral flexion (whole of cervical spine). Rotation is the movement most commonly affected. **When are x-rays indicated?** (see p716 for imaging) Follow the Canadian c-spine rules. Use the NICE 2014 head injury guidance to see if imaging of the neck is needed in head injury (p790). If x-rays are normal but patient still complains of midline tenderness, then consider CT imaging. **Is full immobilization truly possible?** ◆✲ There is no evidence that applying cervical collars reduces c-spine injury, in fact some evidence suggests collars actually cause more harm.[67] The incidence of significant cervical spine injuries in high-risk trauma patients is 0.7%, but application of a collar can inhibit airway management (think of vomiting and the risk of aspiration) and also place the jugular veins under pressure and subsequently increase the ICP (esp. problematic in head injuries see p790). Have someone apply a collar to you—it's very uncomfortable and doesn't stabilize the neck as much as you would want. A cadaver study demonstrated that application of collars in cadavers with inflicted cervical injuries increased the fracture separation by 7mm![68] **A revolution in trauma care?** ◆✲ A prehospital care unit in Norway have removed the collar from routine practice and only utilize it temporarily during extrication (see p808). Many other countries are adopting this proposal that optimal immobilization avoids collars and just uses spinal board, head blocks with straps, and ideally a spinal vaccuum mattress. Transporting patients in the lateral trauma position has also been proposed.[69] **So what should I do now?** For now, you must follow the local protocol of practice and work within the accepted practice of your employer. New hypotheses are always popping up and guidelines are only ever established once safe, evidence-based practice is identifed. Hopefully we have challenged you to reflect on current practice in any speciality and not just take what has 'always been done' as gospel. See also p782.

Further reading

Sansam KAJ (2006). Controversies in the management of traumatic spinal cord injury. *Clin Med* 6:202-4.

Sundstrøm T *et al.* (2014). Prehospital use of cervical collars in trauma patients: a critical review. *J Neurotrauma* 31(6):531-40.

The spinal cord originates from the brainstem at the base of the skull and terminates at L1 where the cauda equina starts (see p681). Most SCI do not completely sever the cord, instead the ability of the cord to function is compromised to varying degrees. The ASIA scale can be used to describe the completeness of the injury. Someone without an initial SCI does not receive an ASIA grade. Determining the neurological level of injury (NLI) refers to the most caudal segment of the cord with intact sensation and >3 muscle function strength.

A	Complete; no sensory or motor function is preserved in the sacral segments S4–S5
B	Sensory incomplete. Sensory but not motor function is preserved below the NLI (includes S4–S5)
C	Motor incomplete. Motor function is preserved at the most caudal sacral segments for voluntary anal contraction (VAC) and less than half of key muscle functions below the single NLI have a muscle grade ≥ 3
D	Motor incomplete but at least half (half or more) of key muscle functions below the single NLI having a muscle grade > 3
E	Normal motor and sensory function

International Standards of Neurological Standards of Spinal Cord Injury, updated 2015. www.asia-spinalinjury.org [ASIA=American Spinal Injury Association]

Sacral sparing is confirmed by flexion of the great toe and a PR to assess perianal sensation and anal tone. Preservation of sacral funtion (S4–5) is a prognostic indictor confirming the integrity of the cord and can be the only neurological finding to help differentiate between incompete and complete SCI.

Does this patient have a spinal cord injury?

At the accident In any unexplained trauma, suspect cord injury if:
- Responds to pain only above clavicle.
- Dermatomal pattern of sensory loss.
- Breathing—diaphragmatic without use of accessory respiratory muscles.
- Muscles—hypotonic, including reduced anal tone (do a PR).
- Reflexes—hyporeflexic.
- Absence of movement in both legs.
- Slow pulse and ↓BP, but in the presence of normovolaemia.
- Priapism[12] or urinary retention.
- Unexplained ileus.
- Clonus in an unconscious trauma patient without decerebrate rigidity.

Use this 2-page work sheet from the 'International Standards for Neurological Classification of Spinal Cord Injury' to formally assess spinal cord injuries:

http://www.asia-spinalinjury. org/elearning/isncsci_ worksheet_2015_web.pdf

Fig 12.40 Cross-section of the spinal cord. The only neurons to decussate at (or near) their spinal cord level are those in the spinothalamic tract. Pyramidal tract fibres decussate in the medulla and the dorsal column fibres decussate after the gracile and cuneate nuclei of the medulla.

Adapted from Donaghy, M. *Oxford Core Texts: Neurology* (2008) with permission from Oxford University Press.

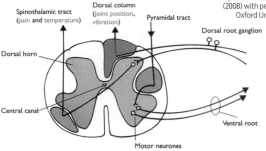

Spinothalamic tract (pain and temperature)

Dorsal column (joint position, vibration)

Pyramidal tract

Dorsal root ganglion

Dorsal horn

Central canal

Ventral root

Motor neurones

Trauma

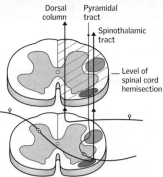

Fig 12.41 *Brown–Séquard* syndrome (*OHCM*, p710). In this rare injury pattern, there is hemisection of the spinal cord (more often seen after penetrating rather than blunt trauma), causing ipsilateral loss of dorsal column sensation and motor function below the lesion and contralateral loss of spinothalamic sensation from a few levels below the lesion.

NB: spinothalmic tract fibres ascend for a few levels on the same side as cord entry before they decussate.

Adapted from Donaghy, M. *Oxford Core Texts: Neurology* with permission from Oxford University Press.

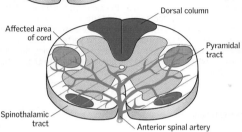

Fig 12.42 Anterior cord syndrome. There is infarction of the spinal cord in the distribution of the anterior spinal artery, causing complete loss of motor function and pain and temperature sensation below the lesion. Vibration and joint position sense are retained. This injury pattern has the worst prognosis of the incomplete injuries.

Adapted from Donaghy, M. *Oxford Core Texts: Neurology* with permission from Oxford University Press.

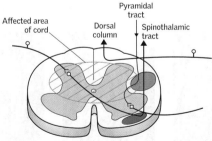

Fig 12.43 Central cord syndrome. Usually seen after a hyperextension injury in someone with pre-existing spinal canal stenosis (most often in the cervical region). There is greater loss of motor power in the upper extremities compared to the lower extremities combined with varying patterns of sensory loss and sphincter dysfunction.

Adapted from Donaghy, M. *Oxford Core Texts: Neurology* with permission from Oxford University Press.

12 *Priapism* is when pathologic stimuli (eg cervical cord lesions) cause prolonged erection (>4h), or when normal stimuli occurring under pathologic circumstances, eg stasis from sickle-cell disease or leukaemia with leucostasis (wcc↑↑) cause prolonged erections. As it can cause permanent damage, get help. Bilateral shunting between the corpus cavernosum and corpus spongiosum may be needed.

Priapism is named after Priapus, the son of Aphrodite (the goddess of love). He, though, is ugly in most depictions—with a penis so large that he is generally relegated to the position of a scarecrow in the fields. From this position he is happy to be the god of gardens, bees, goats, sheep—and fertility.

The area of 'tightest fit' between cord and canal is in the thoracic spine; this region also has the poorest blood supply. These facts explain why thoracic lesions are more likely to be complete than cervical or lumbar lesions. Ischaemic injury often spreads below the level of the mechanical injury. Neurological symptoms often increase in the hours following injury, so repeat examinations are essential. For the segment of the cord involved with injury at a specific vertebra, see below.

Cord compression For causes, see MINIBOX. Root pain (p680) and lower motor neuron signs occur at the level of the lesion with upper motor neuron signs and sensory changes below the lesion (spastic weakness, brisk reflexes, upgoing plantars, loss of co-ordination, joint position sense, vibration sense, temperature and pain).

Causes:
• Bone displacement
• Disc prolapse
• Local tumour
• Abscess
• Haematoma

Cord anatomy (p754) is such that dorsal column sensibilities (light touch, joint position sense, vibration sense) are affected on the same side as the insult, but spinothalamic tract interruption affects pain and temperature sensation for the opposite side of the body 2–3 dermatome levels lower than the affected sensory level. As the cord ends at L1, compression at this vertebral level affects information in the cord relating to lower dermatomes. To determine the cord level affected behind a given vertebra, add the number in blue to that of the vertebra concerned, thus:

• C2–7: **+1**
• T1–6: **+2**
• T7–9: **+3**
• T10 has L1 and L2 levels behind it
• T11 has L3 and 4
• L1 has sacral and coccygeal segments.

It can be difficult to determine the level: MRI will help clarify this (fig **12.44**).

Lower lumbar problems can cause cauda equina compression (▶▶BOX, p681) characterized by muscular pain, dermatomal sensory changes (if the lowest sacral dermatomes are affected the genitals are anaesthetic), and retention of urine ± faeces. ▶*These signs indicate urgent neurosurgical referral with imaging*, eg to confirm or exclude a tumour or extradural abscess.

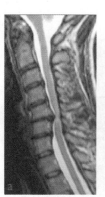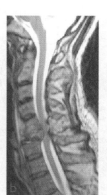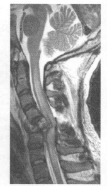

Fig 12.44 Cord compression. Because of different technical settings, MRI images can be called T1 or T2 weighted. These images can be recognized as T2 weighted because the CSF is white (see *OHCM* p749). Compression of the cord has occurred as a result of: (a) disc protrusion, (b) metastatic deposit, and (c) trauma.   Courtesy of Prof Peter Scally.

Trauma

Restoring lost function: is it possible?

Inducing repair of the spinal cord must take into account the complex patho-physiology involved during spinal cord damage. Primary injury is the direct mechanical damage to the neural elements, the resultant oedema and vascular disruption triggers secondary damage. Secondary injury is the delayed and prolonged response to neurotoxins and subsequent apoptosis; this secondary injury can be minimized with prompt emergency care. The four key principles of spinal cord repair are:
• Neuroprotection (to protect the surviving cells from further damage)
• Regeneration (targeting the correct neuronal connections)
• Replacement (of damaged nerve cells)
• Retraining CNS circuits to restore body functions.[70]

Novel therapies aim to optimize the environment both to minimize further damage and encourage repair. Often these options seem a long way off, but note that only 10% of damaged neurons need to be replaced to enable useful locomotion.

Segment injury—a guide to possible subsequent function

C4	Can use electric chairs with chin control; type with mouthstick; use a 'Possum' environmental control system to turn on lights & open doors.
C5	With special devices, he can feed, wash face, comb hair, and help with dressing the upper body. He may be able to push a wheelchair along the flat, if pushing gloves are worn, and there are capstan rims on the wheels. The NHS will supply an electric wheelchair (indoor use only). Unable to transfer from wheelchair to toilet.
C6	Still needs a strap to aid feeding and washing. Dresses top half of body; helps dress lower half. Can drive with hand controls.
C7	Can transfer, dress, feed himself.
C8	Independent wheelchair life.

Spinal shock A transient physiological loss of function, often due to haemorrhage. There is anaesthesia and flaccid paralysis of all segments, and muscles innervated below the level (hence areflexia) and there is retention of urine. A 'stage of reorganization' then occurs (reflex emptying of bladder and rectum; sweating). Later, flexion at hip and knee may be induced by stimuli (notably cold), often with emptying of the bladder and rectum (Head and Riddoch's mass reflexes). The legs may become permanently fixed in a drawn-up position, with dorsiflexion of the ankles (spastic paraplegia in flexion). Over months, tendon reflexes return, and proprioceptive stimuli give rise to 'mass extension'.[71]

> **Spinal or neurogenic?**
> ▶NB: **Don't** confuse *spinal shock* with *neurogenic shock*: the latter is BP↓ without tachycardia, caused by impairment of the descending spinal sympathetic pathways. caused by lesions above T6.

Spinal shock has been well recorded throughout history and the full recovery is often dramatically portrayed in media as the soldier who returns miraculously manages to walk at a critical point in the plot months after the injury. In reality, the temporary loss of sensory and motor function tends to recover within days but exact duration is not predictable.

Further reading
www.spinal-research.org
www.ninds.nih.gov

Approximately 0.4% of the population in the USA reported paralysis due to spinal cord injury.[72] These numbers are increasing as we continue to improve care for long-term neurological conditions.

Autonomic dysreflexia In those with lesions above the sympathetic outflow (ie above T6) any noxious stimulus may result in sympathetic overactivity below the level of the lesion. There is vasoconstriction and hypertension (potentially life-threatening as may cause seizures/intra-cranial haemorrhage and death). The patient may have a headache, a feeling of anxiety, sweaty/blotchy skin above the lesion with pale, dry skin below the level of lesion. The carotid baroreceptors are stimulated causing reflex vagal bradycardia, but the signals which would normally produce relieving vasodilatation are unable to pass down the cord. The most common cause is bladder distension (eg with a blocked catheter), followed by bowel distension (eg with constipation).[73] Other stimuli which may produce this effect include UTI, calculi, ejaculation, and bladder/colonic irrigation. Ensure good bowel and bladder care. *Treatment:* Sit the patient upright and give **nifedipine** (10mg—bite the capsule) with **glyceryl trinitrate** 0.5mg (not if patient has used sildenafil in the prior 24h).

Bladder dysfunction Genitourinary complications are among the commonest causes for rehospitalization in spinal cord injury patients. Key problems include urinary incontinence, reflex detrusor activity (after acontractility in the period of spinal shock) and the presence of residual urine. This predisposes to infection and ureteric reflux. These are major causes of renal failure, morbidity, and mortality. The most common method of bladder drainage is intermittent self-catheterization but no method has shown superiority.[74] *Urinary infection:* Historically used to be a serious cause of mortality (along with infected skin ulceration).[75] It may be prevented by a high fluid intake, ensuring effective bladder emptying, and acidification of the urine (eg **ascorbic acid** 1g/6h PO).

Pressure ulcers can develop quickly in skin with reduced sensation in patients unable to physically shift their positions. Skin is made more vulnerable when moist; from perspiration or urinary incontinence. Regular skin inspections are essential with good lifting techniques; avoid sliding patients across the bed as this stretches the skin. Healing of an ulcer requires months of pressure-relieving strategies and monitoring for infection.

Bowel dysfunction in lesions below L1, arises from cord compression of the conus and results in reduced peristalsis (and subsequent constipation) and a lax anal sphincter leading to faecal incontinence. Lesions at or above L1 result in an UMN picture with increased anal tone and subsequent retention of faeces and constipation. From the second day of injury, gentle manual evacuation using plenty of lubricant is needed. A flatus tube may be helpful in relieving distension once the ileus of spinal shock has passed. Remember, bowel health affects QOL and increases risk of autonomic dysreflexia—use laxatives wisely. See p248 *OHCM*.

Respiratory function depends on phrenic nerve involvement (C3, C4, C5). For lesions above C3 the diaphragm loses innervation and no respiratory effort can be made without a ventilator and tracheostomy. Even those with lesions below C5 encounter respiratory complications as their ability to cough forcefully and ventilate the lung bases is inhibited by lack of abdominal musculature. This predisposes patients to repeated pneumonia; a leading cause of death in this patient population. Mucolytics and physiotherapy to assist coughing can help clear respiratory secretions.

Spasticity (see p760)

Further reading
www.christopherreeve.org

Trauma

►Sexual counselling is an integral part of rehabilitation. It is important in itself, but we should recognize that sexuality interacts with important determinants of our patients' quality of life, eg levels of dependency, aggression, self-esteem, and autonomy. Don't be shy and don't be shocked: for help with discussing sexual issues, see p385. ►Given a knowing and patient partner, most people with spinal injury can enjoy a satisfying sex life. In some studies, locomotor impairment and autonomic dysreflexia were more frequently given as causes of reduced sexual pleasure than specific sexual dysfunctions.[76] Bowel and bladder incontinence is a frequent concern, but these can be anticipated if sexual activity is planned. It is equally important to assess the partner's needs and responses to the injury. This takes time. Be aware that sexuality encompasses more than physical attractiveness and intercourse. With spinal cord injury, use of sexual imagery and concentration on body areas that retain sensation have especial importance, as does a certain inventiveness and readiness to experiment.

When helping these patients it is important to distinguish sexual drive and sexual satisfaction from fertility and parenting needs. Both need addressing in a systematic way within the broader contexts of psychosocial, emotional, and relationship aspects. Living with a sci can be tough, there are a whole host of reasons why sexual satisfaction is not met; not just neurogenic.

Sexual health in men The first question will likely be; can I still get an erection? This depends on the site of injury. There are two types of erection: psychogenic erections are modulated by impulses from the brain and are the result of audiovisual stimuli or fantasy. Reflexogenic erections are governed by spinal reflexes (s2–s4) and arise from tactile stimuli to the genital area.[77] The latter type is most likely to be preserved in sci, patients with complete sci are unlikely to experience psychogenic erections. Erectile dysfunction is common and a source of distress.[78] In men with lesions between t6 and l5, 75% can expect improvement in erections with use of sildenafil. Fertility issues in men centre around performance and sperm quality, which may be reduced by scrotal hyperthermia, retrograde ejaculation, prostatic fluid stasis, and testicular denervation. Electro-ejaculation and intracytoplasmic sperm injection have useful roles.

Sexual health in women is less affected, largely because, anatomically, a woman can still engage in intercourse. Alternative positioning due to spasticity and additional lubrication may be required. Women can still bear children, but autonomic dysreflexia and the prothrombotic state are serious risks. Only 17% of women with complete lower motor neuron dysfunction affecting the s2–s5 spinal segments can achieve orgasm, compared with 59% of women with other levels and degrees of injury. Evidence suggests the potential for orgasm is there, but patients are disheartened by the lack of sensation.[79]

Talk about sex, it's important!

'Never underestimate the difference you can make' (C. Reeve)

Christopher Reeve was an actor who fractured his c1 and c2 after falling from a horse. Made famous on screen through playing the role of Superman, his time after the injury was heroically dedicated to helping establish a foundation to aid sci research. The most recent breakthrough in research is epidural electrical stimulation of the spinal cord. By applying continuous electrical current to the lumbosacral spinal neurons, the spinal cord 'wakes up' and can function at a basic level to allow the repetitive movements which it used to do. This revolutionary treatment enabled a young male with complete motor sci to stand independantly whilst being electrically stimulated in 2011. It has just been reproduced in 4 more patients in 2014 and is definitely an area of research to keep your eye on.[80,81]

Personal qualities in therapists are almost as important as exact anatomic lesion. There may be big mood swings from euphoria to despair as the patient accustoms himself to his loss and his new body image.

The occupational therapist (OT) is a key person in maximizing the levels of achievement. They can arrange a home visit with a member of the spinal injuries team and a community liaison nurse. The aim is to construct a plan with local services, so that the patient's (and his family's) hopes can be realized to the fullest extent. They can arrange the necessary home modifications, and give invaluable advice about the level of independence which is realistic to strive for. As ever, the aims of the OT extend into augmenting self-esteem, and helping the patient come to terms with loss of role, and loss of confidence, and to mitigate the effects of disability by arranging for as much purposeful activity as possible, in the realms of both work and leisure. They will also be able to make plans for acquiring social skills to assist the patient in his new way of life.

Nursing & physiotherapy • *The chest:* Regular physio with coughing and breathing exercises prevents sputum retention and pneumonia which are likely to follow diaphragmatic partial paralysis (eg C3–4 dislocation). If the lesion is above the T10 segmental level, there is no effective coughing.
• *The straight lift:* (for transferring patients) One attendant supports the head with both hands under the neck so that the head lies on the arms. 3 lifters standing on the same side insert their arms under the patient, one at a time, starting at the top. After the lift, withdraw in the reverse order.
• *Posture:* Place joints in a full range of positions. Avoid hyperextensions. Keep the feet flexed at 90° with a pillow between soles and bed-end.
• *Wheelchairs:* The patient should be kept sitting erect; adjust the footplates so that the thighs are supported and there is no undue pressure on the sacrum. ▸Regular relief of pressure on sacral and ischial areas is vital.
• *Standing and walking:* Using a 'tilt table', or the Oswestry standing frame, the tetraplegic patient can become upright. If the injury level is at L2–4, below-knee calipers and crutches enable walking to take place. If the lesion is at T1–8, 'swing to gait' may be possible. The crutches are placed a short distance in front of the feet. The goal is to promote re-establishment of functional connections in neuronal networks and shaping the motor patterns that they generate.[82]
• *Sport:* Consider archery, darts, snooker, table tennis, and swimming for those with paraplegia. Many other sports may also be suitable. There are interesting and important factors to consider such as the optimal heart rate (eg with lesions above T4 there is severely diminished cardiac acceleration, and a maximal rate of ~130bpm) and the reduction in bone density below the lesion.[83]

Spasticity arises from UMN lesions and is defined as increased muscle tone which tends to develop after the initial phases of spinal shock. Symptoms can manifest as spasms, pain, contractures, or abnormal tone.[84] >80% of SCI patients develop some form of spasticity.[84] ▸Changes in spasticity can herald new changes in the spinal cord (eg post-traumatic syringomyelia). *Treatment:* Intensive physiotherapy with passive stretching exercises to keep muscles supple and exercises to strengthen the spastic and synergistic muscles. Antispastic medication include baclofen, diazepam, and tizanidine. IM botulinum toxin inhibits ACH release, the clinical effects appear ~24 hours afterwards and can last 2–6 months depending on dose.[84] Surgery is reserved for those where severe spasms significantly affects activities of daily living. Orthopaedic surgery targets tendon release or transfers for contractures. Neurosurgical intervention includes ablation of motor nerves and rhizotomy which severs the dorsal sensory roots responsible for spasticity.

---

13 *The Alexander technique* aims to improve posture and movement. Classes teach gentle lying, sitting, and standing exercises which eliminate unecessary muscle tension and improve balance. In addition to chronic neck and back pain, evidence suggests patients with Parkinson's disease benefit (www.alexandertechnique.com).

Pathological fractures

Definition A # that occurs in diseased or abnormal bone. Disruption of bony structural integrity means that even trivial forces can produce a fracture, so suspect a pathological # if the energy of the trauma is abnormally low for the resulting injury. Common sites include the subtrochanteric femur and the proximal humeral shaft (fig 12.45).

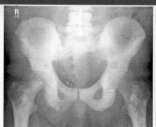

Fig 12.45 Diffuse bony sclerotic lesions, putting the patient at risk from pathological fracture.

Causes The commonest causes are osteoporosis (so-called 'fragility' fractures) and bony metastases (eg from breast or prostate primaries). Rarer causes include osteomalacia, bone infection, primary bone tumour, and osteogenesis imperfecta.

ΔΔ: Metastasis from prostate and breast, and rarely GI carcinoma; primary lymphoma; multiple myeloma.

Management If the underlying diagnosis is unclear, then do rigorous directed investigation, eg in a search for a primary cancer. Without treating the bone metastases, the chances of healing are nearly zero.

►Remember to image the whole femur if a proximal pathological fracture is identified—the forces through any fixation device could snap any other surrounding infiltrated bone.

Courtesy of The Norfolk and Norwich University Hospitals (NNUH) Radiology Dept.

Trauma

Overuse phenomena at work

Activity requiring repetitive actions, particularly those associated with prolonged muscle contraction, may lead to chronic symptoms. Those who use vacuum cleaners, assemble cars, or play stringed instruments may all develop overuse phenomena, as can sports players. Employers have a duty to provide a safe working environment and well-designed chairs and tools. Changes of posture and activity help to reduce work-related 'non-specific arm pain'. The cost of these injuries in suffering, and hours lost from work, is considerable as treatment of established symptoms is often difficult and may necessitate change in employment—if one is available.

Compensation is a vexed issue, and recent court judgments have gone in favour of employers in some instances, and in favour of patients in others. Some people argue that the condition does not exist as a separate medical entity, emphasizing lack of histopathology. It should be noted that this is not a prerequisite for a disease (see *Sudden infant death*, p148)—and in any case, histopathology is sometimes demonstrable. Treatments tried include splinting (may prolong the problem), physiotherapy, β-blockers for relaxation, and the Alexander technique for posture re-education.[13]

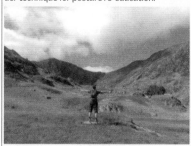

Fig 12.46 Why is the term repetitive strain injury a fallacy? Just because anginal chest pain can be provoked by walking up hills, hill walking does not cause coronary artery stenosis (although the idea for some may be enough to cause a little heart flutter). And so, because use of the arm may provoke the symptoms of an underlying condition (eg carpal tunnel syndrome, OA at the base of the thumb, de Quervain's disease), it does not mean that it is the cause of the underlying condition.

© Nina Hjelde.

Fig 13.1 Emergency medicine feels the pressure of time; patients are waiting for you, targets need to be met, and life-saving decisions need to be made. Salvador Dali's melting clocks, however, remind us that time is neither relative nor fixed; attempting to forcibly manipulate time beyond your abilities can disrupt the natural progression. Look up his painting 'Soft watch at the moment of explosion (1954)'. Dali was particularly inspired by spirals (especially the double helix of DNA) and his exploding clock shows time spiralling and twisting out of control. The department will always seem chaotic. Take the time you need to ensure that neither you nor the patient spirals out of control.[1]   © Gillian Turner.

Once people hear that you are an emergency medic, they will expect great things in times of pressure. Knowing the basics (p780) is key. The situation can quickly spiral out of control and become overwhelming. Take control. Use common sense by removing dangers, call for help, and position your patient well until more help arrives.

If your patient is unconscious with a patent airway, place them in the recovery position (fig 13.2). This ensures their airway remains patent and encourages vomitus to be expelled rather than aspirated. Place the patient's nearest arm at 90° on floor and the dorsum of the other hand on the nearest cheek. Bend the knee furthest from you to a right angle and pull on this to roll the patient towards you. Their arm will help keep the chin tilted. Check pockets for keys or other objects which might be painful to lie on before rolling!

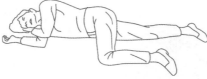

Fig 13.2 Recovery position.
Reproduced with permission from Randle J, et al. (eds). *Oxford Handbook of Clinical Skills in Adult Nursing*. Copyright © Oxford University Press 2009, with permission from Oxford University Press.

We thank our Specialist Reader Dr Simon Rendell for his help. Thanks also to Dr Kenneth Anderson for his help and support.

Emergency medicine is a relatively new specialty, and prior to 1952 it was informally led by junior surgical staff. The lack of dedicated senior staff resulted in poor quality of care and abysmal staffing levels. By the 1970s, consultants dedicated to emergency medicine were recruited. Significant progress has since been made, culminating in the establishment of the College of Emergency Medicine in 2006, from early incarnations since 1993, with dedicated training programmes and full-time staff. In 2015, the college was awarded a royal charter. A doctor working in emergency medicine is expected to maintain a good general knowledge of all specialties and expertise in trauma to enable them to deliver emergency care and ensure that each patient receives appropriate ongoing care. The ethos of delivering emergency care is to ensure good flow of patients through the department and necessary treatment initiated. It is important to recognize this and understand how the Emergency Department fits in together with other specialties for the good of the patient.

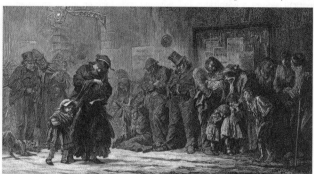

Fig 13.3 Waiting in a queue for admission to the Casual Ward.
Although it doesn't feel like it on a busy Saturday night, waiting room conditions have improved!
Mary Evans Picture Library.

Casualty, A&E, or emergency departments?

Historically, the term 'casual ward' was used as travellers and workers could seek medical attention on a casual basis rather than by formal appointment (fig 13.3). 'Casualty' was of military origin, indicating a severely injured patient. Early departments treated both these casual attenders and those acutely injured. In 1962, Sir Henry Platt moved to change the name to Accident and Emergency (A&E) as the service received both medical and surgical emergencies beyond purely trauma. In an attempt to discourage inappropriate non-emergent attendance, the term emergency department (ED) is now preferred. For emergency physicians, this battle of nomenclature is a sensitive subject as they have fought hard to establish their specialty over the years. One author even received a smack on the bottom (!) from her consultant for answering the phone using the older term 'Casualty'.

Further reading

Exadaktylos AK *et al.* (2008). Emergency medicine and acute care surgery: a modern 'Hansel and Gretel' fairytale? *Emerg Med J* 25(6):321–2.

Platt H (1962). *Report Of The Standing Medical Advisory Committee, Accident And Emergency Services*. London: HMSO.

Sakr M *et al.* (2000). Casualty, accident and emergency, or emergency medicine, the evolution. *J Accid Emerg Med* 17:314–19.

From our point of view, the ideal scenario is to have a pristine, ever-ready but empty trauma department with the doctors and nurses educating themselves in the coffee room, occasionally being called out by paramedics to save a few lives in a brief display of energy and technical brilliance. This is not how the public sees our role. All EDs are abused—because it is always doctors who define what abuse is. Up to 70% of users have been deemed inappropriate in some studies. This figure dwindles down to nothingness if abuse is defined as those consultations where all 3 parties to the visit (the doctor, the patient + family, and the patient's GP), on reflection, concur that it was inappropriate.

Overcrowding and 'exit-block' is a major problem in EDs the world over—partly reflecting centrally determined reductions in acute bed provision and availability, and partly reflecting access problems from populations seeking prompt help with immediate (and sometimes chronic) problems. If the inpatient side of a hospital is full, patients will stack up in the ED awaiting admission; this increases mortality. If overcrowding is cumulative, ambulances may be redirected to other hospitals (adding to delay and danger) and patients with genuine needs may, catastrophically, decide they cannot wait any more hours for help. At first glance, emergency physicians can be perceived as ruthless and brisk, yet it is essential they maintain a fast pace and delegate tasks to more specialized services.

BREACH! Since 2010, EDs must see, treat, and admit/discharge 95% of their patients by 4 hours. Efficient patient flow to specialities is dependent on staffing levels, access to specialty services, and inpatient beds in order to prevent a 'breach' of this target; a term which can have significant financial impacts on a hospital. When working in the ED, bear this timing in mind and observe how all the services knit together towards the common goal. This target is welcomed in theory as it encourages efficient patient flow, yet it has raised concerns that this time pressure could compromise patient care.

Another busy shift?

In the middle of any horrendous ED shift, you may be forgiven for wondering what on earth is happening outside to prompt such a heave in the number of attendances. It can be tempting to drop your work and shuffle out to the waiting room with your hands held up in defeat and announce to the multitude of bewildered patients; 'We give up ... You win!'

Rumours circulate that sunshine means that children are out in force at the local playgrounds, or rain means that old ladies will be slipping up on the kerb. Perhaps late on a Friday night you despair at the number of alcohol-related incidents. Similarly, you hear that because the World Cup is on, the shift is going to be a quiet one ... until the game finishes and people are out celebrating (or drowning their losses). Factors that have been suggested to be correlated with an increase in the number of ED attendances include:

- Warm, dry, and sunny weather conditions
- Local music festivals (despite on-site facilities)
- National sport teams winning at home (sadly, for assault)
- Major natural disasters (eg a hurricane, though with an understandable reduction on the day of disaster)
- And yes ... Mondays.

Studies have also suggested reduced attendances during major televised sporting events. From personal experience, trying to predict how busy your shift will be rarely seems to help. Ultimately, the aim of such epidemiological studies is to help in ED staffing and logistics, and one clear message remains: ▸▸Don't despair, all of these factors are well beyond your control!

How to cope with inappropriate attendance

Triage by a trained nurse can help offer simple advice that may guide patients to more appropriate care. If the most urgent patients are seen first, the prolonged wait will cause many unnecessary attendances to drift away.

Employing primary care facilities within the ED helps divert non-life-threatening issues to more appropriate services. GPs working alongside ED doctors has been successful because they use resources more sparingly and are used to dealing with mismatches between patients' expectations and reality. GPs treating people with semi-urgent problems investigated less (by 20%), referred to other hospital services less (by 39%), admitted fewer patients (by 45%), and prescribed more often (by 43%).[2] There were no differences in measures of outcome. However, it is not clear whether their more economical style was to do with being a GP, or because these doctors were older and more experienced than their emergency medi-

Hospital vs community
- Easy access at a time which suits patient
- Perception that quality of care is superior
- Difficulties obtaining a GP appointment
- Poor understanding of alternative community services.

cine counterparts. An NHS report showed that 1 in 10 people attending the ED admitted their problem did not warrant ED level of care.[3] Yet attendances to the ED are increasing annually as the public choose hospital services over community (see MINIBOX). In response, public health campaigns such as 'Choose Well' have encouraged users to explore community services thus reserving the ED for acute illness (fig 13.4).

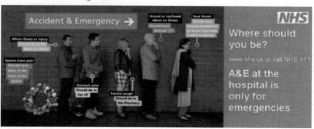

Fig 13.4 The NHS Choose Well campaign. © NHS, Department of Health.

Crying wolf in the ED

You know when you have become part of the team when you start to recognize the frequent attenders. This cohort of patients typically have medically unexplained symptoms associated with chronic disease, alcohol abuse, or mental health issues. Studies have emphasized the importance of case management strategies in partnership with community alcohol and drug services.[4] They typically have complex presentations, which subsequently result in 38.5% higher admission rates.[5] This latter number is frustrating, yet understandable. You are about to see a patient with cardiac-sounding chest pain yet the nursing staff whisper that he presents with this every weekend. The department is really busy with many unwell patients still waiting to be seen. You see he has had multiple troponin requests in the past year; all negative. It is 2am with no seniors about who know the patient. Would you consider it safe practice to send him home without admitting him to assess his troponin levels?

Further reading

The Royal College of Emergency Medicine. *Exit Block Campaign*. http://www.rcem.ac.uk/Shop-Floor/Policy/Campaigns/

Emergency medicine

The majority of burns are minor; non-specialist staff will see very few major burns. Their task should be to ensure the rapid and safe transfer to burns units (with ITU resources and access to burn surgery) experienced in their care. Staff should be familiar with ATLS and EMSB protocols (Early Management of Severe Burns).[6]

Only a small percentage of burns presenting to the ED are major burns. Those of over 15% BSA (burn surface area) in an adult and 10% BSA in a child will require formal resuscitation and referral to a burns specialist unit. All suspected inhalational injuries and any burn to face, hands, feet, or genitalia should be referred to a burns unit regardless of the size of burn.

First aid should be started on-scene and consists of removing all burnt clothing and irrigating the burn for 10 minutes with cool sterile saline. This is to stop the burn process. Chemical burns will require continuous irrigation. Burns should be kept clean, covered with cling film (do not wrap circumferentially). ▶▶Cool the burn and warm the patient to prevent shock.

Airway and breathing ▶▶Formal airway assessment by an ICU anaesthetist is advisable. ▶▶Give high-flow O₂. Inhalational injury can be thermal or chemical. Accurate history is vital and there must be a high index of suspicion for any injury sustained in a closed space.

- *Signs of inhalational injury:* Direct injury to face/neck, singed nasal hair, carbonaceous sputum, voice changes, dyspnoea, soot around nose or mouth.
- Systemic oedema is rare at time of presentation to ED but will increase rapidly once formal fluid resuscitation is underway.
- ▶▶Give *high-flow O₂*. Give 100% O₂ until *carboxyhaemoglobin (COHb)* levels are known. Continue on 100% until satisfied that COHb is normal, if raised then continue until COHb levels are less than 10% for more than 6 hours. High levels of COHb are likely to be associated with high *cyanide (CN)* levels which comes from burning foam. It is not readily measured in the clinical situation—suspect where there is persistent evidence of tissue poisoning (mechanism of toxicity is cytochrome inhibition). The effects of *CO* and *CN* are often overestimated. (See p804 for antidotes, and OHCM, p854.)
- ▶▶Formal *airway assessment* by an anaesthetist is advisable. Early intubation is likely to be required for the majority of major burns prior to transfer. If unsure, seek advice from the receiving burns unit. If intubation is required then it is vital to use an *uncut* endotracheal tube with an internal diameter of more than 7.5mm to allow passage of a bronchoscope. A nasogastric tube should be passed at the time of intubation as this will be difficult once swelling progresses and early feeding is essential.
- *c-spine and chest injuries* eg tension pneumothorax or flail chest may be caused by the event (eg force of explosion, running/jumping to safety).

Circulation The extreme inflammatory response seen in major burn injuries means that large volumes of fluid are needed for resuscitation. Hartmann's solution, should be given according to the *Parklands formula:*[1]

| Vol in millilitres = 4 × body weight (kg) × BSA (%) of burn |

Give 50% of this in the first 8h from the time of burn, the other ½ in the next 16h. This formula only calculates fluid requirements for the burn resuscitation, other fluid requirements for maintenance or other losses will be in addition.
Colloids should be avoided in the first 24h (due to colloid permeability).
Blood and clotting products should be given as required. IV access should be through unburnt skin where possible. Arterial monitoring and central venous access will be required prior to transfer. All fluids should be warmed and all efforts made to prevent any drop in body temperature.

We thank Dr Jo Rogers for help with this page.

The Parkland formula is a guide to the minimum fluid required for the burn, resuscitation should be targeted to urine output of minimum 0.5mL per kg and a Hct of <40%. The aim of fluid 'resuscitation' in burns is to anticipate and prevent shock.

Burn surface area (BSA) can be estimated by the rule of nines (MINIBOX) or using the palmar aspect of the patients own hand which will be 1% of their BSA. A Lund and Browder chart is time-consuming, but more accurate (fig 13.5).

Wallace rule of nines
• Arm (all over) 9%
• Leg (all over) 18%
• Front 18%
• Back 18%
• Head (all over) 9%
• Genitals/perineum 1%

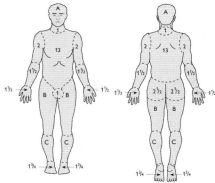

Relative percentage of body surface area affected by growth

Area	Age 0	1	5	10	15	Adult
A: half of head	9½	8½	6½	5½	4½	3½
B: half of thigh	2¾	3¼	4	4¼	4½	4¾
C: half of leg	2½	2½	2¾	3	3¼	3½

Fig 13.5 The Lund and Browder chart.

Reproduced from Longmore, Wilkinson, Baldwin, Wallin, *Oxford Handbook of Clinical Medicine*, 9e, 2014, with permission from OUP.

Assessing burn depth

Many burns, especially scalds in children, are mixed depth. Also, burns can evolve for up to 48h. In ED, the most important aspect of assessing burn depth is *erythema*; to avoid overestimating burns, don't count mild redness, blisters, or oedema. Simple erythema can be discounted.

• *Superficial burns* are red, painful with blistering but hair follicles will be intact.
• *Deep dermal burns* are red, painful , peeling sheets more common than blistering and few hair follicles are intact.
• *Full-thickness burns* are pale and charred black or grey. There is no erythema , there are no hairs intact, and the skin is insensate. It is leather-like and can cause constriction if circumferential.

Paediatric burns Standard estimation of area cannot be applied: Wallace's rule of nines must be modified but is then rather unwieldy, and specific burn charts are more reliable.

Other considerations[6] Analgesia should be given as required, burns are extremely painful. Burnt limbs should be elevated to reduce the risk of compartment syndrome and peripheral pulses need to be monitored. Major burns carry a high mortality so good communication is essential between teams and in discussions with relatives. Predictors of mortality are pre-morbid conditions, surface area of burn, presence of inhalational injury, and age .

1 In electric shock injuries, higher volumes of fluid may be needed; see p769.

Emergency medicine

Emergency medicine

Drowning is the 3rd leading cause of unintentional injury or death worldwide and increasingly recognized as a worldwide public health problem. Injuries account for nearly 10% of total global mortality. Low- and middle-income countries account for 95% of drowning deaths; drowning death rates are highest in Africa (10× higher than the UK). Children <5 are at greatest risk. Adult drowning is often associated with alcohol.

The term 'distress' signifies pending danger as a person is struggling but still able to keep afloat and shout for help. A person 'drowning' is already starting to suffocate. The classic media portrayal of people drowning shows distressed swimmers loudly thrashing about; in reality, drowning is typically silent and quick. Drowning is classified by outcome into: death, morbidity, and no morbidity.

Management

	Key concerns

- Do not attempt CPR in water, compressions are only effective against hard ground.
- Try to maintain c-spine immobilization throughout—there may be trauma here through cause or effect.
- Surrounding water exerts pressure on venous return and helps maintain cardiac output; place patient in prone position to minimize circulatory collapse when lifted from water.
- Cardiac arrest occurs 2° to hypoxaemia and correction is critical to obtaining return of spontaneous circulation. Give 100% oxygen to mitigate hypoxia—water in alveoli will dilute surface surfactant and increase atelectasis. Intubation with high PEEP increases survival.
- Suspect hypothermia (use a low-reading rectal thermometer).

Key concerns
- Cardiac arrest
- Hypothermia (OHCM p860)
- Pulmonary oedema

Does he need admission? Always observe patients after a drowning event as the risk of aspiration can lead to pulmonary oedema. Monitor for haemoptysis, basal crackles, CXR changes, and hypoxia on room air. If asymptomatic 4h post-event then he can be discharged home. Advise out-patient follow-up with CXR in 2 weeks to check for atypical infection from infected water. Prophylactic antibiotics are not advocated.

When should prolonged resuscitation take place?

▶▶Prolonged resuscitation is usually needed in hypothermia; be prepared for this.

Deciding when to discontinue resuscitation efforts in hypothermia is notoriously difficult. If the victim was submersed in water <5°c the rapid development of hypothermia may offer protection against hypoxia due to the mammalian diving reflex. Severe hypothermia can mimic clinical signs of death with no pulse, respiratory effort, and muscle rigidity. Aggressively resuscitate all patients until rewarmed and further investigations performed at hospital. Hyperkalaemia = poor prognosis. Use ECG monitoring and end-tidal CO_2 to help diagnose cardiac arrest. *No hypothermic patient should be pronounced dead, until warm and dead.*

Case study A fit, young Norwegian woman was cross-country skiing with friends when she fell down a gully and became trapped in water beneath the ice. Frantic efforts were made to extract her, but after 40 minutes all movements ceased. Her body was eventually recovered, 1 hour 19 minutes later, through a hole cut in the ice downstream. She was pronounced dead at the scene, but given CPR throughout the flight back to hospital, where her rectal temperature was recorded as 13.7°c. Her body was rewarmed by means of an extracorporeal membrane oxygenator. After 35 days on a ventilator and a further 5 months of rehabilitation, she was able to resume her job as a hospital doctor.

Accounts for 1000 deaths per year in USA, for every death there are 2 serious injuries and >30 reported electric shocks. Utility workers and those working with electricity lines are the most commonly affected. Injuries at home are usually due to using improperly earthed appliances or using electrical appliances near water. Electrical current causes cellular physiological changes, thermal tissue destruction, and secondary damage from muscle spasms and falls.

Factors that increase the severity of injury

1 *Type of current:* Alternating current (AC) is more dangerous than direct current (DC) of the same magnitude, causing muscle spasm that may make it impossible for the victim to let go of the source. DC usually produces a single large muscular contraction. DC usually causes asystole, and AC causes VF.

2 *Energy delivered:* This is a product of the applied voltage and subsequent current. Extreme heating of tissues may occur, causing internal and external burns and coagulation necrosis.

3 *Current pathway:* The route that the current takes through the body is an important factor. If it passes through the head or chest (eg entry in one arm and exit from the other), fatal injury is more likely.

4 *Resistance encountered:* Fluid and electrolyte-rich tissues conduct electricity well. Bone is the most resistant tissue, whereas skin thickness (∴ resistance) can limit the amount of current passing through the body. Tissues designed to conduct electricity—heart and nerves—do badly, and they may sustain preferential damage when other tissues remain intact. ►Check carefully for nerve damage, even if surface appearances are mild.

5 *Contact duration:* The briefer, the better!

Treatment of electric shock

• Ensure the source of current is turned off before attempting rescue.
• Use paradoxical triage: resuscitate the apparently 'dead' before attending to the living. Using standard resuscitation techniques, resuscitate long and aggressively—remarkable recoveries have been reported.
• Burns (p766), more fluid replacement is required than for normal thermal burns as electrical burns may penetrate deeper (start at 7mL/kg/% and adjust to urine output of 1–2mL/kg/h). ►Check for rhabdomyolysis.
• Treat arrhythmias conventionally.
• Occult internal damage can lead to compartment syndrome, most frequently in the legs. See p727.

Lightning strikes

• Lightning strikes ~30,000 times a year in UK. 30–60 people are struck by lightning each year, only ~10% of which are fatal. Types of lightning strike: 1 *Direct* Lightning strikes and enters ground through patient. Outdoor enthusiasts (such as golfers) are especially at risk. 2 *Side flash* Lightning hits another object, such as a tree, and jumps sideways. 3 *Ground strike* Lightning strikes nearby and travels through the ground to patient.
• Despite cinematic belief, lightning strikes are often unwitnessed and the patient is typically found confused with tattered clothing + tympanic membrane rupture. It is safe to touch patients immediately after! Conduct full trauma assessment. Document visual acuity as electrical cataract formation is frequently missed. Immediate effects may involve asystole which only persists if secondary hypoxic arrest develops. Generalized muscle aches and any neurological deficit tend to resolve over 24h.

Further reading

Cooper MA *et al.* (2007). Lightning injuries. In Auerbach PS (ed) *Wilderness Medicine* (5th ed), pp.67–108. St. Louis, MO: Mosby.

Royal Society for the Prevention of Accidents: www.rospa.com

Rull G (2012). *Electrical Injuries and Lightning Strikes*. http://www.patient.co.uk/doctor/Electrical-Injuries-and-Lightning-Strikes.htm

Emergency medicine

WHO estimates that 140 million people live at altitudes >2500m and 40 million lowland dwellers travel to high altitude each year to ski, trek (fig 13.6) or work. High-altitude illness refers to conditions afflicting individuals ascending to altitudes faster than their bodies can acclimatize. It chiefly[2] comprises: 1 Acute mountain sickness (AMS) 2 High-altitude cerebral oedema (HACE) 3 High-altitude pulmonary oedema (HAPE). The latter two may be rapidly fatal if untreated.

Acclimatizing to high altitudes During ascent, partial pressure of O_2 in blood falls as barometric pressure drops. Carotid body and medullary chemoreceptors respond to this hypobaric hypoxia by ↑ rate and depth of ventilation. The kidneys respond to the ensuing respiratory alkalosis over a period of days by excreting bicarbonate and reabsorbing hydrogen ions. A true ↑ in the red cell count (RCC) resulting from renal erythropoietin secretion takes weeks to develop. Acclimatization does not return the body to its sea level state.[8] There is considerable variation in the rate and extent of altitude acclimatization. Above 3000m, each night's sleeping altitude should be no higher than 300m above the previous night, with a rest day every 2-3 days or 1000m ascended. High-altitude mental and physical deterioration occurs during prolonged stays at extreme altitude (>5500m).

Acute mountain sickness (AMS) Mild AMS is common at altitudes of >2500m. It may result from ↑ cerebral blood flow and mild cerebral oedema with an input from oxidative stress mediated by oxygen free radicals. Mild AMS is managed conservatively with rest, hydration, analgesia, and antiemetics. For management of severe AMS (inability to walk, care for oneself, disturbed consciousness) see TABLE.

Risk factors for AMS
• Rate of ascent
• Absolute altitude
• Blunted ventilatory response to hypoxia (unreliable sign)[9]
• Level of exertion (NB: physical fitness does not protect)
• Permanent home at <900m
• Previous AMS
• Concurrent URTI
• Neck irradiation or surgery

High-altitude cerebral oedema (HACE) HACE is a potentially rapidly fatal encephalopathy with a change in mental status ± ataxia which is usually preceded by AMS. It may co-exist with HAPE. The exact incidence varies between studies but may be as much as 0.5–1%. It arises from vasogenic cerebral oedema caused by disruption of the blood–brain barrier ± cytotoxic oedema. HACE requires a greater degree of descent than HAPE and recovery takes longer.

High-altitude pulmonary oedema (HAPE) HAPE is more common than HACE and may accompany AMS, typically 2–4 days after ascent to altitudes of >3000m.

Symptoms: Cough, dyspnoea at rest, haemoptysis, extreme lethargy.

Signs: Tachycardia, tachypnoea, cyanosis ± crackles (often right middle lobe; listen in the axilla). HAPE arises from patchy pulmonary vasoconstriction leading to stress failure of pulmonary capillaries and pulmonary oedema. People with a strong hypoxic pulmonary vasoconstrictor response, concurrent respiratory infection, or congenital absence of a pulmonary artery are most susceptible.

Using acetazolamide Acetazolamide is a carbonic anhydrase inhibitor that causes ↑bicarbonate excretion by the kidneys, thus accelerating acclimatization.
• It does *NOT* hide symptoms of AMS.
• It may be used as prophylaxis at a dose of 250mg/12h PO (until 1 day after the maximum altitude is reached) in those with past severe AMS, or those making a forced rapid ascent.
• It can also aid sleep by ↓periodic breathing (dose: 125mg PO 1h before bed).
• Contraindication: sulfa allergy. Give a test dose prior to travel.

We thank Dr Gerard Flaherty for supplying figure 13.5 and compiling this page for us.

2 Other high-altitude illnesses: retinal haemorrhage (common; rarely problematic); chronic mountain sickness (polycythaemia, headache, somnolence, depression); subacute mountain sickness. NB: harmless swelling of extremities, more common in females, does not predict AMS.

Golden rules at high altitude

- 'Climb high, sleep low' to promote acclimatization.
- Avoid undue exertion at high altitude.
- Avoid alcohol, sedating antihistamines, or sedative-hypnotics.
- Feeling unwell at altitude=altitude illness until proved otherwise.
- Never ascend with AMS symptoms.
- Never leave someone with AMS alone.
- If you are worsening, or developing HACE or HAPE...▶▶descend immediately.

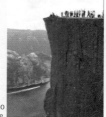

Fig 13.6 Preikestolen in Norway attracts base jumpers who notoriously require difficult rescue missions. © Nina Hjelde.

Lake Louise consensus criteria for the diagnosis of AMS

AMS is defined as the presence of headache plus at least one of the following symptoms occurring several hours after reaching a higher altitude:
- Gastrointestinal upset
- Fatigue or weakness
- Dizziness or light-headedness
- Difficulty sleeping.

▶▶Emergency management of severe high-altitude illness

Severe AMS (acute mountain sickness)			
DESCENT	Acetazolamide 250mg/8h po	Dexamethasone 4mg/6h po	Trekkers should *NOT* ascend on dexamethasone

HACE (high-altitude cerebral oedema)			
DESCENT	Acetazolamide 250mg/8h po	Dexamethasone 8mg IM then 4mg/6h po	Portable hyperbaric chamber (fig 13.7) Consider O₂ 4L/min

HAPE (high-altitude pulmonary oedema)			Role unclear
DESCENT	Portable hyperbaric chamber Consider O₂ at 4L/min	Nifedipine SR 20mg/12h po	Acetazolamide 250mg/8h po	Inhaled salmeterol
			Dexamethasone 8mg IM then 4mg/6h po	Sildenafil by mouth

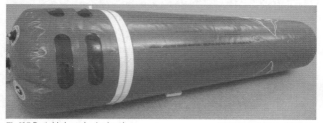

Fig 13.7 Portable hyperbaric chamber.   Courtesy of Dr Gerard Flaherty.

Further reading

Patients on intensive care endure significant levels of hypoxia. Research at high altitude has improved understanding of the physiological responses to hypoxia; including taking an arterial blood gas at the top of Everest! www.extreme-everest.co.uk contains a summary of their findings and it's worth watching their BBC documentary: 'Doctors in the Death Zone' (2007) (available on youtube). Can you guess the PaO_2 of a climber at the top of Everest?

Principles of management Where possible, convert dirty ragged wounds into clean wounds that can be reconstructed simply.

Important points in the management of wounds

1 Irrigation, irrigation, and more irrigation with 0.9% saline or clean tap water. It is vital to clean the wound well as soon as possible particularly if the patient is referred to specialist care that could incur further delay.

2 Infiltrate with **lidocaine** 3mg/kg plain or 7mg/kg with adrenaline. Lidocaine is a vasodilator (∴ increases its own systemic clearance). **Adrenaline** is used where vasoconstriction to reduce bleeding is useful and if the predicted dose of lidocaine needed would exceed 3mg/kg. 1 in 200,000 adrenaline is most suitable for daily use (1:1000 is 1mg/mL). Use the minimum strength for job. Local anaesthesia (LA) will still work at dilute concentrations but you will need to wait for longer; for suturing 1% provides a good effect with less toxicity (fig 13.9, p773). Infiltrate through devitalized tissue of the wound using a small volume to avoid distorting the tissues.

3 Remove debris, foreign bodies, and necrotic tissue; ragged or shelved skin edges may need trimming. Avoid excessive tissue resection on the face where reconstruction may be difficult. Abrasions need to be scrubbed thoroughly otherwise permanent tattooing will occur after re-epithelialization.

4 Use absorbable subcutaneous sutures (Vicryl®/PDS®) to bring skin edges together and avoid skin tension. Use interrupted monofilament (nylon/Prolene®) on the skin in most cases for optimal apposition 6'0 for the face, 5'0 or thicker for other areas. Avoid skin tension and wound inversion. Vicryl Rapide® or other absorbables may be considered as skin sutures in non-cosmetic areas: brush suture knots away after a week (OHCM p572).

5 Remove sutures at the correct time to minimize risk of unsightly permanent stitch marks: face 5 days, upper limb/body 7–10 days, lower limb 14 days.

Suture alternatives *Steri-Strips®:* Good for non-hairy skin that is unlikely to get wet. Avoid too much traction. They may be combined with buried dermal absorbable sutures. *Glues:* (eg **Dermabond®**) After haemostasis, place directly on top of accurately apposed and dried skin edges. Avoid thick layers as the exothermic reaction may hurt. Allow to dry for 30sec, then apply another thin layer. Avoid getting the glue inside the wound as it is cytotoxic. Post-op: 'you can shower, but don't soak or scrub'.[10]

Antibiotics Often not needed,[11] unless human/animal bite, hand wound.[12]

Tetanus Prophylaxis is vital. A full course (p151) provides good immunity. Vaccinate those who have not completed their schedule or where there is uncertainty.

Pre-tibial lacerations

The shin (esp. if elderly) has poor blood supply. It is vulnerable to flap wounds (fig 13.8). **Treatment** Try hard to iron out all the flap, repositioning it carefully. The important thing is to evacuate the haematoma to prevent tension (tension → breakdown → plastic surgery). Skin closure with adhesive strips (eg Steri-Strips®) is better than sutures, as they can be loosened if the tissues swell. Wound glue may be better still. Dress, and advise a support bandage, and leg elevation. Review to check for infection, wound tension, and necrosis

Before
Flap retracts back

Good
No tension in flap.
Held with adhesive
sutures.

Bad
Flap stretched tight
and likely to necrose.

Fig 13.8 Flap wounds

Calculating lidocaine (= lignocaine) doses

For more information on local anaesthetic doses, toxicity, and onset and duration times (see p632). For lidocaine doses (*without adrenaline*):

Percentage	Concentration (mg/mL)	Approx. allowable volume (mL/kg)
0.25%	2.5	1.12
0.5%	5	0.56
1%	10	0.28
2%	20	0.14

Lidocaine blocks voltage-gated Na^+ channels to prevent depolarization.

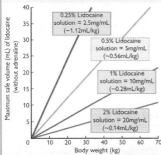

0.25% Lidocaine solution = 2.5mg/mL (~1.12mL/kg)

0.5% Lidocaine solution = 5mg/mL (~0.56mL/kg)

1% Lidocaine solution = 10mg/mL (~0.28mL/kg)

2% Lidocaine solution = 20mg/mL (~0.14mL/kg)

Fig 13.9 Maximum safe volume of plain lidocaine by body weight.

Max. safe dose of lidocaine *without adrenaline:* 3mg/kg; *with adrenaline:* 7mg/kg. *Use different strengths for different jobs:* 0.25–0.5% for infiltration & IV regional anaesthesia; 1% for nerve blocks, epidural anaesthesia, and IV regional anaesthesia; 2% for nerve blocks. NB: 1%=10mg/mL. See p632 for types of local anaesthetics.

Emergency medicine (side tab)

Wound healing and associated problems

Wound healing is a fascinating but complex web of physiology: to attempt to explain it in detail would be unflattering to such a remarkable process (fig 13.10).

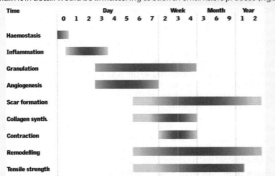

Fig 13.10 The diagram outlines the important and overlapping stages during the wound healing process—NB: milestones are variable.   Courtesy of Dr Tom Turmezei.

Wound healing problems Wound healing capability ↓ with ↑age, malnutrition, DM, steroid therapy, smoking (p719), peripheral vascular disease, and irradiation. Wound infection worsens scarring and so topical **chloramphenicol** can be used to reduce the risk of cosmetic insult (eg on face). *Keloid scarring* is exaggerated scarring (from excess collagen production, especially type III) to beyond the confines of the initial wound and can appear progressively and after a delay. *Hypertrophic scarring* is exaggerated scarring within the confines of the initial wound, is often associated with a wound across a joint surface, and tends to regress. Both are more common in dark-skinned individuals.

▶When in doubt, ask the ED nurse: she will have seen it all before.

'I've hammered my finger, doctor' This usually causes a subungual haematoma—relieved by expressing the blood through a hole trephined in the nail, using a 19G needle. No force is needed. Simply twiddle the needle vertically on the nail: the cutting edge will make a suitable hole (see fig 12.24 p733).

'I've swallowed a fish bone and it's stuck' Always examine the throat and tonsils carefully. Often the bone has only grazed the mucosa. Use a good light, and grip the tongue with gauze to move it out of the way before removing any visible bones with forceps. If you fail, refer to ENT. See FB ingestion (BOX, p777).

'My fish hook has barbed my finger' Infiltrate with plain lidocaine and push the hook on through the finger, provided no important structures are in its way. Once the barb is through, cut it off. Remove the hook where it entered.

'My tooth has been knocked out' Try to replace permanent teeth. Send deciduous teeth to the tooth fairy. If the former, after the patient sucks it clean (do not use water) transport in milk—or reinsert it, stabilizing with finger pressure (or biting). Go to a dentist for splinting.

Plaster 'backslabs' (for undisplaced forearm fractures).
• Remove anything which impairs finger circulation (eg rings).
• Protect yourself and your patient with a plastic apron.
• Measure the length for the back slab—from knuckles to just below elbow, so that the fingers and elbow will remain mobile.
• Cut a piece of plaster-impregnated bandage 5 times longer than the desired length. Fold it into 5-ply. Then see fig 13.11. ①.
• Cut off one corner so that it does not impinge on the thumb.
• Cut a wedge off the other end when the wedge's thick end on the same side as the thumb. This aids elbow movement. ②
• Roll stockinette over the forearm, to well above the elbow.
• Wind a roll of wool padding over the stockingette (turns must overlap by 50%, so protecting flesh from the hard plaster). ③
• Immerse the plaster bandage in tepid water and apply it to the dorsum of the arm—without pitting it with your finger tips. ④
• Reflect the stockinette down from the elbow and up from the wrist making comfortable top and bottom ends to the plaster. ⑤
• Place a bandage right around the forearm to keep everything in place, securing its end with a strip of wet plaster. ⑥
• Setting takes place over 4min: sooner if warm water is used.
• Put the arm in a sling for 1 day—after which encourage movement of shoulder, elbow, and fingers to prevent stiffness. ▶*Cautions for the patient:* **1** Return immediately to ED if the fingers go blue, swell, or you cannot move them. **2** Do not get the plaster wet. **3** Do not lift heavy weights with the hand. Give the patient a plaster care information card.

Removing a tight ring from a swollen finger Not only encountered in trauma, remember your pregnant friends too. Pass a No.4 silk suture through the ring from distal to proximal. Wind the distal end around the finger in a distal direction. Then unwind from the proximal end distally (should pull the ring over the coil). Lubrication + compression + traction may also make for success and a relieved patient. If not, try using a ring cutter (not for brass or steel).

'I've caught my penis in my zip' Failing copious lubrication with mineral oil, the most elegant method is to cut the bridge from the slider of the zip with strong wire-cutters as shown in fig 13.12. The zip then falls apart and all that is needed is a new zip. (Beware the bridge flying off at speed: hold gauze by it.) What if the trousers are of immense value? Try the Savile Row technique: infiltrate the skin with 1% lidocaine (no adrenaline!); carefully manipulate the prepuce along the side of the slider by an unzipping movement.

Emergency medicine

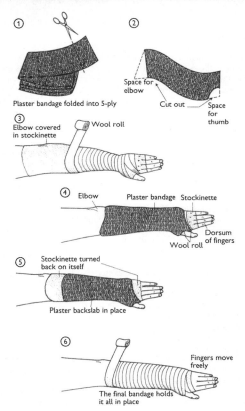

① Plaster bandage folded into 5-ply

② Space for elbow · Cut out · Space for thumb

③ Elbow covered in stockinette · Wool roll

④ Elbow · Plaster bandage · Stockinette · Dorsum of fingers · Wool roll

⑤ Stockinette turned back on itself · Plaster backslab in place

⑥ Fingers move freely · The final bandage holds it all in place

Fig 13.11 Plaster backslab.

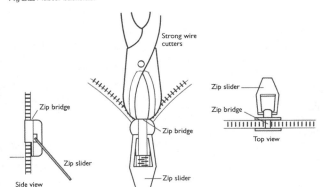

Strong wire cutters

Zip bridge · Zip slider · Side view

Zip bridge · Zip slider

Zip slider · Zip bridge · Top view

Fig 13.12 Solution to the zipped penis problem.

Mammal bites All animal bites are contaminated, especially those of human animals: *everything that comes out of the human mouth is poison.* John Steinbeck *Cannery Row.* Clean well with soap and water, debriding if needed. See p772. ▸Avoid suturing unless cosmetically essential. Give antibiotics covering anaerobes unless very trivial and not high risk (risk↑ if: ♀, >50yrs, immunosuppressed, wound is to the hand, face, or foot, delayed presentation, penetration of underlying structures, crush wound), eg co-amoxiclav 500/125 8h po (clindamycin 300mg/6h po if allergic to penicillin). Bites from monkeys (specifically macaques) require treatment with valaciclovir to prevent transmission of *Cercopithecine herpesvirus 1* which in humans leads to a fatal encephalitis. NB: dog bites may lead to crush injuries, so x-ray to check no underlying fracture or foreign body, bites from cats may not be as trivial as they look: they carry *Pasteurella multocida*, streps, and fusibacteria. Assess tetanus status. Consider rabies if bitten outside UK. See post-exposure rabies prophylaxis guidelines.[3]

Snake bites The WHO considers envenomation to be a neglected tropical disease (see p461), with >10,000 envenomations occurring in India alone. Australia has ~3000 bites per year, with 1–2 fatalities. Britain's only poisonous snake, the adder, is very rarely lethal. There are about 100 bites per year in the UK and only 12 people have died during the last 100 years (last fatality was in 1975.) Adder bites will mostly occur during summer in people walking through long grass. ℞: Immobilize limb and transfer to hospital. Incisions and wound sucking are discouraged, as are bandages and tourniquets as can often be too tight. Identify the species if possible. Treat ABCs—respiratory paralysis, hypotension, cardiac arrest, and seizures can occur. Check clotting time (many venoms are anticoagulant), renal function, CK, D-dimer, FBC, urine for myoglobinuria. Venom detection kits exist—use if there are clinical signs (nausea, reduced GCS, ptosis, weakness, coagulopathy, muscle pain) or abnormal biochemistry. In the UK, give European viper venom antiserum (see BNF). Have adrenaline to hand (p237). If the bite is from a foreign snake or spider, the relevant antivenom may be held in London or Liverpool UK—they are available via www.toxbase.org. For adder bites, observe for at least 2 hours, admit those with evidence of localized swelling or systemic symptoms. Localized pain, swelling, and blistering can occur. Adder toxin continues to damage tissue for 4–5 days so advise rest; typically treated with antihistamines to reduce swelling and antibiotics to prevent secondary infection.

Lesser weever fish stings eg in barefoot UK bathers. It is not serious. Immerse leg for 5–20min in water which is as hot as can be tolerated (eg <45°c).

Scorpion venom *Signs:* BP ↓ or ↑, renal failure, LVF. ℞: Lidocaine SC at the site relieves pain. Antidotes prepared from animal antisera are effective against some species of scorpion. Prazosin & levocarnitine 660mg/8h po *may* help.

Airgun pellets These are common, and can be hard to remove. Get 2 x-ray views to position the foreign body. Ultrasound guidance may also help localize the pellet, but be aware that only shadow or reverberation artefact may be visible, and not the pellet itself. If it has just penetrated the skin, inject local anaesthetic carefully so that you can still palpate it: if you cannot remove it easily, leave it *in situ* rather than risk extensive tissue destruction trying to find it; give antibiotics. Pellets tracking subcutaneously, or which have penetrated deeply, must be sought.

Other foreign bodies ▸*Always do an x-ray if there may be glass/metal/ stone in a wound.* Tiny shards may be left *in situ*. Even large shards can be hard to find, needing exploration under GA to remove. Ultrasound may be useful. ▸Always do orbit x-ray for a high-velocity metallic foreign body that cannot be seen (eg grinding/hammering injury).

3 www.gov.uk/government/publications/rabies-post-exposure-prophylaxis-management-guidelines

Ingestion of a foreign body

Mostly a paediatric problem and rarely affects adults (except those intellectually impaired, mental illness, prisoners, and 'body-packers' who ingest packets of drugs for smuggling). **Children** will often be accompanied by a concerned witness and be asymptomatic at presentation. Always x-ray as, luckily, most commonly ingested items include coins/toys etc which tend to be radio-opaque. If the x-ray shows a FB below level of diaphragm then the patient can go home but advise parents to monitor for signs of obstruction (once in the stomach there is an 80% change of passage). ▶▶Button battery ingestions have a high risk of oesophageal necrosis and require urgent x-rays and referral for removal of object. Suspect chronic oesophageal impaction if presenting with poor feeding, FTT, stridor, PUO or repetitive aspiration pneumonias. **Adults** typically ingest chicken and fish bones; <50% are visible on x-ray, and endoscopic removal is often required. Urgent endoscopy is neccessary if food bolus stuck (? carcinoma).

Failure to pass the FB can range from vague abdominal symptoms, subacute obstruction, to acute obstruction or perforation (causing mediastinitis or peritonitis depending on level).[13]

Examination is often unremarkable but must include examination of abdomen and neck. ▶▶Respiratory assessment is essential; always suspect FB inhalation! If displaying neck/upper airway symptoms then do a lateral CXR which enables differentiation between GI and respiratory tract.

Management Most patients will pass the FB asymptomatically, urgent airway assessment may be needed in upper oesophageal obstruction. Foley catheters and bougienage can be used in stable cooperative patients by experienced practitioners. Endoscopy can remove impacted oesophageal FBs.

Bee stings

Scrape them out gently with a knife or credit card *quickly*. This technique is better at removing a sting than pinching it out, because bee stingers are barbed (fig 13.13), whereas wasp stingers are smooth. As a consequence, the stinger is left in the skin, still attached to the poison sac and tip of the abdomen, meaning that her first sting will likely be her last.[4] Pheromones released from the expiring bee attract more bees, but you may be able to outrun them if you see them coming. NB: although always fatal to the bee, a single sting almost never kills you (risk <1 in 1,000,000; ~4 deaths/yr in UK). Fatalities are more likely if you get >200 stings (but >1000 is survivable). Ice ± calamine lotion help itch. Give antihistamines for severe swelling/itch. Venom allergy is most common cause of anaphylaxis.[14] *Killer bee stings:* (Africanized honeybees: *Apis mellifera scutellata.*) Despite treatment on ITU (antihistamines, corticosteroids, bronchodilators, vasodilators, bicarbonate, mannitol, and ventilation), deaths occur ~1–3 days after the attacks (>100 stings), from ARDS, BP↑↑, hepatic and subendocardial necrosis, haemolysis, rhabdomyolysis, acute tubular necrosis, and DIC.

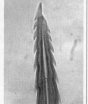
Fig 13.13 Bee stinger (×40).
Courtesy of Jeff Beck

Sidebar: Emergency medicine

Further reading

Munter DW (2014). *Gastrointestinal Foreign Bodies Clinical Presentation.* Medscape. http://emedicine.medscape.com/article/776566-clinical#showall

The primary clinical toxicology database of the National Poisons Information Service: www.Toxbase.org

4 Bees that sting are ♀. The stinger is a vestigial ovipositor that has subsequently become a stinging organ, evolved for defence purposes (against both other bees and larger, thicker-skinned interferers).

Emergency medicine

Major trauma is defined as multiple, serious injuries which could result in serious disability or death. Incidence ~20,000 cases each year in England but trauma is the 6th major cause of death globally (10% of all deaths annually) and the 5th major cause of significant disability. Males aged 17–45 are more affected, probably due to their interest in high-risk sports. The elderly are less commonly affected by trauma but will suffer more as their physiology fails to compensate as effectively.[15]

Although these injuries are quite rare (0.1% of total ED activity)[16] these events create a significant work load as a full trauma team is needed to receive the patient: ED, anaesthetics, surgery, orthopaedics, and radiology. Other specialist members include neurosurgery, plastics, cardiothoracics, maxillofacial, and vascular surgery. Continued care is usually a joint effort on ITU or trauma wards. Intensive rehabilitation and physio starts early in hospital and continues in the community. Pain and disability management is a priority as >50% of trauma patients report impaired quality of life due to pain >2 years post-injury.

Deaths from trauma were originally described by Trunkey[17] in 1983 as following the 'trimodal distribution' where the first peak occurred within minutes due to major neurovascular disruption (rarely treatable). The second peak was attributed to injuries to head, thorax, limbs, or abdomen causing haemorrhage; these patients benefit from early intervention. Days later, the third peak was due to sepsis and organ failure. Improved trauma care has now greatly diminished this last peak, although frequency of first peak/immediate deaths remains similar. Trauma deaths are now largely bimodal, immediate (on scene) 61%, and early (<4h from injury) 29%.[18] Intentional injuries and alcohol intoxication were independent predictors of immediate death.

Trauma scoring

Quantifying the severity of injury and predicting outcome after trauma is a complex field from which multiple scoring systems have arisen. Although perhaps initially intended to be used on-scene to assess injuries and influence patient transfer, scoring systems are now used mainly as research and audit tools to enable trauma centres to evaluate their performance. Anatomical and physiological data is analysed retrospectively using various statistical formulas to calculate expected vs actual survivors. No score is universally accepted or without limitations. Note that trauma scoring in children is especially problematic.

Glasgow Coma Scale (GCS)

This is a subjective way of quantifying the conscious state of a person in response to defined stimuli. It was originally introduced as a method to communicate the consciousness of patients with acute brain injury. It is now widely used for the initial and continuing assessment of any actely unwell patient with altered conscious levels. You can access self-tests here: http://www.glasgowcomascale.org/

Best motor response	Best verbal response	Eye opening
6 Obeying commands	5 Oriented	4 Spontaneous eye opening
5 Localizing response to pain	4 Confused conversation	
4 Withdraws to pain	3 Inappropriate speech	3 Eye opening (to speech)
3 Flexor response to pain	2 Incomprehensible speech	2 Eye opening (to pain)
2 Extensor posturing to pain		
1 No response to pain	1 None	1 No eye opening

Trauma networks

A national audit in 1989 (Trauma Audit and Research Network) www.tarn.ac.uk stated that a proportion of trauma deaths could have been prevented by implementing a more structured approach to care delivered on-scene through to rehabilitation. In response, regional trauma networks were created to channel patients towards major trauma centres equipped with the full MDT services required to cater for the complex needs of a trauma patient. A pivotal tool in trauma care is fast access to a CT scanner for prompt diagnosis. Patients used to wait 7–10 days before transfer to specialist care, TARN now reports that >90% are transferred within 2 days. The focus of trauma care has massively shifted to follow the mantra 'Getting the right patient to the right hospital at the right time' where it is now recognized that despite a longer ambulance trip, getting patients to a major trauma centre not only saves lives, but improves long-term outcome. This shift in the delivery of trauma patients to major centres has fired the development of PHEM (p797) as the need for medical intervention on scene and ensuring patient stability throughout transfer is rising. Although trauma remains the leading cause of death in <40 year olds, the establishment of trauma networks has allowed a 20% increase in survival in patients who would have previously died from severe injuries. However, it remains essential that smaller hospitals retain an understanding of trauma care too.

Emergency medicine

What we take for granted

A staggering 85% of all RTC-related deaths worldwide in 1998 were from developing countries. Developed countries have the advantage of robust transport & infrastructure, political stability, healthcare education, and financial support (fig 13.14). It may seem strange that, despite the long-term existence of specialist hospital care, development of pre-hospital services are still in their early phases. To fully appreciate the large-scale cooperation and resources required to set up national ambulance networks, take a moment to reflect on the difficulties pre-hospital services face. Availability of transport and safe infrastructure are aspects taken for granted in developed countries.

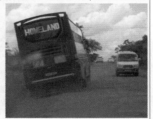

Fig 13.14 Bumpy roads make emergency patient transport very difficult.
© Nina Hjelde.

We rarely think about our patient's journey upon their arrival to hospital, in fact we take it for granted that our patient will be delivered to our door step safely. One of our authors visited Uganda recently in order to teach a trauma course. A story about the local service inspired horror and disbelief in equal measure. A villager suffered a serious leg injury and his neighbours enthusiastically grouped together to borrow a pick-up van which could facilitate prompt transfer to the local hospital. The van sped along the bumpy rural road and arrived hours later. Staff dashed out to help but found no patient. On the drive home they discovered the patient in a ditch. It would seem that he had been catapulted out of the van by a pothole and passed away from a simple airway obstruction following being knocked unconscious. It is a sobering thought that this patient died of something so preventable despite the enthusiasm of his friends. This illustrates the importance of basic safety in transport and simple ABC interventions; foundations upon which our modern ambulance services have taken years to build.

The WHO have generated excellent resources adapted for care facilities staff in developing countries. They outline a sustainable education programme of primary trauma care.   www.primarytraumacare.org

Synonyms Artificial respiration; cardiopulmonary resuscitation (CPR).

Definition BLS is the provision of life support—expired air (your own) ventilation and external chest compressions, without any equipment. The algorithm in fig 13.15 assumes you are the only rescuer present. Ensure the scene is safe to approach. See recovery position (fig 13.2 p762).

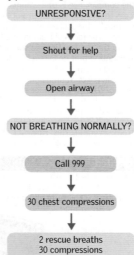

UNRESPONSIVE?

↓

Shout for help

↓

Open airway

↓

NOT BREATHING NORMALLY?

↓

Call 999

↓

30 chest compressions

↓

2 rescue breaths
30 compressions

Fig 13.15 Adult basic life support.

Reproduced with the kind permission of the Resuscitation Council (UK).

Automated chest compression devices?

The delivery of quality compressions with minimal interruptions, consistently adequate depth (at least 5cm) and rate (at least 100bpm), whilst allowing full recoil of the chest wall is difficult, labour intensive, and tiring. The use of automated devices therefore seems attractive, yet there is a paucity of convincing data to support their widespread adoption. A randomized controlled trial (n=4471) involving out-of-hospital cardiac arrest patients showed no evidence of improvement in 30-day survival when compared with manual compression. However, it may be that we see these devices slowly enter select services for particular patient populations as staff become more familiar with their use and more robust studies can be conducted.[19]

Choking in adult patients

Typically sudden onset whilst eating. Early recognition is key and ask patient 'Are you choking'?

Mild obstruction Encourage patient to cough.

Severe obstruction in conscious patient Lean patient forwards with supporting hand on their chest and administer 5 sharp back blows (with heel of hand between shoulder blades) and then 5 abdominal thrusts (stand behind patient with arms wrapped around and fists clenched into epigastrium). Continue alternating between 5 back blows and 5 abdominal thrusts until successful or unconsciousness.

Unconscious choking patient Begin BLS (even in the presence of pulse).

In 1976 (after a light aircraft crash in which he lost his wife), the reflections of the pilot, a Nebraskan orthopaedic surgeon Dr JK Styner, drove him to create the means of disseminating education to optimize care of trauma patients to those for whom trauma did not play a major part in everyday medical practice. By 1978, the ATLS® course became an international standard of care for all trauma patients. The programme also promotes the value of leadership and teamwork. Now in its 9th edition, the course aims to equip non-specialists with the basic skills of providing life-saving trauma care. The ATLS® principles give an excellent structure to the trauma team, but watch out for new research proven to improve outcomes as it can take years for the ATLS® manuals to be updated internationally. ATLS® encourages the ABCDE mantra for every patient. It prioritizes direct treatment according to the most life-threatening injury identified and avoids delay.

▸▸Remember to act immediately. ~10% of trauma deaths arise from airway obstruction.

Primary survey

A: Airway + o₂ + cervical spine. (see c-spine immobilization p782). Assess airway; use jaw thrust in trauma to protect the c-spine. Give 100% o_2. Patients talking to you are unlikely to have significant A or B compromise.

B: Breathing + ventilation. Check air entry with auscultation; also auscultate the heart; inspect, palpate, and percuss the chest wall for further evidence of injury. Check RR. Chest trauma, p788.

C: Circulation + haemorrhage control. Skin perfusion, BP, & pulse. Control any visible haemorrhage with local pressure, and consider possible sources of occult haemorrhage if no source identified but the patient is shocked (see p784). NB: blood loss estimates from the scene of injury are unreliable. Obtain 2 separate points of venous access (take bloods first from one—including pregnancy test). Crossmatch and overestimate the amount of blood lost. RBC replacement will be needed with >1.5L blood loss. Remember the possibility of cardiac or neurogenic shock with a low BP and HR or if unresponsive to fluid resuscitation. Young, fit patients have excellent reserves, and so haemodynamic instability may represent extreme compromise. Abdo trauma, p792. Pelvic trauma, p794. Limb trauma, p734.

Although the ATLS® mantra dictates 1L warmed Ringer's lactate solution/ Hartmann's solution/0.9% normal saline, current evidence supports the use of hypotensive resuscitation (see p784). cABC: The main deaths from trauma arise from CNS complications and catastrophic blood loss.

D: Disability. Check GCS/AVPU, pupillary reflexes, gross evidence of a lateralizing injury or spinal cord level. Also check BM. Head injury, p790.

E: Exposure. Check and maintain body temperature with rewarming methods. Totally undress the patient, cutting all clothes off if necessary. Hypothermia, *OHCM* p860. ▸▸If there is any change in the state of the patient OR if there has been a problem identified and treated during the primary survey, begin the primary survey over again—eg laparotomy may even precede 'D'. Secondary survey (see p786). Now that the patient is stabilized, every inch must be scrutinized for another injury, working from scalp to toe.

▸▸Remember tetanus—p772.

Further reading

Advanced Life Support Group: www.alsg.org/uk

American College of Surgeons (2012). *Advanced Trauma Life Support® (ATLS®)* (9th ed). Chicago, IL: ACS.

Resuscitation Council (UK): www.resus.org.uk

Adjuncts to the primary survey can add life-saving information: a CT scan should ideally be performed within 30 minutes (max 60 minutes) of arrival and have largely superseded the initial CXR, lateral c-spine x-ray and pelvic x-rays. The CT should be reported within 60 minutes.[20] Peripheral x-rays tend to take place during the secondary survey. Urinary catheters can accurately assess urine output (▶▶exclude urethral injury first). NGT insertion (▶▶not in presence of facial #). ABG can accurately assess oxygenation in cold patients where pulse oximetry fails to get a signal.

Airway management in trauma patients

When to intubate is always a tricky question in the stable, moderately injured patient, since the risk of aggravating an occult c-spine injury must be weighed against hypoxia. Even jaw thrust/chin lift techniques can cause distraction of at least 5mm in a cadaver with C5/6 instability.[21] Yet, delayed intubation is associated with increased mortality in patients who were initially stable but later required intubation.[22] This deterioration can be predicted by the presence of rib fractures.

Indications to intubate in trauma often extend beyond ability to oxygenate and ventilate: •GCS <9 •Sustained seizure activity •Facial or airway trauma •High aspiration risk• Flail segments or respiratory failure.

▶▶ Manual inline stabilization is essential (hard collars interfere with procedure) (see p753 for current thoughts on immobilisation of the c-spine).

Logrolling a patient

The ATLS® logrolling technique is used to examine the back or move a patient to another bed. Staff are positioned strategically to ensure that the spine remains immobilized. ▶▶Remember to warn patient as their cooperation is paramount. Remove items in patient's pockets to minimize discomfort and risk patient movement. The person holding the head must lead the roll and use commands familiar to the whole team.

Some studies advocate against incorporating the logroll within the primary survey as it can disrupt internal clots, induce spinal and pelvic movement, and heighten patient distress.[23] Identification of spinal fractures through palpation during a logroll has only shown a 60% success rate (slightly more useful than tossing a coin). Obviously the back must be inspected in penetrating trauma, but prompt CT scanning will identify life-threatening injuries without aggravating existing injury. Moving supine patients in a scoop is suggested as an alternative. ATLS® no longer advocates PR exam as it frequently fails to provide any useful information, rarely alters managment, and distresses the patient. Use of the logroll continues in clinical practice, but perhaps reconsider the value of it prior to CT scanning which can swiftly identify life-threatening issues.

c-spine protection

Protection of the c-spine is the utmost priority in trauma (see also 'Spinal cord injury', p752). ATLS teaches c-spine immobilization should take place simultaneously to airway assessment. Once adequately immobilized, one can focus on life-saving interventions within ABC (see BOX, p753).

▶▶ Always assume the presence of spinal injury in any trauma patient.

Preserving c-spine integrity is time critical; clearing it is not.

The ambulance call to warn you that a young patient in cardiac arrest is due to arrive. ETA 2 minutes. No peripheral venous access obtained, so you know no cardiac drugs have been given yet. *What do you do?* Would you spend precious minutes looking for a vein? Even though the patient has an endotracheal tube in situ, UK resuscitation guidelines no longer use the endotracheal route for drug administration. You've heard of the venous cut-down but it will be time-consuming.

In emergency situations where obtaining IV access will delay treatment, intraosseus (IO) access is desirable.[24] Initially the IO approach was restricted to military and paediatric medicine, but increasingly it is being embraced into adult emergencies (eg trauma, DKA, severe burns) and could potentially play a role in mass casualty CBRN events.[25]

How does it work? Fluids, blood, and all medications commonly used in resuscitation can be pushed into the bone matrix to infuse through the bone marrow cavity and into the systemic circulation. Flow rates up to 200mL/min with pressure are possible. Take a quick sample of bone marrow for glucose, venous blood gas, electrolytes, and haemoglobin before connecting the fluids. Remember to check with the lab beforehand to ensure that they can process such samples.

How do I insert it? The FAST1 device is used for the sternum and the Big Injection Gun (BIG) used for proximal tibia and humerus. The EZ-IO is most commonly used in the UK and accesses proximal and distal tibia and humerus (fig 13.16). It is a battery-operated hand-held drill with different needle sizes dependent on patient's age and tissue depth over the landmarks. To insert the EZ-IO into the tibia, palpate

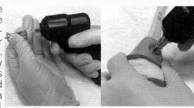

Fig 13.16 The EZ-IO.
Image reprinted with permission from Mark P. Brady, PA-C, and Medscape Drugs & Diseases (http://emedicine.medscape.com/), 2015, available at: http://reference.medscape.com/features/slideshow/intraosseous-access

the tibial tuberosity and place the needle 2.5cm below on the anteromedial aspect of the tibia. Hold the knee in flexion and insert the needle at 90° through subcutaneous tissue until it is stopped by the bone, start drilling through the bone until a loss of resistance is felt (more pronounced in adults). Remove the central trochar and aspirate bone marrow to confirm position. The embedded cannula protrudes out and will require dressings for support.

What can go wrong? IO access is relatively easy to use, with a high success rate and always available in the shocked patient. Contraindications include previous failed attempts, infections or trauma at the insertion site, and previous surgery near site (to avoid hitting prosthetic devices). Complications are rare and largely comprise of fractures from insertion and local extravastation of drugs and fluids; this may lead to compartment syndrome. To minimize osteomyelitis remove IO line as soon as practical after more robust IV access secured. Although pain is significant, patients are most often unconscious.

Further reading

Mayglothling J *et al.* (2012). Emergency tracheal intubation immediately following traumatic injury: an Eastern Association for the Surgery of Trauma practice management guideline. *J Trauma Acute Care Surg* 73(5 Suppl 4):S333-40.

Resuscitation Council (UK) (2015). *Adult Advanced Life Support*. https://www.resus.org.uk/resuscitation-guidelines/adult-advanced-life-support/

Emergency medicine

Initial fluid resuscitation for critically injured patients with suspected major haemorrhage now relies on the concept of **'Damage control resuscitation':**[26]

1 Early haemostasis with surgery, splintage, or angiography
2 Awareness and treatment of the lethal triad (p786)
3 Reduce excessive crystalloid/colloid use
4 Early use of RBCs, plasma, and platelets in 1:1:1 ratio
5 Hypotensive resuscitation.

Surgeons form a key part of the trauma team as the need for internal haemorrhage control is critical. IV tranexamic acid (1g over 10min, then 1g over 4h) within 3h of injury has antifibrinolytic properties and reduces risk of death from bleeding. Crystalloid fluids are avoided in modern trauma resuscitation as they contribute to hypothermia and haemodilution of clotting factors and Hb,[27] thus worsening coagulopathy in trauma already exacerbated by haemorrhage and the looming lethal triad. Permissive hypotension is encouraged as we struggle between worsening tissue hypoxia versus the risk of clot disruption through the hydrostatic forces from BP. ▶▶Only give aliquots of 250mL aiming for: 70–80mmHg in penetrating trauma, 90mmHg in blunt trauma, and simply cerebration in the awake patient. These targets are difficult to achieve in reality and prompt surgical intervention may be needed. Definitive resuscitation takes place after haemostasis has been achieved.

Which fluids to use? Colloids may be superior (FIRST trial)[27] but this is disputed and we don't bleed saline.[29] Blood products facilitate volume expansion that augments coagulation. Use a combination of FFP, platelets, and RBCs (ratio 1:1:1), there is a tendency to only remember RBC but you are reliant on the coagulation factors present in FFP. Warm fresh whole blood (WFWB) contains a full complement of platelets, clotting factors, and fibrinogen leading to improved outcome when compared to 1:1:1 component therapy,[30] but WFWB is typically only used by the military as blood components are difficult to store and good donor availability hinders the <24h shelf-life. Fibrinogen is key to clotting and early replacement may improve outcomes.

Trauma-induced coagulopathy can be challenging to identify so treat on clinical suspicion (see 'The lethal triad', p786). Standard lab tests fail to demonstrate the clotting derangements unique to trauma; especially evaluation of clot strength critical to assessing internal haemorrhage. Trauma patients are typically young and their physiological reserve will readily compensate despite significant blood loss and tissue hypoxia; this 'cryptic shock' is associated with increased mortality. Although the ATLS® course suggests how basic physiological parameters can aid the estimation of blood loss, these values have been disputed[31] and further prove that physiological markers cannot be solely relied upon. Metabolic assessment of lactate, base excess, and central venous oxygenation can also be indicators of blood loss.

As it becomes increasingly obvious that correcting coagulopathies improves mortality rates, 'Point-of-care coagulation' testing allows rapid (~20min) assessment of clotting profiles and in theory will enable early targeted blood component therapy. This is still in early phases of implementation into clinical practice.

Deciding when and which blood products to use can be confusing and there is conflicting research on what is needed in trauma. Every hospital has a 'major haemorrhage protocol', once initiated blood bank promptly delivers predetermined ORh –ve blood components until full cross-matching takes place. Consider Beriplex® early on if a patient on warfarin is actively bleeding. Ask for haematology specialist advice if needed (*OHCM* p.342).

On the floor and four more

Hypovolaemia is the main cause of shock in trauma and sources of blood loss are 'on the floor and 4 more': Chest—treat haemothorax with chest drain. Abdomen — might need surgical intervention. Do not underestimate the value of splinting the long bones and pelvis for haemorrhage control. Note non-haemorrhagic causes of shock include spinal injury (neurogenic shock), cardiac tamponade, drug effects, and tension pneumothorax.

Occult blood loss
• Long bones (0.75 L) (p811)
• Pelvic # (several L)
• Abdomen (all) needs surgical intervention
• Chest (all) treat with chest drain (see fig 13.17)

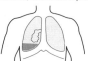 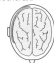 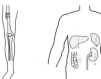

Fig 13.17 Where to look for occult blood loss.

Emergency ultrasound

Physical examination of trauma patients may yield equivocal results and investigations are often required, especially in blunt abdominal trauma (p792). **Focused assessment with sonography with trauma (FAST)** evaluates the presence of free fluid in the peritoneum or pericardium—which in the context of trauma is assumed to be blood (fig 13.18). Free fluid is black and typically collects around organs or gravity-dependent recesses. FAST can detect ~200mL intraperitoneal fluid with 90% sensitivity, smaller volume identification possible with more experienced operators. (NB: free fluid can also be urine from bladder rupture, ascites, peritoneal dialysis). It is not sensitive at detecting liver and spleen tears or hollow viscous injuries.

Extended FAST (eFAST) can also identify haemo- and pneumothoraces; demonstrated to have a greater sensitivity for small pneumothoraces than CXR, especially in the supine trauma patient. It is especially useful in the hypotensive patient with no obvious source of bleeding—within minutes the team can know to focus on thorax, mediastinum, or abdomen. Also useful in stable patients with no indication yet for exposure to CT radiation, but presenting with worrying mechanisms of injury.

In ATLS®, sonography is performed immediately after the primary survey as resuscitation can be ongoing throughout. It is rapid, reproducible, and non-invasive; rendering the diagnostic peritoneal lavage (DPL) obsolete.[5]

Fig 13.18 Shown are the 4 transducer positions in FAST: (1) pericardial (2) right and (3) left upper quadrant and (4) pelvis.

Reproduced from Scott A. LeMaire, MD, Raja R. Gopaldas, MD. Organ Systems. 'Cardiac System'. In: Ashley SA, editor. *Scientific American Surgery* [online]. Hamilton (ON): Decker Intellectual Properties; July 2015. Available at: http://www.sciamsurgery.com

Further reading

Dutton RP (2008). Pathophysiology of traumatic shock. *ITACCS* 18:12–15. http://www.trauma-care.org/traumacare/archive/2008_vol18_no1/Pathophysiology_of_Traumatic_Shock_Itaccs_vol18no1-4.pdf

Harris T et al. (2012). Early fluid resuscitation in severe trauma. *BMJ* 345:e5752.

Reardon R. *Ultrasound in Trauma - The FAST Exam.* http://www.sonoguide.com/FAST.html

5 Diagnostic peritoneal lavage: insertion of a catheter into peritoneum. If no free fluid can be aspirated, then 1L warmed normal saline was infused for 5min then drained and sent for analysis. Presence of blood, WCC or faecal material was indication for laparotomy. Largely replaced by FAST in UK as it is time-consuming and technically difficult so rarely used.

The 'lethal triad' describes the interaction of three physiological parameters seen in major trauma, their presence is predictable and associated with high mortality rates (fig 13.19). The cascade of inflammatory mediators (clinically producing SIRS) and neuroendocrine compensatory mechanisms can ultimately lead to multiple organ failure *even after* the initial insult has been corrected in severely injured patients.[32]

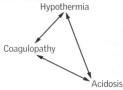

Fig 13.19 The lethal triad.

Hypothermia is traditionally defined as T°<35°c, but is defined at T°<36°c in trauma since it has been associated with especially poor outcomes.[33] The elderly, intoxicated, burnt, and exposed patients are esp. at risk. Hypothermia dampens the CVS compensatory mechanisms against hypovolaemic shock thus worsening tissue hypoxia. **Acidosis** arises from tissue hypoperfusion and subsequent lactic acid production, further exacerbated by respiratory acidosis arising from hypoventilation (flail chest, opiates/alcohol, COPD). Temperature and pH heavily influence clotting and platelet function; even subtle physiological disruptions can contribute to life-threatening coagulopathies as the patient continues to haemorrhage, which in turn depletes clotting factors and platelets. **Coagulopathy** develops in ~25% of severely injured patients and is associated with 4× increase in mortality rates; its presence demands respect.[34] Coagulopathy in trauma was, until recently, thought to arise mainly from haemorrhage and haemodilution from excessive fluid resuscitation; but coagulopathy has been noted to develop within minutes of injury causing reduced tissue perfusion. Note pre-existing medical conditions that alter clotting (liver failure) or oral anti-coagulants (warfarin, dabigatran).

▸▸Simple early interventions against hypothermia and haemorrhage control can help stave off this lethal triad. Optimizing the patient's physiological state should be a priority; this starts with basic care on-scene. It is estimated that ~20% of trauma deaths could be prevented with better haemorrhage control.[35] Enthusiastically search for all bleeding points and apply pressure; this includes a pelvic binder for internal haemorrhage. Always assume your patient is becoming colder—this is easy to forget as you sweat from working. Apply blankets, use a Bair Hugger™ and warmed fluids.

Secondary survey

The secondary survey is a thorough head-to-toe examination following completion of ABCDE once the patient is responding to initial resuscitation. It includes taking a more complete history and further imaging (US, angiography, etc.). Continuous reassessment of ABCDE is still expected. It is often poorly performed and documented in the aftermath of an adrenaline-filled ABCDE assessment. It is especially important in the unconscious patient who is unable to report a finger fracture or testicular rupture.

A mnemonic was proposed to help add focus to this assessment (see MINIBOX).[36]

Mnemonic	Secondary survey
• Has	• Head/skull
• My	• Maxillofacial
• Critical	• Cervical spine
• Care	• Chest
• Assessed	• Abdomen
• Patient's	• Pelvis
• Priorities	• Perineum
• Or	• Orifices (PR/PV)
• Next	• Neurological
• Management	• Musculoskeletal
• Decision?	• Diagnostic tests/ definitive care

Emergency medicine

Your assessment of the patient starts the moment you approach the scene. Remember that clinical signs of injury may not manifest on-scene, largely due to circulating catecholamines. Understanding the mechanism of injury is critical to diagnoses made in major trauma. It's a bit like taking a history as reading the wreckage creates a picture of anticipated injuries. Become suspicious when your predictions are not found. Appreciation of which injuries might have been sustained also helps extrication methods (see p808). Hospital staff receive patients already packaged by the ambulance crew; it can be difficult to appreciate the severity of the trauma scene without a good handover. Pictures from the scene can be useful here.

There are 4 components leading to injury from motor vehicle crashes:
- Impact of vehicle with object
- Occupants hit inside of vehicle
- Organs jerked to a halt (risk of ruptured liver/torn aortic arch, esp. if >40mph)
- Impact from unrestrained objects/occupants

NB: Modern cars are made safer with airbags, crumple zones, and seatbelts.

Motor cyclists have 4 points of injury:
- Impact of vehicle with object
- Pelvic and femoral fractures from impact with handlebars and fuel tanks
- Impact of landing
- Organs jerked to a halt.

Questions to ask Airbag deployed? Car written off? Other passengers? Damage sustained to car? Major bodywork distortion—assume major injury. Seatbelt worn? What type of seatbelt (right/left shoulder strap, lap belt)? Relate the damage of the vehicle to potential injuries.

'Bulls-eye' on windscreen Suggests facial fractures and internal head injuries (often due to lack of seatbelt). Rear view mirror may also cause damage.

Impact onto steering wheel Suspect severe chest injuries or abdominal compression (may result in diaphragmatic rupture). If wearing a seat belt, clavicle and sternal injuries are common and bruising from belt across abdomen may suggest internal organ damage (such as rupture of small bowel).

Intruding dashboard may compress femur and dislocate hip posteriorly (thigh will be abducted and internally rotated with left knee held in fixed flexion deformity). Look for patellar injury.

Intruding engine compartment Look for tibia/fibula injuries or trapped feet.

Lateral impact Vehicles are better designed to tolerate frontal impacts over lateral. Associated with 44% of all RTA-induced aortic dissections and lateral chest, abdominal and pelvic compression injuries.

Rear impact Lower back and whiplash injuries.

Fall from height Injuries are dependent on height and type of surface. Landing on heels leads to a characteristic pattern of injury following the transmission of force through the body; calcaneum #, Pilon ankle # (p738), tibial plateau #, hip injury, spinal compression at any level, base of skull #.

Further reading

Calland V *et al.* (2013). Scene safety and assessment. In Nutbeam T, Boylan B (eds) *ABC of Prehospital Emergency Medicine*, pp13–17. Chichester: Wiley-Blackwell. P. 14 ABC of trauma /pre hospital care

Gerecht R (2014). *Trauma's Lethal Triad of Hypothermia, Acidosis & Coagulopathy Create a Deadly Cycle for Trauma Patients.* http://www.jems.com/article/patient-care/trauma-s-lethal-triad-hypothermia-acidos

Hodgetts *et al.* (2008). *Trauma Rules 2: Incorporating Military Trauma Rules* (2nd ed). Oxford: Blackwell.

Hypoxia is the most serious feature of chest trauma: ▸▸Start 15L O_2 in non-rebreather bag in all patients. ATLS® teaches that the **Primary survey** will identify the following life-threatening injuries 'ATOM FC' and these should be corrected as they are identified. ▸▸Assume all patients have a c-spine injury until proven otherwise.

Airway obstruction is associated with trauma to neck, face, and larynx. Laryngeal injury and posterior dislocations of the clavicular head can directly obstruct the airway. Listen for noisy breathing, stridor, or altered voice quality. ▸▸High risk of vomiting and aspirating; have suction quickly available. *Tension pneumothorax* develops when penetrating injury creates a 'one-way valve' forcing air from lung or through chest wall into thoracic cavity. The affected lung is collapsed, and mediastinum displaced away, resulting in ↓ venous return and compression of the opposite lung. ▸▸Immediate decompression of affected side with large-bore cannula inserted into 2nd intercostal space midclavicular line. Definitive treatment involves chest tube insertion. *Open pneumothorax* (sucking chest wound) arises from large chest wall defects and necessitates immediate occlusion with sterile dressings taped on 3 sides to create a flutter-valve effect; complete the seal upon chest drain insertion. *Massive haemothorax* accumulation of >1500mL blood/fluid in hemithorax can cause shock. Wounds of intercostal vessels, great vessels, or heart can cause massive haemorrhage; haemopnuemothoraces are common. Treat with large-bore chest drain (32G) and simultaneous IV fluid/blood replacement. Consider auto-transfusion of blood. Thoracotomy may be needed. *Flail chest* describes a segment of fractured ribs with no bony continuity with the rest of the chest wall; resulting in disrupted chest wall movement and pulmonary contusions of underlying lung, causing serious hypoxia. Give high-flow O_2. The need for intubation and ventilation depends on respiratory distress and P_aO_2. Pulmonary contusions may also occur in blunt injury and are frequently missed; suspect if significant hypoxia persists with no other obvious cause. *Traumatic cardiac tamponade* 15% of deep chest injuries involve the heart. *Diagnosis:* Clinical diagnosis using Beck's triad (rising JVP, falling BP, muffled HS)(+ pulsus paradoxus) is difficult in the trauma situation. (Portable US is more reliable—black stripe around heart indicates fluid.) ▸▸Pericardial aspiration may buy time before thoracotomy. *Procedure* (OHCM p787): Insert an 18G needle to the left of the xiphoid (preferably under US guidance). Aim at the left shoulder but with needle angled downwards at 45°. Elevate legs to help venous return. Emergency needle pericardiocentesis is only a temporizing measure and may fail due to clotted blood, pericardotomy is the definitive treatment. These patients need urgent cardiothoracic input, frequent ECHOs, and invasive monitoring in ITU.

Secondary survey tends to identify more subtle injuries and relies on adjuncts. *Simple pneumothorax:* (OHCM p182.) Observe for progression to tension pneumothorax. *Simple haemothorax:* (<1500mL blood.) Lacerations in lung or blood vessels tend to be self-limiting and do not require surgery. Large-calibre (36 French) chest tube if haemothorax large enough to visualize on CXR. If not fully evacuated, residual blood can clot and cause lung entrapment or infection. *Tracheobronchial tree/aortic disruption* tends to cause death at scene and requires urgent surgical intervention. Suspicion based on mechanism of injury and CXR findings (widened mediastinum, altered tracheobronchial anatomy). Missing a diagphragmic injury can cause insidious respiratory distress or bowel strangulation. *Blunt cardiac injury:* Significant injury is quite uncommon as most die on-scene. May result in life-threatening arrhythmias so consider careful ECG monitoring and US. Troponin rise in blunt injury may indicate cardiac contusion.[37] *Oesophageal rupture:* Consider if disproportionally unwell when compared to apparent injury. Typically associated with left pleural effusions and/or pnuemomediastinum.

Blast injury may be encountered in domestic (eg gas explosion), industrial (eg mining) accidents or military/terrorist bombings. Typically will have multiple casualties (see p813 for mass casualty). There are 4 recognized phases of a blast, each is associated with a unique pattern of injury:

Primary injuries are characterized by an absence of external features; the resultant internal injuries are often missed or their severity under-estimated. The wave of overpressure generated by the explosion compresses gas-filled spaces such as ears (deafness should prompt thoughts of significant blast injury), intestinal perforation and haemorrhage, and fatal air embolism affecting coronary or cerebral arteries. Pulmonary barotrauma 'blast lung' is the most common cause of death in those who survive the explosion. Intra-alveolar haemorrhage causes acute respiratory distress syndrome (*OHCM* p178) and may be delayed (up to 48h).

Secondary injuries arise from missiles and projectile debris striking the victim causing a combination of blunt and penetrating injuries. These are the most common injuries.

Tertiary injuries caused by the victim being thrown by the blast wind and striking the surrounding objects.

Quaternary other injuries caused by the explosion—eg burns, asphyxia, crush injuries. Consider toxic substance exposure (eg radiation, co, or cyanide poisoning is associated with burning buildings).

Psychological support is essential. Acute fear and panic is the aim of the terrorist. Later, chronic intrusive thoughts, anxiety, and poor concentration may form the basis of post-traumatic stress disorder (p353).

▶▶Do not approach the scene until the possibility of a secondary device has been excluded and it has been declared safe to approach.

Also remember that you are at a forensic scene, do not disturb the environment (or any dead bodies) unless necessary to treat the patient.

Gun shot injuries

Deaths by firearms must be influenced by other factors other than their availability since WHO report that Switzerland has a high gun ownership (46 guns per 100 residents; USA 90; UK 6), but a relatively low homicide rate (0.5 per 100,000; USA 4.1; UK 0.1) and high gun suicide rate (5.8 per 100,000; USA 6.1; UK 0.2). Gun violence is hyped by the media but it causes only 0.5% of UK trauma. Gunshot wounds (GSWs) to the head are the most lethal (90%), followed by myocardium (80%). Gunshots to chest commonly cause a haemopneumothorax.

GSWs are typically divided into ↓velocity (<1000ft/sec eg most handguns, will lacerate and crush tissues) and ↑velocity (>1000ft/sec eg military rifles, are more destructive due to cavitation and the associated shock wave).
- Unremarkable surface examination may hide much deeper internal injuries.
- Factors influencing internal injury: weapon used, bullet speed and distance, trajectory, yaw, and tumble.

The GMC (www.gmc-uk.org) and BMA (www.bma.org.uk) offer legal guidance on how to liaise with police (as they conduct risk assessments for patient/public and will seek patient details) in potentially difficult medico-legal situations including patient consent.

Further reading

Born CT (2005). Blast trauma: the fourth weapon of mass destruction. *Scand J Surg* 94:279–85.

The Trauma Audit & Research Network: www.tarn.ac.uk

Emergency medicine

Primary traumatic brain injury occurs at the time of impact. Secondary injury arises mins–days later from neurophysiological consequences and anatomical damage incurred by the primary insult eg ↑ intracranial pressure (ICP), cerebral oedema, expanding haematomas, seizures, and infection.

Assaults (~40%), falls (~30%), and RTAs (~25%) account for the majority of minor head injuries, whilst RTAs take the lead in moderate–severe head injuries. Alcohol complicates up to 65% of presentations; is it alcohol that is causing vomiting/confusion or is it a serious head injury? Would you subject a young person to the radiation just to make sure? A CT head equates to 8 months of background radiation, increased to 16 months if repeated with contrast.[38]

Cranial injuries
• Skull fracture
• c-spine fractures
Intracranial injuries
• Diffuse axonal injury
• Extradural bleed*
• Subdural bleed*
• Subarachnoid bleed#
• Intracerebral bleed
• Cerebral contusion
(See images: *OHCM p487; #p483)

Assessment follows the ABCDE mantra, paying particular attention to GCS (p778) trends, pupil sizes, and c-spine protection (BOX, p753). Document all neurological trends meticulously. Unequal pupils are less important if conscious, but a grave sign in coma. Look for localizing neurological long tract signs ie assess power, tone, reflexes, and all sensory modalities, comparing right side vs left, upper body vs lower. Check for priapism and anal tone which can suggest spinal cord damage, although priapism is more likely to arise from pelvic or penile injury. Remember that spinal shock will also cause transient neurological features (see p752). Low BP together with inappropriately low pulse rate indicates sympathetic disruption in cervical spinal cord.

▶▶The clinical imperative is to prevent/minimize secondary brain injury by optimizing ABC; do not neglect other injuries leading to ↓BP, hypoxia, etc.

Imaging is guided by the 2014 NICE guidelines.[39] Note there are different guidelines for <16-year-olds. See also 'The neck', p753. Patients presenting with head injury and reduced GCS need a CT head within the first hour of injury with a written report available within 1h of scan. If no identified risk factors (see BOX) all patients on warfarin/known coagulopathy should have a CT head within 8h (see BOX). Note that NICE does not take into account the newer anticoagulants and only mentions warfarin; you should treat all anticoagulants as you would warfarin.

▶▶Always consider possibility of c-spine damage in patients with head injury.

Urgent CT head if:[39]	And add cervical spine (CT) if:[39] (see p717)
• GCS <13 at initial assessment	• GCS <13 at initial assessment
• GCS <15 at 2h post injury	• Intubation
• Open or depressed skull or basal skull fracture	• Definitive diagnosis of c-spine injury is required urgently (eg before surgery)
• Post-traumatic fit	• Other areas are being scanned for head injury
• Focal CNS deficit	or multi-region trauma.
• >1 episode of vomiting.	The patient is alert and stable, there is a suspicion of c-spine injury and any of the following are present:
CT head if any LOC/amnesia &	
• Age >65 years	• Age >65
• Dangerous mechanism of injury	• Dangerous mechanism of injury
• Coagulopathy	• Focal CNS deficit
• Retrograde amnesia >½h.	• Paraesthesia in upper or lower limbs.

If CT is abnormal, GCS <15, or significant symptoms or signs you must admit 'under a consultant with specialist training in managing head injured patients'. Tertiary referral to neurosurgical services should be according to agreed local guidelines. Those patients with no concerning features can be discharged with *head injury advice leaflets*.

Older patients presenting with unwitnessed falls and patchy histories are an important subgroup of patients presenting with minor head injury. It is becoming increasingly recognized that symptomology and INR values cannot predict intracranial haemorrhage (ICH) (even a sub-therapeutic INR does not appear to offer protection). In response, a key change in the NICE guidelines is that all warfarinized patients presenting with head injury should receive a CT scan within 8h. Further updates (Royal College of Emergency Medicine) state that all warfarinized head injuries should be scanned within 1 hour. ▶▶Consider early reversal of high INR (even before CT head/INR results) if strong suspicion of ICH. Minimizing haematoma expansion is key to improving morbidity and mortality rates.[40] Risk of ICH is higher in patients on clopidogrel (12%) than warfarin (5%).[41]

Discharging patients on anticoagulants It can be tempting to observe these patients in hospital for features of delayed ICH, yet this complication is rare (0% in clopidogrel, <1% in warfarin). These patients can be sent home with comprehensive written advice.

Physiology of head injury management

Intracranial pressure (ICP) is raised if >20mmHg. The normal occupants of the cranium are CSF, blood, and brain tissue (90%). The Monro–Kellie doctrine explains how the presence of an intracranial mass can initially be accommodated by displacing venous blood and CSF, but a limit is quickly reached where ICP will ↑ and restrict cerebral perfusion pressure (CPP), thus worsening cerebral ischaemia. Key principles in management include enhancing cerebral perfusion by normalizing ICP and monitoring the mean arterial pressure (MAP) since CPP = MAP − ICP. Target MAP to ~90mmHg to ensure CPP>60mmHg.

Medical managment of head injury

The aim is to prevent secondary brain injury and optimize recovery by optimizing physiological parameters (see OHCM p840):

- *Avoidance of hypotension:* Keep systolic BP>90. Even a single episode of low BP is associated with worse outcomes in severe traumatic brain injury. Normovolaemia with isotonic solutions are favoured. Do not overload (risk of cerebral oedema). Do not use glucose preparations (damage brain tissue).
- *Avoidance of hypoxia and hypercapnia:* Keep P_aO_2>11 KPa and P_aCO_2 between 4.5–5.0 KPa in order to optimize CPP. Hyperventilation will reduce P_aCO_2, resulting in cerebral vasoconstriction which reduces the effects of ↑ICP. Only use as a temporizing measure for the reduction of acute elevations of ICP since vasoconstriction may also lead to ↑ischaemia thereby worsening neurological injury.
- *Opiates* can be used to mitigate the stress response from intubation and prevent a surge in ICP.
- *Mannitol:* 0.25–1g/kg of 20% mannitol solution causes osmotic diuresis, aiming to reduce ICP in the acute situation (such as impending herniation eg dilated, non-reactive pupil). Avoid systemic hypotension.
- *Seizure control:* Treat aggressively with IV lorazepam/buccal midazolam as the stress with ↑ICP. Prophylactic anti-epileptics may mitigate early seizures, but there is no evidence they reduce occurrence of late seizures.
- *Raise head 30°* to improve jugular venous return.
- *Avoidance of hyperglycaemia and hyperpyrexia.*
- *Urgent neurosurgical input* if mass amenable to surgery.

Further reading

Olson DA (2014). *Head Injury: Treatment & Management.* Medscape. http://emedicine.medscape.com/article/1163653-treatment

SIGN (2009). *Early Management of Patients with a Head Injury* (SIGN 110). http://www.sign.ac.uk/guidelines/fulltext/110/

Diagnosis of abdominal injury in trauma patients can be difficult; maintain a high index of suspicion. ▶▶Early surgical review is essential. Remember that the abdomen extends from nipples (T4) to groin anteriorly and to iliac crests posteriorly—although diaphragmatic rupture may also expose abdominal contents to injury in the chest. **Key questions** Is the peritoneum breached? Are the intra-peritoneal organs damaged? ▶▶Do not deny analgesia on finishing your assessment, simply for fear of masking signs.

Penetrating injuries from high-velocity missiles (gunshots, shrapnel, etc.) are more difficult to predict compared to stab wounds (see 'Gunshot injuries' p789). Most penetrating injuries require prompt laparotomy/laparoscopy if the posterior rectus sheath is breached; all but the most superficial injuries will require exploration. Liver is the most commonly injured abdominal organ in penetrating trauma (MINIBOX).

Stab involvement
Liver (40%)
Small bowel (30%)
Diaphragm (20%)
Colon (15%)

Blunt trauma Deceleration forces may tear bowel from mesentery, liver from vena cava, bladder from bladder neck, pancreas from retroperitoneum, and aorta from itself. The spleen is the most commonly injured abdominal organ in blunt trauma (MINIBOX). ▶▶Suspect a ruptured spleen in the presence of shock, abdominal tenderness /distension, left shoulder tip pain, and an overlying rib #.

Blunt involvement
Spleen (~50%)
Liver (~40%)
Small bowel (~10%)
Retroperitoneal (15%)

Unstable patients (BP; shock; GI, GU, or PR bleeding; evisceration; peritonitis) warrant immediate laparotomy to identify source of injury and bleeding. Initial FAST scan (p785) can demonstrate haemoperitoneum. Obtaining a CT should not delay operative intervention, but portable CXR can be achieved quickly. Cross-match >6 units blood. Hypotensive resuscitation (p784).

Stable patients must still be treated with a high index of suspicion, systolic BP doesn't fall consistently until >30% of blood volume is lost. There is no substitute for monitoring vital signs and examining the abdomen often with repeated FAST scans. 10% of injuries in trauma are initially missed and ~30% of patients with significant abdominal trauma have unremarkable initial assessments. CVP measurements, CT, and US may all mislead. Consider diagnostic laparoscopy to evaluate damage to peritoneum and diaphragm rather than exploratory laparotomy. Observe for a minimum of 24 hours as pancreatic and hollow viscus injury may not initially be seen radiologically.

Asymptomatic stable patients with anterior abdominal stab wounds

Historicallly, all stab wounds were evaluated with routine laparoscopies, this practice is no longer accepted. >25% of anterior abdominal stab wounds do not penetrate the abdominal cavity and only 50% of penetrating wounds require surgical intervention. Wound assessment which can demonstrate an intact rectus fascia has been found to be reliable in excluding peritoneal penetration. Comprehensive wound exploration can facilitate the safe and early discharge of 25% of patients with an abdominal stab wound from the ED, thus reducing unnecessary hospital admissions and surgical interventions.

Use local anaesthetic and you may need to extend the wound for better views. When in doubt or end point of wound track not clearly defined, further investigation with FAST scans and serial clinical examinations (preferably by the same clinician) can aid identification of injuries not immediately apparent. *Caution:* Exploration of lower chest wounds incurs risk of iatrogenic pneumothorax. Wounds tracking posteriorly are more difficult to assess due to increased musculature and contrast CT is advised. Increased BMI or uncooperative patients can make exploration more unreliable.

No longer the doughnut of death?

Once described as the 'doughnut of death', the CT scanner was frequently skipped in favour of direct transport to the operating theatre. However, as imaging becomes faster and safer for unstable patients, and resources more available, trauma care is becoming increasingly reliant on radiological imaging such as CT, FAST, and angiography.

Interventional radiology in trauma

Unrecognized haemorrhage, especially in the abdomen, and subsequent delay in treatment contribute to most preventable deaths in trauma. Early resuscitation is key to prevent the lethal triad (p784). Prompt surgical intervention has historically been advocated in these patients, however the rise of interventional radiology has successfully used transcatheter embolization to block bleeding vessels and stents to realign them; these minimally invasive techniques aim to stop the bleeding without the physiological stress of surgery.

Haemodynamically, patients with solid organ injuries (liver, kidney, spleen) are increasingly being managed with endovascular techniques. Embolization of splenic injuries has similar survival rates, yet may help avoid the impaired immunity associated with splenectomy. Stent grafting in the management for traumatic rupture of thoracic aorta is well established.

Severe injuries causing haemodynamic instability, which would typically have skipped CT in preference for immediate operation, are now only considered a relative contraindication for interventional radiology (see *Pelvic injury*, p794). Emerging evidence is supporting additional indications for endovascular approaches to those haemodynamically unstable and thus continue to reduce the need for surgery.

The current evidence base in trauma management is insufficient to create conclusive guidelines as to when surgical or radiological intervention is most appropriate, and institutional resources must be considered. ▸▸Management of the bleeding trauma patient should always involve expertise from both trauma surgeons and interventional radiologists. The RAPTOR (resuscitation with angiography, percutaneous techniques, and operative repair) suite is a novel concept incorporating interventional radiology, surgery, and resuscitation equipment in one location in order to minimize transfer times and optimize resuscitation without interruption (fig 13.20).

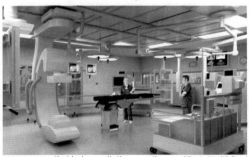

Fig 13.20 RAPTOR—the ideal resuscitation room.[42]   Alberta Health Services.

Further reading

Morris CS (2015). *Interventional Radiology for Vascular and Solid Organ Trauma*. Medscape. http://emedicine.medscape.com/article/423295

Zealley IA *et al*. (2010). The role of interventional radiology in trauma. *BMJ* 340:c497.

Emergency medicine

Rang's aphorism: *The pelvis is like a suit of armour: after damage there is much more concern about its contents than about the structure itself.*[43]

Owing to the ring structure of the pelvis, single fractures from eldery falls are often stable (see BOX) and just need a few weeks' rest. In contrast, ≥2 fractures in the pelvis (with one above the level of the hip) renders the ring unstable and is a serious injury, more than 25% have internal injuries.

> ### The stability of pelvic fractures
>
> 'Rocking the pelvis' is no longer recommended as it may disturb the tamponading effect of any retroperitoneal haematoma, thus exacerbating haemorrhage. The pelvis may be gently compressed (once, preferably by the most senior doctor present) to assess stability. Multiple systems exist. Most useful is the Tile classification (fig 13.21).
>
>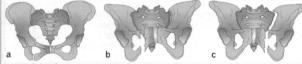
>
> Fig 13.21 Pelvic fractures. (a) Vertically stable, rotationally stable eg isolated pubic rami # or iliac wing fractures. (b) Vertically stable, rotationally unstable eg ipsi-or contralateral ('bucket handle' type) lateral compression #; 'open-book' fracture (look for widening at the SI joints and diastasis (=separation) of the pubic symphysis). (c) Vertically unstable, rotationally unstable; eg # through ipsilateral SI joint and pubic rami. Includes Malgaigne's fracture (20% of all pelvic #s, 60% of unstable ones)—disruption of the pelvis anteriorly and posteriorly with displacement of a fragment containing the hip joint. NB: a clue to the presence of vertical instability is superior migration of the pelvic fragment.

Signs of pelvic fracture Leg length discrepancy, abdominal distension, loin bruising, perineal or scrotal haematoma, PV bleeding, palpable haematoma or # line on PR/PV exam (rectal injury is common 5% and associated with sepsis risk).

Signs of GU injury Urethral injury occurs in up to 15% of males (typically with type B & C fractures). Extra-peritoneal bladder rupture can give false +ve FAST scan. Blood at urethral tip (signifying ruptured urethra), frank or microscopic haematuria, PR exam to assess bowel integrity and presence of blood. Seek urology opinion if suspicion of urethral damage (retrograde urethrography must be performed before catheterization if urethral injury is suspected). Suprapubic catheterization may be necessary.

Reduce blood loss Have a low threshold to apply pelvic splints. These are placed firmly over the greater trochanters (preferably at the site of accident). Do not over compress the pelvis to less than normal circumference. Avoid log-rolls, use orthopaedic scoops which minimize pelvic disruption. ▶▶Check foot pulses and urine output often. Shock in pelvic fracture carries a mortality of 14–55%.[44]

Associated injury? >25% of patients have internal injuries in B & C fractures. In one series there were splenic lesions (37%), diaphragm (21%) and bladder ruptures (24%), liver lacerations (19%), urethral lesions (17%), intestinal lesions (17%), and kidney rupture (9%).

Radiology FAST scan can quickly assess the presence of intraperitoneal fluid (can miss retroperitoneal collections); see p793. Only do pelvic x-ray if no indication for CT. Endovascular embolization for haemorrhage control in pelvic fractures is well established as surgical exploration is technically challenging and fraught with complications. The pelvic fracture is temporarily immobilized and can be fixed later when the patient is fitter for surgery.

▸▸Alert both obstetric and trauma teams who must work in unison, not sequentially. Trauma is the leading cause of maternal death and an important complication in pregnancy as it affects 1 in 12 pregnancies. Road safety is key, see p798 on the importance of public health. Educate on safe use of seatbelts (fig 13.22). Pregnant women are more prone to falls due to weight gain and joint laxity. Blunt trauma (often RTAs) commonly causes placental abruption with a high risk of feto-maternal haemorrhage (p56) whilst penetrating trauma is typically associated with poor foetal survival and better maternal outcomes. Fetal death is mostly associated with hypoxia secondary to cardiovascular disruption.

▸▸Maintain all women beyond 3rd trimester in a left lateral tilt position (15–30 degrees) to prevent aortocaval compression. Left displacement of the uterus increases cardiac output by 30%.

▸▸Rh –ve mothers must be given IM anti-D (see BOX, p11) promptly within 72 hours after abdominal trauma.

Although the primary trauma survey is identical, differences in maternal and fetal physiology (p6) must be acknowledged. In addition to the routine secondary survey, assessment in pregnancy should include vaginal/perineal/rectal examination and continuous fetal monitoring. Think of the fetus as an end-organ; fetal distress is an early sign of hypovolaemia in a relatively asymptomatic mother. Try to establish the gestational age quickly as this will help you predict anatomical damage and physiological changes. Blood loss is typically underestimated. The general approach is that resuscitation of the mother will in turn resuscitate the fetus. Do not undertreat maternal trauma out of fear for fetal welfare.

Indications for caesarean section[45]
• Laparotomy needed to assess internal organs
• Uterine rupture
• Fetal distress with viable fetus
• Maternal cardiac arrest within 5min of CPR (to save mother as delivery of fetus facilitates improved CPR compression technique, reduction of O_2 consumption, assessment of internal organs, and access for internal cardiac massage).

Pelvic # is not an absolute indication and women can attempt vaginal delivery in stable #s.

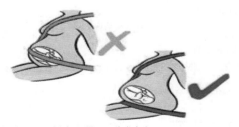

Fig 13.22 How to appropriately position seatbelt during pregnancy.
© RoadDriver http://www.roaddriver.co.uk/safety-tips/driving-safety-tips-for-pregnant-women

Further reading
Crawford Mechem C (2015). *Pelvic Fracture in Emergency Medicine*. Medscape. http://emedicine.medscape.com/article/825869
Summerton DJ *et al.* (2014). *Guidelines on Urological Trauma*. Arnhem: European Association of Urology.

14 Pre-hospital care

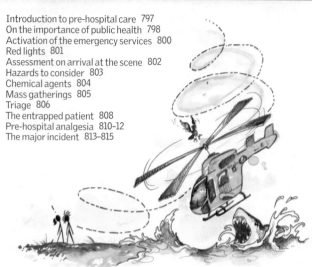

Fig 14.1 As the helicopter spirals down to the rescue, there are dangers to consider to ensure the safety of both crew members and patients. © Gillian Turner.

Pre-hospital care introduces a new world of fast-paced acronyms

BASICS British Association for Immediate Care

CBRN Chemical, Biological, Radiological, and Nuclear (incidents)

CCS Casualty Clearing Station (established near site of major emergency to treat & stabilize patients)

ETA Estimated Time of Arrival

HART Hazardous Area Response Teams

HEMS Helicopter Emergency Medical Service

MERIT Medical Emergency Response Incident Team

PHEM Pre-Hospital Emergency Medicine

RTC Road Traffic Collision

USaR Urban Search and Rescue.

Sources

The following books give a comprensive overview with many practical points from real experiences in the field:

Nutbeam T, Boylan B (eds) (2013). *ABC of Prehospital Emergency Medicine*. Chichester: Wiley-Blackwell.

Skinner DV, Driscoll PA (eds) (2013). *ABC of Major Trauma* (4th ed). Chichester: Wiley–Blackwell.

The MIMMS (Major Incident Medical Managment and Support) course is essential for any team member of major incidents.

Website for Intercollegiate Board for Training in Pre-hospital Emergency Medicine: http://www.ibtphem.org.uk/

We thank our Specialist Reader Dr Robert Anderson for reviewing this chapter. We also thank Mr Drew Carroll, Dr Kenneth Anderson, and Laura Summersell for their kind help and support.

Introduction to pre-hospital care

Pre-hospital care is the delivery of medical attention beyond the realms of established medical centres. The scenarios encountered can vary from aspects of first aid to medical emergencies. As we strive to spiral deep inside our patient in order to understand them more, we must also reach out towards the very start of a patient's journey at the original event. The aim of this chapter is not to provide an account of any patient prior to hospitalization—this is largely the province of the GP. Rather, our aim here is to highlight the doctor's role and how we can work together with paramedics effectively to save lives in the community. Military pre-hospital care is not covered here.

Prior to the creation of the NHS in 1948, ambulances were manned by volunteers and simply transported patients to hospital. In 1964, ambulances started to initiate treatment prior to arrival at hospital,[1] and the training of professional paramedics was introduced in the 1980s. Today paramedics form an essential part of the pre-hospital care team. Pre-hospital care is a field which truly relies on the multi-disciplinary approach to ensure a prompt and appropriate medical response. Traditionally, the focus has been on swift and safe transfer of patients to hospital. However, the recent shift towards centralizing trauma care now necessitates the transport of patients across further distances and thus increasing levels of early intervention are being performed in order to optimize the patient prior to arrival at hospital. Pre-hospital care providers range from technicians, paramedics, and nurses to doctors. They are required to work in challenging environments with long hours of work without food, sleep, or toilet breaks; it is each staff member's professional responsibility to look after themselves and remain fit for duty.

The essence of pre-hospital care staff

'Our patients did not choose us. We chose them. We could have chosen another profession, but we did not. We have accepted responsibility for patient care in some of the worst situations: when we are tired or cold; when it is rainy and dark; when we cannot predict what conditions we will encounter. We must either embrace this responsibility or surrender it. We must give to our patients the very best care that we can-not while we are daydreaming, not with unchecked equipment, not with incomplete supplies and not with yesterday's knowledge.'

NAEMT, PHTLS: Prehospital Trauma Life Support, 2011: Jones & Bartlett Learning, Burlington, MA. www.jblearning.com. Reprinted with permission

Pre-hospital emergency medicine (PHEM) was approved by the GMC in 2010 as a sub-speciality open to all doctors in emergency medicine and anaesthetics (acute medicine and intensive care are less common). Their duties encompass care on-scene and in-transit for patients requiring transfer either to or between hospitals. PHEM practitioners are largely involved with the subset of acutely unwell patients in need of intensive care. The majority of unwell patients fall under the remit of paramedics. Ambulance control organizes the services based on advice from the paramedics on scene (p800).

Pre-hospital Trauma Life Support Committee of the National Association of Emergency Medical Technicians in co-operation with the Committee on Trauma of the American College of Surgeons.

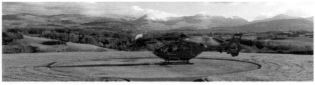

Fig 14.2 In mountainous areas such as Snowdonia (UK), pre-hospital care relies heavily on helicopters to travel vast distances quickly. Landing sites are ideally at the back of the hospital with easy access to the emergency department. © Nina Hjelde.

Public health seems a far throw from the emergency rescue missions you expected when exploring this chapter, yet we all agree that it is better to encourage prevention than resorting to the cure (which is you). It is through enthusiastic public health campaigns and continuous health & safety assessments that accidents are now being termed 'preventable occurrences' as we start to recognize all processes are subject to laziness, haste, ignorance, bad design, poor maintenance, false economy, and failure to apply existing knowledge.

'*I trust this sort of nonsense will never happen again*' was the conclusion of the coroner present at the enquiry of the first RTA fatality in 1896 (London, UK). The driver was described to be travelling at 'tremendous speed' yet was reported to only be driving at 4mph. The 44-year-old pedestrian died within minutes from a head injury.[2]

There are five well recognized risk factors in road safety (speed, drink-driving, motorcycle helmets (fig 14.3), seat-belts, and child restraints), yet only 28 countries (representing 7% of the world's population) have adequate legislation which comprehensively addresses these key areas.[3]

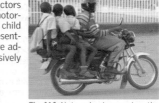

Fig 14.3 Note who is wearing the helmet.

© Nina Hjelde.

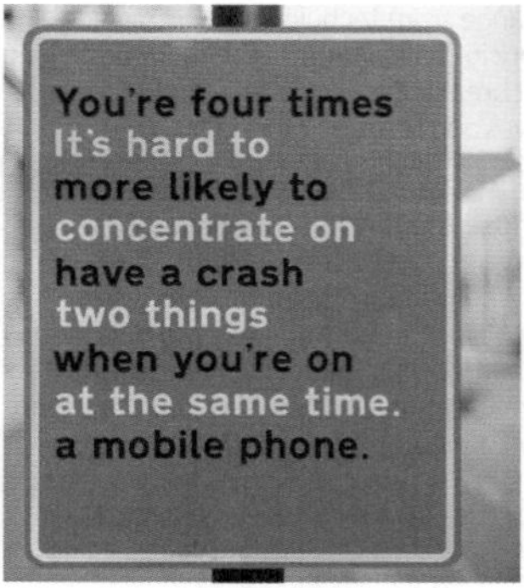

You're four times It's hard to **more likely to** concentrate on **have a crash two things** when you're on **at the same time. a mobile phone.**

Fig 14.4 Public health advertising.
© Department for Transport.

Globally, the 8th leading cause of death is RTAs and it is predicted to become the 5th leading cause by 2030. RTAs affect 1 in 4 people in their lifetime. Each day ~3400 people die and >50,000 are injured on the world's roads. 90% of fatalities are in low- and middle-income countries, even though they contain <50% of the world's vehicles.[3]

Through intensive road safety health campaigns in the UK, the public are well educated on the dangers involved with driving (fig 14.4). Health education posters picturing tragic consequences to loved ones are successful. We almost take it for granted and assume that most mishaps on the road can be avoided if all the rules are followed. Human error is to be considered. In 2009, most accidents involving young drivers occurred during the rush-hour on Fridays. Few drivers remember details about the drive during their commute; do you also switch into automatic mode? Failure to 'look properly' was the main cause of car accidents.

A decade of road safety[3]

In 2013, the WHO reported that road-related incidents caused approximately 1.24 million deaths every year and a further 20–50 million non-fatal injuries. In response, the WHO declared the period of 2011 to 2020 as the 'Decade of Road Safety'. World governments have collaborated to improve safety for all users. So far, there has been no overall reduction in fatalities, but importantly it has prevented the feared rise (which is impressive considering the 15% global surge in motorized vehicles).

The observation that pedestrians and cyclists account for 27% of all road traffic deaths is a very sobering thought. It raises the issue that public health initiatives must encompass all road users beyond simply addressing the five key risk factors mentioned on p798 which are more heavily associated with drivers. NICE has published guidelines urging the public to embrace the health benefits of cycling, yet the fear of traffic forces nervous cyclists back to their cars. Could you justifiably advise your patient to pursue healthier forms of travel on the roads with the knowledge that it may well lead to major trauma?

Mobile phone usage whilst driving was originally associated with a quadrupled risk of crashes (1997). Although more recent studies (2012) have cast doubt over such an explicit relationship, we cannot ethically allow (nor afford) to wait until a more robust study is performed. In this situation we must simply take for granted that distraction whilst driving can only result in negative outcomes. After several years, public health campaigns successfully stamped 'drink-driving' as a negative social stigma; this is the attitude that *must* be adopted towards mobile phones too[4] (see p526 for fitness to drive).

The most dangerous sport?

Each year in the UK, 30,000 people suffer an out-of-hospital cardiac arrest. Despite the recognized benefits of regular exercise for golfers, the high incidence of cardiac arrests on the golf course has pushed golf into becoming one of the most lethal sports (fig 14.5). This is mainly because golfers are typically males in their 60s who are spending their morning hours (most MIs are recorded to happen between 6–11am) walking across large stretches of remote ground. The isolation means that discovery is delayed and access to the patient is limited. In the US, a golf course is the 5th most common place to have a cardiac arrest. **Automatic external defibrillators (AEDs)** have now been enthusiastically introduced across golf clubs as the chance of survival falls by 7–10% for every minute without compressions and defibrillation. The Resuscitation Council of the UK recommends that although layperson training in the use of AEDs is to be encouraged, it is not necessary for their use by members of the public.

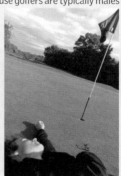

This is an inspiring example of a how public health initiatives have been embraced by a population, yet simple interventions such as good hydration, healthy lifestyle choices, and picking a partner who knows CPR remain the best prophylaxis.

Fig 14.5 A 'hole in one' is a rare occurrence, like an out-of-hospital cardiac arrest, but it happens.

© Nina Hjelde.

▶▶ *How to use an AED* Place one pad to the right of the sternum, below the clavicle, and the other in the left mid-axillary line approximately over the position of the v6 ECG electrode. Whilst most pads are labelled left and right (or have a picture indicating position) it does not matter if their positions are switched. Laypeople should then follow the AED voice/visual prompts, ensuring that if a shock is indicated nobody is touching the victim.

Further reading

Department for Transport (2013). *Reported Road Casualties: Great Britain 2012*. https://www.gov.uk/government/uploads/system/uploads/attachment_data/file/269601/rrcgb-2012-complete.pdf

WHO (2013). *Global Status Report On Road Safety: 2013*. http://www.who.int/violence_injury_prevention/road_safety_status/2013/en/

Pre-hospital care

▶▶ The cornerstone of pre-hospital care is forward planning and organisation with prompt activation and organized distribution of resources. These processes start with the skilled management of 999 calls and appropriate deployment of pre-hospital services. Calls are prioritized into RED (immediately life-threatening), AMBER (urgent), or GREEN (routine). Call-centre staff follow protocols which can provide interim first-aid instructions. The more complex calls are passed onto PHEM practitioners (see p797) who are better placed to assess the need for a more advanced response.

Immediate dispatch criteria for PHEM practitioners[5]
Fall from >20 ft
Fall or jumped in front of train RTA*
Ejection from vehicle/another vehicle occupant has died
Explosions/industrial incidents*
Amputation above wrist or ankle
Trapped under vehicle (not motorcycle) Drowning* Shooting/stabbing*   * Need discussion with PHEM team first

There are several factors influencing which type of emergency service is deployed. **Land vehicles** are not limited by weather conditions and function well in urban areas. Land vehicles are used for shorter distances and vehicles can be parked strategically to help protect the scene.

Helicopters can cover large areas and quickly access remote locations. Air ambulances are manned by paramedics whilst HEMS (Helicopter Emergency Medical Service) also include doctors. Helicopters may be restricted to daylight hours (although increasingly transfers of the critically ill patient are being performed at night), appropriate landing sites, and fair weather. Arrival by helicopter to a major incident allows a unique overview of the scene and helps identify hazards and patient location. The risks of patient transport must be carefully weighed. One must consider the physiological needs of a cold, tired, and hungry crew in addition to the clinical implications of travel for the patient. A full bladder can distract attention from monotonous monitors. You won't be able to hear monitor alarms during the flight. Equipment should be robust with audible alarms and easily manipulated in poor lighting or turbulent flights; consider drawing up drugs in advance. Know your equipment packs well, there is NO opportunity to 'fetch more from the storeroom' in-flight. Checklists to ensure all equipment is present onboard are frequently used: www.ukhems.co.uk

Effects of transport[6]	Clinical implications
Vestibular dysfunction	Fatigue, nausea
Temperature changes	Fatigue, coagulopathies
Linear acceleration	Haemodynamic instability Patient positioning affects fractures/injuries Angle of flight affects ICP in head injury (p790)
Noise and turbulence	Clot disruption
Poor space and lighting	Limited access to patient/equipment
Altitude	Risk of hypoxia, alterations in acid–base balance Gas volumes increase with altitude (due to decreasing pressure) causing problems in body cavities (bowel, lung, cranium) *Consider decompression of gas-filled cavities or equipment prior to flight*

It is a common misconception that emergency vehicles can legally power straight through red lights when on their way to an emergency scene. They are obliged to treat red lights as 'give-way' signs and turn off flashing lights and sirens when approaching another vehicle who would not be safely able to move out of the way. Revalidation for emergency drivers is relentless and thorough, but equally the public must be educated to only move out of the way when it is safe to do so.

Consider the following scenarios:

• *Breaking and entering:* Doctors and paramedics cannot legally force entry to a private address, but you would be unlikely to face repercussions if doing so in an attempt to save a life.

• *Driving:* For example, as long as appropriate sirens/lights are used, you: *can* exceed the statutory speed limit by 20mph; *can* use bus lanes; *can* stop and park on clearways; *can* treat red lights as 'give way'; *cannot* ignore one-way signs; *cannot* cross double white lines; *cannot* ignore stop signs.

• *Consent:* This is too large a topic to cover here. If there is a situation where obtaining informed consent may be an issue (eg unconscious, mental health issues, <16yrs old in absence of parent or guardian) life-saving treatment can probably be administered without fear of repercussion. Further non-life-saving treatment beyond this may raise problems. See also OHCM p570.

• *Restraint:* Unless restraining an aggressive or violent individual for safety reasons, medical practitioners have no right to restrain an individual: to do so would constitute assault. Always act in the patient's best interests. Continuously attempt to calm the patient and re-assess capacity if needed.

• *Confidentiality:* Be aware that the open environment of a pre-hospital setting is more vulnerable to breaches in confidentiality in the form of both verbal and written communication. Fire fighters will quickly erect screens to maintain confidentiality. PHEM staff must remain acutely aware of social media; there should be no images shared which could identify the scene.

▶Check that you have the appropriate *clinical indemnity* to cover your practice. As you become more senior, your scope of practice changes. Coroners will also investigate cases in prehospital care to ensure all practitioners are held accountable for their actions. See www.aace.org.uk.

Be prepared

Preparation is key for coordinating a successful response in an emergency; desperately searching for essential equipment is time-consuming and frustrating. Various processes have been employed, but in this growing world of checklists and bureaucracy, visual reminders are successful. One approach is to place pictures of the equipment on the back wall of the resuscitation room, thus when a piece is missing you instantly see the underlying picture (figs 14.6 & 14.7).

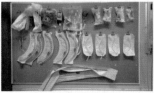

Fig 14.6 Airway equipment in the resuscitation bay.

© Nina Hjelde.

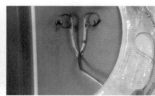

Fig 14.7 The picture on the wall alerts a busy team to the missing Magill forceps.

© Nina Hjelde.

Further reading

BlueLightAware video: http://www.bluelightaware.org.uk/
British Association for Immediate Care: http://www.basics.org.uk

►►The number one priority is you—is the scene safe to approach? Admittedly risks in the pre-hospital environment frequently cannot be removed, but make efforts to diminish the dangers. Wear personal protective equipment (PPE) to protect eyes, ears, heads, and hands with high-visibility clothing. Consider life-vests for water rescue and harnesses for rescues involving height. PPE is your responsibility, treat it with respect and include it in training. Donning PPE for chemical protection can be intimidating and difficult—practise regularly! Resuscitators working in PPE quickly become warm and can easily underestimate how cold the immobile patient is becoming, bear this in mind. HARTs (Hazardous Area Response Teams) are specifically trained for rescue in dangerous environments.

Scene safety is everyone's responsibility and requires continuous reassessment as conditions change quickly. A reckless rescuer can become a casualty and a hindrance rather than help. Park obliquely prior to the incident ('fend off position'), place high-visibility cones, and leave hazard lights on.

Communications Liaise with the police (they are in overall command), fire service (for any hazards, they are invaluable for patient extrication (see p808), and paramedics. Inform the receiving hospital by radio or telephone using pre-determined codes for escalation. Relay number of casualties and severity of injuries to enable the most appropriate medical response.

Always consider the possibility of a CBRN risk (Chemical, Biological, Radiological, Nuclear). Remain upwind/uphill and do not approach fire or chemical hazards until the fire service have made the area safe. Patient care in CBRN events is sometimes significantly delayed in order to ensure scene safety first.

New European regulations on classification, labelling, and packaging of substances and mixtures came into force in June 2015.[7] (See figs **14.8** to **14.15**.)

Fig 14.8 Acute toxicity (contact is fatal). **Fig 14.9** Corrosive (eg drain cleaners). **Fig 14.10** Unstable explosive (eg fireworks). **Fig 14.11** Gas under pressure.

Fig 14.12 Health hazard (contact may be fatal). **Fig 14.13** Environmental hazard (eg pesticides). **Fig 14.14** Flammable (eg petrol). **Fig 14.15** Oxidizing (eg oxygen cylinders).

Some CBRN agents cannot easily be detected by sight or smell; this makes detection of CBRN events challenging. It is therefore recommended that standard precautions are employed for all mass casualty scenarios of unknown cause. Consider also when strange smells or tastes are reported. Public Health England now have an algorithm for diagnosis and early management of chemical incidents that starts with the time-critical questions 'Could this be cyanide?', then 'Could this be organophosphates?' followed by other typical chemical culprits.[8]

Fire <5% of road crashes result in fire and <1:500 result in significant burns. The deadliest pile-up was the Salang Tunnel Fire (Afghanistan, November 1982) which involved a petrol tanker explosion with an estimated 1100–2700 killed. Car fires are more likely to be deliberate, 1 in 12 reported stolen vehicles will be burnt out.

Electricity Overhead lines are typically uninsulated and if objects get too close then electricity can 'jump' and be lethal. Call the power company to ensure the power is off before approaching.

Rail An electrified rail can be short-circuited by a bar carried by the fire service or rail authority. Cutting power lines does not stop diesel locomotives that may operate on the same line. Trains may be stopped by signal lights, red flags, or a series of charges placed on the rail—the noise warns the driver.

Underground/tube/metro In addition to rail hazards above, underground scenarios are complicated by lack of lighting and ventilation, cramped conditions, and difficult access to site.

Chemical CBRN events require particular processes to ensure scene safety. Vehicles carrying hazardous loads must clearly display an orange 'HAZCHEM' board (white boards indicates the load is non-toxic). This provides instructions to the rescue services on how to fight the fire, what PPE to wear, if the chemical can be safely washed down sewage drains, and whether to evacuate the area. The 'Kemler' plate is the European version containing only the UN product number and a numerical hazard code (which, if doubled, means intensified hazard) (fig 14.16).

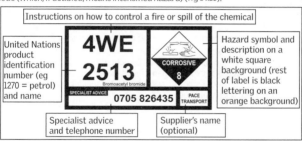

Instructions on how to control a fire or spill of the chemical	
United Nations product identification number (eg 1270 = petrol) and name	**4WE** **2513** Bromoacetyl bromide — SPECIALIST ADVICE — 0705 826435 PACE TRANSPORT — CORROSIVE 8	Hazard symbol and description on a white square background (rest of label is black lettering on an orange background)
	Specialist advice and telephone number — Supplier's name (optional)	

Fig 14.16 The Kemler plate. Understanding the labelling helps you treat spillages.

Radiological casualties have varied presentation based on the source whilst **nuclear** casualties have been exposed to sudden high levels of radiation, often associated with injuries from explosion. Radiation disrupts gastrointestinal, nervous, skin, and cardiac systems. The priority is prompt decontamination, after which there is minimal risk to care providers.

Biological Often difficult to identify due to delayed presentation and multiple symptoms. Consider if multiple patients present with unusual symptoms for that season or geographical area.

Decontamination processes are essential for all CBRN events Prompt removal of all clothing followed by a series of rigorous rinsing. This takes place in specialized decontamination tents. Further casualties can quickly arise if primary cases are not adequately decontaminated. A few chemical agents have particular anti-dotes (p804). HART will take an active role in organizing safe decontamination.

Further reading

Health and Safety Executive (2015). *Chemical Classification*. http://www.hse.gov.uk/chemical-classification/index.htm

Health and Safety Executive (2015). *Health and Safety Statistics 2014/15*. http://www.hse.gov.uk/statistics/

Pre-hospital care

The four major classes of chemical agents

Organophosphates are used in pesticides, consider *nerve agents* (Eg sarin) if no occupational exposure or occurs in public place (see TABLE on p805 for mass casualty incidents). Effects produced by inhibition of acetylcholinesterase resulting in parasympathetic cholinergic overdrive because acetylcholine is not degraded. *SLUDGEM* syndrome: **S**alivation, **L**acrimation, **U**rination, **D**efecation, **G**astrointestinal upset, **E**mesis, **M**iosis. High doses cause respiratory muscle paralysis, seizures, and death. Specific antidotes are **atropine 0.6–4mg** IV (muscarinic antagonist to block action of acetylcholine peripherally) and **pralidoxime 2–30mg/kg** IV over 4min (regenerates acetylcholinesterase) are available as autoinjectors for pre-hospital purposes. Give **atropine** every 10–20min (max 20mg) to control secretions and bradycardia, do not rely on reversal of miosis for dose titration.

Cyanides Muscle twitching and excess secretions help distinguish organophosphates from cyanide. Cyanide binds to mitochondria and disrupts cellular anaerobic respiration. Symptoms arise within seconds to minutes with severe dyspnoea and respiratory arrest. These patients are unlikely to survive, prehospital providers will more frequently encounter moderate exposure causing metabolic acidosis (due to exaggerated anaerobic respiration) with confusion and hyperventilation. The most common source of cyanide poisoning is from smoke inhalation in house fires. Rapid administration of antidote (hydroxocobalamin or sodium thiosulfate often combined with sodium nitrate) is time-critical if respiratory symptoms present.

Pulmonary agents (chlorine, phosgene) affect eyes and respiratory system causing progressive airway irritation. No specific antidote, ventilatory support and effective decontamination to mitigate corrosive effects.

Vesicants (agents that cause characteristic blisters to skin and mucosal membranes) include mustard gas and Lewisite. Cause damage to DNA and subsequent cell death at exposed membranes. Ocular irritation is quickly followed by blistering and respiratory symptoms. No specific antidote, ventilatory support and burns management.

Also see acute poisoning in *OHCM* p850–7.

Further reading

Nutbeam T, Boylan B (eds) (2013). *ABC of Prehospital Emergency Medicine*. Chichester: Wiley-Blackwell.

Public Health England: www.gov.uk/government/organisations/public-health-england

It is easy to only plan medical kit for the performers or athletes at a big event; the challenge is to ensure the crowd is catered for. Needless to say, when a large number of people gather within a restricted area there is an increased risk of multiple casualties should anything happen. Over the past 60 years, football matches have suffered the most mass casualty incidents yet music concerts and political gatherings are also of concern. Use of alcohol and drugs add further risk. The level of health-care staff required to be on stand-by can be determined by models which take into account the nature of event, venue, spectator profile and numbers, duration, and geographical location (see TABLE).

Risk scoring for mass gatherings[9]			
Nature of event		**Nature of venue**	
Country show	2	Indoor	1
Classical performance	2	Outdoor park	2
Motor sport	4	Streets	4
Bonfire/fireworks	4	Includes overnight camping	5
Pop/rock concert	5	**Nature of seating**	
New Year celebration	7	Seated	1
Rave/disco	8	Mixed	2
Political demonstration	Low risk = 2 Opposing factions = 9	Standing	3
Spectator profile		**Season (outdoor events)**	
Family groups	2	Summer	2
Mostly young adults	3	Autumn	1
Mostly children & teenagers	4	Winter	2
Mostly elderly	4	Spring	1
Profile of nearby hospitals		**Proximity to nearest ED**	
Choice of Emergency Departments (ED)	1	<30min by road	0
Large ED	2	>30min by road	2
Small ED	3		

Example calculation

An *OHCS* music festival (3) has a spectator profile of all ages (but not families) (3) who will be standing (3) for an outdoor event lasting more than 12 hours (3) in the summer (3) with overnight camping (5) and a street theatre (1). The closest suitable hospital is 45min drive away (2) with a small ED (3). Plastering (−2) and suturing (−2) facilities will be onsite. There is an expected attendance of 200,000 (50).

The resultant risk score is 76, but the presence of some facilities onsite reduces risk to 72 which places the event into a lower staffing category. This event would therefore require:
- 6 ambulances
- 48 BLS providers
- 6 ALS providers
- 3 doctors
- 3 nurses
- 1 coordinator.

If you are the first on the scene, the following tasks (which assumes a highly organized response) will seem impossible on a dark night, alone. So, the first priority is to raise awareness to prevent further causalities and get help. You may be surprised in how short a time it all becomes organized. Requesting the fire service when dialling 999 may be the quickest way to get a dozen trained first-aiders to the scene with unrivalled skills in extrication.

Sorting through history

Triage From the French '*trier*'; to sort. First used in medical terms during the Napoleonic Wars when Napoleon's Chief Surgeon, Baron Dominique-Jean Larrey, recognized that the casualty load far exceeded their limited medical services. His triage system aimed to use the resources wisely in order to effectively categorize patients on the battlefield and treat as many as possible. He was a pioneer in trauma surgery as he encouraged amputation of limbs to take place immediately after injury on the battle field, rather than weeks later, whilst the body remained in a state of adrenaline-induced vasoconstriction and numbness. Speed was of the essence in the absence of analgesia and sedation. His methods famously paid no regard to rank, and officers and soldiers were treated purely on the basis of need.

Modern triage systems have followed in his footsteps and are used widely in healthcare to optimize care for each individual patient. In contrast, the emphasis in triage during mass casualty scenarios shifts to delivering the best possible outcome for the greatest numbers of patients. The chart in fig 14.17 is a simple system; its main virtue is speed. It starts by relocating the 'walking wounded' by encouraging casualties to walk towards medical aid, followed by prompt assessment of remaining immobile. Each patient is assigned a colour code (see BOX p807).

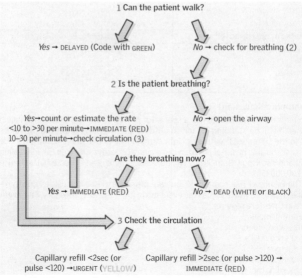

Fig 14.17 The triage sieve. This is a simple system: its main virtue is speed. Once a patient is allocated a triage category, you must move immediately onto the next patient.

When faced with a train crash with unknown numbers of casualties, it becomes essential to first identify those patients who can be saved with simple manoeuvres. *Resist temptation to 'stop and treat'* the first patient in distress; if the paramedic's attention is trapped by the screaming child (demonstrating a very patent airway) then three patients only needing a simple airway adjunct might miss their precious windows (upgrading the patient from a red to orange). ~13% of RTC deaths result from an obstructed airway. The process of mass casualty triage requires a stone heart as some may be *'expectant'*; those who will certainly die and attempting to treat them may delay you helping the salvageable. In contrast, if a single expectant patient arrived to hospital, resuscitation attempts would be worthwhile. Attempting to 'ignore' these expectant patients is understandably an emotional decision to make amidst the chaos of a trauma scene. Over-triage is common, especially in children, and this can put pressure on already limited resources.

Triage categories

Distribution of trauma deaths was classically described as trimodal. *Immediate* (aortic deceleration injury, head injury), *early* (hypoxia and hypovolaemia) and *delayed* (sepsis, multiple organ failure—see p778). However, improved resuscitation care has significantly reduced the 'delayed' peak of deaths.

Colour code	Category	Expectancy
■	Immediate	Few minutes
■	Urgent	1–2h
■	Delayed	>4h
■	Expectant	Moments
□ or ■	Dead	N/A

Fig 14.18 Triage labels.
© Nina Hjelde.

Use triage labels (fig 14.18) to categorize patients into **IMMEDIATE** (colour-code RED, will die in a few minutes if no treatment, eg obstructed airway, tension pneumothorax); **URGENT** (YELLOW, may die in 1–2h if no treatment, eg hypovolaemia); and **DELAYED** (GREEN, can wait eg >4h, eg minor fractures). Those who will certainly die are labelled **EXPECTANT**—to treat them may delay you helping the salvageable, who then die unnecessarily. However, should the expectant patient be your sole casualty (as they would in the ED as an ambulance standby) then approach them as you would a red patient.

Each patient is labelled with a triage-tag to alert others of this patient's needs. Do not forget to label the dead (WHITE OR BLACK), otherwise emergency personnel may repeatedly take a doctor to the same victim, so wasting time and resources. Certification of death on scene must be performed by a doctor in the presence of a police officer.

Note that triage is dynamic It starts with rapid assessment but all casualties should be reassessed when time and resources allow. Triage categories may change whilst waiting and after treatment. Triage in children is even more specialist, and depends on factors such as height, age, or weight. Once more resources arrive, secondary triage systems (eg Triage Sort) are employed. Senior clinicians further triage patients by incorporating GCS, injury severity, and BP.

Further reading

Gunst M *et al.* (2010). Changing epidemiology of trauma deaths leads to a bimodal distribution. *Proc (Bayl Univ Med Cent)* 23(4):349–354.

The fire service are unrivalled in their extrication skills and will often take the lead alongside a senior medical officer. Each trauma scene is different and teams must be coordinated and ready to adapt in the face of unexpected challenges. Think about how you would approach a RTC involving a convertible car versus a mini-van. Reading the wreckage (see p787) helps guide what type of emergency response is needed and where to look for casualties; don't forget to look for patients who may be ejected out of rolled vehicles.

▶▶**SAFETY IS PARAMOUNT** Start with simple measures such as making the vehicle safe: turn off ignition, immobilize the battery, swill away any petrol. Be wary of un-deployed airbags. Padding and wedges will stabilize the vehicle. The extrication team works to physically release the patient from the wreck and will work to create space to mobilize the patient safely. Think simple: the easiest way to enter a car is through the door—try this before removing the windscreen or roof! Remove the wreckage from around the casualty, don't try to awkwardly remove a casualty through too small a hole.

The medical team attempts to assess and stabilize the patient. They work in unison with continuous communication as the state of vehicle and patient is closely related. Rapid extrication (termed *B-plan*) is required in face of immient environmental danger (eg fire) or urgent medical concerns (eg airway obstruction). In a more controlled situation (the *A-plan*), greater care can be paid to spinal stabilization, clot preservation, and the avoidance of potential hazards (eg loose wires, glass shards). A sudden shift to B-plan may need to take place if the scene suddenly deteriorates, so always make a solid B-plan before embarking on your A-plan. It can be an intimidating decision; this is the time for clear and confident decisions.

Resist the temptation to set-up complex monitoring during the early phases as the many wires/tubes can hinder the extrication processes. Stick to the essentials whilst the patient remains trapped. Do consider analgesia as this may aid the movement of painful limbs rather than having to spend time dismantling the crushed vehicle. A spinal board[1] is applied as soon possible, often with patient still partially in vehicle. Prior to transport away from the scene, carry the patient to a designated medical post ~20 metres from the scene to reassess.

Take care to not disturb aspects of the scene which could be used for evidence (such as tyre marks, paint scrapes) by the accident investigators. For this complex system of extrication and patient management to work, regular joint training between branches of the rescue services is invaluable. The fire service must have an appreciation of basic medical principles and the medical team must be educated in the intricate methods of extrication so as not to hinder each other. The two processes cannot function in isolation.

Think about your approach

Minimizing a trauma patient's c-spine movement starts as you enter the scene; if possible, approach the patient in line with their vision to avoid brisk neck movements as the patient strains to see you.

Handover is a skill to be honed, and especially important in the pre-hospital environment where treatment moves fast. ATMIST—Age; Time of injury; Mechanism of injury; Injuries; vital Signs; Treatment—is a useful mnemonic. Always give an ETA to the receiving hospital. *Example handover with succinct information:* 35-yr-old female driver of motorcycle. High-speed impact with stationary bus and ejected 9 metres. GCS 3. Tubed and ventilated on scene. Head, facial, pelvic, and femoral injuries. Peripheral pulses intact. Sats 98% RR 24 HR 140 BP 95/60 250mL Normal saline given. ETA 16 minutes.

---

1 Spinal boards are now only used as extrication devices. Patients are always transported to hospital on a scoop.

In 2003, Aron Ralston's forearm became trapped under a fallen boulder. He spent 5 days surviving off dwindling levels of water and food until delirium and desperation drove him to the only possible escape route: self-amputation of his arm. He survived to write an inspiring autobiography which was the basis of the film '127 Hours'.

He recognized the key principle of 'life over limb'; when the peripheries must be sacrificed if it will facilitate survival. Most limb entrapments are due to RTCs but can arise after building collapses or major transport crashes. The need for pre-hospital amputation is exceptionally rare; ensure regular training and practise on carcasses in order to both prepare mentally and technically. Could you amputate a limb in time of need? Often the decision is eased by the realization that the limb is often non-salvageable after severe impaction.

There are four main indications for pre-hospital limb amputation:

1 Quick extrication critical for medical management
2 Structural collapse/environmental hazards
3 Extrication is likely to be impossible
4 Patient currently stable but is unlikely to survive a prolonged extrication.

The procedure is basic and designed for non-surgical specialists in a difficult environment. Firstly sedate appropriately and apply a tourniquet (never over a joint) to tighten until bleeding stops. Note this time. Wash the area and, using a scalpel, divide the soft tissues as distally as possible. A battery-powered bone cutter is ideal, but confined spaces only allow space for a wire saw. Leave the tourniquet *in situ*, additional measures may be needed to ensure haemostasis. Generously apply saline-soaked gauze and bandages to the stump. Transport the limb in a clean plastic bag with patient.

'Golden Hours' and 'Platinum Minutes'? The debate is over

A driving force behind the current trauma care systems has been the 'Golden Hour'; a concept famously coined by Dr Cowley in 1975 who felt that patients should be evacuated to a definitive care facility within the first hour after injury. This approach has since been questioned as not only is this arbitrary timing lacking in evidence, it also encouraged a culture where speed became the priority. Pre-hospital teams then developed the 'Platinum Ten' which advised that critically injured patients should be stabilized and evacuated within 10 minutes of the medical team arriving on-scene. This was in response to military statistics which showed that most battlefield fatalities occur within 10 minutes of wounding.

However, despite these ideal timings, the pre-hospital environment is unpredictable and obstructive. These two concepts were based on the obselete debate over 'Scoop and run versus stay and play'. You do neither. These issues have faded as ambulances and PHEM teams offer more than just a taxi with a bed. You should initiate life-saving interventions on scene and continue resuscitation during transport. Extrication of the patient must be dictated by scene safety (both for you and your patient), physical barriers, and the patient's condition. Use of the 'Platinum Ten' is more as guidance to encourage efficient decision-making processes and optimizing the patient's situation within the constraints of the working environment. With the rise of trauma centres (see p799), value is placed on getting the *right* patient to the *right* place at the *right* time, rather than arbitrarily allocating golden timings. Taking the time to cannulate on scene may seem stressful at the time, yet immensely worthwhile when the patient later deteriorates en route. Each trauma patient is unique, facial trauma may only have a few Golden minutes compared to the Golden days of a fractured wrist. Yet every patient deserves the same Golden treatment through rapid assessment and efficient evacuation.

Pain has a huge psychological component which is acutely exacerbated in emergencies when a terrified patient can become very difficult to assess. Physiologically, the catecholamines released with pain may further reduce peripheral perfusion and oxygen delivery in hypovolaemic shock. Prompt control of acute pain will not only aid physiological assessment, but will also inspire confidence in the rescuers and thus help to settle a distressed casualty. Your confident approach and calming presence is a strong analgesic; do not underestimate these non-pharmacological approaches (fig 14.19).

Beecher noted in 1944 at Anzio[1] that soldiers were indifferent to pain from serious injury. This is unlikely in road crashes; those soldiers were released from war horrors by their injuries, but a crash victim is just beginning his nightmare. So the question is never *why*, but *when* should analgesia be given (see p812)? In the chaos of pre-hospital scenes, pain is frequently overlooked as rescuers focus on extrication and treatment plans. Unless all hope of life and rescue has been abandoned, the priorities of securing an airway and stabilizing c-spine, and optimizing ABC should come before analgesia.

Assessment of pain can be difficult in impaired GCS; but do not assume that this equates to absence of pain perception. Use visual analogues and pain scoring for rapid assessment, but note that it is the trend in the pain reported that must guide treatment.

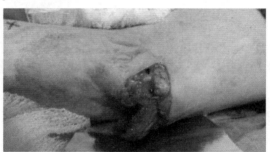

Fig 14.19 ▶▶Photography of a wound will prevent excessive dressing removals which aggravates pain and increases infection risk, but do remember to annotate pictures appropriately as it can be difficult to locate the anatomy.[2]

© Nina Hjelde.

Pharmacological approaches to analgesia The options can be mind-boggling, but rather than attempting complex polypharmacy, stick to familiar combinations that work for you. ▶Documentation is key to preventing iatrogenic overdose.

IV paracetamol is frequently used for all patients, especially the elderly trauma patient. Use the plastic 100mL IV bottles and give over 5–10 minutes. PO paracetamol is offered to those who can be discharged from scene.

NSAIDs are excellent for longer-lasting relief of musculoskeletal pain, rarely used in severe injuries, and typically used for those discharged from scene.

See p812 for ketamine, opioids, and Entonox® use.

1 Anzio, 33 miles south of Rome, was a crucial Allied beachhead in recapturing of the 'Eternal City' (5/6/44).
2 Open ankle fracture with dorsalis pedis 'X' marked by paramedics with pen to prove a pulse was present when they assessed patient.

Splintage and manipulations: back to basics

NH was called to see an elbow fracture as the patient was noted to be tachycardic and hypertensive. As I was chatting to the patient she seemed comfortable at rest and well in herself. The elbow in question was protectively held by her other arm. I cheerfully reassured her when I felt her pulse to be 85. I then witnessed a nurse diligently check for the painful side and apply the BP cuff to her other arm; failing to notice the grimace of pain on our stoical patient's face as her self-splinting was temporarily abandoned. No wonder her BP shot up.

Our patient recognized this pain was temporary and remained uncomplaining, to the detriment of her overall care as x-rays and analgesia became less important in the face of tachycardia. We can sometimes be blinded by numbers and forget the basic skills. Splinting of soft-tissue injuries will support and protect the injury to help alleviate pain and prevent further damage.

Splinting of limbs is synonymous with fractures, yet we urge you to apply the benefits of joint immobilization in all limb injuries. Splinting aims to immobilize and potentially realign fractured or dislocated bone segments to neutral position to reduce pain and further injury to soft tissues. No limb injury should be transported before splinting takes place (see fig 14.20).

Simple splints can be improvised from clothing; an uninjured leg can splint the injured one. Use inflatable jacket splints to immobilize ankle, tibial, and forearm fractures. Femoral shaft fractures can be splinted using a Kendrick splint in the pre-hospital environment, once in hospital they may require Thomas splints which offer more powerful traction. Pelvic splints (p794) are essential for controlling blood loss in addition to providing pain relief. Splint hands by rolling a bandage in the fist with overlying straight fingers. Simple slings can splint an arm to the chest. Pad (eg with blankets) bony prominences to maintain skin integrity (esp. for immobile patients). Splints should cover the joint above and below the fracture site to ensure minimum movement of bone ends. Attempt to splint the joint in neutral anatomical position unless realignment is met with significant resistance or will compromise circulation.

Reduction of an injured limb is indicated when faced with deformity which could lead to soft-tissue ischaemia or neurovascular compromise; apply traction to gently restore normal anatomical alignment. Timely reduction of deformity will improve the neurovascular outcomes. Distal perfusion must be evaluated before and continuously after manipulation.

Estimated blood loss caused by fractures [10]	
Site of fracture	**Estimated blood loss (litres)**
Humerus	0.5-1.5
Tibia	0.5-1.5
Femur	1-1.25
Pelvis	1-4

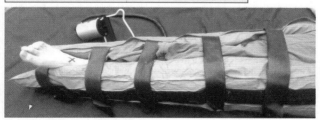

Fig 14.20 Splint fractures distal to the knee in a vaccum splint. The pump pictured functions to suck the air out to create a stiffened splint moulded to the patient's lower limb. Notice the dorsal pedis pulse has been marked for palpation both prior to and after the application of the splint. © Nina Hjelde.

Gaseous Nitrous oxide is mixed with 50% o_2 as Entonox® in blue cylinders with a white top (store horizontally to prevent gas separation). Fast onset and offset of effect; used to fill time whilst IV access is established or additional short bursts of analgesia are needed (ie moving injured limb). Do not use in decompression sickness, pneumothorax (may tension), acute head injury or bowel obstruction.

Opioids Morphine is effective and frequently used. Give 0.1mg/kg (1-10mg) in 2mg aliquots titrated against pain and patient (less needed in elderly). **Fentanyl** is as effective as morphine, easier to titrate due to faster onset of action, and can be given by nasal and buccal routes. Drawbacks of opiates include the impracticality of patiently titrating to pain amidst the chaos of an accident scene with variable patient responses to opiates and typical time to maximal effect of 20 minutes. Respiratory depression is avoided with careful titration but naloxone should always be available (0.2-0.4mg IV repeated every 2min as necessary). Be careful not to over administer naloxone as it will reverse analgesic effect. Consider anti-emetics, studies have shown that 50mg IV cyclizine or 4mg ondansetron may be more efficacious than the traditional 10mg metoclopramide.[11] **Ketamine** is becoming increasingly popular, especially for use in trauma patients. At sub-anaesthetic doses (0.25-0.5mg/kg IV or IO) ketamine is a potent, short-acting analgesic with rapid onset and amnesic effects. A large therapeutic index and less adverse effects on breathing makes it relatively safe in prehospital care. Ketamine in adults can cause profound hallucinations and unpleasant trips or 'emergence phenomenon'; have **midazolam** 1mg IV available in case patient becomes difficult to manage (but administration is rarely needed). It can cause tachycardia (usually minimal) and hypertension (but in practice this has little effect on cardiovascular stability or haemorrhage control); do not automatically attribute tachycardia to drug effect—your patient might be shocked. **Peripheral nerve blocks** are attractive as they can offer excellent analgesia with no sedation, yet this is rarely achievable in the pre-hospital care setting due to time constraints, need for splinting, and multiple injuries requiring opioids. **Procedural sedation** is mostly reserved for fracture-dislocation injuries which must be reduced (eg causing neurovascular compromise) on scene. Also consider for painful (extrication of trapped limb) or invasive (chest drain insertion) interventions. A combination of **ketamine** (sedation dose is 0.5-1mg/kg) IV/IO and **midazolam** (1-2mg/kg) can be used with continuous monitoring attached. Only sedate your patient if you are competent in intubation should anaesthesia be induced.

Intra-nasal (IN) analgesia

IN analgesia has long been used in paediatric emergencies where gaining IV access would cause even more distress. The pre-hospital environment does not lend itself to gaining easy IV access and IN delivery is often used (and can be used for adults too). In hospital, adults tend to be given Entonox® or undergo injections or cannulation just for analgesia, even when resuscitation is not required. Although the majority of studies are in children, interest for IN analgesia in adults is growing which, if you think about it, makes sense as IN has attractive advantages: rapid onset similar to IV opiates, unskilled delivery technique makes it quickly and ubiquitously available, higher bioavailability than oral as it passes directly into blood stream.

IN fentanyl and diamorphine are most commonly used. Dosing can be intimidating since you often need double the IV dose (and sometimes more!) of fentanyl for therapeutic effect, clinicians failing to give proper doses initially halted the popularity of IN techniques. The trick is to use highest concentration available and titrate to pain (as you would do in IV opiates). **Fentanyl** 2mcg/kg and **diamorphine** 0.1mg/kg, administer half dose into each nostril to maximize absorptive surface area. Reassuringly, naloxone can also be administered IN.[3]

▶▶The major incident 1

Mass casualty incidents (MCIs) do unfortunately happen and the media are quick to draw our attention to death counts, yet consider these events and the large-scale emergency responses needed to cope with those injured. *Those* are the patients we can salvage (see p807, 'Triage').

Examples of mass casualty incidents [1,2]			
Type	Location	Deaths	Injured
Tsunami	Japan	15,534	5364
Attack on World Trade Centre	USA	2993	8700
Train bombings	Madrid	191	1900
Theatre siege	Moscow	168	Unclear
Multiple bombings	London	52	650
Shooting	Norway	77	153
Sarin gas	Japan	13	1100

When do major incidents become complex emergencies?

• If the context involves administrative, political, or economic anarchy.
• If the incident sparks a self-perpetuating chain of violence.
• If the incident is not a random event, but focused on one ethnic group.
• If competition for wholly inadequate resources compounds their inadequacy.
• If the incident leads to displacement of children.
• If the incident promotes a state of war.

Hospital response in major incidents

Ideally medical staff on-scene should not be from the local hospital due to receive the casualties, however this may be unavoidable in rural areas. The hospital clinician in command should be of a non-trauma-related speciality as these services will be in demand. Although care standards must be maintained throughout, once the receiving hospital declares a major incident then elective procedures should be delayed, discharges facilitated to free bed space, and spare staff recruited to busier areas. The usual case-load of patients attending the emergency department should continue to be treated and appointments opened up in local GP surgeries.

Keeping records

In the controlled bustle of activity at a pre-hospital emergency scene, the same focus that is applied to care provision also needs to be applied to recording of the care given. Recording procedures and drugs is vital for safe, and therefore good, practice

Essence of keeping records
• Good practice = safe practice
• Treat first, then make records
• Use well-known formats

(see MINIBOX). On arrival at hospital, a full dose of morphine given on top of an unknown administration in the field can be enough to lead to overdose.

Care provision will inevitably have to come first, but then it is vital to create accurate records (and dare we say, 'undoctored') in retrospect. Importantly, if using a pre-prepared sheet, use those that are widespread and not your own customized layout, which may cause confusion from delay in interpretation. Good record keeping is also vital for trauma scoring (p810 and fig 14.19).

Handing over to emergency services is an essential skill (p808).

Further reading

Department of Health (2013, updated May 2015). 2010 to 2015 *Government Policy: Health Emergency Planning*. www.gov.uk/government/publications/2010-to-2015-government-policy-health-emergency-planning

Pre-hospital care

Major incidents (MIs), either man-made or natural, are simply defined as situations where the immediate health resources are overwhelmed by the casualty load. This varies with geography: 5 casualties in a car crash may strain rural resources, whilst a large city hospital could easily cope. Equally, situations requiring specialist interventions (paediatrics, burns) can quickly overwhelm larger centres too. Escalation to MCIs if >100 casualties involved (p813).

The general management of MIs follow the principles of **CSCATT (Command, Safety, Communications, Assessment, Triage, Treatment)** (as taught by the MIMMS course) which guides a highly structured chain of events (fig 14.21).

Flow of **Command** is dependent on time of arrival, with responsibility shifting as more senior staff arrive. Overall scene control is police-led, with help from incident commanders representing each emergency service; only the control vehicle for each service leaves their flashing lights on. Each person must report to the scene commander on arrival. Police will also organize bystanders, coordinate media and local authority responses. Organization of the scene must be established early in order to optimize service delivery.

Scene **Safety** (see p807) is largely the domain of the fire service who work towards mitigating hazards.

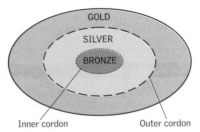

Fig 14.21 The outer cordon is defined and patrolled by the police who control access to the scene. The silver area lies within the inner cordon and hosts the incident commanders of each emergency service and the Casualty Clearing Station (CCS); a place of safety close to the incident where MERIT physicians stabilize patients for transport. See p815. The bronze area defines the inner cordon directly surrounding the incident; medical intervention here is limited to triage and extrication processes.

Communication is often a problem at MCIs due to environmental restrictions, although radio use is the primary form of communication, consider written messages and runners in busy times. Codes and call signs must be pre-determined and staff should be familiar with radio communication. Good communication allows coordination between the services and sensible reassignment of staff after completed tasks. It is a skill to strike a balance between under- and over-communicating! *Handover* in a major incident uses: METHANE (**M**ajor incident declared, **E**xact location, **T**ype of incident, **H**azards (present and future, see p802), **A**ccess (remember to consider a safe route in and out), **N**umber, type and severity of casualties, **E**mergency services now present and those required (see p808 for handover skills).

Further reading

Major incident planning and the required cordons are described well here: www.wiltshire.police.uk/departments/major-incident-planning/interactive-major-incident-schematic

Assessment of the scene and recruitment of the support needed to cope with an MI is dependent on the first responders acting quickly and having the confidence to declare an MI; an intimidating call for a junior to make. Seek prompt senior support.

CSCATT (p814) is completed by closely related phases of medical management:

Triage (p806) The ambulance first on-scene should initiate the triage process rather than treat the first casualties spotted. It is continuously revised as more staff arrive.

Treatment Excessive medical intervention must be avoided in the initial stages, except life-saving treatments, until the scene has been adequately assessed and casualties triaged. (Ambulance personnel coordinate these initial phases.) Permissible interventions could include placing casualties in the recovery position, simple airway adjuncts, or tourniquets for haemorrhage. The MERIT (formerly 'Mobile Medical Team') consisting of a team of doctors, nurses, and paramedics who perform secondary surveys on casualties in the CCS may be recruited to help with triage and extrication. MERIT members should arrive equipped with kit bags containing limited equipment to support ABC including rapid sequence intubation and orthopaedic splints. In contrast, HART comprises of medical staff trained to provide life-saving interventions within the hazardous inner cordons to salvageable patients not able to reach the CCS. HART kitbags will carry antidotes. Involvement of voluntary aid organizations, eg Red Cross, is useful for those minimally injured.

Transport will usually be coordinated by the ambulance services, though consider taxis/buses for ambulant patients who require hospital attention to avoid saturating ambulance resources. Secondary triage systems are typically employed to categorize patients prior to transfer. Transport to an on-site morgue must also be considered. Certification of death on-scene, in the UK, must be in the presence of both a doctor and police officer.

Peering over the edge

The very nature of a spiral is that it repeats itself continuously, many lessons in clinical practice will continue to present themselves and your ability to deal with each one grows as you nurture your journey through medicine. Peering over the edge of this whirlwind can be intimidating for those afraid of heights, for those afraid to look back over their mistakes that can now be seen so clearly spiralling below them, as the benefit of hindsight is granted through reflection after an event. But only by applying those lessons from past steps can we hope to learn anything. Madness can be defined as trying the same thing over and over again, and expecting a new, or different, outcome. Planning is essential to ensure smooth action which satisfies the public's high expectations of emergency responses in major incidents; the media continues to raise these expectations. The intricate infrastructure required to deal effectively with MIs is dependent on extensive training and pre-planning to create algorithms which facilitate coordinated deployment of the appropriate rescue teams. And thus we spiral back towards preventative medicine to empower the public to deal with the unpredictable. Effective pre-hospital care lies in the hands of the public at the very beginning of their desperate dash through emergency care. In response to the July 2005 London bombings, over 200 major transport hubs in England now have emergency dressing packs strategically positioned in order to equip bystanders and first responders with materials to control catastrophic haemorrhage.

Pre-hospital care

The helix, the spiral, and a penultimate point

Spirals and helices, beautiful (p534) and deadly (p99), are weaving their way through this book—to what central point? Unlike the circle, the spiral never returns us to our starting place, and recognizes that the person who set out reading this book is not the same as the person who, now exhausted and probably filled-to-bursting, has reached this penultimate point. So reflect on your spiritual journey, and guess its direction—in towards the centre, concentrating on ever finer, but vital detail—or away from the centre, towards infinity?

The last word

It is a pleasure to end this work with a chapter which is really a new beginning: the patient on his way to hospital. So far we have concentrated on what we can bring to the patient. Now let us turn to what the patient brings to us. All too often, time and circumstance lead us to the view that patients are tireless devourers of our energies, and that for all practical purposes, we must go on giving until we die, or give up the unequal struggle with Nature and her diseases. This is to negate the view of patients as food: not just in the sense of giving us our daily bread and butter, but also in the sense of nourishing our personalities. They do this by telling us about ourselves. You may think that you are kind and wise, or clumsy and inadequate, and it takes our patients to disabuse us of these illusions, and to show us that some days we are good, and some days we are bad. Thanks to our patients, we never stay the same. After practising medicine for a few decades, our minds become populated by the ghosts of former patients, beckoning us, warning us, reminding us of the things we cannot control—and the ideals to which we aspire.

We are lucky to work in a profession in which experience counts for more than knowledge, and it is to augment this thirst for experience that we urge our readers to turn away from learning by rote: let us read novels, cultivate our friends, travel far—and try to keep forever curious, for then, if we are lucky, we stand to gain that priceless therapeutic asset: a rich and compassionate personality, and we will be all the more inclined to reformulate this tiresome and inconvenient patient who now confronts us into a lovable series of imperfections, which match and reflect, and reveal our own foibles.

Abbreviations: i refers to an image; t refers to a table; syn.=syndrome; dis.=disease.

Schematic example of a Snellen chart

Be sure to use a proper Snellen chart. The above is just to give an idea of what a Snellen chart looks like.

Ishihara colour deficiency test
selected plates

NB: These plates should *not* be used for diagnostic purposes.
See numbered notes for plate descriptions.
The Plates of 'Ishihara Test for Colour deficiency' reproduced with permission, The Public Interest Incorporated Foundation Isshinkai, Tokyo, Japan.

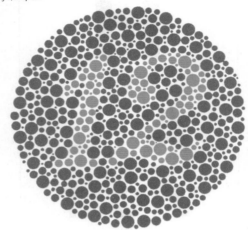

1

2

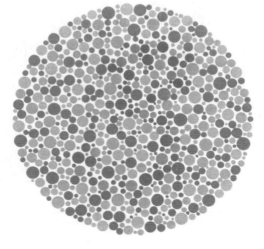

1. Demonstration plate: everyone should read '12'.
2. Normal vision read '3'; red–green deficiency read '5'.
3. Normal vision read '42'; in protanopia (blindness to red) and protanomalia (insensitivity to red) only '2' is read (or '2' is clearer than '4' in mild protanomalia); in deuteranopia and deutranomalia (blindness/insensitivity to green) only '4' is read (or '4' is clearer than '2' in mild deuteranomalia).
4. Normal vision read '6'; the majority with colour vision deficiency cannot read a number or read it incorrectly.

3

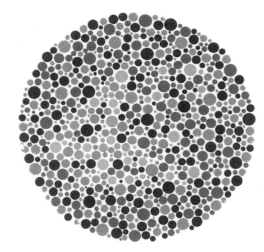

4

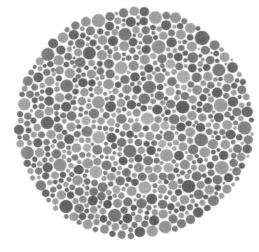

Reference intervals—biochemistry

See p220 for children and p15 for obstetric reference intervals

►*All laboratory discourse is probabilistic.* ►Drugs may interfere with any chemical method; as these effects may be method-dependent, it is difficult for us to be aware of all possibilities. If in doubt, discuss with the lab.

Substance	Specimen	Normal value	Your hospital
Adrenocorticotrophic hormone	P	<80ng/L	
Alanine aminotransferase (ALT)	P	5–35IU/L	
Albumin	P¶	35–50g/L	
Aldosterone	P**	100–500pmoL/L	
Alkaline phosphatase	P¶	30–300IU/L (adults)	
α-fetoprotein	S	<10ku/L	
α-amylase	P	0–180 Somogyi u/dL	
Angiotensin II	P**	5–35pmol/L	
Antidiuretic hormone (ADH)	P	0.9–4.6pmol/L	
Aspartate transaminase	P	5–35IU/L	
Bicarbonate	P¶	24–30mmol/L	
Bilirubin	P	3–17μmol/L (0.25–1.5mg/100/mL)	
Calcitonin	P	<0.1μg/L	
Calcium (ionized)	P	1.0–1.25mmol/L	
Calcium (total)	P¶	2.12–2.65mmol/L	
Chloride	P	95–105mmol/L	
*Cholesterol (see p654)	P	3.9–7.8mmol/L	
VLDL (see p654)	P	0.128–0.645mmol/L	
LDL	P	1.55–4.4mmol/L	
HDL	P	0.9–1.93mmol/L	
Cortisol	P	a.m. 450–700nmol/L midnight 80–280nmol/L	
Creatine kinase (CK)	P	♂ 25–195IU/L; ♀ 25–170	
Creatinine (*related to lean body mass*)	P¶	70–≤150μmol/L	
Ferritin	P	12–200μg/L	
Folate	S	2.1μg/L	
Follicle-stimulating hormone (FSH)	P/S	2–8u/L (luteal): ovulatory peak 8–15 follicular phase, & ♂: 0.5–5 postmenopausal: >30	
Gamma-glutamyl transpeptidase	P	♂ 11–51; ♀ 7–33IU/L	
Glucose (fasting)	P	3.5–5.5mmol/L	
Glycated (glycosylated) haemoglobin	B	5–8%	
Growth hormone	P	<20mu/L	
Iron	S	♂ 14–31μmol/L; ♀ 11–30	
Lactate dehydrogenase (LDH)	P	70–250IU/L	
Lead	B	<1.8mmol/L	
Luteinizing hormone (LH)	P/S	premenopausal: 3–13u/L follicular: 3–12 ovulatory peak: 20–80 luteal: 3–16 postmenopausal: >30	
Magnesium	P	0.75–1.05mmol/L	
Osmolality	P	278–305mosmol/kg	
Parathyroid hormone (PTH)	P	<0.8–8.5pmol/L	
Phosphate (inorganic)	P	0.8–1.45mmol/L	
Potassium	P	3.5–5.0mmol/L	
Prolactin	P	♂ <450u/L; ♀ <600u/L	
Prostate specific antigen	P	0–4 nanograms/mL	
Protein (total)	P	60–80g/L	
Red cell folate	B	0.36–1.44μmol/L (160–640μg/L)	
Renin (erect/recumbent)	P**	2.8–4.5/1.1–2.7pmol/mL/h	